Levangie & Norkin's

JOINT STRUCTURE & FUNCTION

A Comprehensive Analysis

Seventh Edition

Levangie & Norkin's

JOINT STRUCTURE & FUNCTION

A Comprehensive Analysis

Seventh Edition

Michael D. Lewek, PT, PhD
Professor
Division of Physical Therapy
Department of Health Sciences
University of North Carolina at Chapel Hill
Chapel Hill, North Carolina

Pamela K. Levangie, PT, DPT, DSc, FAPTA
Professor Emerita
Department of Physical Therapy
School of Health and Rehabilitation Sciences
MGH Institute of Health Professions
Boston, Massachusetts

F.A. DAVIS
Philadelphia

F.A. Davis Company
1915 Arch Street
Philadelphia, PA 19103
www.fadavis.com

Printed in the United States of America

Last digit indicates print number: 10 9 8 7 6 5 4 3 2 1

Editor-in-Chief: Jean Rodenberger
Acquisitions Editor: Jennifer A. Pine
Director of Content Development: George W. Lang
Developmental Editor: Laura Horowitz
Content Project Manager: Elizabeth Stepchin
Senior Manager of Art and Design: Carolyn O'Brien

As new scientific information becomes available through basic and clinical research, recommended treatments and drug therapies undergo changes. The author(s) and publisher have done everything possible to make this book accurate, up to date, and in accord with accepted standards at the time of publication. The author(s), editors, and publisher are not responsible for errors or omissions or for consequences from application of the book, and make no warranty, expressed or implied, in regard to the contents of the book. Any practice described in this book should be applied by the reader in accordance with professional standards of care used in regard to the unique circumstances that may apply in each situation. The reader is advised always to check product information (package inserts) for changes and new information regarding dose and contraindications before administering any drug. Caution is especially urged when using new or infrequently ordered drugs.

Library of Congress Cataloging-in-Publication Data

Library of Congress Control Number: 2026941875

Preface

With publication of the seventh edition of *Joint Structure and Function*, we continue on a journey started nearly 45 years ago. This text began as a collaboration between Drs. Cindy Norkin and Pamela Levangie, who both joined the faculty of the Physical Therapy Program at Boston University, Sargent College of Allied Health in 1973. After co-teaching Functional Anatomy for several years, Dr. Norkin had the vision to turn their course materials into a textbook. The first edition came out several years later. Drs. Norkin and Levangie continued their close and productive collaboration through the second, third, fourth, and fifth editions. I had the pleasure of joining them for the sixth edition. *Joint Structure and Function* has strongly influenced the professional journey of more than 200,000 students through the years.

The text initially targeted a substantive void in the evidence-based kinesiologic foundations upon which an understanding of typical and impaired movement should be based. With continuing advances in research and information technologies, there are innumerable ways to access and use the explosion of information available. Our goal in the seventh edition is to be responsive to the needs and preferences of our contemporary audience while continuing the tradition of being an accessible, well-referenced, and preferred resource for those seeking current concepts in kinesiology.

The seventh edition reflects changes in an understanding of adult learning and in learning preferences.

- We have enhanced the images that support the underlying concepts.
- We have retained and expanded the boxed features—named *Foundational Concepts*, *Expanded Concepts*, and *Patient Applications*—to facilitate the reader's ability to prioritize content. Additionally, we have included a new box entitled *Clinical Applications*. This box is intended to showcase the "why" so that readers understand the clinical utility of the information.
- Chapter outlines that include page numbers at the beginning of each chapter allow more efficient chapter navigation to seek the information needed.
- We have retained the *Anatomy Overview* tables at the beginning of each joint complex chapter to provide a quick review of the musculature.
- A new chapter has been added, Chapter 15, Aquatics: Biomechanical Principles. This chapter provides a much-needed look at how movement occurs in aquatic environments, and how this differs from movement on land. As clinicians are increasingly using pools as therapeutic modalities, this chapter is instrumental in helping readers understand the foundations of how movement and forces might change in the water.
- New chapter contributors reflect a commitment to engaging a new generation of clinical and researcher educators.

Although our learners—and the technology that supports their learning—are evolving, *Joint Structure and Function* remains committed to providing a strong, contemporary, and evidence-based foundation in the principles of human structure and function while also being as accessible and concise as possible. We very much appreciate our opportunity to contribute to the health of society by assisting in the professional development of the students and providers who are our readers.

Michael D. Lewek

Pamela K. Levangie

Acknowledgments

The seventh edition of *Joint Structure and Function* is made possible only by the continued and combined efforts of many people and groups. We are, first and foremost, grateful for the time, effort, and expertise of our esteemed and growing group of contributors with whom it has been a pleasure to work. Our thanks, therefore, to Drs. Sam Ward, David Berry, Behar Shahidi, William Thompson, Gary Chleboun, Diane Dalton, Sean Lowers, Dan Cerniglia, Pam Ritzline, Jenna York, Paula Ludewig, John Borstad, Jane Fedorczyk, Mia Erickson, RobRoy Martin, Yongni Zhang, Elanna Arhos, Miriam Hazlett, Laura Schmitt, Lindsay Carroll, Dana Judd, Chris Hurt, Tara Pearce, and Emily Paul. We would also like to acknowledge and thank our colleagues and students who continue to pass along their welcomed suggestions through the years.

We extend our continuing gratitude to F.A. Davis for their investment in the future of *Joint Structure and Function*. Particular thanks go to our Developmental Editor, Laura Horowitz (York Content Development), as well as to Jennifer Pine (Acquisitions Editor at F.A. Davis), who provided great support. As always we must thank the artists who, through the years, provided the images that are so valuable to the readers. These include artists of past editions, Joe Farnum, Timothy Malone, and Dragonfly Media Group, all of whom have helped us take our figures to a new level.

Finally, we acknowledge and thank our colleagues and families, without whose support this work could not have been done and to whom we are eternally indebted. We hope that readers will appreciate the late nights and weekends sacrificed to bring this text to completion.

Contributors

Elanna K. Arhos, PT, DPT, PhD
Assistant Professor
Physical Therapy and Human Movement Sciences
Feinberg School of Medicine
Northwestern University
Chicago, Illinois

David B. Berry, PhD
Assistant Professor
Department of Orthopaedic Surgery
Associate Director for High Field Animal MRI
Center for Functional Magnetic Resonance Imaging
University of California San Diego
San Diego, California

John Borstad, PT, PhD
Clinical Professor
Department of Physical Therapy
OSU-Cascades
Bend, Oregon

Lindsay A. Carroll, PT, DPT, PhD
Board Certified Clinical Specialist in Orthopaedic Physical Therapy
Assistant Professor
Division of Physical Therapy
Shenandoah University
Winchester, Virginia

Dan Cerniglia, PT, DPT
Clinical Supervisor
Rehabilitation Services
UNC Hospitals
Chapel Hill, North Carolina

Gary Chleboun, PT, PhD
Professor Emeritus of Physical Therapy
Department of Physical Therapy
Ohio University
Athens, Ohio

Diane Dalton, PT, DPT
Board Certified Clinical Specialist in Orthopaedic Physical Therapy
Clinical Associate Professor
Sargent College of Health & Rehabilitation Sciences
Boston University
Boston, Massachusetts

Mia Erickson, PT, EdD
Certified Hand Therapist
Professor
Department of Physical Therapy
Midwestern University
Glendale, Arizona

Jane Fedorczyk, PT, PhD, FAPTA
Certified Hand Therapist
Professor Emerita
College of Rehabilitation Sciences
Thomas Jefferson University
Philadelphia, Pennsylvania

Miriam F. Hazlett, PT, DPT, MBA
Health and Rehabilitation Sciences PhD Program
School of Health and Rehabilitation Sciences
Ohio State University
Columbus, Ohio

Christopher P. Hurt, PhD
Associate Professor
Department of Physical Therapy
Program Director Disability Studies and Rehabilitation Science
The University of Alabama at Birmingham
Birmingham, Alabama

Dana L. Judd, PT, DPT, PhD
Associate Professor and Associate Program Director
Department of Physical Medicine and Rehabilitation
Physical Therapy Program
University of Colorado Anschutz Medical Campus
Aurora, Colorado

Sean Lowers, PT, DPT
Board Certified Clinical Specialist in Cardiovascular and Pulmonary Physical Therapy
Assistant Professor
Division of Physical Therapy, Department of Health Sciences
University of North Carolina at Chapel Hill
Chapel Hill, North Carolina

Paula M. Ludewig, PT, PhD, FAPTA
Professor, Division of Physical Therapy & Rehabilitation Science
Department of Family Medicine and Community Health
University of Minnesota
Minneapolis, Minnesota

RobRoy L. Martin, PT, PhD
Professor
Department of Physical Therapy
Duquesne University
Pittsburgh, Pennsylvania

Emily Paul, PT, DPT, ATC
Clinical Specialist and Clinic Coordinator
Adjunct Assistant Professor UNC Division of Physical Therapy
UNC Therapy Services at Meadowmont
Chapel Hill, North Carolina

Tara S. Pearce, PT, DHS
Director of Clinical Education
Associate Professor
Department of Physical Therapy
The University of Alabama at Birmingham
Birmingham, Alabama

Pamela D. Ritzline, PT, EdD
Dean, College of Health Professions
Professor, Physical Therapy
University of the Cumberlands
Williamsburg, Kentucky

Laura C. Schmitt, PT, PhD, FAPTA
Professor
Division of Physical Therapy
School of Health and Rehabilitation Sciences
Ohio State University
Columbus, Ohio

Bahar Shahidi, PT, DPT, PhD
Associate Professor
Department of Orthopaedic Surgery
University of California San Diego
San Diego, California

William R. Thompson, PT, DPT, PhD, FASBMR
Associate Professor and Director of Research, Physical Therapy
School of Health & Human Sciences
Co-Director, Musculoskeletal Health PhD Program
Indiana Center for Musculoskeletal Health
Adjunct Associate Professor of Anatomy, Cell Biology, and Physiology
Indiana University
Indianapolis, Indiana

Samuel R. Ward, PT, PhD, FAPTA
Vice Dean of Research, School of Medicine
Professor of Orthopaedic Surgery & Radiology
Affiliate Professor of Bioengineering
Vice Chair of Research and Innovation—Orthopaedic Surgery
Director, Device Acceleration Center, Altman Clinical Translational Research Institute
University of California San Diego
San Diego, California

Jenna York, PT, DPT
Board Certified Clinical Specialist in Orthopaedic Physical Therapy
Clinical Assistant Professor, Physical Therapy Program
Walsh University
North Canton, Ohio

Yongni Zhang, PT, PhD
Duquesne China-Health Institute
Duquesne University
Pittsburgh, Pennsylvania

Contents in Brief

Section 1 **Joint Structure and Function: Foundational Concepts** 1

Chapter 1 **Biomechanical Applications to Joint Structure and Function** 2
Samuel R. Ward, PT, PhD, FAPTA
Bahar Shahidi, PT, DPT, PhD
David B. Berry, PhD

Chapter 2 **Complexity of Human Joint Design** 46
William R. Thompson, PT, DPT, PhD, FASBMR

Chapter 3 **Muscle Structure and Function** 83
Gary Chleboun, PT, PhD

Section 2 **Axial Skeletal Joint Complexes** 111

Chapter 4 **The Vertebral Column** 112
Diane Dalton, PT, DPT, OCS

Chapter 5 **The Thorax and Chest Wall** 167
Sean Lowers, PT, DPT, CCS
Dan Cerniglia, PT, DPT

Chapter 6 **The Temporomandibular Joint** 184
Pamela D. Ritzline, PT, EdD
Jenna York, PT, DPT, OCS

Section 3 **Upper Extremity Joint Complexes** 203

Chapter 7 **The Shoulder Complex** 204
Paula M. Ludewig, PT, PhD, FAPTA
John Borstad, PT, PhD

Chapter 8 **The Elbow Complex** 242
Jane Fedorczyk, PT, PhD, CHT, FAPTA

Chapter 9 **The Wrist and Hand Complex** 269
Mia Erickson, PT, EdD, CHT

Section 4 **Lower Extremity Joint Complexes** 309

Chapter 10 **The Hip Complex** 310
Yongni Zhang, PT, PhD
RobRoy L. Martin, PT, PhD, CSCS

Chapter 11 **The Knee** 351
Elanna K. Arhos, PT, DPT, PhD
Miriam F. Hazlett, PT, DPT, MBA
Laura C. Schmitt, PT, PhD, FAPTA

Chapter 12 **The Ankle and Foot Complex** 397
RobRoy L. Martin, PT, PhD, CSCS
Lindsay A. Carroll, PT, DPT, PhD, OCS

Section 5 **Integrated Function** 441

Chapter 13 **Posture** 442
Dana Judd, PT, DPT, PhD

Chapter 14 **Gait** 469
Christopher P. Hurt, PhD
Tara S. Pearce, PT, DHS

Chapter 15 **Aquatics: Biomechanical Principles** 512
Emily E. Paul, PT, DPT, ATC

Index 525

Contents

Preface v
Acknowledgments vi
Contributors vii
Contents in Brief ix

Section 1 **Joint Structure and Function: Foundational Concepts** 1

Chapter 1 **Biomechanical Applications to Joint Structure and Function** 2

Samuel R. Ward, PT, PhD, FAPTA
Bahar Shahidi, PT, DPT, PhD
David B. Berry, PhD

INTRODUCTION 3
DESCRIPTIONS OF MOTION 4
- Types of Displacement 4
- Location of Displacement in Space 5
- Direction of Displacement 6
- Magnitude of Displacement 6
- Rate of Displacement 6

INTRODUCTION TO FORCES 8
- Definition of Forces 8
- Force Vectors 9
- Force of Gravity 10

INTRODUCTION TO STATICS AND DYNAMICS 13
- Newton's Law of Inertia 13
- Newton's Law of Acceleration 14

TRANSLATORY MOTION IN LINEAR AND CONCURRENT FORCE SYSTEMS 14
- Linear Force Systems 14
- Concurrent Force Systems 15
- Newton's Law of Reaction 16

ADDITIONAL LINEAR FORCE CONSIDERATIONS 19
- Tensile Forces 19
- Joint Distraction 20
- Revisiting Newton's Law of Equilibrium 21
- Shear and Friction Forces 22
- Considering Vertical and Horizontal Linear Equilibrium 23

TORQUE, OR MOMENT OF FORCE 24
- Parallel Force Systems 25

MUSCLE FORCES 28
- Total Muscle Force Vector 28

TORQUE REVISITED 30
- Changes to Moment Arm of a Force 30
- Angular Acceleration With Changing Torques 31
- Moment Arm and Angle of Application of a Force 32

LEVER SYSTEMS, OR CLASSES OF LEVERS 33
- Mechanical Advantage 35
- Limitations of Analysis of Forces by Lever Systems 35

FORCE COMPONENTS 36
- Resolving Forces Into Perpendicular and Parallel Components 36
- Perpendicular and Parallel Force Effects 36
- Translatory Effects of Force Components 40
- Rotary Effects of Force Components 41

MULTISEGMENT (CLOSED-CHAIN) FORCE ANALYSIS 41
SUMMARY 44
STUDY QUESTIONS 44
REFERENCES 45

Chapter 2 **Complexity of Human Joint Design** 46

William R. Thompson, PT, DPT, PhD, FASBMR

INTRODUCTION 46
- Form Follows Function 46

THE COMPLEXITY OF HUMAN JOINT DESIGN 48
- Joint Classification 48
- Joint Motion 54

MATERIALS FOUND IN HUMAN JOINTS 59
- Composition of Connective Tissue 59
- Specific Connective Tissue Composition 61

BEHAVIORAL PROPERTIES OF CONNECTIVE TISSUE 66

Structural and Material Properties 67
Viscoelasticity 70
Time-Dependent and Rate-Dependent Properties 70
Properties of Specific Tissues 72
GENERAL CHANGES WITH DISEASE, INJURY, IMMOBILIZATION, EXERCISE, AND OVERUSE 73
Disease 74
Injury 74
Immobilization (Stress Deprivation) 74
Exercise 76
Overuse 77
SUMMARY 78
STUDY QUESTIONS 79
REFERENCES 79

Chapter 3 **Muscle Structure and Function** 83
Gary Chleboun, PT, PhD
INTRODUCTION 83
ELEMENTS OF MUSCLE STRUCTURE 83
Composition of a Muscle Fiber 83
The Contractile Unit 84
The Motor Unit 87
Muscle Structure 88
Muscle Architecture: Size, Arrangement, and Length 89
Muscular Connective Tissue 90
MUSCLE FUNCTION 92
Muscle Tension 92
Classification of Muscles 98
Factors Affecting Muscle Function 100
EFFECTS OF IMMOBILIZATION, INJURY, AND AGING 104
Immobilization 104
Injury 105
Aging 106
SUMMARY 106
STUDY QUESTIONS 106
REFERENCES 107

Section 2 **Axial Skeletal Joint Complexes** 111

Chapter 4 **The Vertebral Column** 112
Diane Dalton, PT, DPT, OCS
INTRODUCTION 115
STRUCTURE AND FUNCTION OF THE VERTEBRAL COLUMN 115
Structure 115
Function 124
REGIONAL STRUCTURE AND FUNCTION 129
Structure of the Cervical Region 129
Function of the Cervical Region 134
Structure of the Thoracic Region 138
Function of the Thoracic Region 140
Structure of the Lumbar Region 140
Function of the Lumbar Region 145
Structure of the Sacral Region 148
Function of the Sacral Region 151
MUSCLES OF THE VERTEBRAL COLUMN 152
The Craniocervical/Upper Thoracic Regions 152
Lower Thoracic/Lumbopelvic Regions 156
Muscles of the Pelvic Floor 161
EFFECTS OF AGING ON THE LUMBAR SPINE 162
SUMMARY 164
STUDY QUESTIONS 164
REFERENCES 164

Chapter 5 **The Thorax and Chest Wall** 167
Sean Lowers, PT, DPT, CCS
Dan Cerniglia, PT, DPT
INTRODUCTION 167
STRUCTURE AND FUNCTION OF THE THORAX 167
Structure 167
Function 172
LIFE SPAN AND CLINICAL CONSIDERATIONS 180
Differences Associated With the Neonate 180
Differences Associated With the Elderly 181
Pathological Changes in Structure and Function 181
SUMMARY 183
STUDY QUESTIONS 183
REFERENCES 183

Chapter 6 **The Temporomandibular Joint** 184
Pamela D. Ritzline, PT, EdD
Jenna York, PT, DPT, OCS
INTRODUCTION 186
STRUCTURE AND FUNCTION OF THE TM JOINT 186
Structure 186
Function 190
Relationship to the Cervical Spine and Posture 195
Dentition 196
LIFE SPAN AND CLINICAL CONSIDERATIONS 197
Age-Related Changes in the TM Joint 197
Clinical Considerations 197
Inflammatory Conditions 197
Osseous Mobility Conditions 198
Degenerative Conditions 199
SUMMARY 200
STUDY QUESTIONS 200
REFERENCES 200

Section 3 **Upper Extremity Joint Complexes** 203

Chapter 7 **The Shoulder Complex** 204

Paula M. Ludewig, PT, PhD, FAPTA

John Borstad, PT, PhD

INTRODUCTION 207

SHOULDER COMPLEX JOINTS AND STRUCTURES 207

- Sternoclavicular Joint Structure 207
- Acromioclavicular Joint Structure 209
- Scapulothoracic Joint Structure 210
- Glenohumeral Joint Structure 211
- Coracoacromial Arch and Bursae 215

SHOULDER JOINT FUNCTION 216

- Sternoclavicular Motion 216
- Sternoclavicular Stability 217
- Acromioclavicular Kinematics 218
- Acromioclavicular Stability 219
- Scapulothoracic Kinematics 220
- Scapulothoracic Stability 223
- Glenohumeral Kinematics 223
- Static Glenohumeral Joint Stability in the Dependent Arm 225
- Dynamic Glenohumeral Joint Stabilization 225

INTEGRATED FUNCTION OF THE SHOULDER COMPLEX 229

- Integrated Joint Function 229
- Integrated Shoulder Muscle Function: Elevation 233
- Integrated Shoulder Muscle Function: Depression 236

LIFE SPAN AND CLINICAL CONSIDERATIONS 238

- Life Span Considerations 238
- Structural Dysfunction 238

SUMMARY 239

STUDY QUESTIONS 239

REFERENCES 239

Chapter 8 **The Elbow Complex** 242

Jane Fedorczyk, PT, PhD, CHT, FAPTA

INTRODUCTION 244

STRUCTURE AND FUNCTION OF THE HUMEROULNAR AND HUMERORADIAL ARTICULATIONS 244

- Structure 244
- Joint Articulations 244
- Joint Capsule 246
- Function 250

STRUCTURE AND FUNCTION OF THE PROXIMAL AND DISTAL RADIOULNAR ARTICULATIONS 254

- Structure 254
- Function 257
- Stability 258

MOBILITY AND STABILITY OF THE ELBOW COMPLEX 260

- Functional Activities 260
- Relationship to the Hand and Wrist 260

LIFE SPAN AND CLINICAL CONSIDERATIONS 260

- Effects of Age 261
- Injury 261

SUMMARY 265

STUDY QUESTIONS 266

REFERENCES 266

Chapter 9 **The Wrist and Hand Complex** 269

Mia Erickson, PT, EdD, CHT

INTRODUCTION 272

STRUCTURE AND FUNCTION OF THE WRIST JOINT 272

- Joints of the Wrist 273
- Ligaments of the Wrist 275
- Muscle Function 277
- Wrist Kinematics 281
- Wrist Kinetics 284

STRUCTURE AND FUNCTION OF THE HAND COMPLEX 284

- Digits 2–5 284
- Muscles of the Digits 289
- The Thumb 297

PREHENSION 300

- Power Grip 301
- Lateral Prehension 302
- Precision Grip 302

FUNCTIONAL POSITION OF THE WRIST AND HAND 304

SUMMARY 304

STUDY QUESTIONS 304

REFERENCES 305

Section 4 **Lower Extremity Joint Complexes** 309

Chapter 10 **The Hip Complex** 310

Yongni Zhang, PT, PhD

RobRoy L. Martin, PT, PhD, CSCS

INTRODUCTION 312

STRUCTURE AND FUNCTION OF THE HIP JOINT 312

- Structure 312
- Function 325

HIP JOINT FORCES AND MUSCLE FUNCTION IN STANCE 337

- Bilateral Stance 337
- Unilateral Stance 338

HIP PAIN ACROSS THE LIFE SPAN 344

- Femoroacetabular Impingement Syndrome 344

Acetabular Dysplasia 345
Hip Osteoarthritis 345
SUMMARY 346
STUDY QUESTIONS 346
REFERENCES 346

Chapter 11 **The Knee** 351
Elanna K. Arhos, PT, DPT, PhD
Miriam F. Hazlett, PT, DPT, MBA
Laura C. Schmitt, PT, PhD, FAPTA
INTRODUCTION 353
TIBIOFEMORAL JOINT STRUCTURE AND FUNCTION 353
Structure 353
Function 368
PATELLOFEMORAL JOINT 380
Tibiofemoral (Knee) Joint Motion and Patellar Contact 380
Motions of the Patella 381
Patellar Function 384
Patellofemoral Joint Stress 384
Quadriceps Strengthening Exercises and Patellofemoral Pain 386
Patellar Motion and Medial/Lateral Patellar Restraints 387
Lateral Bias of Patellar Motion 388
LIFE SPAN AND CLINICAL CONSIDERATIONS 390
Tibiofemoral Joint Injury 390
Patellofemoral Joint Injury 390
SUMMARY 391
STUDY QUESTIONS 391
REFERENCES 391

Chapter 12 **The Ankle and Foot Complex** 397
RobRoy L. Martin, PT, PhD, CSCS
Lindsay A. Carroll, PT, DPT, PhD, OCS
INTRODUCTION 400
DEFINITIONS OF MOTION 400
JOINT STRUCTURE 401
The Ankle Joint 401
The Subtalar Joint 405
Transverse Tarsal Joint 406
Tarsometatarsal Joints 408
Metatarsophalangeal Joints 408
Interphalangeal Joints 409
JOINT FUNCTION 409
The Ankle Joint 409
The Subtalar Joint 412
Transverse Tarsal Joint 418
Tarsometatarsal Joints 423
Metatarsophalangeal Joints 424
PLANTAR ARCHES 427
Structure of the Arches 427
Function of the Arches 428
Muscular Contribution to the Arches 430
MUSCLES OF THE ANKLE AND FOOT 430
Extrinsic Musculature 431
Intrinsic Musculature 433
LIFE SPAN AND CLINICAL CONSIDERATIONS 433
Foot and Ankle Problems Revisited 434
SUMMARY 435
STUDY QUESTIONS 436
REFERENCES 436

Section 5 **Integrated Function** 441

Chapter 13 **Posture** 442
Dana Judd, PT, DPT, PhD
INTRODUCTION 442
POSTURE AND BALANCE DEFINED 442
Posture 442
Balance 443
The Role of Sensorimotor Motor Control in Posture and Balance 444
Control of Posture in Static Positions 445
Control of Posture During Movement 447
KINETICS AND KINEMATICS OF POSTURE AND POSTURAL CONTROL 448
Joint and Ground Reaction Forces 448
THE ROLE OF POSTURAL ASSESSMENT IN PHYSICAL THERAPY 449
EXPECTED STANDING ALIGNMENT 449
Analysis of Standing Posture 449
Analysis of Standing Posture: Sagittal Plane View 450
Analysis of Standing Posture: Frontal Plane 452
EXPECTED SITTING POSTURES 454
COMMON DEVIATIONS FROM EXPECTED ALIGNMENT 455
The Role of Pain 455
Scoliosis 455
Additional Spinal Abnormalities 457
Shoulder and Scapulothoracic Joint Abnormalities 457
Lumbopelvic and Hip Abnormalities 458
Knee Joint Abnormalities 458
Ankle, Feet, and Toe Abnormalities 460
Neurological Conditions That Influence Posture 462
POSTURAL CONTROL CHANGES ACROSS THE LIFE SPAN 462
Adults and Older Adults 462
Pregnancy 463
DYNAMIC POSTURAL CHANGES: KINEMATICS AND KINETICS 464
Sit to Stand 464
Jumping 464

DYNAMIC POSTURE ASSESSMENT AND CLINICAL REASONING 465
SUMMARY 465
STUDY QUESTIONS 465
REFERENCES 465

Chapter 14 **Gait** 469
Christopher P. Hurt, PhD
Tara S. Pearce, PT, DHS
INTRODUCTION 469
Gait Analysis 469
Major Tasks of Gait 470
Phases of the Gait Cycle 470
GAIT TERMINOLOGY 472
Time and Distance Terms 472
Kinematic Terms 474
Kinetic Terms 474
Electromyography 477
CHARACTERISTICS OF TYPICAL GAIT 477
Time and Distance Characteristics 477
Sagittal Plane Joint Angles 477
Frontal Plane Joint Angles 478
Ground Reaction Force and Center of Pressure 478
Sagittal Plane Moments 482
Frontal Plane Moments 482
Sagittal Plane Powers 485
Frontal Plane Powers 488
Muscle Activity 489
Gait Initiation and Termination 495
Trunk and Upper Extremities 495
TREADMILL, STAIR, AND RUNNING GAITS 496
Treadmill Gait 496
Stair Walking 497
Incline Walking 498
Running Gait 499
EFFECTS OF AGE ON GAIT 502
ATYPICAL GAIT 504
Structural Impairment 504
Functional Impairment 504
Pain 505
TREATMENT OF GAIT DISORDERS 506
Assistive Devices 506
Orthoses 506
Gait Retraining 506
SUMMARY 507
STUDY QUESTIONS 508
REFERENCES 508

Chapter 15 **Aquatics: Biomechanical Principles** 512
Emily E. Paul, PT, DPT, ATC
INTRODUCTION 512
PROPERTIES OF WATER 512
Buoyancy 512
Viscosity, Drag, and Turbulence 516
Hydrostatic Pressure 516
Relative Density/Specific Gravity 517
Refraction 518
Thermodynamics 520
APPLICATIONS OF NEWTON'S LAWS IN WATER 520
EFFECT OF AGE, SEX, AND BODY MASS ON CENTERS OF GRAVITY AND BUOYANCY 521
HYDROSTATICS AND HYDRODYNAMICS 521
SUMMARY 523
STUDY QUESTIONS 524
REFERENCES 524

Index 525

SECTION 1

Joint Structure and Function: Foundational Concepts

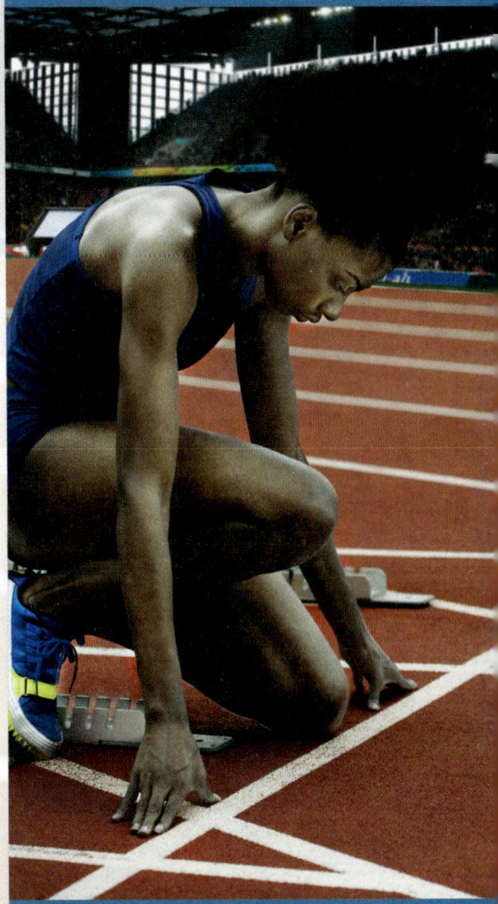

CHAPTER 1 Biomechanical Applications to Joint Structure and Function 2

CHAPTER 2 Complexity of Human Joint Design 46

CHAPTER 3 Muscle Structure and Function 83

CHAPTER 1

Biomechanical Applications to Joint Structure and Function

Samuel R. Ward, PT, PhD, FAPTA | Bahar Shahidi, PT, DPT, PhD | David B. Berry, PhD

CHAPTER OUTLINE

INTRODUCTION 3

PART 1: KINEMATICS AND INTRODUCTION TO KINETICS 4

DESCRIPTIONS OF MOTION 4

Types of Displacement 4

Translatory Motion 4

Rotary Motion 4

General Motion 5

Location of Displacement in Space 5

Direction of Displacement 6

Magnitude of Displacement 6

Rate of Displacement 6

INTRODUCTION TO FORCES 8

Definition of Forces 8

Force Vectors 9

Force of Gravity 10

Segmental Centers of Mass and Composition of Gravitational Forces 11

Center of Mass of the Human Body 12

Center of Mass, Line of Gravity, and Stability 12

INTRODUCTION TO STATICS AND DYNAMICS 13

Newton's Law of Inertia 13

Newton's Law of Acceleration 14

TRANSLATORY MOTION IN LINEAR AND CONCURRENT FORCE SYSTEMS 14

Linear Force Systems 14

Determining Resultant Forces in a Linear Force System 14

Concurrent Force Systems 15

Determining Resultant Forces in a Concurrent Force System 16

Newton's Law of Reaction 16

Gravitational and Contact Forces 17

ADDITIONAL LINEAR FORCE CONSIDERATIONS 19

Tensile Forces 19

Joint Distraction 20

Joint Compression and Joint Reaction Forces 21

Revisiting Newton's Law of Equilibrium 21

Vertical and Horizontal Linear Force Systems 22

Shear and Friction Forces 22

Static Friction and Kinetic Friction 22

Considering Vertical and Horizontal Linear Equilibrium 23

PART 2: KINETICS—CONSIDERING ROTARY AND TRANSLATORY FORCES AND MOTIONS 24

TORQUE, OR MOMENT OF FORCE 24

Parallel Force Systems 25

Determining Resultant Forces in a Parallel Force System 25

Identifying the Joint Axis About Which Body Segments Rotate 26

Bending Moments and Torsional Moments 27

MUSCLE FORCES 28

Total Muscle Force Vector 28

Anatomic Pulleys 28

Anatomic Pulleys, Action Lines, and Moment Arms 28

TORQUE REVISITED 30

Changes to Moment Arm of a Force 30

Angular Acceleration With Changing Torques 31

Moment Arm and Angle of Application of a Force 32

Changing the Gravitation Moment Arm by Changing the Center of Mass 32

LEVER SYSTEMS, OR CLASSES OF LEVERS 33

Mechanical Advantage 35

Limitations of Analysis of Forces by Lever Systems 35

FORCE COMPONENTS 36

Resolving Forces Into Perpendicular and Parallel Components 36

Perpendicular and Parallel Force Effects 36

Determining Magnitudes of Component Forces 37

Force Components and the Angle of Application of the Force 39

Manipulating External Forces to Maximize Torque 39

Translatory Effects of Force Components 40

Rotary Effects of Force Components 41

MULTISEGMENT (CLOSED-CHAIN) FORCE ANALYSIS 41

SUMMARY 44

STUDY QUESTIONS 44

REFERENCES 45

Introduction

Humans possess the remarkable ability to perform an almost limitless range of postures and movements. These actions depend on the body's ability to both generate and respond to forces that initiate and control the motion of its joints. Although it is not possible to capture all the kinesiologic factors that contribute to human musculoskeletal function at any given moment, a foundational understanding of the physical principles that govern the body's response to both active and passive stresses is essential for understanding normal and impaired human movement.

In this chapter, we will examine the complexities of human musculoskeletal function by examining the roles of the bony segments, joint-related connective tissue structures, and muscles, as well as the external forces applied to those structures. The goal is to develop a conceptual framework for understanding the stresses placed on the body's major joint complexes and how those joints respond to such stresses. Case examples and clinical scenarios will be used to ground the reader's understanding in relevant applications of the presented principles. The objective is to cover the key biomechanical principles necessary to understand individual joints and their interdependent functions in posture and locomotion. Although we acknowledge the role of the neurological system in motor control, we leave it to others to develop an understanding of the theories that govern the roles of the controller and feedback mechanisms.

This chapter will explore the biomechanical principles that must be considered in the examination of the internal and external forces that produce or control movement. The focus will be largely on rigid body analysis; the next two chapters explore how forces affect deformable connective tissues (Chapter 2) and how muscles create and are affected by forces (Chapter 3). Subsequent chapters then examine the interactive nature of force, stress, tissue behaviors, and function through a regional exploration of the joint complexes of the body. The last group of chapters will integrate the function of the joint complexes into the comprehensive tasks of posture (Chapter 13) and gait (Chapter 14) and then discuss how the forces imposed on the body may be altered in aquatic environments (Chapter 15).

To maintain our focus on clinically relevant applications of the biomechanical principles presented in this chapter, the following patient application will provide a framework within which to explore the relevant principles of biomechanics.

Patient Application 1–1

John Alexander is 20 years old, 5 ft 9 in. (1.75 m) in height, and weighs 165 pounds (~75 kg or 734 N). John is a member of the university's lacrosse team. He sustained an injury when another player fell onto the posterior-lateral aspect of his right knee. Physical examination and magnetic resonance imaging (MRI) resulted in a diagnosis of a tear of the medial collateral ligament, a partial tear of the anterior cruciate ligament (ACL), and a partial tear of the medial meniscus. John agreed with the orthopedist's recommendation that a program of knee muscle strengthening was in order before moving on to more aggressive options such as surgery. The initial focus will be on strengthening the quadriceps muscle **(Fig. 1–1)**. The fitness center at the university has a leg-press machine **(Fig. 1–1A)** and a heavy ankle cuff weight **(Fig. 1–1B)** that John can use.

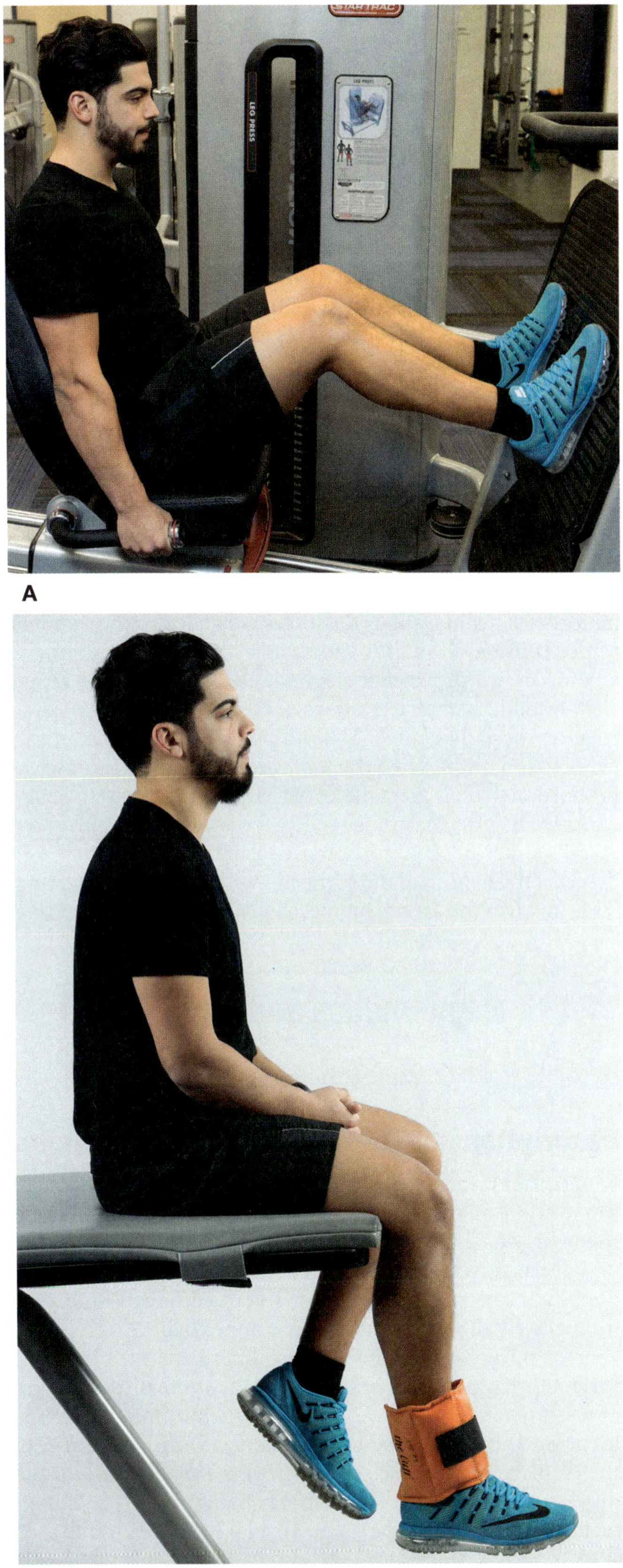

Figure 1–1 **A.** Leg-press exercise apparatus for strengthening hip and knee extensor muscles. **B.** Ankle weight for strengthening knee extensor muscles.

As we move through this chapter, we will consider the biomechanics of each of these rehabilitation exercise options in relation to John's injury and strengthening goals.

Human motion is inherently complex, involving multiple segments (bony levers) and forces that are most often applied to two or more segments simultaneously. To develop a conceptual model that can be understood and applied clinically, the common strategy is to focus on one segment at a time. For the purposes of analyzing John Alexander's issues, the focus will be on the leg-foot segment, treated as if it were one rigid unit acting at the knee joint. **Figure 1–2** is a schematic representation of the leg-foot segment in the leg-press and ankle weight scenarios. The leg-foot segment is the focus of the figure, although the contiguous components (distal femur, footplate of the leg-press machine, and the ankle weight) are maintained to give context. In some subsequent figures, the femur, footplate, and ankle weight are omitted for clarity, although the forces produced by these segments and objects will be shown. This limited visualization of a segment (or a selected few segments) can be referred to as a **free body diagram** or a **space diagram.** If proportional representation of all forces is maintained as the forces are added to the segment under consideration, it is known as a "free body diagram." If the forces are shown but a simplified understanding rather than graphic accuracy is the goal, then the figure is referred to as a "space diagram."[1] We will use space diagrams in this chapter and text because the forces are generally not drawn in proportion to their magnitudes for purposes of space efficiency.

As we begin to examine the leg-foot segment in either the ankle weight or leg-press exercise scenario, the first step is to describe the motion of the segment that is or will be occurring. This involves the area of biomechanics known as **kinematics.**

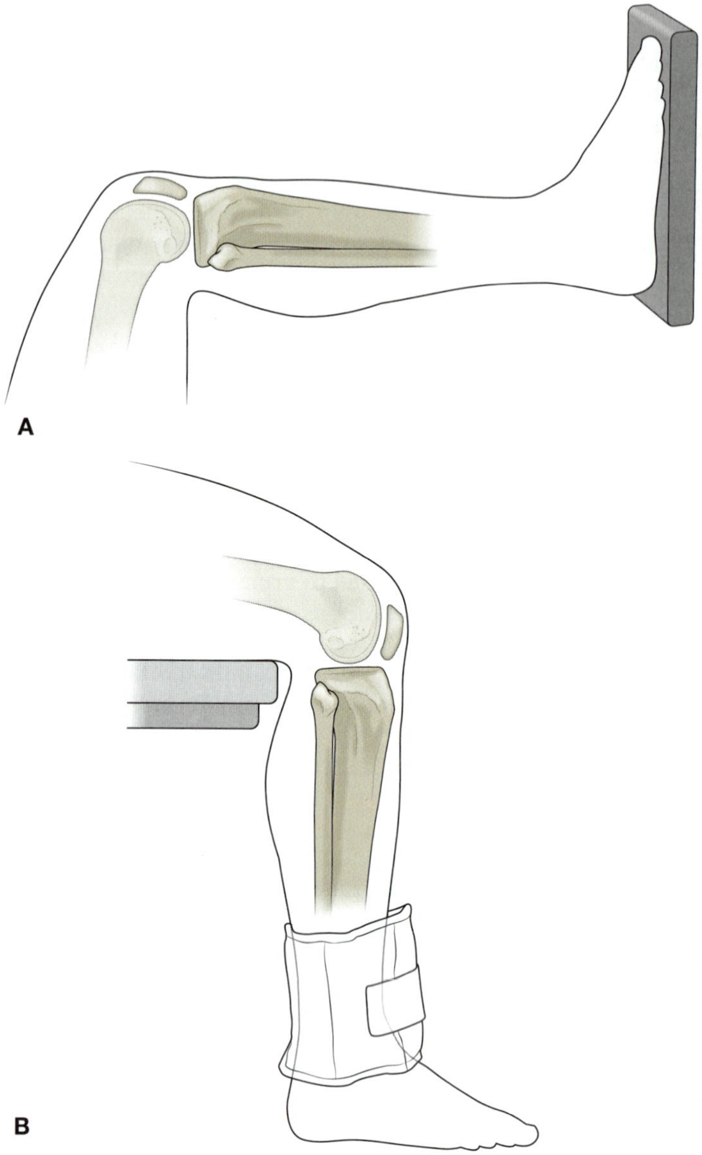

Figure 1–2 **A.** The leg-foot segment on the leg-press footrest. **B.** The leg-foot segment with an ankle weight.

PART 1: Kinematics and Introduction to Kinetics

Descriptions of Motion

Kinematics refers to the branch of mechanics that describes the motion or **displacement** (the change in position) of a segment over time, without regard to the forces that produce or influence that movement. The human skeleton is, quite literally, a system of segments or levers. Although bones are not truly rigid, we will assume that bones behave as rigid levers for purposes of simplification. There are five kinematic variables that fully describe the motion, or the displacement, of a segment: (1) the **type** of displacement (motion), (2) the **location** in space of the displacement, (3) the **direction** of the displacement of the segment, (4) the **magnitude** of the displacement, and (5) the **rate** of change in displacement (velocity) or the rate of change of velocity (acceleration).

Types of Displacement

Translatory and rotary motions are the two basic types of movement that can be attributed to any rigid segment. General motions are achieved by combining translatory and rotary motions.

Translatory Motion

Translatory motion (linear displacement) is the movement of a segment in a straight line. In human movement, isolated translatory movements are rare. However, a clinical example of an attempt at isolated translatory motion occurs during joint mobilization, whereby a clinician imposes a near linear motion (sliding) between two articular surfaces such as sliding the tibial plateau on the femur at the knee joint. In fact, translation of a body segment at an intact joint rarely occurs in human motion without some concomitant rotation (rotary motion) of that segment (even if the rotation is barely visible).

Rotary Motion

Rotary motion (angular displacement) is movement of a segment around a fixed axis **(center of rotation [CoR])** in a curved path. In true rotary motion, each point on the segment moves through the same angle, at the same time, at a constant distance from the center of rotation. True rotary motion can

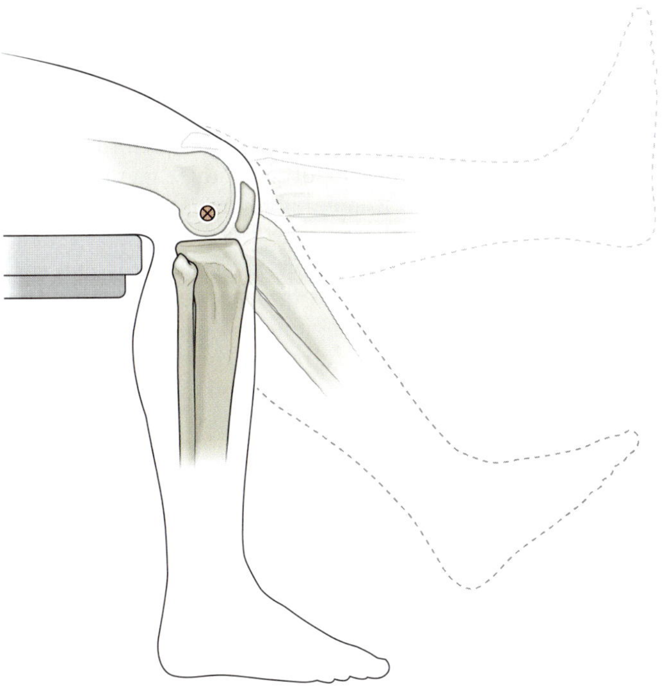

Figure 1–3 Rotary motion. Each point in the leg-foot segment moves through the same angle, at the same time, at a constant distance from the fixed (or relatively fixed) center of rotation or axis.

occur only if the segment is prevented from translating and is forced to rotate about a fixed axis. This rarely happens in human movement. In the example in **Figure 1–3**, all points on the leg-foot segment appear to move through the same angle at the same time around what appears to be a fixed axis. In actuality, none of the body segments move around truly fixed axes; all joint axes shift at least slightly during motion because segments are not sufficiently constrained to produce pure rotation.

General Motion

When nonsegmented objects move, their motion typically involves a combination of rotation and translation, referred to as **general motion.**

Curvilinear motion (also called **plane** or **planar motion**) designates a combination of translation and rotation of a segment in *two dimensions* (parallel to a plane with a maximum of three degrees of freedom).[2-4] When this type of motion occurs, the axis about which the segment moves is not fixed but rather shifts in space as the object moves. The axis around which the segment appears to move at any point in its path is referred to as the **instantaneous center of rotation (ICoR),** or **instantaneous axis of rotation (IaR).** An object or segment that travels in a curvilinear path may be undergoing rotary motion around a fixed but quite distant CoR[2,4]; that is, the curvilinear path can be considered one portion of a much larger circle with a distant axis.

Three-dimensional motion is a general motion in which the segment moves across all three dimensions (planes). Just as curvilinear motion can be considered to occur around a single distant center of rotation, three-dimensional motion can be considered to be occurring around a **helical axis of motion (HaM),** or **screw axis of motion.**[4]

As already noted, the motion of a body segment is rarely sufficiently constrained by the ligamentous, muscular, or other bony forces acting on it to produce isolated rotary motion. Instead, there is typically at least a small amount of translation (and often a secondary rotation) that accompanies the primary rotary motion of a segment at a joint. Most joint rotations, therefore, take place around a series of instantaneous centers of rotation. The "axis" that is generally ascribed to a given joint motion (e.g., knee flexion) is typically a midpoint among these instantaneous centers of rotation rather than a truly fixed center of rotation. Because most body segments actually follow a curvilinear path, the true center of rotation is the point around which true rotary motion of the segment would occur and is generally quite distant from the joint.[2,4]

Location of Displacement in Space

The rotary or translatory displacement of a segment is commonly located in space by using the three-dimensional Cartesian coordinate system as a useful frame of reference. In describing human movement, the intersection of the x-axis, y-axis, and z-axis of the coordinate system is traditionally located at the **center of mass (CoM)** of the human body, assuming that the body is in **anatomic position** (facing forward in standing with palms forward) **(Fig. 1–4).** According to the common system described by Panjabi and White, the x-axis runs side to side in the body and is labeled as the **coronal axis;** the y-axis runs front to back in the body and is labeled as the **anteroposterior (A-P) axis;** and the z-axis runs up and down in the body and is labeled as the **vertical axis.**[4] Motion of a segment can occur either *around* an axis (rotation) or *along* an axis (translation). An unconstrained segment can either rotate or translate around each of the three axes, resulting in six potential options for motion of that segment. The options for movement of a segment are also referred to as **degrees of freedom.** A completely unconstrained segment always has six degrees of freedom because it can rotate around the three axes (three degrees of freedom) as well as translate along the three axes (three additional degrees of freedom). Segments of the body, of course, are not unconstrained and—consequently—often have less than six degrees of freedom.

Rotation of a body segment is described as occurring around one of three possible axes, but also as moving in or parallel to one of three possible **cardinal planes** (see Fig. 1–4). As a segment rotates *around* a particular axis, the segment also moves in a plane that is perpendicular to its axis of rotation. Rotation of a body segment *around* the x-axis (coronal axis) occurs in the **sagittal plane.** Sagittal plane motions are most easily visualized as front-to-back motions of a segment (e.g., flexion/extension of the upper extremity at the glenohumeral joint).

Rotation of a body segment *around* the y-axis (A-P axis) occurs in the **frontal plane.** Frontal plane motions (also referred to as *coronal plane motions*) are most easily visualized as side-to-side motions of the segment (e.g., abduction/adduction of the upper extremity at the glenohumeral joint). Rotation of a body segment *around* the z-axis (vertical axis) occurs in the **transverse plane.** Transverse plane motions are most easily visualized as motions of a segment parallel to the ground (e.g., medial/lateral rotation of the lower extremity at the hip

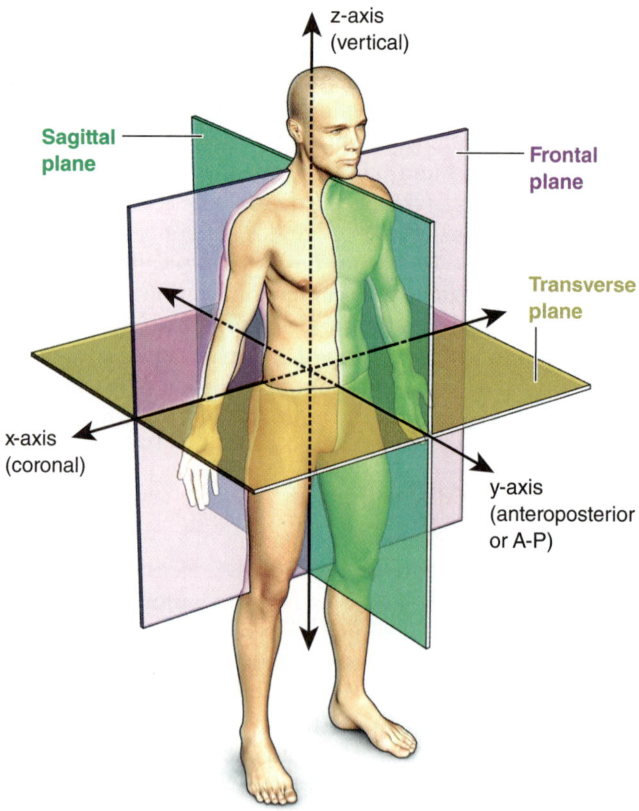

Figure 1–4 Body in anatomic position showing the x-axis, y-axis, and z-axis of the Cartesian coordinate system (for motion in the sagittal, coronal, and transverse planes, respectively).

joint). Transverse plane motions at a joint often occur around an axis that passes through the length of the rotating long bone, resulting in an axis that is not truly vertically oriented. Consequently, the term **longitudinal axis** (or **long axis**) is often used instead of "vertical axis."

The rotation and translation of body segments are not confined to movement along or around cardinal axes or within the cardinal planes. In fact, cardinal plane motions are the exception rather than the rule. Use of cardinal planes and axes is helpful for describing joint movements in a simplified manner, but tends to oversimplify the complexity of human motions. In reality, body segments typically move in three dimensions and often exhibit two or more degrees of freedom simultaneously.

Direction of Displacement

Even if displacement of a segment is confined to a single axis, the rotary or translatory motion of a segment around or along that axis can occur in two different directions **(Fig. 1–5)**. For rotary motions, the direction of movement of a segment around an axis can be described as occurring in a clockwise or counterclockwise direction.

Flexion and **extension** are motions of a segment occurring around the same axis and in the same plane (uniaxial or uniplanar) but in opposite directions **(Fig. 1–5A)**. Flexion and extension generally occur in the sagittal plane around a coronal axis, although exceptions exist (e.g., carpometacarpal flexion and extension of the thumb). **Abduction** and **adduction** of a segment occur around the A-P axis and in the frontal plane in opposite directions to each other (although carpometacarpal abduction and adduction of the thumb again serve as exceptions; **Fig. 1–5B**). Anatomically, abduction brings the segment away from the midline of the body, whereas adduction brings the segment toward the midline of the body. When the moving segment *is* part of the midline of the body (e.g., the trunk or the head), the rotary movement is commonly termed **lateral flexion** (to the right or left).

Medial (or **internal**) **rotation** and **lateral** (or **external**) **rotation** are opposite motions of a segment that generally occur around a vertical (or longitudinal) axis in the transverse plane **(Fig. 1–5C)**. Anatomically, medial rotation occurs as the segment moves parallel to the ground and the anterior surface moves toward the midline, whereas lateral rotation occurs opposite to that. When the segment is part of the midline (e.g., the head or trunk), rotation in the transverse plane is simply called *rotation to the right* or *rotation to the left*. The exceptions to the general rules for naming motions must be learned on a joint-by-joint basis.

Magnitude of Displacement

The magnitude of rotary motion (or angular displacement) that a body segment can move through is known as its **range of motion (ROM).** The most widely used standardized clinical method of measuring available joint ROM is goniometry, with units given in degrees. If an object rotates through a complete circle, it has moved through 360°.

Translatory motion (displacement) of a segment is quantified by the linear distance through which the object or segment is displaced. The units for describing translatory motions are the same as those for length. The unit for the *Système International* system (SI) is the meter (or millimeter or centimeter); the corresponding unit in the U.S. system is the foot (or inch). This text will use the SI system but include a U.S. conversion when this appears to facilitate understanding (1 in. = 2.54 cm). Linear displacements of the entire body are often measured clinically. For example, the 6-minute Walk Test[5] (a test of functional status in an individual's gait) measures the distance in feet or meters that someone walks in 6 minutes.

Rate of Displacement

Although the magnitude of displacement is important, the rate of change in position of the segment (the displacement per unit time) is equally important. Displacement per unit time, regardless of direction, is known as **speed,** whereas displacement per unit time in a given direction is known as **velocity.** If the velocity is changing over time, the change in velocity per unit time is termed **acceleration.**

Linear velocity (velocity of a translating segment) is expressed as meters per second (m/sec) in SI units or feet per second (ft/sec) in U.S. units; the corresponding units for acceleration are meters per second squared (m/sec^2) and feet per second squared (ft/sec^2). Angular velocity (velocity of a rotating segment) is expressed as degrees per second (deg/sec), whereas angular acceleration is given as degrees per second squared (deg/sec^2).

An electrogoniometer or a three-dimensional motion analysis system can be used for documentation of the changes

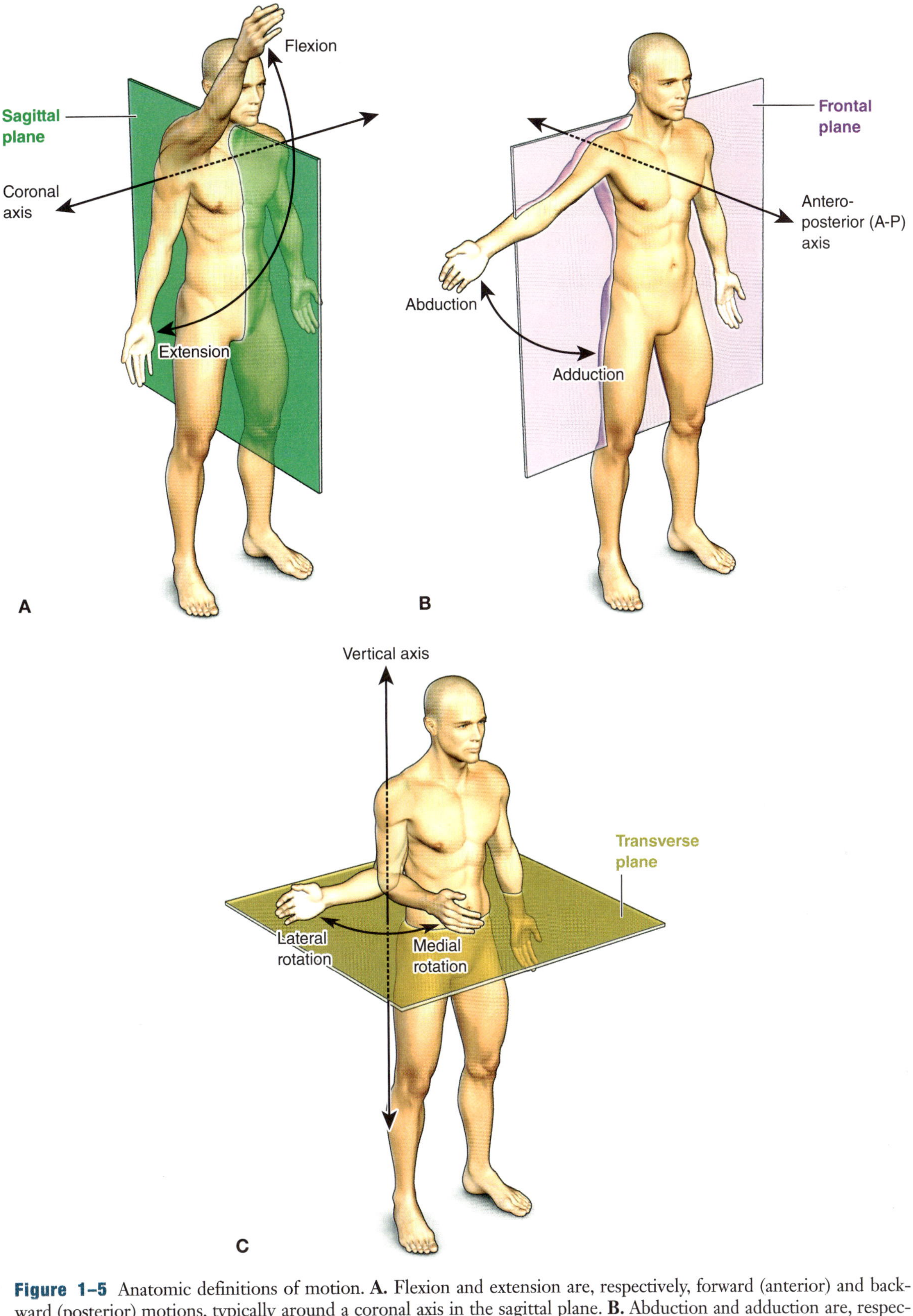

Figure 1–5 Anatomic definitions of motion. **A.** Flexion and extension are, respectively, forward (anterior) and backward (posterior) motions, typically around a coronal axis in the sagittal plane. **B.** Abduction and adduction are, respectively, movements away from the midline of the body and movement toward the midline of the body, typically around an A-P axis in the frontal plane. **C.** Medial and lateral rotation are, respectively, a "rolling" toward and away from the midline of the body, typically around a vertical (or longitudinal) axis in a transverse plane.

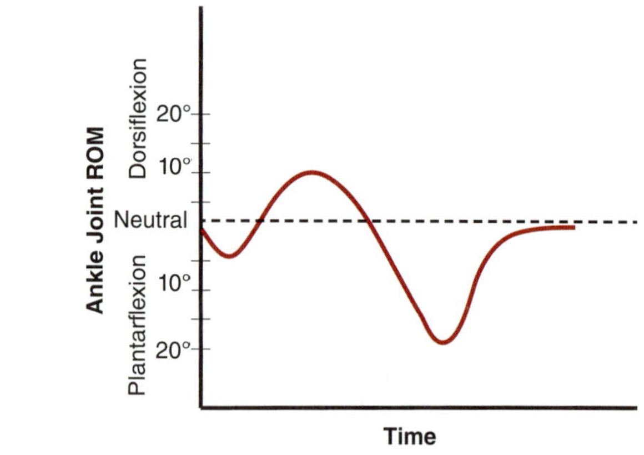

Figure 1–6 When a joint's range of motion is plotted on the y-axis (vertical axis) and time is plotted on the x-axis (horizontal axis), the resulting time-series plot portrays the change in joint position over time. The slope of the plotted line reflects the velocity of the joint change.

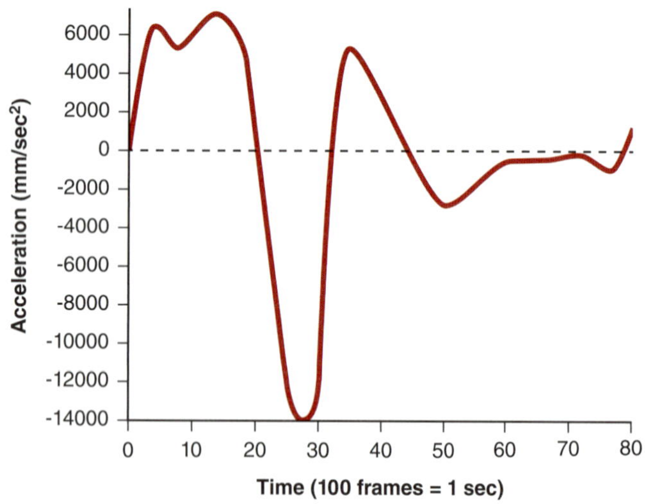

Figure 1–7 Movement of a point on a segment can be displayed by plotting the acceleration of the segment (y-axis) over time (x-axis). The slope and trend of the line represent increases or decreases in magnitude of acceleration as the movement continues. *(Courtesy of Fetters L. Boston University, 2003.)*

in displacement over time. The outputs of such systems are increasingly encountered when summaries of displacement information are presented. A computer-generated time-series plot, such as that in **Figure 1–6**, graphically portrays the angle between two bony segments (or the rotation of one segment in space) at each point in time as well as the direction of motion. The steepness of the slope of the graphed line represents the angular velocity. **Figure 1–7** plots the linear acceleration of a body segment (or a point on the body segment) over time without regard to changes in joint angle.

Introduction to Forces

Definition of Forces

Kinematic descriptions of human movement allow us to visualize and describe motion; however, they do not explain *why* that motion occurs. This requires a study of forces. Whether a body or body segment is in motion or at rest depends on the forces acting upon it.

In its simplest form, a *force* can be defined as a push or a pull exerted by one object or substance on another. Whenever two objects contact each other, they will either push or pull on each other with some magnitude of force. The unit for a force (a push or a pull) in the SI system is the **newton (N);** the unit in the U.S. system is the **pound (lb).** The concept of a force as a push or pull can readily be used to describe the forces encountered in evaluating human motion.

Foundational Concepts 1–1
A Force

Although a force is most simply described as a push or a pull, it is also described as a "theoretical concept" because only its effects (e.g., acceleration) can be measured.[2] A force (F) on an object is directly proportional to both the acceleration (a) and to the mass (m) of that object; that is,

$$\text{Force} = (\text{mass})(\text{acceleration})$$

$$\text{or } F = (m)(a)$$

Because mass is measured in kilograms (kg) and acceleration in m/sec^2, the unit for force is actually kg·m/sec^2 or, more simply, the newton (N). A newton is the force required to accelerate 1 kg at 1 m/sec^2; the pound is correspondingly the amount of force required to accelerate a mass of 1 slug at 1 ft/sec^2. A "slug" is a rarely used term for a unit of mass in the U.S. system.

External forces are pushes or pulls on the body that arise from sources outside the body. **Gravity (g),** the attraction of the earth's mass to another mass, is an external force that under normal conditions constantly affects all objects. The **weight (W)** of an object is the pull of gravity on the object's mass with an acceleration of 9.8 m/sec^2 (or 32.2 ft/sec^2) in the absence of any resistance; that is:

$$\text{weight} = (\text{mass})(\text{gravity})$$

$$\text{or } W = (m)(g)$$

Because weight is a force, the appropriate unit is the newton (or pound). It is common to see weight given in **kilograms (kg),** although this is technically incorrect because the kilogram is a unit of mass. In the U.S. system, the pound is commonly used to designate mass and is appropriately a force unit (1 kg = 2.2 lb).

Expanded Concepts 1–1
Force and Mass Unit Terminology

Force and mass units are often used incorrectly in the vernacular. The average person using the metric system expects a scale to show weight in kilograms rather than in newtons. In the United States, the average person correctly thinks of "weight" in pounds but also—incorrectly—considers the pound to be a unit of mass. Because people commonly tend to think of mass in terms of weight (the force of gravity acting on the mass of an object), the pound is often (incorrectly) used to represent the mass of an object in the United States.

One attempt to maintain common usage while clearly differentiating force units from mass units for scientific purposes is to designate "lb" and "kg" as mass units and to designate the corresponding force units as "lbf" (pound-force) and "kgf" (kilogram-force).[2,4] When the kilogram is used as a force unit:

$$1 \text{ kgf} = 9.8 \text{ N}$$

When the pound is used as a mass unit:

$$1 \text{ lb} = 0.031 \text{ slugs}$$

These conversions assume an unresisted acceleration of gravity of 9.8 m/sec^2 or 32.2 ft/sec^2, respectively. It might be obvious to the reader who is unfamiliar with the kgf and the slug that these terms have not come into common usage.

The distinction between a measure of mass and a measure of force is important because mass is a scalar quantity (without action line or direction), whereas the newton and pound are measures of force and have vector characteristics. In this text, we will consistently use the terms *newton* and *pound* as force units and the term *kilogram* as the corresponding mass unit. The term *slug* is not in common usage and will not be used further in the text.

Because gravity is the most consistent and predictable force acting on the body, it should be the first consideration when analyzing the potential forces influencing a body segment. However, gravity is only one of an infinite number of external forces that can affect the body and its segments. Examples of other external forces that may exert a push or pull on the human body or its segments are wind (the push of air on the body), water (the push of water on the body), other people (the push or pull of an examiner on John Alexander's leg), and other objects (the push of the floor on the feet, the pull of an ankle weight on the leg). A critical point is that the forces on the body or any one segment must come from something that is touching the body or segment. The major apparent exception to this rule is the force of gravity. However, we can circumvent this exception by using the notion that gravity (the pull of the earth) "contacts" all objects on earth, thereby allowing a standing rule that *all forces on a segment must come from something that is contacting that segment* (including gravity). The opposite also holds true: *Anything that contacts a segment must create a force on that segment*, although the magnitude may be small enough to disregard.

Foundational Concepts 1–2
Primary Rules of Forces

- All forces on a segment must come from something that is contacting that segment.
- Anything that contacts a segment *must* create a force on that segment (although the magnitude may be small enough to disregard).
- Gravity can be considered to be "touching" all objects.

Internal forces are those forces that act on structures of the body and arise from the body's own structures (i.e., the contact of two structures within the body). A few common examples are the forces produced by the muscles (the pull of the biceps brachii on the radius), the ligaments (the pull of a ligament on the bones to which it attaches), and the bones (the push of one bone on another bone at a joint). Both internal and external forces can either facilitate or restrict movement. Internal forces, however, are most readily recognized as essential for *initiation* of movement. It should be apparent that internal forces also control or counteract movement produced by external forces, as well as counteracting other internal forces. Much of the presentation and discussion in subsequent chapters of this text relate to the interactive role of internal forces in producing or controlling joint rotations as well as in maintaining the integrity (stability) of joint structures against the effects of external forces and other internal forces.

Force Vectors

All forces, regardless of the source or the object acted on, are **vector** quantities. A force is represented by an arrow (vector) that (1) has its base on the object being acted on (the point of application), (2) has a shaft and arrowhead in the direction of the force being exerted (direction/orientation), and (3) has a length representing the amount of force being exerted (magnitude). As we begin to examine force vectors (and at least throughout this chapter), the *point of application* (*base*) of each vector in each figure will be placed on the segment or object to which the force is applied—which is generally also the object under discussion.

The contact of a coffee cup on the forearm-hand and the pull of a muscle on the forearm-hand serve as examples of external and internal forces, respectively. **Figure 1–8** shows a forearm-hand segment with the hand holding a coffee cup (an external force). Because the cup contacts the forearm-hand segment, the cup must exert a force (in this case, downward) on the segment. The force, called cup-on-forearm/hand (CFh), is represented by a vector. The point of application on the forearm-hand segment is at the hand where the cup exerts its pull; the action line and direction indicate the direction of the pull and the angle of pull of the cup in relation to the forearm-hand; and the length is drawn to represent the magnitude of the pull (equivalent to the weight) of the cup. The force CFh is an external force because the weight of the cup is not part of the body, although it contacts the body. **Figure 1–9** shows the force of an elbow flexor (an internal force) pulling on the forearm-hand segment. The point of application is at the attachment of the muscle on the forearm, and the orientation and direction are toward the center of the muscle (a "pull" is always toward the source of the force). The force

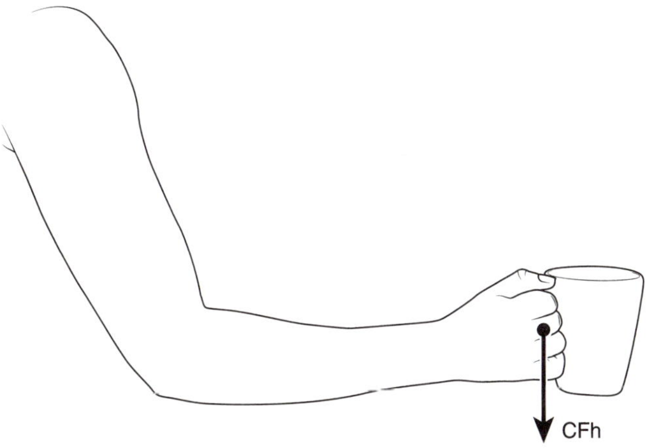

Figure 1–8 Vector representation of the pull of the weight of the cup on the forearm-hand segment (cup-on-forearm/hand [CFh]), with a magnitude proportional to the mass and equivalent to the weight of the cup.

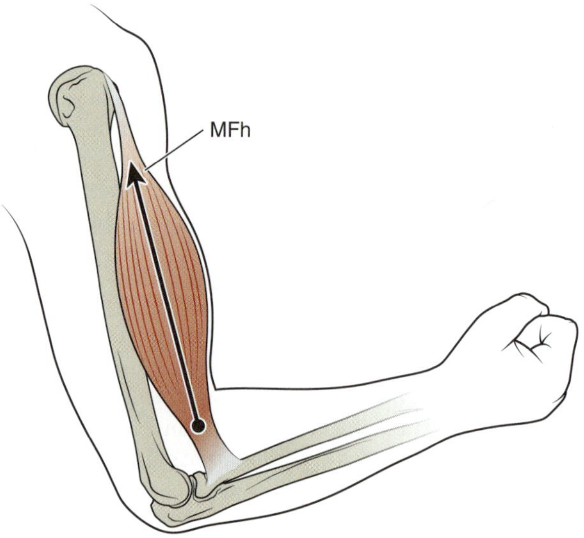

Figure 1–9 Vector muscle-on-forearm/hand (MFh) represents the pull of a muscle on the forearm-hand segment.

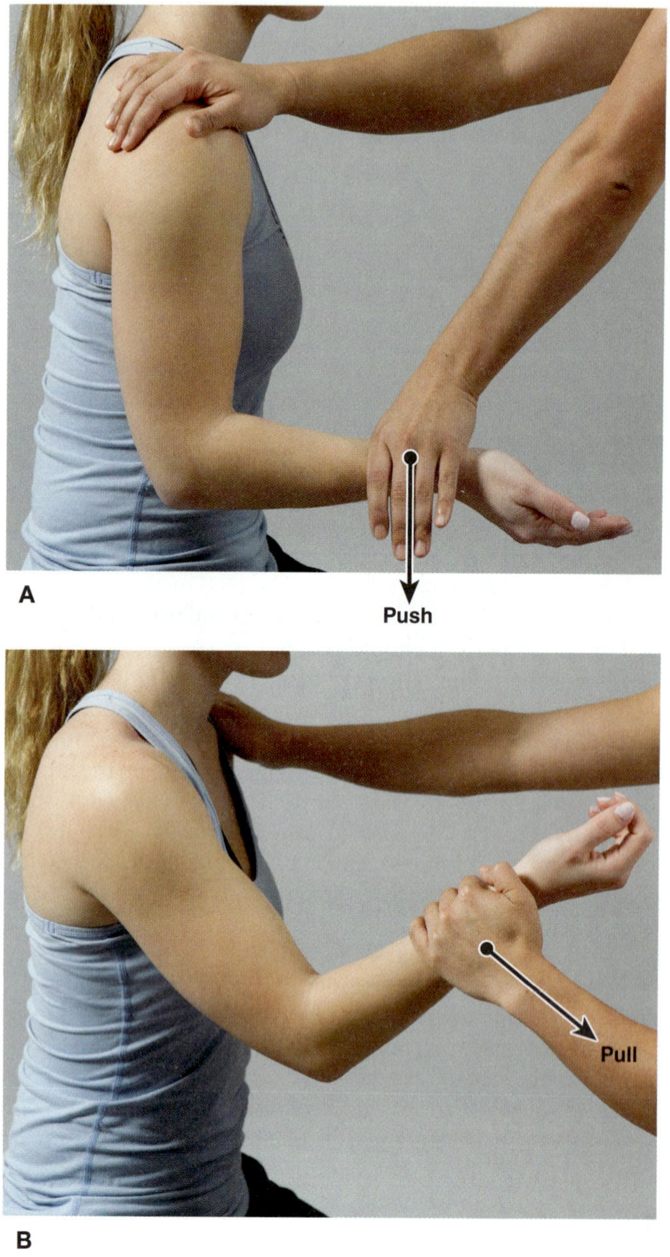

Figure 1–10 Push vs. pull forces. **A.** The clinician's manual resistance to the forearm is applied as a push, whereas in **B.** the clinician's manual resistance is applied to the forearm as a pull. Both vectors look similar and would be indistinguishable as a push vs. a pull if the clinician's hand was removed from each photo.

is called muscle-on-forearm/hand (represented by the vector MFh). Although the designation of a force as "external" or "internal" may be useful in some contexts, the rules for drawing (or visualizing) forces are the same for external forces, such as the cup, and internal forces, such as the muscle.

Vectors can represent either a push or a pull on a segment depending on the point of application and the source of the force. **Figure 1–10** shows the force vector of both a *push* and a *pull* of an external resistance on the forearm. In **Figure 1–10A**, the push vector is directed away from the source of the manual resistance; in **Figure 1–10B**, the pull vector is directed toward the source of the manual resistance. Whether a push or a pull, the vectors are similar and would have an identical effect on the forearm-hand segment if the magnitudes of the force were the same.

Foundational Concepts 1–3
Force Vectors

Force vectors are characterized by:

- A **point of application** *on the object acted upon.*
- An action line and **direction/orientation** indicating a *pull toward* the source object or a *push away from* the source object, at a given angle to the object acted upon.
- A length that represents, and may be drawn proportional to, its **magnitude** (the quantity of push or pull).
- A length that may be extended to assess the relation between two or more vectors or to assess the relation of the vector to adjacent objects or points.
- A force **name** that uses the *"X-on-Y"* where the first part of the force name ("X") will always identify the *source* of the force and the second part of the force name ("Y") will always identify the object or segment that is acted upon.

Force of Gravity

As already noted, gravity is one of the most consistent and influential forces that the human body encounters in posture and movement. For that reason, it is useful to consider gravity first when examining forces. As a vector quantity, the force of gravity can be fully described by point of application, action line/direction/orientation, and magnitude. The force of gravity acting on an object or segment is considered to have its point of application at the center of mass (CoM) or **center of gravity (CoG)** of that object or segment—the hypothetical point at which all the mass of the object or segment appears to be concentrated. Every object or segment can be approached as if it had a single center of mass.

In a symmetrical object, the center of mass is located in the geometric center of the object. In an asymmetrical object, the center of mass will be located toward the heavier end because the mass must be evenly distributed around the center of mass. In cases where the center of mass conceptually lies outside the object, it is still the point from which the force of gravity *appears* to act. The center of mass of an object can be approximated by thinking of it as the balance point of the object (assuming you could balance the object on one finger).

Although the direction and orientation of most forces vary with the source of the force, the force of gravity acting on an object is *always* vertically downward toward its source—the center of the earth. The gravitational vector is commonly referred to as the **line of gravity (LoG).** The length of the line of gravity can be drawn to scale (as in a free-body diagram where length is determined by the magnitude of the force) or it may be extended (like any vector) when the relationship of the vector to other forces, points, or objects is being explored. The line of gravity can best be visualized as a string with a weight on the end (a plumb line), with the string attached to the center of mass of the object.

Segmental Centers of Mass and Composition of Gravitational Forces

Each segment in the body can be considered to have its own center of mass and line of gravity **(Fig. 1–11)**. **Figure 1–11A** shows the gravitational vectors acting at the centers of mass of the arm, the forearm, and the hand segments (vectors GA, GF, and GH, respectively), with the hand treated as a single solid segment. It is often useful, however, to consider two or more segments as a single rigid segment (such as the leg-foot segment in the patient application). In **Figure 1–11B**, the gravitational forces on the forearm and hand have been combined into a single vector (GFH) acting at the combined center of mass of these two segments. In **Figure 1–11C**, the gravitational force for all three segments is represented by a single vector (GAFH) applied at the center of mass of all three segments taken together.

When the masses of two segments are combined (e.g., forearm and hand segments as in Figure 1–11B or the arm and forearm-hand segments as in Figure 1–11C), the new point of application (the new center of mass) will be located between and in line with the original two segmental centers of mass. When the linked segments are not equal in mass, the new center of mass will lie closer to the heavier segment. The new vector will have the same effect on the combined segment(s) as on the original vectors and is known as the **resultant force.** The process of combining two or more forces into a single resultant force is known as **composition of forces.** When segments are rearranged as in **Figure 1–11D**, the rule for identifying the

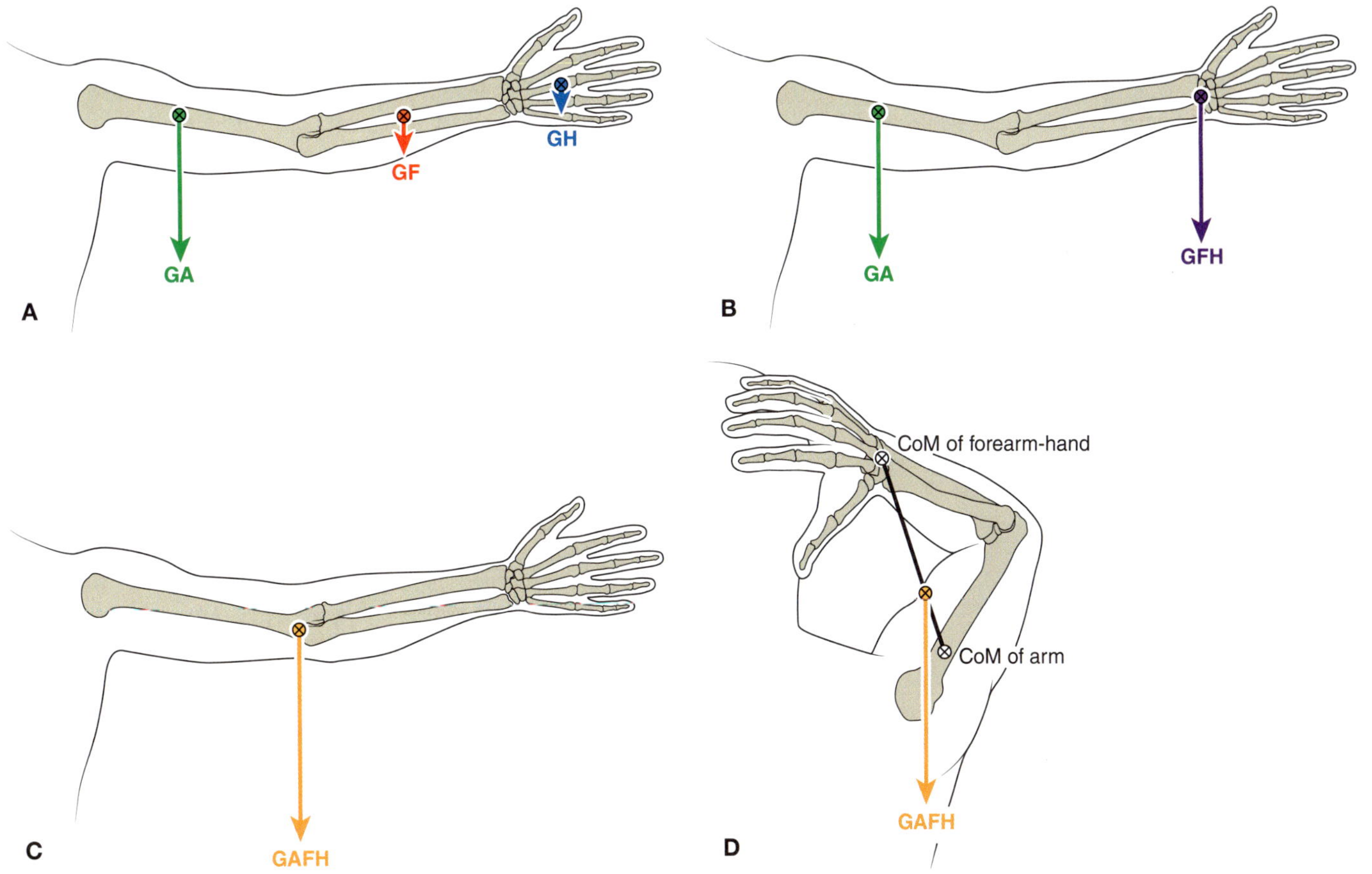

Figure 1–11 Gravity acts at the center of mass of each segment—or may be shown acting at a center that combines the mass of two or more segments taken together. **A.** Gravity is shown acting separately at the centers of mass of the arm (GA), forearm (GF), and hand (GH) segments. **B.** Gravity acting on the combined masses of the forearm and hand can be shown as a single resultant vector, GFH, with a point of application at the new combined center of mass of those two segments. **C.** Gravity acting on the combined masses of the arm-forearm-hand segment is shown as a single resultant vector, GAFH, applied at the new center of mass of all three segments. **D.** When the masses of the arm and forearm-hand segments are rearranged, the point of application of the gravitation vector, GAFH, shifts to the new center of mass that still lies in between and along a line connecting the original centers of mass.

location of the combined center of mass (point of application of GAFH) remains the same but may actually lie outside the body; the magnitude of GAFH remains unchanged.

Center of Mass of the Human Body

When all the segments of the body are combined and considered as a single rigid object in anatomic position, the center of mass of the body lies approximately anterior to the second sacral vertebra (S2). The precise location of the center of mass for a person in the anatomic position depends on the proportions (weight distribution) of that person. In **Figure 1–12**, the line of gravity is between the person's feet **(base of support [BoS])** as the person stands in anatomic position; the line of gravity is parallel to the trunk and limbs. If the person is lying down (still in anatomic position), the line of gravity projecting from the center of mass of the body will lie perpendicular to the trunk and limbs rather than parallel as it does in the standing position. In reality, of course, a person is not rigid and does not remain in anatomic position. Rather, a person is constantly moving, resulting in rearrangement of the various body segments in relation to each other. With each rearrangement of body segments, the location of the individual's center of mass will potentially change.

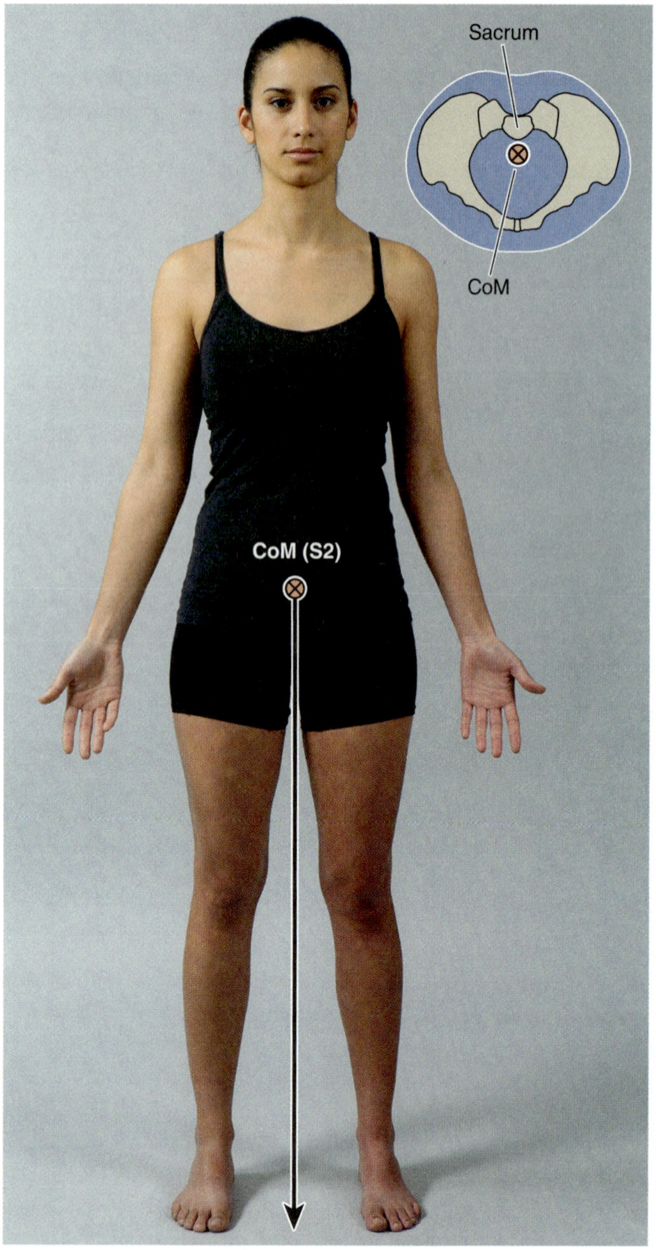

Figure 1–12 The center of mass (CoM) of the human body lies approximately at S2, anterior to the sacrum (inset). The extended line of gravity (LoG) lies within the base of support (BoS) between the feet.

Example 1–1
Altering Center of Mass Location

If a person is considered to be composed of a rigid upper body (**head-arms-trunk** [**HAT**]) and a rigid lower limb segment, both segments will have their own center of mass. If the trunk is inclined forward **(Fig. 1–13)**, the segmental masses remain unchanged but the composite center of mass of the rearranged body segments shifts from its original location (within the pelvis just anterior to S2) to a new location on a line between the original two centers of mass. Because the head, arms, and trunk together typically have twice the mass of the lower extremities, the new center of mass will be closer to HAT. The relocated center of mass is physically located outside the body, with the line of gravity correspondingly shifted forward within the base of support.

Center of Mass, Line of Gravity, and Stability

In Figure 1–13, the line of gravity shifts toward the front of the feet that serve as the base of support. For a static object to be stable, *the line of gravity must fall within the base of support.* When the line of gravity is outside the base of support, the object will be unstable and will start falling.

When an object's base of support is large, the line of gravity is less likely to be displaced outside the base of support and the object, consequently, is more stable. When a person stands with their legs spread apart **(Fig. 1–14)**, the base is wide and the trunk can move side to side a good deal without displacing the line of gravity from the base of support and without the person falling over. Whereas the center of mass remains in approximately the same place within the body as the trunk shifts to each side, the *line* of gravity moves within the wide base of support. It is useful here to think of the line of gravity as a plumb line. As long as the plumb line does not leave the base of support, the person should not fall over.

Just as an object is more stable when the base of support is large, an object is also stable when its center of mass is low (close to the ground). When the center of mass is low, the vertical line of gravity projecting from the center of mass to the base of support will be shorter and, therefore, less likely to "swing" outside the base of support.

Foundational Concepts 1–4
Stability of an Object or the Human Body

- The larger the base of support of an object, the greater the stability of that object.
- The closer the object's center of mass is to the base of support, the more stable the object.
- A static object cannot be stable unless its line of gravity is located within its base of support.

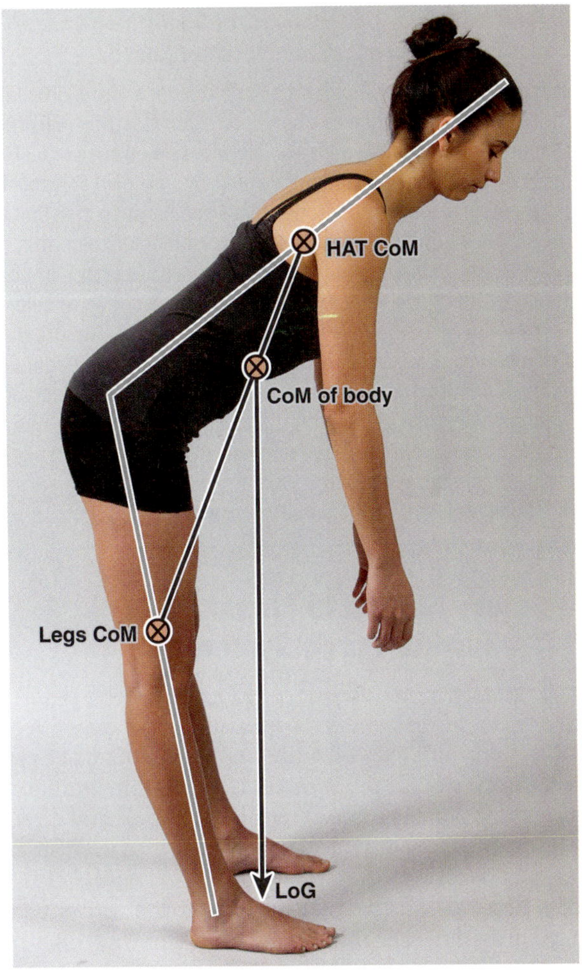

Figure 1–13 Rearrangement of the head, arms, and trunk (HAT) in relation to the lower extremities (legs) relocates the center of mass (CoM) and shifts the line of gravity (LoG) forward in the base of support.

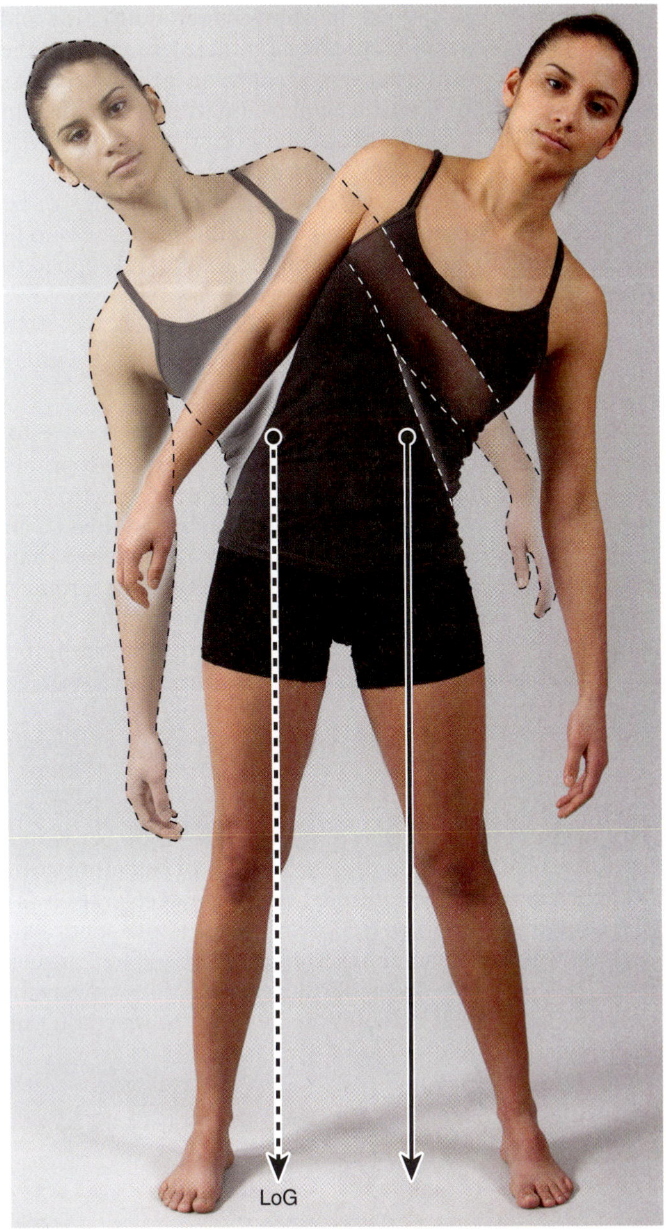

Figure 1–14 A wide base of support permits a wide excursion of the line of gravity (LoG) without the LoG falling outside the base of support (the two widely spaced feet).

Introduction to Statics and Dynamics

The primary concern when looking at forces acting on the body, or a particular segment of the body, is the effect that those forces will have on the body or segment. If all the forces acting on a segment are "balanced" (a state known as **equilibrium**), the segment will remain at rest or in uniform motion. If the forces are not "balanced," the segment will accelerate. **Statics** is the study of the conditions under which objects remain at rest or in uniform motion. **Dynamics** is the study of the conditions under which objects accelerate. Isaac Newton's first two laws govern whether an object is static or dynamic.

Newton's Law of Inertia

Newton's first law, the **law of inertia,** identifies the conditions under which an object is in equilibrium. **Inertia** is the property of an object that resists both the initiation of linear motion and a change in linear motion and is directly proportional to its mass. Similarly, **moment of inertia** is the property of an object that resists rotary motion and changes in rotary motion. The term *moment* (also known as torque) refers to the magnitude of a force's tendency to cause an object to rotate. The law of inertia states that an object will remain at rest or in uniform motion unless acted on by an unbalanced force (producing translation) or torque (producing rotation). If the forces or torques acting on an object are balanced, the object can be motionless (**static equilibrium**). However, an object acted upon by balanced forces or torques may also be in uniform motion, that is, moving with a constant speed and direction. Velocity (rate of change) is a vector quantity that describes both speed and direction/orientation. An object in equilibrium can have a velocity of any magnitude, but its velocity must remain unchanged. When the velocity of an object is constant but not zero, the object is moving and is in **dynamic equilibrium.** An object in dynamic equilibrium can be moving linearly (translatory motion), around an axis (rotary motion), or in a combination of both translation and rotation (e.g., general or curvilinear motion). In joints of the body, dynamic equilibrium occurs infrequently. Therefore, within the scope of this text, equilibrium will be simplified to mean an object at rest (in static equilibrium) unless otherwise specified.

Newton's law of inertia (or law of equilibrium) can be restated thus: For an object to be in equilibrium, the sum of all the forces (F) and the sum of all the torques (τ) applied to that object must be zero.

$$\Sigma F = 0$$

$$\Sigma \tau = 0$$

The equilibrium of an object is determined only by forces or torques *applied to that object*—that is, with points of application on that object. There is no restriction on the number of forces or torques that can be applied to an object in equilibrium, although there must be more than one force or torque. If one (and only one) force or torque is applied to an object, the sum of the forces or torques cannot be zero. When the sum of the forces or torques acting on an object is not zero ($F \neq 0$ or $\tau \neq 0$), the object *must* be accelerating.

Newton's Law of Acceleration

The magnitude of acceleration of a moving object is defined by Newton's second law, the **law of acceleration.** Newton's second law states that the linear acceleration (a) or angular acceleration (α) of an object is proportional, respectively, to the net unbalanced forces (F_{unbal}) or torques (τ_{unbal}) acting on the object. Further, acceleration is inversely proportional to the mass (m) or moment of inertia (I) of that object:

$$a = \frac{F_{unbal}}{m}$$

$$\alpha = \frac{\tau_{unbal}}{I}$$

Note that the concept of "moment of inertia (I)" is far less intuitive than the concept of mass. Moment of inertia is defined as $I = mr^2$, where m is the mass of an object and r is the distance that mass lies from the axis of rotation. Therefore, resistance to rotary motion is dependent both on the total mass of an object *and* on the spatial distribution of that mass. In other words, a heavy object has more rotary inertia than a lighter object, and an object with mass farther from the axis of rotation will have more rotary inertia than an object with mass focused closer to the axis of rotation.

An object acted upon by a net unbalanced force or torque *must* be accelerating, and the acceleration of the object will be in the direction of the net unbalanced force or torque. A net unbalanced *force* will produce translatory motion; a net unbalanced *torque* will produce rotary motion; and a combination of unbalanced force and torque will produce general (e.g., curvilinear) motion.

Foundational Concepts 1–5
Applying the Law of Acceleration (Inertia)

To put the law of acceleration into simple words: a large, unbalanced push or pull (F_{unbal}) applied to an object of a given mass (m) will produce more linear acceleration (a) than a small, unbalanced push or pull. Similarly, a given magnitude of unbalanced push or pull on an object of large mass or moment of inertia will produce less acceleration than that same push or pull on an object with smaller mass or moment of inertia. From the law of acceleration, it can be seen that inertia (a body's or object's resistance to change in velocity) is also the resistance to acceleration and is proportional to the mass of the body or object. The greater the mass or moment of inertia of an object, the greater the magnitude of net unbalanced force or torque needed either to get the object moving or to change its motion. A very large woman in a wheelchair has more inertia than a small woman in a wheelchair; an aide must exert a greater push on a wheelchair with a large woman in it to get the chair in motion than on the wheelchair with a small woman in it.

Translatory Motion in Linear and Concurrent Force Systems

The composition, or addition, of forces is used to determine whether a net (unbalanced) force exists on a segment because this will determine whether the segment remains at rest or moves. Furthermore, the direction/orientation and location of the net unbalanced force determines the type and direction of motion of the segment. The process of composition of forces was oversimplified in Figures 1–11 and 1–13. The process depends on the relationship of the forces to each other; that is, whether the forces are in a linear, concurrent, or parallel force system. When force vectors applied to the same segment have action lines that lie in the same plane, and act in the same line (collinear and coplanar), these two vectors are part of a **linear force system.** If two forces are collinear but not coplanar (parallel to each other) or coplanar but not collinear (lying at angles to each other), the forces are not part of the same linear force system.

Linear Force Systems

A linear force system exists whenever two or more forces acting *on the same segment* lie in the same line (collinear) and in the same plane (coplanar) **(Fig. 1–15)**. If their action lines were extended, they would completely overlap **(Fig. 1–15A)**. Forces in a linear force system are assigned positive or negative signs. Forces applied up (z-axis), anteriorly (y-axis), or to the right (x-axis) will be assigned positive signs, whereas forces applied down, posteriorly, or to the left will be assigned negative signs.

Determining Resultant Forces in a Linear Force System

The resultant, or net effect, of all forces that are part of the same linear force system can be composed into a single resultant (net) vector **(Fig. 1–15B)**. The resultant vector has an action line in the same line and plane as that of the original composing vectors; the magnitude is equivalent to the arithmetic sum of the composing vectors and is in the direction of the net force. Because the vectors in the same linear force system are all collinear and coplanar, the point of application

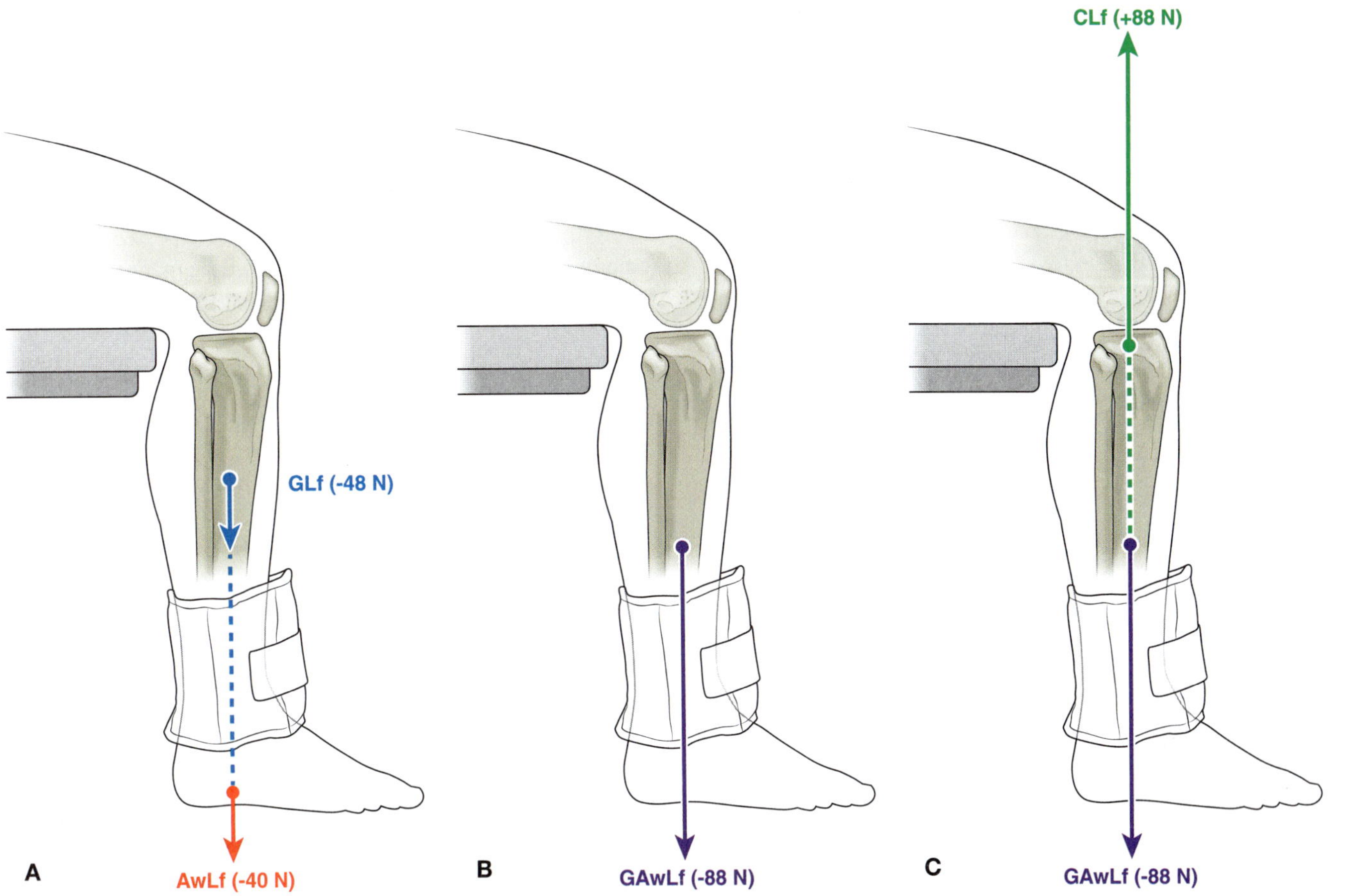

Figure 1–15 Resultant forces in a linear force system. **A.** The forces of gravity-on-leg/foot (GLf) and ankle weight-on-leg/foot (AwLf) are in the same linear force system because they are applied to the same object and are both collinear and coplanar. **B.** GAwLf is the resultant of GLf and AwLf, with a magnitude of 88 N (the sum of the original two forces of 48 N and 40 N) and with a point of application between those of GLf and AwLf (slightly toward the force of greater magnitude). **C.** An opposing force such as capsule-on-leg/foot (CLf) must exist so that the sum of the linear forces is zero and the leg-foot segment is at rest.

of the resultant vector will lie along the common action line of the composing vectors.

A net force that moves a bony segment away from its adjacent bony segment is known as a **distraction force.** A distraction force tends to cause a separation between the bones that make up a joint. In Figure 1–15B, GAwLf is the only force shown acting on the leg-foot and would appear to indicate that the leg-foot segment is accelerating downward away from the femur. At least one additional force must act on the leg-foot segment for it to be at rest because an object cannot be at rest unless the sum of the forces is zero. That force must come from something that is touching the leg-foot segment.

The two bones in a synovial joint (e.g., the knee joint) are connected (and, therefore, "touched") by a joint capsule made of connective tissue. Although we are oversimplifying for now, the force of the capsular ligaments (capsule-on-leg/foot) can pull up on the leg-foot segment **(Fig. 1–15C)** along the same line as GAwLf and with a force that is equal in magnitude and opposite direction to GAwLf; thus, the net of forces acting on the leg-foot segment is zero and the leg-foot segment will be in equilibrium.

The joint capsule does not exert the simplified pull on the bone shown in Figure 1–15C. In reality the capsule *surrounds* the adjacent bones in three dimensions, acting like a sleeve that surrounds the joint, with the sleeve attaching circumferentially both to the proximal joint segment (femur) and the distal joint segment (tibia). The force of the capsule, therefore, would be a set of forces applied around the periphery of the adjacent articular surfaces. **Figure 1–16** shows a schematic drawing of the capsule of a generic synovial joint on cross section. The vector arrows for the pulls of the anterior and posterior capsules must follow the fibers of the capsule at their respective points of application on the tibia and continue in a straight line. *A vector is always a straight line*; the vector continues in the same straight line even if the fibers of the capsule change direction beyond their bony attachment. Even in this two-dimensional representation, it is apparent that the anterior and posterior fibers of the capsule will pull (capsules cannot "push") on the distal segment at different places with forces that lie at angles (rather than in line) with each other. The forces shown in Figure 1–16 are part of a **concurrent force system.**

Concurrent Force Systems

It is quite common (and perhaps nearly universal in the human body) for forces to be applied to the same object but with action lines that lie at angles to each other. To understand the net effect (resultant) of two or more forces acting on a segment in

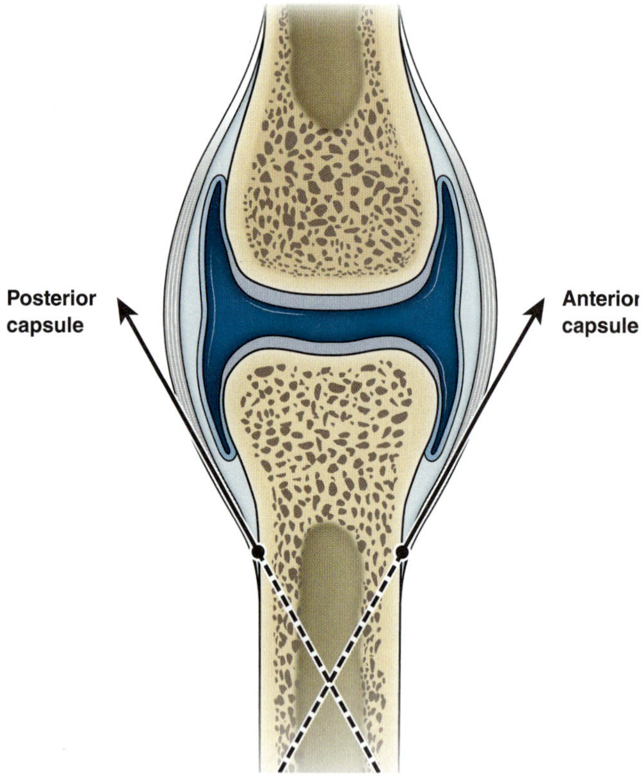

Figure 1–16 This schematic cross section of a generic synovial joint shows the pull of the anterior and posterior capsule on the distal segment of the joint. The two forces are applied to the same object but lie at angles to each other and, if extended, intersect. These forces form a concurrent force system.

a concurrent force system, a different method of composition of forces is needed than is used for composition of forces in a linear force system. Any two forces in a concurrent force system can be composed into a single resultant force through a graphic process known as **composition by parallelogram.**

Determining Resultant Forces in a Concurrent Force System

In composition by parallelogram, two forces that are part of the *same* concurrent force system (more than one can exist on an object) are taken at a time **(Fig. 1–17). Figure 1–17A** shows John Alexander's leg-foot segment with the resultant GAwLf as shown in Figure 1–15B, with the addition of the forces of the anterior capsule on leg-foot (AcLf) and posterior capsule on leg-foot (PcLf). Vectors AcLf and PcLf are extended to identify their common point of application and their relationship to each other. In **Figure 1–17B**, vectors AcLf and PcLf (now starting from their common point of application) form two sides of a parallelogram, with the parallelogram completed by adding dotted lines *parallel* to AcLf and to PcLf as shown in the figure. The resultant (CLf) is the diagonal of the parallelogram with the same point of application as the original vectors and with its length determined by the intersection of the two dotted lines. Note that the resultant CLf in Figure 1–17B is essentially identical to CLf in Figure 1–15C, indicating that the simplification used in that earlier figure was a reasonable representation of the combined pulls of the anterior and posterior fibers of the joint capsule on the leg-foot segment, albeit still an oversimplification of the pull of a circumferential capsule.

The magnitude of the resultant force of two concurrent forces is proportionally related to the magnitudes and the angle between the original forces. The relationship is dependent both on the magnitudes of the composing vectors *and* the angle (orientation of) the intersecting vectors. The magnitude of the resultant of two concurrent forces will always be smaller than the sum of the magnitude of the composing forces (e.g., CLf < AcLf + PcLf in Fig. 1–17B) because a single push or pull is more efficient than two divergent pushes or pulls, although the net effect is the same.

The concept of composition by parallelogram can provide an understanding (and, perhaps, a visualization) of the net effect of two concurrent forces. If the magnitudes of the composing forces and the angle at which the composing forces intersect are known, trigonometric functions can be used to determine the magnitude of the resultant. Because the angle values are rarely known outside a research setting, the mathematic (trigonometric) solution is conceptually valuable but not as practical in a clinical situation as the potential "visual" solution of composition by parallelogram.

Expanded Concepts 1–2
Trigonometric Solution to Composition by Parallelogram

Let us assume that AcLf and PcLf (originally shown in Fig. 1–17A) each have a magnitude of 51 N and that the vectors are at a 60° angle (θ) to each other (**Fig. 1–18**). A parallelogram still needs to be drawn and is completed by forming two lines parallel and opposite to AcLf and PcLf ($AcLf_1$ and $PcLf_1$, respectively); the resultant (CLf) is drawn as the diagonal of the parallelogram. That diagonal vector will divide the parallelogram into two equal triangles. The magnitude of the resultant vector (CLf) can be determined using the law of cosines, permitting calculation of the length of the side of a triangle that is opposite to the known angle (when the triangle is not a right triangle).

The reference triangle (shaded) is formed by PcLf, $AcLf_1$, and CLf. To apply the law of cosines, angle β must be known because vector CLf (whose length we are solving for) is the "side opposite" that angle. We already identified the angle (θ) in Figure 1–18 as 60°. If PcLf is extended (as shown by the red dotted line in Fig. 1–18), the angle θ is replicated because $AcLf_1$ is parallel to AcLf so that it has the same angular relationship to PcLf. Angle β will be the complement of angle α, or:

$$\beta = 180° - 60° = 120°$$

By substituting the variables given in the example, the magnitude of the resultant, CLf, can be solved for by using the following equation:

$$CLf = \sqrt{PcLf^2 + AcLf^2 - 2(PcLf)\,(AcLf)\,(\cos\beta)}$$

If the value of 51 N is entered into the equation for both PcLf and AcLf and an angle of 120° is used, vector CLf = 88 N.

Newton's Law of Reaction

Newton's third law (the law of reaction) is commonly stated as follows: For every action, there is an equal and opposite

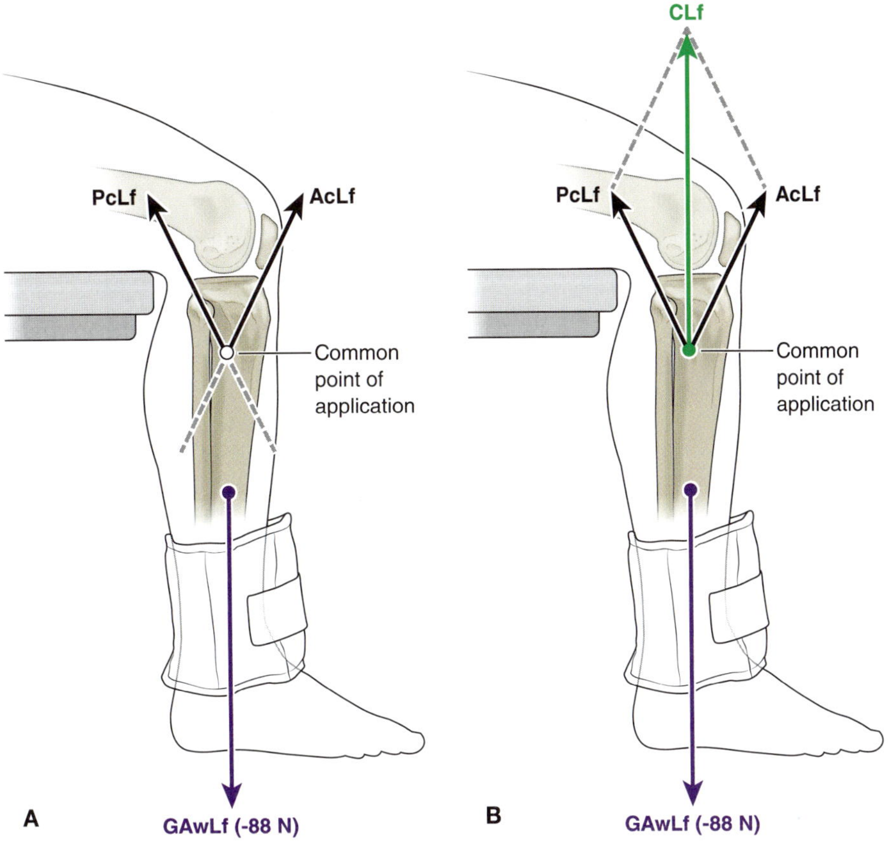

Figure 1–17 Composition of concurrent forces. **A.** The vectors of the anterior capsule (AcLf) and posterior capsule (PcLf) acting on the leg-foot segment can be extended to identify their common point of application. **B.** With AcLf and PcLf shown now as acting from their common point of application, the remaining two sides of the parallelogram are drawn. The resultant pull of AcLf and PcLf is the diagonal of the parallelogram (CLf). Capsule on the leg-foot (CLf) has the same effect on the leg-foot segment as do the combined forces of AcLf + PcLf.

reaction. In other words, when an object applies a force to a second object, the second object *must* simultaneously apply a force equal in magnitude and opposite in direction to the first object. These two forces that are applied to the two contacting objects are an **interaction pair** and can also be called **action-reaction** (or simply **reaction**) **forces.**

Expanded Concepts 1–3
Action-Reaction Pairs

In Figure 1–17B we see the force vector of capsule-on leg/foot (CLf) that is due to the pull of the capsule on the leg-foot segment. If the capsule is touching the leg-foot segment and pulling on the leg-foot segment, the leg-foot segment must also be touching and pulling on the capsule, introducing the force of leg/foot-on-capsule (LfC). CLf and LfC are an action-reaction pair, coexisting because two objects touch *each other*. Because we have been limiting our interest to forces on the leg-foot segment, we could theoretically ignore LfC. However, John has injured his medial collateral ligament, which is closely associated with the knee joint capsule and has a similar line of pull. We will subsequently need to consider the forces pulling on the capsule (and its associated ligaments) to understand the effect of the exercises on John's injured knee structures.

Reaction forces always act along the same line but are applied to different, contacting objects in opposite directions. The directions of reaction forces are always opposite to each other because the two touching objects either pull or push on each other. Because the points of application of reaction forces are never on the same object, reaction forces are never part of the same force system and typically are not part of the same space diagram. However, reaction forces play a critical role in human function, because no body segment operates in isolation; every movement involves the interaction of adjacent segments and external structures (as seen in a space diagram).

Gravitational and Contact Forces

A different scenario can be used to demonstrate the sometimes subtle but potentially important distinction between a force applied to an object and its reaction force. We generally assume when we get on a scale that the scale shows our weight. However, "weight" is the pull of gravity on a person's mass (gravity-on-person or GP) and is not applied to the scale. If GP is not applied to the scale, it cannot act on the scale. What is actually being recorded on the scale is the contact (downward push) of the "person-on-scale" (PS) and not

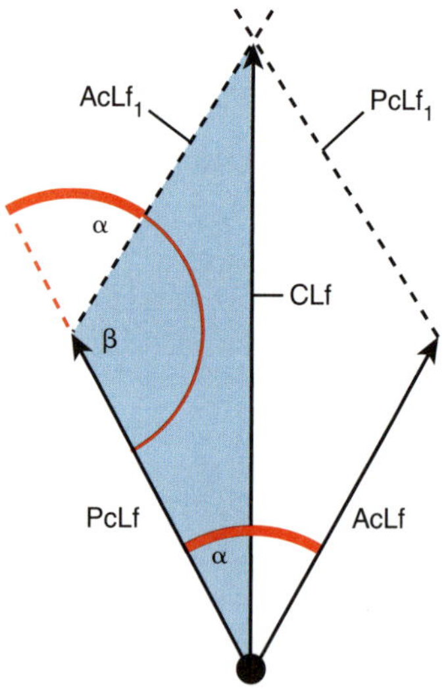

Figure 1–18 The law of cosines for triangles is used to compute the magnitude of CLf, given the magnitudes of AcLf and PcLf, as well as the angle of application (α) between them. The relevant angle (β) is the complement of angle α (180° – α).

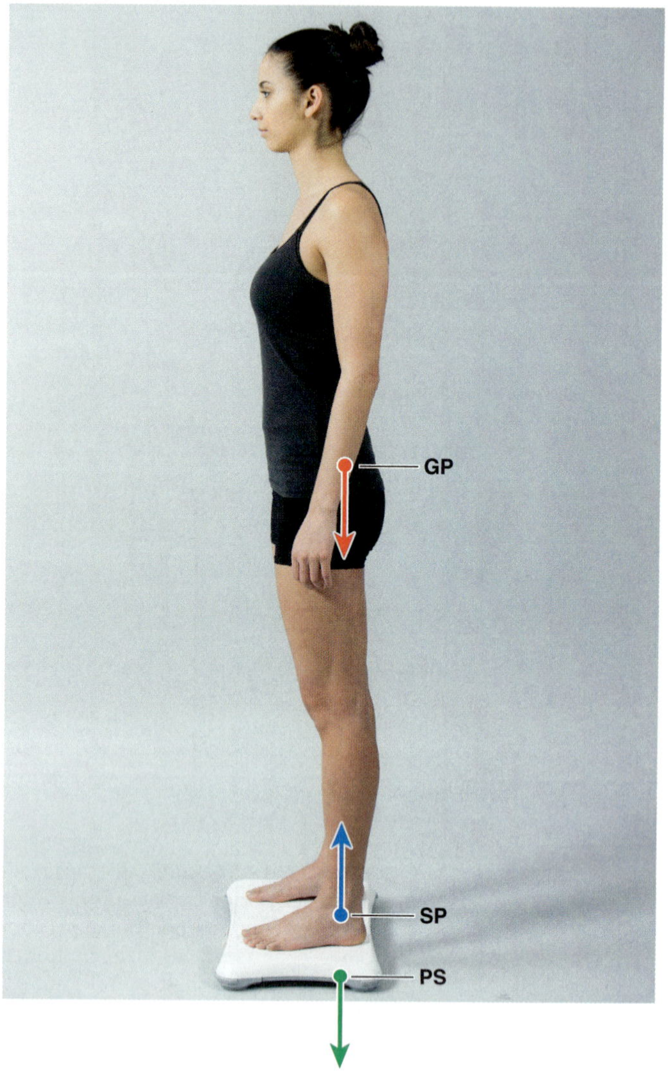

Figure 1–19 Although a scale is commonly thought to measure the weight of the person standing on the scale (gravity-on-person, or GP), it actually measures the contact of person-on-scale (PS). Because nothing else is touching the person in this figure but gravity and the scale, the push of scale-on-person (SP) must be equal in magnitude and opposite in direction to gravity-on-person (GP) for the sum of the forces on the static person to equal zero. Per Newton's second law, SP has a reaction force of person-on-scale (PS) that is equal in magnitude, opposite in direction, and applied to the scale. As long as nothing else is touching the person, then the magnitudes of GP, SP, and PS are all equivalent. That is, the "weight" of the person (GP) is equal to the person's contact with the scale (PS).

"gravity-on-person." The distinction between these forces and the relation between these two forces can be established by using both Newton's first and third laws.

The person standing on the scale **(Fig. 1–19)** must be in equilibrium ($\Sigma F = 0$) because the person is not moving. If the gravity-on-person vector (GP) is acting down with a magnitude of –734 N (the person's weight), there must also be an upward force of equal magnitude acting on the person for the person to remain motionless. The only other object, besides gravity, that appears to be contacting the person in Figure 1–19 is the scale. The scale, therefore, must be exerting an upward push on the person (scale-on-person, or SP) with a magnitude equal and opposite to the pull of gravity-on-person, thus +734 N. Per Newton's third law, if the scale is pushing on the person, the person must also be pushing on the scale. As is always true for reaction forces, the reaction force to scale-on-person will be equal in magnitude (734 N) and opposite in direction (down) but applied to the scale (person-on-scale, or PS in Fig. 1–19). In this scenario, the magnitude of the person's weight (GP) and the magnitude of the person's push on the scale (PS) are equivalent in magnitude *although applied to different objects.*

The distinction is not always made between gravity-on-person and its reaction force of person-on-scale. However, it can be very important if something else is touching the person or the scale. If the person is holding an object while on the scale, the person's body weight does not change, but the contact forces between the person and the scale will increase. Similarly, a gentle pressure down on the bathroom countertop as a person stands on the scale will result in an apparent body weight reduction as the person contacts a new surface. Situations are frequently encountered in which the contact of an object with a supporting surface and the weight of the object are used interchangeably. A recognition of the difference between gravity's pull on a body or segment (weight) and the force of contact a surface makes with that body or segment permits more flexibility in understanding how to modify these forces, if necessary.

The reaction forces of person-on-scale (PS) and scale-on-person (SP) occur as a result of two contacting surfaces *pushing* on each other. When reaction forces arise from the *push* of contacting surfaces, the force pair are often referred to as **contact forces (F_C).** When contact forces are perpendicular to the surfaces that produce them, the term **normal force (F_N)** is also used.[5-9] Contact forces, therefore, are a subset of reaction forces.

Foundational Concepts 1–6
Action-Reaction Forces

- Whenever two objects or segments touch, the two objects or segments exert a force on each other. Consequently, every force has a reaction or is part of an action-reaction pair.
- The term *contact force* is commonly used to label one or both of the forces in an action-reaction pair where the "touch" of contacting objects is a push (rather than a pull).
- Reaction forces are *never* part of the same force system and cannot be composed (cannot either be additive or offset each other) because the two forces, by definition, are applied to different objects.
- The static or dynamic state of an object cannot be affected by another object that is not touching it or by a force that is not applied to it.
- The reaction to a force should be acknowledged but may be ignored graphically and conceptually *if* the object to which it is applied and the other forces on that object are not of interest.

Additional Linear Force Considerations

To return to John Alexander's leg-foot segment as he sits with the dangling ankle weight, equilibrium in the leg-foot segment is dependent on the upward pull of the capsule (and its associated ligaments) on the leg-foot segment (CLf) with a force equal in magnitude to the downward pull of gravity and the ankle weight (GAwLf) **(Fig. 1–20)**. We now know that if the capsule pulls on the leg-foot segment with a magnitude of 88 N, Newton's third law (law of reaction) stipulates that the leg-foot segment must also be pulling on the capsule (leg/foot-on-capsule, or LfC) with an equivalent 88 N force. John sustained an injury to his medial collateral ligament. The medial collateral ligament reinforces the knee joint capsule and has a similar line of pull to that of the capsule. Therefore, a pull on the capsule could be creating a pull on the injured medial collateral ligament. To understand how the pull of the leg-foot on the capsule affects the capsule (and its associated ligaments), we need to explore **tensile forces** and how they are produced.

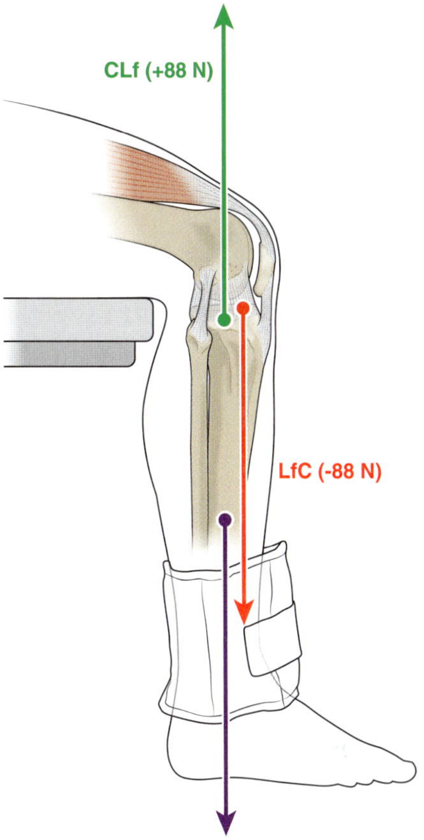

Figure 1–20 The pull of the capsule on the leg-foot segment (CLf) is needed to offset the pull of gravity and ankle weight (GAwLf) for the leg-foot segment to remain at rest. Newton's third law (law of reaction) says that if the capsule is pulling on the leg-foot segment (CLf), the leg-foot segment must also be pulling on the capsule (LfC) with a force equal in magnitude and opposite in direction. *[Note: Vectors CLf and LfC are effectively collinear and coplanar although applied to different objects. The vectors are separated in the figure so that each can be seen.]*

Tensile Forces

Tension in a joint capsule, just like tension in any passive structure (including relatively solid materials such as bone), is created by pulls in opposite directions on the same object. If there are not two opposite pulls on the object (each of which is a tensile force), there cannot be tension in the object.

We established that the leg-foot segment is pulling on the capsule (LfC) with 88 N of force. Newton's first law (law of inertia) tells us that the capsule cannot be in equilibrium (at rest) if LfC is the only force acting on the capsule. Therefore, there must be at least one other force on the capsule, and it must come from something "touching" the capsule. Because the capsule is attached both to the leg-foot segment distally and to the femur proximally, the femur is also touching the capsule (femur-on-capsule, or FC) **(Fig. 1–21)**. If the capsule is in equilibrium, FC must also have a magnitude of 88 N (LfC + FC = 0). The forces of leg/foot-on-capsule and femur-on-capsule are pulls in opposite directions that create tension in the capsule (each of which, then, is a tensile force). We can analogize the joint capsule to thin pieces of rope holding the two bones together. Like a rope in a tug-of-war, the capsule is getting pulled in opposite directions by forces of equal magnitude and will be under equal tension throughout. For a joint capsule and its associated ligaments to do the job of holding the bones of a joint together, the capsuloligamentous tissues must have sufficient tissue integrity to be able to withstand the tensile stresses imposed by the pulls of the contiguous bones.

Foundational Concepts 1–7
Tension and Tensile Forces

- Tensile forces (or the resultants of tensile forces) on an object are always equal in magnitude and opposite in direction.
- Tensile forces are collinear, coplanar, and applied to the same object; therefore, tensile vectors are part of the same linear force system.
- Tensile forces applied at either end to a flexible or rigid structure of homogenous composition create the same tension at all points along the long axis of the structure (in the absence of additional contact and friction).

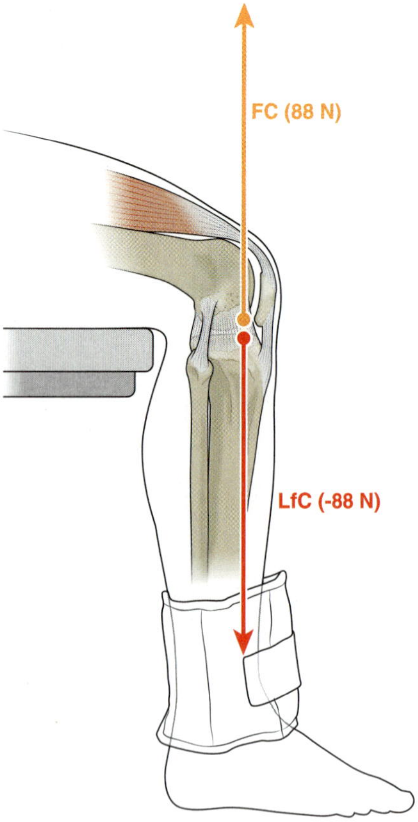

Figure 1–21 For the knee joint capsule to be in equilibrium, there must be a second force on the capsule coming from something touching the capsule. Because the femur is the only other "object" touching the capsule, femur-on-capsule (FC) must be equal in magnitude (88 N) and opposite in direction to leg/foot-on-capsule (LfC). Because both FC and LfC are pulling on the capsule in opposite directions, these forces create tension in the capsule and are considered to be tensile forces.

Joint Distraction

Joint capsules and ligaments are not always under tension. John's capsuloligamentous structures are under tension because of the downward pull of gravity and the ankle weight on John's leg-foot segment must be offset as John's unsupported leg-foot segment dangles (see Fig. 1–20). If John's foot was supported by someone's hand pushing upward on the bottom of John's foot (hand-on-leg/foot) with a force of 88 N, the tension in the capsule (and ligaments) would be eliminated because the upward pull of the capsuloligamentous structures is no longer necessary. In fact, the capsuloligamentous structures can become slack. If the upward support of the hand is gradually removed (and assuming the capsuloligamentous structures are initially slack), there would be at least a small net unbalanced force downward that would cause the leg-foot segment to accelerate away from the femur with the small acceleration proportional to the net unbalanced force (law of acceleration). The movement of one bony segment away from another is known as **joint distraction.**[4] As the distraction increases with the decreasing support of the hand, the tension in the capsule will concomitantly increase until, once again, the tension in the capsule completely offsets the 88 N downward pull of gravity and the ankle weight on the leg-foot segment; equilibrium is restored once again to the leg-foot segment.

The pulls of gravity and the ankle weight (separately or together) on the leg-foot segment in this scenario can be referred to as **distraction forces**[4] or **joint distraction forces.** A distraction force is directed away from the joint surface to which it is applied, is perpendicular to its joint surface, and leads to the separation of the joint surfaces. It is important to note that here the term *distraction* refers to separation of rigid nondeformable bones. Distraction across or within a deformable body is more complex and will be considered in Chapter 2 as tensile loading.

Expanded Concepts 1–4
Acceleration in Joint Distraction

Although not feasible in a clinical setting, the acceleration of the leg-foot segment downward can be calculated.

Gravity and the pull of the ankle weight together is 88 N. To calculate acceleration ($a = F_{unbal} \div m$), however, the mass (not the weight) of the leg-foot segment and ankle weight must be known. Recalling that 1 N is the amount of force needed to accelerate 1 kg at 1 m/sec^2, weight (in newtons or equivalently in kg·m/sec^2) is mass (in kilograms) multiplied by the acceleration of gravity, or:

$$W = (m)(9.8\ m/sec^2)$$

Solving for mass, a force of 88 N is equivalent to 88 kg·m/sec^2 ÷ 9.8 m/sec^2 = 8.97 kg. Consequently, the leg-foot segment and ankle weight together have a mass of approximately 9 kg. Assigning some arbitrary values, assume that a downward force of –88 N is offset in this static example by an upward push of the supporting hand of 50 N and a capsular tensile force of 10 N. The net unbalanced force on the leg-foot segment is –28 N (–88 + 50 + 10). Therefore:

$$a = \frac{-28\,kg - m/sec^2}{9\,kg}$$

$$a = -3.11/sec^2$$

In the human body, the acceleration of one or both segments away from each other in joint distraction (the dynamic phase) is very brief unless the capsule and ligaments (or muscles crossing the joint) fail. John's leg-foot segment will not accelerate away from the femur for very long (milliseconds) before the distraction forces applied to the leg-foot are balanced by the tensile forces in the capsule. Presuming that John is relaxed as the ankle weight hangs on his leg-foot segment (we have not asked him to do anything yet), the limitation to joint distraction will fall entirely to tension in the capsuloligamentous structures. John presumably has a ligamentous injury that is likely to cause pain with tension in these pain-sensitive connective tissues.

Foundational Concepts 1–8
Joint Distraction and Distraction Forces

- Distraction forces create separation of contiguous joint surfaces.
- Joint distraction requires a minimum of one (or one resultant) distraction force on adjacent joint segment, with each distraction force perpendicular to the joint surfaces, opposite in direction to the distraction force on the adjacent segment and directed away from its joint surface.

- Joint distraction can be dynamic (through unequal or opposite acceleration of segments) or static (when the tensile forces in the tissues that join the segments are balanced by distraction forces of equal or greater magnitude).

Joint Compression and Joint Reaction Forces

Supporting John Alexander's leg-foot segment with a hand underneath his foot can minimize or eliminate the tension in his injured capsuloligamentous structures. If the supporting upward push of the hand on the leg-foot segment increases to 90 N while the magnitude of the downward pull of gravity and the ankle weight remains at –88 N, the sum of these forces will result in a net unbalanced *upward* force on the leg-foot segment of 2 N. If the 90 N support of the hand continues, the leg-foot segment will undergo a slight acceleration upward until a new downward force is encountered. The new force will emerge when the leg-foot segment contacts ("touches") the femur that lies above the tibial plateau. The upward acceleration of the leg-foot segment will stop when the new contact force, femur-on-leg/foot (FLf), reaches a magnitude of –2 N, at which point equilibrium of the leg-foot segment is restored.

When the two bony segments of a joint are pushed together and "touch" each other, the resulting reaction (contact) forces are also referred to as **joint reaction forces.**[4] Joint reaction forces are contact forces that result whenever there is contact between contiguous joint surfaces. Joint reaction forces are dependent on the existence of one force on each of the adjacent joint segments because the two bones must push on each other. Those forces will be perpendicular to and directed *toward* the joint surfaces. The two forces that cause joint reaction forces on each segment are known as **compression forces.** Compression forces push joint surfaces together to produce joint reaction forces, just as distraction forces separate joint surfaces to produce capsuloligamentous tensile forces. In the example we have been using, the push of the hand on the leg-foot segment is a compression force. Although there also must be a compression force on the femur to allow the femur to push on the leg-foot segment, our analysis does not require that we account for it.

Foundational Concepts 1–9
Joint Compression and Joint Reaction Forces

- Joint compression forces create contact between joint surfaces.
- There must be a minimum of one (or one resultant) compression force on each contiguous joint segment, with each compression force perpendicular to and directed toward the segment's joint surface and opposite in direction to the compression force on the adjacent segment.

Expanded Concepts 1–5
Close-Packing of a Joint

Capsuloligamentous structures are typically not under tension when there are *net* compressive forces (and no shear forces) across a joint. There is an important exception, however. With sufficient twisting of the capsuloligamentous structures of a joint caused by active or passive joint rotation, the adjacent articular surfaces can be drawn together into contact by the capsuloligamentous structures. This is called "close-packing" of the joint. Although considered an "Expanded Concept" in Chapter 1, this concept will be elaborated upon in Chapter 2 and in the examination of individual joint complexes in subsequent chapters. In those chapters, the concept of close-packing becomes a "Foundational Concept."

Revisiting Newton's Law of Equilibrium

It would appear that the ankle weight is a poor option for John, given the potential tensile forces created in his injured capsuloligamentous structures, unless we plan to continue supporting his leg-foot segment with a hand (or, perhaps, a bench). Let us explore the option of the leg-press exercise to see how the change in exercise might change the forces at the knee joint **(Fig. 1–22)**.

In the leg-press exercise **(Fig. 1–22A)**, the leg-foot segment is still acted upon by a –48 N gravitational force (GLf), but the change in orientation of the leg-foot segment means that the orientation of gravity has changed as well. The leg-foot segment is also contacted by the footplate (footplate-on-leg/foot, or FpLf) with a force of unknown magnitude. Because GLf and FpLf are not part of the same linear force system in this scenario (neither collinear nor coplanar), no assumptions can be made about the magnitude of footplate-on-leg/foot

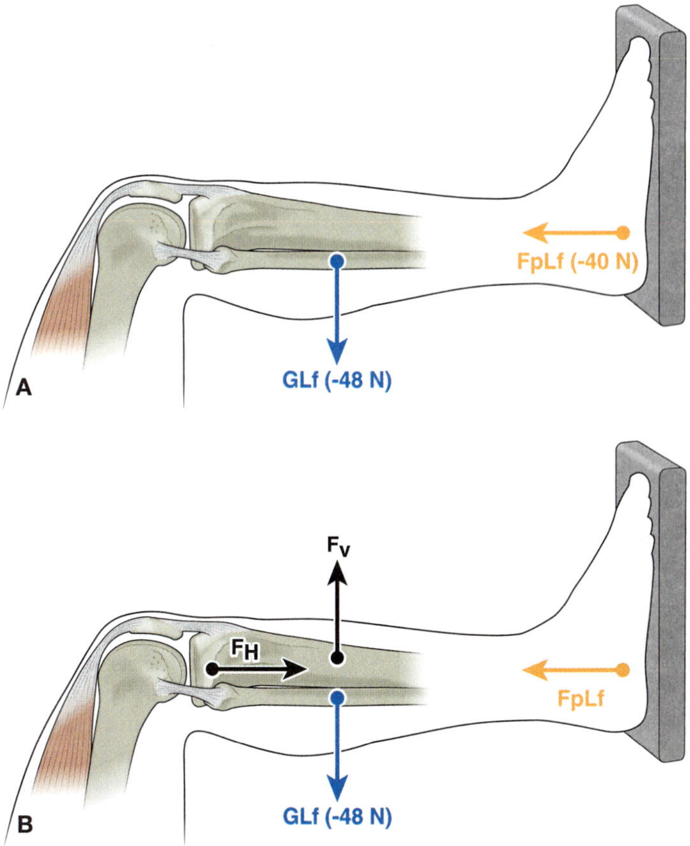

Figure 1–22 **A.** Before John begins the leg-press exercise, the leg-foot segment is contacted by gravity (GLf) and by the footplate (footplate-on-leg/foot, or FpLf). GLf and FpLf are not part of the same linear force system; the leg-foot segment cannot be in equilibrium with only these two forces. **B.** One additional vertical force (F_V) and one additional horizontal force (F_H) must exist on the leg-foot segment so that the sum of the vertical forces and the sum of the horizontal forces on the leg-foot are zero.

based on what we know about gravity-on-leg/foot. Elaboration on Newton's law of inertia can assist us.

Vertical and Horizontal Linear Force Systems

As Newton's law of inertia was already defined, the sum of the forces on an object in equilibrium must be zero ($\Sigma F = 0$). We now can refine Newton's law of inertia to state that the sum of the **vertical forces (F_V)** acting on an object in equilibrium must total zero ($F_V = 0$) and, independently, the sum of the **horizontal forces (F_H)** acting on that same object must total zero ($F_H = 0$). To meet this more specific set of conditions, there must be at least one additional vertical force (F_V) and one additional horizontal force (F_H) acting on John's leg-foot segment that are equal in magnitude and opposite in direction to gravity-on-leg/foot and footplate-on-leg/foot, respectively **(Fig. 1–22B)**. The sources of F_V and F_H are not yet established.

We know that the femur and capsule are both contacting and potentially creating forces on the leg-foot segment. Given these possibilities, F_H is likely to be the push of the femur on the leg-foot segment because the footplate can push the leg-foot segment into contact with the femur, creating a femur-on-leg/foot force. The source of the F_V is difficult to ascertain because the joint capsule (still touching the leg-foot segment) is an unlikely candidate; nothing else appears to be contacting the leg-foot segment. To identify F_V, we must acknowledge an additional property of all contact forces. Whenever there is contact between two objects, the potential exists for friction forces on both contacting surfaces. The friction forces will have magnitude, however, only if there are concomitant opposing shear forces on the contacting objects.

Shear and Friction Forces

A **shear force (F_S)** is any force (or component of a force) that has an action line parallel to contacting surfaces (or tangential to curved surfaces) that creates or attempts to create a sliding movement between surfaces, with its direction in the direction of potential movement. *[Note: The discussion here is about shear forces between two rigid (nondeformable) structures (e.g., bones).]*

A **friction force (Fr)** potentially exists on an object whenever there is a contact force on that object. Friction forces are always parallel to contacting surfaces (or tangential to curved surfaces) and have a direction that is opposite to potential movement. For friction to have magnitude, a net shear force must exist that creates or attempts to create movement between two contacting objects. Shear and friction forces share the common property that both are forces parallel to contacting surfaces, but shear forces are always applied in the direction of movement (or potential movement) whereas friction forces are always applied in the direction opposite to movement or potential movement. To understand the magnitude of a frictional force, we need to further explore the force of friction.

Static Friction and Kinetic Friction

The magnitude of a friction force on an object is always a function of the magnitude of contact between the objects and the slipperiness or roughness of the contacting surfaces. When two contacting objects (with a net shear force on each) are not moving on each other (objects are static), the magnitude of the **force of static friction (Fr_s)** on each object is less than or equal to the product of a constant value known as the **coefficient of static friction (μ_S)** and the magnitude of the contact force (F_C) on each object; that is,

$$Fr_S \leq \mu_S F_C$$

The coefficient of static friction is a constant value for given materials. For example, μ_S for ice on ice is approximately 0.05; the value of μ_S for wood on wood is as little as 0.25.[6] As the contacting surfaces become softer or rougher, μ_S increases. As the magnitude of contact (F_C) between objects increases, so too does the potential magnitude of friction. The greater the contact force on an object and the rougher the contacting surfaces, the greater the maximum potential force of friction. When you use friction to warm your hands, the contact of the hands warms both of them (friction forces exist on both the right and left hands). If you wish to increase the friction, you press your hands together harder (increase the contact force) as you rub. Pressing your hands together harder increases the contact force between the hands and increases the maximum value of friction (the coefficient of friction remains unchanged because the surface remains skin on skin). It is commonly thought that the magnitude of friction between two surfaces is related to the amount of surface area in contact. However, the only contributing factors are the magnitude of contact and the coefficient of friction of the contacting surfaces.[3]

In **Figure 1–23**, a large box weighing 445 N (~45 kg or 100 lb) is resting on the floor. The floor must push on the box (FB) with a magnitude equal to the weight of the box (GB) because the box is not moving, therefore $\Sigma F_V = 0$. Because nothing is attempting to move the box parallel to the contacting floor (no shear forces), there will be no friction on either the box or the floor **(Fig. 1–23A)**. However, as soon as the man begins to push on the box **(Fig. 1–23B)**, a shear force (man-on-box, or MB) is created, with a concomitant resulting force of friction-on-box (FrB). *[Note: Although the example works,* **Figure 1–23B** *is oversimplified because it appears that all the forces are acting at the same point. Although floor-on-box does act through the center of mass of the box, it is applied at the bottom of the box; the force of friction-on-box would also act at the bottom of the box rather than as shown.]* Assuming that the shear force of man-on-box is not sufficient to move the box, the maximum potential magnitude of friction-on-box can be calculated.

The maximum friction force on the box when the box is not moving is a product of the coefficient of static friction of wooden box on wood floor (0.25) and the magnitude (445 N) of the upward contact of floor-on-box:

$$FrB \leq (0.25)(445\ N)$$

$$FrB \leq 111.25\ N$$

The magnitude of the friction-on-box force will be equal to that of the shear force (man-on-box) *as long as the box is not moving* because $\Sigma F_H = 0$. As the man increases his push on the box without moving it, the magnitude of friction will simultaneously increase by the same amount, up to a maximum of 111.25 N, as calculated in this example. The magnitude of static friction will change in response to the magnitude of

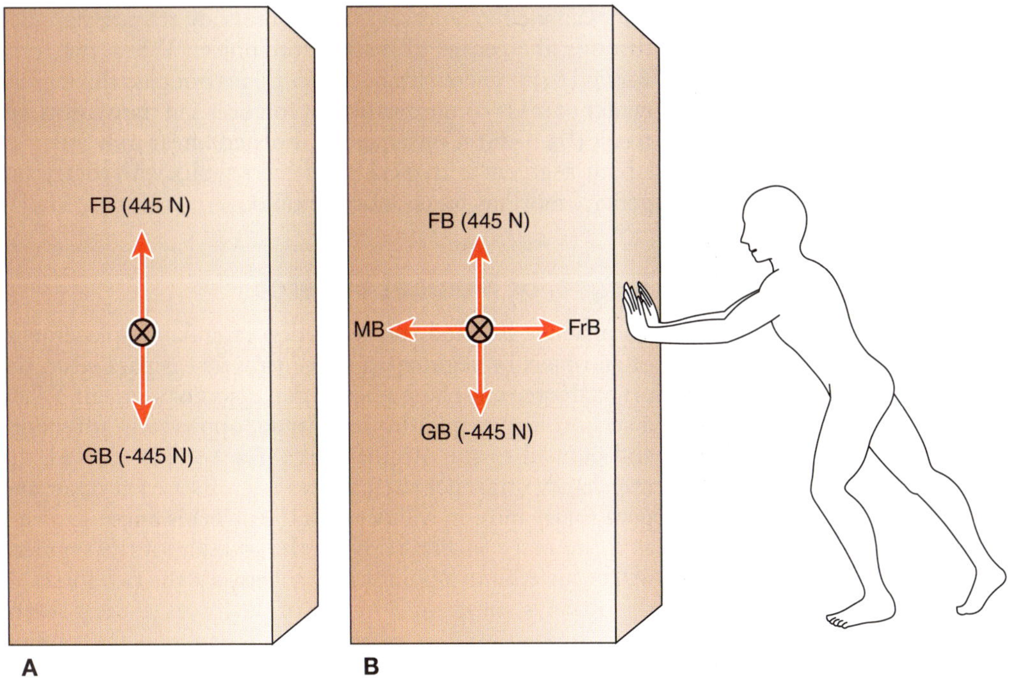

Figure 1–23 **A.** The box is acted on by the forces of gravity (GB) and the contact of floor-on-box (FB). The force of friction has no magnitude (so it is not shown) because there is no attempted movement. **B.** The force of the man-on-box (MB) causes an opposing friction force (FrB).

shear force on the object, but static friction cannot exceed its calculated maximum force.

If the push of the man on the box exceeds 111.25 N, the box will begin to move because friction cannot have a magnitude greater than 111.25 N; there will be a net unbalanced force in the direction of the man's push. Once an object is *moving*, the magnitude of the **force of kinetic friction (Fr_K)** must be calculated. Unlike static friction, kinetic friction between surfaces is constant in magnitude and equal to the product of the contact force (F_C) and the **coefficient of kinetic friction (μ_K):**

$$Fr_K = (\mu_K)(F_C)$$

The coefficient of kinetic friction (μ_K) is always smaller in magnitude than the coefficient of static friction (μ_S) for any set of contacting surfaces. Consequently, the magnitude of the force of friction is always greatest immediately before the object is about to move (when the shear force has the same magnitude as the *maximum* value of static friction). Once the shear force exceeds the maximum value of static friction and the object begins to move, the value of friction drops from its maximum static friction value to its smaller kinetic friction value, resulting in a sudden increase in the net unbalanced force on the object even if the push of the man is the same. The sudden drop in magnitude of friction results in the classic situation in which the man pushes harder and harder to get the box moving along the floor and then suddenly finds himself and the box accelerating too rapidly.

Foundational Concepts 1–10
Friction and Shear Forces

- Shear and friction forces potentially exist whenever two objects touch.
- A shear force is any force (or force component) that lies parallel to the contacting surface (or tangential to a curved surface) of an object, attempts movement between the contacting objects, and is applied in the direction of movement or potential movement.
- A friction force lies parallel to the contacting surface (or tangential to the curved surface) of any object but always in a direction opposite to potential or relative movement between contacting surfaces.
- Friction has magnitude only when there is a net (resultant) shear force applied to an object.
- The magnitude of static friction can change with an alteration in the net shear force applied to the object; the magnitude of kinetic friction between contiguous moving objects remains the same regardless of the magnitude of the shear force or forces on the object or the speed of the moving object.
- The magnitude of friction can never exceed the magnitude of the net shear force it opposes.
- Shear and friction forces are always parallel to contacting surfaces, whereas the contact force (or contact force component) that must exist concomitantly is perpendicular (normal) to the contacting surfaces. Consequently, shear and friction forces are perpendicular to a contact force (or, more correctly, the component of a contact force that is "normal" to the contacting surfaces).[4]

Considering Vertical and Horizontal Linear Equilibrium

We can now return to John and the leg-press example. An understanding of shear and friction forces can be used to identify the source of the friction-on-leg/foot force (F_V) in Figure 1–22B and to calculate the magnitudes of FpLf, F_V, and F_H.

Because the force of gravity (GLf) lies parallel to the footplate and has the potential to slide the leg-foot segment down on the footplate (see Fig. 1–22B), GLf is a shear force (lies parallel to contacting surfaces). If there is a net shear force between the vertically aligned footplate and leg-foot segment, there will also be a friction force that is vertical and in a direction opposite to the net shear force (GLf). Therefore, the unknown F_V in Figure 1–22B is likely to be friction-on-leg/foot from contact with the footplate as GLf pulls the leg/foot segment downwardly.

The leg-foot segment in Fig. 1-22B is in equilibrium and there are only two identified vertical forces. Therefore, the magnitude of the friction-on-leg/foot force (F_V) must be equal to the magnitude (although opposite in direction) to the 48 N shear force (GLf). If the coefficient of static friction between the sole of John's shoe and the metal footplate is estimated at $\mu_S = 0.6$ (slightly rougher than wood-on-wood),[6] we can determine the magnitude of footplate-on-leg/foot (FpLf) given that friction-on-leg/foot (F_V) is 48 N:

$$48\ N = (0.6)(F_C)$$

$$F_C \text{ or } FpLf = 80\ N$$

If the calculated magnitude of the contact force footplate-on-leg/foot vector (FpLf) in Figure 1–22B is –80 N (directed to the left), then the magnitude of the femur-on-leg/foot force must be +80 N (directed to the right), because the sum of the horizontal forces must be zero for the leg-foot to be in equilibrium.

PART 2: Kinetics—Considering Rotary and Translatory Forces and Motions

As we begin exploring rotary and general motion, we will continue to confine the discussion and examples to two-dimensional analyses to facilitate an understanding of the concepts. Subsequent chapters will superimpose the third dimension conceptually, although rarely mathematically.

When an object is completely unconstrained (not attached to anything), a single force applied at or through the center of mass of the object will produce linear displacement regardless of the angle at which the force is applied **(Fig. 1–24)**. However, forces applied to bony segments in the body are rarely applied through the center of mass of the object. When the force applied to an unconstrained object does not pass through its center of mass, a combination of rotation and translation will result **(Fig. 1–25)**. Consequently, isolated linear movement of a bony segment is atypical (if it occurs at all), with rotary and general motions much more common.

Torque, or Moment of Force

To produce isolated rotary motion (angular displacement) of an object or segment, a *second force* that is parallel to the original force must be applied to that object or segment. When a second force equal in magnitude, opposite in direction, and parallel to the original force **(Fig. 1–26)** is applied, the translatory effects of these forces will offset each other and pure rotary motion will occur. If the object is unconstrained, as is the block in Figure 1–26, the rotation of the segment will occur around a point midway between the two forces. If the object is constrained by one of the forces (if the point of application of FB_2 is fixed, making it like an axis), the rotation will occur around the point of application of the constraining force **(Fig. 1–27)**. Two forces equal in magnitude, opposite in direction, parallel, and applied to the same object at different points are known as a **force couple.** A force couple acting at some distance from each other on the same object will always produce a **moment of force,** or torque (τ). Torque (used interchangeably with moment of force or "moment") is the product of the magnitude of one of the forces in a force couple and the shortest perpendicular distance to the axis (or other arbitrarily chosen point), referred to as the **moment arm (MA):**

$$\tau = (F)(MA)$$

Because torque is directly proportional to both the magnitude of the applied force (the magnitudes of the forces in a force couple are equivalent) and the distance between the force couple (which creates an axis in this case), torque can be thought of as the strength of rotation. Therefore, the greater the magnitude of the force couple, the greater the strength

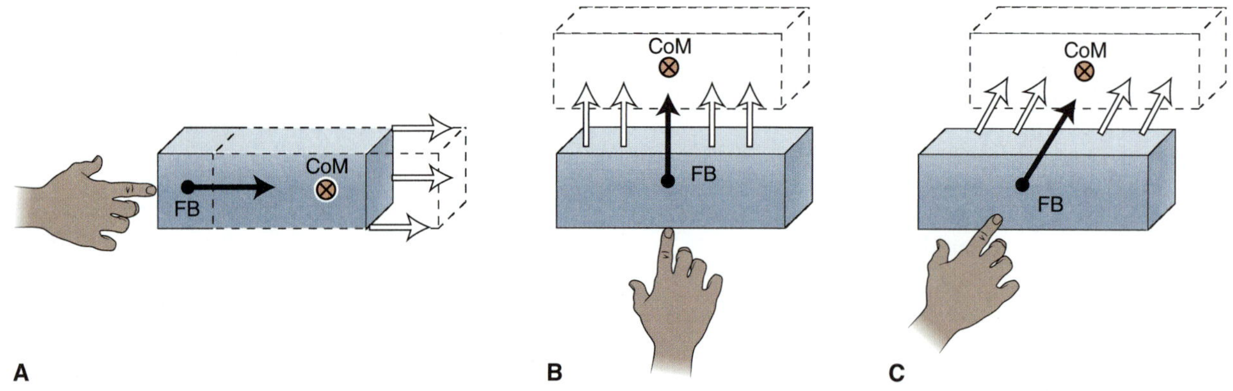

Figure 1–24 An isolated force (finger-on-block, or FB) applied to the block that passes through its center of mass (CoM) will produce linear displacement (translatory motion) of the block in the direction of the unbalanced force regardless of the direction from which the force is applied.

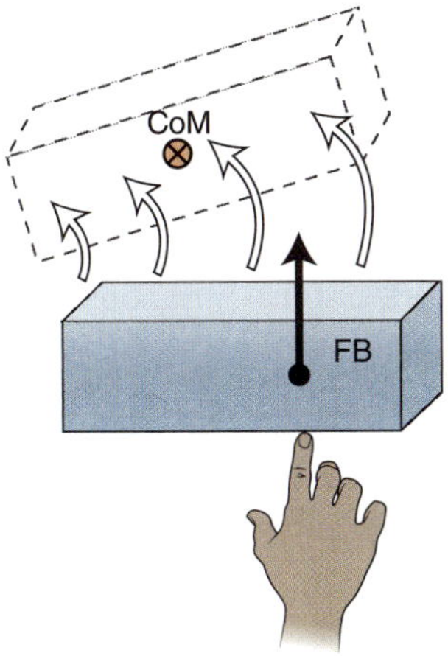

Figure 1–25 When an isolated force (finger-on-block, or FB) that does not pass through the center of mass (CoM) is applied to the block, a combination of rotary and translatory motion of the block will occur (general motion).

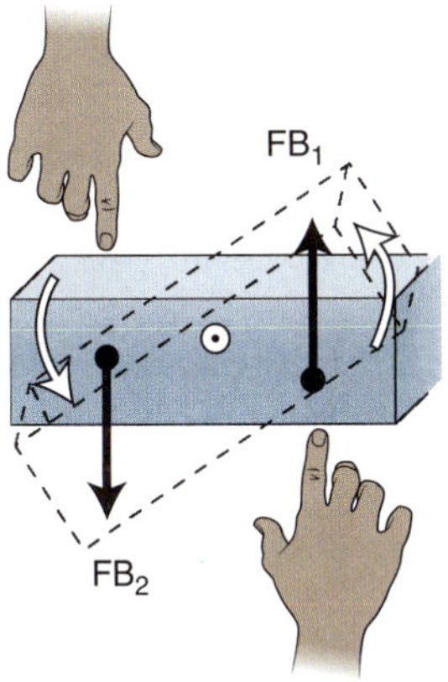

Figure 1–26 Two forces of finger-on-box (FB_1 and FB_2) that are equal in magnitude are applied to the block in opposite directions. FB_1 and FB_2 constitute a force couple and will create isolated rotation about a point midway between the forces, presuming no constraints on the object.

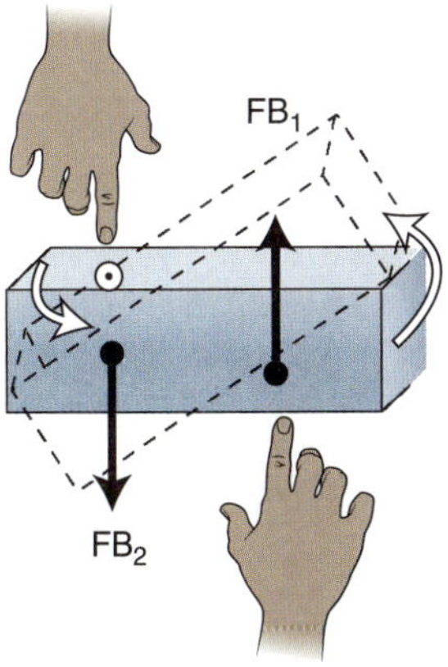

Figure 1–27 Two forces of finger-on-box (FB_1 and FB_2) that are equal in magnitude are applied to the block in opposite directions. However, the point of application of FB_2 is fixed, creating an axis. FB_1 and FB_2 constitute a force couple with isolated rotation occurring around the fixed point of application of FB_2.

of rotation; the farther apart the forces of a force couple (the greater the MA), the greater the strength of rotation.

Force is measured in newtons and distance in meters; therefore, the unit for torque is the **newton-meter (N·m)** (or the foot-pound in the U.S. system). The direction of potential rotation or torque at a joint segment can also be labeled by using the terms *flexion/extension*, *medial/lateral rotation*, or *abduction/adduction*. Consequently, a torque in the direction of joint flexion may be referred to either as a **flexion moment** or a flexion torque.

Parallel Force Systems

Because the forces in a force couple are parallel to each other, the two forces are part of a **parallel force system,** which exists whenever two or more forces applied to the same object are parallel to each other. The torque generated by each of the parallel forces is determined by multiplying the magnitude of the force by its moment arm, with the moment arm being the shortest distance from the force to either the point of constraint of the segment or to an arbitrarily chosen point on the segment (as long as the same point is used for each of the parallel forces).

Determining Resultant Forces in a Parallel Force System

The net or resultant torque produced by forces in the same parallel force system can be determined by adding the torques contributed by each force, considering their positive or negative signs. By convention, clockwise torques are considered negative whereas counterclockwise torques are considered positive.

Three forces are applied to an unconstrained segment in **Figure 1-28**. The magnitudes of forces F_1, F_2, and F_3 are 5 N, 3 N, and 7 N, respectively. The shortest distance (moment arms) between F_1, F_2, and F_3 and an arbitrarily chosen point on the object are 0.25 m, 0.12 m, and 0.12 m, respectively. F_1 and F_2 are applied in a clockwise direction, whereas F_3 is applied in a counterclockwise direction (in relation to the chosen point of rotation). The net (resultant) torque would be:

$$\tau_{net} = (0.25\ \text{m})(-5\ \text{N}) + (0.12\ \text{m})(-3\ \text{N}) + (0.12\ \text{m})(+7\ \text{N})$$

$$\tau_{net} = -0.77\ \text{N·m}$$

That is, there will be a net rotation of the segment in a clockwise direction with a magnitude of 0.77 N·m.

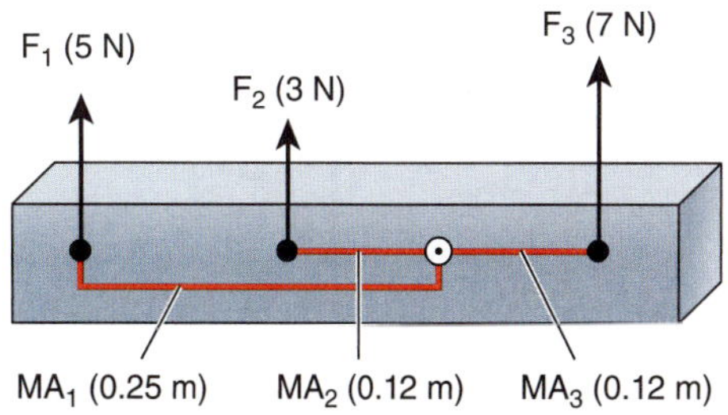

Figure 1–28 The resultant of three parallel forces is found by the sum of the torques, with the torques being the product of each force (F_1, F_2, and F_3) and its moment arm (MA; distance from the specified point of rotation).

Because the net torque in Figure 1–28 is calculated around a point that is *not* at the center of mass of the segment, the segment will not only rotate but will also translate. This is evident when we consider that all three forces (F_1–F_3) are upward vertical forces; these forces not only produce rotation (torque) but also produce translation. The sum of the vertical forces yields a net upward translatory force of 15 N, with that upward translation occurring concomitantly with the net torque of -0.77 N·m.

Foundational Concepts 1-11
Revisiting Newton's Law of Equilibrium

Using Newton's law of inertia, $\Sigma F = 0$ for an object or segment in equilibrium. More specifically, for an object or segment to be in equilibrium, $\Sigma F_V = 0$ and $\Sigma F_H = 0$. Additionally, for an object or segment to be in equilibrium, $\Sigma\tau = 0$. All three conditions must be met for an object or segment to be in equilibrium such that:

$$\Sigma F_V = 0$$

$$\Sigma F_H = 0$$

$$\Sigma\tau = 0$$

If the goal in Figure 1–28 is to rotate rather than translate the segment (as is the goal of joints in the human body), the unwanted upward translation of the segment must be eliminated by the addition of a new force. However, let us first simplify by composing F_1 and F_2 into a single resultant force, given that both are producing clockwise rotation of the segment. In **Figure 1–29**, forces F_1 and F_2 have been composed into resultant force $F_{1\text{-}2}$, and a new vector (F_4) has been added. *[Note: Force F_4 might be easier in this particular figure to visualize as a push downward, as shown by the dotted gray arrow. However, we will continue to use the convention that the base of the arrow is on the point of application, as shown for the vector labeled F_4.]*

In Figure 1–29, force F_4 has been assigned a magnitude of –15 N. With the addition of F_4, the sum of vertical forces ($F_{1\text{-}2}$, F_3, and F_4) is now zero. Force F_4 passes through the hypothetical point of rotation for the segment. Because it passes through that point, it is applied at 0 m from the point; the torque produced by F_4, therefore, is zero (–15 N x 0). Any force applied *through* a reference point or point of rotation will not produce torque. Although the addition of vector F_4 results in vertical equilibrium, the net torque is still –0.77 N·m. The offsetting effect produced by the addition of F_4 is what happens in the human body. A body segment will translate (with or without a concomitant rotation) until an equal and opposite constraint is encountered, at which point the translatory forces on the segment are balanced and pure rotation is produced.

Identifying the Joint Axis About Which Body Segments Rotate

Figure 1–30A shows John's leg-foot segment in the same position as in the leg-press exercise but without the contact of the footplate. If John is still relaxed, his leg-foot segment

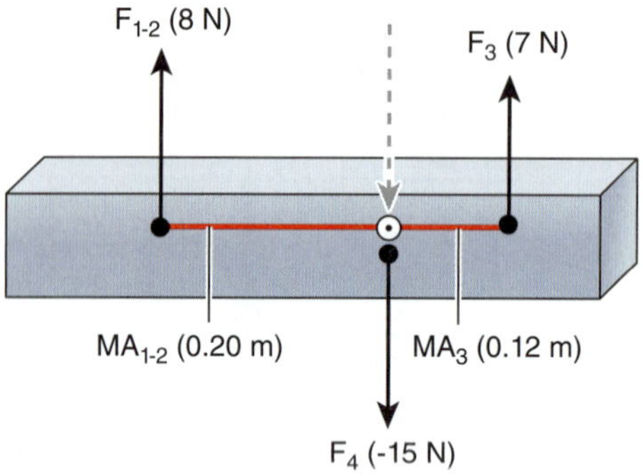

Figure 1–29 Forces F_1 and F_2, originally shown in Figure 1–28, have been composed into force $F_{1\text{-}2}$. The addition of F_4, applied through the point of rotation, will produce vertical equilibrium without producing any additional torque because F_4 passes through the axis (has no moment arm). The block will now rotate around a fixed axis in the direction of unbalanced torque.

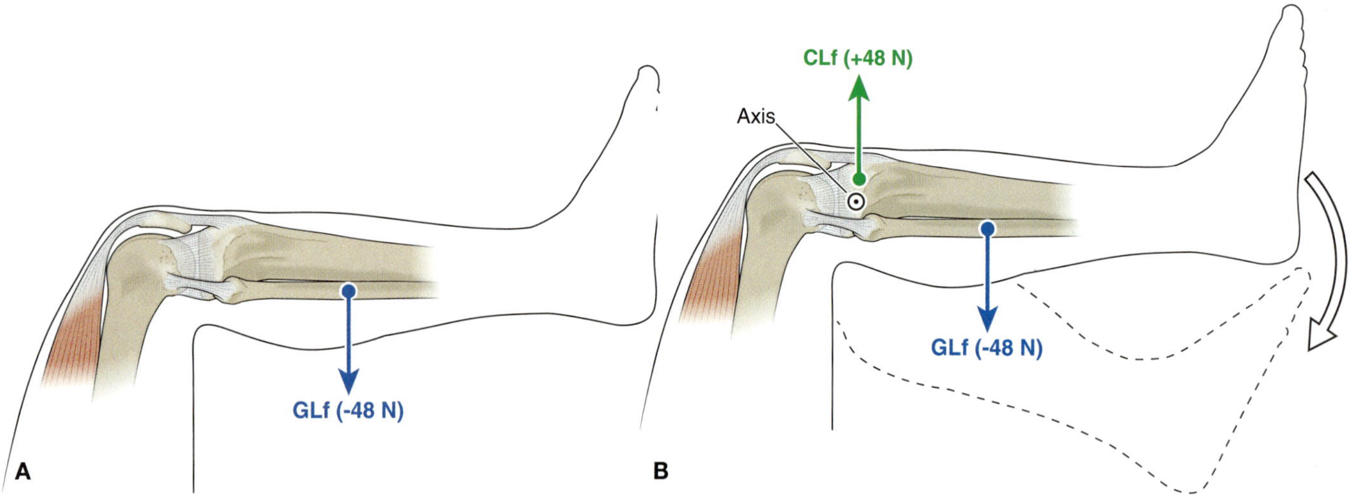

Figure 1–30 **A.** Gravity-on-leg/foot alone would cause downward translation of the leg-foot segment. **B.** As the leg-foot segment translates downward, the capsuloligamentous structures of the knee joint (CLf) become increasingly tight. When CLf reaches 48 N and constrains further downward movement, CLf and GLf form a force couple that produces clockwise rotation of the knee joint around the point of application of the constraining force, CLf.

cannot remain in equilibrium. Initially, the leg-foot segment would translate downward linearly given the effect of the downward force of gravity (GLf). Gravity here is considered a shear force because it lies parallel to the contacting surfaces of the femoral condyles and the tibial plateau. Although a shear force has the potential to generate an opposing friction force, the very small coefficient of friction that exists in a synovial joint (with estimates as low as 0.005) means that the magnitude of friction would be negligible.[4] The leg-foot segment without frictional resistance would translate downward as the knee joint capsule increased in tension, creating the force of capsule-on-leg/foot (CLf) **(Fig. 1–30B)**. As the leg-foot segment translates downwardly, the magnitude of tension in the capsule would increase until CLf reached 48 N. We can now see that capsule-on-leg/foot (CLf) forms a force couple with the gravity-on-leg/foot (GLf). Motion of the leg-foot segment then continues as isolated rotation around the point of constraint (axis) of the tensile capsule-on-leg/foot force.

In the human body, the motion of a segment at a joint is ultimately constrained by the articular structures, either by joint reaction forces resulting from bony contact or through capsuloligamentous forces in the surrounding connective tissues. The point of application of the joint reaction or capsuloligamentous force that constrains further translation becomes the fixed pivot point for rotation (one half of a force couple). The net effect of translation (to the point of constraint) followed by rotation (around the point of constraint) is a subtle curvilinear motion of the segment. Because the motion is curvilinear, the axis shifts slightly during the motion. If the normal articular constraints at a joint are inadequate (as for damaged tissues), there will be excessive translatory motion; an excessive shift in the instantaneous center of rotation can occur.

Although it is acknowledged that the instantaneous center of rotation of a joint shifts with motion of a body segment, it is common practice to identify the joint axis as a fixed point about which the joint rotation *appears* to occur. This is most often assumed to be approximately in the center of the sequential instantaneous centers of rotation. It must be acknowledged, however, that this practice somewhat oversimplifies the assessment of torques on a body segment.

Bending Moments and Torsional Moments

When parallel forces are applied to a rigid object in such a way that the object remains in equilibrium without either rotation or translation, the resulting torques (moments of force) applied to a specific point on the object can also be labeled as **bending moments (Fig. 1–31)**.[2,4]

In **Fig. 1-31A**, parallel forces F1 and F2 with a magnitude of 10 N each are applied to a block; the block will rotate around the fixed point of rotation (point of application of F1) because F1 and F2 are a force couple. Introducing a new force (F3) as in **Figure 1–31B** can restore equilibrium to the block, with F2 and F3 each having half the magnitude of F1 ($\Sigma F_V = 0$). Although the segment is neither rotating nor translating, F2 and F3 would tend to "bend" a *rigid* segment around the apex of the triangle (point of application F1); hence, force couples in an equilibrium situation (when the segment cannot rotate) can also be considered to be bending moments. Because it took all three parallel forces to create the bending effect, bending moments may also be referred to as **three-point bending.** Occasionally, a bony segment is constrained in a way that results in substantial bending forces that cause damage, that is, fracture. Bone strength is often tested in experimental conditions using three-point bending **(Fig. 1–31C)**.

A **torsional moment** is sometimes considered a special case (or subcategory) of a torque or moment of force **(Fig. 1–32)**. A torsional moment is produced when a force is applied tangential to the periphery of a segment and at a distance from the segment's axis of rotation, creating (or tending to create) rotation *within a segment* around its long axis **(Fig. 1–32A)**. A common example of the result of such a

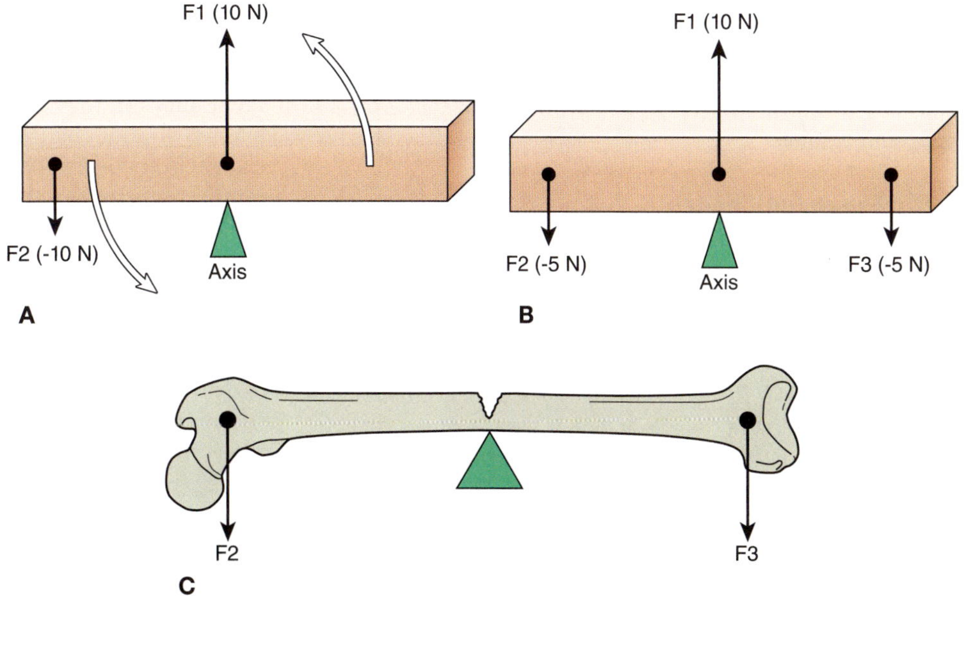

Figure 1–31 **A.** A force couple (F_1 and F_2) will produce rotation around the fixed force (F_1). **B.** A bending moment is created when a third force (F_3) is added to a force couple (F_1 and F_2), resulting in rotary and translatory equilibrium but tending to "bend" the object around the point of application of the fixed force (F_1). **C.** The principle of bending moments (or three-point bending) is often used in biomechanical testing of long bones (e.g., the femur).

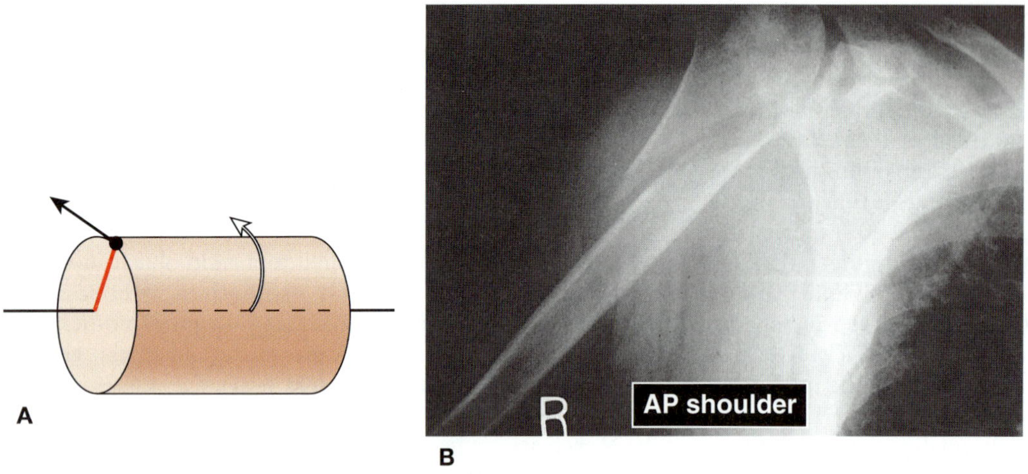

Figure 1–32 **A.** A tangential force applied to the periphery of a long segment (at some distance from the axis that passes longitudinally) produces a "torsional moment" that is directly proportional to the magnitude of the force and its distance from the longitudinal axis. **B.** A spiral fracture of a humerus results from a torsional moment on the bone.

torsional moment is a spiral fracture in a long bone of the body **(Fig. 1–32B)**.

Muscle Forces

Total Muscle Force Vector

The force applied by a muscle to a bony segment is actually the resultant force of many individual forces (muscle fibers) pulling on a common point of application. Each fiber in the muscle can be represented by a force vector that converges with the other fiber vectors at the muscle's attachment, forming a concurrent force system with a resultant represented by the total muscle force vector (Fms) **(Fig. 1–33)**. The vector of a muscle force can be approximated by drawing an action line through the middle of the muscle's fibers in the direction of the middle of the muscle. The direction of pull for any muscle is *always* toward the *center of the muscle*. Every muscle exerts a force (a pull) of equal magnitude on each of its attachments simultaneously. Therefore, every muscle creates a minimum of two force vectors, one on each of the two (or more) segments to which the muscle is attached; each of the two (or more) vectors is directed toward the middle of the muscle. The type and direction of motion that results from an active muscle contraction depends on the net forces and net torques acting on each of the bony segments to which the muscle is attached. The muscle will rotate a segment in its direction of pull only when the torque generated by the muscle exceeds opposing torques.

Expanded Concepts 1–6
Measuring Muscle Force

The magnitude of a muscle force in a living human is typically estimated because the actual magnitude (the pull of a muscle on its attachment) cannot be determined in a person without invasive (implanted) measurement tools. Electromyography (EMG) measures the electrical activity of a muscle. The electrical activity is directly proportional to the motor unit activity which, in turn, is directly proportional to isometric muscle force (see Chapter 3). However, neither electrical activity nor the number of motor units is a measure of absolute muscle force because muscle is exquisitely sensitive to its mechanical environment (e.g., length, velocity). The clinical "strength" of a muscle is measured by using devices such as weights, force transducers, or isokinetic devices. However, what is actually being measured directly or indirectly is the torque being applied to the joint. Although the net internal torque on the segment can be estimated if the moment arms of the known external forces (gravity, weights, and so on) are known, the magnitudes of individual internal forces contributing to the net internal torque are difficult, if not impossible, to quantify. Even if a single muscle is active (which is almost never the case), it would be difficult to separate out the influence of forces such as joint reaction forces, capsuloligamentous forces, and small intra-articular friction forces. The result is that the actual magnitude of pull of a single muscle cannot be assessed in a living person (in vivo) without surgically implanting a device directly onto the tendon, which may itself alter the force normally produced by a muscle. It should be noted that individual muscle forces are often approximated using mathematical models of varying levels of sophistication. The outputs of these models are the best estimates of muscle force.

In a space diagram, we will often draw only the pull of the muscle on the segment under consideration. However, it should be recognized that we are purposefully ignoring that same muscle's concomitant pull on the other segment(s) to which it is attached.

Anatomic Pulleys

Frequently, the fibers of a muscle or muscle tendon wrap around a bone or are deflected by a bony prominence. When the direction of pull of a muscle is altered, the bone or bony prominence causing the deflection forms an **anatomic pulley.** Pulleys (if they are frictionless) change the direction of a force without changing the magnitude. As we will see, the change in action line produced by an anatomic pulley will have implications for the ability of the muscle to produce torque.

Anatomic Pulleys, Action Lines, and Moment Arms

The function of any pulley is to redirect a force to make a task easier. The "task" in human movement is to rotate a body segment. Anatomic pulleys (in many instances) make this task easier by deflecting the action line of the muscle farther from the joint axis, thus increasing the moment arm of the muscle force. By increasing the moment arm (MA) of a muscle force, a force (F) of the same magnitude will produce greater torque (remembering that $\tau = F \times MA$).

Sesamoid bones lie where tendons pass over joints and function to change the direction of a muscle or tendon action line, resulting in increased ability of a muscle to produce torque

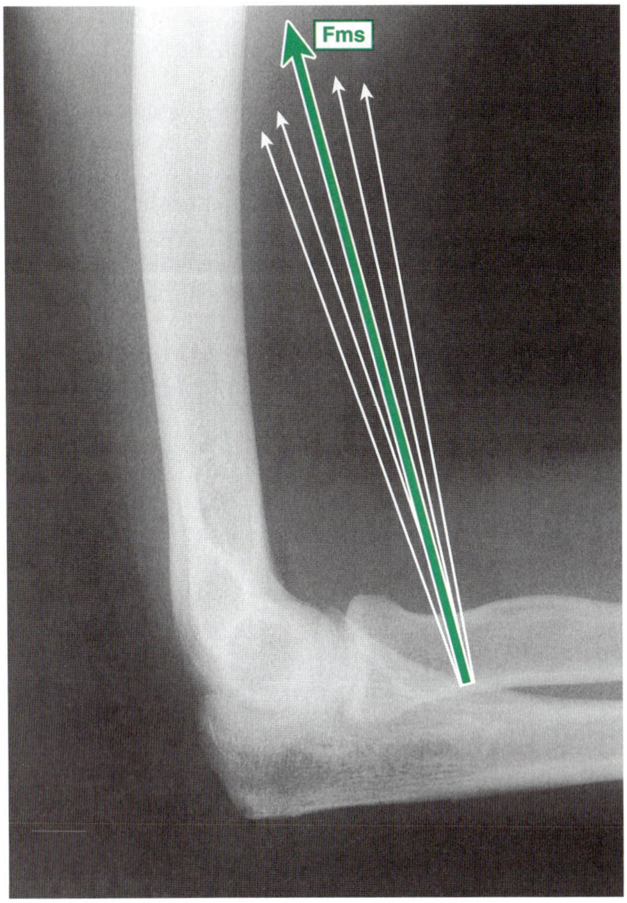

Figure 1–33 A representative sample of brachialis muscle fibers converge on the ulna, with the total muscle force (Fms) being the resultant of all the individual muscle fiber pulls.

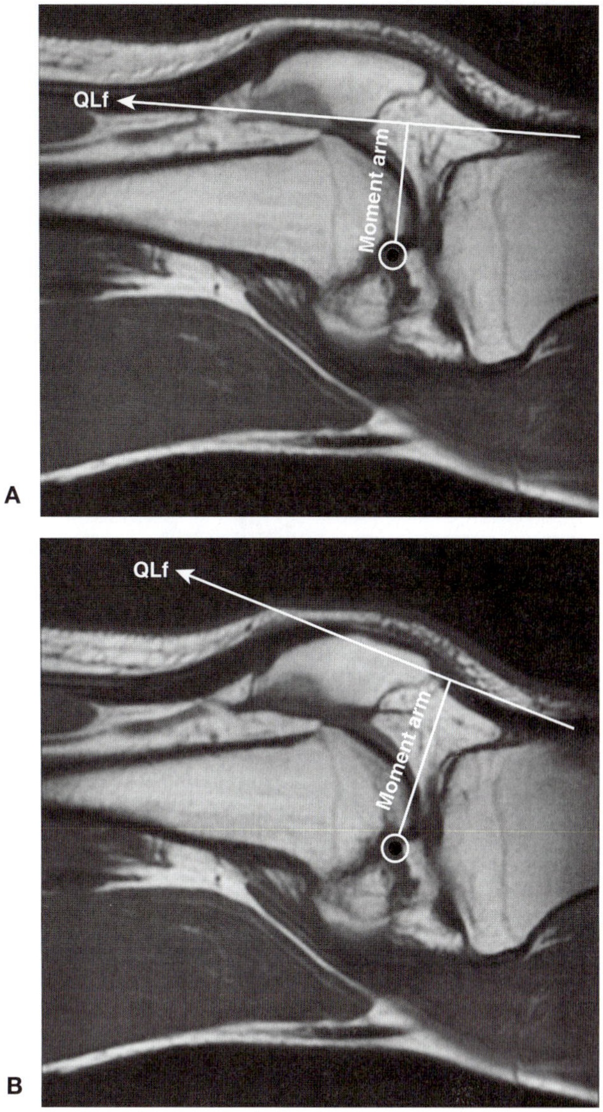

Figure 1–34 Sagittal T1-weighted MRIs of the knee. **A.** The line of pull and moment arm of the quadriceps muscle without the patella. **B.** With the patella's pulley effect, the line of pull of the muscle is deflected away from the joint axis, increasing the moment arm of the muscle force.

around one or more of the joint's axes. There are several sesamoid bones in the human body, the largest being the patella.

Example 1–2
The Patella as an Anatomic Pulley

The classic example of an anatomic pulley is that formed by the patella **(Fig. 1–34)**. The quadriceps muscle belly lies parallel to the femur. The tendon of the muscle passes over the knee joint and attaches to the tibia via the patellar tendon at the tibial tuberosity. For knee joint extension, the joint axis is considered to be located through the femoral condyles. The moment arm for the quadriceps muscle force (QLf) is the shortest perpendicular distance from the vector (QLf) to the joint axis. Without the patella, the line of pull of the quadriceps muscle on the leg-foot segment (tibia) would follow the patellar tendon at the tibial tubercle and would lie parallel to the leg-foot segment **(Fig. 1–34A)**. However, the patella is embedded in the quadriceps tendon and pushes the tendon away from the femur, changing the angle that the patellar tendon makes with the tibia, deflecting the line of pull of the quadriceps muscle away from the knee joint axis **(Fig. 1–34B)**. Changing the line of pull of the quadriceps muscle on the tibia increases the moment arm. Given an increased moment arm, the same magnitude of quadriceps force will produce greater torque (and potentially greater angular acceleration) in Figure 1–34B than in Figure 1–34A.

Foundational Concepts 1–12
Muscle Force Vectors

- Active *or passive* tension in a muscle creates a force (pull) on all segments to which the muscle is attached, although one may choose to consider only one segment at a time.
- The point of application of a muscle force vector is located at the point of attachment on a segment.
- The muscle action line is in the direction of the fibers or tendon *at the point of application.*
- Muscle vectors (like all vectors) are represented by a straight line. Once the direction of the muscle's action line at its point of application is identified, the vector continues in a straight line regardless of any change in direction of muscle fibers or tendons beyond the point of application.
- The magnitude of a muscle force is generally a hypothetical or theoretical value because the absolute force of a muscle's pull on its attachments in an individual isn't realistically measurable.

Torque Revisited

We are now ready to add the quadriceps muscle force to the leg-foot segment at the point at which knee extension will be initiated in the ankle weight example; that is, it is time for John Alexander to attempt to extend his knee **(Fig. 1–35)**.

Changes to Moment Arm of a Force

To understand the effect of initiating a quadriceps contraction on John Alexander's leg-foot segment, we need to identify the moment arms for the relevant forces. **Figure 1–35A** shows the pull of the quadriceps muscle (QLf) on the leg-foot segment as well as the resultant pull (GAwLf) of both gravity and the ankle weight. For some vectors, finding the shortest (or perpendicular) distance (moment arm) between a force and a joint axis requires that the force vector be extended. The effect of a force is not changed by extending the vector graphically—nor should it be considered to change the magnitude of the force. When GAwLf is extended in **Figure 1–35A** (dashed line), the force still has a magnitude of –88 N, but its moment arm

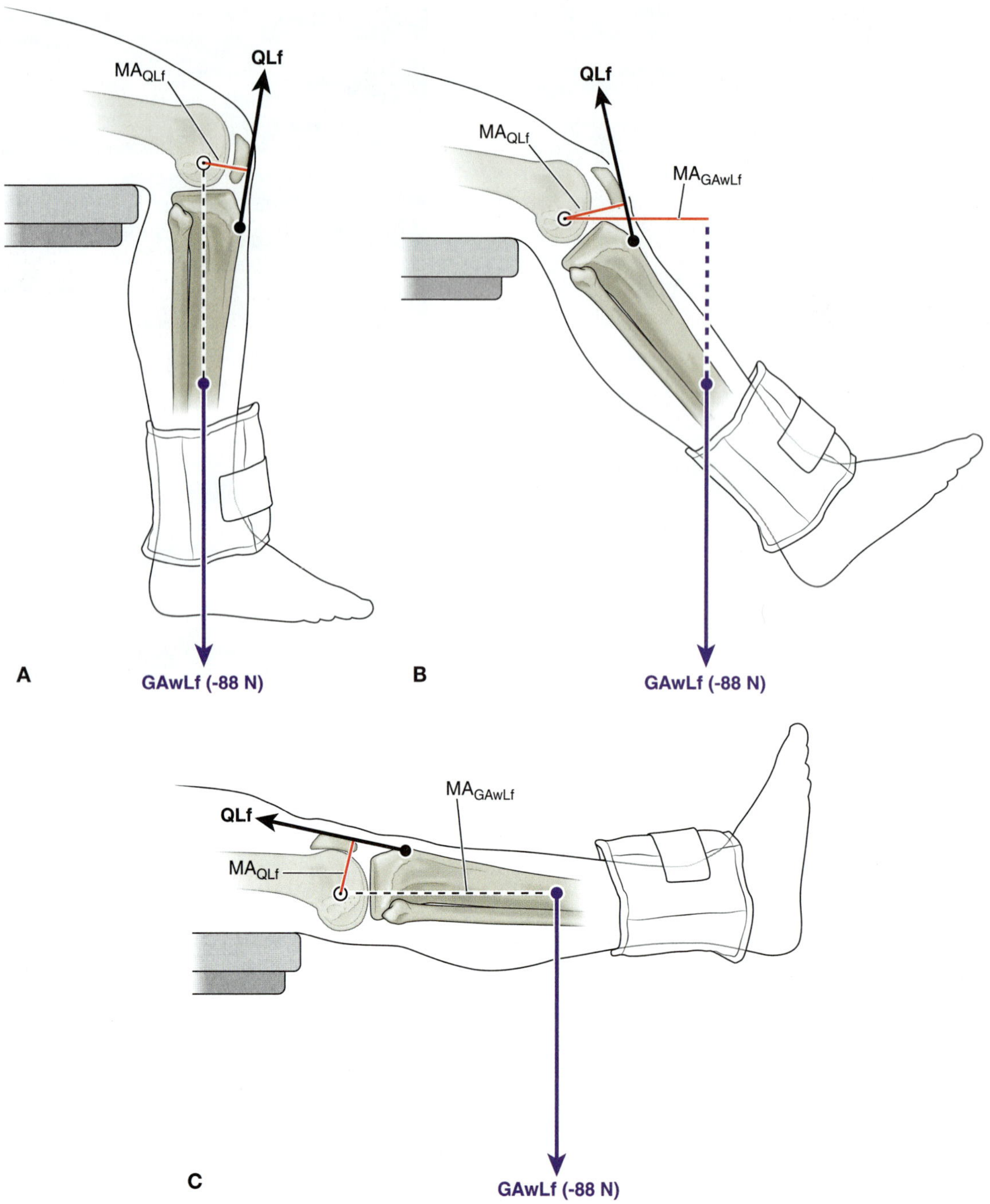

Figure 1–35 **A.** At 90° of knee flexion, the moment arm (MA_{QLf}) for the quadriceps (QLf) is shown. The moment arm for GAwLf is effectively zero because the extended vector (dashed line) passes through the knee joint axis. **B.** At 45° of knee flexion, MA_{QLf} increases slightly but the moment arm for GAwLf (MA_{GAwLf}) increases substantially, thus considerably increasing the torque against which the quadriceps must now work to extend the knee. **C.** At 0° of knee flexion, MA_{QLf} has gotten slightly smaller whereas MA_{GAwLf} has increased substantially. The quadriceps will now have to increase the force of its contraction tremendously to generate sufficient torque to maintain the knee at full extension.

(MA) is effectively zero because the extended vector passes through the knee joint axis (MA ≈ 0). Therefore, gravity and the ankle weight create negligible torque on the leg-foot when the knee joint is still at 90° of knee flexion. Given that GAwLf produces no torque in this knee joint position, a relatively small force by the quadriceps muscle (applied through its relatively larger moment arm estimated in this example to be 0.03 m) will yield a net resultant torque in the direction of knee extension. The scenario will change as soon as the knee is no longer at 90° because the torques created by the forces applied to the leg-foot segment will change as the orientation of the leg-foot segment changes.

In **Figure 1–35B**, the leg-foot segment has been brought farther into knee extension (~45°of knee flexion). As the segment moves in space, the relationship between the forces applied to the segment and the segment itself changes. The gravitational force (GAwLf) now lies at a substantially greater distance from the knee joint axis, increasing the moment arm. The quadriceps muscle force also has a larger moment arm (increasing the estimated distance from 0.03 to 0.05 m), although minimal compared to the increase in the moment arm of GAwLf (increased from 0 m to an estimated 0.27 m). The magnitude of the quadriceps force necessary to continue knee extension from this new point in the ROM is now considerably greater.

If the moment arm for GAwLf in **Figure 1–35B** is 0.27 m, then a force of 88 N would create a clockwise (knee flexion) torque of 23.76 N·m. For John to hold the knee in the new position, the quadriceps muscle would have to create a counterclockwise (extension) torque of 23.76 N·m to maintain rotary equilibrium. If the moment arm for the quadriceps muscle is 0.05 m, the quadriceps force would have to be 475.2 N (~107 lb) just to hold the leg-foot segment at 45°. For John to continue to extend the knee, the quadriceps force must be greater than 475.2 N to create a net unbalanced torque into further extension.

Figure 1–35C shows the leg-foot segment at the end of knee extension (0° of knee flexion). GAwLf is now perpendicular to the leg-foot segment and farther away from the joint axis (its moment arm increasing to an estimated 0.36 m). The line of pull of the quadriceps is now closer to the joint axis than when the knee was at 45°, decreasing its moment arm. The magnitude of GAwLf remains unchanged at 88 N. However, GAwLf now creates a clockwise (flexion) torque of 31.68 N·m. If the reduced moment arm for the quadriceps is now 0.01 m, the muscle will have to generate a force of 3,168 N (712 lb) to maintain this fully extended knee position in rotary equilibrium.

Whenever any force is applied at 90° to the long axis of a segment (as GAwLf is in Fig. 1–35C), the length of the moment arm for that force is maximal. The moment arm will lie parallel to the long axis of the segment (the lever) and, under these conditions, can also be referred to as the **lever arm** of the force. Because the moment arm of a force is greatest when that force is at 90° to the segment, the torque *for a given magnitude of force* will also be greatest when the force is applied at 90° (or as close to 90° as possible for that force). As John Alexander uses his quadriceps to extend his knee, the quadriceps will have to exert the most force on the fully extended knee, making this the hardest knee position to maintain.

Foundational Concepts 1–13
Moment Arms and Torque

- As the moment arm of a force increases, its potential to produce torque increases.
- The moment arm of a force is at its maximum when the force is applied at 90° to its segment.
- The moment arm of a force is zero when the action line of the force passes through the center of rotation of the segment to which the force is applied.
- A gravitational force (line of gravity) will always be applied at 90° to a segment when that segment is horizontal to the ground and will be applied at 0° when the segment is vertical.
- When the moment lies parallel to the segment, the term *lever arm* may also be used to describe the shortest distance from the force vector to the joint axis.

Expanded Concepts 1–7
Work, Energy, and Power

Work, energy, and power are combinations of kinematic and kinetic variables. Although these terms are not the focus of this chapter, these important concepts in biomechanics are related to muscle force production and warrant brief discussion. **Work** is the transfer of energy that takes place when a force is applied through some linear or angular distance and is expressed in units of joules (or N·m).

$$W = F \times D$$

If an examiner applied a load of 10 N to the distal forearm when testing elbow flexion (see **Fig. 1–10**) and the distal forearm moved 2 cm at the point of application of the force, the examiner would have completed 0.2 J (10 N × 0.02 m) of linear work. **Power** is the *rate* of work production and is expressed in watts (or J/sec).

$$P = W \div \text{time}$$

If the examiner created the 2-cm movement of the distal forearm over a 2-second period, 0.1 watt of power would be generated. Although this concept may seem trivial, power is frequently misused when talking about force. Power is the rate of work production and is much more complicated than simple force production due to the time element. The final concept is energy. **Energy** is the ability to perform work and is expressed in the same units as work (joules).

Angular Acceleration With Changing Torques

We approached our analysis of the ankle weight exercise in Figures 1–35A, B, and C as a series of freeze-frames or single points in time. Human motion, of course, is not a series of points of equilibrium but involves rotation of the bony segment around a joint axis with a changing rotary (angular) acceleration as the segment moves through its arc of motion.

We established that the quadriceps muscle would need to contract with a force of approximately 3,168 N at full knee extension to hold the limb against the flexion torque of the weight of the limb and ankle weight (Fig. 1–35C). If a quadriceps contraction of 3,168 N was also generated at 90° of knee flexion as in Fig. 1–35A), the ankle weight and weight of the limb (GAwLf) at that point provide almost no flexion torque because of the small moment arm. There would be a large net extension torque ($\Sigma\tau$) produced by the quadriceps contraction. The net torque would produce a substantial angular acceleration of the leg-foot segment. *[Note: Newton's law of acceleration states that linear acceleration is directly proportional to the net unbalanced force, and that angular (rotary) acceleration is proportional to the net unbalanced torque.]* If the quadriceps muscle continues to contract with a force of 3,168 N as John's knee extends, the net unbalanced extension torque will decrease as the flexion torque generated by GAwLf increases due to its increasing moment arm as the knee approaches full extension. As the net unbalanced extension torque decreases, so too does the angular acceleration of the leg-foot segment. The angular acceleration will reach zero at the point of full knee extension when tightening posterior knee structures contribute to checking further knee extension; full equilibrium of the leg-foot segment is restored when $\Sigma\tau = 0$ and $\Sigma F = 0$). In this example, the changing torque is attributable to the changes in moment arms of GAwLf and the quadriceps because the magnitudes of both forces remain unchanged. *[Note: It is a characteristic of the quadriceps muscle that its moment arm is greatest in, approximately, the middle of the knee ROM. The point in the joint ROM where the moment arm of a muscle is largest, thereby producing its greatest potential torque, is essentially unique to each muscle and is not predictable by any rules.]*

Moment Arm and Angle of Application of a Force

We have seen that the moment arm of a force can change as a segment rotates around its joint axis and as the segment changes its orientation in space. The length of the moment arm is directly related to the **angle of application of the force** on the segment. The angle of application of a force is the angle made by the intersection of the force vector and the segment to which it is applied *on the side of the joint axis under consideration.* Any time a force is applied to a segment, at least two angles are formed. The viewer's eye will automatically tend to find the acute (rather than the obtuse) angle. To identify the angle of application of a force, the angle *on the side of the joint axis* is the angle of interest, regardless of whether that angle is acute (less than 90°) or obtuse (greater than 90°).

Figure 1–36 shows a force vector (e.g., brachialis) at four different angles of application to the forearm. It can be seen how the angle of application of the force affects the size of the moment arm. When the angle of application of a force is small (~35°), the moment arm will be small **(Fig. 1–36A)**. As the angle of application for the force increases (~70°), the moment arm increases because the vector lies farther from the joint axis **(Fig. 1–36B)**. When the angle of application of the force is at 90°, the moment arm is as large as it can get **(Fig. 1–36C)**. When the angle of application moves beyond 90° (e.g., 145°) **(Fig. 1–36D)**, the moment arm is measured from the extended tail of the vector. The extended tail swings closer to the joint axis as the angle of application of the force continues to increase beyond 90°. As the moment arm of a muscle force changes, so too does its ability to generate torque, as we saw already with the quadriceps in Figures 1–35A, B, and C.

In Figures 1–36A, B, C, and D, the moment arms and torques changed as the segment moved through ROM. There will also be a change in moment arm and angle of application of the line of gravity as a segment moves through its joint ROM. However, the basis for the change in angle of application of a gravitational force is different than for a muscle. A gravitational force is always vertically downward. Consequently, it is the orientation of the *segment in space* rather than the joint angle that causes a change in the angle of application of gravity.

In **Figure 1–37A**, the elbow joint is at 90° and the forearm is parallel to the ground (horizontal). Therefore, gravity-on-forearm will be applied at 90° to the forearm and the moment arm of gravity-on-forearm will be at its greatest. In **Figure 1–37B**, the elbow joint is still at 90° but the forearm is no longer parallel to the ground. Consequently, the moment arm for gravity-on-forearm (and its torque) will be less. Because the *magnitude* of the gravitational force on a segment does not change as the segment moves through space, the torque produced by the weight (G) of a segment is a function of the position of the segment in space rather than the joint angle.

Unlike gravity that has a fixed center of mass in an unsegmented object, other external forces (e.g., a manual resistance, mechanical resistance, or applied load) may be able to change the point of application on the body segment. When the point of application of an external force on the segment changes, so too does its moment arm (and torque) of that force. As a manual resistance to a joint motion is shifted farther from the joint axis, production of the same torque requires less manual force because of its larger moment arm.

Foundational Concepts 1–14
Moment Arms and Angle of Application

For all forces (internal and external):

- The moment arm of a force is greatest when the force is applied at, or as close as it will get to, 90° (perpendicular) to the segment it is acting on.
- The moment arm of a force is smallest when the force is applied at, or as close as it will get to, either 0° or 180° (parallel) to the segment.
- The angle of application (and moment arm) of a muscle force will vary with the angle of the joint it is crossing because the segment moves in space.
- The angle of application (and moment arm) of gravity will vary with the orientation of the segment in space, regardless of the joint angle.
- Most muscles are aligned approximately parallel to the bony segments to which they attach; consequently, muscles that have an angle of application that comes close to 90° are the exception rather than the rule.

Changing the Gravitation Moment Arm by Changing the Center of Mass

Figure 1–38 shows three graded exercises for the abdominal muscles. The vertebral interspace of L5 to S1 is considered here to be a hypothetical axis about which the head-arms-trunk (HAT) rotates. In each figure, the arms are positioned slightly different, resulting in a rearrangement of mass and a shift in the center of mass. In **Figure 1–38A**, the arms are raised above the head. As a result, the center of mass of the HAT is located closer to the head (cephalad), with a line of gravity that is farther from the axis of rotation (greater moment arm) than when the arms are in the other two positions. The torque generated by gravity is counterclockwise (a trunk extension

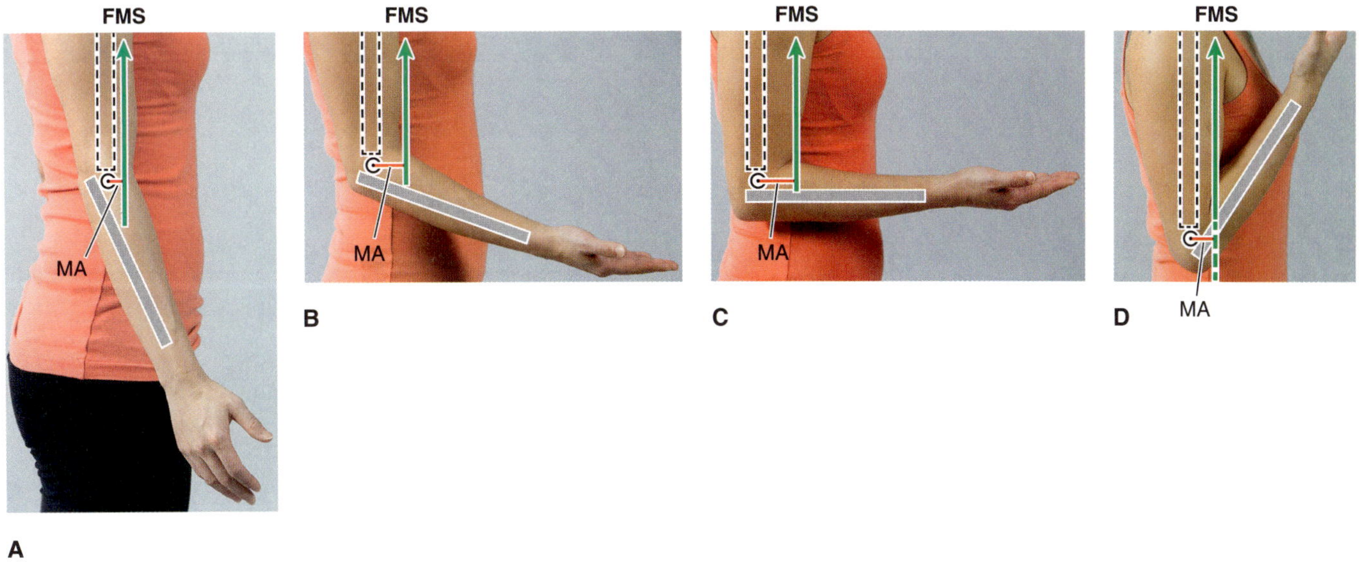

Figure 1–36 Changes in the angle of application of the force (the angle between the force vector and lever *on the side of the axis*) on the forearm result in changes to the moment arm (MA) of the force (Fms). **A.** The moment arm is smallest when the angle of application is smallest (~35°). **B.** As the angle of application of Fms increases (70°), the MA increases. **C.** The MA is maximal when the force is applied at 90° to the segment. **D.** When the angle of application of Fms is greater than 90° (145°), the vector must be extended to find the length of the MA.

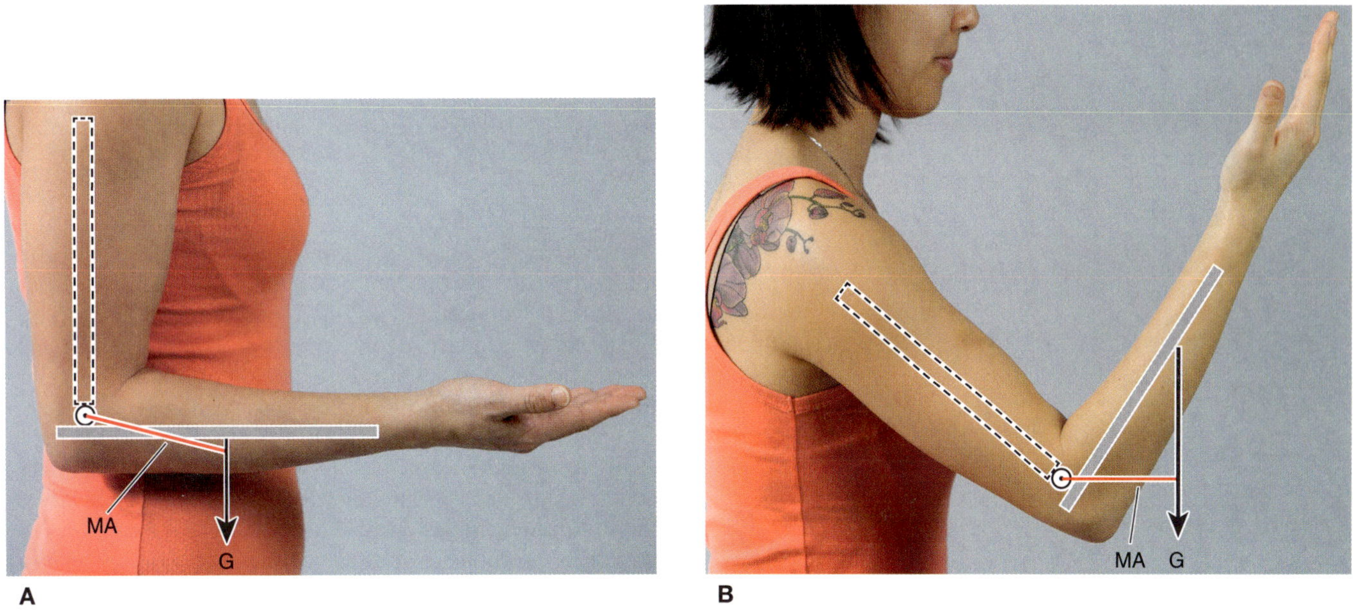

Figure 1–37 **A.** When the forearm is parallel to the ground (horizontal), gravity (G) will always have an angle of application of 90° and the moment arm (MA) for the force will be as large as it can get. **B.** Although the elbow is still at 90° of flexion, the angle of application of G is now applied at 45° to the forearm and the MA is smaller than in position A.

torque or moment). To maintain rotational equilibrium in this position, the abdominal muscles must generate an equal torque in the opposite direction (an equivalent flexion moment). In **Figures 1–38B** and **C**, the center of mass moves caudally as the arms are lowered. The relocation of the center of mass of the HAT brings the line of gravity closer to the axis. Because the weight of the upper body does not change when the arms are lowered, the magnitude of torque applied by gravity to the upper body diminishes because of the reduction in the moment arm. The decreased gravitational torque requires less opposing torque by the abdominal muscles to maintain equilibrium. Consequently, it is easiest to maintain the position in Figure 1–38C and hardest to maintain the position in Figure 1–38A.

Lever Systems, or Classes of Levers

One perspective used to assess the relative torques of internal and external forces is that of **lever systems,** or **classes of levers.** Although applying the terminology of lever systems to human movement requires some important oversimplifications, the terms (like those of the cardinal planes and axes) provide a useful frame of reference and a common terminology that permit us to break complex kinetics into describable component parts.

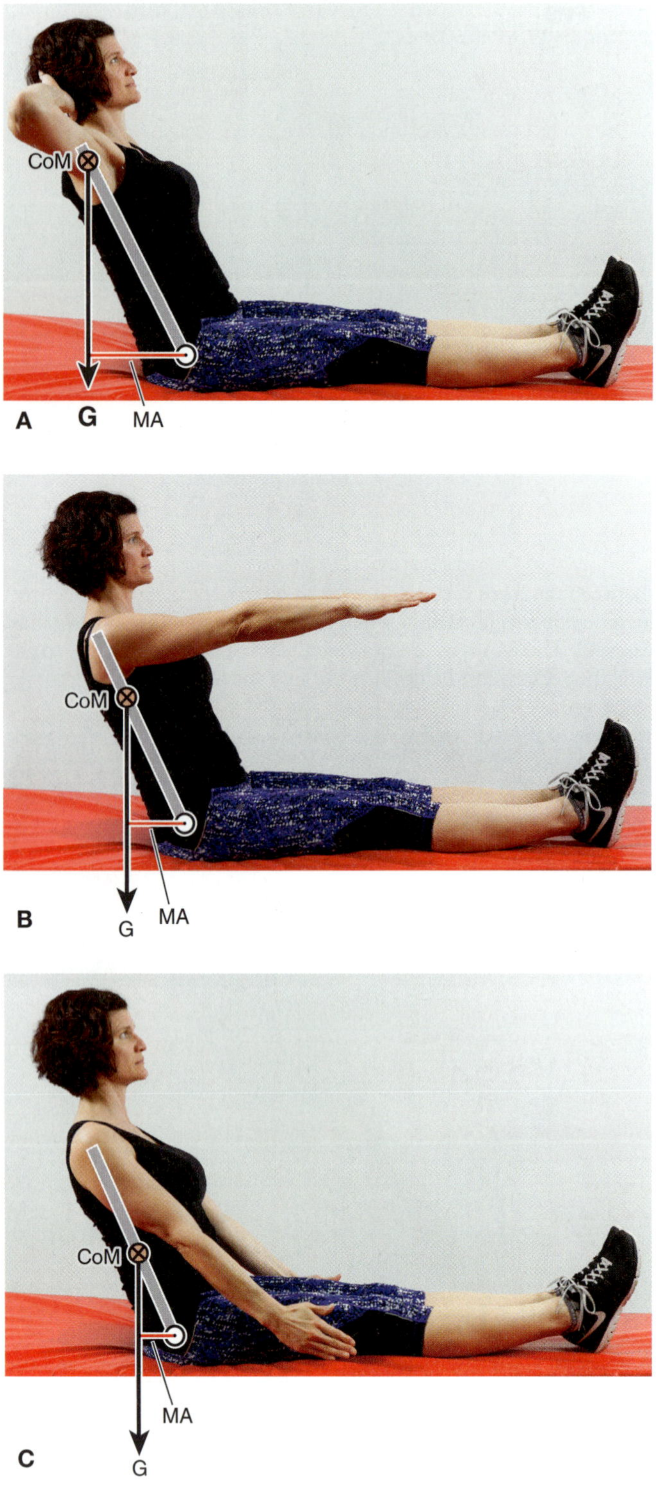

Figure 1–38 Changes in arm position in a sit-up cause the center of mass (CoM) of the upper body segment to move, the moment arm (MA) to change, and the torque due to gravity (G) to decrease from position A to position C.

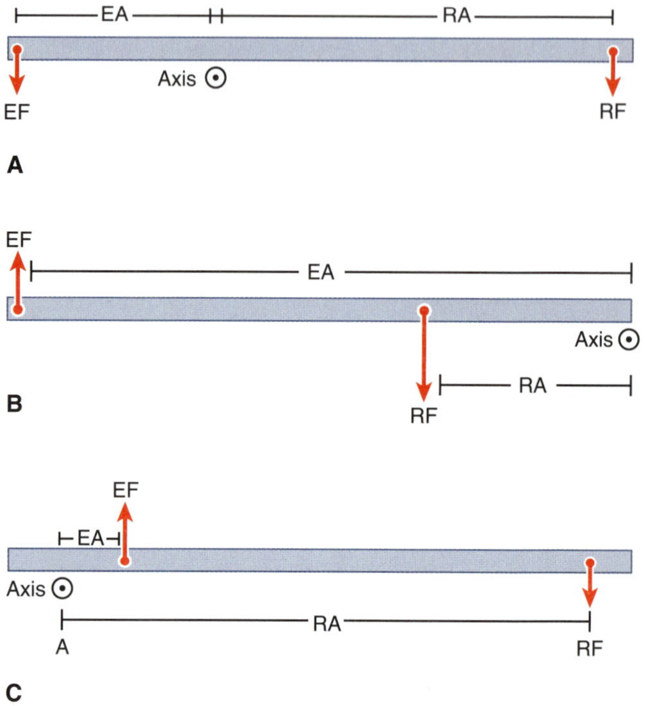

Figure 1–39 **A.** First-class lever: The axis lies between the effort force (EF) and the resistance force (RF). **B.** Second-class lever: The RF lies between the axis and the EF so that the effort arm (EA) is always larger than the resistance arm (RA). **C.** Third-class lever: The EF lies between the axis and the RF so that RA is always larger than EA.

A lever is any rigid segment that rotates around a fulcrum. A lever system exists whenever two forces are applied to a lever in a way that produces opposing torques. To apply concepts of levers to a bony segment, we must also consider the joint axis of the bony segment to be relatively fixed (a problematic assumption, as we have already discussed). However, it is common to apply the concepts of levers to bony segments when looking at the net rotation produced by two forces, typically (1) a muscle force and (2) a gravitational or external force.

In a lever system, the force that is producing the resultant torque (the force acting in the direction of rotation) is called the **effort force (EF).** Because the other force must be creating an opposing torque, it is known as the **resistance force (RF).** Another way to think of effort and resistance forces acting on a lever is that the effort force *is always the winner* in the torque game, and the resistance force *is always the loser* in producing rotation of the segment. The moment arm for the effort force is referred to as the **effort arm (EA),** whereas the moment arm for the resistance force is referred to as the **resistance arm (RA).** Once the effort and resistance forces are identified and labeled, the position of the axis and relative sizes of the effort and resistance arms determine the class of the lever (**Fig. 1-39**).

A **first-class lever** is a lever system in which the axis lies somewhere between the point of application of the effort force and the point of application of the resistance force (**Fig. 1-39A**). A **second-class lever** is a lever system in which the resistance force has a point of application between the axis and the point of application of the effort force (**Fig. 1-39B**); this always results in the effort arm being larger than the resistance arm. A **third-class lever** is a lever system in which the effort force has a point of application between the axis and the point of application of the resistance force (**Fig. 1-39C**); this always results in the resistance arm being larger than the effort arm.

Foundational Concepts 1–15
Muscles in Lever Systems

- When a muscle is contracting **concentrically** (actively shortening), the muscle must be moving the segment to which it is attached in the direction of the muscle's pull. Therefore, the muscle is "winning" and will be the effort force. In most instances, concentrically contracting muscles are acting on third-class levers because the muscular effort force attaches closer to the joint axis than the resistance force.
- When a muscle is contracting **eccentrically** (actively lengthening), the muscle is pulling in a direction opposite to the motion of the segment; that is, the muscle is "losing" and is the resistance force. When a muscle is contracting eccentrically, it generally serves to *control* (slow down) the acceleration of the segment produced by the effort force and, in most instances, is acting on a second-class lever because what is now the muscular resistance force is closer to the joint axis than the effort force.
- When a lever is in rotational equilibrium, the muscle acting on the lever is contracting **isometrically.** In such a case, labeling the muscle as the effort or resistance force is arbitrary, so the class of lever on which the muscle is acting depends on the choice in labeling.
- There are a few muscles that lie on one side of an axis while the center of mass of the limb being moved by the muscle acts on the other side of the axis. In the human body, these muscles act on infrequently identified first-class levers.

Mechanical Advantage

Mechanical advantage (M Ad) is a measure of the mechanical efficiency of the lever system (the relative effectiveness of the effort force in comparison with the resistance force). Mechanical advantage is related to the classification of a lever and provides an understanding of the relationship between the torque of an external force (which we can roughly estimate) and the torque of a muscular force (which we only can estimate in relation to the external torque). Mechanical advantage of a lever is the ratio of the effort arm (EA; moment arm of the effort force) to the resistance arm (RA; moment arm of the resistance force), or:

$$\text{M Ad} = \frac{\text{EA}}{\text{RA}}$$

When the effort arm is larger than the resistance arm it is in a second-class lever (Fig. 1–39B), and the mechanical advantage will be greater than one. When the mechanical advantage is greater than one, the magnitude of the effort force is working through a larger moment arm and therefore can be smaller than the magnitude of the resistance force while still creating enough torque to "win." The "advantage" is that a small force can defeat a larger force.

When the effort arm is smaller than the resistance arm as it is in a third-class lever (Fig. 1–39C), the mechanical advantage will always be less than one. A third-class lever is "mechanically inefficient" or is working at a "disadvantage" because the magnitude of the effort force *must* always be *greater* than the magnitude of the resistance force for the torque of the effort force to "win" (produce a greater torque) while working through a smaller moment arm.

It is important to note the mechanical advantage of a lever is determined by the lengths of the moment arms and not by the *magnitudes* of the effort and resistance forces. If an effort force is winning (as it must be to earn the "effort force" label) and has a magnitude smaller than that of the resistance force, the muscle *must* be working through a larger moment arm than the resistance or it couldn't "win." However, if the moment arm of the effort force is larger than that of the resistance (e.g., acting on a second-class lever), the magnitude of the effort force is *not necessarily* smaller than that of the resistance force. If both the magnitude of the effort force and the moment arm of the effort force are larger than those of the resistance force, the net torque and angular acceleration will be large.

Foundational Concepts 1–16
Mechanical Advantage and Classes of Levers

- In all second-class levers, the mechanical advantage (M Ad) of the lever will always be *greater than one*. The magnitude of the effort force can be (but is not necessarily) less than the magnitude of the resistance.
- In all third-class levers, the mechanical advantage of the lever will always be *less than one*. The magnitude of the effort force must be greater than the magnitude of the resistance for the effort to produce greater torque.
- The mechanical advantage of a first-class lever can be greater than, less than, or equal to one. However, it is often true of first-class levers in the body that the moment arm of the muscle will be shorter than the moment arm of the external force, thus rendering the lever inefficient.
- When the muscle is the effort force in a lever with a mechanical advantage of less than one, the necessary expenditure of energy to produce sufficient muscle force to "win" is offset by the need for minimal linear displacement and velocity of the muscle's length, which produces proportionally greater angular displacement and angular velocity of the distal portions of the segment.
- When an external force is the effort force in a lever with a mechanical advantage greater than one (e.g., a second-class lever), the magnitude of the effort force can be small in comparison with the resistance force, but less is gained in angular displacement and velocity.

Most muscles have a moment arm that is smaller than that of the external force(s) against which they are working because most muscles lie close to joint axes than most opposing external forces. Consequently, the muscle must be able to create large forces not only to "win" (work concentrically as the effort force) but also to eccentrically control external forces when the external force is "winning." As shall be shown in Chapter 3, a muscle is typically structured to optimize production of the large force required to produce sufficient torque when working through a small moment arm, whether functioning eccentrically as a resistance force or concentrically as an effort force.

Limitations of Analysis of Forces by Lever Systems

Although the conceptual framework of lever systems described here provides useful terms and some additional insights into rotation of segments and muscle function, there are distinct limitations to this approach. Our discussion of lever systems ignored the established fact that the rotation of a lever requires at least one force couple. An effort force and a resistance force are *not* a force couple because effort and resistance forces produce rotation in the opposite direction (whereas a force couple works together to produce rotation in the same direction). The second force in the "couple" is generally an articular constraint (a joint reaction force or capsuloligamentous force) that may serve as the pivot point for the rotation. Consequently, a simple lever-system approach to analyzing human motion requires oversimplification that fails to take into consideration key elements that affect human function and structural integrity. Torques on human segments are not simply produced by one muscle group and one external force but result from many forces *including* vertical and horizontal translatory forces that are typically ignored in a simple lever approach.

Force Components

In the analysis of the quadriceps force producing an extension torque on the leg-foot segment (see Fig. 1–35A–C), we did not identify the second part of the force couple that is actually required to produce the knee extension torque. We also did not identify the mechanism by which translatory equilibrium ($\Sigma F_V = 0$ and $\Sigma F_H = 0$) of the leg-foot segment was established—a necessary condition for rotation of a joint around a relatively fixed axis. To examine the degree to which these conditions are met (net extension torque and translatory equilibrium), we need to understand how to resolve forces into their component parts.

To review, a force of constant magnitude produces its greatest torque when the force is applied at 90° to the lever. At other angles of application for that same force, the torque will be less, even if the magnitude of the force is unchanged. However, if the *same* magnitude of force produces *less* torque when the angle of application is not 90°, some of that force must be doing something other than producing rotation. Torque, in fact, is typically considered to be produced only by that *portion* of the force that contributes to rotation. When the force is applied to a lever at some other angle (greater or less than 90°), the component of force that *is* applied at 90° to the lever is the portion that contributes to rotation. Consequently, the portion of a force that is applied at 90° to the segment is known as the **perpendicular** (**rotary** or **"y"**) **component** of the force **(Fy).** The rotary component is the "y" component because the long axis of the body segment is usually the reference line, serving as the x-axis. Consequently, the component that is perpendicular to the segment is the y-axis.

The magnitude of Fy can be found graphically by the process of **resolution of forces.** In resolution of forces, the original (or **total**) **force (F_{TOT})** is broken down into two components that are perpendicular *to each other*. Just as two concurrent forces can be composed into a single resultant vector (composition by parallelogram), a single vector (F_{TOT}) can be resolved into two concurrent components. In this instance, the components will be specifically constructed so that one component (Fy) lies perpendicular to the segment and the second component (Fx) is drawn parallel to the segment, thus perpendicular to each other.

Resolving Forces Into Perpendicular and Parallel Components

In **Figure 1–40**, three steps are shown to resolve the quadriceps force (QLf or F_{TOT}) into its perpendicular (Fy_{QLf}) and parallel (Fx_{QLf}) components:

Step 1 (see **Fig. 1–40A**). A line with the *same point of application* as the original force (F_{TOT} or QLf in this example) is drawn perpendicular to the long axis of the lever in the direction of the original force (this is the "draft" line of component Fy). A second line with the *same point of application* as QLf is drawn parallel to the long axis of the lever in the direction of the original force (this is the "draft" line of component Fx). The draft Fx and Fy component lines should be drawn long enough to reach or go past the arrowhead of the original vector QLf.

Step 2 (see **Fig. 1–40B**). The rectangle is completed (closed) by drawing (from the arrowhead of the F_{TOT} or QLf vector) lines that are parallel to each of the draft Fx and Fy components.

Step 3 (see **Fig. 1–40C**). All the lines are "trimmed," leaving only the completed rectangle with QLf (F_{TOT}) as its diagonal. Components Fy (the rotary component) and Fx (the translatory component) each form one side of the rectangle, have a common point of application, and have arrowheads at the corners of the rectangle. It is important that the lengths of vectors Fy and Fx are "trimmed" to make QLf a perfect diagonal, thereby maintaining a fixed proportional relation among Fx, Fy, and F_{TOT} at a given angle of application of F_{TOT}. This proportional relation will permit determination of the predominant and relative effects of F_{TOT}.

Perpendicular and Parallel Force Effects

Focusing on the components of the quadriceps force (Fy_{QLf} and Fx_{QLf} in Fig. 1–40C) rather than on the quadriceps "total" force (QLf), it can be seen more readily that the components of QLf have the potential to create three different motions of the leg-foot segment: vertical motion, horizontal motion, and rotary motion. Component Fx_{QLf} (Fig. 1–40C) will tend to create vertical translatory motion, while component Fy_{QLf} will both create rotation and tend to create horizontal translation. Because a force component (e.g., Fy_{QLf}) may create both rotation and translation, labeling components as "rotary" and "translatory" can be confusing. For the remainder of this chapter, therefore, we will refer to Fy and Fx exclusively as the components perpendicular and parallel to the lever, respectively; the effects of Fy and Fx (rotation or translation) will depend on the scenario.

We have already established that determining whether a segment is in equilibrium or not requires assessment of ΣF_V, ΣF_H, and Σ_τ (Newton's law of inertia). Consider, however, that a force that is perpendicular to the segment and also horizontally oriented in space (e.g., Fy_{QLf} in Fig. 1–40C), may become vertically oriented in space while still remaining perpendicular to the segment (e.g., as the knee moves toward full extension). The same shift in spatial orientation may happen with an Fx component. Because the relationship of the force or force component to the segment is the critical factor in understanding the effect of the force(s) on the joint

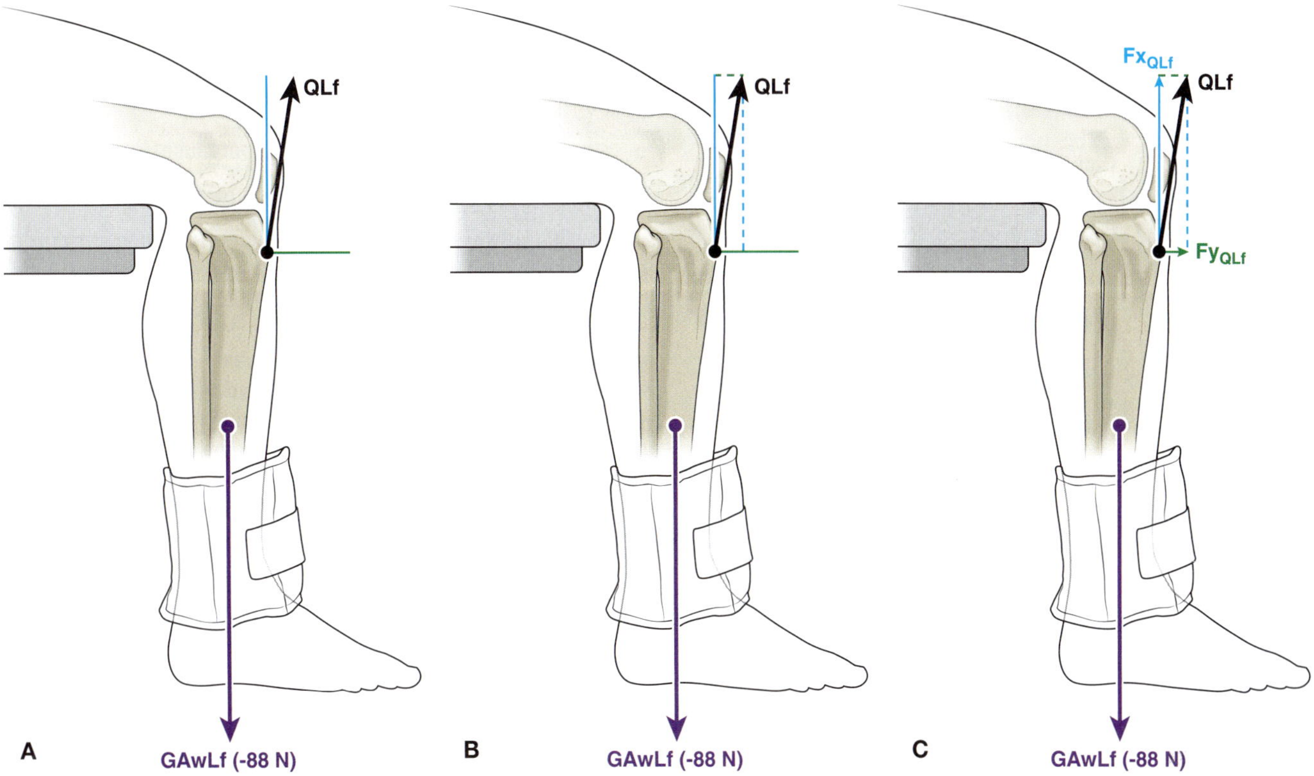

Figure 1–40 When a force (e.g., QLf) is resolved into its components, **A.** two lines that are perpendicular and parallel to the long axis of the bone are drawn from the point of application of the original QLf force; **B.** a rectangle is completed by drawing parallel lines from the arrowhead of the original QLf force; and **C.** the perpendicular (Fy) and parallel (Fx) component vectors are the adjacent sides of the rectangle that have a common point of application with the original force. The original force (QLf) is the diagonal of the rectangle.

(not whether a force is vertical or horizontal in space), we will proceed to assess translatory equilibrium of a body segment by considering the sum of the Fx (ΣFx) and Fy (ΣFy) components. The rotary equilibrium of the body segment will be assessed by determining the sums of the torques (Σ_τ) contributed by the forces or force components.

Determining Magnitudes of Component Forces

In a figure drawn to scale, the relative vector lengths can be used to estimate the net unbalanced forces. If the vectors are not drawn to scale, the relative magnitudes of Fy and Fx must be determined by using trigonometric functions of sines (sin) and cosines (cos).

Component forces Fx and Fy are always two sides of a rectangle that is divided into two right triangles by their resultant force (F_{TOT}). Based on the example of the quadriceps force (QLf) in **Figure 1–41A**, the quadriceps vector (QLf) and its components are shown in isolation and enlarged. The shaded half of the rectangle is the triangle of interest because the angle (θ) is the angle of application of the quadriceps (the angle between QLf and the long axis of the leg-foot segment on the side of the knee joint axis). Vector QLf is the hypotenuse (longest side) of the triangle and is now assigned an arbitrary magnitude of 1,000 N. The angle of application θ is 25° in this example. Vector Fx is the side adjacent to angle θ, and vector Fy is the side opposite angle θ. **Figure 1–41B** shows the same rectangle as in Figure 1–41A, but it is reoriented to one more commonly seen when assessing elements in a right triangle. It should be noted that the "side

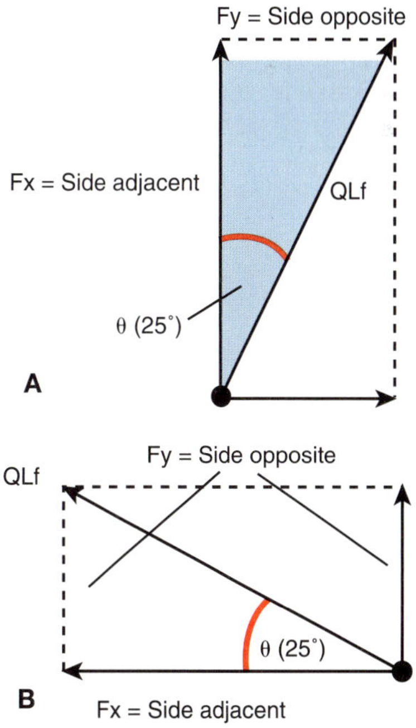

Figure 1–41 Review of trigonometry. **A.** Vector QLf and its Fx and Fy components are replicated (although enlarged) in the same orientation shown in Figure 1–40C. The reference triangle (shaded) shows that QLf is the hypotenuse, Fx is the side adjacent to angle θ, and Fy (or its equivalent length) is the side opposite to angle θ. **B.** The same figure is reoriented in space to provide an alternative visualization.

opposite" the angle θ is not the perpendicular component (Fy) as we *initially* labeled it. However, the side of the rectangle opposite to the original Fy is identical in magnitude (see Fig. 1–41B) because opposite sides of a rectangle are equivalent in length.

Trigonometry now can be used to solve for the magnitudes of Fx (Fx_{QLf}) and Fy (Fy_{QLf}), where the angle of application θ is given as 25° and QLf is 1,000 N. *[Note: The interested reader is referred to Expanded Concepts 1–8 for details of the trigonometric solution.]*

Fx_{QLf} = (cos 25°)(1,000 N) = (0.91)(1,000 N) = **910 N**

Fy_{QLf} = (sin 25°)(1,000 N) = (0.42)(1,000 N) = **420 N**

It should be recognized that the sum of the magnitudes of the Fx and Fy components will always be greater than the magnitude of the resultant force (F_{TOT}). As with composition of forces, the resultant is more "efficient." However, analysis of the translatory or rotary effects of any set of forces will produce mathematically equivalent results, whether the total force or the force components are used in appropriate analyses.

Expanded Concepts 1–8

Trigonometric Resolution of Forces

The relation between the lengths of the three sides in a right (90°) triangle is given in the Pythagorean theorem: $A^2 + B^2 = C^2$, where C is the length of the hypotenuse of the triangle (the side opposite the 90° angle) and A and B are, respectively, the lengths of the sides adjacent to and opposite the angle θ **(Fig. 1–42A)**. This equation is useful when the lengths (magnitudes) of *at least two* of the three sides of the triangle are known. In resolution of internal and external forces, we typically know, at best, the length of the hypotenuse and one angle. In these cases, the sine and cosine rules allow the unknown lengths in the triangle to be computed:

sin θ = Side opposite/hypotenuse

cos θ = Side adjacent/hypotenuse

These formulas may be used to solve for the length of the adjacent side (Fx) or opposite side (Fy) when angle θ (the angle of application of the force) and the hypotenuse (the magnitude of the resultant force) are known:

side opposite = (sin θ)(hypotenuse)

side adjacent = (cos θ)(hypotenuse)

The values of the sine and cosine functions in trigonometry are not arbitrary numbers. The sine and cosine values reflect a fixed relationship between the lengths of the sides of a triangle for any given angle. In **Figure 1–42B**, a right triangle with an angle θ of 25° is drawn. The large triangle is divided into two smaller triangles. The hypotenuses of the smallest to largest triangle are assigned scaled values of 10 cm, 15 cm, and 20 cm, respectively. The corresponding values of Fy (side opposite θ) will be 4.2 cm, 6.3 cm, and 8.5 cm, respectively; the corresponding values of Fx (side adjacent to θ) will be 9.1 cm, 13.6 cm, and 18.1 cm, respectively. The ratio of any two sides of one of these 25° triangles will be the same, regardless of the size of the triangle, and that ratio will be the value of the trigonometric function for that angle.

1. Given the lengths of the side opposite θ and the hypotenuse for each of the three right triangles, the sin of 25° is **0.42** for each of the differently sized triangles [(4.2/10 = **0.42**); (6.3/15 = **0.42**); and (8.5/20 = **0.42**)].
2. Similarly, the cos of 25° is **0.91** for all three triangles [(9.1/10 = **0.91**); (13.6/15 = **0.91**); and (18.1/20 = **0.91**).
3. Lastly for each of the three triangles, the value of the tangent (tan, or sin÷cos) of 25° is **0.46** [(4.2/9.1 = **0.46**); (6.3/13.6 = **0.46**); and (8.5/18.1 = **0.46**).

This is the "proof" that, for a given angle of application of F_{TOT}, Fx and Fy have a fixed proportional relationship to F_{TOT} *and* a fixed proportional relationship to each other regardless of the magnitude of F_{TOT} (and regardless of the orientation of the segment in space or whether the force is internal or external).

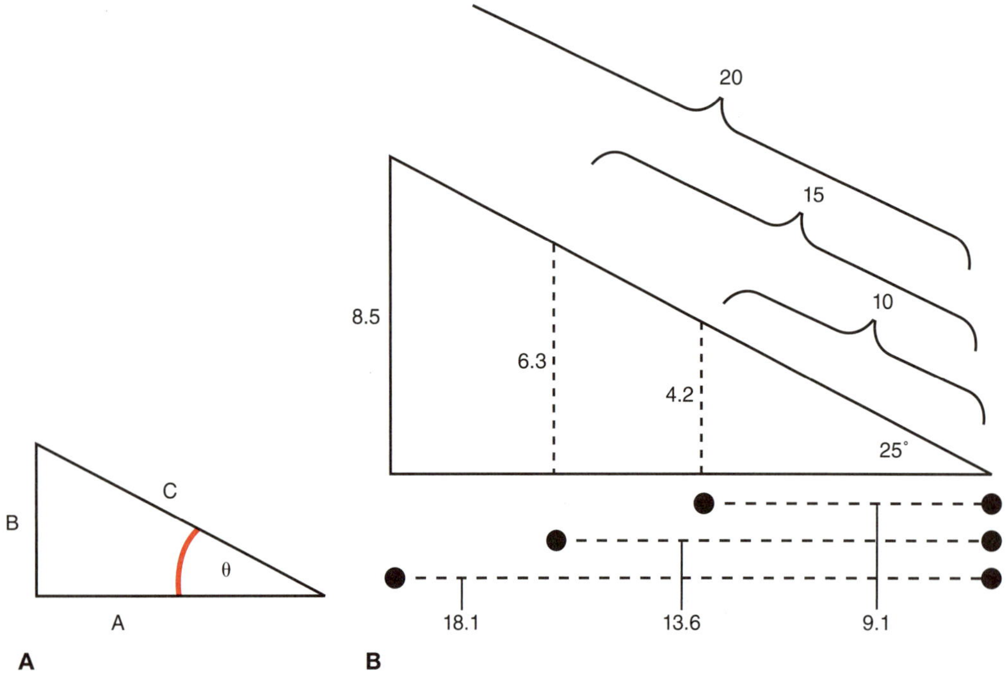

Figure 1–42 Review of trigonometry. **A.** The Pythagorean theorem states that $A^2 + B^2 = C^2$, where A, B, and C are the lengths of the sides of a right triangle. **B.** For a given angle θ (e.g., 25°), the lengths of the side opposite and side adjacent to the angle will have a fixed relationship to each other and to the original force, regardless of the size of the triangle.

Force Components and the Angle of Application of the Force

We have established that the moment arm (and, therefore, the torque) of a force of constant magnitude will change as the segment rotates around its joint axis, and that the change in the moment arm of that force is a function of the change in the angle of application of that force as the segment rotates. Because the perpendicular component (Fy) of a force is effectively the portion of the total force that produces all the torque, a change in torque produced by a force of constant magnitude must mean that the magnitude of Fy is changing. This is quite logical because the magnitude of Fy is a function of the angle of application of the force ($Fy = [\sin \theta][\text{hypotenuse}]$) and we have already established that the angle of application of a force changes as the segment moves around its joint axis.

When a force is applied at 90° to the segment, we have established that the moment arm is as large as it can be for a force. Similarly, the Fy component will be as large as it can be and is equivalent in magnitude to the total force (F_{TOT}); a line drawn perpendicular to the segment (Fy) at the point of application of F_{TOT} will coincide completely with F_{TOT} whenever F_{TOT} is applied at 90° to the segment. Consequently, both moment arm and Fy have their greatest magnitude when a force is applied at 90° to a segment. Importantly, there will also be a proportional decrease in Fx as Fy increases. As the angle of application of F_{TOT} gets closer to 90° (perpendicular to the segment), its perpendicular component (Fy) will get longer and its parallel component (Fx) will get shorter. Correspondingly, as F_{TOT} gets closer to an angle of application of 0° or 180° (parallel to the segment), its parallel component (Fx) will get longer and its perpendicular component will get shorter. That is, the magnitudes of Fx and Fy are inversely proportional.

The majority of muscles in the body: (1) lie nearly parallel to the segment to which they attach, (2) have relatively small angles of pull (Fx is greater than Fy) regardless of the joint angle, and (3) almost always pull toward (in the direction of) the joint axis given the uncommon scenario where the angle of application of a muscle is greater than 90°. The effect of this arrangement of muscles is that a muscle force generally has a relatively small Fy component contributing to rotation, with a larger Fx component that is nearly always compressive. Therefore, most of the force generated by a muscle contributes to joint *compression*, rather than joint *rotation*. This arrangement enhances joint stability but means that a muscle must generate a large total force to produce sufficient torque to move the lever through space.

The generalizations that can be made about the majority of muscle forces do not apply to external forces. Gravity is constrained in its direction (always vertically downward) and therefore, has some predictability (the torque of gravity is always greatest when the limb segment is parallel to the ground). Other external forces (e.g., manual resistance) have few if any constraints and, therefore, most often do not have predictable relationships to or effects on a segment. However, the *principles* of forces in relation to the angle of application and the consequential magnitudes of the moment arm, Fy component, Fx component, and torques apply to any and all forces, including those commonly encountered in clinical situations.

Manipulating External Forces to Maximize Torque

In **Figure 1–43**, a manual external force (hand-on-leg/foot [HLf]) is applied to two different points of application on the leg-foot segment with the same amount of force and same angle of application in each case. When the goal is to require the quadriceps to work as hard as possible, thus maximizing its extension force to strengthen the muscle, one probably wishes to *minimize* the effort on the part of the person applying the opposing flexion force while the leg-foot maintains $\Sigma_\tau = 0$; one strategy (of the first two offered) has distinct advantages over the other. In **Figure 1–43A**, HLf has a substantially smaller moment arm than does HLf in **Figure 1–43B** because the resisting hand is placed closer to the knee joint. By moving the resisting hand down (distally on) the leg-foot segment (Fig.1–43B), the moment arm of HLf is substantially increased. The flexion torque produced by HLf in Figure 1–43B is going to be much greater than the flexion torque produced by the same magnitude of force shown in Figure 1–43A. The joint angle and angle of pull of the quadriceps is the same in both scenarios, thus its moment arm does not change; the muscle must increase its force of contraction in Figure 1–43B to produce the greater extension torque needed to maintain equilibrium of the leg-foot segment against the increased torque of HLf. A similar manipulation of the resistance force (and corresponding quadriceps force) can take place by modifying the angle of application of the manual resistance. If the resisting hand (HLf) in Figure 1–43B was applied to the leg at 45° (rather than 90°) as in Figure 1-43C, only about half HLf would contribute to a flexion rotation. At a 45° angle of application, $Fy_{HLf} \approx \frac{1}{2}$ HLf; a manual resistance applied at 90°, $HLf = Fy_{HLf}$. An understanding of the ability to manipulate both moment arm and angle of application of an external manual force will allow the person applying the force to either increase or decrease the challenge to the quadriceps muscle (and to the person applying the resistance), depending on the goal of the quadriceps exercise.

Foundational Concepts 1–17
Components of Muscle Forces

- The angle of application (angle of pull) for the majority of muscles is small, with an action line more parallel than perpendicular to the bony lever.
- The parallel (Fx) component of a muscle force is larger than the perpendicular (Fy) component for most muscles.
- The parallel component (Fx) of most muscle forces contributes to joint compression, making muscles important joint stabilizers.

Foundational Concepts 1–18
Manipulating External Forces to Maximize Torque Production

- The torque from an external force can be increased by adding to the magnitude of the applied force.
- The torque from an external force can be increased by applying the force perpendicular (or closer to perpendicular) to the lever.
- The torque from an external force can be increased by increasing the distance of the point of application of the force from the segment's joint axis.

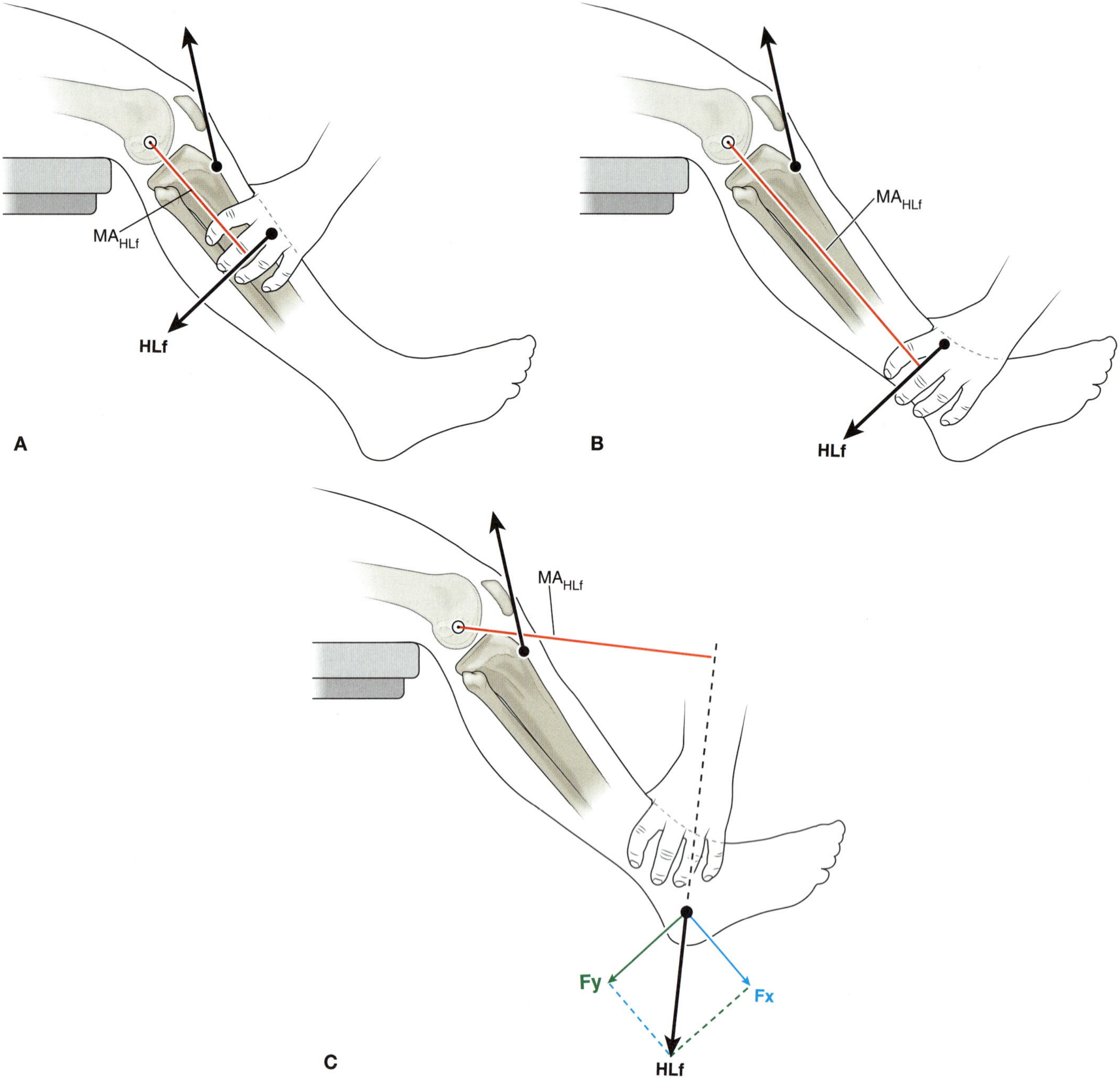

Figure 1–43 **A.** A manual force (HLf) is applied at 90° to the leg-foot segment but at a point relatively close to the knee joint axis. **B.** A manual resistance of the same magnitude produces substantially greater torque when the point of application of HLf is farther from the knee joint axis because the moment arm (MA) is substantially larger. **C.** When the manual resistance of the same magnitude is applied at an angle to the segment, then all of the applied force does not go toward producing joint torque.

Translatory Effects of Force Components

Let us return once again to John and the ankle weight exercise. The goal is to have the segment in translatory equilibrium ($\Sigma Fx = 0$ and $\Sigma Fy = 0$) while having the quadriceps muscle produce a net extension torque to extend the knee. To understand the complex interaction of forces, we must identify the translatory effects of the forces already applied to the leg-foot segment, as well as determine what additional forces, if any, are necessary to create translatory equilibrium.

In **Figure 1–44**, the forces of gravity and the ankle weight on the leg-foot segment (GAwLf) and the Fx component of the quadriceps (Fx_{QLf}) are both parallel to the leg-foot segment, in opposite directions and sufficiently coplanar and collinear to be considered as part of a linear force system. GAwLf is a joint distraction force because it is away from the knee joint, whereas vector Fx_{QLf} is a joint compression force because it is applied toward the knee joint. Given the magnitude of GAwLf (–88 N) and that of Fx_{QLf} (determined by our earlier trigonometric calculation to be 910 N for this angle of application of the quadriceps force), there is an apparent net unbalanced parallel force of 822 N (upward). Given this upward pull of the quadriceps, the leg-foot will translate upward until it contacts the adjacent

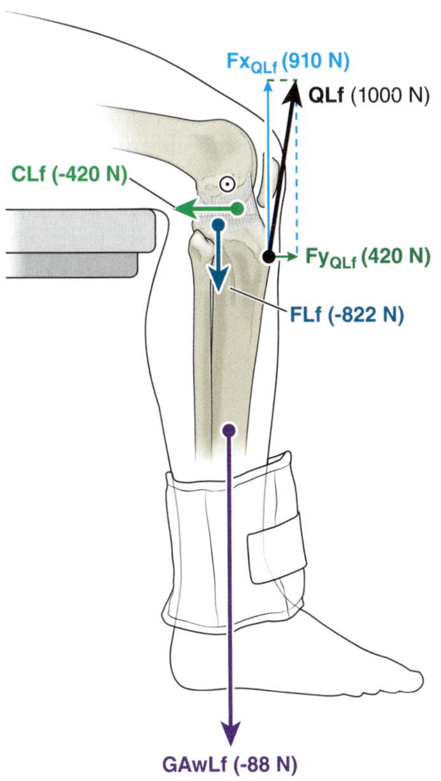

Figure 1–44 The forces of GAwLf and Fx_{QLf} (–88 N and 910 N, respectively) are both applied parallel to the leg-foot segment with a net upward force of 822 N. *The leg-foot segment will translate upwardly* until it hits the femur, at which point the femur-on-leg/foot (FLf) will push down with a force of –822 N. The perpendicular force of Fy_{QLf} (420 N) will translate the leg-foot segment to the right (anteriorly) until tension in the capsuloligamentous tissues (CLf) checks further translation. When CLf reaches 420 N of force, CLf and Fy_{QLf} will constitute a force couple and the leg-foot segment will pivot (rotate) around the point of constraint of the capsuloligamentous structures.

femur (joint reaction force), resulting in a femur-on-leg/foot (FLf) force that is in a similar line and should be able to offset the net upward pull of the quadriceps, thus FLf = –822 N.

Fy_{QLf} was calculated trigonometrically to be 420 N to the right. In **Figure 1–44**, there must be another force (or forces) of 420 N to the left before Fy_{QLf} can produce rotation rather than translation. The most obvious source of that force is the pull of capsuloligamentous structures on the leg-foot segment (CLf) that are positioned to check translation of the tibia out from under the femoral condyles. *[Note: There are other possible forces that might be the source of the missing Fy component(s), but the key here is to recognize that additional forces are needed for translatory equilibrium rather than to identify the source(s).]*

Rotary Effects of Force Components

In **Figure 1–44**, CLf and Fy_{QLf} are perpendicular to the leg-foot segment. As is true for any forces perpendicular to a segment, these forces will contribute to rotation of the segment if translation is prevented. These two forces qualify as a force couple because they are applied to the same segment in opposite directions, have equal magnitudes (albeit not drawn proportionally), and produce rotation of the leg-foot segment in the same direction (extension). Once the tension in the capsule reaches 420 N (after a small movement of the tibial plateau to the right, that is, anteriorly), rotation of the leg-foot segment will be initiated around the pivot point of the capsular attachment.

Thus far in this chapter, torque has been computed as F × MA (or F_{TOT} × MA). When a force is *not* applied at 90° to the segment (as is true for the quadriceps force in Fig. 1–44), the torque can equivalently be computed as Fy × MA, although the moment arm (MA) for the Fy component is not the same as the moment arm for F_{TOT} (other than when Fy = F_{TOT}). In Figure 1–44, it can be appreciated that the shortest distance between QLf (F_{TOT}) and the knee joint axis is different than the shortest distance between Fy_{QLf} and the joint axis. Regardless of whether the torque of a force is computed using F_{TOT} × MA or using Fy × MA, the product (magnitude) of torque will be the same. If the moment arm of Fy_{QLf} is 0.06 m, Fy_{QLf} would generate a torque of 25.2 N·m (420 N × 0.06 m).

$$(F_{TOT} \times MA_{FTOT}) = (Fy \times MA_{Fy})$$

Expanded Concepts 1–9
Rotation Produced by Parallel (Fx) Force Components

Typically, only forces (or force components) that are perpendicular to a bony segment produce torques on that segment. However, *any force* (including an Fx component) with an action line that lies at some distance from a joint axis will produce rotation around that axis (including Fx_{QLf} in Fig. 1–44). Because the contribution of an Fx component to torque (as opposed to its contribution to translation) for any given force is generally small (or smaller than that of Fy), estimating torque based on Fy alone is generally considered to be a reasonable (albeit conservative) estimate of torque produced by the total force.

Foundational Concepts 1–19
Force Components and Joint Motion

- Segmental rotation around a joint axis in a human requires that $\Sigma Fx = 0$. If $\Sigma Fx \neq 0$, there will be an initial translatory motion of the segment (alone or in combination with rotation) in the direction of the Fx resultant until the translation is checked either by a capsuloligamentous force or by a joint reaction force.
- Rotation around a joint axis requires that the *translation* produced by an Fy component be checked ($\Sigma Fy = 0$). If $\Sigma Fy \neq 0$, there will be an initial translatory motion of the segment (alone or in combination with rotation) in the direction of the net Fy resultant until the translation is checked either by a capsuloligamentous force or by a joint reaction force. Once translation is checked, rotation produced by Fy will take place (there is now a force couple).
- The majority of torques on a segment will be produced by forces or force components that are applied at 90° to the segment (Fy) and at some distance from the joint axis.
- Whenever the goal is the rotation of a joint, a net unbalanced torque in the direction of desired movement ($\Sigma_\tau \neq 0$) is necessary.
- The greater the net unbalanced torque on a segment, the greater the angular acceleration of the segment.

Multisegment (Closed-Chain) Force Analysis

The primary difference between John Alexander's ankle weight and leg-press exercises is that the leg-foot segment is "fixed," or weight-bearing at both ends when using the leg press. The distal end of the leg-foot segment is constrained by its contact with the footplate and is not free to move in space; the proximal end is connected to the femur and also is not free to move in space. Whenever one end of a segment or set of segments is free to move in space, this is referred to as an **open chain.** When *both* ends of a segment or set of segments are constrained in some way (and not free to move in space), this is referred to as a **closed chain.**

Expanded Concepts 1–10

Open and Closed Chains

The adjectives "kinetic" or "kinematic" are often used to modify the terms *open chain* and *closed chain.* Although either might be justified, there is no consensus about which is preferred. At this juncture, the terms "open chain" and "closed chain" are now in such common use that modifiers no longer seem necessary. What is necessary, however, is to avoid *misuse* of the term "closed chain" as equivalent to "weight-bearing" (unfortunately, a commonly used but inappropriate synonym). A segment *may* be fixed at both ends by proximal joint attachments and distal weight-bearing. However, a segment or set of segments can be weight-bearing *without* being fixed at both ends (and without being subjected to the constraints of a closed chain). The effects of open and closed chains on two or more segments will be encountered in subsequent chapters because there are substantial implications for understanding forces that create or limit human movement.

When the leg-foot segment is in a closed chain leg-press exercise, the analysis of forces becomes substantially more complex. In a closed chain, motion of one segment in the chain can be produced by forces applied elsewhere in the chain. **Figure 1–45** is an oversimplified representation of the leg-press exercise, showing *only* the force of the gluteus maximus muscle acting on the femur. The femur is in a closed chain *with* the leg-foot segment because the femur is attached proximally to the pelvis and the leg-foot segment is attached distally to the footplate, with the hip and knee joints in between. In this example, we shift the segment of interest from the leg-foot segment to the femur.

In **Figure 1–45**, the perpendicular component of the gluteus maximus (Fy_{Gm}) will tend to create clockwise rotation of the femur. The gluteus maximus is a large muscle that can apply a force of considerable magnitude to the femur, with an Fy component that lies at a considerable distance from the knee joint axis (has a large moment arm). That is, Fy_{Gm}—although not crossing the knee joint—will create a substantial clockwise rotation (torque) of the femur around the knee joint axis (knee extension); this occurs in a closed chain because clockwise rotation of the femur will cause the femur to contact the leg-foot segment and push the leg-foot segment to the right (the goal of the leg-press exercise). In the leg-press exercise, both the quadriceps force on the leg-foot and the gluteus maximum force on the femur will create simultaneous knee extension torques. *[Note: Given the limitations on the figure proportions in Figure 1–45, the magnitude of the gluteus maximus vector and its components are substantially underestimated by the length of the vectors in the figure. Furthermore, the actual point of application of the gluteus maximus on the femur is more proximal (further to the left) than is shown because the correct point of application is beyond the limits of the figure. Consequently, the effect of* Fy_{Gm} *on the femur and knee joint is markedly underestimated in the figure.]*

Because the leg-press exercise involves forces on the femur as well as on the leg-foot segment, a complete analysis would involve (at a minimum) identification of the sources, magnitudes, and effects of all forces (and their components) on both the leg-foot *and* femur segments—a task beyond the scope or intent of this chapter. However, the complexity of the closed chain leg-press exercise means that John Alexander will be using his gluteus maximus as well as his quadriceps, although the target is the quadriceps. It is nearly impossible for John to isolate the exercise to the quadriceps muscle alone. This is an important concept in designing exercises to strengthen a muscle or muscle group. Although weight-bearing exercises may appear more "functional" (more closely approximating activities of daily living), the combinations of forces that may be used to perform such exercises are large in number and not always predictable (or controllable). That is, the person may avoid the use of a weak or injured muscle (or muscles) simply by shifting the load to another muscle or muscle group.

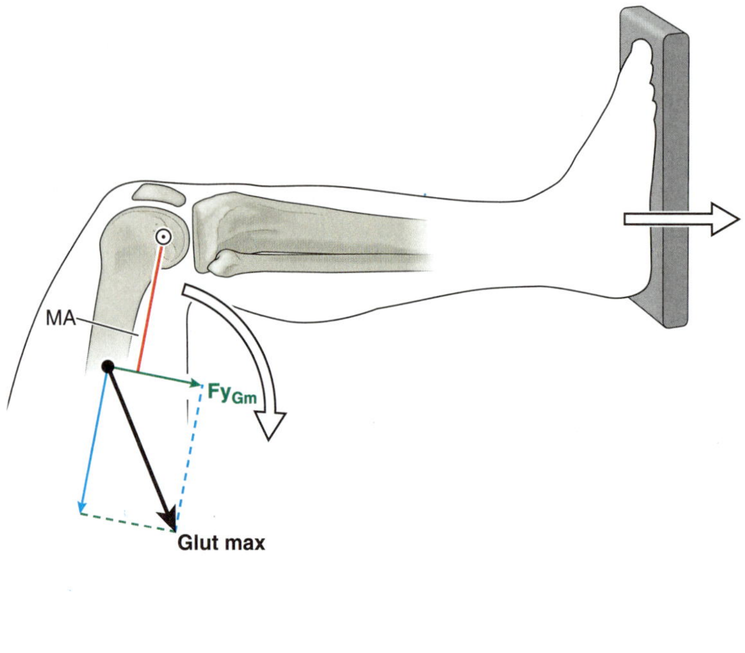

Figure 1–45 The force of the gluteus maximus muscle (Glut max) is applied to the femur in a closed chain. The resulting extension of the hip from component Fy_{Gm} will push the leg-foot segment to the right against the footplate and create an extension torque at the knee joint.

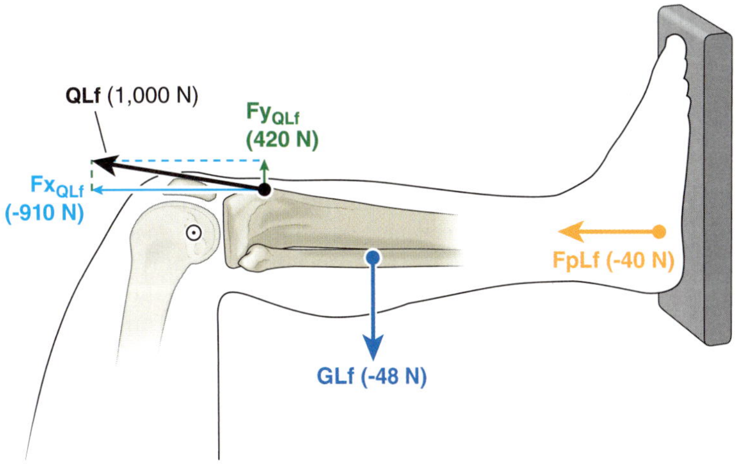

Figure 1–46 The forces of quadriceps muscle (QLf) and its components, gravity (GLf), and the footplate (FpLf) on the leg-foot segment are shown for the leg-press exercise at 90° of knee flexion. Although a friction force might exist between the foot and the footplate (opposing the net upward shear), its magnitude would be minimal and is, therefore, omitted from the figure.

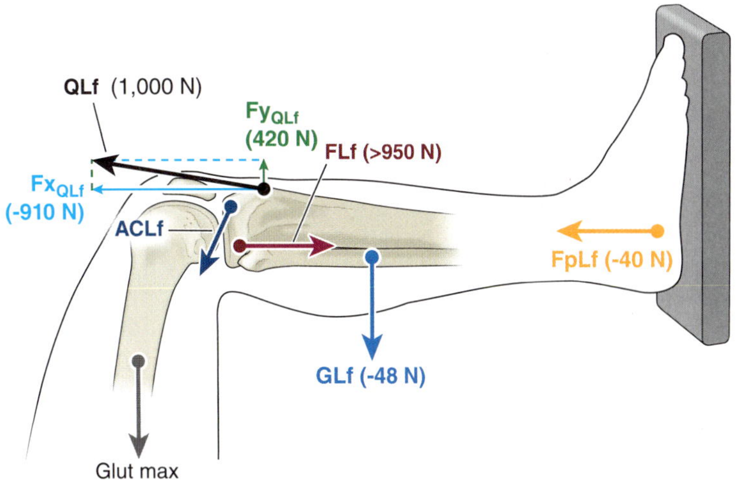

Figure 1–47 The contact of the femur with the leg-foot segment (FLf) and its components have been added to the force analysis, along with the force of the anterior cruciate ligament and the joint capsule on the leg-foot segment (ACLf). The force of the gluteus maximus (Glut max) on the femur is shaded and remains only as a reminder of one of the potential sources of FLf.

The larger moment arm and force-generating capability of the gluteus maximus as compared with the quadriceps would make it likely that the gluteus maximus will contribute more knee extension torque in the leg-press exercise than will the quadriceps. However, we will proceed with an analysis of the leg-press exercise as if the quadriceps were the prime mover because this assumption simplifies the presentation while quite adequately conveying the important principles.

Figure 1–46 shows the leg-foot segment in the leg-press exercise once again. Gravity (GLf) is acting on the leg-foot segment with a magnitude of 48 N. The quadriceps muscle (QLf) is shown generating the same 1,000 N contraction with the same Fx_{QLf} and Fy_{QLf} components shown for the ankle weight exercise (see Fig. 1–44) because the angle of application of the quadriceps remains the same as long as the knee joint is at 90°. The footplate is contacting and creating a force on the leg-foot segment (footplate-on-leg/foot, or FpLf). Let us assume that there is a 40 N weight on the leg-press machine (the same weight that was used in the ankle weight exercise). The push of the footplate on the leg-foot segment (FpLf) cannot be greater than the amount of weight on the machine, so FpLf is assigned a magnitude of 40 N. Although a friction force might exist between the foot and the footplate (opposing the net upward shear), its magnitude would be minimal and is, therefore, not included. We will identify any additional forces acting on the leg-foot segment by balancing the forces already in place.

Figure 1–46 indicates a net compressive force of −950 N (ΣFx), given the magnitudes of Fx_{QLf} and FpLf as −910 N and −40 N (to the left), respectively. There is a net upward force of 372 N (ΣFy), given the magnitudes of Fy_{QLf} and GLf, which are 420 N and −48 N, respectively. These net Fx and Fy forces would result in the leg-foot segment moving to the left and upward. The goal, however, is to move the leg-foot segment to the right against the resistance of the footplate without any upward sliding (shear) between the tibial plateau and femoral condyles. Therefore, some additional forces must be applied to the leg-foot segment for John Alexander to get the job done.

Given the net Fx component of −950 N, the leg-foot will translate to the left until it hits the femur, at which point there will be a femur-on-leg/foot (FLf) force **(Fig. 1–47)**. Although an FLf force of 950 N will be sufficient to prevent the footplate from pushing the leg-foot to the left, the magnitude of FLf must *exceed* 950 N to actually translate (push) the footplate to the right as is appropriate for this exercise. *[Note: The force of* *the gluteus is shown in Figure 1–47 as a shaded vector to remind the reader that the analysis is more complicated than we are showing.]*

There is a net upward (Fy) force of 372 N in Figure 1–47. Assuming again that friction between the foot and footplate is of insufficient magnitude to help, we must now identify a structure that will prevent this anterior slide (upward shear) of the tibial plateau on the femoral condyles. The possible source is a capsuloligamentous force—more specifically, tension in the anterior capsule and in the anterior cruciate ligament (ACL). Consequently, a composite capsuloligamentous force of anterior cruciate/capsule-on-leg/foot (ACLf) has been added to the figure. Although no attempt has been made to resolve ACLf into its components, its Fy component (posterior displacement) should be approximately 588 N. There will also be an Fx component of ACLf, with a magnitude that will depend on the angle of pull but will contribute further to the 950 N joint compression force already created by Fx_{QLf} and FpLf. The joint compression in the leg-press exercise, therefore, will substantially exceed the 822 N compression estimated for the ankle weight exercise at the same knee joint position and with the same magnitude of quadriceps muscle contraction.

Although we did not estimate the net torques that would result from all the forces on the leg-foot segment (to confirm that there is a net knee extension torque), the example was sufficient for demonstrating the complexity of force analyses even in very oversimplified situations. It also demonstrates that applying the principles of Newton's laws is fairly straightforward if approached very methodically.

In spite of very rough estimates of angles of application of forces (and concomitant Fy components and moment arms), our findings with regard to net effects for both the ankle weight and leg press are reasonably in line with findings from at least one group of researchers (although we used a minimum resistance in both the weight boot and leg-press exercises, in comparison with their substantially heavier loads).[7,8] This group of researchers also demonstrated the imprecise nature of biomechanical analyses (even using sophisticated instrumentation) because they found differing results (e.g., magnitudes of joint compression and joint shear forces) using the same data from the same subjects on the basis of different mathematical modeling variables. Their results also contradicted some of the findings in at least one previous study.[9]

SUMMARY

- The goal of this chapter was to use the John Alexander example to introduce key biomechanical principles that form a conceptual framework for analyzing the forces acting on segments and joints—and the effects of those forces—at various points in a joint's range of motion. This approach relied primarily on a simplified two-dimensional approach and utilized static rather than dynamic analyses to explore these principles.
- We identified many, but not all, of the limitations in this conceptual framework when applied to the complex phenomena of human function, while laying the foundation for understanding dysfunction. Particular attention was given to the interdependence of muscular forces, gravitational forces or other external forces, and articular constraints, highlighting how these components influence segment or joint behavior and movement.
- The need for articular constraints (joint reaction forces or capsuloligamentous forces) to accomplish joint rotation is too often underappreciated. At best, these constraints are assessed only when there are problems with joint stability and ignored when they are effective in their function. To avoid this omission, we will next explore the structural composition and properties of the articular constraints (bone, cartilage, capsule/ligament/fascia), as well as those of the muscles and their tendons (Chapters 2 and 3, respectively).
- The composition and mechanical behavior of various tissues are essential to understanding the stresses (force per unit area) that these tissues impose on surrounding structures or must respond to during movement.
- With chapter concepts in hand, the reader should understand the basis of both normal and abnormal function at each of the presented joint complexes.

STUDY QUESTIONS

1. Name three types of motion and provide examples of each.
2. In what plane and around what axis does rotation of the head occur?
3. Is naming the plane of motion considered part of kinetics or part of kinematics? Why?
4. How does a center of rotation (or instantaneous center of rotation) differ from a fixed axis? How does the distinction apply to motion of human joints?
5. What is the definition of a force, what are the units of measure for force, and what are the sources of forces applied to a segment?
6. What are the characteristics that are common to all force vectors? What characteristics are common to all gravitational vectors?
7. What generalizations can be made about the line of gravity (gravity vector) of all stable objects?
8. What happens to the center of mass and line of gravity of a rigid object when the object is moved around in space?
9. What happens to the center of mass and line of gravity of the body when the body segments are rearranged? What happens to the body's center of mass if the right upper extremity is amputated? Provide a simple drawing to support your answer.
10. A student is carrying all of their books for the fall semester courses in their right arm. What does the additional weight do to the center of mass? To the line of gravity? How will the body most likely respond to this change?
11. Give the name, point of application, magnitude, and direction of the contact force applied to a man weighing 90 kg as he lies on a bed.
12. Are the two forces of an action-reaction pair (reaction forces) part of the same linear force system? Defend your answer.
13. What conditions must exist for friction on an object to have magnitude? What are the conditions under which the magnitude of the force of friction is always greatest?
14. How does a contact force, shear force, and friction force differ?
15. A man who weighs 90 kg (882 N, or ~198 lb) is lying on a bed in cervical traction with a weight of 5 kg (49 N, or ~12 lb), suspended from a horizontal rope. Assuming that

the entire body is a single unsegmented object and that the body is in equilibrium, identify all the forces acting on the body (assuming that μ_S for skin on bed is 0.25).

16. A man who weighs 90 kg (882 N, or ~198 lb) is lying on a bed. A nurse standing at the foot of his bed has grasped his ankles and is pulling him down toward the foot of the bed. Treating the man as a single unsegmented object, determine the minimum force that the nurse must apply to the man to *initiate* the movement (assuming that μ_S for skin on bed is 0.25).
17. Assuming now that the leg-foot segment of the man in Question 16 is joined to the rest of his unsegmented body by capsuloligamentous structures at his knee, what must be the magnitude of tension in the knee joint capsuloligamentous structures just as the man begins to be pulled toward the foot of the bed by the nurse? What are the names of the forces causing tension in the capsuloligamentous structures? What are the names of the forces causing distraction of the knee joint segments?
18. How do you graphically determine the net (resultant) effect of two forces applied to the same segment that intersect at an angle to each other? What is this process called?
19. What are the *minimum* requirements to produce rotation of a segment? What are the terms used to refer to the magnitude of rotation?
20. Define *moment arm*. How does moment arm affect the ability of a force to rotate a segment?
21. If two forces exist on a body segment on the same side of the joint axis but in opposite directions, how does one determine which is the effort force and which is the resistance force?
22. How do anatomic pulleys affect the magnitude and direction of a muscle force (Fms)?
23. Muscle "strength" and muscle "power" are often used interchangeably. What is the difference between these two terms?
24. What factors can cause the net torque on a segment to change?
25. What kind of contraction is a muscle performing when that muscle is the effort force on a rotating segment? What kind of contraction is a muscle performing when it is the resistance force on a rotating segment?
26. What are the benefits of a mechanical advantage greater than one? Do muscles most often work on levers with or without mechanical advantage? What challenges does this present to muscle function?
27. Using the values below, identify the class of the lever, its mechanical advantage, what kind of contraction the muscle is performing, and the point of application of the resultant force of gravity-on-forearm and ball-on-forearm (the hand will be considered part of the forearm). Here Fms = muscle force, MA = moment arm, G = gravity-on-forearm, and B = ball-on-forearm (assume that all forces are applied perpendicular to the forearm lever):

    Fms = 500 N (counterclockwise), MA = 2 cm

    G = 32 N (clockwise), MA = 18 cm

    B = 20 N (clockwise), MA = 28 cm

28. Describe how the perpendicular component of a force and the moment arm of that force are related. When is the moment arm of any force applied to a segment potentially greatest?
29. Describe how you would position the leg-foot segment in space so that gravity exerts the least torque on the leg-foot segment. How would you position the leg-foot segment so that gravity exerts the greatest torque?
30. A muscle (Fms) is rotating a segment around a joint against the resistance of gravity (G). Identify at least one force other than Fms and G that *must* be applied to the segment for rotation of the segment to occur.
31. If not all of a muscle's force is contributing to rotation, what happens to the "wasted" force?
32. What effects at a joint may a perpendicular force have on a segment other than rotation?
33. When a force is applied at 135° to a segment, what proportion of the force will rotate the segment? What proportion of the force will translate the segment, and will the direction of that force be compressive or distractive?
34. The quadriceps muscle is acting on the free leg-foot segment with a force of 500 N at an angle of 45° (unrealistic, but simplified). Identify the forces (not the magnitudes or locations) that would be required for the leg-foot segment to successfully extend at the knee joint.

REFERENCES

1. LeVeau B: Williams and Lissner's Biomechanics of Human Motion (ed 3). Philadelphia, PA, WB Saunders, 1992
2. Brinckmann PF, Frobin W, Leivseth G: Musculoskeletal Biomechanics. New York, NY, Thieme, 2002
3. Hall S: Basic Biomechanics (ed 3). Boston, MA, WCB/McGraw-Hill, 1999
4. Panjabi MW, White A: Biomechanics of the Musculoskeletal System. Philadelphia, PA, Churchill-Livingstone, 2001
5. Hamilton DM, Haennel RG: Validity and reliability of the 6-minute walk test in a cardiac rehabilitation population. J Cardiopulm Rehabil 20:156-64, 2000
6. Cromer A: Physics for the Life Science (ed 2). New York, NY, McGraw-Hill, 1994
7. Escamilla RF, Fleisig GS, Zheng N, et al: Biomechanics of the knee during closed kinetic chain and open kinetic chain exercises. Med Sci Sports Exerc 30:556-69, 1998
8. Zheng N, Fleisig GS, Escamilla RF, et al: An analytical model of the knee for estimation of internal forces during exercise. J Biomech 31:963-7, 1998
9. Lutz GE, Palmitier RA, An KN, et al: Comparison of tibiofemoral joint forces during open-kinetic-chain and closed-kinetic-chain exercises. J Bone Joint Surg Am 75:732-9, 1993

CHAPTER 2

Complexity of Human Joint Design

William R. Thompson, PT, DPT, PhD, FASBMR

CHAPTER OUTLINE

INTRODUCTION 46
Form Follows Function 46
THE COMPLEXITY OF HUMAN JOINT DESIGN 48
Joint Classification 48
Fibrous Joints 48
Cartilaginous Joints 49
Synovial Joints 49
Joint Motion 54
Osteokinematics 54
Arthrokinematics 54
Range of Motion 57
Kinematic Chains 57
MATERIALS FOUND IN HUMAN JOINTS 59
Composition of Connective Tissue 59
Cells 59
Extracellular Matrix (ECM) 59
Specific Connective Tissue Composition 61
Ligaments 61
Tendons 62
Cartilage 63
Bone 65
BEHAVIORAL PROPERTIES OF CONNECTIVE TISSUE 66
Structural and Material Properties 67
Load, Force, and Elongation 67
Stress and Strain 68
Viscoelasticity 70
Time-Dependent and Rate-Dependent Properties 70
Creep 70
Stress-Relaxation 70
Strain-Rate Sensitivity 70
Properties of Specific Tissues 72
Bone 72
Tendons 72
Ligaments 73
Cartilage 73
GENERAL CHANGES WITH DISEASE, INJURY, IMMOBILIZATION, EXERCISE, AND OVERUSE 73
Disease 74
Injury 74
Immobilization (Stress Deprivation) 74
Effects on Ligament and Tendon 74
Effects on Articular Surfaces and Bone 75
Exercise 76
Bone Response to Exercise 76
Cartilage Response to Exercise 77
Tendon Response to Exercise 77
Ligament Response to Exercise 77
Overuse 77
SUMMARY 78
STUDY QUESTIONS 79
REFERENCES 79

Introduction

Form Follows Function

The joints of the human body, like those used in the construction of buildings, furniture, and machines, connect different segments together and often allow movement between those segments. The design of the joint reflects similar demands. The dictum *form follows function*, coined by the American architect Louis Sullivan and promoted by the Bauhaus school of design of post–World War I Germany,[1] suggests that the appearance (form) of an object or building is governed by its function. Although a wooden stool and a chair with a padded seat, arms, and back are both used for sitting, the differences in form hint at the intended functions, respectively, of short-term versus longer-term support. The function of a stepstool is to support weight, so the elements are joined to serve stability and can be made of a sturdy material such as hardwood. However, if the step ladder needs to be portable and collapsible while still stable when opened, the design and material composition will become much more complex. An aluminum step ladder is lighter than wood and has a metal strut with a locking device as well as hinges at the intersection of the two sides of the ladder **(Fig. 2–1)**. The ladder can be folded when the brace is unlocked; when the brace is locked **(Fig. 2-1A)**, the ladder is still stable. If the ladder is opened but the brace is not locked **(Fig. 2-1B)**, stability is compromised by excessive mobility. Human joints that must meet both stability and mobility demands are more complex than joints that favor stability alone. The more complex the demands on and design of a human joint, the more stresses the joint must withstand and the more at risk the joint is for failure.

Form includes an object's structure as well as its composition, and a change in either structure or materials (or both) can influence function. The prosthetic foot shown in **Figure 2–2** reflects the relationship between physical form (structure and composition) and function. The design of the curved foot allows the structure to bend as body weight is applied, whereas the heel extension provides stable support. The bending of the foot can both absorb shock and provide an elastic recoil that contributes to the subsequent propulsion. Alterations in the material from a typical carbon fiber composite affect the amount of elastic recoil. A person with a lower extremity amputation can order limbs made of different materials, depending on their functional demands. Springier materials that are harder to stretch and have more recoil are used for activities with large loads and high speeds (e.g., running, jumping), whereas materials with less elastic recoil are used for walking. A track athlete with lower extremity amputations can use feet that are less stable (no heel extension) but have greater recoil for increased mobility (speed) **(Fig. 2–3)**.[2]

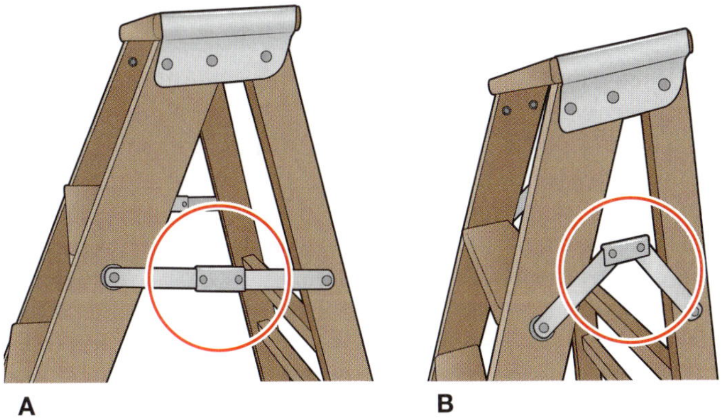

Figure 2–1 Folding stepladder joint. **A.** The sides of the step ladder are prevented from moving when the brace is engaged, providing necessary stability **B.** The sides of the step ladder are free to move (mobile) when the brace is unlocked, resulting in a less stable ladder.

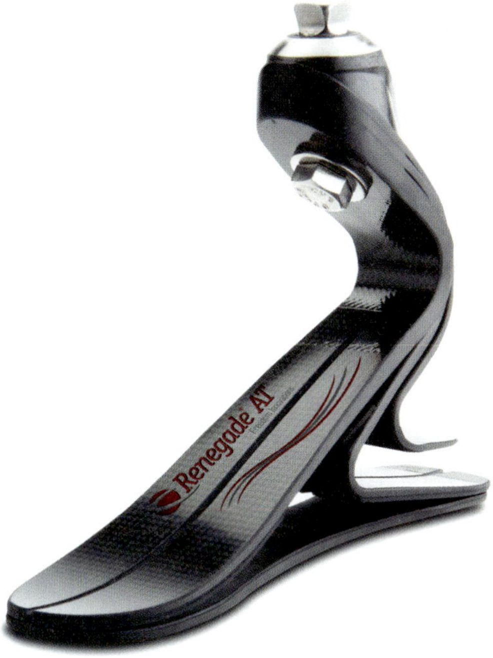

Figure 2–2 The design of this prosthetic foot facilitates gait through its design and composition. The curved blade bends during loading and then assists with propulsion as the blade recoils. The heel piece increases stability. *Photo courtesy of Freedom Innovations.*

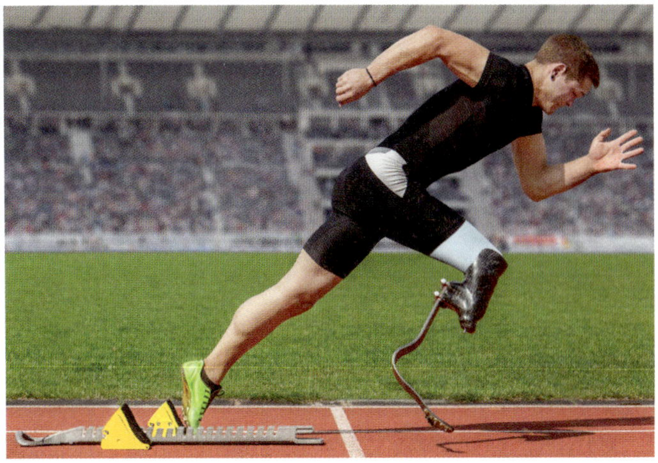

Figure 2–3 The form of a prosthetic foot changes when the goal is to maximize mobility (speed), even at the expense of stability. With running blades, the heel can be eliminated and the elastic recoil of the foot is increased for stronger propulsion. *(filrom/iStock/Thinkstock)*

Human structural forms are relatively static. When a stepladder is collapsed, the shapes of all the component parts remain unchanged. Structure, function, and form in humans are dynamic and interactive. Cellular composition and the structure of a tissue will affect the form that a tissue will take which, in turn, is affected by the type and amount of stresses applied to a tissue. Stresses are determined by the functional demands placed on a tissue. As function is altered, the stresses on the tissue will change and may signal cells and extracellular elements to alter composition and shape and, therefore, the form that the tissue takes **(Fig. 2–4)**.

Changes in the material properties of tissues and shapes of human joints occur as we develop and can result from demands imposed during typical and atypical movement. This relationship is illustrated in the case of developmental hip dysplasia. The structural elements of the hip joint develop before birth. The mature shape of the head of the femur and the acetabulum is determined by the functional interaction between these two structures over time. Decreased contact between the acetabulum and femoral head during fetal development may lead to a shallow acetabulum or less spherical femoral head (alteration in form), as well as to deficiencies in the acetabular cartilage (alteration in composition)[3,4] **(Fig. 2–5)**. Changing the stresses across the hip joint in the infant by creating a deeper acetabulum or repositioning the femoral head in the acetabulum (e.g., through surgical intervention) generally will lead to adaptive changes in the femoroacetabular joint structure and composition;[5] the changes will lead to improvements in both the mobility and stability of the hip joint. Julius Wolff described the adaptation of bone to changes in stresses in the late 1800s (now known as *Wolff's law*).[6] However, the interaction between form and function is not unique to bone but is common to all living tissues.

All the elements of human joints—including bones, cartilage, ligaments, muscles, and tendons—adapt their appearance and composition in response to functional demands. These demands can change with immobilization, inactivity, or training. Knowing the functional demands and the tissues' responses to those demands, therapists can modify the functional demands

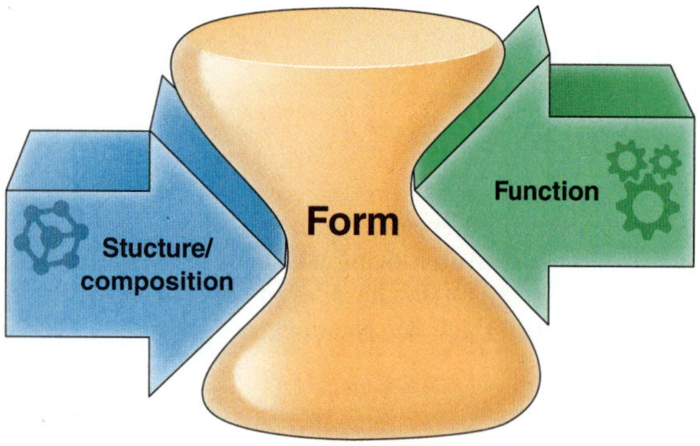

Figure 2–4 The form of human tissues is determined both by the overall composition and structure of the connective tissues and by functional use. The size of the tissue and its composition will determine the types of loads the tissue can bear. However, tissues may adapt to altered functional demands in response to shifting stresses that lead to cellular and extracellular events affecting the form of the tissue.

(stresses) on joint structures during rehabilitation to optimize targeted tissue structure and function.

Foundational Concepts 2–1
Interaction of Joint Function, Structure/Composition, and Form

- The form that a joint takes is dependent upon the function the joint is serving as well as its structure (design) and composition (materials).
- Most human joints serve a dual purpose of stability and mobility, although one purpose may predominate.
- As demands for both mobility and stability increase, the design and composition of the joint become more complex.
- The elements of structure/composition, function, and form in human tissues and joints are dynamic and interactive; changes in one element can affect one or more of the other elements.

The Complexity of Human Joint Design

An appreciation of the complexities of human joint design may be gained by considering the nature of the bony components and the functions that the joints must serve. The human skeleton has about 200 bones that are connected by joints. Bones vary in size from the pea-sized distal phalanx of the little toe to the long femur of the thigh. The shape of the bones varies from round to flat, and the contours of the ends of the bones vary from convex to concave. It is a considerable engineering problem to design joints that are capable of working together to provide both mobility and stability for the total structure.

Joint designs in the human body vary from simple to complex. Simple human joints usually have stability as a primary function; more complex joints usually have mobility as a primary function without sacrificing stability—a combination know as *dynamic stability*. Stability joints may be contoured either to fit snuggly into each other or to lie flat against each other with relatively little motion between. As joints require increasing amounts of mobility without fully sacrificing stability, additional structural elements such as joint capsules, ligaments, and accessory joint structures help make the compromise between mobility and stability demands. Classifications of human joints are named based on the structure of the joint or amount of movement. Structurally, joints can be classified as **fibrous, cartilaginous,** or **synovial,** with each referring to the connective tissue that binds the bony elements together or the presence or absence of a synovial joint cavity. The joint categories of **synarthrosis, amphiarthrosis,** and **diarthrosis** refer to the degree of movement afforded by a joint. Synarthrosis joints are those that have little or no movement, amphiarthrosis joints allow minimal to moderate movement, and diarthrosis joints are freely moveable joints. The two different classification schemes actually have considerable overlap because joints with little movement (synarthroses) typically are united by fibrous tissue, those with moderate movement are typically united directly by **hyaline (articular) cartilage** or **fibrocartilage,** and those with a lot of movement (diarthrodial) are united by a synovial joint structure. Consequently, we will identify joint classifications using the simpler structural nomenclature where both structure and function (movement) for each classification are described.

Joint Classification

Examples of fibrous, cartilaginous and synovial joints are illustrated in **Figure 2–6**.

Fibrous Joints

The bony components of a fibrous joint are joined together by fibrous interosseous connective tissue that directly unites one bone to another. This creates a solid connective tissue-bone interface that allows for little or no movement, thus classifying them functionally as synarthroses. Three different types of fibrous joints are found in the human body: sutures (e.g., between the frontal and parietal bones of the skull), gomphoses (e.g., between each tooth and the mandible), and syndesmoses (e.g., between the distal tibia and fibula) (see Fig. 2–6).

A suture joint is one in which two bony components are united by a collagenous sutural ligament or membrane. The ends of the bony components are shaped so that the edges interlock or overlap one another. This type of joint is found exclusively in the skull early in life and allows a small amount of movement between the bones of the skull. Fusion of the two opposing bones in suture joints occurs later in life and leads to the formation of a bony union.

A gomphosis joint is one in which the surfaces of bony components join each other like a peg in a hole and are connected by fibrous connective tissue. The only gomphosis joint that exists in the human body is the joint between a tooth and either the mandible or maxilla.

A syndesmosis joint is a type of fibrous joint in which two bony components are joined directly by an interosseous ligament, a fibrous cord, or an aponeurotic membrane. These joints usually allow a small amount of motion and can be seen between the shafts of the radius and ulna and the shafts of the tibia and fibula.

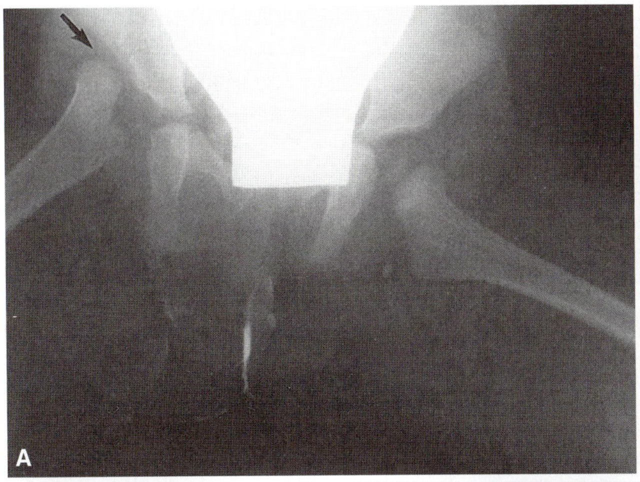

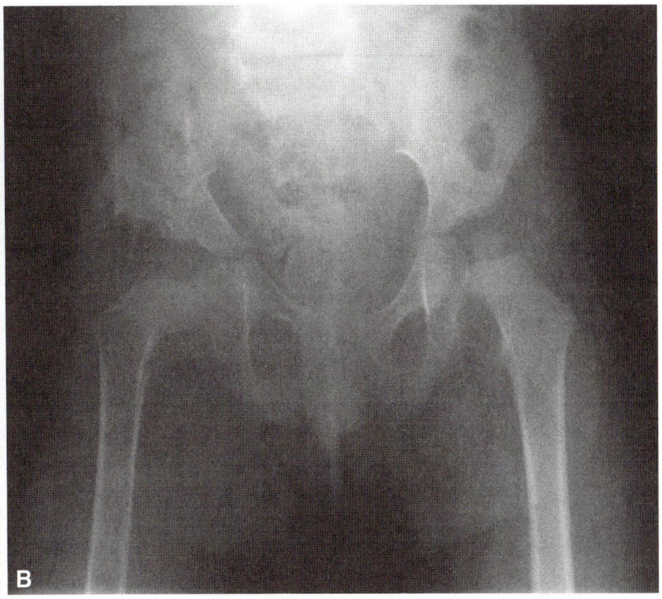

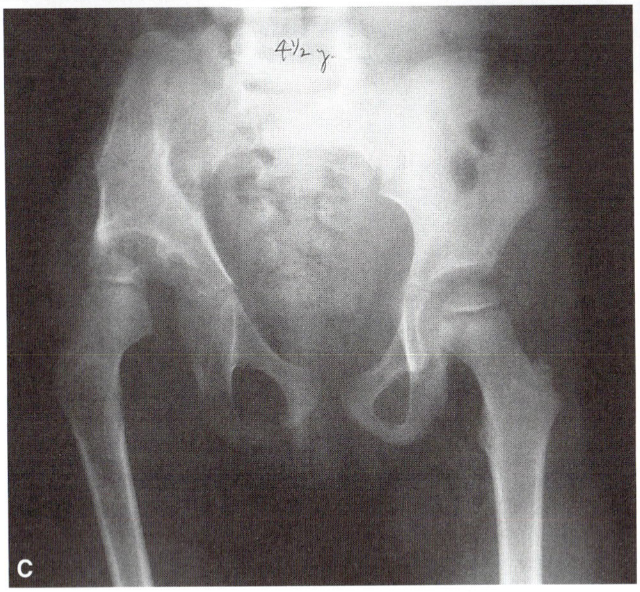

Figure 2–5 Developmental dysplasia of the hip in a toddler. **A.** Arrow points to the congenital deformity of the right hip joint seen preoperatively in this 16-month-old boy. For comparison, note the configuration of the child's normal left hip joint in the same film (much of the femoral head and acetabulum are cartilage, so they are transparent on radiograph). **B.** A film 6 months after surgical creation of an acetabular fossa (posterior iliac osteotomy) shows improved location of the femoral head relative to the new acetabulum. **C.** At 4½ years old, the femoral head is sufficiently seated in the now rounded acetabulum to support all ambulatory activities.

Cartilaginous Joints

The materials connecting the bony components in cartilaginous joints are fibrocartilage or hyaline cartilage. These materials directly unite one bony surface to another, creating a bone-cartilage-bone interface that allows for some movement between the bones. The two types of cartilaginous joints are symphyses and synchondroses (see Fig. 2–6).

In symphysis joints, the two bony components are covered with a thin lamina of hyaline cartilage and directly joined by fibrocartilage in the form of discs or pads. Examples of symphysis joints include the intervertebral joints between the bodies of the vertebrae, the joint between the manubrium and the body of the sternum, and the symphysis pubis in the pelvis.

A synchondrosis joint is one in which hyaline cartilage connects two bony components. An example would be the articulation of the first seven ribs with the sternum. Synchondroses also refer to the hyaline cartilage bond between two ossifying centers of bone in a developing skeleton. In **Figure 2–5C**, the cartilaginous ossification centers appear as spaces between the femoral head and femoral neck. Epiphyseal growth plates near the ends of long bones as well as in the pelvis are also synchondrosis unions. Epiphyseal synchondroses permit bone growth while also providing stability and allowing a very small amount of mobility. When bone growth is complete, these joints ossify and convert to bony unions.

Foundational Concepts 2–2
Fibrous and Cartilaginous Joints

- Fibrous joints include sutures, gomphoses, and syndesmoses.
- The two types of cartilaginous joints are symphyses and synchondroses.
- Bones directly connected by fibrous or cartilaginous connective tissue afford less movement and greater stability than do synovial joints, with cartilaginous joints typically being somewhat more moveable than fibrous joints.

Synovial Joints

The joint construction in synovial joints differs from that found in fibrous and cartilaginous joints. In synovial joints, the ends of the bony components are free to move in relation to one another because no connective tissue directly unites the adjacent bony surfaces. The bony components are indirectly

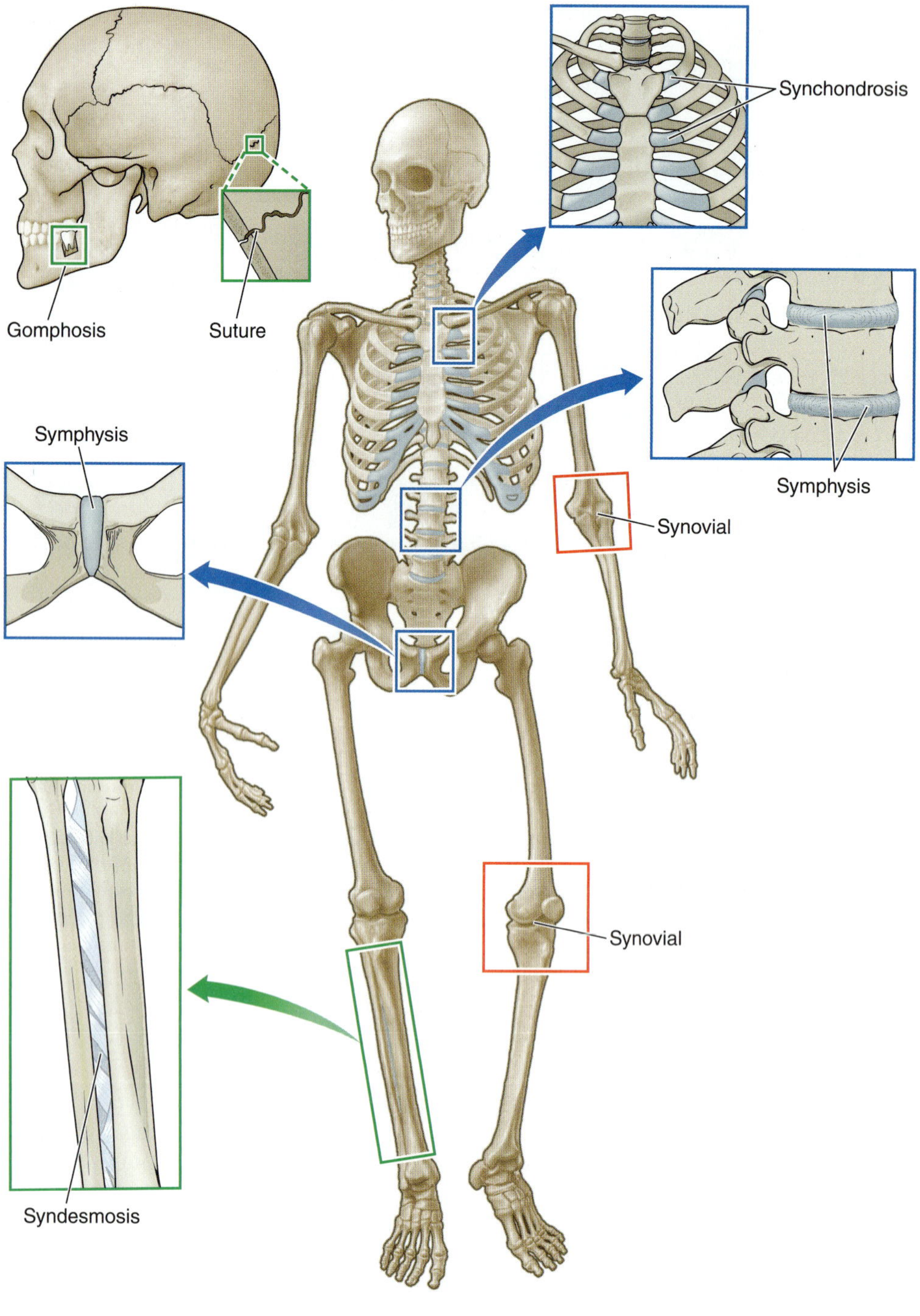

Figure 2–6 Fibrous joints allow for little or no movement between the bones; examples (outlined in green) include sutures (e.g., between the frontal and parietal bones of the skull), gomphoses (e.g., between each tooth and the mandible), and syndesmoses (e.g., between the distal tibia and fibula). Cartilaginous joints (outlined in blue) directly unite one bony surface to another via hyaline or fibrocartilage; examples include symphyses (e.g., between the vertebral bodies and between the pubic bones) and synchondroses (between the first 7 ribs and the sternum). In synovial joints (outlined in red) such as the knee and elbow joints, the bones are indirectly united by a fibrous capsule lined with synovium.

connected to one another by means of a fibrous synovium-lined joint capsule that encloses the joint. Examples of synovial joints include the elbow and knee joints (see Fig. 2–6). Synovial joints are constructed in a similar manner to each other **(Fig. 2–7)** and have the following common features numbered in red in Figure 2-7: (1) a **joint cavity** that is enclosed by (2) **a fibrous joint capsule** that surrounds the joint; (3) a **synovial membrane** that lines the inner surface of the fibrous capsule; (4) hyaline cartilage that covers the articular surfaces of the contiguous bones; and (5) synovial fluid that forms a film over the joint surfaces within the capsule.[7] Synovial joints may also include associated structures (numbered in blue in Fig. 2-7) such as capsular ligaments that reinforce the capsule, bursae to reduce friction between structures, fibrocartilaginous accessory structures (discs, menisci, plates, or labrums) that typically contribute to joint stability while minimizing loss of mobility, and fat pads where cushioning is needed. All synovial joints are crossed by muscles or their associated tendons. The capsule and other structures associated with a synovial joint typically keep joint surfaces aligned and can guide motion. Stabilization by the passive joint structures and active stabilization by muscles and their associated tendons will limit joint distraction and excessive translation of the contiguous bones.[8]

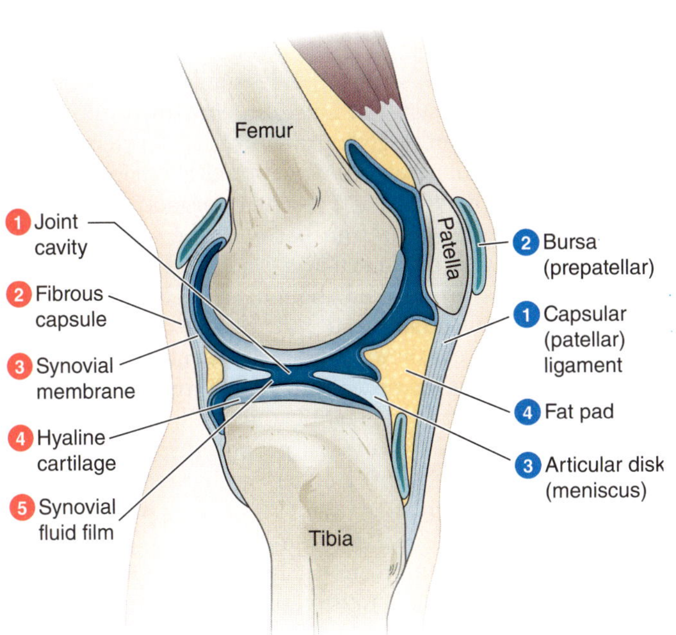

Figure 2–7 Elements of a synovial joint such as the knee joint will always include (listed in red): (1) a joint cavity that is enclosed by (2) a fibrous joint capsule that surrounds the joint; (3) a synovial membrane that lines the inner surface of the fibrous capsule; (4) hyaline cartilage that covers the articular surfaces of the contiguous bones; and (5) synovial fluid that forms a film over the joint surfaces within the capsule. A synovial joint may also include associated structures (as the knee does) such as (listed in blue): (1) capsular ligaments, (2) bursae, (3) accessory structures such as menisci, discs, plates, or labra, and (4) a fat pad.

Patient Application 2–1

Sione Tanielu is a 16-year-old football player who hyper-dorsiflexed his ankle when another player tackled him from behind. He tore the ligaments supporting his distal tibiofibular joint. This joint is structurally classified as a fibrous joint (syndesmosis) and is supported by anterior and posterior tibiofibular ligaments as well as the interosseous membrane. The structures allow relatively small but important movements between the distal tibia and fibula. The stability of this joint is even more critical because the tibia and fibula together form the proximal segment of the synovial (diarthrodial) talocrural (ankle) joint. Disruption (hypermobility) of Sione's distal tibiofibular joint will greatly affect the stability of the talocrural joint, limiting if not completely preventing effective weight-bearing.

JOINT CAPSULE

The synovial joint cavity is an area between two bones that is enclosed by a joint capsule that consists of two layers: an outer fibrous layer and an inner synovial layer (see Fig. 2–7). The outer fibrous layer inserts circumferentially around the ends of the articulating bones. Its primary functions are to provide an enclosure for the joint cavity and enhance joint stability through its passive restraints.[9] The inner synovial layer lines the joint cavity, providing lubrication and nutrition to the articular cartilage.[10] Both layers of the capsule house sensory nerve fibers that provide important information to the central nervous system about, for example, position sense and the need for active muscular support of the joint.

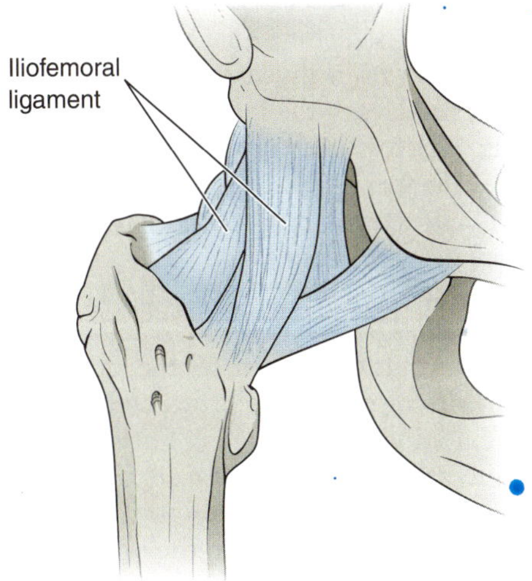

Figure 2–8 The iliofemoral ligament reinforces the anterior hip joint capsule, providing added passive restraint to strong hip joint extension torques.

The fibrous layer of the joint capsule is composed of dense irregular connective tissue with varying thickness and composition from joint to joint, thus affording different amounts of passive restraint. For example, the hip joint capsule is thick and dense, providing stability to this weight-bearing joint that undergoes considerable stress. Other joint capsules such as that of the glenohumeral joint are thin and loose, providing less stability while allowing increased mobility. The thickness, fiber orientation, and composition of the fibrous capsule depend on the stresses placed on it, illustrating the dynamic nature of the joint capsule. In patients with shoulder instability (a chronically subluxing glenohumeral joint), the joint capsule is subjected to repeated tensile stresses that alter tissue composition, such as capsular collagen fibrils and elastin fibers that are larger and denser when compared with typical capsules. These adaptations may increase capsular strength and resistance to stretching deformations.[8] In contrast, portions of an articular capsule that are subjected to repeated compression forces may show development of fibrocartilaginous tissue.[9,11]

Capsular ligaments are localized thickenings of the capsule with distinct fiber orientation that distinguish it from the capsule. These passive tissues provide additional joint stability or restraint to movement based on their orientation, with that orientation influenced by typical stresses at that joint. For example, the iliofemoral ligament of the hip reinforces the anterior joint capsule as it runs from the anterior inferior iliac spine and fans out to attach to the intertrochanteric line of the femur **(Fig. 2–8)**. The ligament forms an inverted Y shape as the ligament fans into superior and inferior bands.[12] This reinforcement of the anterior capsule of the hip provides needed extra restraint to hip extension that enhances passive joint stability and reduces the need for active hip flexor activity to oppose strong extension torques that occur at the hip.

The synovial layer of the capsule is the inner lining of the fibrous joint capsule. The synovium does not cover the articular cartilage or menisci/disks (if present), but it will line other intra-articular structures that may be present (e.g., the cruciate ligaments within the knee joint). The synovial layer is divided into two layers: the intima and the subintima. The **intima** consists of a thin layer of surface cells that line the joint space.[10] These cells are responsible for the removal of debris from the joint cavity, structural repair of the synovium, response to antigens and tissue destruction, and synthesis of hyaluronic acid (a component of synovial fluid).[10] The intima is richly endowed with capillary vessels, lymphatic vessels, and nerve fibers. The **subintima** lies outside (superficial to) the intima and is a loose network of highly vascularized fibrous connective tissue that allows the membrane to move freely. The subintima supports the intima and merges on its external surface with the fibrous capsule. The blood vessels in the subintima transport oxygen, nutrients, and immunologic cells to the joint.

Branches of nearby sensory nerves and branches of nerves from muscles near the joint penetrate the joint capsule through the fibrous layer.[9] Large-diameter sensory efferent nerves and thinly myelinated nerves are present in the fibrous capsule; nonmyelinated C-type fibers are found in the synovium.[13] The joint receptors found in the fibrous joint capsule are sensitive to stretching or compression of the capsule, as well as to any increase in internal pressure due to increased production of synovial fluid (joint swelling). Using the knee joint and its capsule as an example, most of the joint receptors are located in the subintima layer of the capsule close to the insertions of the anterior cruciate ligament (ACL). Mechanoreceptors (predominantly Ruffini receptors) in the subintima capsule and ACL respond primarily to the stretch (e.g., with terminal knee extension). Pacini receptors are reported less frequently and are thought to be activated by compression. Free nerve endings are more numerous than mechanoreceptors and function as nociceptors that react to inflammation and pain stimuli (Table 2–1).[14,15] Together, sensory stimuli, among other functions, contribute to active joint stability by regulating resting muscle tension and initiating reflexive changes in muscular contractions.[13]

SYNOVIAL FLUID

Synovial fluid, a thin film that covers the inner surface of the synovial membrane of the joint capsule and the articular cartilage, helps to keep the joint surfaces lubricated and reduces friction.[16,17] Synovial fluid also provides nourishment for the hyaline cartilage that covers articular surfaces as the fluid moves in and out of the cartilage with joint compression and release.

The composition of synovial fluid is similar to that of blood plasma, except that synovial fluid also contains hyaluronate (hyaluronic acid) and a glycoprotein called lubricin.[18] The hyaluronate component of synovial fluid is responsible for the viscosity of the fluid and is essential for joint lubrication. Hyaluronate reduces friction between the synovial folds of the capsule and the articular surfaces.[10] Lubricin is the component of synovial fluid thought to be responsible for cartilage-on-cartilage lubrication.[10,16,19,20]

The minimal wear shown by normal articular cartilage, despite varied loads, is the result of the structure of the cartilage matrix and the presence of a lubricating fluid.[17,19,20] Although a number of models have been proposed to explain how synovial joints are lubricated under varying load conditions (e.g., "boundary lubrication" and "fluid-film lubrication"), the general consensus is that no single model is adequate to explain human joint lubrication.[16] It is recognized, however, that changes in the concentration of hyaluronate or lubricin in the synovial fluid will affect the overall lubrication and the amount of friction that is present in the joint. Many experiments have confirmed that articular coefficients of friction in synovial joints are far lower than those created by currently available manufactured lubricants.[17] The lower the coefficient of friction, the lower the resistance to movement. There is some evidence to support the use of injections of hyaluronate and lubricin (and their synthetic derivatives) to alleviate symptoms of hip or knee osteoarthritis.[21,22]

Normal synovial fluid appears as a clear, pale yellow, viscous fluid present in small amounts at all synovial joints.[19] There is a direct exchange between the vasculature of the synovial layer and synovial fluid in the intracapsular space, whereby nutrients are supplied and waste products can be taken away from the joint space by diffusion. When a joint is injured or diseased, the volume of synovial fluid increases in the joint and is related to reports of pain.[23] The synovial fluid, like all viscous substances, resists shear loads.[16]

Changes in the synovial layers of the joint capsule are seen in inflammatory arthritic conditions, such as rheumatoid arthritis, and are associated with articular cartilage degeneration. Increased levels of inflammatory cells hinder the lubricating features of synovial fluid. The synovial layer of the capsule hypertrophies and develops *pannus*, invasive granulation tissue that further destroys the joint articular cartilage. Rheumatic

Table 2–1 Joint Receptors

TYPE	NAME	SENSITIVITY	LOCATION
I	Ruffini	Stretch, usually at extremes of extension	Fibrous layer of joint capsules on flexion side of joints, periosteum, ligaments, and tendons[10]
II	Pacini or pacini-form	Compression or changes in hydrostatic pressure and joint movement[10]	Located throughout joint capsule, particularly in deeper layers and in fat pads
III	Golgi, Golgi-Mazzoni	Pressure and forceful joint motion into extremes of motion	Inner layer (synovium) of joint capsules, ligaments, and tendons[10]
IV	Unmyelinated free nerve endings	Non-noxious and noxious mechanical stress or biomechanical stress	Located around blood vessels in synovial layer of capsule and in adjacent fat pads and collateral ligaments, tendons, and the periosteum

diseases are systemic and will affect more than one joint in the body. As a result, they ultimately lead to decreased mobility, functional capacity, and quality of life.[24]

HYALINE CARTILAGE

Hyaline cartilage, from the Greek word *hyalos*, meaning "glass," forms a relatively thin (1 to 7 mm) layer on the ends of the bones in synovial joints. It provides a smooth, resilient, low-friction surface and is important for bearing and distributing forces over a person's lifetime. Detailed discussion of its composition and function will be discussed later in the section on Specific Connective Tissue Composition in this chapter. Hyaline cartilage is commonly referred to as *articular cartilage*.

Patient Application 2–2

Enid Brown is a 50-year-old woman who was recently diagnosed with rheumatoid arthritis. She has been experiencing episodes of stiffness and soreness in her hands, right knee, and neck over the last year. Recently, she realized that the joints in her fingers were red and swollen in both hands. She had pain and crepitus when she tried to grab anything, especially when she tried to twist the lids off jars. Her primary care physician referred her to a rheumatologist, who diagnosed rheumatoid arthritis. Rheumatoid arthritis is an autoimmune disease that is characterized by inflammation, swelling, and hypertrophy of the synovial lining of synovial joints, which leads to the symptoms described by Enid. The disease is progressive, and the inflammatory response will ultimately affect the health of the articular cartilage and surrounding connective tissues, such as joint capsules and ligaments.

Foundational Concepts 2–3
Synovial Joint Capsule

The synovial joint capsule:

- Provides an enclosure for the joint cavity
- Contributes to passive joint constraints and stability via the fibrous layer
- Provides lubrication and nutrition to intra-articular joint structures via the synovial layer
- Has sensory receptors in both the fibrous and synovial layers that provide information regarding joint position, movement, and pain

SYNOVIAL JOINT–ASSOCIATED STRUCTURES

Fibrocartilaginous menisci, labrums, plates, and discs help to increase joint congruence ("fit"), absorb compressive joint forces, increase stability, and facilitate motion. For example, the wedge-shaped fibrocartilage medial and lateral menisci of the knee deepen the relatively flat tibial plateau, providing increased congruence of the tibia with the large convex femoral condyles. That greater contact area not only increases stability of the joint but also allows for distribution of joint compressive forces across a larger surface area, thus decreasing joint stress. In fact, it has been estimated that the menisci of the knee bear 45% to 70% of the load across the knee depending on joint angle.[25] In another example, fibrocartilage labra deepen and extend the articular concave surface to which they attach. The acetabular labrum attaches around the entire periphery of the pelvic acetabulum, enhancing joint stability both by deepening the acetabulum and by creating negative pressure that holds the femoral head in the acetabulum.[26] In some instances a fibrocartilage articular disc extends all the way across a joint and actually divides the joint into two separate cavities. The articular disc of the sternoclavicular joint transects the joint and is attached in such a way that it increases joint stability while serving as a pivot point for motions. In each instance, the fibrocartilage accessory joint structure provides increased joint stability with little or no sacrifice of mobility.

Ligaments play an important role in keeping joint surfaces aligned as well as both guiding and restraining motion. Excessive separation or translation of joint surfaces is limited by passive tension in ligaments, as well as by the fibrous joint capsule and muscle tendons that cross the joint. As described previously, ligaments may blend with the joint capsule and appear as thickenings in the capsule (e.g., the iliofemoral ligament, the glenohumeral ligaments). Other ligaments are distinct from the capsule and may consist of dense white bands or cords of connective tissue (e.g., ACL, lateral collateral ligament of the knee). Ligaments are typically named descriptively according to their location, shape, bony attachments, and relationship to one another. The anterior longitudinal ligament of the spine derives its name from both location (anterior) and shape (longitudinal). The medial and lateral collateral ligaments of the elbow and knee joints are examples of ligaments named for location. Ligaments such as the coracohumeral ligament that connects the coracoid process of the scapula to the humerus, and the radioulnar ligaments that connect the radius to the ulna are named for their bony attachments. The deltoid ligament at the ankle joint is named for its shape. Occasionally, ligaments are named for the individuals who first identified them (e.g., the Y-ligament of Bigelow—an older name for the iliofemoral ligament).

The primary task of a tendon is to transmit forces developed by muscles to their bony attachments to create or limit bony rotation; however, active and passive musculotendinous forces also may stabilize the joint by creating joint compression or by restricting excessive or unwanted translatory movement between bony segments. Shapes and configurations of tendons vary throughout the body.[27-29] They may be round and ropelike structures such as the biceps brachii tendon at the elbow or the tibialis posterior tendon as it wraps around the medial malleolus. Tendons can also be flat like the tendons of the supraspinatus, latissimus dorsi, and pectoralis major muscles. Very broad, flattened tendons are often referred to as **aponeuroses.** Tendons can also lie *within* a muscle to allow short muscle fibers to connect to a central tendon, as is seen in the soleus and deltoid muscles.[27]

Bursae are flat, dense, irregular connective tissue sacs lined with a synovial membrane in which the inner sides of the sacs are separated by a fluid film. Bursae are found where structures in tight approximation to each other might move on each other (thus producing friction forces), such as between tendon and bone, bone and skin, muscle and bone, or ligament and bone. Bursae located between the skin and bone (such as the prepatellar bursa at the knee) are called *subcutaneous bursae*.[30] Subtendinous bursae lie between tendon and bone, and submuscular bursae lie between muscle and bone.

Foundational Concepts 2–4
Synovial Joint Stability

In general, synovial joints offer the greatest amount of movement between two contiguous bones as compared with fibrous or cartilaginous joints. However, that increase in mobility can come at the expense of stability. There are several features that can be associated with synovial joints to enhance stability without seriously affecting functional mobility:

- Ligaments are passive stabilizers of the joint that can blend in with the capsule or appear as individual structures.
- Fibrocartilage menisci, labrums, plates, and discs provide passive joint stability by deepening articular surfaces and increasing joint congruence.

CLASSIFICATION OF SYNOVIAL JOINTS

Synovial joints can be divided into subclassifications based on the shape and configuration of the ends of the bony components.[31] These classifications describe simple geometric surfaces and include **plane, ball-and-socket, condyloid, saddle, hinge,** and **pivot** **(Fig. 2–9)**. It is important to keep in mind that joint surfaces and geometry are more complex than the labels may imply, but those labels provide a simplified description of the orientation and function of the articulating surfaces.[32] Synovial joints within these classifications also can be categorized based on the number of axes about which "gross visible" rotary motion at the joint occurs: **uniaxial, biaxial,** and **triaxial.**[33-35] The actual direction and magnitudes of motion at a joint are dictated not only by joint geometry, but also by surrounding articular structures.

Uniaxial (also known as **uniplanar**) joints are those with visible rotation of the bony components in one plane around a single axis (one degree of freedom). Hinge and pivot joints are uniaxial. A hinge joint mechanically resembles a door hinge, with a cylindrical component fitting into a concave component. The humeroulnar articulation of the elbow joint is an example of a hinge joint, formed by the trochlea on the distal end of the humerus and the trochlear notch on the proximal end of the ulna (see **Fig. 2–9A**). A pivot joint mechanically has a cylindrical component that rotates within a ring-shaped component. The proximal radioulnar joint is an example, with the annular ligament and radial notch on the ulna forming a ring within which the head of the radius rotates (see **Fig. 2–9B**).

Biaxial (also known as **biplanar**) joints are those with visible rotation of the bony components in two planes around two axes (two degrees of freedom). Condyloid and saddle joints are biaxial. The term **ellipsoid** is often used interchangeably with condyloid. The radiocarpal joint is an example of a condyloid joint—formed by convexities of the scaphoid, lunate, and scapholunate ligament in both the sagittal and frontal planes with corresponding concavities on the distal radius (see **Fig. 2–9C**). A saddle joint has a complex configuration where both segments are convex in one plane and concave in a perpendicular plane. The shape is similar to that of a horse saddle where an anterior to posterior concavity runs perpendicular to a medial to lateral convexity. The carpometacarpal joint of the thumb is an example of a saddle joint formed by the trapezium's articulation with the base of the first metacarpal (see **Fig. 2–9D**). The convexity of the base of the first metacarpal moves on the concavity of the trapezium in flexion/extension, whereas the concavity of the metacarpal moves on the convexity of the trapezium in abduction/adduction.

Triaxial or **multiaxial** joints are those in which the bony components are free to rotate in three planes around three axes (three degrees of freedom). The two types of joints in this category are plane joints and ball-and-socket joints. Plane joints are articulations between two relatively flat surfaces. The opposing surfaces can have a variety of configurations with slight but mostly inconsequential curvatures that permit both rotation and sliding between two or more bones. Examples of these joints can be seen in intercarpal articulations such as that between the capitate and hamate (see **Fig. 2–9E**). Ball-and-socket joints are formed by a ball-like convex surface that fits into a concave socket. An example of a ball-and-socket joint is the hip (femoroacetabular) joint, formed by the concave head of the femur and convex acetabulum (see **Fig. 2–9F**). The rotary motions of the flexion/extension occur in the sagittal plane around a coronal axis; abduction/adduction occurs in the frontal plane around an anteroposterior axis and medial/lateral rotation occurs in the transverse plane around a longitudinal axis.

Joint Motion

In the descriptions of the subclassifications of synovial joints, joints were categorized according to the "visible" motions around one (uniaxial), two (biaxial), or three (triaxial/multiaxial) axes of motion. The rotatory movement of the bony segments at a synovial joint are known as **osteokinematics.** During osteokinematic movement of the bony levers at a joint, the contiguous articular surfaces within a joint modify their points of contact with each other; this shifting in points of articular contact within a joint is known as **arthrokinematics.**

Osteokinematics

Osteokinematics refers to the rotary movement of the bony levers in space during physiological joint motion. These movements are typically described by the plane in which the motion occurs (sagittal, frontal, and transverse planes), the axis about which they occur (coronal, anteroposterior, and longitudinal or vertical), and by the direction of movement (flexion/extension, abduction/adduction, and medial/lateral rotation).

Arthrokinematics

Often during osteokinematics, one of the joint surfaces is relatively stable and serves as a base for the motion, whereas the other segment moves on that stable base. The terms **roll, slide,** and **spin** are used to describe the different types of changes in articular contact that the moving segment can make on the more stable segment.[17,33-35] These changes in articular contact are known as arthrokinematic, or accessory, motions **(Figure 2–10)**. Unlike osteokinematic motions, arthrokinematics cannot be volitionally isolated under normal conditions.[33,35]

A **roll** refers to the rolling of one joint surface on another, as in a tire rolling on the road. During a pure rolling motion, there is a linear progression of points of contact between

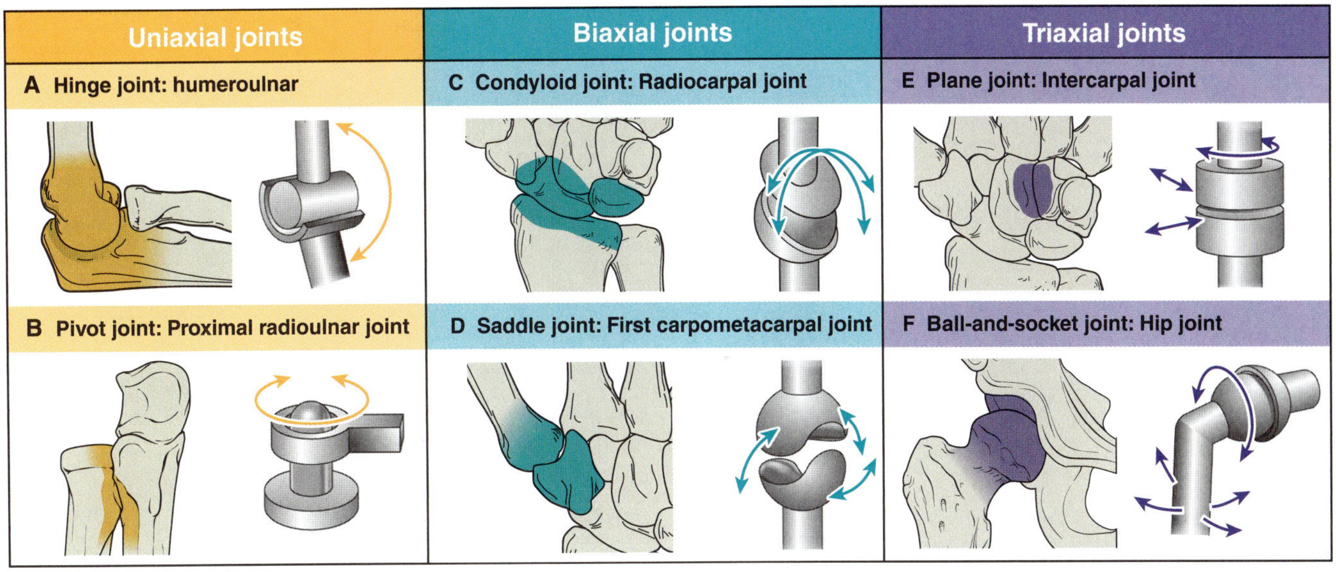

Figure 2–9 Synovial joints can be subclassified both by joint geometry and by the number of axes around which visible motion of the bony segments can take place at the joint. A sample of each type of joint is accompanied by a mechanical representation of its movement.

both the moving and the stable surfaces **(Fig. 2–10A)**. Sliding, also commonly known as **gliding**, refers to the linear translation of one component on another, as when a braked wheel skids **(Fig. 2–10B)**. In pure sliding, a fixed point on the sliding surface moves over changing points of contact in the stable component. Combinations of rolling and sliding usually occur together during most physiological movements. **Spin** refers to rotation of the moving component, as when a top spins. In a pure spin around a fixed axis, the point of contact changes for the moving component but the point of contact on the stable component does not **(Fig. 2–10C)**. A spin around a relatively fixed axis may also result when a roll and a slide occur in opposite directions and in approximately equal amounts **(Fig. 2–10D)**. When rolling and sliding occur disproportionately, the resulting "spin" may take place about an axis that is not fixed but shifts as the motion continues (an instantaneous axis of rotation).

Uniaxial, biaxial, and triaxial joints are referred to as having one, two, and three degrees of freedom, respectively. White and Panjabi[35] referred to joint motions and their associated intra-articular (arthrokinematic) components as having the potential for six degrees of freedom: three degrees of rotation around three axes, and three degrees of translation along those same three axes. The section on Descriptions of Motions in Chapter 1 and other chapters in this text also refers to the potential for six degrees of freedom. The six degrees of freedom and three degrees of freedom models are not really in conflict because the White and Panjabi model is an elaboration of the simpler model. The White and Panjabi model is the foundation of at least some of the manual therapy approaches to joint interventions.

During human joint motion, rolling and sliding often occur together in differing proportions to maintain joint integrity. Whereas rolling of the articular surface of a moving lever occurs in the *same* direction as the osteokinematic motion of the lever (see Fig. 2–10A), the osteokinematic/arthrokinematic relationship can differ depending on the shape of the moving and stable articular surfaces. This shift in relationship is commonly referred to as the **convex-concave rule.**[36]

When a convex joint surface moves on a relatively stable concave surface, the convex surface *rolls* in the *same direction* as the osteokinematic movement of the bony lever. However, *sliding* of the convex surface will occur in the *opposite direction* to the roll to maintain optimum contact. Elaborating on the example shown in Figure 2–10D, the initial stage of weight-bearing knee flexion occurs with the convex femoral condyles rolling posteriorly on the fixed tibial plateau in the same direction as the posteriorly rotating (flexing) femur **(Fig. 2–11)**. After this initial rolling, the femoral condyles must slide anteriorly while continuing to roll posteriorly so that the femoral condyles do not roll off the posterior tibial plateau **(Fig. 2–11A)**. This roll-and-slide combination in the flexing knee approximates a pure spin of the femoral condyles on the posterior tibial plateau only toward the end of knee flexion. This is in contrast to what is seen when a concave articulating surface is moving on a stable convex surface. Although *rolling* still occurs in the *same direction* as the osteokinematic movement of the segment, *sliding* typically occurs in the *same direction* as rolling of the articular surface. During extension of the tibia (as in a seated position), the slightly concave tibial plateau rolls anteriorly in the same direction as the anteriorly rotating (extending) tibia. The tibial plateau must also slide anteriorly in the same direction as the roll to fully extend the tibia while maintaining contact of the tibial plateau with the femoral condyles **(Fig. 2–11B)**. The ability of a joint to move through its full osteokinematic (physiological) range of motion (**ROM**) is dependent upon the ability of the contacting articulating segments to roll, slide, or spin based on the demands of the shape of the moving surface and appropriate constraints from the surrounding tissues.

For articular surfaces to be free to move in the appropriate direction (arthrokinematics) as the bony lever rotates (osteokinematics), the joint must have a certain amount of **"joint play."** This freedom of movement of one articular surface on another can be tested by an examiner when the joint is in a **loose-packed** position, typically tested as the amount of

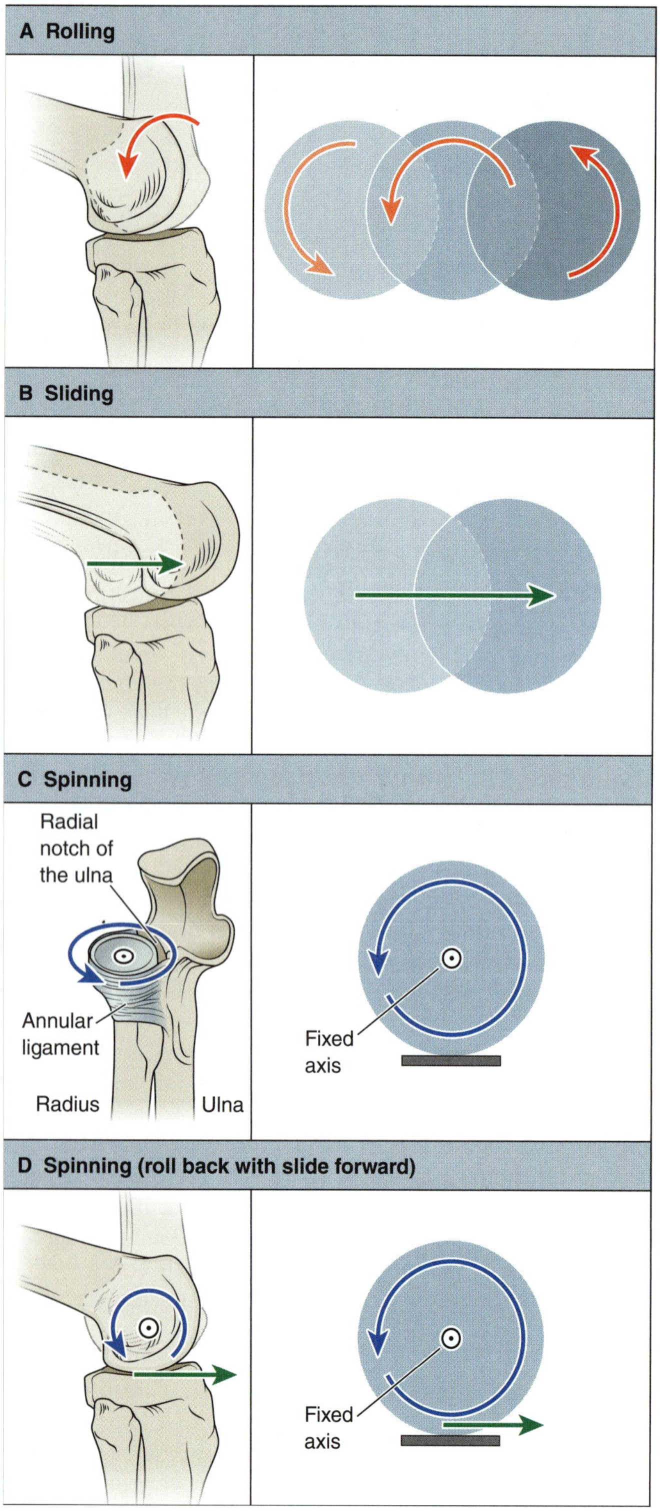

Figure 2–10 Arthrokinematic joint motions include **A.** rolling (femur rolls posteriorly on the tibial plateau), **B.** sliding (femur slides anteriorly on the tibial plateau), and **C.** spinning (of the radial head within the annular ligament). **D.** When the femur simultaneously rolls posteriorly and slides anteriorly on the tibial plateau, the effect appears to be a spin of the femoral condyles around a relatively fixed axis.

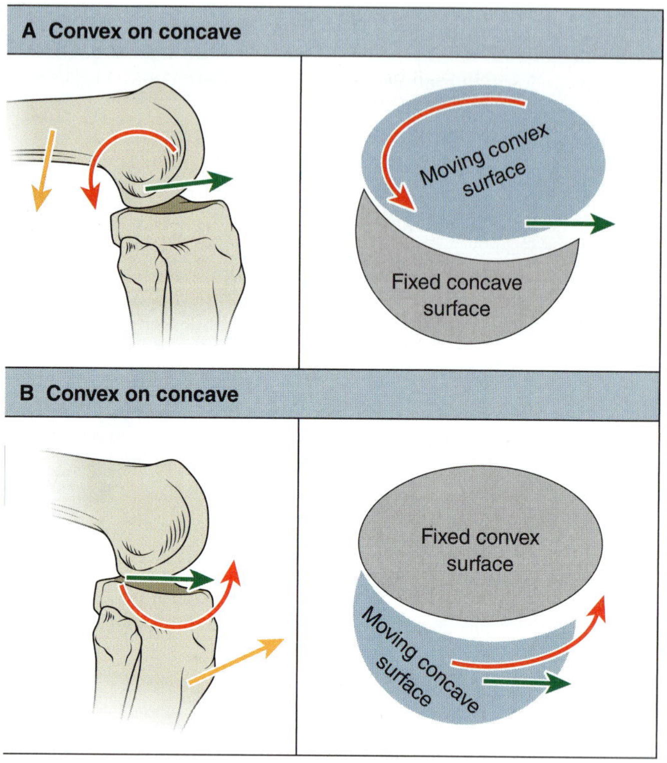

Figure 2–11 Convex/concave rule. **A.** During flexion of the *femur*, the convex femoral condyles move on a fixed concave surface; the convex femoral condyles roll posteriorly (red arrow) in the same direction as the flexing femur (orange arrow), while sliding anteriorly (green arrow) in a direction opposite to the roll. **B.** During extension of the *tibia*, the concave tibia plateau rolls anteriorly (red arrow) in the same direction as the extending tibia (orange arrow) and slides anteriorly (green arrow) in the same direction as the roll.

available passive (manual) sliding of one surface upon the other. The loose-packed position of a joint most often is described as the point in the joint's range where the capsule and ligaments provide the least restraint to passive sliding. If the supporting joint structures are excessively lax (e.g., stretched or torn), the joint may have too much play and become unstable. If the joint structures are excessively tight (e.g., adaptively shortened or hypertrophic), the joint will have too little movement between the articular surfaces; movement of the bony lever will be restricted because the appropriate intra-articular movement will not accompany the physiological movement of the bony lever.

For most synovial joints, there is a point in the ROM where minimal or no joint play between the articular surfaces is expected. This is referred to as the **close-packed** position for a joint and is the point in the ROM where the ligaments and capsule are maximally taut. The close-packed position is usually (but not always) at the end of a joint's ROM, is the position of greatest joint stability, and is most resistant to any distraction forces that have the potential to cause separation of the joint surfaces. In the close-packed position, little or no joint play is possible. The position of full extension is the close-packed position for the knee and interphalangeal joints.[33] For many joints the close-packed position of a joint can also be referred to as the "locked" position, as is true for the knee.

Patient Application 2–3

James Connelly, a 62-year-old man, fell off a stepladder and fractured his tibial plateau. He was placed in a long leg cast from his thigh to his ankle that kept his knee in 20° of flexion for 6 weeks. Upon removal of his cast, his ability to actively flex or fully extend his knee was very limited, although there is evidence that the tibial plateau fracture healed without any disruption to the tibial plateau. Although the knee joint musculature is understandably weak after prolonged casting, immobilization changes to the joint capsule and joint ligaments are significant factors in James' joint motion issues. If arthrokinematics (roll, slide, and spin) of the femoral condyles or tibial plateau are excessively constrained by shortened capsuloligamentous structures, the osteokinematic motions of flexion and extension of the tibia (or of the femur) will be limited. Beginning James' treatment by facilitating the arthrokinematic motions typically expected of the tibia at the knee through manual joint mobilization techniques (increasing joint play) may be more effective and safer initially in restoring knee joint ROM than forcing the tibia into flexion or extension.

Range of Motion

The anatomic or physiological ROM of a joint refers to the amount of *passive* rotation available to a joint in a given direction within the anatomic limits of the joint structure.[33] The extent of the anatomic range (osteokinematic motion) is determined by a number of factors, including the shape of the joint surfaces, the joint capsule, ligaments, muscle bulk, contiguous bony structures, and surrounding musculotendinous tissues, any of which can affect arthrokinematics and osteokinematics of the joint. In some joints, there are no bony limitations to motion and the ROM is limited only by soft tissue structures. Other joints have definite bony restrictions to motion in addition to soft-tissue limitations. The humeroulnar joint at the elbow is limited in extension by bony contact of the olecranon of the ulna with the olecranon fossa of the humerus, whereas flexion is limited most often by approximation of the forearm with the elbow flexor muscle bellies. The sensation experienced by the examiner performing passive movements to the end of physiological ROM at each joint is referred to as the *end-feel.* Using terminology first promoted by Kaltenborn,[36] a motion that is limited by approximation of soft tissues (as is typical of elbow flexion) is considered to have a **soft end-feel;** a motion limited by capsuloligamentous restraints (as is typical of knee extension) is considered to have a **firm end-feel;** and a motion with a bony limitation (as is typical of elbow extension) is considered to have a **hard end-feel.**

A joint ROM is considered to be atypical when motion either exceeds or fails to reach the typically expected anatomic (osteokinematic) limits of motion. When a passive ROM exceeds the expected limits, the joint can be labeled as **hypermobile.** When the passive ROM is less than what would typically be permitted at the joint, the joint can be labeled as **hypomobile.** Either hypermobility or hypomobility of a joint may have negative consequences not only at the affected joint but also on adjacent joint structures. Increased joint stresses may result in further changes to joint structures and can lead to activity and participation limitations.

Hypermobility may be caused by a failure of bony elements or soft tissues, including weak musculature, to restrain the motion. Inadequate joint restraints can lead to excessive joint play and instability. For example, the ACL is a major stabilizing ligament of the knee, preventing, among other movements, excessive anterior sliding of the tibial plateau on the femoral condyles. Rupture of this ligament can lead to knee joint instability if the surrounding muscles (e.g., hamstrings) and remaining articular structures (capsule, ligaments, and menisci) cannot adequately substitute for the torn ligament. The result may be avoidance of activities that stress the now unstable knee joint, as well damaging other joint structures.

Hypomobility of a joint may be caused by bony or cartilaginous blocks to motion or by the inability of the capsule, ligaments, or muscles to elongate sufficiently to allow a typical ROM. For example, the hip joint typically extends during the terminal stance phase of gait as the body passes over the supporting limb. With hip osteoarthritis, hip extension can be limited both by the resulting overgrowth or unevenness of the articular surfaces and by excessive tension in the hip flexors that is a physiological response to hip pain. Step length will be shortened because of the lack of hip extension. The person may compensate by increasing lumbar extension (increasing lordosis) in terminal stance to increase step length and facilitate forward progression. This adaptive change, over time, can have negative consequences on the low back. A **contracture** is a shortening of soft-tissue structures around a joint with accompanying fibrotic changes. A contracture can be another cause of hypomobility or may be a consequence of sustained hypomobility over time.

Foundational Concepts 2–5
Joint Motion

- Osteokinematics: rotary movement of the bony lever(s) of a joint around one or more axes in the associated planes
- Arthrokinematics: rolling, sliding, or spinning of one contiguous joint surface on another
- Convex-concave rule: a convex joint surface that moves on a stable concave surface generally rolls in one direction and slides in the *opposite* direction; a concave joint surface that moves on a stable convex joint surface generally rolls and slides in the *same* direction
- Physiological ROM: the typical amount of expected passive joint rotation in one plane within the anatomic limits of the joint structure as a function of both osteokinematic and arthrokinematic factors
- End-feel: the soft, firm, or hard sensation experienced by the examiner at the end of the available passive ROM at each joint due to structure(s) that check further motion

Kinematic Chains

The concepts of open and closed chains were introduced in Chapter 1 in the section on Multisegment (Closed-Chain) Force Analysis to identify how forces applied to one segment can affect another segment. The concepts are also relevant to understanding the interdependence of how segments move through space. Engineers originally described a so-called "kinematic" chain as a series of rigid segments linked together by a series of pin-centered joints (as, literally, in a length of large-linked chain). In an **open chain,** one end of the series of segments is free to move while the other is fixed **(Fig. 2–12A).** Movement in an open chain can take place at one link (joint) without causing motion at other links (joints) in the chain, although the attached segments will move in space. In a

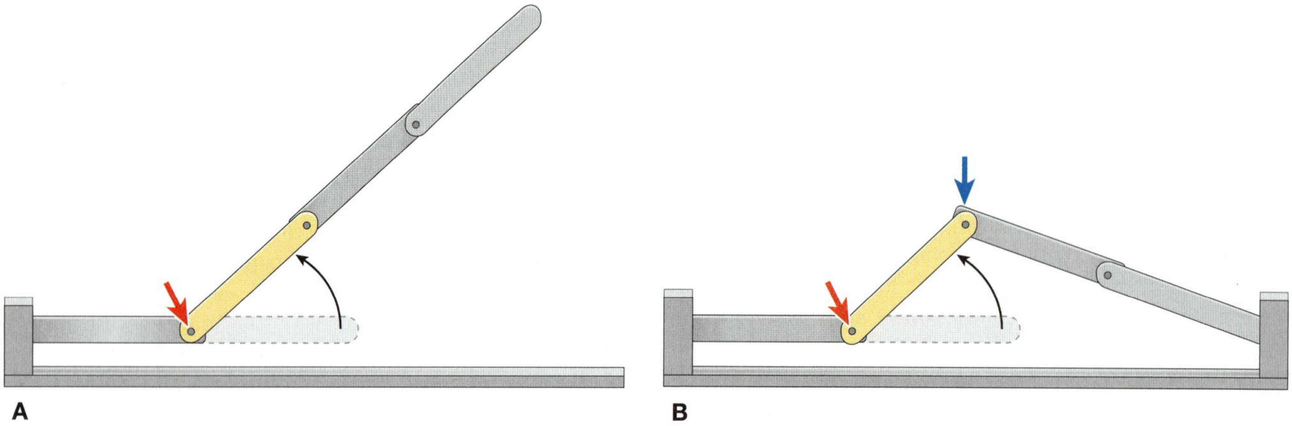

Figure 2–12 Mechanical open and closed chains. **A.** In an open four-segment chain (fixed at only one end), rotation of one segment can occur around a single axis (red arrow) without causing rotation at another link (joint). **B.** In a closed four-segment chain (fixed at both ends), rotation of the same segment as in A. causes rotation not only around the same axis (red arrow) but around at least one other axis (blue arrow) as well.

closed chain, both ends of the chain are fixed **(Fig. 2–12B)**. Movement at one link (joint) not only moves one or more attached segments in space but will also create movement in one or more other links (joints) in the chain.[33]

Human movements can take place in either open chain or closed chain systems. For example, the term *closed chain* has often been applied to human movements that take place under weight-bearing conditions, where the distal segment of a limb is "fixed" on the supporting surface (see Expanded Concepts 1–10 in Chapter 1). Under weight-bearing conditions, motion at one joint generally is accompanied by motion at one or more other joints for the body to remain stable. In contrast, the term *open chain* is often applied to movements that occur in non–weight-bearing conditions, with the distal segment free to move in space. For instance, under open-chain (non–weight-bearing) conditions, the right foot is not fixed on the ground; right knee flexion can occur independent of motion at the contiguous hip and ankle joints **(Fig. 2–13A)**. When both feet are weight-bearing and "fixed" on the ground, knee flexion will occur bilaterally and result in simultaneous hip flexion and ankle dorsiflexion if the head is to remain upright and eyes forward, as well as maintaining the line of gravity within the base of support **(Fig. 2–13B)**. In this instance (and as is common in bilateral weight-bearing), the closed chain includes all joints between the right foot, up the right lower extremity, across the pelvis, and down the left extremity to the left foot. The closed chain may also be thought of as extending from the weight-bearing feet to the head that is relatively fixed in space (eyes oriented vertically and over the base of support). Although *weight-bearing* and *closed chain* are sometimes used synonymously, the person in Figures 2–13A and B is weight-bearing in both instances. *Weight-bearing* and *closed chain* are synonymous *only* when both ends of the chain are fixed, whether by bearing weight or through some other constraint or adaptive mechanism.

In human movement, body segments, especially the upper extremities, are frequently free to move distally (or at one end) in an open chain. Motion of bony segments in an open chain may function either independently of each other or in a myriad of combinations limited only by degrees of freedom and ranges of available motion of each joint in the chain. If one joint in an open chain is immobilized by an atypical structural constraint, the lost motion may be made up by motions at more proximal or distal joints in the chain. In Figure 2–12A, immobilization of the joint at the red arrow would not prevent full ROMs from occurring at the more distal joints. Motions of joints in a closed chain are more predictable because the

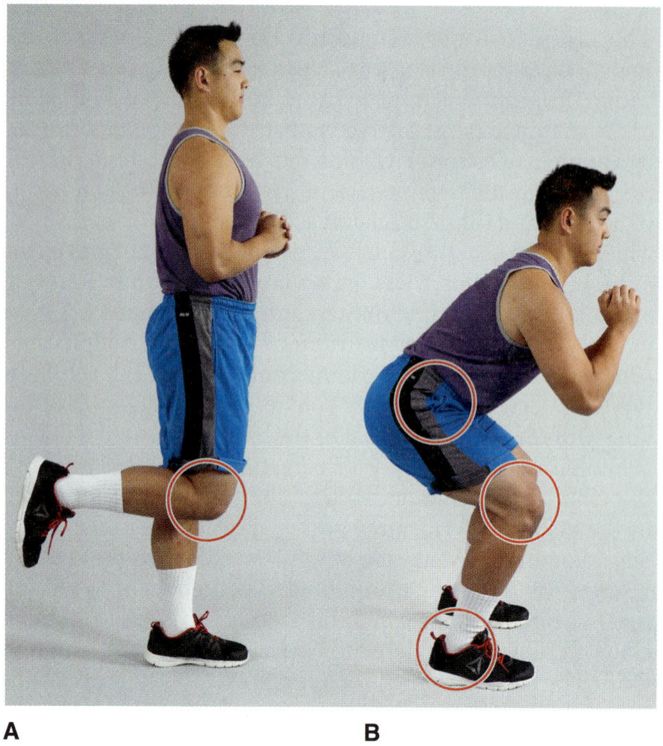

Figure 2–13 Open and closed chains in human motion. **A.** Knee flexion in an open chain may occur without motion at the contiguous hip and ankle. **B.** In a closed chain, knee flexion must be accompanied by hip flexion and ankle dorsiflexion to keep the head upright and the line of gravity within the base of support.

interdependence of the contiguous segments reduces the available options. If one joint in a closed chain is immobilized, motion at contiguous joints may also be functionally limited. In Figure 2–12B, immobilization of the joint at the red arrow would prevent any motion at the next joint (blue arrow) and probably at the next joint axis as well. The concept of open and closed chains is valuable for understanding both kinematic and kinetic concepts of human motion, effects of therapeutic exercise, and consequences of injury and disease on the interrelated joints of the body. Therefore, the concepts of open and closed chains will be referenced throughout this text to understand the extent of functional loss that might occur with joint injury or disease.

Patient Application 2–4

George Chen is a 40-year-old electrician and business owner who caught his skate on another player's stick when playing ice hockey. George ended up with a bimalleolar (tibial and fibular malleolar) fracture that was treated with open reduction and internal fixation. A plate and screws were placed along the distal fibula; additional screws were placed to secure the tibia's medial malleolus and to stabilize the distal tibiofibular joint. He was non–weight-bearing on crutches for a period of time, followed by a walking boot. When the walking boot was discontinued, George had only 5° dorsiflexion and 20° plantarflexion, as well as restricted subtalar motion. George's current foot/ankle limitations will affect the entire lower extremity chain when his affected ankle is weight-bearing. With his ankle ROM limitations and without mobility in the subtalar joint to accommodate, George's knee and hip flexion will be limited sufficiently to affect weight-bearing activities such as walking (especially on sloped surfaces), stair climbing, sitting in low chairs, and squatting to help his daughter tie her shoes. With manual joint mobilization, the subtalar mobility (largely impaired by the immobilization rather than by injury) can be restored, but the hardware in the tibia and fibula may limit restoration of tibiofibular, and therefore ankle, joint function.

Materials Found in Human Joints

Having described the structures that make up fibrous, cartilaginous, and synovial joints and the factors that influence movements available to those joints, this section focuses on the tissues that make up those joint structures: connective tissue. Human joints are comprised of living tissues that change their structure in response to changing environmental or functional demands. Tissues require nourishment and some amount of stress to survive; they can adapt to imposed stresses or demands but may also become injured if the tissues' adaptation fails. The ability of the tissues to adapt can be challenged by a variety of factors including injury, disease, and aging. An understanding of the composition of tissues and how they respond to stresses and strains is necessary to understand how tissues adapt or fail to adapt to imposed stresses.

Composition of Connective Tissue

The joint structures that were discussed thus far in this chapter are all composed of connective tissues, including bones, bursae, capsules, cartilage, discs, labrums, menisci, plates, ligaments, and tendons. These joint structures fall into three primary categories of connective tissue; bone, cartilage, and **dense connective tissue.** Although there are other classifications of connective tissues, this chapter will detail primarily these three. The gross anatomic structure and microarchitecture, composition, and biomechanical behavior of connective tissues is under continual investigation as changes in technology improve our ability to understand these tissues. Despite the variations among connective tissue types, there are common elements among them. Connective tissues are characterized by widely dispersed cells and a large volume of **extracellular matrix (ECM).** At the microscopic level, the extracellular matrix has both **interfibrillar components** (also known as the **ground substance**) and **fibrillar** (fibrous) **components.** Whereas tissues such as nerve and muscle depend predominantly on cell structure to determine function, all connective tissues are strongly influenced by extracellular components.

Cells

The cells of all connective tissues function primarily (although not exclusively) to synthesize the extracellular matrix of connective tissue. The **fibroblast** is the basic cell of most connective tissues. Depending on its mechanical and physiological environment, fibroblasts can differentiate into **chondroblasts** (cartilage), **tenoblasts** (tendon), or **osteoblasts** (bone). As each of these cell types further differentiate, they become more specialized cells including **fibrocytes, chondrocytes, tenocytes,** and **osteocytes,** respectively. The distinction between a "blast" and a "cyte" is based primarily on appearance, which reflects cell synthetic activity. Generally, "blasts" are more metabolically active in secreting both fibrillar and interfibrillar components of the extracellular matrix, whereas "cytes" are more mature cells that maintain the interfibrillar component of the extracellular matrix. Given the appropriate environment or stimuli, differentiated connective tissue cells can "de-differentiate" and change the type of extracellular matrix they produce. For example, tendon cells can produce a cartilage-like (rather than tendon-like) tissue when subjected to prolonged compressive forces.[37-39] Such findings suggest that connective tissue structure can be modified by changes in loading conditions; therefore, it might be possible to manipulate the mechanical environment to cause connective tissues to synthesize somewhat different materials that might enhance their function.

Extracellular Matrix (ECM)

The extracellular matrix is the part of connective tissues outside the cells. It comprises almost the entire volume of connective tissue and determines the tissue's function. The extracellular matrix primarily contains proteins and water and is organized into its fibrillar and surrounding interfibrillar components. The extracellular matrix can also be modified by nonorganic components that influence structure, such as the addition of mineralized hydroxyapatite, in the case of bone.

FIBRILLAR COMPONENT OF THE ECM

The fibrillar, or fibrous, component of the extracellular matrix contains two major classes of structural proteins: collagen and elastin.[11] **Collagen,** the main substance of most connective tissues, is found in all multicellular organisms. The most abundant protein in the human body, it accounts for 25% to 30% of all protein in mammals.[40] Collagen has a tensile strength similar to steel and is responsible for the functional integrity of connective tissue structures and the resistance of connective tissue to tensile forces.[40-48]

Many types of collagen have been identified, but the functions of all are not yet well understood.[40-44] The fibril-forming collagens (types I, II, and III) are the most common. Type I collagen accounts for 90% of the total collagen in the body and is found in most connective tissues, including tendons, ligaments, menisci, fibrocartilage, joint capsules, synovium, bones, labrums, and skin.[40-46] Type I collagen appears to be responsible for the tensile strength of tissues. Type II collagen is found mainly in cartilage and intervertebral discs where compressive forces are common.[41,42] Type III collagen is found in skin, joint capsules, muscle and tendon sheaths, and in healing tissues where, like type I, tensile stresses are common.[41,47]

The basic building block of collagen is a triple helix of three polypeptide chains called the **tropocollagen molecule.** The tropocollagen molecules aggregate in groups to form **microfibrils**; the microfibrils in turn combine to form **fibrils** (fibers) of varying sizes[46,47] **(Fig. 2–14)**. Cross-links stabilize and strengthen the fibrils, with the cross-links being either intramolecular (between peptide chains within a collagen molecule) or intermolecular (between molecules of adjacent fibrils).[49] Fibrils enlarge as more collagen is added to them and as more cross-linking occurs among neighboring molecules; thus, older fibrils are larger and contain more cross-links, making them stronger. Generally, the organization of type I collagen in both tendons and ligaments continues to follow a hierarchical structure whereby fibrils collect to form successively larger aggregations or bundles. Specific descriptions and nomenclature for successive bundles vary across resources but all appear to agree on a hierarchical pattern.[27,46] As seen in Figure 2–14, collagen fibrils bundle together to form the **collagen fiber.** Cross-links formed between the collagen fibers may be arranged in many different ways and vary in size and length. In most relaxed tissues, the collagen fibers have a wavy configuration called a **crimp**. Similar to a wrinkled shirt, when collagen fibers are stretched, the crimp disappears. Collagen fibers bundle to create successively larger bundles that ultimately constitute the tendon or ligament.

In a tendon, bundles of collagen fibers are enclosed in loose connective tissue sheaths called **endotenons** (see Fig. 2–14). These sheaths enclose the nerves, lymphatic vessels, and blood vessels supplying the tendon and include cross-links to adjacent fibers.[46] The **epitenon** encircles the tendon as a whole and is connected to the endotenon on its inferior surface. Many tendons are also covered by a **paratenon** on its outermost layer. For additional protection, tendons that wrap around bones and are those without a paratenon are covered by a tendon sheath with a synovial lining that interfaces with the tendon to reduce friction.[27]

Elastin is also found in many connective tissues but, unlike collagen, the molecule consists of single alpha-like strands without a triple helix.[11] The alpha-like strands are cross-linked to each other to form rubberlike elastic fibers **(Fig. 2–15)**. Each elastin molecule uncoils into a more extended formation when the fiber is stretched **(Fig. 2–15A)**, recoiling spontaneously when the stretching force is removed **(Fig. 2–15B)**. Elastin fibers branch freely and are found in all joint structures including the skin, the tracheobronchial tree, and the walls of arteries. Elastin fibers typically are a much smaller component of the extracellular matrix than collagen fibers. As one might expect, tissues that require "give" contain more elastin. The aorta contains approximately 30% elastin and 20% collagen (percentage of the tissue dry weight), the ligamentum nuchae of the cervical spine has 75% elastin and 15% collagen, whereas the Achilles tendon contains only 4.4% elastin and 86% collagen.

INTERFIBRILLAR COMPONENT OF THE ECM

The interfibrillar component of connective tissue, often referred to as the ground substance, contains primarily water and proteins called **proteoglycans (PGs)** with attached **glycosaminoglycans (GAGs)**.[50-52] A PG can contain up to approximately 100 GAGs, which extend from its protein core forming a shape like a bottle brush.[53,54] Hyaluronan is a GAG that does not attach to a protein core but exists either as a free GAG chain of variable length (e.g., in a tendon or ligament) or a core molecule to which large numbers of PGs are attached (e.g., in cartilage) **(Fig. 2–16)**.

One large cartilage PG is called **aggrecan.** As shown in Figure 2-16, the protein core of aggrecan has GAGs (such as

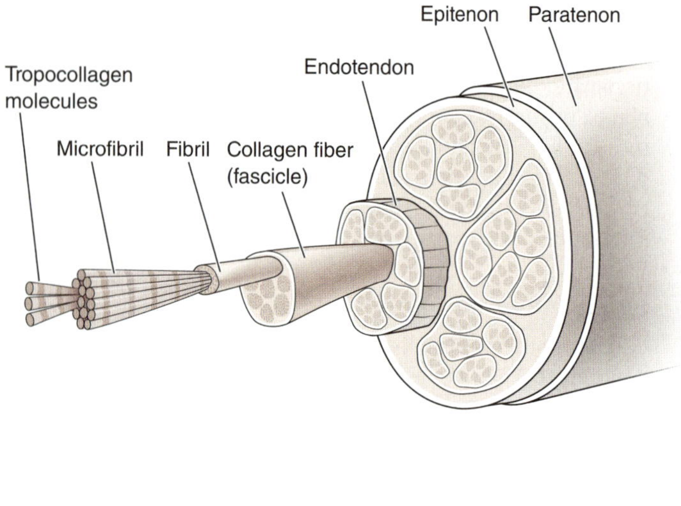

Figure 2–14 Dense connective tissues, using the tendon as an example here, have a hierarchical structure beginning with the tropocollagen molecule (left) and building to the composed tissue (right), with successive bundles enclosed in an endotendon sheath and, ultimately, the epitenon or paratenon.

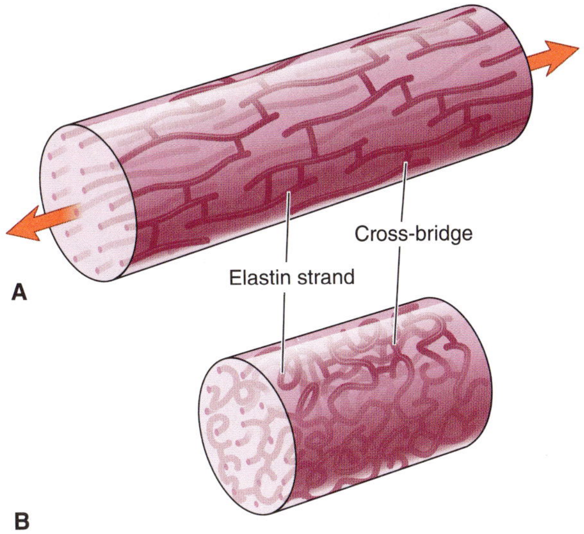

Figure 2–15 **A.** When an elastin fiber is under tension (stretched), the strands straighten out and the fiber lengthens, with the length limited in part by cross-linking of the strands. **B.** When tension on the elastin fiber is released, the strands recoil, and the elastin fiber shortens.

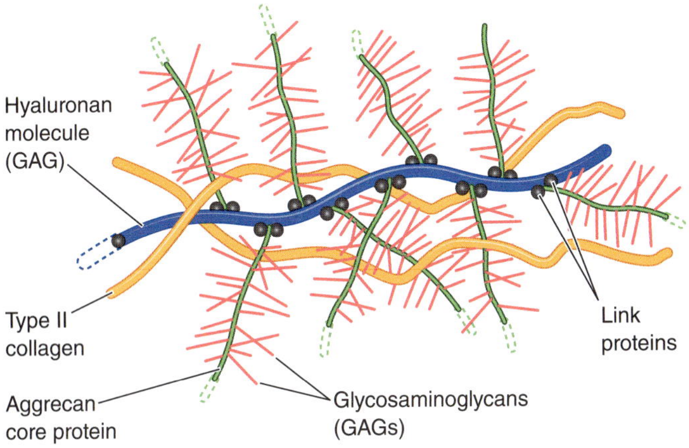

Figure 2–16 The extracellular matrix of articular cartilage includes the large aggrecan proteoglycan (in green) with glycosaminoglycans (GAGs) (in red) attached to its protein core. The aggrecan protein core is stabilized on the hyaluronan filament (in blue) by link proteins (in black). These interfibrillar components will lie between, in this example, type II collagen fibers (in orange).

chondroitin sulfate and keratin sulfate) bristling out from its length; the protein core attaches to a hyaluronan chain via separate link proteins.[53] These large hydrophilic aggregates of PGs, with their attached GAGs, are largely responsible for the water-binding that characterizes the extracellular matrix of cartilage and gives articular cartilage the ability to withstand compression. Some of the GAGs associated with articular cartilage (hyaluronan, chondroitin sulfate, and glucosamine) are used as injectables or supplements to treat osteoarthritis, although their efficacy remains unproven.[55]

The PGs in the extracellular matrix of a connective tissue (bone, cartilage, tendon, or ligament) affect its hydration through their attached GAGs.[54] The GAG chains attract water into the interfibrillar matrix, creating a tensile stress on the surrounding fibrillar collagen network, much like filling up a water balloon. The collagen fibers resist and contain the swelling, thus increasing the rigidity of the extracellular matrix. This increased rigidity allows the tissue to resist compressive forces. The PGs also form a reservoir for nutrients and growth factors that may play a role in directing or limiting the size of collagen fibers. The amount and type of PGs in a tissue is another example of the form/function interaction of connective tissues because tissues that are subjected to high compressive forces (like cartilage) have more PGs and different GAGs than tissues that resist tensile forces.[38,39] Table 2–2 provides a synopsis of the variations in extracellular composition found in connective tissues associated with synovial joints.

Foundational Concepts 2–6
Connective Tissue Composition

Whether a connective tissue is bone, cartilage, or dense connective tissue such as a tendon or ligament is determined by its cellular and extracellular composition. Cellular composition may shift depending on the demands placed on the tissue (form/function interaction):

- Cells
  - Fibroblasts/cytes: the basic cell forms that can differentiate into other cell types and are the predominant cell in ligaments; fibroblasts produce the extracellular matrix
  - Tenoblasts/cytes: found in tendons
  - Chondroblasts/cytes: found in cartilage
  - Osteoblasts/cytes: found in bone
- Extracellular matrix
  - Interfibrillar components: water, PGs, and GAGs
  - Fibrillar components: collagen (mainly type I or II) and elastin

Specific Connective Tissue Composition

The following sections provide brief overviews of the more distinguishing elements in the composition of connective tissue structures that are associated with synovial joints.

Ligaments

Ligaments are heterogeneous structures containing only a small number of cells (about 10% to 20% of the tissue volume, primarily as fibroblasts) and a large amount of extracellular matrix (about 80% to 90% of tissue volume). In most ligaments, the fibrillar component of the extracellular matrix is composed mainly of type I collagen with varying amounts of elastin. One notable exception is the ligamentum flavum of the spine, which has a distinctly yellowish color and contains a large amount of elastin (75% of the tissue's dry weight).[11] The type I collagen fibrils in ligaments are densely packed with a relatively low concentration of interfibrillar proteoglycans. Most ligaments have a similar hierarchical structure to that of tendons[56] (see Fig. 2–14), with fiber bundles arranged in line with the applied tensile forces. The arrangement of the collagen fibers and the collagen/elastin fiber ratio varies among ligaments, depending on the relative abilities of these structures to meet or respond to changing stability and mobility needs of a particular joint.

Table 2–2 Composition of Extracellular Matrix for Selected Connective Tissues

TISSUE	WATER CONTENT*	COLLAGEN†	PG/GAG†	COMMENT
Bone	25%	25%–30% Mainly type I	Mainly CS	65%–70% dry weight is inorganic
Cartilage	60%–85%	10%–30% >90% type II	8%–10% aggregating PGs	Cells are 10% of total weight
Ligament	70%	75% 90% type I Mainly DS 10% type III	<1% Mainly DS	20% dry weight unknown
Tendon	60%–75%	80% 95% type I <5% type III	0.2%–1% Mainly DS	More linear collagen fibrils than a ligament contains
Capsule	70%	90% Mainly type I	CS, DS	Some elastin
Menisci	70%–78%	60%–90% Mainly type I	<10%	Fibrocartilage
Anulus of IV disc	65%–70%	50%–60% Types I and II	20% CS, KS	
Nucleus of IV disc	65%–90%	20%–30% Mainly type II	65% aggregating PGs	

*Water content is percentage of total tissue weight.

†Collagen and PG content is percentage of tissue dry weight after water has been removed.

CS, chondroitin sulfate (associated with compressive stresses); DS, dermatan sulfate (associated with tensile stresses); GAG, glycosaminoglycan; KS, keratan sulfate (common in cartilage); PG, proteoglycan; IV, intervertebral.

Ligaments are subjected to varying directions of tensile forces depending on the joint angle, so the collagen fibers in ligaments run in many directions—enabling the ligament to resist forces in more than one direction. For example, the posterior fibers of the medial collateral ligament of the knee may be stressed by extension, while the middle fibers are under tension when a varus stress is applied to the knee joint.

The appearance and composition of ligaments change near their **entheses** where the ligament attaches to bone. Ligaments may insert directly into bone via fibrocartilage or indirectly via fibrous attachments.[57] With fibrous attachments, the collagen fibers blend into the **periosteum** of the bone, which is in turn attached to the underlying cortical bone via **Sharpey's fibers.** These fibrous attachments of a ligament to bone have been likened to trees that are rooted in the ground, with Sharpey's fibers serving as the "roots" for the ligament (as well as a tendon). The stiffening of the ligament-bone interface at direct fibrocartilage insertions decreases the likelihood that the ligament will give way at the enthesis; however, it is a common site for degenerative change, usually in the underlying bone.[57-59]

Tendons

Tendons and ligaments have a similar composition and basic structure although the cells in tendons are predominantly tenoblasts and tenocytes, with the proportions and organization of the components of a tendon's extracellular matrix differing slightly from that of a ligament.[52] A tendon's collagen is 95% type I collagen, with type III in the tendon sheaths.[44,59] Tendons contain slightly more type I collagen and slightly less type III collagen than ligaments (see Table 2–2). The increased type I collagen in tendons (compared with ligaments) is thought to be an adaptation to larger tensile forces because type I collagen is considered stronger than type III collagen.[44]

The collagen fibrils of the tendon form successively larger bundles surrounded by sheaths as described in Figure 2–14.[48] The loose connective tissue sheath of the endotenon contains mostly type III collagen fibrils and encloses the nerves, lymphatic vessels, and blood vessels that supply the tendon.[44] Each fascicle of the tendon is associated with a discrete group of muscle fibers or motor units at the muscle-tendon junction.[60,61] Several fascicles may form a larger bundle that also is enclosed in the endotenon. The epitenon sheath encloses the entire tendon. The paratenon is a double-layered sheath of areolar tissue that is loosely attached to the outer surface of the epitenon. The epitenon and paratenon together are sometimes called the **peritendon.** The peritendon may become a synovium-lined sheath called the **tenosynovium** (or **tendon sheath**) in tendons that are subjected to high levels of friction such as where tendons pass over bony prominences or through fibrous tunnels. The paratenon protects the tendon by allowing it to freely slide past adjacent structures, and provides a source of replacement cells if the tendon is injured. The tensile forces on tendons are created by a muscle's contractile force. In contrast to ligaments, forces in tendons tend to be applied in primarily one direction, so the collagen fibers in tendons are straighter and more parallel. The tendon attaches to bone at one end and to the muscle at the other, each with unique attachment structures.

Tendons, like ligaments, can attach to bone in one of two ways: either a fibrocartilaginous or a fibrous enthesis.[57] The fibrocartilaginous attachment of tendon to bone involves gradual changes in the tendon structure over a length of about

1 mm, divided into four zones based on histological observation (Fig. 2–17).[57] The first zone of the enthesis consists of tendon proper that is continuous with the midsubstance of the tendon. The second zone contains uncalcified fibrocartilage and marks the beginning of the transition from tendon to bone. The third zone contains calcified fibrocartilage, and the fourth zone is bone. The changes in tissue are gradual and continuous, presumably to aid in effective load transfer between the very different tendon and bone materials. A **tidemark** frequently appears between the calcified and uncalcified parts of the enthesis, representing the boundary between hard and soft tissues; however, the tidemark is not an absolute line of demarcation. Dramatic changes in connective tissue composition occur in the different zones, suggesting that the tendon insertion is subjected to both compressive and tensile forces.

The fibrous entheses may be further divided into two categories: periosteal and bony.[57,58] At the periosteal enthesis, the tendon fibers attach to the periosteum, which provides an indirect attachment of tendon to bone. With bony entheses, the tendon attaches directly to the bone. There can be a mixture of the two types of attachment, with periosteal attachments sometimes converting to bony attachments with age. Examples of these mixed attachments include the attachments of the deltoid muscle to the humerus, scapula, and clavicle. When a tendon is surgically reattached to a bone the new enthesis initially will be fibrous, although a fibrocartilage attachment may form over time.[57]

At its opposite end, a tendon attaches to its muscle at the **myotendinous junction (MTJ)** via highly folded membranes where the muscle fibers interdigitate with the tendon[60,61] (Fig. 2–18). There are direct connections between the muscle fiber cell membrane and the fibroblasts, PGs, and collagen of the tendon. The endotenon and epitenon of the tendon blend into the endomysium and epimysium of the muscle, respectively, forming a meshwork of connective tissue around the muscle fibers. The interdigitating configuration of the musculotendinous junction is essential for normal function of the musculotendinous unit that is very sensitive to mechanical conditions and tends to become flatter and less infolded when loads are decreased. Decreased stresses on a tendon weakens the junction and may make the junction more susceptible to injury. Thus, when muscle and tendon loading begins after a period of immobilization, loads should begin at a lower level and progress gradually to reduce risk of injury.

Foundational Concepts 2–7
Tendon and Ligament Connective Tissues

- Contain mostly type I collagen that has the greatest tensile strength of any collagen types
- Reflect the stresses placed on them through alignment of collagen, with tendons having a more parallel alignment from linear muscle pulls than ligaments that may be required to resist stresses in multiple directions at the joint
- Have collagen that is organized in a hierarchical structure that aligns with the applied forces to accommodate the high tensile forces experienced by these tissues
- Attach to bone through a gradual transition in tissue composition that "diffuses" the load at the tissue-bone interface, perhaps helping prevent injury[57]
- Have attachment sites that are highly sensitive to changes in loading, especially declines in loading

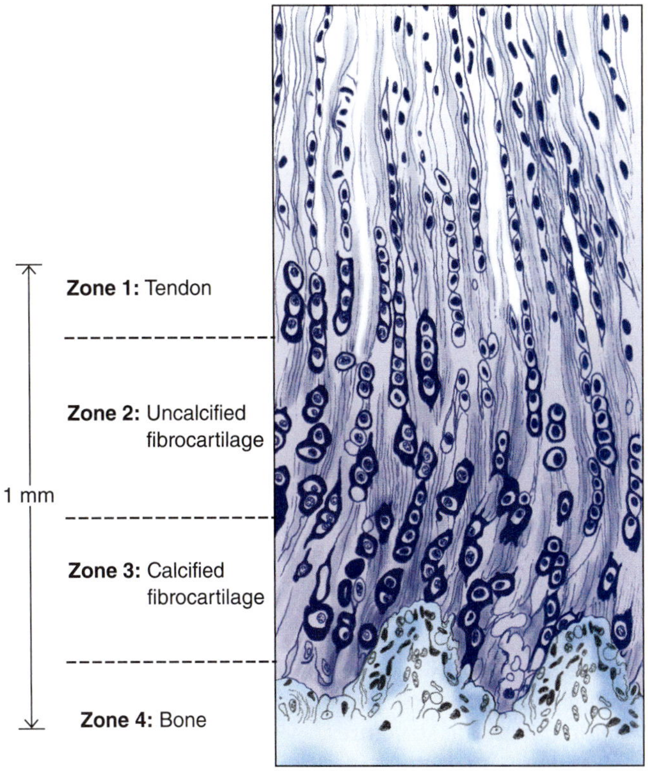

Figure 2–17 The bone-tendon fibrocartilaginous junction. There are four zones, from pure tendon (zone 1) to bone (zone 4). In between zones 1 and 4, the material gradually transitions from fibrocartilage (zone 2) to mineralized fibrocartilage (zone 3).

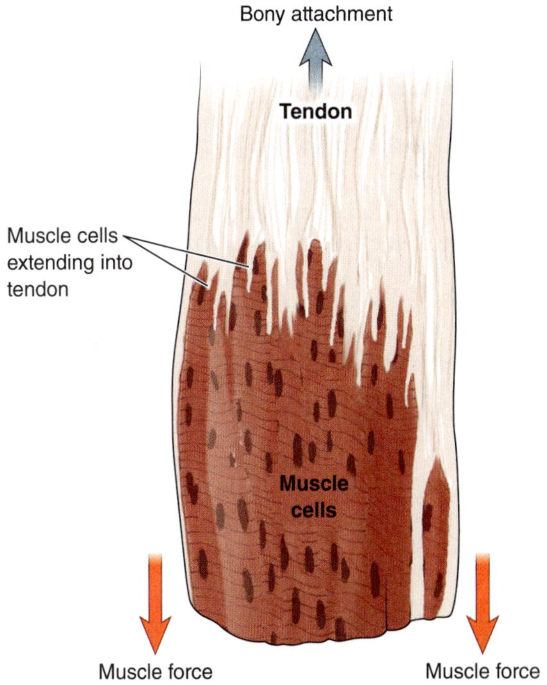

Figure 2–18 The musculotendinous junction. The muscle cells interdigitate with the tendon.

Cartilage

Cartilage is usually divided into the following types: fibrocartilage, hyaline (articular) cartilage, and elastic cartilage.[62] Hyaline cartilage lines the articulating ends of bones and is one of the distinguishing features of a synovial joint. Fibrocartilage forms the bonding material in many cartilaginous joints, such as at the interbody articulations in the spine and the costosternal joints. Fibrocartilage may also be present in some synovial joints in forms such as intraarticular discs or plates. Elastic cartilage is found in the ears and epiglottis and has more elastin than fibrocartilage.[62] Elastic cartilage will not be discussed further because it does not occur in or around joints.

HYALINE CARTILAGE

Hyaline (articular) cartilage composition includes chondroblast and the more mature chondrocyte cells, and has an extracellular matrix with much more interfibrillar material than that of tendons and ligaments.[63] The chondroblasts produce collagen, PGs (mainly aggrecan), and GAGs, all of which are extruded into the extracellular matrix. The fibrillar component of the extracellular matrix includes some elastin and other types of collagen, but type II collagen accounts for about 90% to 95% of the hyaline collagen content.[63] Collagen is dispersed throughout the interfibrillar component of the extracellular matrix,[51] forming a meshwork that surrounds and compresses the PGs and their attached water molecules.[51,63] Hyaline (articular) cartilage contains much more PG content than do other joint structures.

Three distinct layers (zones) of articular cartilage are found on the ends of the bony components of synovial joints[64] **(Fig. 2–19)**. In the outermost layer (zone 1: tangential zone), type II collagen fibers are arranged parallel (tangential) to the joint surface. This layer faces the joint cavity that lies within the joint capsule. This smooth outer layer helps reduce friction between opposing joint surfaces and distributes forces across the joint surfaces. In the next layer (zone 2: middle or transitional zone), type II collagen fibers form an open meshwork. The collagen network keeps the interfibrillar PG and water contained, giving the cartilage its ability to absorb compressive forces. In the third layer (zone 3: radial zone), collagen fibers lie perpendicularly (radially) to the bony surface, crossing the interface between uncalcified and calcified cartilage to establish a secure hold in the calcified cartilage.[30,51] The calcified layer of cartilage, sometimes referred to as the fourth zone, lies adjacent to subchondral bone and anchors the cartilage securely to the bone.[63] This calcified layer is impervious, limiting the ability of nutrients to cross into the cartilage from the vascular bone underlying it.[65] The interface between the calcified and uncalcified cartilage is the tidemark[62,63]—similar to that found between the calcified and uncalcified areas in the fibrocartilaginous connection of tendon to bone.

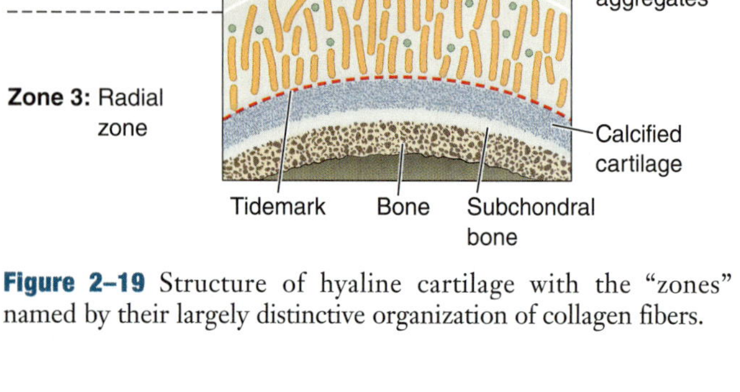

Figure 2–19 Structure of hyaline cartilage with the "zones" named by their largely distinctive organization of collagen fibers.

Hyaline cartilage is thought to have virtually no cellular turnover, based on the facts that the tissue: (1) is hypocellular and avascular; (2) relies on diffusion for its nutrient supply; and (3) contains only tenocyte and tenoblast cells that cannot de-differentiate. Normally, replacement of the calcified layer of articular cartilage with bone occurs by **endochondral ossification.** The calcification front advances toward the noncalcified area of cartilage slowly, in equilibrium with the rates of absorption of calcified cartilage and, perhaps, new extracellular matrix formation by cells.[66,67] In aging, the balance changes as deeper layers of cartilage (e.g., zone 3) are gradually replaced with bone, resulting in cartilage thinning more superficially. In injuries that involve microfractures to the subchondral bone, a secondary ossification center in the bone may be activated to produce new bone growth, which expands into the calcified layer of cartilage, advancing the tidemark and thinning the noncalcified layer.[68]

The design of articular cartilage is a remarkable example of the interaction between form and function. Aggregating PGs attract a large volume of water, creating an osmotic swelling pressure in the cartilage.[69] With compression of the articular cartilage (e.g., in weight-bearing), swelling pressure creates tension in the hoops of the collagen network, which in turn creates an opposing force that keeps the PGs and water contained; when the swelling pressure and load on the joint reach equilibrium, the articular cartilage deformation stops.[70] Cartilage resistance to compressive forces thus depends on two features: (1) a large volume of aggregating PGs, and (2) an intact collagen network. During joint motion, or when the cartilage is compressed, some of the fluid content of the cartilage exudes into the joint space through pores in the outermost collagen layer (zone 1).[69-71] The fluid then flows back into the cartilage after the compressive load is removed, carrying nutrients from synovial fluid in the joint space to support the chondrocytes. Because hyaline cartilage is devoid of blood vessels, its nourishment is derived solely from this synovial flow of fluid. Thus, the free flow of fluid is essential for the survival of hyaline cartilage.

Fluid flow in cartilage is affected by the magnitude and duration of an applied force.[71] If the force is either excessive or sustained over a long period, the lack of compression and release reduces fluid flow.[69] Diminished flow also occurs with decreased loading. Hyaline cartilage can thus undergo degenerative changes due to inadequate nutrition as fluid flow is diminished after either prolonged loading or unloading.[72] Cartilage health thus appears to depend on alternating cycles of moderate compressive forces.[73]

Damage to the superficial collagen layer of articular cartilage through excessive frictional forces or trauma can damage the meshwork that resists the swelling pressure of the PGs. Initially, the articular cartilage swells and becomes thicker as the PGs attract more water without the opposing force of the now-damaged superficial collagen network.[74] Eventually, fluid movement slows, reducing both cell nutrition and the ability to synthesize new extracellular matrix. Without the containment of the superficial collagen meshwork, PGs begin to escape into the synovial fluid, gradually eroding and thinning the cartilage. This is the sequence that occurs during the development of osteoarthritis.[74]

FIBROCARTILAGE

Fibrocartilage composition is different from that of hyaline cartilage. The cellular composition includes fibroblasts, fibrocytes, and, on occasion, fibrochondrocytes. When compared with hyaline cartilage, fibrocartilage has a smaller percentage of water and proteoglycans, with a greater percentage of collagen. Type I collagen is more prevalent in fibrocartilage, although type II collagen is present,. The density of these collagen fibers helps trap and retain water. Fibrocartilage primarily uses collagen structure to keep water in the tissue, whereas hyaline cartilage utilizes structure and chemical attraction of the PGs.[75]

Collagen fiber organization has been described as varying across regions in fibrocartilage and is thought to be related to the function of the region. For example, collagen fibers are randomly aligned in the superficial layer of the meniscus of the knee and circumferentially arranged in the deep zone; radially-oriented fibers are observed throughout the deep zone and on the periphery.[75] Tension in the circumferential fibers resists the deformation caused by compression of the cartilage, and radial fibers are thought to prevent longitudinal splitting of the circumferential fibers.[76]

Whereas fibrocartilage has some blood supply (unlike hyaline cartilage), vascularity is still limited. Blood supply to fibrocartilage is typically found only in more peripheral regions that lie adjacent to the attachments of the vascularized joint capsule.[26,75] Therefore, diffusion through loading, as occurs in hyaline cartilage, is still necessary for exchange of nutrients and waste products for much of the fibrocartilaginous structure.

Patient Application 2–5

Katie is a 17-year-old soccer player who tore the medial meniscus in her knee. After 5 weeks of physical therapy, she continues to have pain, swelling, and some catching as she flexes her knee. With continuing symptoms, Katie discusses surgical options with her doctor. Katie is told that repairing the meniscus is possible, but is only feasible if the tear is in the periphery of the meniscus where there is a blood supply. If the tear is into the center portion of the meniscus, surgery carries more risks. The central portion of the meniscus has no blood supply, which is needed for the meniscus to heal. The surgeon would therefore have to remove, rather than repair, a portion of a centrally-torn meniscus. The meniscus normally dissipates some of the weight-bearing load on the articular cartilage of the knee (especially the flatter tibial plateau); removal of a portion of the meniscus could increase load as well as deformation of the articular cartilage, reducing fluid flow through the avascular articular cartilage and putting Katie's knee at risk for osteoarthritic changes over time. Consequently, surgery is only recommended if the meniscal tear is isolated to the outer portion of the meniscus, where repair and healing of this slightly vascularized portion may be feasible.

Foundational Concepts 2–8
Cartilage

- Hyaline (articular) cartilage contains mostly type II collagen as well as an extracellular matrix with a relatively high proportion of PGs and water, both contributing to resistance to compressive forces.
- Fibrocartilage typically contains both type I and II collagen, indicating that the tissue is undergoing both compressive and tensile stresses.
- Hyaline cartilage is completely avascular; fibrocartilage has a limited blood supply that is restricted to areas that are adjacent to the synovial capsule.
- Avascular hyaline cartilage and any portion of fibrocartilage with limited or no vascularity depend on synovial fluid exchange to supply nutrients and remove waste through application and removal of compression.

Bone

Bone is the hardest of all the connective tissues. The extracellular matrix is composed of organic fibers, mainly type I collagen, and inorganic mineral crystals, primarily **hydroxyapatite,** that fill in around the fibers.[11,30] The organic material gives bone its flexibility and tensile strength, whereas the inorganic material gives bone its compressive strength.[77] The cellular composition of bone includes fibroblasts, osteoblasts, osteocytes, osteoclasts, and progenitor cells that can differentiate into osteoblasts. The fibroblasts produce type I collagen and other extracellular matrix components. The osteoblasts are the primary bone-forming cells that are responsible for the synthesis of bone and its deposition of inorganic materials and mineralization. Osteoblasts also secrete **procollagen** (the precursor of type I collagen) into the surrounding matrix. Osteoclasts, large monocyte-derived polymorphous cells, are responsible for bone resorption. The balance between bone formation and resorption is tightly regulated by nutrition, hormonal influences, and mechanical loading.[77]

Bone is organized into two types: a dense type that typically forms the bone's outer shell, and a spongier type found in the inner portion of bone.[30] The spongy bone is called **cancellous** (also **trabecular** or **spongy**) **bone;** the outer shell is called **compact** (also **cortical**) **bone** **(Fig. 2–20).** In cancellous bone, the calcified tissue forms thin plates called **trabeculae** that are laid down in line with stresses placed on the bone. It has been suggested that the loading history of the trabeculae, including loading from multiple directions, influences the distribution of bone density and trabecular orientation.[78] Increases in bone density in some areas and decreases in density in other areas occur in response to the loads placed on the bone.[79] The cancellous bone is covered by a layer of dense, compact cortical bone organized in concentric layers. The relative percentage of cortical versus trabecular bone, and the areas in which those bone types form, provide specific bones with varying degrees of mechanical resistance, and account for variations in density.

Expanded Concepts 2–1
Strength of Bone

The compressive strength of compact bone is about 250 megapascals (MPa), greater than that of concrete (approximately 4 MPa) or wood (100 MPa), but less than that of steel (400 to 1,500 MPa). Bone is about as strong as cast iron (140 to 300 MPa) but weighs much less. Bone is not as strong in tension as it is in compression, with its strength dependent on density (mineralization) as well as the orientation of the trabeculae in relation to the load. If the load is applied along the long axis of the bone, the bone is much stronger.

The periosteum (see Fig. 2-20) is a fibrous layer that covers the entire surface of each bone, except for the articular surface. Collagen fibers from ligaments and tendons blend into the periosteum, and Sharpey's fibers from attaching tendons and ligaments pass from the periosteum to deeper layers of bone. The periosteum houses cells that are precursors to osteoblasts and osteoclasts and includes many capillaries that provide nourishment. The periosteum thus acts as a reservoir for the cells needed for growth and repair. If the periosteum and underlying bone are damaged by trauma or surgery, the healing capacity of the bone will be decreased.

At the microscopic level, both cortical and cancellous bone have two distinct types of bone architecture: **woven bone** and **lamellar bone.** In woven (primary) bone, collagen fibers are irregularly arranged to form a pattern of alternating coarse and fine fibers that resemble woven material. Woven bone is young bone and is formed rapidly without an underlying framework. It is often found in newborns, fracture calluses, and metaphyseal regions of long bones. Lamellar bone requires an extracellular matrix framework to form, is organized into parallel layers, and is the older bone that constitutes most of the adult skeleton.

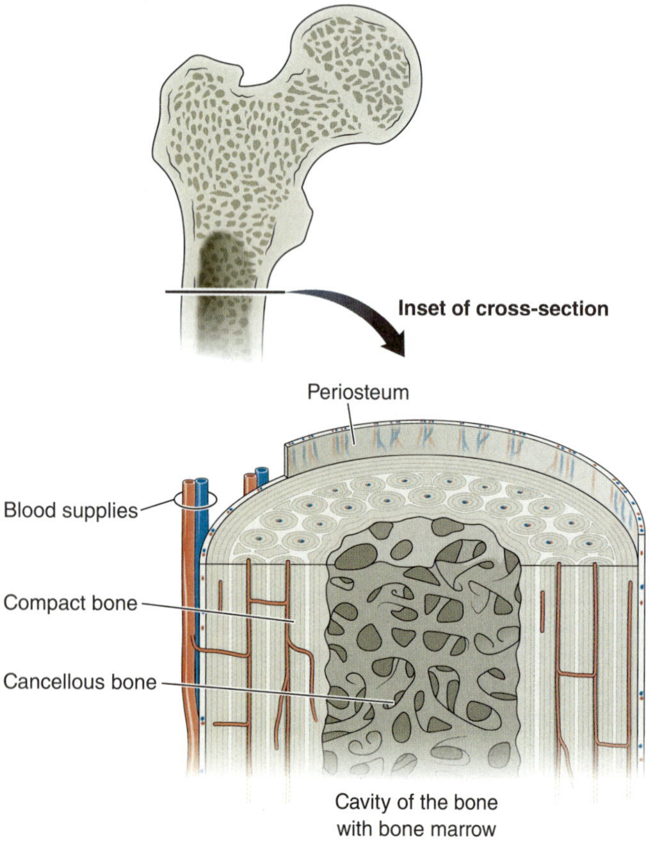

Figure 2–20 Using the femur to represent a typical long bone, a cross-section of the shaft of the femur is shown (inset). The dense outer layer of compact (cortical) bone surrounds the core of cancellous bone with its trabecular plates. The entire outer surface of the bone (exclusive of articular surfaces) is surrounded by a thin fibrous periosteum that carries the blood vessels to and from the bone.

Bone is dynamic and remodels throughout life as it responds to changes in forces, such as an increased pull of tendons with strengthening, changes in body weight, or change in stresses from new activities.[80] As noted earlier in the chapter, the change in bone shape and form to match function is known as Wolff's law. The application of new or increased forces causes osteoblast activity to increase, and as a result, bone mass increases. With reduction of usual forces, osteoclast activity predominates and bone mass decreases. Internal influences, such as aging, nutritional status, metabolic processes, and disease, among others, also may affect bone remodeling because bone is interdependent with both physiological and mechanical functions.[77,81]

An imbalance between bone synthesis and resorption, in which osteoclasts break down or absorb the bone at a faster rate than the osteoblasts can remodel or rebuild the bone, results in a condition called **osteoporosis.**[82] In osteoporosis, bones have decreased mineral density (mass per unit volume) compared with normal bone and thus are weaker and more susceptible to fracture. **Osteopenia** is considered an earlier stage of decreased bone mineralization whereby osteocytes can still synthesize other elements of the extracellular matrix. Bones that have been immobilized are frequently osteopenic.

Patient Application 2–6

June Sabato was diagnosed with multiple sclerosis at age 56. During a recent exacerbation of her symptoms, her physician placed her temporarily on glucocorticoids, a type of steroid, to decrease her symptoms. June's symptoms subsided with the steroids, and June wondered why the doctor did not give her a prescription for regular use. Her doctor explained that steroids affect the cells responsible for bone health and could make her osteoporotic. If a drug impairs osteoblast function and increases osteoclast formation, as a steroid can do, the balance between bone formation and degradation results in greater bone degradation and weaker bones that are at risk for fracture.[81]

Expanded Concepts 2–2

In Vitro Tissue Growth

Connective tissues can be grown under laboratory conditions for later implantation to replace damaged tissues. For example, new chondrocytes can be grown and later injected into areas of cartilage degeneration (autologous cartilage implantation).[83] The starting point is fibroblasts (often taken from damaged cartilage that can be regrown in vitro), usually seeded in some sort of extracellular mesh or scaffold.

Behavioral Properties of Connective Tissue

Homogeneous materials such as steel display the same mechanical behavior no matter the direction in which forces are applied and are called **isotropic** materials. In contrast, heterogeneous materials, such as connective tissues, behave differently depending on the size and direction of applied forces and are called **anisotropic.** Connective tissues are called *heterogeneous* because they are composed of a mixture of different solid and semisolid components. The behavior of the tissue therefore depends on the properties of the different components, the varying proportions of each component in the structure, and the interactions among these components.[33,34,84]

Structural and Material Properties

Human joint components experience changing forces during ordinary daily activities and must have the ability to withstand these forces to provide support and protection. The mechanical behavior of these components dictates how different structures and tissues provide support. Mechanical behavior is described with respect to both structural and material properties. Structural properties take into consideration such characteristics as the cross-sectional area and length. Material properties provide information about the component properties of the tissue itself.

Load, Force, and Elongation

The term **load** refers to a force or forces applied to a structure. Many examples are discussed in Chapter 1, including the forces exerted by the ankle weight, the leg-press footplate, and gravity on a leg-foot segment. The magnitude, direction, and rate of force application, as well as the size and composition of the tissue, will all affect the tissue's response to load.

When a force acts on an object, it produces a **deformation** (a change in shape). A tensile load produces elongation; a compressive force produces compression. The **load-deformation curve** is the result of plotting the applied load (force) against the deformation, providing information about the strength properties of a particular material or structure.[85-87] The load-deformation curve of connective tissue reflects the **toe, elasticity, plasticity, ultimate strength,** and **stiffness** of the material **(Fig. 2-21)**, as well as the amount of energy (given by the area under the load-deformation curve) that the material can absorb before it fails.

When a load (for example, a tensile force) is first applied to the tissue, it takes very little force for the crimp (waviness or laxity) in the tissue to cause the fibers to straighten out (see the change from Fig. 2-15A to Fig. 2-15B). This is referred to as the **toe region** of the curve. After the fibers straighten out, there is an area where the relationship of the load and deformation is linear; an increase in load will produce a proportional (but not necessarily equal) increase in deformation. This is known as the **elastic region.** The slope of this linear region represents the stiffness of the material (stiffness being the change in length over change in force). The inverse of stiffness is **compliance.** If a large increase in load results in a proportionally small increase in deformation, the slope of the load-deformation curve is steep, with the material exhibiting high stiffness and low compliance. If a relatively small load results in a proportionally large increase in deformation, the slope of the curve is less steep with the material exhibiting low stiffness and high compliance. If loading is confined to the elastic region, the deformation of the material will not be permanent; the structure will return to its original dimensions after the load is removed. At the end of the elastic region, the **yield point** is the beginning of the point in the deformation curve where the material will no longer return to its original state when the load is removed. Although the structure will appear to be intact after the load is removed, the material will not recover its original length or shape; the deformation is permanent. The portion of the load-deformation curve between the yield point and overt tissue failure is the **plastic region.** Any recovery of the original structure in a material deformed into the plastic range probably could only occur through the synthesis and reorganization of new tissue components as occurs in some ligament sprains. If loading continues to deform the tissue through the plastic region, the material will reach the **ultimate failure point.** The load being applied when this point is reached is the **failure load** (e.g., a torn ligament).

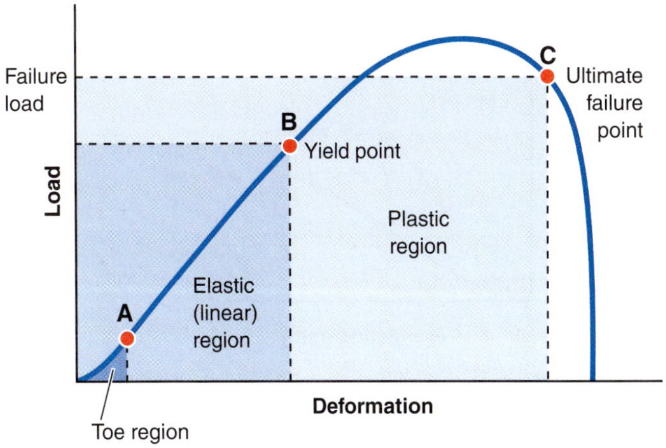

Figure 2–21 Load-deformation curve for a connective tissue tested in tension. Initially, the crimp straightens with application of very little force (toe region). Actual stretching of collagen fibers takes place in the elastic region that is characterized by its linearity (A to B). After the elastic region ends at the yield point (B), further force application causes deformation that results in a residual change in tissue structure (plastic region). Continuation of or increase in load beyond the plastic region may cause the tissue to rupture at its ultimate failure point (C), at which point the material can no longer sustain the load. *(From Butler DL, Grood ES, Noyes FR, et al: Biomechanics of ligaments and tendons. Exerc Sport Sci Rev 6:144, 1978, with permission from Lippincott Williams & Wilkins.)*

Force values on the load-deformation curve depend on both the size of the structure and its composition **(Fig. 2-22)**. A structure with a greater cross-sectional area can withstand more force with less deformation than a structure of the same length with less cross-sectional area **(Fig. 2-22A)**. A longer structure deforms more when a given force is applied than does a shorter structure of similar cross section under the same force **(Fig. 2-22B)**. If two tissues are composed of the same material, the tissue with the greater cross-sectional area will have more tensile strength (stiffness), and the longer tissue will be less stiff. Because the forces and deformations measured during testing are so dependent on the structural features of the tissue (cross-sectional area and length), the load-deformation curve is said to reflect the "structural properties" of the structure being tested. Tensile force is measured in newtons (N), compressive force (pressure) is measured in pascals (Pa), and elongation or compression is measured in units of length such as millimeters (mm) or micrometers (μm).

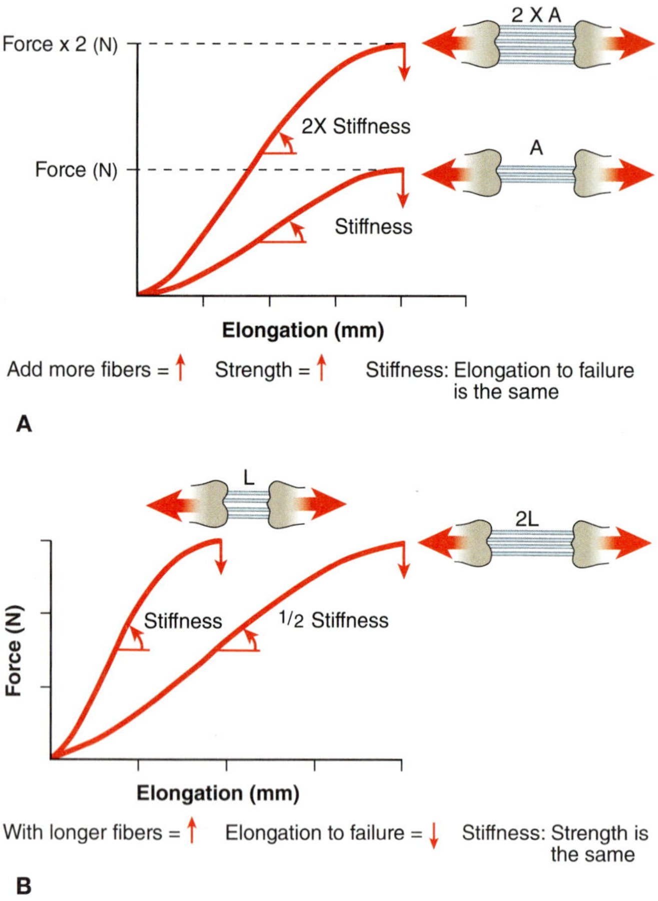

Figure 2–22 Changes to cross-sectional area or length of two similarly composed tissues will affect its overall response to load (force). **A.** Doubling cross-sectional area means that the tissues can withstand more force at any given length before failure (it is stiffer). **B.** Doubling length means that it will elongate farther under the same loading conditions (it is less stiff). Stiffness is reflected by the slope of the linear portion of the curves. *(Adapted from Butler DL, Grood ES, Noyes FR, et al: Biomechanics of ligaments and tendons. Exerc Sport Sci Rev 6:144, 1978, with permission from Lippincott Williams & Wilkins.)*

Stress and Strain

When loads (forces) are applied to a structure or material, there are resulting forces generated within the material that oppose the applied forces. These forces within the material depend on the composition of the material. If we account for the mechanical effect of the tissue structure (cross-sectional area and length), testing can tell us something about the tissue's material properties. We can control for tissue length or cross-sectional area by converting the magnitude of the applied force into a quantity that is independent of tissue size referred to as **stress.** Stress is the force applied to a cross-sectional unit of material, and can be expressed mathematically with the following formula, where F = applied force and A = area:

$$\text{Stress} = F/A$$

Stress is expressed in units of pascals ($P = N/m^2$) or megapascals ($MPa = N/mm^2$). These are the same units used to measure pressure, or force per unit area. However, pressure is produced by a compressive force applied perpendicular to the surface of the material. The percentage change in the length (or cross section) of a structure or material is called **strain.**[88,89] Like stress, strain cannot be measured directly but is calculated mathematically with the following formula, where L1 = original length and L2 = final length:

$$\text{Strain} = (L2 - L1) \div L1$$

Strain is expressed as a percentage and thus has no units.

The type of strain that occurs in human tissue depends on how the load is applied to the tissue **(Fig. 2–23)**. If two forces are applied to a material along the same line but in opposite directions, they create a distractive or tensile load (tensile stress) and cause a tensile strain within the structure or material **(Fig. 2–23A)**.[34,35] If two applied forces act in a line toward each other in the same material, they constitute compressive loading (compressive stress) and cause a compressive strain in the structure **(Fig. 2–23B)**. If two applied forces within a materials are parallel and are applied in opposite directions but are not in-line with one another, they constitute shear loading (shear stress) **(Fig. 2–23C)**. Forces applied perpendicular to the long axis of a structure constitute torsional loading (torsional stress) **(Fig. 2–23D)**. When longitudinal forces are applied to a curved structure such as the femur (slightly curved side to side and front to back), the bending loads create tensile stress on the convex side and compressive stress on the concave side **(Fig. 2–23E)**.[90] Tensile, compressive, shear, and torsional stress may look similar to forces described across the knee joint in Chapter 1. However, in the knee examples, the forces resulted in movement or potential movement at the joint, whereas the stresses described here lie *within* the tissue and may lead to tissue deformation.

The types of stress and strain that develop in human tissues depend on the material, the type of load applied, the point at which the load is applied, the direction and magnitude of the load, and the rate and duration of loading.[90,91] Because stress and strain are independent of length or cross section of the material based on their formulas, the stress-strain curve is said to reflect the **material properties** of the tissue in contrast to the load-deformation curve that reflects the structural properties of the tissue.

A stress-strain curve can be used to compare the strength properties of one material with that of another material or to compare the same tissue under different conditions (e.g., ligaments before and after immobilization). The stress-strain curve contains the same defining points as the load-deformation curve, but the shape of the curve and the amount of stress and strain will vary with the composition of the material **(Fig. 2–24)**. The stiffness of a material under compressive or tensile loading is represented by the slope of the linear portion of the stress-strain curve (elastic region). Stiffness (also known as **Young's modulus** or the **modulus of elasticity**) is found by dividing the change (Δ) in stress by the change (Δ) in strain for any two consecutive sets of points in the elastic range (linear portion) of the curve.

Each material has its own unique stress-strain curve. The stress-strain information for a ligament can be used as an example to better understand the information available in a stress-strain curve shown in Fig. 2–24. A minimal amount of

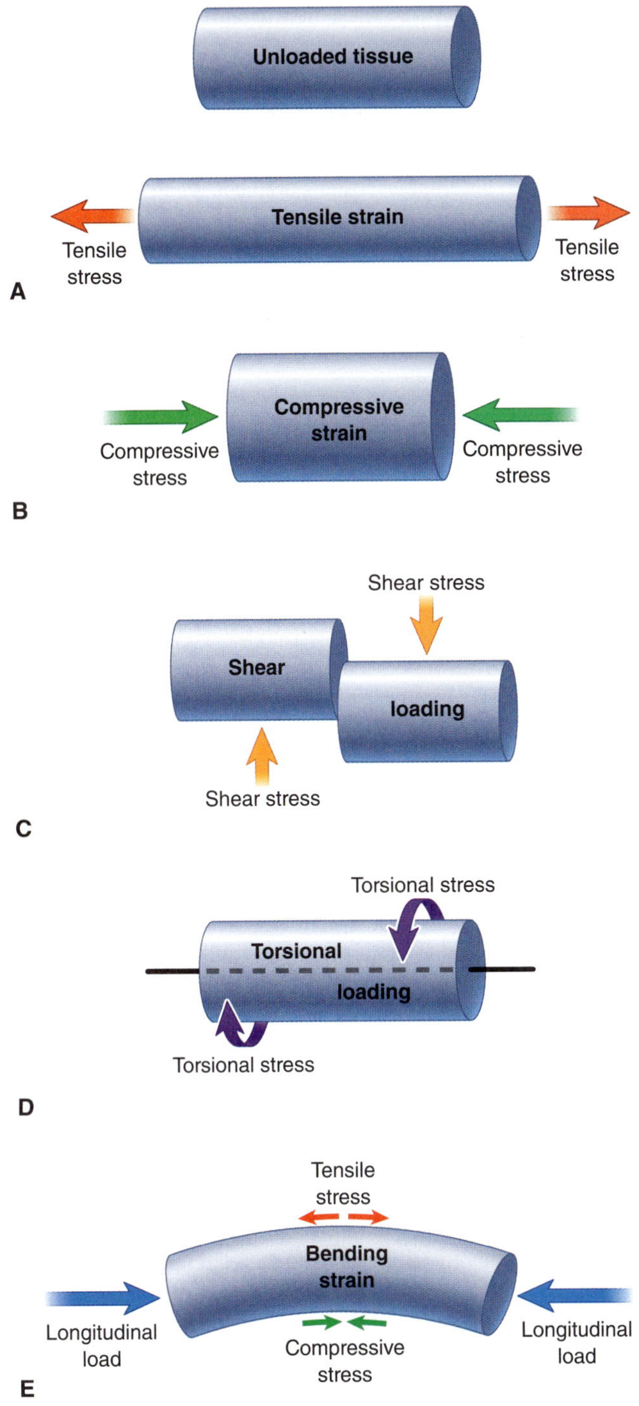

Figure 2–23 The various types of stresses (loads) to which connective tissues can be subjected with resulting deformation (strain). **A.** Tensile stress. **B.** Compressive stress. **C.** Shear loading. **D.** Torsional stress. **E.** Bending stress.

force applied to the ligament produces deformation of the ligament in the toe region; stress is low and the strain (change in length) is typically in the 1% to 2% range. Laboratory tests determine the toe region in a ligament by measuring the force and lengthening of the ligament needed to take up the slack in the ligament's fibrils before the force is transmitted to a bone. In the elastic (linear region) of a stress-strain curve, collagen fibrils are now actually being stretched and are resisting the applied force. The slope of the linear region of the stress-strain curve reflects the type of collagen, the fibril size, and the cross-linking among collagen molecules. When the stress is removed, the ligament will return to its prestressed dimensions, although this return may take some time. Ligamentous stresses that occur with normal activities typically produce up to about 4% strain.[92,93] In the plastic region of a ligament, the failure of collagen fibers (microfailure) begins, after which the ligament is no longer capable of returning to its original length when the force is removed. Clinical examples of microfailure include Grade I and II ligament sprains. Recovery after this level of loading involves aspects of healing such as synthesis of new tissue and cross-linking of collagen molecules to repair the damage. If force continues to be applied beyond the plastic region, the remaining collagen fibrils experience increased stress and rapidly rupture sequentially, creating overt failure (macrofailure) of the tissue. The terms **ultimate stress** and **ultimate strain** describe the stress and strain, respectively, just before the tissue fails. In the case of a ligament or tendon, failure in the middle of the structure by disruption of the connective tissue fibers is called a **rupture**. If the failure occurs at the bony attachment of the ligament or tendon, it is called an **avulsion**. When failure occurs in a bone, it is called a **fracture**. Slow loading rates to failure tend to create avulsions or fractures, whereas fast loading rates to failure create midsubstance tears.

Each type of connective tissue is able to withstand a different percentage of strain before failure. In general, ligaments and tendons are able to deform more than cartilage, and cartilage is able to deform more than bone. However, the total deformation also depends on the size (length, width, or depth) of the structure.

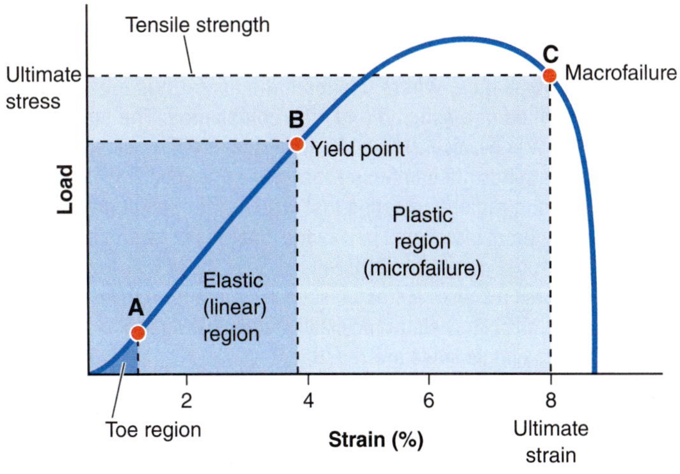

Figure 2–24 An example of a stress-strain curve for collagenous materials. The results are independent of tissue dimensions and thus reflect the material of which the tissue is made. The toe region is the area from initiation of the force to the beginning of fibril stretch, up to about 1% strain (A); the elastic region (A–B) is where there is a proportional (linear) increase in both stress and strain with typical activities causing about 4% strain; and B–C is the plastic region where there is microdamage to (**microfailure** of) the tissue structure. At the point of ultimate stress and strain, the tissue fails completely **(macrofailure)** and the stress in the tissue drops to zero.

Expanded Concepts 2–3

Cortical bone has high stiffness (a high modulus of elasticity) and low compliance, whereas subcutaneous fat has low stiffness (a low modulus of elasticity) and high compliance. The stiffness of cortical bone is between 17 and 25 gigaPascals (GPa), similar to that of wood. As points of comparison, metal (much stiffer than bone) has a steep elastic region indicating that large forces result in relatively little deformation; metal also has a long, flat plastic region indicating that the material deforms extensively at peak loads before failing. In contrast, glass also has a steep elastic region (although not quite as steep as metal) but has almost no plastic region because glass abruptly fails once its elastic limits are reached.[90]

Foundational Concepts 2–9
Ligament Sprains

When a substantial force (stress) is applied to a ligament, the following sequence of events will occur if the force is of sufficient magnitude:

1. The ligament appears to lengthen slightly but there will be no resistance to the increase in length within the tissue (the collagen fibrils are simply straightening out). This is the toe response.
2. The ligament will actually lengthen (collagen fibrils will stretch) because increased stress produces a proportionally greater strain of the ligament. This is an elastic response.
3. Some of the fibers within the ligament will begin to tear, disrupting (among other things) collagen cross-linking. This early plastic response is considered to be a Grade I sprain of the ligament.
4. Further tearing of ligamentous fibers will continue while some continue to remain intact. This response is further into the plastic range, closer to macrofailure, and is considered to be a Grade II sprain of the ligament.
5. The ligament will tear completely (rupture). Macrofailure is considered to be a Grade III sprain of the ligament.

Viscoelasticity

All connective tissues are **viscoelastic** materials; they combine the properties of elasticity and **viscosity,** making their behavior dependent on time, rate, and history.[90,91] The elastic qualities in connective tissues primarily depend on collagen and elastin content and organization and have already been described.

When a material is stretched, positive work is done (work = force × distance) and energy in the stretched material increases. An elastic material stores this energy and readily returns it as negative work so that the stretched elastic material can recoil immediately to its original dimensions. For example, during many functional activities (e.g., walking, running, jumping), the tendon of a lengthening (eccentric) muscle is stretched. the elastic energy stored by the tendon is returned during the subsequent shortening (concentric) contraction of the muscle-tendon unit, thereby contributing to the muscle's ability to generate tension.[92-94]

Viscosity refers to a material's resistance to flow. It is a fluid property and depends on the PG and water composition of the tissue. A tissue with high viscosity will exhibit high resistance to deformation, whereas a less viscous fluid will deform more readily. When forces are applied to viscous materials, the tissues exhibit time-dependent and rate-dependent properties. Viscosity diminishes as temperature rises or loads are slowly applied and increases as pressure increases or loads are rapidly applied.

Expanded Concepts 2–4
Viscosity

Motor oils with different viscosities are used when more or less resistance to deformation is required. When temperatures are high, the oil's resistance will be lower so a more viscous type of oil (10W-30) may be used to maintain lubrication. During the cold of winter, a less viscous oil (5W-30) will still allow the oil to deform (flow, in this case) more readily and coat the engine surfaces.

Time-Dependent and Rate-Dependent Properties

Viscoelastic materials are capable of undergoing a change in shape with application of deforming forces and returning to their original state after removal of the force. However, it is their viscous quality that accounts for the continued deformation after the elastic response of a material under a sustained load, and for the unloaded material to return to its original shape after an initial recoil (time-dependent change in shape). A viscoelastic material possesses characteristics of **creep, stress-relaxation,** and **strain-rate sensitivity** **(Fig. 2–25)**.[91]

Creep

If a force is applied to a viscoelastic tissue, there will be an immediate elastic response; if that same force is maintained after the immediate change in shape, the deformation of the material will gradually continue. This tissue response is known as *creep*. For example, if you hang a weight on the end of an elastic band, you will get an immediate elastic deformation. However, it will also gradually elongate further over time as the weight hangs. Connective tissues also will gradually creep (continue elongation) after an initial elastic response to a constant (e.g., tensile) load and then gradually return to the tissues' original length after the load is removed (recovery). Creep may apply to stretching a shortened tissue in a clinical setting where the clinician maintains a constant force on a tissue while the tissue gradually elongates. For cartilage and bone, compressive loading is used to test creep; the depth of indentation in the material over time is measured as well as the time to recovery once the load is removed **(Fig. 2–25A)**.

Stress-Relaxation

If a viscoelastic tissue is stretched to a fixed length (constant strain), the force (stress) required to maintain that length will decrease over time **(Fig. 2–25B)**. This is called **stress-relaxation.** In a clinical setting, a therapist may perceive this as a reduced resistance to stretch (less force is required to maintain the same tissue length).

Strain-Rate Sensitivity

Most viscoelastic tissues behave differently if loaded rapidly versus slowly, which is called **strain-rate sensitivity.**[95] When a load is applied rapidly, the tissue is stiffer and a larger force is needed to deform the tissue than if the load was applied slowly **(Fig. 2–25C)**. Creep and stress-relaxation also will be greater under conditions of rapid loading.

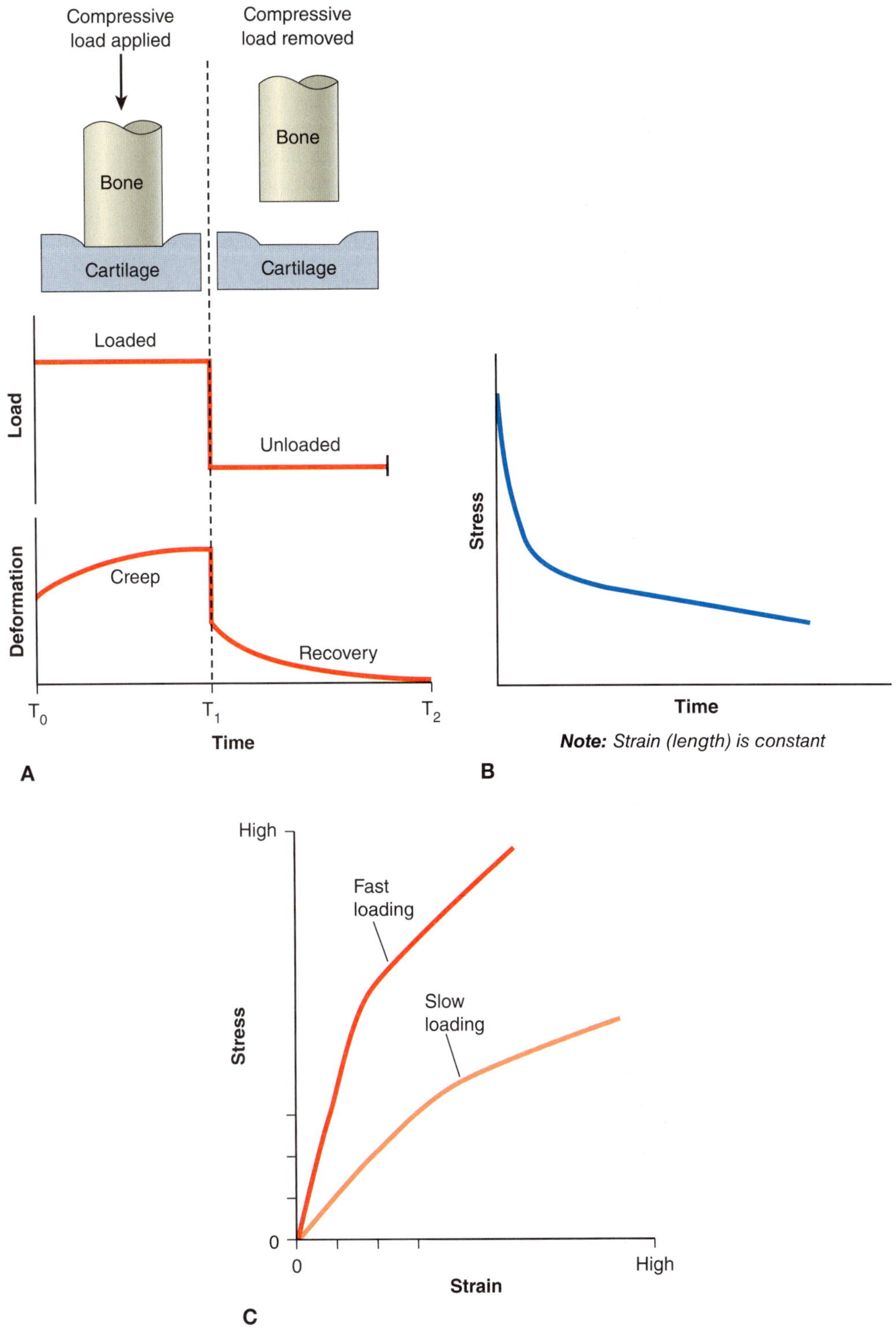

Figure 2–25 Time- and rate-dependent properties of dense connective tissues. **A.** *Creep:* When a connective tissue (e.g., articular cartilage) is loaded with a fixed force (e.g., bony compression within the joint), the original indentation in the cartilage increases as the load is sustained over time (T_0 to T_1); when the load is removed (T_1), the tissue gradually recovers its original shape in a nonlinear manner (T_1 to T_2). **B.** *Stress-relaxation:* If the tissue is stretched to a fixed length and held there (constant strain), the stress needed to maintain this length will decrease with time. **C.** *Strain-rate sensitivity:* If the tissue is loaded rapidly (fast loading), more force (stress) is required to deform (strain) the tissue than is needed when there is slow loading of the same tissue. *(From Oskaya N, Nordin M: Fundamentals of Biomechanics, Equilibrium Motion and Deformation (ed 2). New York, NY, Springer-Verlag, 1999, with permission from the publisher as well as the author, Margarita Nordin.)*

Patient Application 2–7

Angie Bagoda is a 21-year-old woman who underwent surgical repair of a torn ACL. Atypically, she still had not regained full knee extension 1 month after surgery. A course of more aggressive stretching of the knee joint capsuloligamentous structures was recommended. Using an understanding of tissue creep, the therapist applies a manual force against the limited ROM at Angie's knee just short of producing pain. That same manual force is then sustained at that same level over a period of up to 2 minutes to induce creep deformation (elongation) of the tight capsuloligamentous tissues. After a brief rest, the procedure is repeated with a gradual lengthening occurring in the ROM-limiting tissues. The intervention is followed by a cold pack to minimize any inflammation that might result from the necessarily broken cross-links within the collagen fibers of the tissue.

If Angie is not able to tolerate a sustained force sufficient to produce tissue creep, an alternative strategy can be attempted. The therapist can take the joint just to the point of pain and hold the joint at that same point without attempting to stretch the tissues further. That position of the knee is maintained until the manual force needed to hold that position diminishes and Angie feels the reduced tension in the capsuloligamentous tissue (stress-relaxation). After a brief rest, Angie's knee is once again taken to the point of pain to repeat the procedure. It is likely that the capsuloligamentous tissues, after stress-relaxation, will allow slightly greater lengthening before the point of discomfort is again reached. As with the first technique, an application of ice afterward is a reasonable precaution.

Whether using tissue creep or stress-relaxation to lengthen Angie's shortened capsuloligamentous structure, the total length change should probably be no more than 2% to 6% strain to minimize injury (microfailure) in the tight tissues.

Properties of Specific Tissues

Connective tissues change their structure or composition in response to applied forces that may be due to new demands, thus adapting to changes in forces over time. In a tendon, changes in applied compression forces can result in changes in both the amount and type of GAGs and PGs the tissue contains[38,39]; increases in tensile forces can cause increases in type I collagen. This adaptive behavior illustrates the dynamic nature of connective tissue and the strong relationships among structure, composition, and function. The remarkable ability of connective tissues to respond to load alterations is often referred to as the **SAID principle** (*S*pecific *A*daptation to *I*mposed *D*emand). The principles involved in tissue adaptation have been used to create a "physical stress theory" that can be used to guide one's approach to intervention during rehabilitation.[96] Although there are commonalities to adaptive responses, we will also look at the properties of specific types of connective tissues to better understand their unique responses to stress and strains.

Bone

Cortical bone is stiffer than cancellous (trabecular) bone; that is, cortical bone can withstand greater magnitudes of stress with less deformation (strain) than cancellous bone. However, strain in cortical bone that exceeds about 2% results in tissue failure (fracture), whereas cancellous bone can sustain strains of about 15% (but at lower stresses) before failing in vivo.[97] The type of stress and how it is applied to a given tissue also makes a difference. When cortical bone is loaded in compression, longitudinal sections of the bone show the greatest strength (ability to withstand high stress before failure). In tensile testing of the femur, longitudinal sections display twice the stiffness of transverse sections. In general, cortical bone can withstand much higher compressive stresses before failure as compared with tensile stresses, with the same being true of cancellous bone. In other words, bone can withstand greater stress (with less strain) in compression than in tension.[97]

As is true of the strain-rate sensitivity of other tissues, large loads applied to bone over short periods of time will produce high stresses and low strains. Loads applied over longer periods of time will produce lower stresses and higher strains (creep and stress-relaxation). The physiological response of cancellous bone to new sustained increases in loading is to hypertrophy. If loading is decreased or absent over time, the trabeculae in cancellous bone become smaller and weaker. The rate, frequency, duration, magnitude, and type of loading all affect bony adaptation. Frequent loads of low magnitude over time can result in a stress fracture, whereas a single application of a high load can cause failure. Bone loses stiffness and strength with repetitive loading as a result of creep strain. **Creep strain** occurs when a tissue is loaded again (and again) before the tissue has had time to return to its original shape. With each new imposition of the force, the tissue (still in a deformed state) gets pushed farther and farther toward or into the plastic region.

Tendons

Tendons exhibit creep when subject to sustained tensile loading, most often when stress is created via muscle contraction, but can also occur with passive stretch of the entire muscle. With increases in force that bring the tendon into its elastic region, continued deformation may occur through slippage between collagen molecules within fibrils, then interfibrillar slippage between fibrils, and, finally, gross disruption of collagen fibers (plasticity or microfailure). The fibers in the tendon, however, are not perfectly parallel. Those fibers that become straightened at the end of the toe region before others may be the first to fail under increased or sustained forces—or the smaller, weaker fibrils may rupture before larger, stronger fibrils. Most normal activities load tendons in the toe region and in the first part of the linear elastic region.

The physiological response of tendons to intermittent tension is a moderate increase in thickness and strength.[98] Differences in stress-strain curves among different tendons reflect differences in the proportion of type I and type III collagen, differences in cross-linking, maturity of collagen fibers, organization of fibrils, variations in ground substance concentration, and level of hydration. The cross-sectional area, the material, and the length of the tendon determine the amount of force that a tendon can resist and the amount of elongation that it can undergo.[41,99] Under normal conditions, tendons with greater cross-sectional areas should be able to withstand larger forces than tendons with smaller cross-sectional areas, unless the tendon with the greater cross-sectional area is composed of weaker material; thus, it is reasonable to assume that the "thick" Achilles tendon is stronger than the "thin" palmaris longus tendon.[98] Under unusual conditions, this relationship may not be true. For example, an injured tendon may have a much larger diameter than an uninjured tendon, but the injured tendon may contain less collagen, smaller fibrils, or fewer cross-links, rendering it weaker than its smaller counterpart.[99] Tendinosis in the Achilles tendon, a degenerative disorder of the tendon, is characterized by a localized thickening and collagen fiber disorganization that lowers the tendon stiffness, rendering it more susceptible to failure.[100]

Under normal conditions, the tendon is most vulnerable to failure at either end rather than in its midsubstance. Because of the change in composition as the tendon inserts into the bone (with resulting uneven distribution of forces within the tissue), the enthesis is a common site of degenerative changes and injury.[57,58] The myotendinous junction (MTJ) appears to be stronger than the enthesis in spite of the MTJ being a common site for muscle strains and pulls.[101] However, the MTJ depends on the interdigitation of muscle and tendon tissues for its strength so that any injury that distorts the form of the MTJ may decrease its tensile strength and predispose it to further injury.

Healthy tendons rarely rupture under typical conditions and can withstand large tensile forces without injury.[102] However, weakened tendons are more likely to be injured. Tendons subject to immobilization show atrophy at the MTJ, with a loss of infolding and a decrease in collagen concentration and cross-linking.[101-103] Exposure to corticosteroids, nutritional deficiencies, hormonal imbalance, dialysis, chronic loading into the high linear region of the stress-strain curve with inadequate time for recovery, and sudden large loads may predispose the tendon to injury even at physiological levels of loading (levels typically experienced by the tissue); in other words, the same load now produces more deformation in the tendon.

Tendons adapt readily to changes in the magnitude and direction of loading. Tendons subjected to continual compressive forces will alter their composition to what can resemble cartilage, with a resulting decline in tensile strength.[104] Conversely, tendons subjected to tensile loads, especially physiological (apparently safe) loads over long periods of time, will increase in size, collagen concentration, and collagen cross-linking.[105-107] Progressive loading programs are successfully used to treat tendon dysfunction, presumably by inducing changes in tendon composition.[99,108-111]

Ligaments

As noted previously, tendons and ligaments are very similar mechanically. The physiological response of ligaments to intermittent tension, like that of tendons, is an increase in thickness and strength.[85,86] Ligaments must withstand forces in all directions, so they have a more varied orientation of collagen fibrils that renders a ligament slightly less resistant to tensile stress but better able to function within a range of load directions without being damaged. This is another example of form (in this case, collagen fibril orientation) following function.

Cartilage

Three factors interact in cartilage to help resist applied load: (1) stress developed in the fibrillar portion of extracellular matrix (type II collagen), (2) swelling pressures developed in the interstitial fluid (PGs and water), and (3) frictional drag resulting from fluid flow through the extracellular matrix.[51] Compression of cartilage reduces the volume of the cartilage and increases the pressure, causing outward flow of interstitial fluid. Fluid movement through the extracellular matrix creates frictional resistance to the flow within the tissue (frictional drag). Exudation of fluid occurs rapidly at first, causing a concomitant rapid rate of deformation. Subsequently, fluid flow and deformation gradually diminish and cease when compressive stress in cartilage balances the applied load.[68,69,95] Magnetic resonance imaging (MRI) has made it possible to study changes in cartilage volume and thickness in the joints of living subjects. In an MRI study of the knee joints of eight volunteers, Eckstein and colleagues[112] found that up to 13% of the fluid was displaced from the patellar cartilage 3 to 7 minutes after exercise (50 knee bends).

The tensile behavior of cartilage collagen is similar to that of ligaments and tendons but is caused in different ways. Tensile stresses within cartilage are created in the superficial collagen network as the compressed PGs and water push against the collagen fibers.[63] The nonlinear behavior in the toe region of the stress-strain curve for cartilage is thought to be caused by the drag force between the collagen meshwork and the PGs rather than the straightening of collagen fibers seen in tendon and ligament. In the elastic region, straightened cartilage collagen fibers are stretched just as in ligament and tendon fibers. Cartilage specimens from the different zones of cartilage (see Fig. 2–19) show differences in tensile behavior, presumably due to differences in the orientation of the collagen fibers among the zones.[63] Cartilage resistance to shear relies on the amount of collagen present because PGs provide little resistance to shear. Shear stresses are apt to develop at the interface between the calcified cartilage layer and the subchondral bone.

Foundational Concepts 2–10
Effects of Altered Loading on Connective Tissue

- Connective tissues become weaker and lose their typical structure if they are not at least periodically loaded (stressed).
- Changes with decreases in typical loading patterns occur rapidly in connective tissue.
- Recovery of normal structure and function in connective tissues requires gradual and progressive loading.
- Therapeutic loads should be tailored to the targeting type of connective tissue.

General Changes With Disease, Injury, Immobilization, Exercise, and Overuse

Each part of a joint has one or more specific functions that are essential for the overall performance of the joint. Therefore, anything that affects one part of a joint will disrupt the overall function of the joint and its component elements. Likewise, anything that affects joint motion or joint stresses will affect all the structures that constitute that joint. This relationship between form and function is essential for therapists to remember during rehabilitation after injury. For example, when a bone is broken, the fracture may be the primary injury that dictates subsequent treatment, but lack of motion and decreased loading needed for bone healing also will have secondary effects on cartilage, ligaments, joint capsule, tendons, and muscles. The ideal rehabilitation protocol considers the behavior of all the affected structures and includes interventions tailored to induce positive adaptations in each structure. This means understanding the time course and nature of the adaptation of each tissue to changes in loading conditions.

Complex joints are more likely to be affected by injury, disease, or aging than are simple joints. Complex joints have more parts and are subject to more wear and tear because the complexity is typically a response to maximizing ROM while minimizing instability. The function of complex joints depends on a number of interrelated factors. For example, the capsule must produce synovial fluid that also must be of the appropriate composition and of sufficient quantity to lubricate and nourish the joint. The hyaline cartilage must be smooth enough that the joint surfaces can move easily, yet permeable enough to receive nourishment from the joint fluid. The cartilage must undergo periodic compressive loading and unloading to facilitate movement of the fluid, and the collagen network must be intact to retain the fluid attracted to the PGs. The ligaments and capsules must be strong enough to provide sufficient support for stabilization and yet be flexible enough to permit normal joint motion without excessive constraints. Tendons must be able to withstand the forces generated by muscles as they produce movement.

Disease

The general effects of disease, injury, immobilization, and overuse may be illustrated by using the normal function of a joint structure as a basis for analysis. For example, when the synovial membrane of a joint is affected by a disease such as rheumatoid arthritis, the production and composition of the synovial fluid may change, thus affecting joint lubrication. The disease process and the changes in joint structure that occur in rheumatoid arthritis involve far more than just synovial fluid alteration, in part because of the associated effect on other joint structures to reduced lubrication. Osteoarthritis, which may have genetic and/or mechanical origins, is a different disease process where the cartilage is a primary problem. With the erosion and splitting of the cartilage that may occur, friction is increased between the joint surfaces, thus further increasing tissue degradation.

Injury

Joint support is likely to decrease after injury to one or more of the joint components. If a collapsible stepladder (see Fig. 2–1) has an unstable brace between the two sides of the ladder, damage and disruption of function may occur as a result of instability. If a heavy load is placed on the damaged ladder, the two sides will separate excessively under the compressive load and the ladder may collapse, further damaging other components of the ladder, not to mention the person on the ladder.

The effects of decreased support in a human joint are similar to those in a collapsible stepladder. If a joint ligament is torn, separation of the bony surfaces can occur and may result in wobbling or a deviation from the normal alignment of the bony components. Changes in alignment create abnormal joint opening on the side where the ligament is torn. Other ligaments, tendons, and the joint capsule may then be subjected to increased loading, leading them to become excessively stretched or compressed and unable to provide protection. The intact side of the joint may be subjected to abnormal compression during motion or weight-bearing. In canine experiments in which an unstable knee joint is produced by transection of the ACL, morphologic, biochemical, biomechanical, and metabolic changes occur in the articular cartilage shortly after transection.[113] Later, the articular cartilage becomes thicker, shows fibrillation, and the surrounding bone develops osteophytes. The cartilage shows much higher water content than in the opposite knee, and the synovial fluid content of the knee is increased. In addition, a substantial increase in bone turnover occurs, as does a thickening of the subchondral bone.[113] According to van Osch and colleagues, joint instability is a well-known cause of secondary osteoarthritis involving the knee joint.[114] The recognition that joint injuries, especially ligament injuries, lead to osteoarthritis suggests greater efforts are required to prevent and treat ligamentous injuries from sports in young people.

Immobilization (Stress Deprivation)

Any process or event that disturbs the normal function of a specific joint structure will start a chain of events that eventually affects every part of a joint and its surrounding structures. Immobilization is particularly detrimental to joint structure and function and may be externally imposed by a cast, reduced weight-bearing (e.g., bedrest), or denervation.

Immobilization may also be self-imposed as a reaction to pain and inflammation. An injured joint that results in inflammation and swelling will assume a loose-packed position where the capsuloligamentous structures are under least tension to accommodate the increased volume of fluid within the joint space. This position may be referred to as the **position of comfort** because pain is decreased in this position. Each joint has a position of minimum pressure and maximum capsular volume. For the knee and hip joints, the position of comfort is between 30° and 45° of flexion; for the ankle joint, the position is at 15° of plantar flexion.[33] If the joint is immobilized for a few weeks in the position of comfort, the joint capsule will adapt (shorten on one side and lengthen on the other), and contractures[115] can develop in the surrounding muscle-tendon units. Consequently, resumption of a normal range of joint motion upon remobilization will be difficult and may result in additional pathology or functional limitations.

Effects on Ligament and Tendon

Ligaments and tendons adapt to decreased load with reduced collagen content and reduced cross-linking among collagen molecules. Although the overall collagen fiber size may remain the same, the tissue is weakened. Rapid resumption of previously normal loading may cause damaging stress and strain.[85,86] The musculotendinous junction of a tendon loses its interdigitating structure when not loaded, making it weaker.[101] The time course of these adaptations is fairly rapid. Ligaments and tendons show a 50% decrease in tensile strength and stiffness after 8 weeks of immobilization.[85,86] It is assumed that ligaments and tendons eventually recover their mechanical properties, but the time course of this recovery appears to be slow, with the total time for recovery unknown. In general, the time course for the loss of mechanical properties occurs over weeks, whereas recovery can take 12 to 18 months or more.[87] *Gradual* reloading is necessary to restore tendon and ligament strength, with sufficient time between loading episodes to allow the tissue to return to its original shape through both elastic recoil and creep recovery.

Effects on Articular Surfaces and Bone

The effects of prolonged immobilization are not confined to the surrounding soft tissues but may also affect the articular surfaces of the joint and the underlying bone. Biochemical and morphological changes may include: proliferation of fibrofatty connective tissue within the joint space, adhesions between the folds of the synovium, atrophy of cartilage, regional osteoporosis, weakening of ligaments at their insertion sites as a result of osteoclastic resorption of bone and Sharpey's fibers, a decrease in the PG content, and an increase in the water content of articular cartilage.[51,116,117] Thinning and softening of the articular cartilage occurs, and—under compressive test loads—deformation increases up to 42%. As a result of changes in joint structures brought about by immobilization, decreases may be evident in the available joint ROM, the time between loading and failure, and the energy-absorbing capacity of the bone-ligament complex. Immobilization (and swelling) of a joint also inhibits and weakens the muscles surrounding the joint.[118-120] Therefore, the joint is unable to function normally and is at high risk of additional injury.[121] A summary of the possible effects of prolonged immobilization is presented in Table 2–3.

Foundational Concepts 2–11
Deleterious Effects of Immobilization

Joint structures will undergo potentially substantive changes during immobilization:

- Bone: weakened, decreased collagen and mineral content (osteopenia)
- Capsule: shrinking, increased resistance to movement (stiffer)
- Ligament: decreased cross-links, decreased tensile or directional strength (weaker)
- Tendon: decreased cross-links, disorganization of collagen, decreased tensile strength (weaker)
- Muscle: loss of sarcomeres in series, decreased contractile proteins (actin/myosin) resulting in reduced force production
- Cartilage: swelling, decreased PG concentration (softer, weaker)

These changes occur within 8 weeks, but recovery may take 18 months or longer.

Patient Application 2–8

Jamelle Watkins fractured his right femur in a car crash. Once the fracture was stabilized surgically with internal fixation, he was given crutches and told not to bear weight on his leg. Although fracture healing must take place, this type of immobilization is concerning for the health of the joints in his injured leg. Without proper cartilage loading, hyaline cartilage will swell, which will strain the superficial collagen network, reduce nutrient diffusion into the cartilage, and make the superficial collagen layer more susceptible to damage. Jamelle can be instructed in non-weight-bearing activities that will allow for some cartilage loading across the joints via muscle contraction (causing compression across joint surfaces) as well as joint ROM. Joint motion alternately compresses and unloads the joint surfaces, maintaining cartilage nutrition and helping to maintain capsule mobility. Once Jamelle is able to put weight on his leg, the probable changes in hyaline cartilage (as well as other structures) that may have already occurred should be taken into consideration, with weight-bearing resumed gradually. Jamelle was lucky that he did not require full immobilization of his leg. In cases when joint motion and weight-bearing need to be restricted for healing, it is preferable that a removable brace be used rather than a cast so that the patient can remove it for ROM exercise (presuming patient compliance with restrictions can be assumed). When non–weight-bearing and joint immobilization is necessary for bone healing, a postoperative cast is often changed for a cast brace at approximately 3 to 4 weeks once some new bone has started to form.

Table 2–3 Effects of Increased and Decreased Load on Connective Tissues

TISSUE	DECREASED LOAD	INCREASED LOAD
Tendon and ligament	• Decreased collagen concentration • Decreased cross-linking • Decreased tensile strength	• Increased cross-sectional area • Increased collagen concentration • Increased cross-linking • Increased tensile strength • Increased stiffness
Menisci	• Decreased PGs	• Increased PGs
Bone	• Decreased collagen synthesis • Decreased bone formation • Increased bone resorption	• Denser bone • Increased synthesis of collagen and bone
Cartilage	• Thinning of cartilage • Advancing of subchondral bone • Decreased PG synthesis • Fewer PG aggregates	• Increased PG synthesis • Increased volume?
Joint capsule	• Disordered collagen fibrils • Abnormal cross-linking	• Not specifically examined
Synovium	• Adhesion formation • Fibrofatty tissue proliferation into joint space	• Not specifically examined

PG, proteoglycan.

Recognition of the adverse effects of immobilization has led to the development of several strategies to help minimize the consequences. These include: (1) reduction in the duration of casting periods after fractures and sprains, (2) development of dynamic splinting devices to allow joint motion while limiting unwanted motion that may damage healing structures, (3) use of graded loading after immobilization, and (4) extension of the recovery period to months rather than days or weeks.

Exercise

All tissues appear to respond favorably to gradual progressive loading by adapting to meet increased mechanical demands. Exercise influences cell shape and physiological functions and can have a direct effect on matrix alignment. The response to exercise varies among tissues and depends on the nature of the stimulus, including the amount, type, and frequency of loading. The mechanism of connective tissue response to exercise appears to involve detection of tissue strain by cells, then modifying the type and amount of tissue the cells produce. The amount, type, and frequency of deformation are important. Low-frequency compressive loading will increase cartilage formation, whereas higher frequencies can enhance bone synthesis. Higher magnitude or sustained compressive loading will induce fibrocartilage formation, whereas tensile loads induce tissue formation resembling that found in a tendon or ligament. According to Mueller and Maluf's Physical Stress Theory,[96] maintaining the normal mechanical state of connective tissues appears to require repetitive loading beyond a certain (albeit often unknown) threshold level. Below this threshold, immobilization changes can occur rapidly.

Bone Response to Exercise

Bone deposition is increased with weight-bearing exercise and in areas of bone subjected to increased muscle force.[122,123] This response of bone has been known for over 100 years, and exercise is now used as a therapeutic intervention to prevent bone loss.[124] A systematic review showed in 11 of 16 studies, that postmenopausal women demonstrated improvements in bone density with either exercise, or exercise plus calcium or estrogen.[123] Bone formation is very sensitive to strains as well as (or perhaps rather than) the magnitude of the applied load. Very low magnitude (<1 G) high-frequency vibration increases trabecular bone formation by 34% (where 1 G equals the force per unit mass at the earth's surface).[125] This suggests that even very low loads (well below the threshold for physical damage) may increase bone density. Rubin et al. proposed that these far smaller, high-frequency (10 to 30 Hz) mechanical signals that continually barrage the skeleton during longer term activities such as standing and walking are what regulate skeletal architecture.[125-127] Even short durations of loading are effective; just 10 minutes of low-load, high-frequency stimulation limits disuse-induced bone loss.[125] Lanyon suggested that the asymmetrical strains during normal load-bearing activities create an ever-changing strain distribution, with that variety important in inducing bone adaptation through an osteogenic response.[128] He further suggested that exercise regimens designed to control bone architecture can usefully capitalize on this feature of the adaptive (re)modeling response, with each exercise session including as many novel strain distributions as possible—preferably involving high peak strains and strain rates that are repeated daily (or on alternate days).

While some studies suggest that high-magnitude mechanical strains are necessary to induce bone formation,[129] the ability of low-magnitude, high-frequency mechanical signals to influence bone remodeling suggests that such application may be of therapeutic benefit.[130] For example, many patients of advanced age who participate in limited ambulation activities—with few if any activities exerting high magnitude forces (e.g., jumping or running)—are still largely able to maintain their bone density and structure. However, if these individuals are subjected to even a few days of bedrest, bone loss ensues.[131] As such, the forces from frequent low-magnitude mechanical perturbations occurring during short ambulation distances, and the associated pull of muscle on the bone during postural corrections, appear to be sufficient to maintain bone mass and strength when compared to the rapid bone loss that occurs with inactivity.

Increased bone formation requires secretion of matrix from osteoblasts that is later mineralized. Given that the number of osteoblasts regulates the amount of matrix secreted, differentiation of mesenchymal stem cells (MSCs), the precursors to osteoblasts, can influence the amount of bone produced. MSCs can differentiate into several different cell types, including bone and adipose (fat). A variety of factors influence MSC differentiation, including hormones, nutrients, and application of mechanical force. If conditions favor differentiation into fat cells, the pool of available progenitor cells capable of differentiating into bone cells will be depleted. Studies in mice on high-fat diets demonstrate that the resulting increased bone marrow adiposity can be diminished with exercise (running).[132] Further work, using cultured cells, also shows that application of mechanical strain to MSCs restricts adipogenic (fat cell) differentiation, thus maintaining a sufficient pool of progenitor cells available for osteogenesis.[133] In fact, experimental lab cultures demonstrated that the application of mechanical strain to MSCs twice daily, separated by a rest period, produced significantly greater responses compared to a greater overall period of strain applied once daily.[134] This suggests that an initial bout of exercise "primes" the cells, making them more responsive to the second bout of loading. Thus, therapists can tailor therapeutic interventions to maximize cellular, and thus tissue-level, responses to benefit their patients.

MSCs contribute to the total number of osteoblasts, which eventually differentiate into osteocytes. Distinct from the surface-dwelling MSCs and osteoblasts, osteocytes are embedded deep within the bone matrix and secrete factors that bind to osteoblasts and osteoclasts to regulate their function. As such, osteocytes have more recently been considered the "master regulators" of bone.[135] There are several molecules that regulate the ability of osteocytes to sense mechanical force.[137] One of these molecular complexes responsible for mechanosensation of osteocytes binds to a drug called *gabapentin*. Gabapentin is an antiepileptic and neuropathic pain drug, very commonly used for peripheral neuropathy or for pain modulation after surgeries including amputations and joint replacements.[140] A few clinical studies have now shown that chronic gabapentin treatment impairs fracture healing and is associated with increased hip fractures. Furthermore, gabapentin treatment in mice impairs the ability of bone to respond to mechanical loading.[141] The influence of gabapentin on the mechanical attributes of bone is one example of how a drug, which may have beneficial effects on one system (i.e., pain reduction), has negative effects on another. Understanding the effects of such drugs on the musculoskeletal system is essential for physicians and rehabilitation specialists to provide proper care to patients.

Cartilage Response to Exercise

The response of cartilage to immobilization has been described, but its response to increased physiological loading is largely unknown. The health of hyaline cartilage depends on the application and removal of compressive loads. Mechanical forces are transduced into intracellular synthetic activity but the mechanisms by which this transduction occurs and the magnitude and frequency of the loading that will optimize cartilage structure is an area of active research because cartilage injuries heal very poorly. Use of transplanted material to repair cartilage defects is also under active investigation. It is well known that motion enhances tissue formation in cartilage defects, but the tissue formed is fibrocartilage rather than hyaline cartilage.[142] Unlike fibroblasts (in bone, ligament, and tendon), chondrocytes do not readily migrate to and repair areas that have been injured. Defects that extend to subchondral bone are thought to have better healing potential because mesenchymal cells (from bone marrow) can differentiate into chondroblasts under the right loading conditions, hence the use of drilling (creating an artificial defect in the subchondral bone) to surgically treat osteochondral defects.[143] Further, it appears that cyclic low-magnitude, low-frequency (less than 1 Hz) compressive loads may be best for inducing or maintaining cartilage structure. There are no quantitative data available about changes in human articular cartilage after immobilization or exercise, although MRI shows promise in this regard.[144] Studies in rats show that immobilization results in significant decreases in cartilage thickness and collagen density, while exercise prior to immobilization mitigates these losses. This suggests that exercise can prevent degenerative cartilaginous changes induced by knee immobilization.[145]

Tendon Response to Exercise

Tendons respond to increased tensile loads by increasing collagen concentration, collagen cross-linking, tensile strength, and stiffness. Woo et al. showed that after 12 months of physical training, the extensor digitorum tendons of swine increased weight, strength, collagen content, and stiffness to match the normally stronger flexor digitorum longus that showed no change in response to the same program.[107] Similarly, biochemical changes occurred in chicken Achilles tendons after strenuous intermittent running, with increased collagen synthesis, cross-linking, tensile strength, and stiffness, without a concomitant change in tendon size and weight.[146,147] Similar beneficial effects of low-magnitude mechanical forces and chronic loading have shown beneficial effects in structure and material composition.[144-148] Interestingly, exercise also appears to offset some of the changes that occur in connective tissue with age.[152] Progressive tensile loading has been used successfully to treat chronic tendon disorders (thought at one time to be counterproductive) under the assumption that the tendon adapts to the increased loads.[108-111,153] A clinical study found that using a high-loading exercise regimen, defined as training at about 90% of the maximum voluntary isometric plantar flexor strength compared to eccentric training or passive therapy, leads to increased tendon stiffness and cross-sectional area in men with Achilles tendinopathy.[154] Thus, a high-loading intervention may be recommended as an effective protocol for men with Achilles tendinopathy.

Ligament Response to Exercise

The effects of exercise in preventing negative and promoting positive changes in ligaments undergoing repair have been well demonstrated, but the effects of exercise on normal ligaments are less clear.[155-157] Recovery of normal ligament structure and mechanics after immobilization is a slow process that can take months. It appears that exercise may speed up this process, but the volume of loading and the time course of the adaptations are not known.

Expanded Concepts 2–5

Exercise can help facilitate recovery of tissue after immobilization. The types of exercise that may facilitate tissue recovery in the lower extremity include:

- Bone: walking, standing with weight shifts, bouncing, on/off pressure
- Cartilage: moderate loads through available ROM, walking, isometrics
- Ligament: gentle, progressive tensile stress, changes in stress directions
- Tendon: progressive tensile loading, strength training
- Muscle: progressive tensile loading at various speeds (recruit different motor units) and lower load exercise to fatigue (induce metabolic adaptation)
- Capsule: repeated exercise throughout physiological ROM

Although isometric muscle exercises (muscle contraction without joint motion) can be used even during periods of immobilization, it is recommended that large loads be avoided during that period.

Foundational Concepts 2–12
Connective Tissue Adaptation

- All connective tissues will adapt to increased load through changes in structural or material properties (form follows function).
- Newly imposed loads must be gradual and progressive; as the tissue adapts to the new loading conditions, the load must change to induce further adaptation.
- The type of connective tissue formed will match the type and volume of the load:
  - Compression: cartilage or bone
  - Tension: ligament or tendon
- Optimization of load volume and frequency, and the nature of human tissue adaptation, remain largely unknown as yet.

Overuse

Although it is readily recognized that immobilization has negative consequences, both sustained and repetitive loading

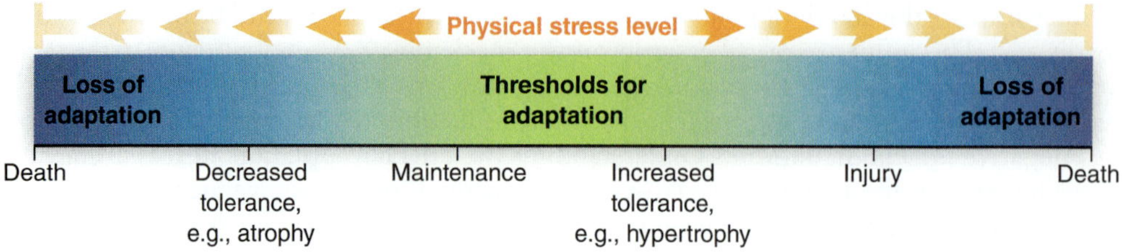

Figure 2–26 The responses to different levels of loading (physical stress level) on connective tissue structures based on Mueller and Maluf's physical stress theory.[96]

of joint structures also may have adverse effects. Damage can occur in one of two ways: (1) sudden application of large loads, and (2) repeated or sustained application of low loads. The former are nonphysiological loads that create large stresses and strains, thus precipitating failure of the tissue on a microscopic or macroscopic scale (e.g., sprains, tendon ruptures, bone fractures). Physiological loads that are typical in magnitude but sustained or repeated while creep is occurring may also result in tissue plasticity or failure. Recovery of normal tissue shape after a load is removed takes an as-yet unknown time. When connective tissue is subjected to imposition of a new load before it has recovered (returned to its original shape), the tissue may enter the plastic range with microfailure. For example, after loss of the ACL, increased load on the posterior knee joint capsule may cause plastic deformation (permanent stretch), leading to increasing knee hyperextension. Cartilage subjected to constant compressive loading will creep and may show evidence of permanent deformation if the load continues long enough. Cell death may occur with rigid sustained pressure at focal points on the cartilage, with permeability and fluid flow further decreased.[62]

An injury resulting from repetitive strain loading may be referred to as an **overuse injury** or **syndrome, repetitive motion disorder,** or **repetitive strain injury.**[7] These disorders have been identified in athletes, dancers, farmers, musicians, and factory and office workers. Such injuries appear to affect a greater proportion of women than men for unknown reasons.[158] Hart and associates hypothesized that intrinsic gender differences may exist in the regulation of connective tissue structures, perhaps related to hormone levels that fluctuate in women during pregnancy and across menstrual cycles.[158] Tendon biopsy material from human subjects undergoing surgery for repetitive motion disorders shows an inflammatory process in some tendons and a degenerative process in others.[159] In view of the findings to date, it appears that simple tissue fatigue is not a sufficient explanation for the cause of repetitive motion disorders and that additional research is needed to determine all of the factors involved in the cause, effect, prevention, and treatment of repetitive motion disorders.

Mueller and Maluf's physical stress theory[96] **(Fig. 2–26)** reflects the concept that physical stress is required for maintenance of tissue health and that tissues have at least limited ability to adapt to changes in stress, showing the interaction of form and function. Tissues may effectively respond to increased or new stresses through adaptations such as hypertrophy, whereas decreased stresses will lead to decreased stress tolerance (e.g., atrophy). With sufficient exposure to *excessive* stress or to stress reduction, tissue failure (death) may occur. The limitation to this stress theory is that the margins between adaptive and nonadaptive stresses are unknown and, as we have already seen in this chapter, are dependent on innumerable interrelated factors across and within different types of connective tissue.

Foundational Concepts 2–13
Chronic Overuse Injuries

- Chronic overuse injuries may involve repeated or sustained loads while the tissue is still in a deformed state.
- Recovery time, not load size, may be the critical variable in susceptibility of tissues to overuse injury.
- The roles of systemic influences (e.g., hormones, nutrition) and neurophysiological factors (e.g., referred pain, focal dystonia) in repetitive injuries remain to be explored.

SUMMARY

- This chapter presents the elementary principles of joint design, a classification system for human joints, and an introduction to the materials found in human joints and their properties, as well as the effects of disease, immobilization, and overuse on joint structures.
- The health, strength, and function of joint structures depend on a threshold amount of stress and strain; this threshold can move up or down, depending on the state of the tissue.
- Nutrition and health of cartilage and bone depend on joint movement and muscle contraction. Cartilage nutrition depends on joint movement through a full ROM to ensure that the entire articular cartilage receives the nutrients necessary for survival.
- Stresses and strains are necessary for ligaments and tendons to maintain or increase their strength. Controlled loading and motion applied early in the rehabilitation process stimulate collagen synthesis and help align collagen fibrils. Bone density and strength increase following the stress and strain created by muscle activity and weight-bearing. In contrast, bone density and strength decrease when stress and strain are absent.
- It appears that tissues have a threshold below which they atrophy and above which they become injured (see Fig. 2–26). This threshold can be modified through progressive load adjustment so that the tissue can withstand changes in forces accompanying new functional activities.
- The inadequacy of cartilage repair mechanisms and the slow recovery of bones, ligaments, and tendons suggest that the prevention of injury to recovering joint structures through the avoidance of excessive reloading is crucial. Gradual, progressive loading is the ideal. The therapist must skillfully load the tissues with the appropriate direction, magnitude, and frequency of forces to prevent weakening or to induce adaptation.

In subsequent chapters, the specific structure and function of each of the major joints in the body will be explored. Knowledge of the basic elements of normal joint structure and function and understanding the changes that function can induce in structures (and vice versa) are necessary to appreciate the complex nature of human joints, as well as for identifying abnormal joint function, and analyzing the effects of injury, disease, or aging on joint structure and function.

STUDY QUESTIONS

1. Is a condyloid joint uniaxial, biaxial, or triaxial? How many degrees of freedom does it have?
2. In the human body, under what conditions will joints form a closed chain? What are the implications of a closed chain on function?
3. What are the common elements of all synovial joints and what is the purpose of each?
4. What is the role of a meniscus or disk at a joint?
5. Describe the osteokinematics and arthrokinematics that take place when the convex end of the lever moves on a fixed concave surface.
6. Define the motions of spin, slide, and roll as they relate to intra-articular joint motions. As the femur flexes on a weight-bearing tibia, which of these motions take place?
7. Describe what it means for a joint to be close-packed and loose-packed. In which position is a joint more stable and why?
8. Define the terms *hypomobility* and *hypermobility* as each refers to human joint motion.
9. What are the common components of which all connective tissues are composed? In what way do these components differ among the primary connective tissues?
10. In what part of connective tissues do proteoglycans (PGs) belong? What is their function?
11. What factors affect the elasticity and point of failure of a tissue?
12. What are the ways by which the capsule, ligament, and tendon attach to bone? Are these tissues more likely to fail at their attachments or at their midsubstance? Why?
13. Describe the differentiating components and arrangement of fibers in the layers (zones) of hyaline cartilage as well as the purpose of each in supporting the function of hyaline cartilage.
14. Which of the following are disruptive to proper nutrition for normal articular cartilage and why: prolonged loading, occasional loading, rare loading?
15. What differentiates bone from other connective tissues and cancellous bone from cortical bone?
16. Define connective tissue *stress*, *strain*, *stiffness*, *yield point*, *plastic region*, and *ultimate failure*.
17. What difference, if any, is there between a load-deformation curve and a stress-strain curve?
18. Differentiate among crimp, elasticity, and creep responses in viscoelastic materials.
19. What happens to viscoelastic tissue when the rate of loading is increased? What happens when the tissue is heated? How does a thicker tissue respond to stress in comparison to a thinner tissue of the same composition?
20. Describe what happens to each of the following tissues when they fail: ligament, tendon, cartilage, and bone.
21. What are the general effects of immobilization on connective tissues? What are the implications for these changes when remobilizing the tissues?
22. Describe how overuse may affect connective tissues.

REFERENCES

1. Michl J: Form follows WHAT? the modernist notion of function. Mag Fac Archit Town Plan 10:2031, 1995
2. Nolan L: Carbon fibre prostheses and running in amputees: a review. Foot Ankle Surg 14:125-9, 2008
3. Dezateux C, Rosendahl K: Developmental dysplasia of the hip. Lancet 369:1541-52, 2007
4. Weinstein SL: Natural history of congenital hip dislocation (CDH) and hip dysplasia. Clin Orthop Relat Res:62-76, 1987
5. Lindstrom JR, Ponseti IV, Wenger DR: Acetabular development after reduction in congenital dislocation of the hip. J Bone Joint Surg Am 61:112-8, 1979
6. Wolf JH: [Julis Wolff and his "law of bone remodeling"]. Orthopade 24:378-86, 1995
7. Allan DA: Structure and physiology of joints and their relationship to repetitive strain injuries. Clin Orthop Relat Res:32-8, 1998
8. Rodeo SA, Suzuki K, Yamauchi M, et al: Analysis of collagen and elastic fibers in shoulder capsule in patients with shoulder instability. Am J Sports Med 26:634-43, 1998
9. Ralphs JR, Benjamin M: The joint capsule: structure, composition, ageing and disease. J Anat 184 (Pt 3):503-9, 1994
10. Smith MD: The normal synovium. Open Rheumatol J 5:100-6, 2011
11. Culav EM, Clark CH, Merrilees MJ: Connective tissues: matrix composition and its relevance to physical therapy. Phys Ther 79:308-19, 1999
12. Wagner FV, Negrao JR, Campos J, et al: Capsular ligaments of the hip: anatomic, histologic, and positional study in cadaveric specimens with MR arthrography. Radiology 263:189-98, 2012
13. Zimny ML: Mechanoreceptors in articular tissues. Am J Anat 182:16-32, 1988
14. Grigg P: Articular neurophysiology, in Zachazewski JE, Magee DJ, Quillen WS (eds): Athletic Injuries and Rehabilitation. Philadelphia, WB Saunders, 1996
15. Hogervorst T, Brand RA: Mechanoreceptors in joint function. J Bone Joint Surg Am 80:1365-78, 1998
16. Armstrong C, Mow V: Friction, lubrication and wear of synovial joints, in Owen R, Goodfellow J, Bullough P (eds): Scientific Foundations of Orthopaedics and Traumatology. Philadelphia, WB Saunders, 1980
17. Goodfellow J, O'Connor J: The design of synovial joints, in Owen R, Goodfellow J, Bullough P (eds): Scientific Foundations of Orthopaedics and Traumatology. Philadelphia, WB Saunders, 1980
18. Fye KH: Arthrocentesis, synovial fluid analysis and synovial biopsy, in Klippel JH, Stone JH, Crofford LJ, et al (eds): Primer on the Rheumatic Diseases. 13. New York, Springer, 2008
19. Jay GD, Torres JR, Warman ML, et al: The role of lubricin in the mechanical behavior of synovial fluid. Proc Natl Acad Sci U S A 104:6194-9, 2007
20. Rhee DK, Marcelino J, Baker M, et al: The secreted glycoprotein lubricin protects cartilage surfaces and inhibits synovial cell overgrowth. J Clin Invest 115:622-31, 2005
21. Brzusek D, Petron D: Treating knee osteoarthritis with intra-articular hyaluronans. Curr Med Res Opin 24:3307-22, 2008
22. Witteveen AG, Hofstad CJ, Kerkhoffs GM: Hyaluronic acid and other conservative treatment options for osteoarthritis of the ankle. Cochrane Database Syst Rev 2015:CD010643, 2015
23. Kraus VB, Stabler TV, Kong SY, et al: Measurement of synovial fluid volume using urea. Osteoarthritis Cartilage 15:1217-20, 2007
24. Oegema T, Lewis J, Mikecz K, et al: Osteoarthritis and rheumatoid arthritis, in Einhorn T, Buckwalter J, O'Keefe R (eds): Orthopaedic Basic Science: Foundations of Clinical Practice (ed 3). American Academy of Orthopaedic Surgeons, 2007
25. Shrive NG, O'Connor JJ, Goodfellow JW: Load-bearing in the knee joint. Clin Orthop Relat Res:279-87, 1978
26. Safran MR: The acetabular labrum: anatomic and functional characteristics and rationale for surgical intervention. J Am Acad Orthop Surg 18:338-45, 2010
27. Benjamin M, Kaiser E, Milz S: Structure-function relationships in tendons: a review. J Anat 212:211-28, 2008
28. Michener LA, Kulig K: Not all tendons are created equal: implications for differing treatment approaches. J Orthop Sports Phys Ther 45: 829-32, 2015

29. Frank C, Shrive N, Lo I, et al: Form and function of tendon and ligament, in Einhorn T, Buckwalter J, O'Keefe R (eds): Orthopaedic Basic Science: Foundations of Clinical Practice (ed 3). American Academy of Orthopaedic Surgeons, 2007
30. Standring S: Gray's Anatomy: The Anatomical Basis of Clinical Practice (ed 41). New York, Elsevier Health Sciences, 2016
31. MacConaill MA: A structuro-functional classification of synovial articular units. Ir J Med Sci 142:19-26, 1973
32. Zatsiorsky VM: Kinematics of Human Motion. Champaign, IL, Human Kinetics, 1998
33. Houglum PA, Bertoti DB: Brunnstrom's Clinical Kinesiology (ed 6). Philadelphia, FA Davis, 2012
34. Gowitzke BA, Milner M: Scientific Bases of Human Movement (ed 3). Baltimore, Williams & Wilkins, 1988
35. White AA, Panjabi MM: Clinical Biomechanics of the Spine (ed 2). Philadelphia, Lippincott, 1990
36. Kaltenborn FM, Evjenth O, Hinsen W: Mobilization of the Extremity Joints (ed 3). Oslo, Olaf Norlis Bokhandel, 1980
37. Covizi DZ, Felisbino SL, Gomes L, et al: Regional adaptations in three rat tendons. Tissue Cell 33:483-90, 2001
38. Vogel KG, Ordog A, Pogany G, et al: Proteoglycans in the compressed region of human tibialis posterior tendon and in ligaments. J Orthop Res 11:68-77, 1993
39. Vogel KG, Thonar EJ: Keratan sulfate is a component of proteoglycans in the compressed region of adult bovine flexor tendon. J Orthop Res 6:434-42, 1988
40. Eyre DR: Collagen: molecular diversity in the body's protein scaffold. Science 207:1315-22, 1980
41. Burgeson RE, Nimni ME: Collagen types: molecular structure and tissue distribution. Clin Orthop Relat Res:250-72, 1992
42. Eyre DR: The collagens of articular cartilage. Semin Arthritis Rheum 21:2-11, 1991
43. Kuivaniemi H, Tromp G, Prockop DJ: Mutations in fibrillar collagens (types I, II, III, and XI), fibril-associated collagen (type IX), and network-forming collagen (type X) cause a spectrum of diseases of bone, cartilage, and blood vessels. Hum Mutat 9:300-15, 1997
44. Myllyharju J, Kivirikko KI: Collagens and collagen-related diseases. Ann Med 33:7-21, 2001
45. Eriksen HA, Pajala A, Leppilahti J, et al: Increased content of type III collagen at the rupture site of human Achilles tendon. J Orthop Res 20: 1352-7, 2002
46. Kannus P: Structure of the tendon connective tissue. Scand J Med Sci Sports 10:312-20, 2000
47. Kastelic J, Galeski A, Baer E: The multicomposite structure of tendon. Connect Tissue Res 6:11-23, 1978
48. Liu SH, Yang RS, al-Shaikh R, et al: Collagen in tendon, ligament, and bone healing: a current review. Clin Orthop Relat Res:265-78, 1995
49. Bailey AJ, Robins SP, Balian G: Biological significance of the intermolecular crosslinks of collagen. Nature 251:105-9, 1974
50. Bosman FT, Stamenkovic I: Functional structure and composition of the extracellular matrix. J Pathol 200:423-8, 2003
51. Cohen NP, Foster RJ, Mow VC: Composition and dynamics of articular cartilage: structure, function, and maintaining healthy state. J Orthop Sports Phys Ther 28:203-15, 1998
52. Rumian AP, Wallace AL, Birch HL: Tendons and ligaments are anatomically distinct but overlap in molecular and morphological features—a comparative study in an bovine model. J Orthop Res 25:458-64, 2007
53. Luo W, Guo C, Zheng J, et al: Aggrecan from start to finish. J Bone Miner Metab 18:51-6, 2000
54. Roughley PJ, Lee ER: Cartilage proteoglycans: structure and potential functions. Microsc Res Tech 28:385-97, 1994
55. Towheed TE, Maxwell L, Anastassiades TP, et al: Glucosamine therapy for treating osteoarthritis. Cochrane Database Syst Rev 2005:CD002946, 2005
56. Tozer S, Duprez D: Tendon and ligament: development, repair and disease. Birth Defects Res C Embryo Today 75:226-36, 2005
57. Benjamin M, Toumi H, Ralphs JR, et al: Where tendons and ligaments meet bone: attachment sites ('entheses') in relation to exercise and/or mechanical load. J Anat 208:471-90, 2006
58. Benjamin M, Kumai T, Milz S, et al: The skeletal attachment of tendons—tendon "entheses." Comp Biochem Physiol A Mol Integr Physiol 133:931-45, 2002
59. Benjamin M, Ralphs JR: Tendons and ligaments—an overview. Histol Histopathol 12:1135-44, 1997
60. Tidball JG, Chan M: Adhesive strength of single muscle cells to basement membrane at myotendinous junctions. J Appl Physiol (1985) 67:1063-9, 1989
61. Trotter JA: Structure-function considerations of muscle-tendon junctions. Comp Biochem Physiol A Mol Integr Physiol 133:1127-33, 2002
62. Walker JM: Cartilage of human joints and related structures, in Zachazewski JE, Magee DJ, Quillen WS (eds): Athletic Injuries and Rehabilitation. Philadelphia, WB Saunders, 1996
63. Ghadially F: Structure and function of articular cartilage. Clin Rheum Dis 7, 1980
64. Izadifar Z, Chen X, Kulyk W: Strategic design and fabrication of engineered scaffolds for articular cartilage repair. J Funct Biomater 3:799-838, 2012
65. Chubinskaya S, Malfait A, Wimmer M: Form and function of articular cartilage, in O'Keefe RJ JJ, Chu CR, et al (eds): Orthopaedic Basic Science: Foundations of Clinical Practice (ed 4). American Academy of Orthopaedic Surgeons, 2012
66. Bullough PG, Jagannath A: The morphology of the calcification front in articular cartilage: its significance in joint function. J Bone Joint Surg Br 65:72-8, 1983
67. Lane LB, Bullough PG: Age-related changes in the thickness of the calcified zone and the number of tidemarks in adult human articular cartilage. J Bone Joint Surg Br 62:372-5, 1980
68. O'Driscoll SW: The healing and regeneration of articular cartilage. J Bone Joint Surg Am 80:1795-812, 1998
69. Mow VC, Holmes MH, Lai WM: Fluid transport and mechanical properties of articular cartilage: a review. J Biomech 17:377-94, 1984
70. Bachrach NM, Mow VC, Guilak F: Incompressibility of the solid matrix of articular cartilage under high hydrostatic pressures. J Biomech 31: 445-51, 1998
71. Mansour JM, Mow VC: The permeability of articular cartilage under compressive strain and at high pressures. J Bone Joint Surg Am 58:509-16, 1976
72. McDonough AL: Effects of immobilization and exercise on articular cartilage—a review of literature. J Orthop Sports Phys Ther 3:2-5, 1981
73. Athanasiou KA, Shah AR, Hernandez RJ, et al: Basic science of articular cartilage repair. Clin Sports Med 20:223-47, 2001
74. Poole AR: An introduction to the pathophysiology of osteoarthritis. Front Biosci 4:D662-70, 1999
75. Sanchez-Adams J, Guilak F: Form and function of the knee meniscus, in O'Keefe RJ JJ, Chu CR, et al (eds): Orthopaedic Basic Science: Foundations of Clinical Practice (ed 4). American Academy of Orthopaedic Surgeons, 2012
76. Beaufils P, Verdonk R: The Meniscus. Berlin, Springer-Verlag, 2010
77. Mankin HJ, Mankin CJ: Metabolic bone disease: an update. Instr Course Lect 52:769-84, 2003
78. Carter DR, Orr TE, Fyhrie DP: Relationships between loading history and femoral cancellous bone architecture. J Biomech 22:231-44, 1989
79. Thompson WR, Scott A, Loghmani MT, et al: Understanding mechanobiology: physical therapists as a force in mechanotherapy and musculoskeletal regenerative rehabilitation. Phys Ther 96:560-9, 2016
80. Warden SJ, Thompson WR: Become one with the force: optimising mechanotherapy through an understanding of mechanobiology. Br J Sports Med 51:989-90, 2017
81. Feng X, McDonald JM: Disorders of bone remodeling. Annu Rev Pathol 6:121-45, 2011
82. Pagnotti GM, Styner M, Uzer G, et al: Combating osteoporosis and obesity with exercise: leveraging cell mechanosensitivity. Nat Rev Endocrinol 15:339-55, 2019
83. Gillogly SD, Voight M, Blackburn T: Treatment of articular cartilage defects of the knee with autologous chondrocyte implantation. J Orthop Sports Phys Ther 28:241-51, 1998
84. Decraemer WF, Maes MA, Vanhuyse VJ, et al: A non-linear viscoelastic constitutive equation for soft biological tissues, based upon a structural model. J Biomech 13:559-64, 1980
85. Noyes FR, DeLucas JL, Torvik PJ: Biomechanics of anterior cruciate ligament failure: an analysis of strain-rate sensitivity and mechanisms of failure in primates. J Bone Joint Surg Am 56:236-53, 1974
86. Noyes FR, Torvik PJ, Hyde WB, et al: Biomechanics of ligament failure. II. An analysis of immobilization, exercise, and reconditioning effects in primates. J Bone Joint Surg Am 56:1406-18, 1974
87. Woo SL, Gomez MA, Woo YK, et al: Mechanical properties of tendons and ligaments. II. The relationships of immobilization and exercise on tissue remodeling. Biorheology 19:397-408, 1982
88. Goldstein SA, Armstrong TJ, Chaffin DB, et al: Analysis of cumulative strain in tendons and tendon sheaths. J Biomech 20:1-6, 1987
89. To SY, Kwan MK, Woo SL: Simultaneous measurements of strains on two surfaces of tendons and ligaments. J Biomech 21:511-4, 1988
90. Nordin M, Frankel VH: Basic biomechanics of the musculoskeletal system (ed 4). Philadelphia, Lippincott Williams & Wilkins, 2012

91. Özkaya N, Nordin M, Goldsheyder D, et al: Fundamentals of Biomechanics: Equilibrium, Motion, and Deformation (ed 3). New York, Springer-Verlag, 2012
92. Alexander RM: Springs for wings. Science 268:50-1, 1995
93. Alexander RM: Tendon elasticity and muscle function. Comp Biochem Physiol A Mol Integr Physiol 133:1001-11, 2002
94. Finni T, Ikegawa S, Komi PV: Concentric force enhancement during human movement. Acta Physiol Scand 173:369-77, 2001
95. Walker JM: Pathomechanics and classification of cartilage lesions, facilitation of repair. J Orthop Sports Phys Ther 28:216-31, 1998
96. Mueller MJ, Maluf KS: Tissue adaptation to physical stress: a proposed "Physical Stress Theory" to guide physical therapist practice, education, and research. Phys Ther 82:383-403, 2002
97. Fyhrie DP, Schaffler MB: Failure mechanisms in human vertebral cancellous bone. Bone 15:105-9, 1994
98. Birch HL, McLaughlin L, Smith RK, et al: Treadmill exercise-induced tendon hypertrophy: assessment of tendons with different mechanical functions. Equine Vet J Suppl:222-6, 1999
99. Curwin S: Tendon injuries: Pathophysiology and treatment, in Zachazewski J, Magee D, Quillen W (eds): Athletic Injuries and Rehabilitation. Philadelphia, WB Saunders, 1996
100. Arya S, Kulig K: Tendinopathy alters mechanical and material properties of the Achilles tendon. J Appl Physiol (1985) 108:670-5, 2010
101. Tidball JG, Salem G, Zernicke R: Site and mechanical conditions for failure of skeletal muscle in experimental strain injuries. J Appl Physiol (1985) 74:1280-6, 1993
102. Barfred T: Kinesiological comments on subcutaneous ruptures of the Achilles tendon. Acta Orthop Scand 42:397-405, 1971
103. Matsumoto F, Trudel G, Uhthoff HK, et al: Mechanical effects of immobilization on the Achilles' tendon. Arch Phys Med Rehabil 84:662-7, 2003
104. Benjamin M, Ralphs JR: Fibrocartilage in tendons and ligaments--an adaptation to compressive load. J Anat 193 (Pt 4):481-94, 1998
105. Kasashima Y, Smith RK, Birch HL, et al: Exercise-induced tendon hypertrophy: cross-sectional area changes during growth are influenced by exercise. Equine Vet J Suppl:264-8, 2002
106. Viidik A: Tensile strength properties of Achilles tendon systems in trained and untrained rabbits. Acta Orthop Scand 40:261-72, 1969
107. Woo SL, Ritter MA, Amiel D, et al: The biomechanical and biochemical properties of swine tendons—long term effects of exercise on the digital extensors. Connect Tissue Res 7:177-83, 1980
108. Silbernagel KG, Thomee R, Thomee P, et al: Eccentric overload training for patients with chronic Achilles tendon pain—a randomised controlled study with reliability testing of the evaluation methods. Scand J Med Sci Sports 11:197-206, 2001
109. Stanish WD, Curwin S, Mandell S: Tendinitis: Its Etiology and Treatment. New York, Oxford University Press, 2001
110. Curwin S: The aetiology and treatment of tendonitis, in Harries M, Williams C, Stanish W (eds): Oxford Textbook of Sports Medicine. New York, Oxford University Press, 1998
111. Kingma JJ, de Knikker R, Wittink HM, et al: Eccentric overload training in patients with chronic Achilles tendinopathy: a systematic review. Br J Sports Med 41:e3, 2007
112. Eckstein F, Tieschky M, Faber SC, et al: Effect of physical exercise on cartilage volume and thickness in vivo: MR imaging study. Radiology 207:243-8, 1998
113. Brandt KD, Schauwecker DS, Dansereau S, et al: Bone scintigraphy in the canine cruciate deficiency model of osteoarthritis: comparison of the unstable and contralateral knee. J Rheumatol 24:140-5, 1997
114. van Osch GJ, van der Kraan PM, Blankevoort L, et al: Relation of ligament damage with site specific cartilage loss and osteophyte formation in collagenase induced osteoarthritis in mice. J Rheumatol 23:1227-32, 1996
115. Perry J: Contractures. A historical perspective. Clin Orthop Relat Res:8-14, 1987
116. Akeson WH, Amiel D, Abel MF, et al: Effects of immobilization on joints. Clin Orthop Relat Res:28-37, 1987
117. Enneking WF, Horowitz M: The intra-articular effects of immobilization on the human knee. J Bone Joint Surg Am 54:973-85, 1972
118. Deandrade JR, Grant C, Dixon AS: Joint distension and reflex muscle inhibition in the knee. J Bone Joint Surg Am 47:313-22, 1965
119. Spencer JD, Hayes KC, Alexander IJ: Knee joint effusion and quadriceps reflex inhibition in man. Arch Phys Med Rehabil 65:171-7, 1984
120. Young A, Stokes M, Iles JF: Effects of joint pathology on muscle. Clin Orthop Relat Res:21-7, 1987
121. Djurasovic M, Aldridge JW, Grumbles R, et al: Knee joint immobilization decreases aggrecan gene expression in the meniscus. Am J Sports Med 26:460-6, 1998
122. Turner CH: Three rules for bone adaptation to mechanical stimuli. Bone 23:399-407, 1998
123. Wolff I, van Croonenborg JJ, Kemper HC, et al: The effect of exercise training programs on bone mass: a meta-analysis of published controlled trials in pre- and postmenopausal women. Osteoporos Int 9:1-12, 1999
124. Todd JA, Robinson RJ: Osteoporosis and exercise. Postgrad Med J 79:320-3, 2003
125. Rubin C, Turner AS, Bain S, et al: Anabolism. Low mechanical signals strengthen long bones. Nature 412:603-4, 2001
126. Rubin C, Turner AS, Mallinckrodt C, et al: Mechanical strain, induced noninvasively in the high-frequency domain, is anabolic to cancellous bone, but not cortical bone. Bone 30:445-52, 2002
127. Rubin C, Xu G, Judex S: The anabolic activity of bone tissue, suppressed by disuse, is normalized by brief exposure to extremely low-magnitude mechanical stimuli. FASEB J 15:2225-9, 2001
128. Lanyon LE: Using functional loading to influence bone mass and architecture: objectives, mechanisms, and relationship with estrogen of the mechanically adaptive process in bone. Bone 18:37S-43S, 1996
129. Robling AG, Turner CH: Mechanical signaling for bone modeling and remodeling. Crit Rev Eukaryot Gene Expr 19:319-38, 2009
130. Thompson WR, Yen SS, Rubin J: Vibration therapy: clinical applications in bone. Curr Opin Endocrinol Diabetes Obes 21:447-53, 2014
131. Baecker N, Tomic A, Mika C, et al: Bone resorption is induced on the second day of bed rest: results of a controlled crossover trial. J Appl Physiol (1985) 95:977-82, 2003
132. Styner M, Thompson WR, Galior K, et al: Bone marrow fat accumulation accelerated by high fat diet is suppressed by exercise. Bone 64:39-46, 2014
133. Thompson WR, Yen SS, Uzer G, et al: LARG GEF and ARHGAP18 orchestrate RhoA activity to control mesenchymal stem cell lineage. Bone 107:172-80, 2018
134. Sen B, Xie Z, Case N, et al: Mechanical signal influence on mesenchymal stem cell fate is enhanced by incorporation of refractory periods into the loading regimen. J Biomech 44:593-9, 2011
135. Bonewald LF: The amazing osteocyte. J Bone Miner Res 26:229-38, 2011
136. Wang B, Lai X, Price C, et al: Perlecan-containing pericellular matrix regulates solute transport and mechanosensing within the osteocyte lacunar-canalicular system. J Bone Miner Res 29:878-91, 2014
137. Wright CS, Robling AG, Farach-Carson MC, et al: Skeletal functions of voltage sensitive calcium channels. Curr Osteoporos Rep 19: 206-21, 2021
138. Wright CS, Lewis KJ, Semon K, et al: Deletion of the auxiliary alpha2delta1 voltage sensitive calcium channel subunit in osteocytes and late-stage osteoblasts impairs femur strength and load-induced bone formation in male mice. J Bone Miner Res 39:298-314, 2024
139. Kelly MM, Sharma K, Wright CS, et al: Loss of the auxiliary alpha(2) delta(1) voltage-sensitive calcium channel subunit impairs bone formation and anabolic responses to mechanical loading. JBMR Plus 8:ziad008, 2024
140. Reyes Fernandez PC, Wright CS, Warden SJ, et al: Effects of gabapentin and pregabalin on calcium homeostasis: implications for physical rehabilitation of musculoskeletal tissues. Curr Osteoporos Rep 20:365-78, 2022
141. Reyes Fernandez PC, Wright CS, Masterson AN, et al: Gabapentin disrupts binding of perlecan to the alpha(2)delta(1) voltage sensitive calcium channel subunit and impairs skeletal mechanosensation. Biomolecules 12, 2022
142. Salter RB: History of rest and motion and the scientific basis for early continuous passive motion. Hand Clin 12:1-11, 1996
143. Vanwanseele B, Lucchinetti E, Stussi E: The effects of immobilization on the characteristics of articular cartilage: current concepts and future directions. Osteoarthritis Cartilage 10:408-19, 2002
144. Wang Y, Wluka AE, Jones G, et al: Use magnetic resonance imaging to assess articular cartilage. Ther Adv Musculoskelet Dis 4:77-97, 2012
145. Maldonado DC, Silva MC, Neto Sel R, et al: The effects of joint immobilization on articular cartilage of the knee in previously exercised rats. J Anat 222:518-25, 2013
146. Curwin SL, Vailas AC, Wood J: Immature tendon adaptation to strenuous exercise. J Appl Physiol (1985) 65:2297-301, 1988
147. Gerriets JE, Curwin SL, Last JA: Tendon hypertrophy is associated with increased hydroxylation of nonhelical lysine residues at two specific cross-linking sites in type I collagen. J Biol Chem 268:25553-60, 1993
148. Thompson WR, Keller BV, Davis ML, et al: Low-magnitude, high-frequency vibration fails to accelerate ligament healing but stimulates collagen synthesis in the achilles tendon. Orthop J Sports Med 3, 2015
149. Keller BV, Davis ML, Thompson WR, et al: Varying whole body vibration amplitude differentially affects tendon and ligament structural and material properties. J Biomech 46:1496-500, 2013

150. Buchanan CI, Marsh RL: Effects of exercise on the biomechanical, biochemical and structural properties of tendons. Comp Biochem Physiol A Mol Integr Physiol 133:1101-7, 2002
151. Hitchcock TF, Light TR, Bunch WH, et al: The effect of immediate constrained digital motion on the strength of flexor tendon repairs in chickens. J Hand Surg Am 12:590-5, 1987
152. Nielsen HM, Skalicky M, Viidik A: Influence of physical exercise on aging rats. III. Life-long exercise modifies the aging changes of the mechanical properties of limb muscle tendons. Mech Ageing Dev 100:243-60, 1998
153. Stanish WD, Rubinovich RM, Curwin S: Eccentric exercise in chronic tendinitis. Clin Orthop Relat Res:65-8, 1986
154. Radovanovic G, Bohm S, Peper KK, et al: Evidence-based high-loading tendon exercise for 12 weeks leads to increased tendon stiffness and cross-sectional area in achilles tendinopathy: a controlled clinical trial. Sports Med Open 8:149, 2022
155. Gomez MA, Woo SL, Amiel D, et al: The effects of increased tension on healing medical collateral ligaments. Am J Sports Med 19:347-54, 1991
156. Vailas AC, Tipton CM, Matthes RD, et al: Physical activity and its influence on the repair process of medial collateral ligaments. Connect Tissue Res 9:25-31, 1981
157. Zuckerman J, Stull GA: Ligamentous separation force in rats as influenced by training, detraining, and cage restriction. Med Sci Sports 5:44-9, 1973
158. Hart DA, Archambault JM, Kydd A, et al: Gender and neurogenic variables in tendon biology and repetitive motion disorders. Clin Orthop Relat Res:44-56, 1998
159. Józsa LG, Kannus P: Human Tendons: Anatomy, Physiology, and Pathology. Champaign, IL, Human Kinetics, 1997

CHAPTER 3

Muscle Structure and Function

Gary Chleboun, PT, PhD

CHAPTER OUTLINE

INTRODUCTION 83
ELEMENTS OF MUSCLE STRUCTURE 83
Composition of a Muscle Fiber 83
Contractile Proteins 83
Structural Proteins 84
The Contractile Unit 84
Organization of the Contractile Unit 84
Cross-Bridge Interaction 84
Types of Muscle Contraction 85
The Motor Unit 87
Organization of the Motor Unit 87
Recruitment of Motor Units 88
Muscle Structure 88
Fiber Types 88
Muscle Architecture: Size, Arrangement, and Length 89
Muscular Connective Tissue 90
Organization of Connective Tissue in Muscle 90
Parallel and Series Elastic Components of Muscle 91
MUSCLE FUNCTION 92
Muscle Tension 92
Passive Tension 92
Active Tension 93
Isometric Length-Tension Relationship 93
Force-Velocity Relationship 95
Types of Muscle Action 96
Production of Torque 96
Interaction of Muscle and Tendon 97
Isokinetic Exercise and Testing 97
Classification of Muscles 98
Based on the Role of the Muscle in Movement 99
Based on Muscle Architecture 100
Based on Length of the Moment Arm 100
Factors Affecting Muscle Function 100
Types of Joints and Location of Muscle Attachments 101
Number of Joints 102
Passive Insufficiency 102
Sensory Receptors 103
EFFECTS OF IMMOBILIZATION, INJURY, AND AGING 104
Immobilization 104
In Shortened Position 105
In Lengthened Position 105
Injury 105
Overuse 105
Muscle Strain 105
Eccentric Exercise–Induced Muscle Injury 105
Aging 106
Fiber Number and Fiber Type Changes 106
Connective Tissue Changes 106
SUMMARY 106
STUDY QUESTIONS 106
REFERENCES 107

Introduction

The skeletal muscles, like the joints, are designed to contribute to the body's need for both mobility and stability. Muscles produce coordinated motion of body segments and constrain extraneous movement to provide stability when needed. Without the ability of muscles to generate force, the body is incapable of either supporting itself against gravity or producing motion.

Human movement is a multifaceted interplay between muscle function and joint lever systems, all intricately regulated by the nervous system. For physical therapy clinicians, a thorough understanding of muscle function is paramount. It serves as the foundation upon which tailored interventions are crafted to restore or optimize patient function. Understanding muscle function begins with a clear picture of the muscle's structure, from the contractile proteins within each muscle fiber to the organization of the fibers in the entire muscle. In this chapter, we will review muscle structure and then examine the basic mechanical properties of muscle fibers, the muscle in its entirety, and groups of muscles. To complete our understanding of muscle function, we will analyze the function of muscles to execute intricate movements essential for everyday activities, occupational demands, athletic pursuits, and recreational endeavours. Patient applications will be used to apply principles related to basic muscle structure and function to selected common muscle injuries.

Elements of Muscle Structure

Skeletal muscles are composed of muscle tissue (contractile) and connective tissue (noncontractile). Muscle tissue has the ability to develop tension in response to chemical, electrical, or mechanical stimuli.[1] Connective tissue elements, on the other hand, develop tension in response to passive lengthening.[2] Properties of the contractile and noncontractile tissues of muscle and the ways in which they are interrelated give muscles their unique characteristics.

Composition of a Muscle Fiber

Contractile Proteins

A skeletal muscle is composed of many thousands of **muscle fibers** (i.e., muscle cells) that are grouped into **fascicles.** Each muscle fiber in a fascicle is composed of numerous **myofibrils,** and each myofibril is composed of numerous stacked myofilaments **(Fig. 3–1)**. The muscle also includes a number

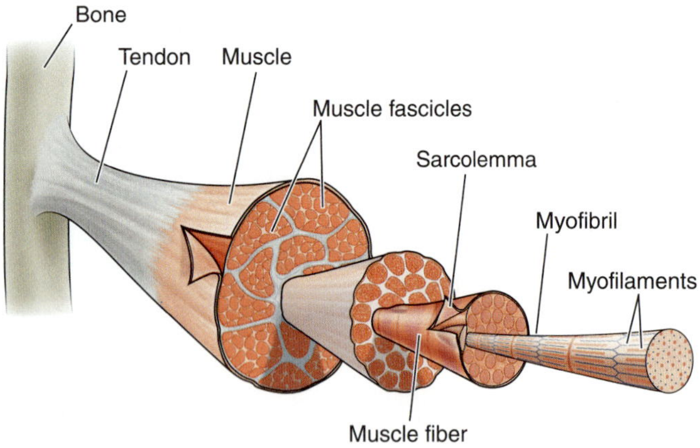

Figure 3–1 Composition of a muscle fiber. Groups of muscle fibers form bundles called *fascicles*. The muscle fiber is enclosed in a cell membrane called the *sarcolemma*. The muscle fiber contains myofibrillar structures called *myofibrils*. The myofibril is composed of thick myosin and thin actin myofilaments.

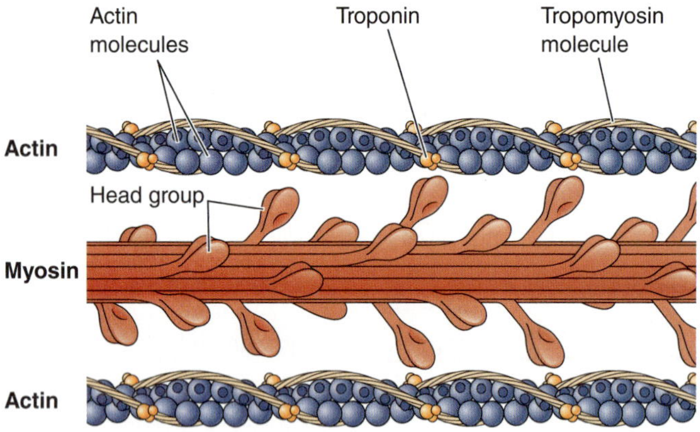

Figure 3–2 Myofilaments. The thin (actin) filament is composed of globular actin molecules (gray) organized in two strands, with globular troponin molecules (orange) located in notches between the two strands. The tropomyosin molecules (orange strands) are thin and are shown lying along grooves in the actin strands. The thick (myosin) myofilament (red) shows head groups that can attach to specific binding sites on the actin molecule.

of different connective tissue elements that we will return to later. The arrangement, number, size, and type of the muscle fibers may vary from muscle to muscle, but every fiber is a single muscle cell that is enclosed in a cell membrane called the **sarcolemma.**[2-4] Like other cells in the body, the muscle fiber is composed of cytoplasm, which in a muscle is called **sarcoplasm.** The sarcoplasm of the cell (fiber) contains myofibrils that are the contractile structures of the muscle fiber as well as nonmyofibrillar structures such as ribosomes, glycogen, and mitochondria that are required for cell metabolism.

A muscle fiber contains many myofibrils bundled together within the fiber. Each myofibril within the fiber is composed of thick (myosin) and thin (actin) **myofilaments** formed by protein molecules of **actin, myosin, troponin,** and **tropomysin** **(Fig. 3–2)**. The interaction of actin and myosin myofilaments is essential for a muscle contraction to occur. Actin myofilaments are formed of two chain-like strings of actin molecules wound around each other. Molecules of the globular protein **troponin** are found in notches between the two actin strings, and the protein **tropomyosin** is attached to each troponin molecule. The troponin and tropomyosin molecules control the binding of actin and myosin myofilaments.

Each of the myosin molecules has globular enlargements called **head groups**[5] (see Fig. 3-2). The head groups, which are able to swivel, are the binding sites for attachment to the actin and play a critical role in muscle contraction and relaxation.

When the entire myofibril is viewed through a microscope, the alternation of thick (myosin) and thin (actin) myofilaments forms a distinctive striped pattern **(Fig. 3–3)**. Therefore, skeletal muscle is also called **striated muscle.**

Structural Proteins

The muscle fiber also consists of several structural proteins.[1,2] Some of these proteins **(intermediate filaments)** provide a structural scaffold for the muscle fiber, whereas others (e.g., **desmin**) may be involved in the transmission of force along the fiber and to adjoining fibers. One protein, **titin,** has a particularly important role in maintaining the position of the thick filament during a muscle contraction and in the development of passive tension.[6-9] Titin is a large protein that is attached along the thick filament and spans the gap from the thick filament to the Z discs **(Fig. 3–4)**. Titin has been implicated as a contributor to a muscle's passive tension, but it also maintains the thick filament in the center of the sarcomere, which is crucial for force production.

The Contractile Unit

Organization of the Contractile Unit

The **sarcomere** is the contractile unit of the muscle and is distinguished by **bands** or **zones** that help to identify the arrangement of thick and thin filaments (see Fig. 3–3A). The portion of a myofibril that is located between any two Z discs along the myofibril is called the **sarcomere.** The Z discs are located at regular intervals along the myofibril, serving not only as boundaries for the serially linked sarcomeres but also to link together the thin filaments of each sarcomere. The portion of the sarcomere that extends over both the length of the thick filaments and a small portion of the thin filaments is called the **anisotropic** or, more commonly, the **A band.** Areas that include only actin filaments are called **isotropic** or, more commonly, the **I bands.**[1,5] The terms anisotropic and isotropic refer to the behavior of these portions of the fibers when light shines on them. The **A band area** (the width of the myosin filaments) has a central area where there is no overlap with the thin filaments, called the **H zone.** The central portion of the H zone, which consists of the wide middle portion of the thick filament, is called the **M line.**

Cross-Bridge Interaction

A muscle contraction is initiated by the interaction of thick and thin filaments within each sarcomere. The interaction is

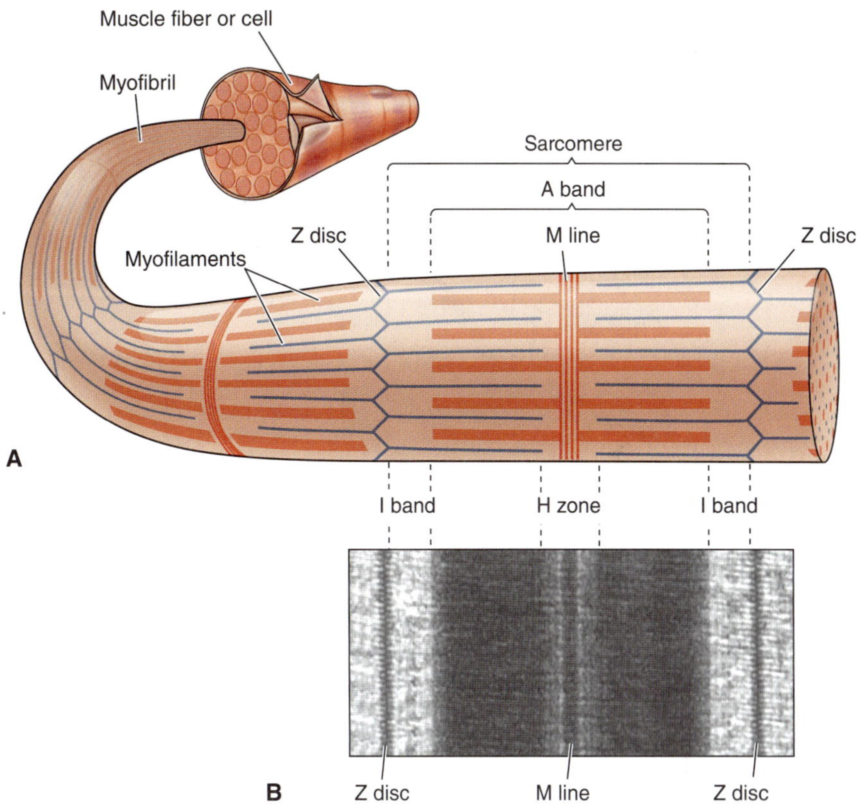

Figure 3–3 Myofibrils in a muscle at rest as shown by **A.** a schematic representation and **B.** electron microscopy. The sarcomere is the portion of the myofibril that lies between the Z discs. The A band portion of the sarcomere contains an overlap of the myosin and actin filaments. The portion of the A band that contains only myosin filaments without overlap is called the *H zone*. The M line, located in the central portion of the H zone, contains transversely oriented myosin filaments that connect one myosin filament with another. The I band portion contains only actin fibers.

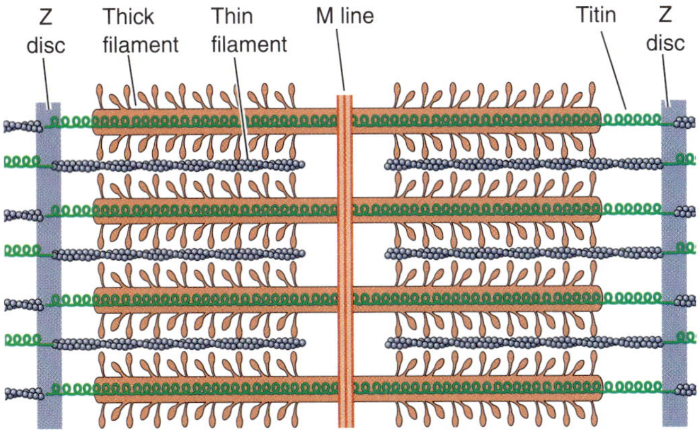

Figure 3–4 The titin molecule is attached along the thick filament and spans the region between the thick filament and the Z disc.

initiated by the arrival of a nerve impulse at the motor endplate, which evokes an electric impulse, or **action potential,** that travels along the muscle fiber.[10] The action potential initiates the release of calcium ions from the sarcoplasmic reticulum.[5] The calcium ions cause troponin to reposition the tropomyosin molecules so that receptor sites on the actin are free, and the head groups of the myosin can bind with actin. This bonding of actin and myosin filaments is called a **cross-bridge.** Tension in the sarcomere is generated with the hydrolysis of **adenosine triphosphate (ATP)** to cock the myosin head, and the release of **adenosine diphosphate (ADP)** and inorganic phosphate from the myosin head during the *power stroke*[1,5,11,12] **(Fig. 3–5)**.

Types of Muscle Contraction

The sliding of the thin filaments toward and past the thick filaments, accompanied by the formation and re-formation of cross-bridges in each sarcomere, results in the shortening of the muscle fiber and the generation of tension **(Fig. 3–6)**. The muscle fiber shortens if a sufficient number of sarcomeres actively shorten and as long as one or both ends of the muscle fiber are free to move. The active shortening of a muscle is called a **concentric** (or **shortening**) **contraction,** whereby the sarcomere length (the distance between the Z discs) decreases as shown by the shift from **Figure 3-6A** to **Figure 3-6B**. In contrast to a concentric contraction in which the thin filaments increasingly overlap the thick filaments, the muscle may undergo an **eccentric** (or **lengthening**) **contraction** whereby the sarcomere length increases as shown by the shift from Figure 3-6A to **Figure 3-6C**. In an eccentric contraction, the thin filaments are pulled away from the thick filaments by a force *external* to the muscle ($F_{external} > F_{sarcomere}$); cross-bridges are broken and re-form as the muscle lengthens. Tension is generated by the muscle as cross-bridges are re-formed. An active muscle fiber will not change length if the force created by the cross-bridge cycling is matched by the external force ($\Sigma F = 0$). The contraction of a muscle fiber without changing length is called an **isometric contraction** where the

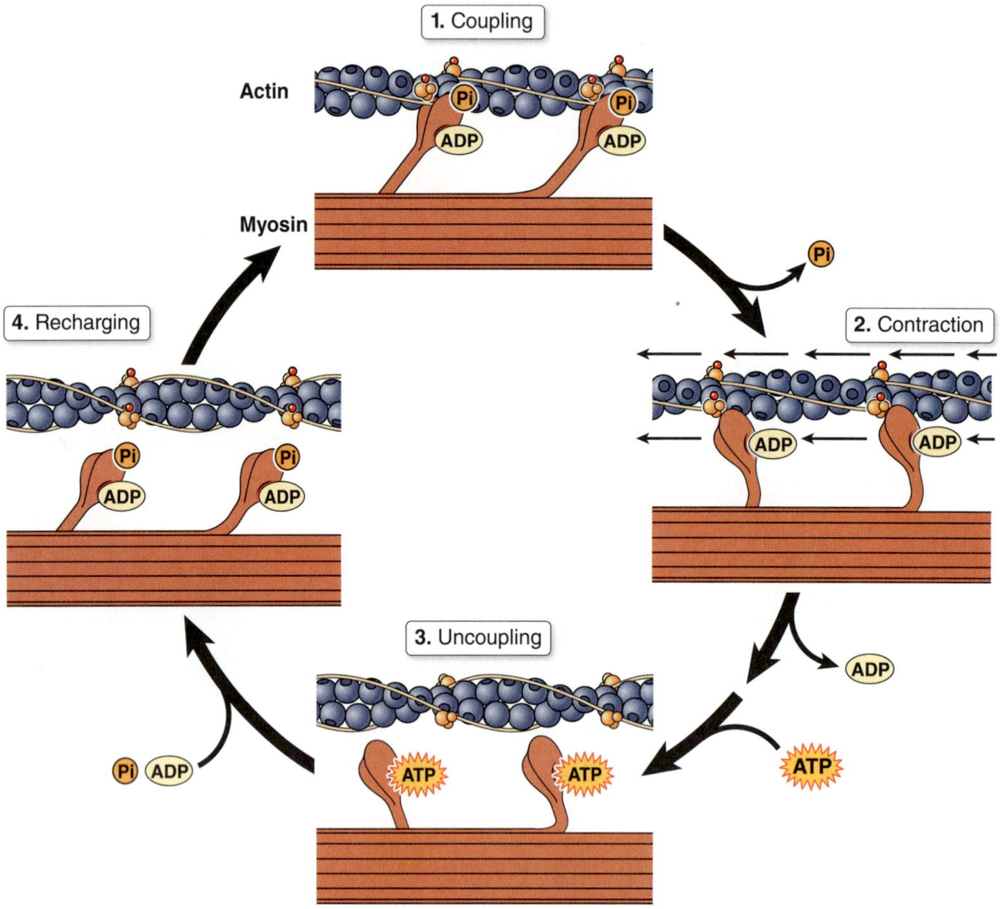

Figure 3–5 Cross-bridge cycle. (1) Coupling: In the presence of calcium ions, the troponin-calcium complex moves to expose the active sites of actin, allowing the cross-bridge to form. (2) Contraction: Adenosine diphosphate (ADP) and inorganic phosphate (Pi) are released, producing the power stroke of the myosin head, thus pulling the thin filament in relation to the thick filament. (3) Uncoupling: ATP binds to the myosin head and the cross-bridge releases from the actin molecule active site. (4) Recharging: ATP hydrolysis occurs, producing ADP and Pi, which are bound to the myosin head, resulting in the cocking of the head to reattach to the actin binding site. The coupling, contraction, uncoupling, and recharging occurs rapidly to allow for a smooth contraction of the muscle.

length of a now active sarcomere (**Fig. 3-6D**) is the same as the length of the resting sarcomere (Fig. 3-6A). See **Expanded Concepts 3–1** for an explanation of muscle contraction terminology.

Expanded Concepts 3–1

Terminology: Muscle Action Versus Muscle Contraction

A potentially more accurate way to describe the types of muscle "contraction" is to use the term *action*. Because the word *contract* means to draw together or shorten, it is an oxymoron to refer to an "eccentric *contraction*" or "lengthening *contraction*." However, during the eccentric contraction, the contractile units (cross-bridges) are attempting to contract/shorten and pull the thin filaments toward the thick filaments, but the forces external to the active muscle are greater than the forces within the muscle, which results in lengthening. Therefore, the term *contraction* implies at least the *attempt* to shorten regardless of the magnitude of other internal and external forces . We have chosen to use the more common term *contraction* in this text, but we realize that muscle *action* is a synonymous term.

Patient Application 3–1

Vik Patel, a 50-year-old man, was playing softball one summer evening. While trying to catch a fly ball, he stepped back with his right foot and slipped slightly. As Vik's foot slipped, the ankle was forced into dorsiflexion despite the active contraction of the ankle plantar flexor muscles as he attempted to push off on the ball of his foot. At the moment his ankle was forced into dorsiflexion, he felt a twinge of pain in his right calf muscle. Because the external moment (torque) created by the dorsiflexion force was unexpectedly greater than the internally generated plantarflexion moment, the plantarflexors contracted eccentrically (lengthened) despite a forceful contraction. This situation is a common mechanism of injury to the muscle or tendon that will result in pain localized to the muscle or tendon.

Foundational Concepts 3–1

Muscle Contraction Facts

The following is a summary of the important facts about muscle contraction at the sarcomere level:

- Tension is generated whenever cross-bridges are formed.
- Calcium influx initiates the muscle contraction.

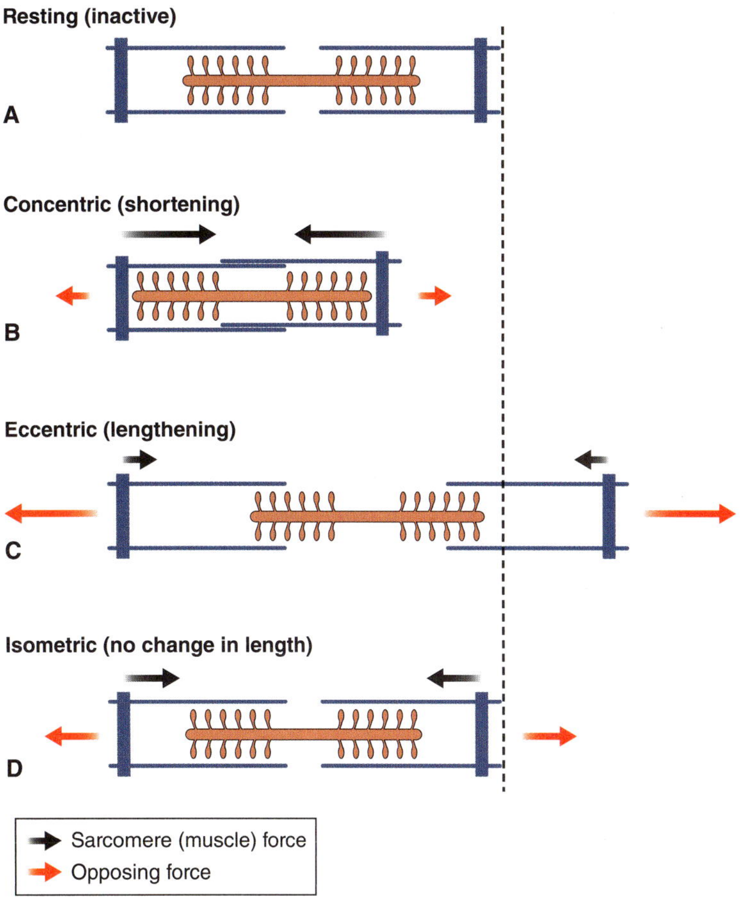

Figure 3–6 Types of muscle contraction from the perspective of change (or lack of change) in sarcomere length during the contraction. **A.** Resting length of the sarcomere. **B.** Concentric or shortening muscle contraction. **C.** Eccentric or lengthening muscle contraction. **D.** Isometric contraction with no change in length.

- ATP hydrolysis fuels the cross-bridge cycle.
- In a concentric contraction, the thin myofilaments are pulled toward the thick myofilaments, and cross-bridges are formed, broken, and re-formed.
- In an eccentric contraction, the thin myofilaments are pulled away from the thick myofilaments, and cross-bridges are broken, re-formed, and broken again.
- In an isometric contraction, the length of the sarcomere is constant.

The Motor Unit

Organization of the Motor Unit

Although the sarcomere is the basic unit of the muscle that produces tension, it is actually part of a larger complex called the **motor unit.** The motor unit consists of the **alpha motor neuron** and all of the muscle fibers it innervates. The contractile process is initiated when the muscle fibers of a motor unit receive a stimulus transmitted through an alpha motor neuron **(Fig. 3–7)**. The cell body of the neuron is located in the ventral horn of the spinal cord. The nerve cell **axon** extends from the cell body to the muscle where it divides into a few or as many as thousands of smaller branches. Each of the smaller branches terminates in a motor endplate that lies in close approximation to the sarcolemma of each muscle fiber. All of the muscle fibers on which a branch of the axon terminates are part of one motor unit, along with the corresponding cell body and axon.

The contraction of the entire muscle is the result of many motor units firing *asynchronously* (not all motor units at the same time) and *repeatedly*. The magnitude of the contraction of the entire muscle may be altered by changing the number of motor units that are activated or the frequency at which they are activated. The number of motor units in a muscle, as well as the structure of these units, varies from muscle to muscle.

Motor units vary according to the size of the neuronal cell body, diameter of the axon, number of muscle fibers, and type of muscle fibers.[5] Each of these variations in structure affects the function of that motor unit. Some motor units have small cell bodies, and others have large cell bodies. Units that have small cell bodies have small-diameter axons. Nerve impulses take longer to travel through small-diameter axons than they do through large-diameter axons. Therefore, in the small-diameter motor units, a stimulus will take longer to reach the muscle fibers than it will in a unit with a large-diameter axon.

The size of the motor unit is determined by the number of muscle fibers that are innervated as well as the size of the motor nerve axon. The number of fibers in a motor unit may vary from two or three to a few thousand. A muscle will have small motor units if the muscle either controls fine movements or is used to make small adjustments to the muscle force. Such motor units generally have small cell bodies and small-diameter axons. Muscles that are used to produce large forces and large movements usually have a predominance of large motor units, large cell bodies, and large-diameter axons. The motor units of the small muscles that control eye motions may contain as few as nine muscle fibers per unit, whereas the

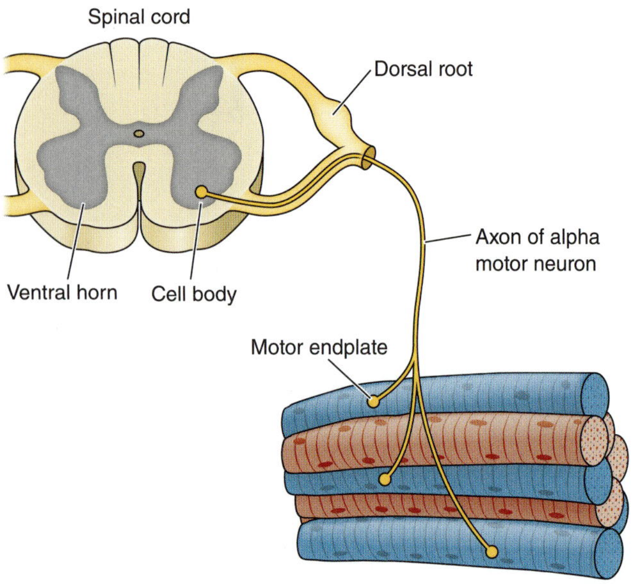

Figure 3–7 An alpha motor neuron. The cell body is in the ventral horn with the motor axon, leaving the ventral root of the spinal cord. Muscle fibers innervated by a single axon are not necessarily contiguous to each other.

gastrocnemius muscles have motor units that each contain about 2,000 muscle fibers. Muscles with a large number of fibers per motor unit usually have a relatively smaller total number of motor units than do muscles that have few fibers per motor unit. The platysma muscle in the neck has relatively small motor units consisting of approximately 25 muscle fibers each, but the muscle has a total of 1,000 of these motor units. The gastrocnemius, on the other hand, has relatively large motor units (2,000 muscle fibers), but the muscle has a relatively small number (600) of such units. In most instances, a muscle has at least some mix of small and large motor units.

Recruitment of Motor Units

Usually, when an isometric muscle action is desired, the motor units with small cell bodies and few motor fibers are recruited first by the nervous system; as force is increased, larger motor units are then recruited.[13,14] This recruitment strategy is referred to as the **size principle of motor unit recruitment.**[13] Small motor units generate less tension than do large motor units and require less energy expenditure; therefore this recruitment strategy is based ultimately on the force required for the motion. In this sense, starting a contraction with small motor units is thought to be energy-conserving. If a few small motor units can accomplish the task, the recruitment of large motor units is unnecessary. If the task demands are such that the small motor units are inadequate, larger motor units can then be recruited. As muscle force purposefully declines, the size principle is also evident, with larger motor units shut off prior to smaller motor units. However, the recruitment strategy may be based not only on energy conservation but also on the nature of the task (a multitask muscle such as the biceps brachii is recruited differently for flexion than it is for supination).[15] Additionally, the type of muscle action (concentric, eccentric, or isometric) may affect the order of motor unit recruitment.[14,16] The recruitment strategy may also vary among the individual muscles of a synergistic group, such as the four muscles of the quadriceps femoris, despite all having a common functional task.[17]

The frequency of a motor unit's firing also affects the force modulation. The relationship between the frequency of firing and force is quite simple in that the greater the frequency of motor unit firing, the greater the muscle force. The contribution of recruitment or firing frequency to the development of muscle force may be different depending on the muscle. Small, distal muscles tend to rely more on the increased frequency of firing, and larger, proximal muscles may rely more on the recruitment of additional motor units.[18] Finally, a more rapid recruitment of motor units may occur during fatiguing contractions in which a constant *position* is maintained than when a constant *force* is maintained.[19-21] For example, when performing a high-velocity eccentric contraction of the plantar flexor muscles, a patient might selectively recruit large motor units first rather than relying on the sequential recruitment of small then large motor units. This may contribute to high muscle forces and an increased chance of injury. It should be obvious from this brief discussion that motor unit recruitment is a complicated and multifaceted topic.

Foundational Concepts 3–2
Active Muscle Tension Summary

Active tension in a muscle may be affected by the following:

1. The number of muscle fibers in a motor unit (which affects the magnitude of the response to a stimulus)
2. The diameter of the axon innervating a motor unit (which determines the conduction velocity of the nerve impulse)
3. The number of motor units that are firing at any one time (which affects the total force response of the muscle)
4. The frequency of motor unit firing (which affects the total force response of the muscle)

Muscle Structure

Fiber Types

Three principal types of muscle fibers are found in varying proportions in human skeletal muscles. These fiber types may be distinguished from one another histochemically, metabolically, morphologically, and mechanically. Although there are different systems of nomenclature used in different texts, in this text the three primary muscle fiber types will be referred to as **type I (slow), type IIA (intermediate),** and **type IIX (fast)** (Table 3–1).[1,4,5] In this classification system (the most common system for human skeletal muscle fiber typing), the myofibrillar ATPase activity under varying acidic and alkaline conditions is used to delineate fiber types. In fact, several intermediate fiber types have been identified through this scheme.

Expanded Concepts 3–2
Another Muscle Fiber Classification Scheme

Another classification scheme uses the response of the muscle to metabolic enzymes to differentiate fiber types. This scheme identifies three main fiber types: fast glycolytic (FG), fast oxidative glycolytic (FOG), and slow oxidative (SO).[4,22,23] This nomenclature is based on the

Table 3–1 Characteristics of Skeletal Muscle Fibers

	TYPE I (SLOW OXIDATIVE)	TYPE IIA (FAST OXIDATIVE GLYCOLYTIC)	TYPE IIX (FAST GLYCOLYTIC)
Diameter	Small	Intermediate	Large
Muscle color	Red	Red	White
Capillarity	Dense	Dense	Sparse
Myoglobin content	High	Intermediate	Low
Speed of contraction	Slow	Fast	Fast
Rate of fatigue	Slow	Intermediate	Fast

combination of reactions of cellular enzymes with substrates to identify myofibrillar ATPase activity (fast versus slow), succinate dehydrogenase activity (oxidative potential), and α-glycerophosphate dehydrogenase activity (glycolytic potential). It is often assumed that the two schemes (FG/SO vs. type I/II) are interchangeable; however, this may not be the case. There appears to be much overlap of metabolic enzyme activity between type IIA and type IIX. The fact that metabolic enzyme activity levels depend on the degree of training of the muscle suggests that these two schemes may not be the same. Another scheme, using immunohistochemical analysis (identification of portions of the myosin molecule using antibodies), has found that types I, IIA, and IIX fibers correspond specifically to different types of myosin molecules (myosin heavy chain [MHC] I, MHC IIA, and MHC IIX).[24] The combination of this scheme and the myosin ATPase system provides an estimate of the contractile properties of the muscle. Whichever classification scheme is used, it should be remembered that, in fact, there is a continuum of fiber types without exact distinctions between types.

Each skeletal muscle in the body is composed of a combination of each of the three types of fibers, but variations exist among individuals in the percentage of each fiber type in similar muscles. The variations in fiber types among individuals are believed to be genetically determined. As identified in postmortem studies, the vastus lateralis, rectus femoris, and deltoid muscles contain about 50% type II and 50% type I fibers;[24] the gastrocnemius contains about 45% type II and 55% type I fibers; and the hamstrings contain about 50% to 55% type II and 45% to 50% type I fibers.[24-27] In studies using muscle biopsy samples from younger subjects, the vastus lateralis tends to be about 54% type II fibers and 46% type I fibers.[28,29] Although the differences may be subtle, fiber types change with age so that a decrease in the number and size of type II fibers occurs. This may account for the differences seen in many of the studies documenting fiber type percentages.

In contrast to the other muscles just identified, the soleus muscle contains up to 80% of type I fibers.[24,29,30] Muscles, such as the soleus muscle, that have a relatively high proportion of type I fibers in relation to type II fibers are able to carry on sustained activity because the type I fibers do not fatigue rapidly. These muscles are often called **stability** or **postural** muscles. The relatively small, slow motor units of the soleus muscle (with small neuronal cell bodies, small-diameter axons, and a small number of muscle fibers per motor unit) are almost continually active during erect standing, making the small adjustments in muscle tension required to maintain body balance and counteract the effects of gravity. Muscles that have a higher proportion of the type II fibers, such as the hamstring and gastrocnemius muscles, are sometimes designated as **mobility** or **nonpostural** muscles. These muscles are involved in producing large ranges of motion (ROMs) of the bony components.[25-27] Type II fibers produce slightly more force per fiber than type I fibers and are able to contract at a significantly higher velocity, thus producing a higher power output than type I fibers.[31] Although muscle fiber type is important in determining the function of a muscle, there are other aspects of muscle structure that also play an important role in determining muscle function.

Patient Application 3–2

Because fiber type is related to muscle function, in certain situations it is reasonable to make assumptions about which muscle may have been preferentially injured. Vik Patel's ankle plantarflexors were excessively loaded as he attempted to run. Because the soleus muscle is composed primarily of type I fibers (postural control) and the gastrocnemius is composed of relatively more type II fibers (power and mobility), the gastrocnemius may be selectively recruited to eccentrically control the large dorsiflexion force and, therefore, is more likely to be the affected muscle in Vik's case.

Muscle Architecture: Size, Arrangement, and Length

Many human muscles have an approximately equal proportion of fast and slow fiber types. Therefore, the determination of muscle function cannot be based solely on this single characteristic. In fact, the architecture of the whole muscle may be more important in determining muscle function than the fiber type.[32,33] The description of skeletal muscle architecture includes the arrangement of the fibers in relation to the axis of force (amount of **pennation**), **muscle fiber length, muscle length, muscle mass,** and the **physiological cross-sectional area (PCSA).** These structural variations affect not only the overall shape and size of the muscles but also the function of the skeletal muscles.

The two most important architectural characteristics that affect muscle function are the muscle fiber length and the PCSA. The fiber length at rest is determined by the number of sarcomeres along the fiber (most often referred to as the number of sarcomeres in series). The amount that the fiber can shorten or lengthen is dependent upon the number of sarcomeres in series; the more sarcomeres, the more a fiber can shorten because the contribution of each sarcomere to shortening is additive. Consequently, a long muscle fiber with

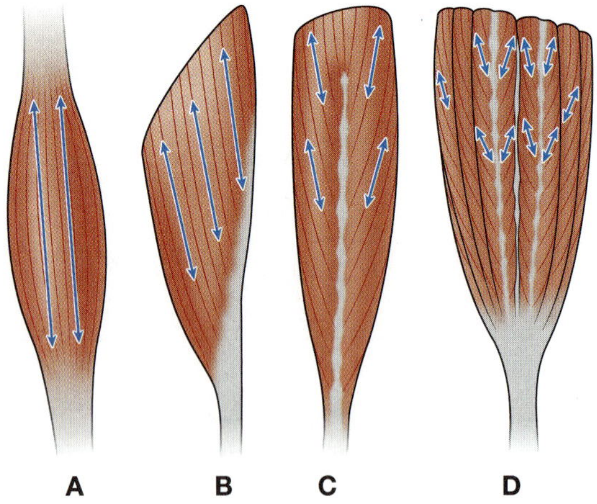

Figure 3–8 Arrangement of fasciculi in a muscle. **A.** Fusiform. **B.** Unipennate. **C.** Bipennate. **D.** Multipennate.

more sarcomeres in series is capable of shortening more than a short muscle fiber. For example, if muscle fibers are capable of shortening to about 50% of resting length, a muscle fiber that is 6 cm long is able to shorten by 3 cm, whereas a fiber that is 4 cm long is able to shorten by only 2 cm. A muscle with long fibers and more shortening capability will be able to move the bony lever to which it is attached through a greater distance than a muscle with short fibers. However, the relationship between the muscle fiber length and the distance that it is able to move a bony lever is not always a direct relationship because, as we shall see, the arrangement of the muscle fibers also affects the length-shortening relationship.

The PCSA is a measure of the cross-sectional area of the muscle perpendicular to the orientation of the muscle fibers. The amount of force that a muscle produces is directly proportional to the number of sarcomeres in parallel (arranged side by side) *within* the muscle fiber (see Fig. 3-1). Therefore, if there is a large number of fibers packed into a muscle (as in a pennate muscle) or if the fiber increases in size (through the addition of myofibrils), the ability of the muscle to produce force will be increased.[32]

A good example of the relationship between muscle architecture and function is the comparison between the quadriceps and hamstring muscles. The quadriceps muscles have a larger PCSA, but the hamstring muscles have longer fibers.[34-37] This architectural arrangement suggests that the quadriceps muscles are designed for force production and the hamstring muscles are designed for movements requiring a larger ROM. Because most of the hamstring muscles cross two joints (hip and knee), it would be expected that the muscle would need longer fibers for the greater excursion required during movements of both the hip and the knee.

The arrangement of fascicles (muscle fiber groups) varies among muscles (**Fig. 3–8**). The fasciculi may be parallel to the long axis of the muscle, as in fusiform-shaped muscles (**Fig. 3–8A**), or at an angle to the long axis in either a **unipennate** (**Fig. 3–8B**), **bipennate** (**Fig. 3–8C**), or **multipennate** (**Fig. 3–8D**) arrangement. Muscles that have a parallel fiber arrangement (parallel to the long axis of the muscle and to each other) are designated as **fusiform** or **strap** muscles. In fusiform muscles such as the sternocleidomastoid or sartorius muscles, the fascicles are long and tend to extend throughout the entire length of the muscle (from one attachment to the opposite attachment). However, in the rectus abdominis, which is also considered a fusiform muscle, the fascicles are divided into short segments by fibrous intersections. In general, fusiform muscles with a parallel fiber arrangement have longer fibers and therefore produce a greater range of motion of a bony lever than will muscles with a pennate fiber arrangement.

Muscles that have a fiber arrangement oblique to the muscle's long axis are called **pennate muscles** because the fiber arrangement resembles that found in a feather. The fibers that make up the fascicles in pennate muscles are usually shorter and more numerous than the fibers in many of the fusiform muscles. In unipennate muscles, such as the flexor pollicis longus, the oblique fascicles fan out on only one side of a central muscle tendon. In a bipennate muscle, such as the biceps femoris and the tibialis anterior, the fascicles are obliquely set on both sides of a central tendon. In a multipennate muscle, such as the soleus or subscapularis, the oblique fascicles converge on several tendons.

The oblique angle of the muscle fibers in a pennate muscle disrupts the direct relationship between the length of the muscle fiber and the distance that the muscle can move a bony lever at the expense of the amount of force that is directed along the long axis of the muscle. Only a portion of the force of the pennate muscles goes toward producing motion of the bony lever. In fact, the more obliquely a fiber lies to the long axis of the muscle, the less force the muscle can exert at the tendon. This decrease in muscle force is a function of the cosine of the pennation angle. Many human muscles have a pennation angle that is less than 30° at rest. Therefore, the muscle force at the tendon will be decreased by a maximum of 13% ($\cos 30° = 0.87$).[4] When a muscle shortens during a contraction, the pennation angle becomes much more oblique, thus potentially affecting the tendon force even more, thus theoretically decreasing the force at the tendon. The loss of force on the tendon from the pennation angle, however, is at least partially negated because pennate muscles usually have a large number of muscle fibers as a result of increased fiber packing, thus increasing PCSA. Therefore, despite the loss of force as a result of pennation, a pennated muscle, such as the soleus, is still able to transmit a large amount of force to the tendon to which it attaches.

Muscular Connective Tissue

Organization of Connective Tissue in Muscle

Muscles and muscle fibers, like other soft tissues in the body, are surrounded and supported by connective tissue (**Fig. 3–9**). The sarcolemma of individual muscle fibers is surrounded by connective tissue called the **endomysium.** Within the muscle fiber, the myofibril is connected to the endomysium via specialized proteins such as intermediate filaments and desmin, which were mentioned previously. Muscle fascicles (groups of muscle fibers) are covered by connective tissue called the **perimysium.** The endomysium and perimysium are continuous with the outer connective tissue sheath called the **epimysium,** which envelops the entire muscle. The **myotendinous junction** is an intricate connection between muscle fibers and the connective tissue of the tendon. Many

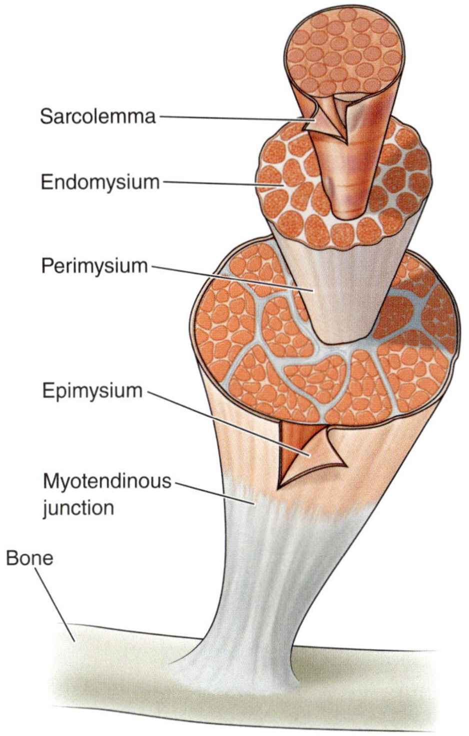

Figure 3–9 Muscular connective tissue. A schematic cross-sectional view of the connective tissue in a muscle shows the endomysium around individual fibers and their individual sarcolemmas, the perimysium surrounding groups of fibers (fascicles), and the epimysium as the outer layer of connective tissue.

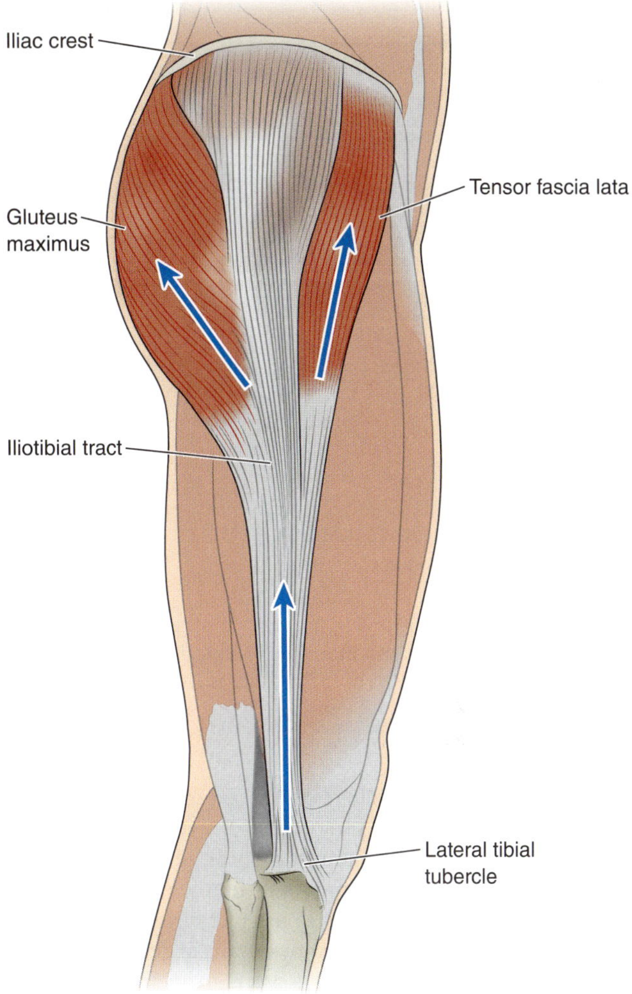

Figure 3–10 Iliotibial tract. A lateral view of the left lower limb showing the deep fascial iliotibial tract extending from the tubercle of the iliac crest to the lateral aspect of the tibia.

special proteins are arranged to make this junction extremely strong. Tendons are attached to bones by Sharpey fibers, which become continuous with the periosteum as noted in the previous chapter. Although the myotendinous junction is designed to be strong and can transmit the large forces from the muscle to the tendon, the myotendinous junction is often the site of muscle strain injuries (microfailure).

Other connective tissues associated with muscles include fasciae, aponeuroses, and sheaths. Fasciae can be divided into two zones: superficial and deep. The zone of **superficial fasciae,** composed of loose connective tissue, is located directly under the dermis (skin). This zone contributes to the mobility of the skin, acts as an insulator, and may contain muscles that connect to skin such as the platysma in the neck. The zone of **deep fasciae** is composed of compacted and regularly arranged collagenous fibers. The deep fasciae attach to muscles and bones and may form tracts, bands, or retinaculae. For example, the deep femoral fascia in the lower extremity forms a tract known as the **iliotibial tract** or **band.** This tract transmits the pull of two of the lower extremity muscles (the tensor fascia lata and the gluteus maximus) to the tibia **(Fig. 3–10).** **Retinaculae** are formed by localized transverse thickenings of fasciae. Each retinaculum forms a loop that is attached at both ends to bone through which tendons pass **(Fig. 3–11).** The retinaculae maintain the relationship of the tendons to their respective joints and joint axes, also preventing tendons from bowing out of position during muscle action. Sometimes deep fasciae are indistinguishable from aponeuroses, which are sheets of dense, white, compacted collagen fibers that attach directly or indirectly to muscles, fasciae, bones, cartilage, and other muscles. Aponeuroses distribute forces generated by the muscle to the structures to which they are attached.[38]

Parallel and Series Elastic Components of Muscle

All of the connective tissues in a muscle are interconnected and constitute the parallel and series **passive elastic components** of a muscle. The connective tissues that surround the muscle, along with the sarcolemma, the elastic protein titin, and other structures (i.e., nerves and blood vessels), form the **parallel elastic component** of a muscle. When a muscle lengthens or shortens, these tissues also lengthen or shorten because they function in parallel with the muscle contractile unit. For example, the collagen fibers in the perimysium of fusiform muscles are slack when the sarcomeres are at rest but straighten out and become taut as the muscle lengthens (either actively or passively) and sarcomere length increases beyond its resting length. As the perimysium is lengthened, it also becomes stiffer (resistance to further elongation increases). The increased resistance of perimysium to elongation may prevent

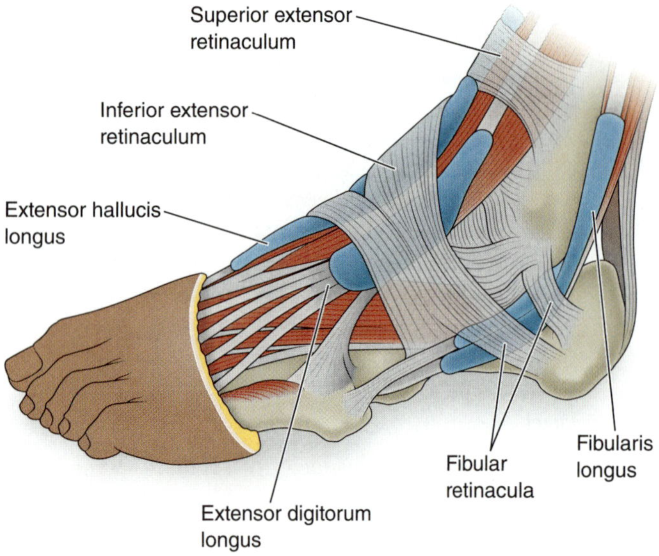

Figure 3–11 The superior and inferior retinaculae and the fibular retinaculae form tunnels for the muscles entering the foot, which maintain the position of each of the tendons relative to the joints and joint axes they cross.

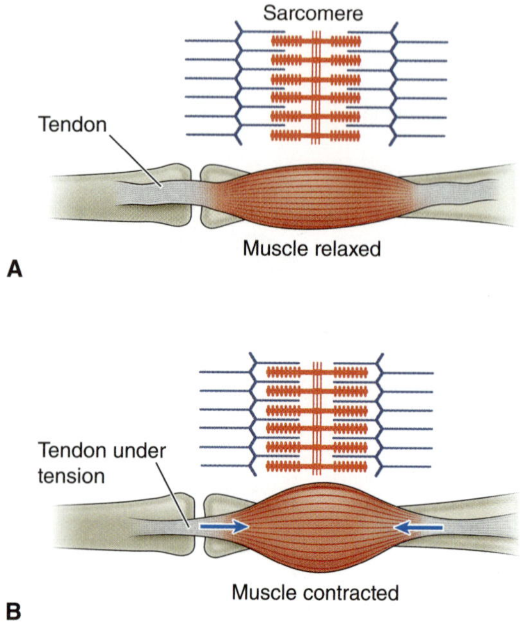

Figure 3–12 Series elastic component. **A.** The muscle is shown in a relaxed state with the tendons slack (crimping or buckling of collagen fibers has occurred). The sarcomere depicted above the muscle shows moderate overlap of thick and thin filaments because the muscle is at resting length. **B.** The muscle in an actively shortened position shows that the tendons are under tension. The sarcomere depicted above the muscle shows extensive overlap of filaments and cross-bridge formation.

overstretching of the muscle fiber bundles and may contribute to the tension the muscle produces at the tendon.[39-42] When sarcomeres shorten from their resting positions, collagen fibers within the parallel elastic component that are slack at rest can **buckle** or **crimp** even further. Whatever tension might have existed in the parallel elastic components at resting length is diminished as the sarcomere shortens from resting length. Because of the many parallel elastic components of a muscle, the increase or decrease in passive tension can substantially affect the total (active plus passive) tension output of a muscle. This relationship between length and tension will be addressed in the next section.

In contrast to the parallel elastic component, the tendon is the primary structure comprising the **series elastic component** of the muscle. The tendon of the muscle is considered to function in series with the contractile elements **(Fig. 3–12)**. When a muscle is at its resting length, the tendon(s) are relaxed and may be crimped (slack) **(Fig. 3–12A)**. The tendon will be under tension when the muscle actively produces tension. When the contractile elements in a muscle actively shorten, they exert a pull on the tendon **(Fig. 3–12B)**. The active pull of the muscle fibers must be of sufficient magnitude to take up the slack (compliance) in the tendon so that the muscle force can be transmitted through the tendon to the bony lever. Fortunately, the **compliance** (or **extensibility**) of the tendon is relatively small (about 3%–5% in human tendons). Thus, although tendons have some stretch to them, most of the muscle force can be used for moving the bony lever and is not dissipated in stretching the tendon. The tendon is also under tension when a muscle is controlling or braking the motion of the lever in an eccentric contraction. A tendon is under reduced tension only when a muscle is completely relaxed while in a relatively shortened position. The role of tendon compliance is revisited below with respect to the entire muscle-tendon unit, as well as in Chapter 14 with respect to gait.

Muscle Function

Muscle Tension

The most important characteristic of a muscle is its ability to develop tension and to exert a force on the bony lever. Muscle tension can be either active or passive, and the **total tension** that a muscle develops includes both active and passive components depending on the length of the muscle. Total tension, which was identified in Chapter 1 as muscle force (Fms), is a vector quantity that has:

1. Magnitude
2. Two points of application (at the proximal and distal muscle attachments)
3. An action line
4. Direction of pull

The point of application, action line, and direction of pull were the major part of the discussion of muscle force in Chapter 1, but we now need to turn our attention to the determinants of the total muscle tension (the magnitude of Fms), which will include a combination of the passive (noncontractile) and active (contractile) elements of a muscle.

Passive Tension

Passive tension refers to tension developed in the parallel elastic components of the muscle. Passive tension in the parallel

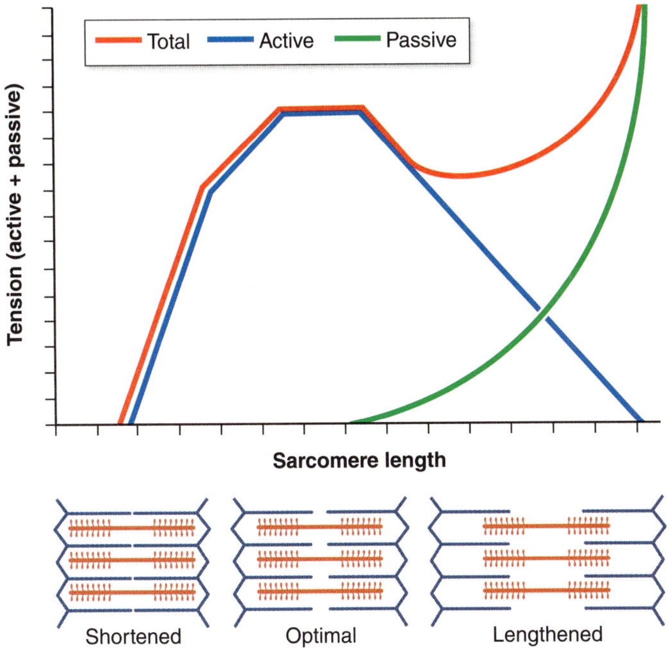

Figure 3–13 The skeletal muscle isometric sarcomere length-tension relationship. The plateau of the active tension curve occurs at optimal sarcomere length. Active tension decreases as the muscle is lengthened because fewer cross-bridges can be formed. Active tension also decreases as the muscle is shortened because of interdigitation of the thin filaments. Passive tension increases (once crimp is picked up) with elongation of the muscle as the parallel elastic elements become increasingly stretched. Passive plus active tension results in the *total tension* developed by the muscle fiber.

elastic components is created by lengthening the muscle beyond the slack length of the tissues, in other words, by stretching the muscle. The parallel elastic components of the muscle will augment the active tension produced by the muscle fibers when the muscle is lengthened and the parallel elastic components are stretched (**Fig. 3–13**). As a muscle shortens, the parallel components will become increasingly less stretched (less tension). Once the parallel elastic elements are slack in a shortened muscle, they will contribute little or nothing to the total muscle tension.

Expanded Concepts 3–3
Passive Muscle Stiffness

Passive muscle stiffness is an important property of skeletal muscle. The passive stiffness of an isolated muscle (not connected to bones and joints) is the slope of the passive length-tension relationship. The steeper the slope, the greater the stiffness in the muscle. The passive stiffness of a muscle attached to bone and crossing a joint is the slope of the torque-angle relationship. Titin and the extracellular matrix of muscular connective tissues are the primary components of the muscle that account for passive stiffness of the muscle (the resistance to stretching throughout joint ROM).[7,43,44] The three classes of proteins in the extracellular matrix (collagens, noncollagenous glycoproteins, and proteoglycans) of the muscle's connective tissue components (endomysium, perimysium, and epimysium) are responsible for muscle stiffness (also known as muscle **extensibility** or **flexibility**), and the extent to which the muscle can be elongated.[40]

Active Tension

Active tension refers to tension developed by the contractile elements of the muscle. Active tension in a muscle is initiated by cross-bridge formation and movement of the thin filaments on the thick filaments. The amount of active tension that a muscle can generate depends on neural factors and mechanical properties of the muscle fibers. The neural factors that can modulate the amount of active tension include the firing frequency, number, and size of motor units that are recruited. The mechanical properties of muscle that influence the amount of active tension are the isometric length-tension relationship and the force-velocity relationship.

Isometric Length-Tension Relationship

One of the fundamental concepts in muscle physiology is the direct relationship between isometric tension development in a muscle fiber and the length of the sarcomeres in a muscle fiber.[45] Identification of this relationship was, and continues to be, the primary evidence supporting the sliding filament theory of muscle contraction. The isometric sarcomere length-tension relationship was experimentally determined with isolated single muscle fibers under very controlled circumstances. There is an optimal sarcomere length at which a muscle fiber is capable of developing maximal total isometric tension (see Fig. 3–13). Muscle fibers develop maximal isometric tension at optimal sarcomere length because the thick and thin filaments are positioned so that the maximum number of cross-bridges within the sarcomere can be formed. If the muscle fiber is lengthened or shortened beyond "**optimal length**" (Fig. 3–13), there is a decrease in the amount of active tension that the muscle fiber can generate.

When a muscle fiber is lengthened beyond optimal length, there is less overlap between the thick and thin filaments, fewer possibilities for cross-bridge formation, and reduced active tension. However, the passive tension in the parallel elastic components may increase as these elements are stretched in the elongating or elongated muscle. This passive elastic tension is added to the active tension produced by the sarcomeres, resulting in greater total tension (Fms) in spite of the decrease in active tension (Fig. 3–13).

When a muscle fiber is shortened from its optimal sarcomere length, there is a similar decrease in potential isometric active tension in the muscle fiber. When the sarcomere is at shorter lengths, the distance between the Z discs decreases and there is interdigitation of the filaments. The interdigitation of the thick and thin filaments may interfere with the formation of cross-bridges from the myosin molecules, thus decreasing the active force. With a shortened muscle fiber, however, the passive parallel elastic components are relatively or completely slack, thus contributing little or nothing to the already reduced active tension of the shortening muscle fiber. The net effect is that the total muscle tension (Fms) is least in a shortened muscle fiber (Fig. 3–13).

It must be remembered that the sarcomere length-tension relationship was determined with isometric contractions and therefore should apply, in the strict sense, only to isometric muscle contraction. In addition, as we will see in the following section, the full range of sarcomere lengthening and shortening may be possible only in experiments with isolated muscle. Sarcomere length obviously changes during dynamic contractions (concentric and eccentric contractions) that affect the tension that can be developed in the muscle. However, during dynamic contractions, *the length-tension relationship must be combined with the force-velocity relationship to determine the effect that both length and velocity have on muscle tension.*

APPLICATION OF THE LENGTH-TENSION RELATIONSHIP

Applying the length-tension relationship to a whole muscle and ultimately to muscle-joint systems is not a simple matter. For example, sarcomere length is not homogeneous throughout the muscle, let alone between muscles with similar functions. This means that, for any particular muscle length at a particular joint position, there may be sarcomeres at many different lengths corresponding to different points on the length-tension relationship. Also, when the muscle is acting at a joint, the torque produced by the muscle is not only a function of the muscle force (which depends on muscle length) but also a function of the moment arm of the muscle. This means that at a certain joint angle, the muscle length may be short (which suggests that force will be low), but the moment arm may be relatively long, thus providing a higher joint torque. These examples clearly show that the sarcomere length-tension relationship is important in our understanding of muscle physiology, but that other important factors cannot be ignored when whole muscle and joint systems are considered.

Only a few experiments have attempted to determine the isometric sarcomere length-tension relationship in intact human muscle.[46-50] In experiments on human wrist and thigh muscles, the range of sarcomere length changes that are seen with normal joint motion is quite small and is located not far from optimal length. This design appears to be quite beneficial in that the muscle is not disadvantaged by being too long or too short. **Figure 3–14** shows the estimated length-tension relationship for the extensor carpi radialis brevis and the biceps femoris long head.[35,48]

One empirical application of the sarcomere length-tension relationship is the observation that a muscle has a diminished ability to produce isometric tension at the extremes of joint motion. This probably occurs only in muscles that cross more than one joint (two-joint or multi-joint muscles) because muscle length excursion is relatively greater for such muscles than for single-joint muscles. A decrease in the torque produced by the muscle may be encountered when the full ROM is attempted simultaneously at all joints crossed by a two- or multi-joint muscle. This decrease in torque production in a position where the whole muscle is shortened is often referred to as **active insufficiency.** Although the decrease in torque can be explained partially by the sarcomere length changes

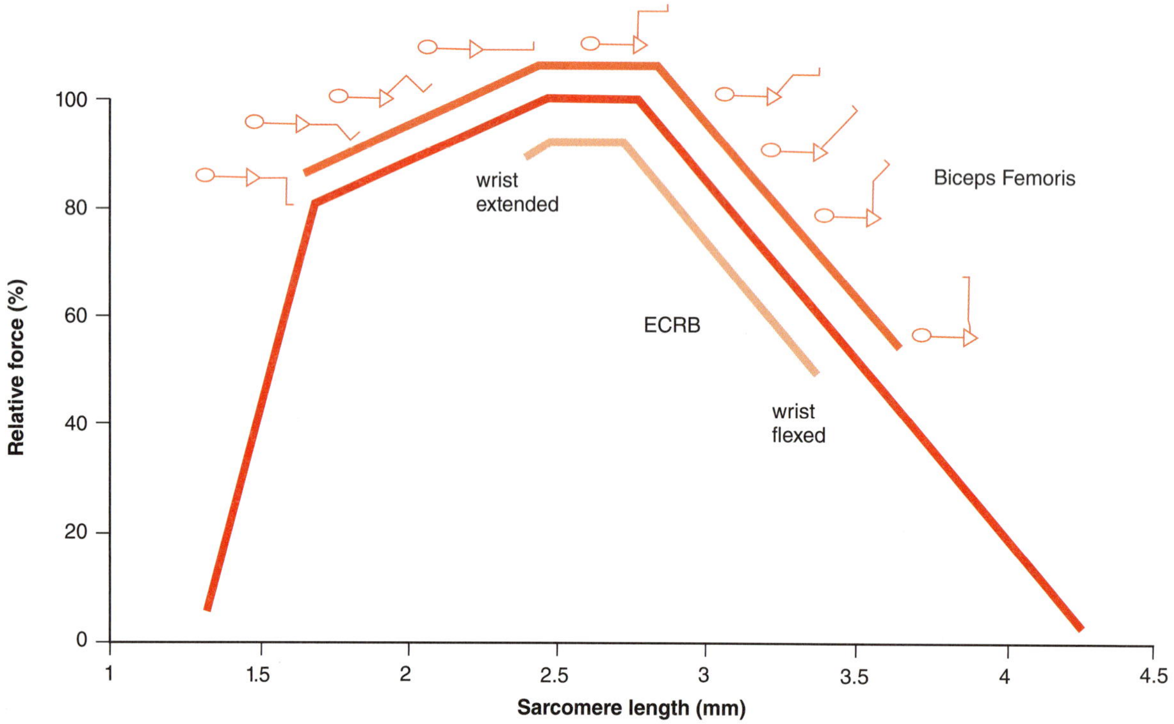

Figure 3–14 The sarcomere length-tension relationship for the human extensor carpi radialis brevis (ECRB) and the long head of biceps femoris is shown, as each contracts from its most shortened position (left) to its most lengthened position (right). The dark red line is the presumed length-tension relationship of the entire muscle in humans, based on the known lengths of human thin and thick filaments. Neither muscle was found to use the full range of that presumed length-tension relationship. The data for the ECRB were determined from intraoperative laser diffraction measurement of the sarcomere length, and the data from the biceps femoris were calculated on the basis of ultrasound measurements of the change in fascicle length with joint position.[35] *(Adapted from Chleboun GS, France AR, Crill MT, et al: In vivo measurement of fascicle length and pennation angle of the human biceps femoris muscle. Cells Tissues Organs 169:401, 2001, with permission.)*

that result in decreased muscle force, other factors, such as the change in the moment arm and the passive restraint of the stretched antagonists, play a substantial role. Because sarcomere length appears to stay close to the optimal length during joint movements, the influences of the moment arm and passive restraint of the antagonists may be more important than once thought.[46-52] Therefore, the term *active insufficiency* refers to a concept that is much broader than just the reduction in active length-tension properties of the muscle.

Patient Application 3–3

Angie Frenden is a 39-year-old woman who sustained a crush injury to her radial nerve resulting from a displaced fracture of the midshaft of her humerus. Although recovery may occur over time, Angie is currently having problems effectively gripping objects with the affected hand caused by the loss of the radially innervated wrist extensors. **(Fig. 3–15)**.

The finger flexors and extensors cross the wrist, carpometacarpal, metacarpophalangeal, and interphalangeal joints. If the intact finger flexors attempt to simultaneously flex all the joints at the same time, the maximally shortened finger flexors will generate less torque and are unlikely to be able to complete the flexion ROM at all joints; this will make grip less effective **(Fig. 3–15A)**. The problem is aggravated by the stretch of the passive finger extensors over all the flexed joints, further restricting motion by creating an opposing passive force.

When Angie's radial nerve recovers, the radial nerve innervated wrist extensors can prevent the finger flexors from flexing the wrist while the fingers flex, thus maintaining a slight stretch of the finger flexors at the wrist. With a more favorable length created by wrist extension, the finger flexors can shorten sufficiently to complete the finger flexion ROM, rendering grip more effective **(Fig. 3–15B)**. The potentially opposing passive tension of the finger extensors is also released somewhat by the wrist extension position.

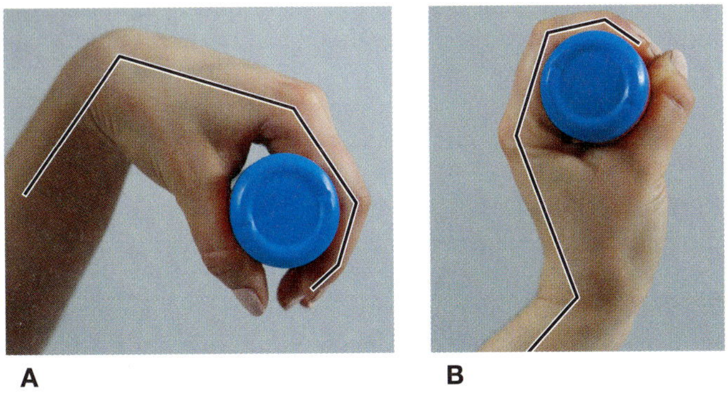

Figure 3–15 Decrease in active tension with muscle shortening. **A.** The individual is attempting to grasp the object but is unable to do so effectively because the finger flexors are attempting to shorten over the flexed wrist as well as over the flexed fingers. In addition, the finger extensors are stretched over the flexed wrist and fingers, potentially restricting flexion range. **B.** By stabilizing the wrist in slight extension, the finger flexors are *stretched* (or at least no longer shortened) at the wrist, enabling the finger flexors to shorten more at the fingers and increasing the effectiveness of grasp. The slight wrist extension also reduces potential resisting passive tension in the opposing finger extensors.

Force-Velocity Relationship

Another factor that affects the development of tension within a muscle is the speed of shortening of the myofilaments. The speed of shortening is the rate at which the myofilaments slide past one another while forming and re-forming cross-bridges. The ability of a muscle to generate force is affected by the speed at which a concentric or eccentric contraction occurs—known as the **force-velocity relationship.**

Based on experiments on isolated muscles, the force-velocity relationship indicates that the velocity of a muscle contraction is a function of the load being lifted.[53] From a clinical perspective, the relationship can be stated with the variables reversed; that is, the force generated is a function of the velocity of the muscle contraction **(Fig. 3–16)**. In a concentric muscle contraction, as the velocity of the contraction decreases (approaches zero), the force production by the muscle *increases*. When the contractile velocity is zero (thus, an isometric contraction), force production is potentially greater than for a concentric contraction. In an eccentric contraction, as the contractile velocity increases, the potential force produced by the lengthening muscle *increases* and then plateaus. The net effect is that the potential for force generation is greatest for an eccentric contraction (regardless of speed) and least for a concentric contraction (regardless of speed). This relationship seen in experimental conditions with isolated muscles lifting a load can also be seen, to some degree, in intact muscles moving bony levers.[54-56] For example, when lifting a dumbbell with the elbow flexor muscles, you are able to move the dumbbell at a higher velocity if the weight is very light. Conversely, if the weight is very heavy, the elbow flexor velocity of shortening is very slow. Lastly, remember that the speed of shortening is

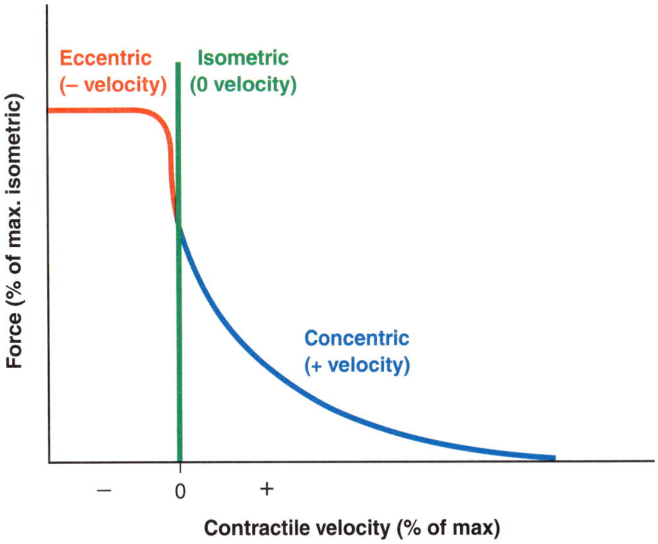

Figure 3–16 The skeletal muscle force-velocity curve. At maximum velocity of muscle shortening (concentric contraction), no force is produced (in other words, maximum velocity of shortening can be attained only with no load on the muscle). As shortening velocity decreases, the force that the muscle can develop during a concentric contraction increases. At zero velocity, the muscle contracts isometrically. Force increases dramatically and then plateaus when the muscle is lengthened actively (eccentric contraction).

related to muscle fiber type as well as to the length (number of sarcomeres in series) of the muscle fiber. Note that muscle strain injuries often occur during high-velocity eccentric muscle actions such as sprinting. In such activities, it is assumed that the force-velocity curve would predict that the muscles were producing high forces, which potentially lead to injury of the muscle or tendon.

It was noted earlier that the length-tension relationship must be combined with the force-velocity relationship to understand force production because both sarcomere length and velocity of contraction affect the development of muscle tension. The length-tension curve data is based on isometric contractions (zero velocity). The fact that most human movements do not occur at a zero velocity of contraction complicates our ability to fully understand force production because the force will vary with changing velocity and changing length.

Foundational Concepts 3–3
Factors Affecting *Active* Muscle Tension

Adding to our understanding of active tension development, the muscle force will be modulated by several additional factors, as follows:

1. The number of muscle fibers in a motor unit affects the magnitude of the response to a stimulus.
2. The diameter of the axon innervating a motor unit determines the conduction velocity of the nerve impulse.
3. The number of motor units that are firing at any one time affects the total force response of the muscle.
4. The frequency of motor unit firing affects the total force response of the muscle.
5. The greater the number of cross-bridges that are formed within sarcomeres, the greater the contribution to tension.
6. Muscles that have large physiological cross sections are capable of producing more tension than are muscles that have small cross sections.
7. Tension increases as the velocity of active shortening decreases and as the velocity of active lengthening increases.

Types of Muscle Action

Isometric, concentric, and eccentric muscle contractions were previously introduced in relation to what was occurring at the sarcomere level. To review: When a muscle fiber is activated so that cross-bridges form, the sarcomeres in the fiber will either stay at constant length, shorten, or lengthen depending on the load that is applied. An isometric contraction occurs when the muscle is activated and the sarcomere does not change length; a concentric contraction occurs when the sarcomere shortens; and an eccentric contraction occurs when the sarcomere lengthens (the load is greater than the force of the sarcomere). An older term, *isotonic contraction*, is not used here because it refers to equal or constant tension, which rarely (if ever) occurs during normal human movements.

What has been observed at the sarcomere or fiber level can be applied to the whole muscle. When the whole muscle is activated and the bones to which it is attached do not move, the muscle action is called an *isometric contraction*. Holding a hand weight without changing the elbow joint angle means that the muscle is contracting isometrically. During an isometric contraction, no mechanical "work" is being done because the joint is not moving. The formula for work is $W = F \times d$, where W is work, F is the force created by the muscle, and d is the distance that the object is moved. Despite the fact that no work is being done, energy is being expended through the hydrolysis of ATP (see Fig. 3–5).

During a concentric contraction, the bones to which the muscle attaches move closer together as the whole muscle shortens. **Positive work** is being done by the muscle because the joint moves through a ROM. Concentric contractions expend the highest amount of energy of the three types of muscle contraction. During an eccentric contraction, the contiguous bones move away from each other as the muscle tries to control the external force that is creating movement of the bony segment(s), with the active muscle elongating (lengthening) as the joint moves through its ROM. The work that is being done during an eccentric contraction is called **negative work;** the work is done *on* the muscle rather than *by* the muscle because the torque from the external force(s) is larger than the torque of the internal muscle force(s). In eccentric contractions, the muscle expends the least amount of energy compared with concentric and isometric contractions.

The amount of tension that can be developed in a muscle varies according to the type of contraction, as was seen in the force-velocity relationship. A greater amount of tension can be developed in an isometric contraction than in a concentric contraction because there is time to recruit more motor units.[57] In general, the tension developed in a maximal eccentric contraction is greater than what can be developed in an isometric or concentric contraction.[58] However, this relationship may not hold true for all muscles at all points in a joint's ROM.[59,60] The greater tension development in a muscle during an eccentric contraction than during a concentric contraction may be due, in part, to mechanical factors in the attachment and detachment of cross-bridges, accompanying increased tension in passive elements, or alterations in the neural activation of the muscle.

We typically think of a muscle contraction as occurring with the proximal segment (so-called "origin") fixed while the distal segment (so-called "insertion") moves. During normal functional activities, however, the proximal segment often moves while the distal segment is stationary. For example, during a pull-up exercise **(Fig. 3–17)**, the brachialis and biceps brachii move the humerus while the forearm (ulna and radius) remain largely stationary. We sometimes refer to this as the **reverse action** of the muscle. Whether the distal or proximal segment moves when a muscle contracts is dependent upon the desired motion, the external forces, and the ability to stabilize other joints. Therefore, in the example of a pull-up, the brachialis and biceps brachii muscles are shortening (concentric contraction) to raise the humeri and the rest of the body to which the humeri are attached.

Production of Torque

Clinicians often assess a patient's muscle strength. Whether strength is assessed using an instrument (such as a handheld dynamometer or an isokinetic device) or by manual resistance,

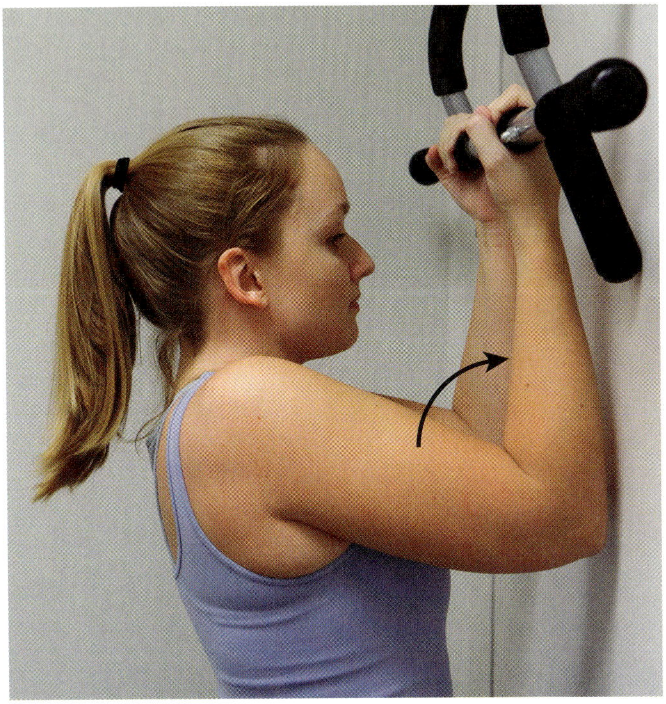

Figure 3–17 In a pull-up exercise, the brachialis and biceps brachii flex the elbow on each side by moving the proximal segment (humerus) toward the distal segment (forearm), sometimes referred to as the "reverse action" of the muscle.

we are actually assessing the amount of joint torque that the muscle can produce. In many physiological experiments on muscle, the muscle is removed from the bone so that the actual muscle force can be measured as the muscle is activated. When the muscle is attached to bones in the body, the muscle still produces a force, but it is the rotational force (torque) on the segment that is being assessed. As already noted, the muscle's ability to produce torque (joint rotation) is a function of both muscle force and the moment arm of the muscle.

By way of review from Chapter 1, if the biceps brachii is producing a consistent 10 N of force, as shown in **Figure 3–18**, the torque (muscle "strength") will be greatest in **Fig. 3–18C** and least in **Fig. 3–18A**. We now know, however, that muscle length is also changing and that the muscle's ability to produce force (total muscle tension or Fms) will not remain constant but will vary as the muscle is lengthened or shortened as the sarcomeres and connective tissues in that muscle lengthen or shorten. In addition, during dynamic movements, the velocity of the shortening or lengthening affects the amount of active force that the muscle produces, thus affecting the total muscle force and torque production.[4,55]

Interaction of Muscle and Tendon

The interaction of muscle and tendon (including the aponeurosis) during muscle contraction and movement also has some important functional implications. Let us begin with a simple example. During an isometric contraction of the whole muscle-tendon unit, the muscle actually shortens slightly and the tendon lengthens slightly (see Fig. 3–12B). In many muscles, the tendon may lengthen by as much as 10% of its resting length during an isometric contraction **(Fig. 3–19)**.[61-65] The compliance of the tendon (or ability to lengthen under load) is important in augmenting the torque production of the muscle. This is the basis for **plyometric exercises,** in which the muscle/tendon complex is stretched before a forceful concentric contraction. The stretch immediately before the concentric contraction helps produce a much greater torque during the concentric contraction. Although the exact mechanism for the increase in torque is debated, evidence shows that the muscle fibers tend to stay at a relatively constant length (isometric) while the tendon lengthens, storing energy to be used during the concentric contraction.[66-70]

Isokinetic Exercise and Testing

Advances in technology have led to the development of testing and exercise equipment that provide for the manipulation and control of some of the variables that affect muscle function. In isokinetic exercise and testing (or a so-called **isokinetic** muscle contraction), the angular velocity of the bony component is preset and kept constant by a mechanical device throughout the joint's ROM.[71] The concept of an "isokinetic contraction" may not be so much a type of muscle action as it is a description of joint motion because the muscle fascicles do not shorten at constant velocity during an isokinetic movement.[72] Because the angular velocity of joint motion is held constant by the isokinetic device, the resistance torque is equivalent to the torque produced by the muscle at all points in the ROM. Therefore, as the torque produced by a muscle changes, the magnitude of the torque of the resistance changes an equivalent amount simultaneously once the limb movement reaches the preset speed. This provides an excellent means of testing muscle strength (torque). Isokinetic devices such as a Biodex are used in many clinics and exercise facilities.

The proposed advantage of isokinetic exercise over free weight-lifting is that isokinetic exercise theoretically accommodates for the changing torque of the muscle (or muscle group) as the muscle's moment arm and length-tension vary throughout the ROM. If the preset speed is achieved, the isokinetic device consistently matches the torque of the muscle through the remaining joint range.[71]

The maximum isokinetic torque for a concentric contraction obtained at high-angular velocities will be less than the torque produced at low-angular velocities. This decline in torque with increasing contraction velocity is expected on the basis of the force-velocity relationship of muscle, described previously. In fact, for any particular point in the joint ROM, isometric torque values are higher than concentric torque values at any velocity for that same point in the joint range. Therefore, the closer the angular velocity of a concentric isokinetic contraction approaches to zero (0 = isometric), the greater the isokinetic torque.[73,74]

Isokinetic equipment is used extensively for determining the amount of joint torque that a muscle can develop at different velocities, for strength training, and for comparing the relative strength of one muscle group with another. Most isokinetic devices also permit quantification of eccentric muscle torque. Isokinetic evaluation of muscle strength has provided important information about muscle function, and isokinetic

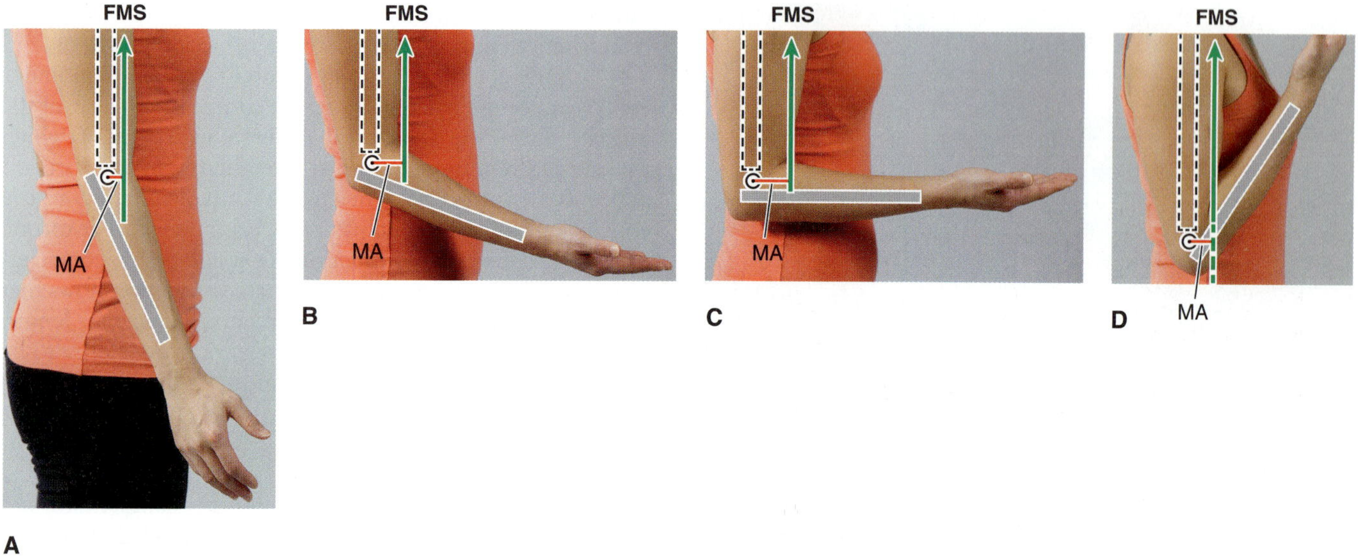

Figure 3–18 The torque generated by the muscle changes as the moment arm of the muscle also changes during joint motion, even if the force production (Fms) remains constant. However, both the active and passive tension will vary with the length of the active muscle, as well as with the type and velocity of the muscle contraction.

exercise is effective for gaining strength. However, there are some limitations to isokinetic evaluation and exercise. For example, at higher speeds the range within which movement is at constant velocity is decreased, and functional movements are rarely performed at constant velocity. Some research shows that isokinetic testing or exercising may differentiate performance in functional tasks or may enhance the training effect for functional activities, and some research shows that it does not.[75-78]

Expanded Concepts 3–4

At various stages of rehabilitation for an injured muscle or muscle group, it is advantageous to limit the force that a muscle produces because we do not want to injure healing muscle or tendon tissue. The most obvious way to decrease muscle force is to decrease the applied resistance. However, based on the discussions in this section, the clinician may choose to exercise the patient on an isokinetic device (or through some other mechanism that provides a constant external resistance) at a higher velocity, which decreases the elicited muscle force. Although this may not be a common choice for exercise training, it may prove useful in certain situations.

Foundational Concepts 3–4
Summary of Intrinsic and Extrinsic Factors Involving Active Muscle Tension

The velocity of muscle contraction is affected by the following:

- *Recruitment order of the motor units:* Units with slow conduction velocities are generally recruited first.
- *Type of muscle fibers in the motor units:* Units with type II muscle fibers can develop maximum tension more rapidly than units with type I muscle fibers; the rate of cross-bridge formation, breaking, and re-formation may vary.
- *The length of the muscle fibers:* Long fibers have a higher shortening velocity than shorter fibers.
- *The magnitude of the resistance:* For a given muscle force production, a greater resistance to the muscle action will result in a slower contraction.

The magnitude of the active tension is affected by the following:

- *Size of motor units:* Larger units produce greater tension.
- *Number and size of the muscle fibers in a cross section of the muscle:* The larger the cross section, the greater the amount of tension that a muscle may produce.
- *Number of motor units firing:* The greater the number of motor units firing in a muscle, the greater the tension.
- *Frequency of firing of motor units:* The higher the frequency of firing of motor units, the greater the tension.
- *Sarcomere length:* The closer the length is to optimal length, the greater the amount of isometric tension that can be generated.
- *Fiber arrangement:* A pennate fiber arrangement gives a greater number of muscle fibers and potentially a larger cross-sectional area, and therefore a greater amount of tension may be generated in a pennate muscle than in a parallel muscle.
- *Type of muscle contraction:* An isometric contraction can develop greater tension than a concentric contraction; an eccentric contraction can develop greater tension than an isometric contraction.
- *Velocity:* As the speed of shortening increases, tension decreases in a concentric contraction. As the speed of active lengthening increases, tension increases in an eccentric contraction.

Classification of Muscles

Individual muscles may be named in many ways based on shape (rhomboids like a rhombus, the deltoid like a delta or triangle), the number of heads (*bi*ceps, *tri*ceps, *quad*riceps), location (biceps *femor*is, *tibia*lis *anterior*), or a combination of location and function (*extensor digit*orum *long*us, *flexor pollicis* [thumb]

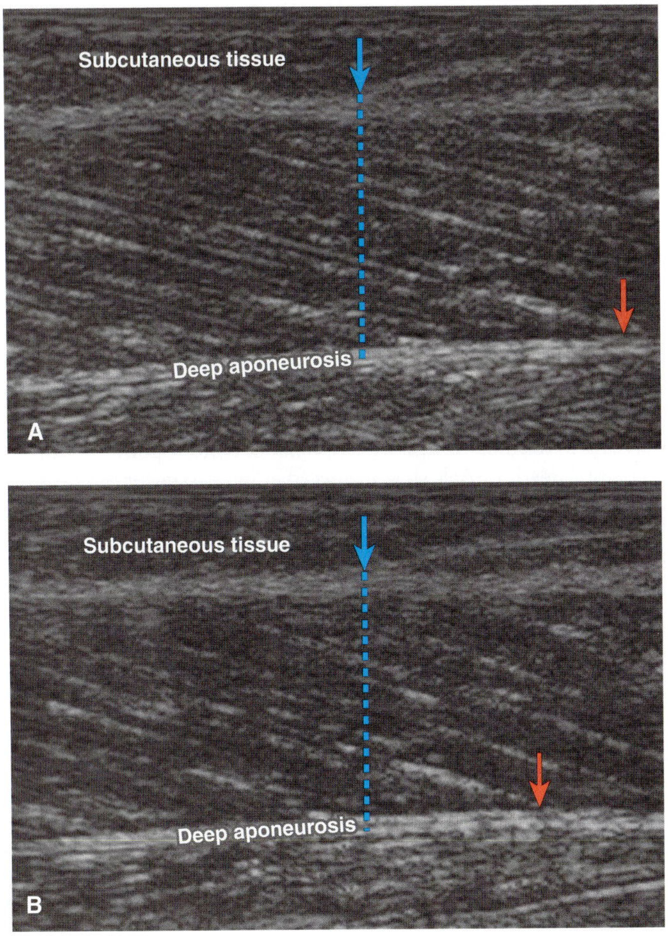

Figure 3–19 Ultrasound image of the medial gastrocnemius. **A.** Relaxed. **B.** During an isometric contraction. In both (A) and (B), the blue arrow and its dotted extension is a fixed reference point in the subcutaneous fat while the red arrow is a fixed point on the aponeuroses of the tendon. Note how the insertion point on the aponeurosis (*red arrow*) in (B) moves to the left (proximally) compared to the same reference point in (A) as the muscle connective tissue and tendon are stretched during an isometric contraction.

brevis). Groups of muscles are categorized either by the actions they perform or the particular role they serve during specific actions. When muscles are categorized by action, they can be considered as flexors, extensors, or rotators. When muscles are categorized according to role, individual muscles or groups of muscles may be referred to as the **agonists, antagonists,** or **synergists** for a particular motion. In this section, we explore the classification of muscle based on the role of the muscle during movement as well as the classification based on muscle architecture and moment arm.

Based on the Role of the Muscle in Movement

The term **prime mover (agonist)** is used to designate a muscle whose role is to produce a desired motion at a joint. If flexion is the desired action, the flexor muscles are the prime movers. However, it is common to limit the term "prime mover" to those flexors that are recruited first or that produce the action with greatest potential force. When flexion is desired, the extensor muscles that would produce the opposite motion are

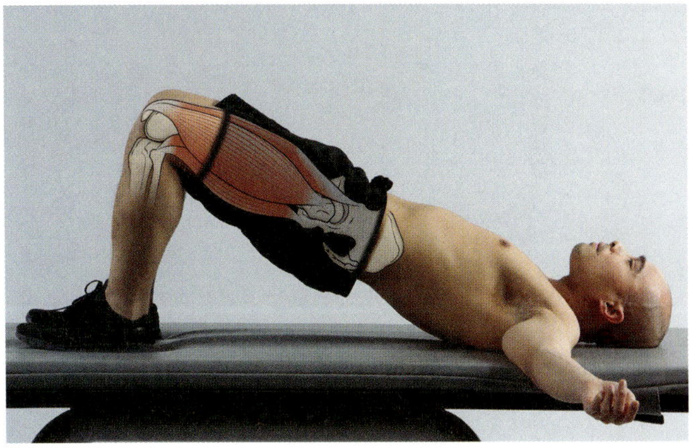

Figure 3–20 Co-contraction of the quadriceps and the hamstrings provide simultaneous extension and flexion torques, respectively, at the knees to stabilize the knees as the hips extend in a bridging exercise.

called the **antagonists.** The desired motion is not opposed by an active contraction of the antagonist(s), but the antagonistic muscles have the *potential* to oppose the action.

Ordinarily, when an agonist (for example, the hamstrings) is called on to perform a desired motion (knee flexion), the antagonist muscle (quadriceps) does not contract concomitantly. If, however, the agonist and the potential antagonist contract simultaneously, then **co-contraction** occurs **(Fig. 3–20)**. Co-contraction of muscles (purposeful simultaneous contraction of an agonist and antagonist) around a joint can help to provide stability for the joint and represents a form of synergy that may be necessary in certain situations. Co-contraction of muscles can be undesirable when a desired motion is prevented by involuntary co-contraction, such as occurs in disorders affecting the control of muscle function (e.g., cerebral palsy). In addition, having muscles active on both sides of the joint during a co-contraction increases the net compressive force through the joint surfaces, enhancing stability.

Muscles that in some way help the agonist (prime mover) to perform a desired action are called **synergists.** The anterior deltoid muscle is a strong flexor of the glenohumeral joint and typically is considered the prime mover. The much smaller coracobrachialis muscle can also produce shoulder flexion but much more weakly. The coracobrachialis muscle, therefore, is sometimes referred to as a synergist or may be referred to as a **coagonist** for shoulder flexion.

Synergists may assist the agonist directly by helping to perform the desired action (such as the coracobrachialis does for the deltoid), or the synergists may assist the agonist indirectly either by stabilizing a segment or by preventing an undesired action. In Figure 3–15B, we saw the example where the wrist extensors worked synergistically with the finger flexors to maintain a more optimal length-tension relationship in the finger flexors to facilitate effective grasp. The wrist extensors prevent unwanted wrist flexion (as in Fig. 3–15A) that would potentially put the finger flexors in a disadvantageous position.

Sometimes the synergistic action of two muscles is necessary to produce a motion that neither could produce alone. The extensor carpi radialis longus and brevis muscles by themselves will produce simultaneous wrist extension and

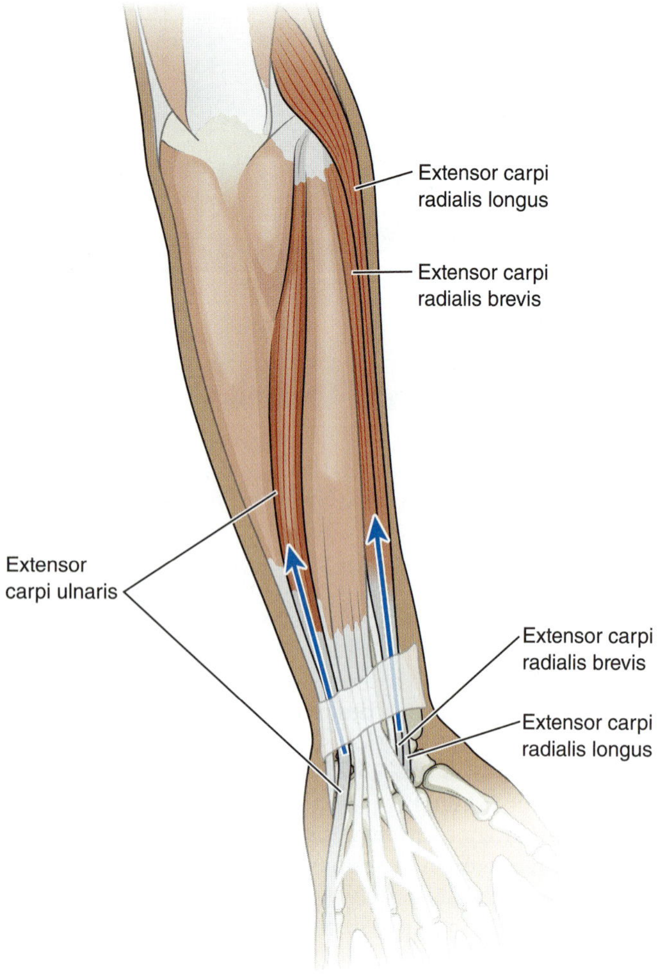

Figure 3–21 Synergistic muscle activity. When the extensor carpi radialis longus and brevis work together with the extensor carpi ulnaris, the radial and ulnar deviations of the wrist, respectively, offset each other and the muscles work synergistically to produce wrist extension.

radial deviation. The extensor carpi ulnaris muscle by itself will produce simultaneous wrist extension and ulnar deviation. Working together, the extensor carpi radialis longus and brevis and the extensor carpi ulnaris produce pure wrist extension, with radial and ulnar deviation components of the muscles cancelling each other out **(Fig. 3–21)**. During wrist extension, the long finger extensors (extensor digitorum communis) may assist with wrist extension as synergists.

Based on Muscle Architecture

Placing muscles into functional categories, such as flexor/extensor or agonist/antagonist, helps to simplify the task of describing the many different muscles and explaining their actions. However, these categories are somewhat arbitrary because muscles can change roles. A potential antagonist in one instance may be a synergist in another situation. Classification of muscles based on their architectural characteristics may provide more meaningful insight into the function of the muscles during movement. For example, muscles that have similar functions also have similar architectural characteristics. This is somewhat intuitive because muscle architecture plays such an important role in determining the potential force and velocity of muscle contraction, and several studies have confirmed that the functional groups of muscles have similar architecture. Examples of this may be seen in experiments with both animals and humans.[4,33,37,79,80]

In the lower extremity, the knee extensors have a larger cross-sectional area compared with knee flexors such as the semitendinosus, semimembranosus, and biceps femoris, but knee extensors and flexors tend to have similar fiber length[37] **(Fig. 3–22)**. Whereas the knee flexors have a decreased ability to produce force compared with the knee extensors, other knee flexors such as the gracilis and sartorius with longer fibers (more sarcomeres in series) can shorten (increased excursion) over a greater ROM and, therefore, have the potential for a greater velocity of contraction. The soleus (a plantarflexor muscle) has a short fiber length (fewer sarcomeres in series) but a large cross-sectional area that sets it apart from the anterior tibialis (an ankle dorsiflexor muscle) that has longer fiber length but a smaller cross-sectional area. Although we can classify many muscles based on architecture, there are obvious exceptions, as seen by some of the knee flexors having similar fiber length to the knee extensors.

Based on Length of the Moment Arm

The relationship of a muscle to the joint has also been used to classify muscles into groups. The length of the muscle's moment arm is an important component of determining the joint torque and, in combination with the fiber length, the range through which the muscle can move the joint.[4] The ratio of the fiber length to the moment arm provides a way of identifying which factor plays a greater role in the production of the joint torque and in determining the resulting ROM at the joint. For example, the ratio of fiber length to the moment arm is much higher in the wrist extensor muscles compared with the wrist flexor muscles. This suggests that wrist extensor fiber length plays a greater role in torque development throughout the ROM than does the moment arm and that the wrist flexor moment arm plays a greater role than fiber length.[48]

Although all skeletal muscles adhere to a general basic structural design, a considerable amount of variability exists among muscles regarding the number, size, arrangement, and type of muscle fibers. Therefore, attempts to classify muscles into only a few groups may be inappropriate. According to the evidence that subpopulations of motor units from a muscle, rather than from groups of muscles, appear to work together for a particular motor task, a more appropriate way of describing muscle action might be in terms of motor units.[18] However, more research needs to be performed in this area before a motor unit classification system can be widely used and accepted.

Factors Affecting Muscle Function

In addition to the large number of factors affecting muscle function that have been examined thus far, a few other factors need to be considered:

- Types of joints and location of muscle attachments
- Number of joints crossed by the muscle
- Passive insufficiency
- Sensory receptors

Figure 3-22 Muscle architectural relationships.[4,33,37] The soleus (a plantarflexor) has a large physiological cross -sectional area (PCSA) (y-axis of the graph) that is off-scale on the graph, with a corresponding ability to produce substantial force that contrasts with the small PCSA and low force production capacity of the anterior tibialis (a dorsiflexor). However, the longer fibers (more sarcomeres in series) of the anterior tibialis (Ant tib, x-axis of graph) give it a greater excursion (ability to shorten). The vastus lateralis (vast lat) is a knee extensor with substantially greater PCSA and force-generating capability than knee flexors such as the semitendinous (semitend), semimembranosus (semimem), gracilis, and sartorius (with the fiber length of the sartorius being off-scale on the graph). However, some of these knee flexors have much greater shortening capability (excursion) that enhances their potential to contract at higher velocities.

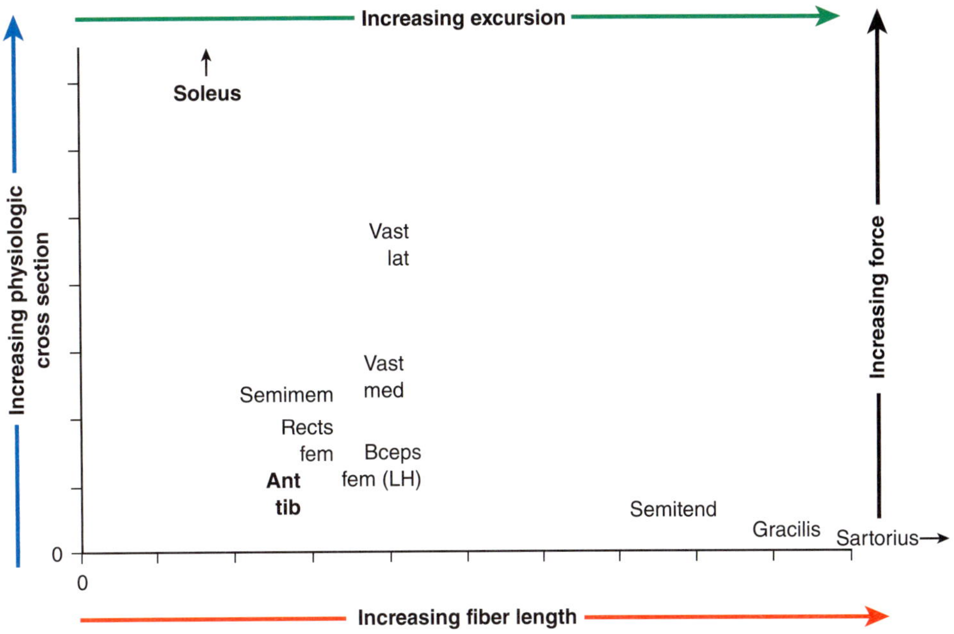

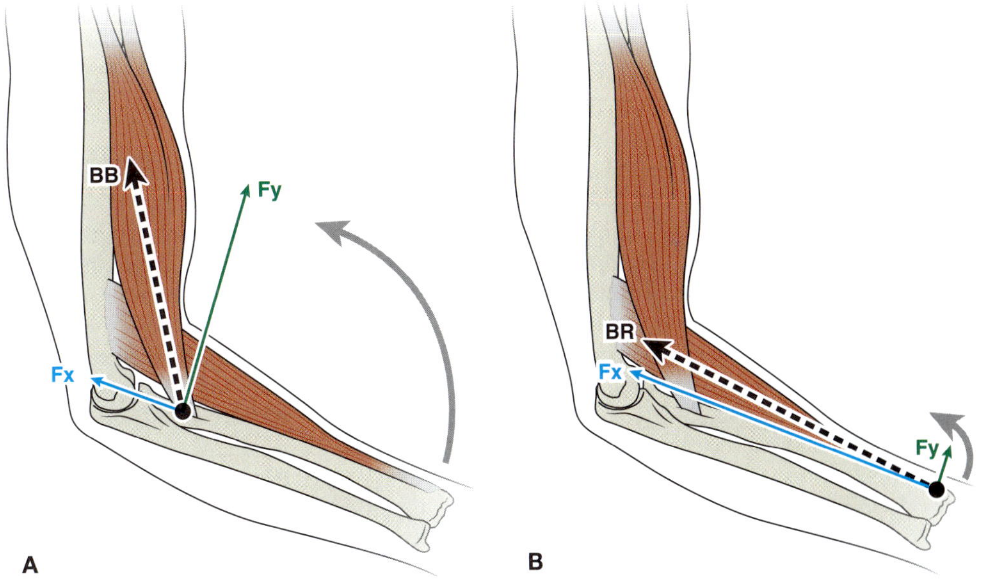

Figure 3-23 Location of muscles. **A.** Because the attachment of the biceps brachii (BB) on the radius lies close to the elbow joint, its substantial rotary component (Fy) will create a large arc of motion for the distal forearm. **B.** The brachioradialis (BR) is attached to the radius far from the elbow joint: Its small rotary component will create only a small arc of motion for the distal forearm. It should be noted, however, that the compressive component of the brachioradialis (Fx) is substantially greater than the compressive component of the biceps, making the brachioradialis a stronger stabilizer.

Types of Joints and Location of Muscle Attachments

The type of joint affects the function of a muscle because the structure of the joint determines the type of motion that will occur (e.g., flexion and extension) as well as the ROM. The muscle's location or line of action relative to the joint axes determines which motion the muscle will perform. In general (but with exceptions), muscles that cross the ventral aspect of joints are flexors, whereas muscles located on the dorsal aspect of joints are typically extensors (with the knee being a notable exception). Muscles located laterally and medially serve as abductors and adductors, respectively, and may also serve as rotators.

Muscles such as the biceps brachii **(Fig. 3-23)**, which has a distal attachment that lies close to a joint axis, have a greater rotatory component (Fy) of its force vector (BB) **(Fig. 3-23A)** than those such as the brachioradialis, which has a distal attachment further from the joint axis **(Fig. 3-23B)**. However, muscles with attachments farther from the joint are designed to provide stability for the joint because most of their force is directed toward the joint ($F_X > F_Y$), producing compression throughout the joint range. As has already been identified in past chapters, the biceps brachii's relative contribution to stability will be less at 90° than when the elbow is in full extension (see Fig. 1-36). At full extension, a greater proportion of the biceps brachii force is directed toward the joint (Fx), resulting in greater compression. A muscle provides maximum joint stabilization at the point at which its compressive component is greatest and, correspondingly, its rotary component is least.

Usually, one group of muscles acting at a joint can produce more torque than another group of muscles acting at the same joint. Disturbances of the normal ratio of agonist-antagonist strength may create a muscle imbalance at the joint and may place the tissues in and around the joint at risk for injury. For example, weakness of the hip external rotators causes a strength imbalance between hip external and internal rotation that may result in excess hip internal rotation during gait. Agonist-antagonist strength ratios for normal joints are often used as a basis for establishing treatment goals after an injury.

Number of Joints

Many functional activities require the coordinated movement of several joints that are controlled by combinations of muscles that cross the joints requiring coordination. To produce a purposeful movement pattern, many believe that motor control mediated by the central nervous system minimizes necessary muscle force to accomplish the task (least motor unit activity) and thus minimizes energy expenditure and muscle fatigue. These strategies of motor control attempt to ensure that movement is done efficiently. There are several theories that attempt to explain differences in how single-joint and multi-joint movements are controlled.[81] This is a current topic of research that will likely continue for several years.

Single-joint muscles tend to be recruited for force and work production, more often as concentric and isometric contractions. Multi-joint muscles, in contrast, tend to be recruited to control the fine regulation of torque during dynamic movements, and involve eccentric actions more often than concentric muscle actions,[82-84] although there are exceptions to these general assumptions. In some animals, for example, the biarticular muscles tend to contract concentrically, producing positive work, whereas the single-joint muscles contract eccentrically.[85] Furthermore, some human biarticular muscles (rectus femoris and biceps femoris) are activated to a greater degree in single-joint knee extension and flexion exercises than in multi-joint exercises such as the leg press that served as exercise options in Chapter 1.[86]

Single-joint and multi-joint muscles may also work together in such a way that the single-joint muscle can assist in the movement of a joint that it does not cross.[82,87] We saw this in Chapter 1 (Fig. 1–45) where the gluteus maximus helped extend the knee. In another example, the movement of standing up from a chair requires simultaneous knee and hip extension. The single-joint knee extensors (vastus medialis, intermedius, and lateralis) may actually "assist" the biarticular hamstrings (and the one-joint gluteus maximus) with hip extension, although the vasti muscles do not cross the hip. Consider that the hamstring muscles are active and are simply attempting to maintain a constant length (e.g., 40 cm) as the person rises from the chair. As the vasti muscles shorten and extend the femur on the weight-bearing tibia, the extending knee will pull on the active hamstring muscles that essentially act as an inextensible rod. With increased knee extension, the hamstrings will pull the pelvis downward posteriorly, resulting in hip extension with little or no shortening of the hamstrings **(Fig. 3–24)**.

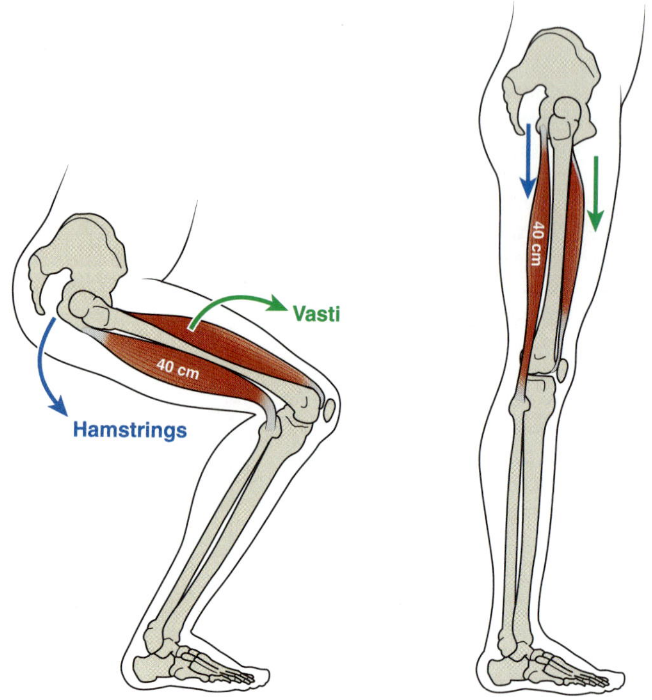

Figure 3–24 Single-joint quadriceps muscles contributing to hip extension. The vasti muscles of the quadriceps extend the knee while the active hamstring muscles maintain a constant length (40 cm, for example); the knee extension action of the vasti muscles pulls on the "inextensible" hamstrings that then pull on the posterior pelvis to produce hip extension.

Passive Insufficiency

If a person's elbow is placed on a table with the forearm in a vertical position and the relaxed hand drops forward into wrist flexion, the fingers tend to extend **(Fig. 3–25A)**. Extension of the fingers occurs because the finger extensors are being stretched over the flexed wrist and are insufficiently long (insufficiently extensible) to permit the fingers to remain flexed. The insufficient length in a passive muscle is termed **passive insufficiency.** If the person moves their wrist backward into wrist extension, the relaxed fingers will tend to flex **(Fig. 3–25B)**. Flexion of the fingers occurs because the finger flexors are stretched over the extended wrist and thus do not have sufficient slack remaining to permit the fingers to remain extended. The "insufficiency" part of passive insufficiency might imply an abnormal situation, but passive insufficiency can, in fact, be quite normal.

Under normal conditions, one-joint muscles rarely, if ever, are of insufficient extensibility to restrict full range of the opposite motion at the joint. Two-joint or multi-joint muscles, however, frequently are of insufficient extensibility to allow full range of the opposite joint motion simultaneously at all joints crossed by these muscles. The passive tension developed in these stretched muscles is sufficient to either cause motion (as shown by finger flexion and extension in Fig. 3–25) or limit motion. For example, the biarticular rectus femoris (a hip flexor and knee extensor muscle) may limit the available range of *knee flexion* if the rectus femoris is stretched over an extended hip. Similarly, the biarticular hamstring muscles (hip extensors and knee flexors) may limit full *knee extension* if the hamstrings

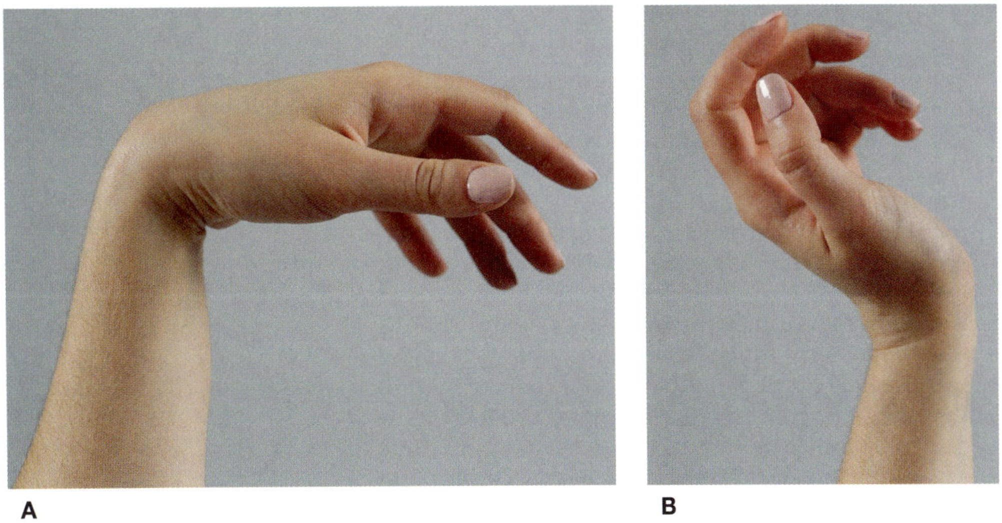

Figure 3–25 Passive insufficiency. **A.** When the wrist is flexed, the inactive finger extensors are stretched over the wrist with enough passive tension to cause the metacarpophalangeal (MCP), proximal interphalangeal (PIP), and distal interphalangeal (DIP) joints to at least partially extend. **B.** When the wrist is extended, the inactive finger flexors are stretched over the wrist with enough passive tension to cause the MCP, PIP, and DIP joints to at least partially flex. These are examples of "passive insufficiency" because the extensibility of the passive muscles and tendons is insufficient to allow fingers to remain flexed (A) or extended (B).

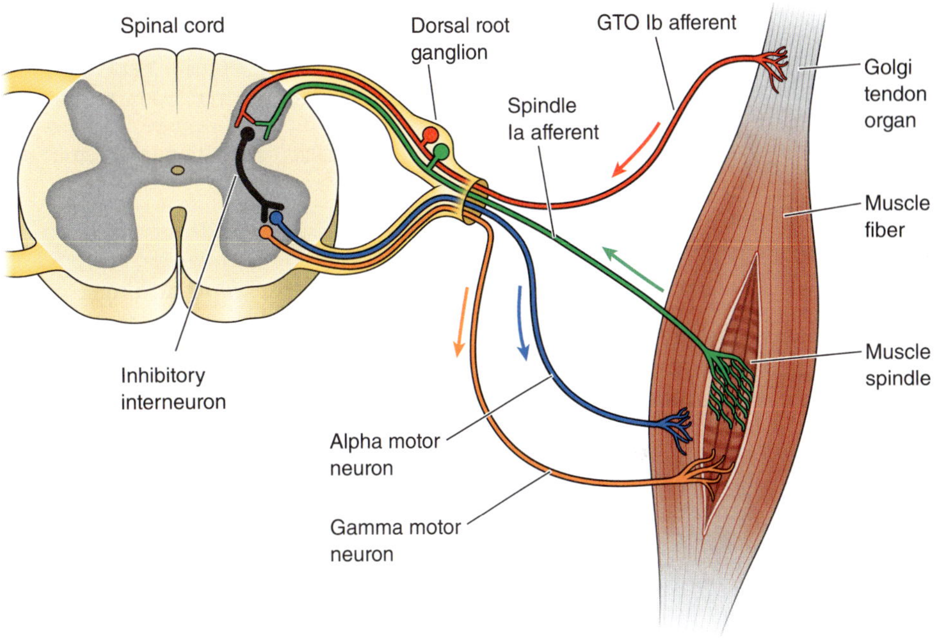

Figure 3–26 The functions of the Golgi tendon organ and the muscle spindle.

are stretched over a fully flexed hip. Passive insufficiency can also occur simultaneously with active insufficiency (although, as mentioned previously, the degree to which the sarcomeres shorten in functional activities is unknown). In Figure 3–15A, the finger flexion ROM was insufficient to allow effective grasp in the wrist flexed position. The finger flexors may have been unable to generate sufficient force because of the shortened position of wrist and finger joint flexion (presumed active insufficiency), but the inactive finger extensors were simultaneously passively stretched, creating enough passive tension to resist the finger flexion (passively insufficient). That is, the finger extensors were not sufficiently extensible to allow full flexion at the joints, resulting in a stretching sensation on the dorsum of the fingers and wrist. Whereas problems with passive insufficiency (with or without concomitant active insufficiency) are typically not encountered in usual activities of daily living, issues with passive insufficiency may be encountered in sports activities that may require unusual combinations of joint motions.

Sensory Receptors

Normal motor control resulting in voluntary movements depends on the coordination of descending motor pathways from the cortex, muscle actions, and a constant flow of sensory information. When performing or participating in athletic events, highly skilled dancers and athletes always seem to make it look so easy. To achieve this level of skill, the movements were practiced frequently, requiring constant sensory information from many systems. Regardless of the intent and skill of a motion, feedback in a muscle comes from two particularly important sensory receptors: the **Golgi tendon organ (GTO)** and the **muscle spindle.** The Golgi tendon organs, located in the tendon at the myotendinous junction **(Fig. 3–26)**, are sensitive to tension and may be activated either by an active muscle contraction or to a lesser extent, by an excessive passive stretch of the muscle. When the Golgi tendon organs are excited, they send a message to the central nervous system via Ib afferent neurons to adjust the muscle tension. The fine-tuning of muscle tension is not accomplished alone, however, because other reflex systems (muscle spindles) are also providing feedback to the muscle.

The muscle spindles consist of 2 to 10 specialized muscle fibers called **intrafusal fibers** and a central group of specialized sensory structures that are enclosed together in a connective tissue sheath and are interspersed throughout the muscle. The sensory structures within the muscle spindle are sensitive to both the length and the velocity of lengthening of the muscle fibers (also known as **extrafusal fibers**). The spindles send messages to the central nervous system about the state of stretch of the muscle. The instantaneous (or current) length of the muscle is sent to the central nervous system via group II afferents, whereas the velocity of lengthening is transmitted by group Ia afferents. For example, when the muscle is passively stretched, the spindles send a message to the spinal cord and central nervous system via the group Ia afferent neurons. Depending upon the extent of this message and the other inputs into the spinal cord, movement may be affected. The sensitivity of the muscle spindle is controlled by efferent signals sent via gamma motor neurons to the intrafusal muscle fibers. Typically, the alpha motor neurons (to the extrafusal fibers) and the gamma motor neurons (to the intrafusal fibers) are coactivated, termed *alpha-gamma coactivation*. Imagine a scenario in which the gamma motor neurons are sending increased signals relative to the alpha motor neurons. In that case, the intrafusal fibers are contracting more than the extrafusal fibers, such that the center of the spindle will be stretched slightly. This increased "load" to the central sensory structures increases the sensitivity of the muscle spindle to any subsequent stretch to the muscle.

The muscle spindle is responsible for sending a message to the central nervous system to provide control for the muscle in which it lies. A common example of this is seen when a muscle contracts when the tendon of that muscle is tapped with a reflex hammer **(Fig. 3–27)**. The tapping of the tendon causes a quick stretch of the muscle, which activates the muscle spindles. The quick change in length is relayed to the central nervous system via the Ia afferents, where it synapses directly on that muscle's alpha motor neuron to trigger a brief contraction. This response is called by various names: for example, **deep tendon reflex (DTR), muscle spindle reflex (MSR),** or simply **stretch reflex.** Both the Golgi tendon organs and the muscle spindles provide constant feedback to the central nervous system during movement so that appropriate adjustments can be made. Consequently, these sensory receptors are thought to help protect the muscle from injury by monitoring changes in muscle length and muscle load.

The presence of the stretch reflex is beneficial for preventing muscle injury but presents a problem in treatment or fitness programs where stretching of a muscle is desirable for improving flexibility and restoring a full range of joint motion. Muscle contraction or reflex activation of motor units during intentional stretching of a muscle has traditionally been thought to create resistance to the stretching procedure, making stretching more difficult and possibly ineffective.[88,89]

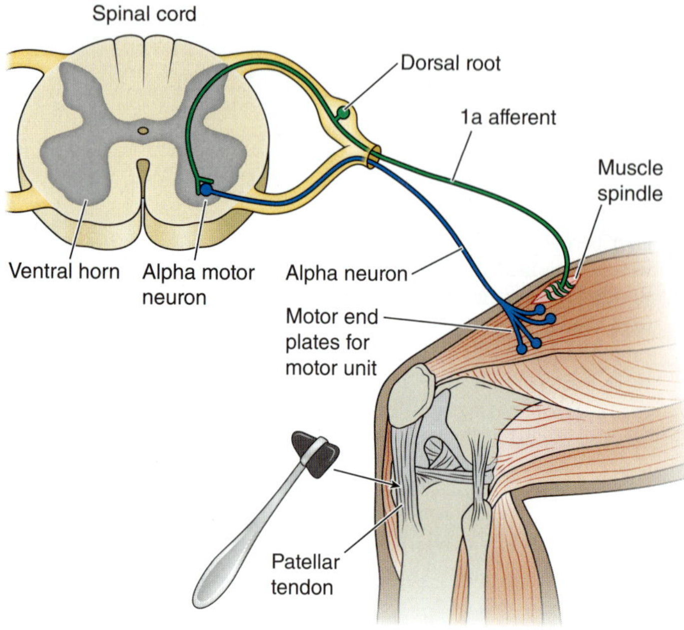

Figure 3–27 The stretch reflex. When the muscle spindle is stretched by the tap of the hammer, the 1a afferent neuron can send a message directly to the alpha motor neuron, which results in contraction of the stretched muscle.

However, more recently it has been suggested that *strengthening* at longer muscle length may increase available ROM to a similar degree as passive stretching.[90] The noncontractile components of a muscle provide resistance to stretching in a relaxed muscle and need to be considered when a muscle-stretching program is implemented.

Receptors that lie in joint capsules and ligaments may have either a positive or a negative influence on muscle activity through their signals to the central nervous system. **Nociceptors** and other receptors in and around the joint can have either excitatory or inhibitory action. For example, even a small joint effusion that is undetectable by the naked eye or pinching of a capsule can cause muscle inhibition and what appears to be weakness.[91-93]

Control of voluntary movements is accomplished not only by feedback systems such as Golgi tendon organs and muscle spindles, but also requires feed-forward control. **Feed-forward control** plays an important role in voluntary movement because it allows for anticipatory control of muscle actions. For example, in preparation for movements of the extremities, the abdominal and pelvic floor muscles contract to stabilize the trunk.[94,95] Feed-forward control relies on sensory input from the visual and auditory systems to learn appropriate movement patterns as well as to anticipate the control of movement.

Effects of Immobilization, Injury, and Aging

Immobilization

Immobilization affects both muscle structure and function. The effects of immobilization on a muscle depend on immobilization position (shortened or lengthened), percentage of fiber types within the muscle, and length of the immobilization period.

In Shortened Position

A muscle that is immobilized in a shortened position adapts to the new resting position through the following structural changes:

- Decrease in the number of sarcomeres with a compensatory increase in sarcomere length[96-98]
- Increase in the amount of perimysium[99]
- Thickening of endomysium[99]
- Collagen fibril orientation becoming more circumferential[100]
- Increase in ratio of connective tissue to muscle fiber tissue
- Decreased muscle mass and muscle atrophy[98,101,102]

Changes in function that result from immobilization in the shortened position are consistent with the structural changes. The decrease in the number of sarcomeres, coupled with an increase in the length of sarcomeres, displaces the length-tension relationship of the muscle so that the maximum tension generated by the muscle now corresponds to the new shortened position rather than the "typical" optimal length for that muscle. Although this altered capacity for developing tension may be beneficial while a muscle is immobilized in the shortened position, the muscle (often referred to as **adaptively shortened**) will not be able to return to typical function immediately after cessation of the immobilization. A muscle that has adapted to its shortened state will resist lengthening, thus potentially limiting joint motion. Furthermore, the overall tension-generating capacity of the muscle is decreased and the increase in connective tissue in relation to muscle fiber tissue results in an increase in resistance to passive stretch.

In Lengthened Position

Muscles immobilized in the lengthened position exhibit fewer structural and functional changes than do muscles immobilized in the shortened position. The primary structural changes are as follows:

- An increase in the number of sarcomeres, resulting in a decrease in sarcomere length at the lengthened position
- Increased endomyseal and perimyseal connective tissue
- Muscle hypertrophy that may be followed by atrophy[98,100,103]

The primary functional changes in a muscle immobilized in a lengthened rather than in a shortened position are an increase in maximum tension-generating capacity and displacement of the length-tension curve close to the longer immobilized position. Passive tension in the muscle (often referred to as **adaptively lengthened**) approximates that of the muscle before immobilization.[98]

Prevention of the effects of immobilization in the shortened position may require only short periods of daily movement. With only 30 minutes of daily ROM activities out of the immobilizer, the negative effects of immobilization in a shortened position were eliminated in animal models.[104,105] This beneficial effect of movement is not apparent when the frequency of movement is decreased to once per week over 3 weeks of immobilization.[106] If daily motion is not possible (e.g., due to fracture), then intensive remobilization with active and passive motion after immobilization can reverse the sarcomere number and connective tissue alterations that occur with immobilization.[107,108] Recall, however, that connective tissue structures are more likely to fail if remobilization is overly aggressive. In summary, a word of caution concerning the interpretation of the response of muscle to immobilization: The studies on sarcomere adaptation to immobilization have all been done with specific muscles in animals. Human skeletal muscle sarcomere numbers may be capable of adaptation similar to that of animals in situations of clinical bone lengthening to compensate for a short limb. When lengthened very slowly over several weeks in a case study, the vastus lateralis muscle adapted with an increase in number of sarcomeres.[109] Despite this one case study, it is not clear whether these changes are apparent in all human muscles and under what conditions.

Injury

Overuse

Overuse may cause injury to muscles as well as to connective tissue elements (tendons, ligaments, bursae, nerves, and cartilage). As noted in Chapter 2, a common etiology of these injuries is repetitive trauma that does not allow time for creep recovery or repair of the tissue. The additive effects of repetitive forces lead to microtrauma which, in turn, triggers the inflammatory process and results in swelling. The tissue most affected by overuse injuries is the musculotendinous unit.[110] Muscle and tendon tissue can fatigue with repetitive submaximal loading, with rapidly applied loads, and when the active (contracting) musculotendinous unit is also stretched by external forces.[111,112] Bursae may become inflamed with resultant effusion and thickening of the bursal wall because of repetitive trauma. Nerves can be subjected to compression injuries by muscle hypertrophy, decreased flexibility, and altered joint mechanics.[113]

Muscle Strain

Muscle strain injuries can occur from a single high-force contraction of the muscle while the muscle is lengthened by external forces (such as body weight). The muscle usually fails at the interface between the muscle and tendon (myotendinous junction).[27,114,115] Subsequently, there is localized bleeding and a significant acute inflammatory response, resulting in swelling, redness, and pain.[116]

Eccentric Exercise-Induced Muscle Injury

Injuries to muscles may occur with even a single bout of eccentric exercise.[117] After 30 to 40 minutes of eccentric exercise (walking downhill) or as few as 15 to 20 repetitions of high-load eccentric contractions, significant and sustained reductions in maximal voluntary contractions occur. Also, a loss of coordination, **delayed-onset muscle soreness (DOMS)**, swelling, and a dramatic increase in muscle stiffness have been reported. The DOMS reaches a peak 2 to 4 days after exercise.[118-120] The DOMS that occurs in muscles after eccentric muscle injury is known to be related to the forces experienced by muscles and may be a result of mechanical strain in the muscle fibers or in their associated connective tissues.[120-124] Morphological evidence shows deformation of the Z disc (Z-disc streaming) and other focal lesions after eccentric activity that induces soreness.[125] Biomechanical and histochemical studies have demonstrated evidence for collagen breakdown and for other connective tissue changes.[119]

Aging

Fiber Number and Fiber Type Changes

As a person ages, skeletal muscle strength decreases due to **sarcopenia** (the loss of muscle mass). Sarcopenia occurs as result of a loss of muscle fibers as well as a decrease in the size of existing fibers. Some muscles (e.g., vastus lateralis) show a 25% to 30% loss of fibers in persons in their 70s and 80s.[126,127] It is commonly thought that there is a gradual decrease in the number and size of type II fibers, leaving the muscle with a proportional increase in type I fibers. But data using immunohistochemical methods of fiber typing (identifying the specific MHC content in the muscle) suggests that the proportion of type I and type II fibers remains relatively constant.[128] The maintenance of the proportion of fiber types may occur to a greater degree in elderly people who stay active, whereas the elderly who are inactive may have a greater proportion of type I fibers.[128] There is also a decrease in the number of motor units, and the remaining motor units have a higher number of fibers per motor unit.[129-132]

Connective Tissue Changes

Aging, as discussed in Chapter 2, also increases the amount of connective tissue, in this case of the endomysium, perimysium, and epimysium within muscles. It is generally assumed that the increased connective tissue results in decreased ROM and increased muscle stiffness,[133,134] although there have been reports that muscle stiffness may not change or may decrease with aging.[135-138] All of these changes in the muscle result in decreased muscle strength and, more importantly, a loss in muscle power. This loss of muscle power, or the ability to contract the muscle with high force and high velocity, may be a contributing factor to falls in the elderly.[139,140] Resistance exercise training in the elderly appears to have positive effects on aging muscles, causing an increase in the size of muscle fibers and an increase in strength and functional performance.[128,141-145] However, the response to resistance training is more limited in the elderly than in the young.[146]

SUMMARY

- There are many factors that affect the function of the muscles. From the individual proteins and whole-muscle architecture that determine the structure of the muscle to the neural and biomechanical relationships that determine the performance of the muscle, the interrelationships between structure and function in muscles are complex and often impossible to differentiate.
- Muscles are more adaptable and, in many ways, more complex than the joints that they serve. Artificial joints have been designed and used to replace human joints, but it is as yet impossible to design a structure that can be used to replace a human muscle.
- All skeletal muscles adhere to the general principles of structure and function that have been presented in this chapter. Muscles produce the forces that power an incredible array of movements. During human movements, muscles not only provide the force to move the limbs but also provide the force for stabilization.

In subsequent chapters, the structure and function of specific muscles and the relationship between muscles and specific joints will be explored. The way in which muscles support the body in the erect standing posture and provide movement during walking will be examined in Chapters 13 and 14 of this book.

STUDY QUESTIONS

1. What are the contractile and noncontractile elements of muscle?
2. How does the relationship between the thick and thin filaments change during isometric, concentric, and eccentric muscle contractions?
3. What is the function of titin in active muscle contraction and in passive muscle lengthening?
4. How is motor unit size related to the production of muscle force?
5. What is the fiber type distribution in the soleus muscle and how does this affect the functional characteristics of the soleus compared with the gastrocnemius muscle?
6. How is the function of the quadriceps similar to or different from the hamstring muscles on the basis of the architectural characteristics of each muscle group?
7. What are the factors that could affect the development of active muscle tension? Suggest positions of the upper extremity that would limit tension development for each of the following muscles: biceps brachii, triceps brachii, and flexor digitorum profundus. What are the positions of the upper extremity in which the same muscles could passively limit motion?
8. Which upper extremity muscles are involved in lowering oneself into an armchair using one's arms? Is the muscle contraction eccentric or concentric? Explain your answer.
9. When testing strength using manual muscle testing, what exactly are we measuring? Other than changes in muscle length, why does muscle strength change at different points in the ROM?
10. Diagram the changes in the moment arm of the biceps brachii muscle from full elbow extension to full flexion. How does the change in moment arm affect the function of the muscle?
11. What are the agonists, antagonists, and synergists in each of the following motions: abduction at the shoulder, flexion at the shoulder, and abduction at the hip?
12. Based on muscle architecture, what is the difference in function between the finger flexors and the finger extensors?
13. How does isokinetic exercise differ from other types of exercise, such as dynamic (free) weight-lifting and isometric exercise?
14. What are the effects of immobilization when the muscle is maintained in a shortened position versus a lengthened position?
15. What adaptations occur in skeletal muscle with aging?

REFERENCES

1. Mukund K, Subramaniam S: Skeletal muscle: a review of molecular structure and function, in health and disease. Wiley Interdiscip Rev Syst Biol Med 12:e1462, 2020
2. Lieber RL, Meyer G: Structure-function relationships in the skeletal muscle extracellular matrix. J Biomech 152:111593, 2023
3. Hesse B, Frober R, Fischer MS, et al: Functional differentiation of the human lumbar perivertebral musculature revisited by means of muscle fibre type composition. Ann Anat 195:570-80, 2013
4. Lieber RL: Skeletal muscle structure and function: implications for rehabilitation (ed 3). Philadelphia, PA, Wolters Kluwer Lippincott Williams & Wilkins, 2010
5. Brooks SV, Guzman SD, Ruiz LP: Skeletal muscle structure, physiology, and function. Handb Clin Neurol 195:3-16, 2023
6. Fukuda N, Granzier HL, Ishiwata S, et al: Physiological functions of the giant elastic protein titin in mammalian striated muscle. J Physiol Sci 58:151-9, 2008
7. Herzog JA, Leonard TR, Jinha A, et al: Titin (visco-) elasticity in skeletal muscle myofibrils. Mol Cell Biomech 11:1-17, 2014
8. Horowits R, Kempner ES, Bisher ME, et al: A physiological role for titin and nebulin in skeletal muscle. Nature 323:160-4, 1986
9. Leonard TR, Herzog W: Regulation of muscle force in the absence of actin-myosin-based cross-bridge interaction. Am J Physiol Cell Physiol 299:C14-20, 2010
10. Dulhunty AF: Excitation-contraction coupling from the 1950s into the new millennium. Clin Exp Pharmacol Physiol 33:763-72, 2006
11. Huxley AF, Simmons RM: Proposed mechanism of force generation in striated muscle. Nature 233:533-8, 1971
12. Muretta JM, Rohde JA, Johnsrud DO, et al: Direct real-time detection of the structural and biochemical events in the myosin power stroke. Proc Natl Acad Sci U S A 112:14272-7, 2015
13. Cope TC, Pinter MJ: The size principle: still working after all these years. Am Phys Soc 10:280-6, 1995
14. Linnamo V, Moritani T, Nicol C, et al: Motor unit activation patterns during isometric, concentric and eccentric actions at different force levels. J Electromyogr Kinesiol 13:93-101, 2003
15. Perot C, Andre L, Dupont L, et al: Relative contributions of the long and short heads of the biceps brachii during single or dual isometric tasks. J Electromyogr Kinesiol 6:3-11, 1996
16. Howell JN, Fuglevand AJ, Walsh ML, et al: Motor unit activity during isometric and concentric-eccentric contractions of the human first dorsal interosseus muscle. J Neurophysiol 74:901-4, 1995
17. Akima H, Takahashi H, Kuno SY, et al: Coactivation pattern in human quadriceps during isokinetic knee-extension by muscle functional MRI. Eur J Appl Physiol 91:7-14, 2004
18. Conwit RA, Stashuk D, Tracy B, et al: The relationship of motor unit size, firing rate and force. Clin Neurophysiol 110:1270-5, 1999
19. Maluf KS, Enoka RM: Task failure during fatiguing contractions performed by humans. J Appl Physiol (1985) 99:389-96, 2005
20. Thomas JS, Ross AJ, Russ DW, et al: Time to task failure of trunk extensor muscles differs with load type. J Mot Behav 43:27-9, 2011
21. Williams PS, Hoffman RL, Clark BC: Cortical and spinal mechanisms of task failure of sustained submaximal fatiguing contractions. PLoS One 9:e93284, 2014
22. Peter JB, Barnard RJ, Edgerton VR, et al: Metabolic profiles of three fiber types of skeletal muscle in guinea pigs and rabbits. Biochemistry 11:2627-33, 1972
23. Staron RS: Human skeletal muscle fiber types: delineation, development, and distribution. Can J Appl Physiol 22:307-27, 1997
24. Johnson MA, Polgar J, Weightman D, et al: Data on the distribution of fibre types in thirty-six human muscles: an autopsy study. J Neurol Sci 18:111-29, 1973
25. Dahmane R, Djordjevic S, Smerdu V: Adaptive potential of human biceps femoris muscle demonstrated by histochemical, immunohistochemical and mechanomyographical methods. Med Biol Eng Comput 44:999-1006, 2006
26. Eriksson K, Hamberg P, Jansson E, et al: Semitendinosus muscle in anterior cruciate ligament surgery: morphology and function. Arthroscopy 17:808-17, 2001
27. Garrett WE, Jr., Califf JC, Bassett FH, 3rd: Histochemical correlates of hamstring injuries. Am J Sports Med 12:98-103, 1984
28. Andersen JL, Aagaard P: Effects of strength training on muscle fiber types and size: consequences for athletes training for high-intensity sport. Scand J Med Sci Sports 20 Suppl 2:32-8, 2010
29. Staron RS, Leonardi MJ, Karapondo DL, et al: Strength and skeletal muscle adaptations in heavy-resistance-trained women after detraining and retraining. J Appl Physiol (1985) 70:631-40, 1991
30. Saltin B, Henriksson J, Nygaard E, et al: Fiber types and metabolic potentials of skeletal muscles in sedentary man and endurance runners. Ann N Y Acad Sci 301:3-29, 1977
31. Bottinelli R, Pellegrino MA, Canepari M, et al: Specific contributions of various muscle fibre types to human muscle performance: an in vitro study. J Electromyogr Kinesiol 9:87-95, 1999
32. Lieber RL, Friden J: Clinical significance of skeletal muscle architecture. Clin Orthop Relat Res:140-51, 2001
33. Lieber RL, Ward SR: Skeletal muscle design to meet functional demands. Philos Trans R Soc Lond B Biol Sci 366:1466-76, 2011
34. Blazevich AJ, Gill ND, Zhou S: Intra- and intermuscular variation in human quadriceps femoris architecture assessed in vivo. J Anat 209:289-310, 2006
35. Chleboun GS, France AR, Crill MT, et al: In vivo measurement of fascicle length and pennation angle of the human biceps femoris muscle. Cells Tissues Organs 169:401-9, 2001
36. Stevens DE, Smith CB, Harwood B, et al: In vivo measurement of fascicle length and pennation of the human anconeus muscle at several elbow joint angles. J Anat 225:502-9, 2014
37. Ward SR, Eng CM, Smallwood LH, et al: Are current measurements of lower extremity muscle architecture accurate? Clin Orthop Relat Res 467:1074-82, 2009
38. Finni T: Structural and functional features of human muscle-tendon unit. Scand J Med Sci Sports 16:147-58, 2006
39. Purslow PP: Strain-induced reorientation of an intramuscular connective tissue network: implications for passive muscle elasticity. J Biomech 22:21-31, 1989
40. Purslow PP: The structure and functional significance of variations in the connective tissue within muscle. Comp Biochem Physiol A Mol Integr Physiol 133:947-66, 2002
41. Tian M, Herbert RD, Hoang P, et al: Myofascial force transmission between the human soleus and gastrocnemius muscles during passive knee motion. J Appl Physiol (1985) 113:517-23, 2012
42. Tijs C, van Dieen JH, Maas H: Effects of epimuscular myofascial force transmission on sarcomere length of passive muscles in the rat hindlimb. Physiol Rep 3, 2015
43. Meyer G, Lieber RL: Muscle fibers bear a larger fraction of passive muscle tension in frogs compared with mice. J Exp Biol 221, 2018
44. Meyer GA, Lieber RL: Elucidation of extracellular matrix mechanics from muscle fibers and fiber bundles. J Biomech 44:771-3, 2011
45. Gordon AM, Huxley AF, Julian FJ: The variation in isometric tension with sarcomere length in vertebrate muscle fibres. J Physiol 184:170-92, 1966
46. Burkholder TJ, Lieber RL: Sarcomere length operating range of vertebrate muscles during movement. J Exp Biol 204:1529-36, 2001
47. Ichinose Y, Kawakami Y, Ito M, et al: Estimation of active force-length characteristics of human vastus lateralis muscle. Acta Anat (Basel) 159:78-83, 1997
48. Lieber RL, Ljung BO, Friden J: Intraoperative sarcomere length measurements reveal differential design of human wrist extensor muscles. J Exp Biol 200:19-25, 1997
49. Lieber RL, Loren GJ, Friden J: In vivo measurement of human wrist extensor muscle sarcomere length changes. J Neurophysiol 71:874-81, 1994
50. Maganaris CN: Force-length characteristics of in vivo human skeletal muscle. Acta Physiol Scand 172:279-85, 2001
51. Ando R, Taniguchi K, Kikuchi S, et al: Sarcomere length of the vastus intermedius with the knee joint angle change. Physiol Rep 9:e14771, 2021
52. Hale R, Dorman D, Gonzalez RV: Individual muscle force parameters and fiber operating ranges for elbow flexion-extension and forearm pronation-supination. J Biomech 44:650-6, 2011
53. Hill AV: First and last experiments in muscle mechanics. Cambridge, UK, Cambridge University Press, 1970
54. Jaric S: Force-velocity relationship of muscles performing multi-joint maximum performance tasks. Int J Sports Med 36:699-704, 2015
55. Perrine JJ, Edgerton VR: Muscle force-velocity and power-velocity relationships under isokinetic loading. Med Sci Sports 10:159-66, 1978
56. Racz L, Beres S, Hortobagyi T, et al: Contraction history affects the in vivo quadriceps torque-velocity relationship in humans. Eur J Appl Physiol 87:393-402, 2002
57. Knapik JJ, Wright JE, Mawdsley RH, et al: Isometric, isotonic, and isokinetic torque variations in four muscle groups through a range of joint motion. Phys Ther 63:938-47, 1983
58. Hollander DB, Kraemer RR, Kilpatrick MW, et al: Maximal eccentric and concentric strength discrepancies between young men and women for dynamic resistance exercise. J Strength Cond Res 21:34-40, 2007
59. Linnamo V, Strojnik V, Komi PV: Maximal force during eccentric and isometric actions at different elbow angles. Eur J Appl Physiol 96:672-8, 2006

60. Yang J, Lee J, Lee B, et al: The effects of elbow joint angle changes on elbow flexor and extensor muscle strength and activation. J Phys Ther Sci 26:1079-82, 2014
61. Bojsen-Moller J, Magnusson SP: Heterogeneous loading of the human achilles tendon in vivo. Exerc Sport Sci Rev 43:190-7, 2015
62. Heinemeier KM, Kjaer M: In vivo investigation of tendon responses to mechanical loading. J Musculoskelet Neuronal Interact 11:115-23, 2011
63. Magnusson SP, Narici MV, Maganaris CN, et al: Human tendon behaviour and adaptation, in vivo. J Physiol 586:71-81, 2008
64. Malliaras P, Kamal B, Nowell A, et al: Patellar tendon adaptation in relation to load-intensity and contraction type. J Biomech 46:1893-9, 2013
65. Wiesinger HP, Kosters A, Muller E, et al: Effects of increased loading on in vivo tendon properties: a systematic review. Med Sci Sports Exerc 47:1885-95, 2015
66. Hauraix H, Nordez A, Guilhem G, et al: In vivo maximal fascicle-shortening velocity during plantar flexion in humans. J Appl Physiol (1985) 119:1262-71, 2015
67. Ishikawa M, Komi PV, Finni T, et al: Contribution of the tendinous tissue to force enhancement during stretch-shortening cycle exercise depends on the prestretch and concentric phase intensities. J Electromyogr Kinesiol 16:423-31, 2006
68. Ishikawa M, Niemela E, Komi PV: Interaction between fascicle and tendinous tissues in short-contact stretch-shortening cycle exercise with varying eccentric intensities. J Appl Physiol (1985) 99:217-23, 2005
69. Kopper B, Csende Z, Trzaskoma L, et al: Stretch-shortening cycle characteristics during vertical jumps carried out with small and large range of motion. J Electromyogr Kinesiol 24:233-9, 2014
70. Kurokawa S, Fukunaga T, Fukashiro S: Behavior of fascicles and tendinous structures of human gastrocnemius during vertical jumping. J Appl Physiol (1985) 90:1349-58, 2001
71. Hislop HJ, Perrine JJ: The isokinetic concept of exercise. Phys Ther 47:114-7, 1967
72. Ichinose Y, Kawakami Y, Ito M, et al: In vivo estimation of contraction velocity of human vastus lateralis muscle during "isokinetic" action. J Appl Physiol (1985) 88:851-6, 2000
73. Burkett LN, Alvar B, Irvin J: Comparing isometric and isokinetic peak strength values using slow speeds on a Cybex 340 isokinetic dynamometer machine. Isokinetics Exerc Sci 8:213, 2000
74. Phillips BA, Lo SK, Mastaglia FL: Isokinetic and isometric torque values using a Kin-Com dynamometer in normal subjects aged 20 to 69 years. Isokinetics Exerc Sci 8:147, 2000
75. Cordova ML, Ingersoll CD, Kovaleski JE, et al: A comparison of isokinetic and isotonic predictions of a functional task. J Athl Train 30:319-22, 1995
76. Guilhem G, Cornu C, Guevel A: A methodologic approach for normalizing angular work and velocity during isotonic and isokinetic eccentric training. J Athl Train 47:125-9, 2012
77. Kovaleski JE, Heitman RH, Trundle TL, et al: Isotonic preload versus isokinetic knee extension resistance training. Med Sci Sports Exerc 27:895-9, 1995
78. Morriss CJ, Tolfrey K, Coppack RJ: Effects of short-term isokinetic training on standing long-jump performance in untrained men. J Strength Cond Res 15:498-502, 2001
79. Burkholder TJ, Fingado B, Baron S, et al: Relationship between muscle fiber types and sizes and muscle architectural properties in the mouse hindlimb. J Morphol 221:177-90, 1994
80. Lieber RL, Friden J: Implications of muscle design on surgical reconstruction of upper extremities. Clin Orthop Relat Res:267-79, 2004
81. Dounskaia N: Control of human limb movements: the leading joint hypothesis and its practical applications. Exerc Sport Sci Rev 38:201-8, 2010
82. Biewener AA: Locomotion as an emergent property of muscle contractile dynamics. J Exp Biol 219:285-94, 2016
83. Sergio LE, Ostry DJ: Coordination of mono- and bi-articular muscles in multi-degree of freedom elbow movements. Exp Brain Res 97:551-5, 1994
84. van Ingen Schenau GJ, Dorssers WM, Welter TG, et al: The control of mono-articular muscles in multijoint leg extensions in man. J Physiol 484 (Pt 1):247-54, 1995
85. Carroll AM, Biewener AA: Mono- versus biarticular muscle function in relation to speed and gait changes: in vivo analysis of the goat triceps brachii. J Exp Biol 212:3349-60, 2009
86. Stien N, Saeterbakken AH, Andersen V: Electromyographic comparison of five lower-limb muscles between single- and multi-joint exercises among trained men. J Sports Sci Med 20:56-61, 2021
87. Kaya M, Jinha A, Leonard TR, et al: Multi-functionality of the cat medical gastrocnemius during locomotion. J Biomech 38:1291-301, 2005
88. Clark L, O'Leary CB, Hong J, et al: The acute effects of stretching on presynaptic inhibition and peak power. J Sports Med Phys Fitness 54:605-10, 2014
89. Trajano GS, Blazevich AJ: Static stretching reduces motoneuron excitability: The potential role of neuromodulation. Exerc Sport Sci Rev 49:126-132, 2021
90. Warneke K, Behm DG, Alizadeh S, et al: Discussing conflicting explanatory approaches in flexibility training under consideration of physiology: A narrative review. Sports Med 54:1785-99, 2024
91. Spencer JD, Hayes KC, Alexander IJ: Knee joint effusion and quadriceps reflex inhibition in man. Arch Phys Med Rehabil 65:171-7, 1984
92. Stokes M, Young A: The contribution of reflex inhibition to arthrogenous muscle weakness. Clin Sci (Lond) 67:7-14, 1984
93. Young A, Stokes M, Iles JF: Effects of joint pathology on muscle. Clin Orthop Relat Res:21-7, 1987
94. Allison GT, Morris SL, Lay B: Feedforward responses of transversus abdominis are directionally specific and act asymmetrically: implications for core stability theories. J Orthop Sports Phys Ther 38:228-37, 2008
95. Sjodahl J, Kvist J, Gutke A, et al: The postural response of the pelvic floor muscles during limb movements: a methodological electromyography study in parous women without lumbopelvic pain. Clin Biomech (Bristol) 24:183-9, 2009
96. Baker JH, Matsumoto DE: Adaptation of skeletal muscle to immobilization in a shortened position. Muscle Nerve 11:231-44, 1988
97. Tabary JC, Tabary C, Tardieu C, et al: Physiological and structural changes in the cat's soleus muscle due to immobilization at different lengths by plaster casts. J Physiol 224:231-44, 1972
98. Williams PE, Goldspink G: Changes in sarcomere length and physiological properties in immobilized muscle. J Anat 127:459-68, 1978
99. Williams PE, Goldspink G: Connective tissue changes in immobilised muscle. J Anat 138 (Pt 2):343-50, 1984
100. Okita M, Yoshimura T, Nakano J, et al: Effects of reduced joint mobility on sarcomere length, collagen fibril arrangement in the endomysium, and hyaluronan in rat soleus muscle. J Muscle Res Cell Motil 25:159-66, 2004
101. Booth FW: Physiologic and biochemical effects of immobilization on muscle. Clin Orthop Relat Res 15-20, 1987
102. Huijing PA, Jaspers RT: Adaptation of muscle size and myofascial force transmission: a review and some new experimental results. Scand J Med Sci Sports 15:349-80, 2005
103. Ponten E, Friden J: Immobilization of the rabbit tibialis anterior muscle in a lengthened position causes addition of sarcomeres in series and extra-cellular matrix proliferation. J Biomech 41:1801-4, 2008
104. Van Dyke JM, Bain JL, Riley DA: Preserving sarcomere number after tenotomy requires stretch and contraction. Muscle Nerve 45:367-75, 2012
105. Williams PE: Use of intermittent stretch in the prevention of serial sarcomere loss in immobilised muscle. Ann Rheum Dis 49:316-7, 1990
106. Gomes AR, Coutinho EL, Franca CN, et al: Effect of one stretch a week applied to the immobilized soleus muscle on rat muscle fiber morphology. Braz J Med Biol Res 37:1473-80, 2004
107. Kannus P, Jozsa L, Kvist M, et al: Effects of immobilization and subsequent low- and high-intensity exercise on morphology of rat calf muscles. Scand J Med Sci Sports 8:160-71, 1998
108. Riley DA, Van Dyke JM: The effects of active and passive stretching on muscle length. Phys Med Rehabil Clin N Am 23:51-7, x, 2012
109. Boakes JL, Foran J, Ward SR, et al: Muscle adaptation by serial sarcomere addition 1 year after femoral lengthening. Clin Orthop Relat Res 456:250-3, 2007
110. Pleacher MD, Glazer JL: Lower extremity soft tissue conditions. Curr Sports Med Rep 4:255-61, 2005
111. Maganaris CN, Narici MV, Almekinders LC, et al: Biomechanics and pathophysiology of overuse tendon injuries: ideas on insertional tendinopathy. Sports Med 34:1005-17, 2004
112. Reinking M: Tendinopathy in athletes. Phys Ther Sport 13:3-10, 2012
113. Herring SA, Nilson KL: Introduction to overuse injuries. Clin Sports Med 6:225-39, 1987
114. Garrett WE, Jr.: Muscle strain injuries. Am J Sports Med 24:S2-8, 1996
115. Liu H, Garrett WE, Moorman CT, et al: Injury rate, mechanism, and risk factors of hamstring strain injuries in sports: a review of the literature. J Sport Health Sci 1:92, 2012
116. Mann G, Shabat S, Friedman A, et al: Hamstring injuries. Orthopedics 30:536-40; quiz 541-2, 2007
117. Proske U, Allen TJ: Damage to skeletal muscle from eccentric exercise. Exerc Sport Sci Rev 33:98-104, 2005
118. Chleboun GS, Howell JN, Conatser RR, et al: Relationship between muscle swelling and stiffness after eccentric exercise. Med Sci Sports Exerc 30:529-35, 1998

119. Clarkson PM, Hubal MJ: Exercise-induced muscle damage in humans. Am J Phys Med Rehabil 81:S52-69, 2002
120. Howell JN, Chleboun G, Conatser R: Muscle stiffness, strength loss, swelling and soreness following exercise-induced injury in humans. J Physiol 464:183-96, 1993
121. Butterfield TA, Herzog W: Effect of altering starting length and activation timing of muscle on fiber strain and muscle damage. J Appl Physiol (1985) 100:1489-98, 2006
122. Lieber RL, Friden J: Muscle damage is not a function of muscle force but active muscle strain. J Appl Physiol (1985) 74:520-6, 1993
123. Warren GL, Hayes DA, Lowe DA, et al: Mechanical factors in the initiation of eccentric contraction-induced injury in rat soleus muscle. J Physiol 464:457-75, 1993
124. Nogueira FRD, Conceiçao MS, Vechin FC, et al: The effect of eccentric contraction velocity on muscle damage: a review. Isokinetics and Exercise Science 21:1-9, 2013
125. Morgan DL, Proske U: Popping sarcomere hypothesis explains stretch-induced muscle damage. Clin Exp Pharmacol Physiol 31:541-5, 2004
126. Charlier R, Mertens E, Lefevre J, et al: Muscle mass and muscle function over the adult life span: a cross-sectional study in Flemish adults. Arch Gerontol Geriatr 61:161-7, 2015
127. Lexell J: Human aging, muscle mass, and fiber type composition. J Gerontol A Biol Sci Med Sci 50 Spec No:11-6, 1995
128. Reeves ND, Narici MV, Maganaris CN: Myotendinous plasticity to ageing and resistance exercise in humans. Exp Physiol 91:483-98, 2006
129. Galea V: Changes in motor unit estimates with aging. J Clin Neurophysiol 13:253-60, 1996
130. McKinnon NB, Montero-Odasso M, Doherty TJ: Motor unit loss is accompanied by decreased peak muscle power in the lower limb of older adults. Exp Gerontol 70:111-8, 2015
131. McNeil CJ, Doherty TJ, Stashuk DW, et al: Motor unit number estimates in the tibialis anterior muscle of young, old, and very old men. Muscle Nerve 31:461-7, 2005
132. Power GA, Dalton BH, Behm DG, et al: Motor unit survival in lifelong runners is muscle dependent. Med Sci Sports Exerc 44:1235-42, 2012
133. Gajdosik RL, Vander Linden DW, Williams AK: Influence of age on concentric isokinetic torque and passive extensibility variables of the calf muscles of women. Eur J Appl Physiol Occup Physiol 74:279-86, 1996
134. Gao Y, Kostrominova TY, Faulkner JA, et al: Age-related changes in the mechanical properties of the epimysium in skeletal muscles of rats. J Biomech 41:465-9, 2008
135. Brown M, Fisher JS, Salsich G: Stiffness and muscle function with age and reduced muscle use. J Orthop Res 17:409-14, 1999
136. Hsu MJ, Wei SH, Yu YH, et al: Leg stiffness and electromyography of knee extensors/flexors: comparison between older and younger adults during stair descent. J Rehabil Res Dev 44:429-35, 2007
137. Oatis CA: The use of a mechanical model to describe the stiffness and damping characteristics of the knee joint in healthy adults. Phys Ther 73:740-9, 1993
138. Winegard KJ, Hicks AL, Vandervoort AA: An evaluation of the length-tension relationship in elderly human plantarflexor muscles. J Gerontol A Biol Sci Med Sci 52:B337-43, 1997
139. de Almeida Nagata C, Hamu T, Pelicioni PHS, et al: Influence of lower limb isokinetic muscle strength and power on the occurrence of falls in community-dwelling older adults: a longitudinal study. PLoS One 19:e0300818, 2024
140. Skelton DA, Beyer N: Exercise and injury prevention in older people. Scand J Med Sci Sports 13:77-85, 2003
141. Reeves ND, Narici MV, Maganaris CN: Musculoskeletal adaptations to resistance training in old age. Man Ther 11:192-6, 2006
142. Caserotti P, Aagaard P, Larsen JB, et al: Explosive heavy-resistance training in old and very old adults: Changes in rapid muscle force, strength and power. Scand J Med Sci Sports 18:773-82, 2008
143. de Labra C, Guimaraes-Pinheiro C, Maseda A, et al: Effects of physical exercise interventions in frail older adults: A systematic review of randomized controlled trials. BMC Geriatr 15:154, 2015
144. Kendrick D, Kumar A, Carpenter H, et al: Exercise for reducing fear of falling in older people living in the community. Cochrane Database Syst Rev 2014:CD009848, 2014
145. Stewart VH, Saunders DH, Greig CA: Responsiveness of muscle size and strength to physical training in very elderly people: a systematic review. Scand J Med Sci Sports 24:e1-10, 2014
146. Brown M: Resistance exercise effects on aging skeletal muscle in rats. Phys Ther 69:46-53, 1989

SECTION 2

Axial Skeletal Joint Complexes

CHAPTER 4 **The Vertebral Column** 112
CHAPTER 5 **The Thorax and Chest Wall** 167
CHAPTER 6 **The Temporomandibular Joint** 184

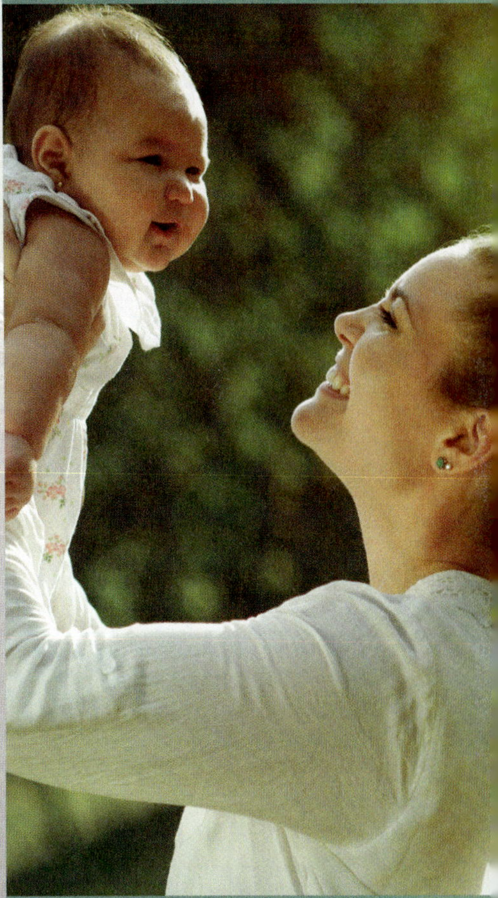

CHAPTER 4

The Vertebral Column

Diane Dalton, PT, DPT, OCS

CHAPTER OUTLINE

INTRODUCTION 115

STRUCTURE AND FUNCTION OF THE VERTEBRAL COLUMN 115
- Structure 115
  - The Mobile Segment 116
  - A Typical Vertebra 116
  - The Intervertebral Disc 119
  - Articulations 121
  - Ligaments and Joint Capsules 122
- Function 124
  - Kinematics 124
  - Kinetics 127

REGIONAL STRUCTURE AND FUNCTION 129
- Structure of the Cervical Region 129
  - Craniovertebral Region 129
  - Articulations 131
  - Craniovertebral Ligaments 131
  - The Lower Cervical Region 132
  - Intervertebral Disc 133
  - Articulations 133
- Function of the Cervical Region 134
  - Kinematics 134
  - Kinetics 137
- Structure of the Thoracic Region 138
  - Typical Thoracic Vertebrae 138
  - Intervertebral Discs 139
  - Articulations 139
  - Ligaments 140
  - Atypical Thoracic Vertebrae 140
- Function of the Thoracic Region 140
  - Kinematics 140
  - Kinetics 140
- Structure of the Lumbar Region 140
  - Typical Lumbar Vertebrae 140
  - Atypical Lumbar Vertebra 141
  - Intervertebral Discs 142
  - Articulations 142
  - Ligaments and Fascia 143
- Function of the Lumbar Region 145
  - Kinematics 145
  - Lumbopelvic Rhythm 146
  - Kinetics 146
- Structure of the Sacral Region 148
  - Sacroiliac Articulations 149
  - Symphysis Pubis Articulation 150
- Function of the Sacral Region 151
  - Kinematics 151
  - Kinetics 151

MUSCLES OF THE VERTEBRAL COLUMN 152
- The Craniocervical/Upper Thoracic Regions 152
  - Posterior Muscles 152
  - Lateral Muscles 154
  - Anterior Muscles 155
- Lower Thoracic/Lumbopelvic Regions 156
  - Posterior Muscles 156
  - Lateral Muscles 159
  - Anterior Muscles 159
- Muscles of the Pelvic Floor 161
  - Structure 161
  - Function 161
  - Squat Lift Versus Stoop Lift 161

EFFECTS OF AGING ON THE LUMBAR SPINE 162

SUMMARY 164

STUDY QUESTIONS 164

REFERENCES 164

ANATOMY OVERVIEW

MUSCLE ACTIONS OF THE VERTEBRAL COLUMN (INTERVERTEBRAL AND CRANIOVERTEBRAL JOINTS)

TABLE KEY: Primary movers Secondary movers

Sagittal Plane	Flexion	Extension
	Rectus abdominis	Splenius cervicis/capitis
	External oblique	Iliocostalis group
	Internal oblique	Longissimus group
	Sternocleidomastoid	Semispinalis group
	Longus capitis	Multifidus
	Longus colli	Rectus capitis posterior major/minor
	Anterior scalene	Oblique capitis superior/inferior
	Rectus capitis anterior	Spinalis
		Rotatores
		Interspinalis
		Intertransversarii
		Levator scapulae
		Trapezius
		Quadratus lumborum

Transverse Plane	Ipsilateral Rotation	Contralateral Rotation
	Splenius cervicis/capitis Internal oblique Longissimus group Iliocostalis group Levator scapulae	External oblique Sternocleidomastoid Trapezius Semispinalis capitis/cervicis Rotatores Multifidus
Frontal Plane	**Lateral Flexion**	
	Iliocostalis group Internal oblique External oblique Semispinalis group Longissimus group Trapezius Multifidi Intertransversarii Quadratus lumborum Splenius capitis/cervicis Scalenes Levator scapulae Sternocleidomastoid	

ANATOMY OVERVIEW

VERTEBRAL COLUMN MUSCLE ATTACHMENTS

Muscles	Proximal Attachment	Distal Attachment
Splenius capitis	Nuchal ligament and spinous processes of C7–T6 vertebrae	Fibers run superolaterally to mastoid process of temporal bone and lateral 3rd of superior nuchal line of occipital bone
Splenius cervicis	Nuchal ligament and spinous processes of C7–T6 vertebrae	Transverse processes of C1–C3 vertebrae
Iliocostalis (erector spinae)	Arises by a broad tendon from posterior part of iliac crest, posterior surface of sacrum, sacroiliac ligaments, sacral and inferior lumbar spinous processes, and supraspinous ligament	Lumborum, thoracis, cervicis; fibers run superiorly to angles of lower ribs and cervical transverse processes
Longissimus (erector spinae)		Thoracis, cervicis, capitis; fibers run superiorly to ribs between tubercles and angles, to transverse processes in thoracic and cervical regions, and to mastoid processes of temporal bone
Spinalis (erector spinae)		Thoracis, cervicis, capitis; fibers run superiorly to spinous processes in the upper thoracic region and to cranium
Semispinalis (transversospinalis)	Transverse processes of C4–T12 vertebrae	Thoracis, cervicis, capitis; fibers run superomedially to occipital bone and spinous processes in thoracic and cervical regions, spanning 4–6 segments
Multifidus (transversospinalis)	Arises from posterior sacrum, PSIS of ilium, aponeurosis of erector spinae, sacroiliac ligaments, mammillary processes of lumbar vertebrae, transverse processes of T1–T3, articular processes of C4–C7	Thickest in lumbar region; fibers pass obliquely superomedially to entire length of spinous processes, spanning 2–4 segments

VERTEBRAL COLUMN MUSCLE ATTACHMENTS		
Muscles	**Proximal Attachment**	**Distal Attachment**
Rotatores: brevis and longus (transversospinalis)	Arise from transverse processes of vertebrae; best developed in thoracic region	Fibers pass superomedially to attach to spinous process of vertebra immediately (brevis) or 2 segments (longus) superior
Interspinalis	Superior surfaces of spinous processes of cervical and lumbar vertebrae	Inferior surface of spinous process of vertebra of proximal attachment
Intertransversarii	Transverse processes of cervical and lumbar vertebrae	Transverse processes of adjacent vertebrae
Quadratus lumborum	Medial 1/2 of inferior border of 12th ribs and lumbar transverse processes	Iliolumbar ligament and lip of iliac crest
Trapezius	Medial 3rd of superior nuchal line, external occipital protuberance, nuchal ligament, spinous processes of C7–T12 vertebrae	Lateral 3rd of clavicle, acromion, and spine of scapula
Levator scapula	Transverse processes of C1–C4 vertebrae	Superior aspect of medial border of the scapula
Anterior scalene	Transverse processes of C3–C6 vertebrae	1st rib
Middle scalene	Transverse processes of C5–C7 vertebrae	Superior surface of 1st rib
Posterior scalene	Transverse processes of C5–C7 vertebrae	External border of 2nd rib
Sternocleidomastoid	Lateral surface of mastoid process of temporal bone and lateral 1/2 of superior nuchal line	Sternal head: anterior surface of manubrium of sternum Clavicular head: superior surface of medial 3rd of clavicle
Rectus capitis posterior major (suboccipital muscles)	Spinous process of C2 vertebra	Lateral aspect of inferior nuchal line
Rectus capitis posterior minor (suboccipital muscles)	Posterior tubercle of posterior arch of C1 vertebra	Medial aspect of inferior nuchal line
Obliquus capitis inferior (suboccipital muscles)	Posterior tubercle of posterior arch of C2 vertebra	Transverse process of C1 vertebra
Obliquus capitis superior (suboccipital muscles)	Transverse process of C1 vertebra	Occipital bone between superior and inferior nuchal lines
Rectus capitis anterior	Base of cranium, just anterior to occipital condyle	Anterior surface of lateral mass of C1 vertebra
Rectus capitis lateralis	Jugular process of occipital bone	Transverse process of C1 vertebra
Longus colli	Bodies of C1–C3 and transverse processes of C3–C6 vertebrae	Bodies of C5–T3 vertebrae; transverse processes of C3–C5 vertebrae
Longus capitis	Basilar part of occipital bone	Transverse processes of C3–C6
Rectus abdominis	Pubic symphysis and pubic crest	Xyphoid process and 5th–7th costal cartilage
Internal oblique	Thoracolumbar fascia, anterior 2/3 of iliac crest	Inferior borders of 10th–12th ribs, linea alba
External oblique	External surfaces of 5th–12th ribs	Linea alba, pubic tubercle, and anterior 1/2 of iliac crest

Introduction

The vertebral column is an amazing and complex structure that must meet the seemingly contradictory demands of mobility and stability for the trunk and extremities while protecting the spinal cord. Although the pelvis is not always considered part of the vertebral column, it will be included in this chapter because of the anatomical and functional interrelationships between the lumbar spine, sacrum, and innominate bones.

Structure and Function of the Vertebral Column

Structure

The vertebral column resembles a curved rod, composed of 33 vertebrae and 23 intervertebral discs. The vertebral column is divided into five regions: cervical, thoracic, lumbar, sacral, and coccygeal **(Fig. 4–1)**. The vertebrae adhere to a common basic structural design but show regional variations in size and configuration that reflect the functional demands of each particular region. The vertebrae increase in size from the cervical to the lumbar regions and then decrease in size from the sacral to coccygeal regions. Twenty-four of the vertebrae in adults are individual bones: Seven separate vertebrae are in the cervical region, twelve in the thoracic region, and five in the lumbar region. Five of the remaining nine vertebrae are fused to form the sacrum, and the remaining four constitute the coccygeal vertebrae. When viewed from the side, four curves are evident **(Fig. 4–1A)**. Curves that have a posterior convexity (anterior concavity) are referred to as **kyphotic curves;** curves that have a posterior concavity (anterior convexity) are called **lordotic curves.** The vertebral column bisects the trunk when viewed from the posterior aspect **(Fig. 4–1B)**.

The four curves of the vertebral column develop through growth and development **(Fig. 4–2)**. The curve of the vertebral column of a fetus exhibits one long curve that is convex posteriorly **(Fig. 4–2A)**. As the child achieves developmental milestones such as crawling **(Fig. 4–2B)** and walking **(Fig. 4–2C)**, the curves of the vertebral column adapt to the demands of upright posture. Four distinct and relatively balanced anteroposterior curves are eventually evident **(Fig. 4–2D)**. The two thoracic and sacrococcygeal curves that retain the original

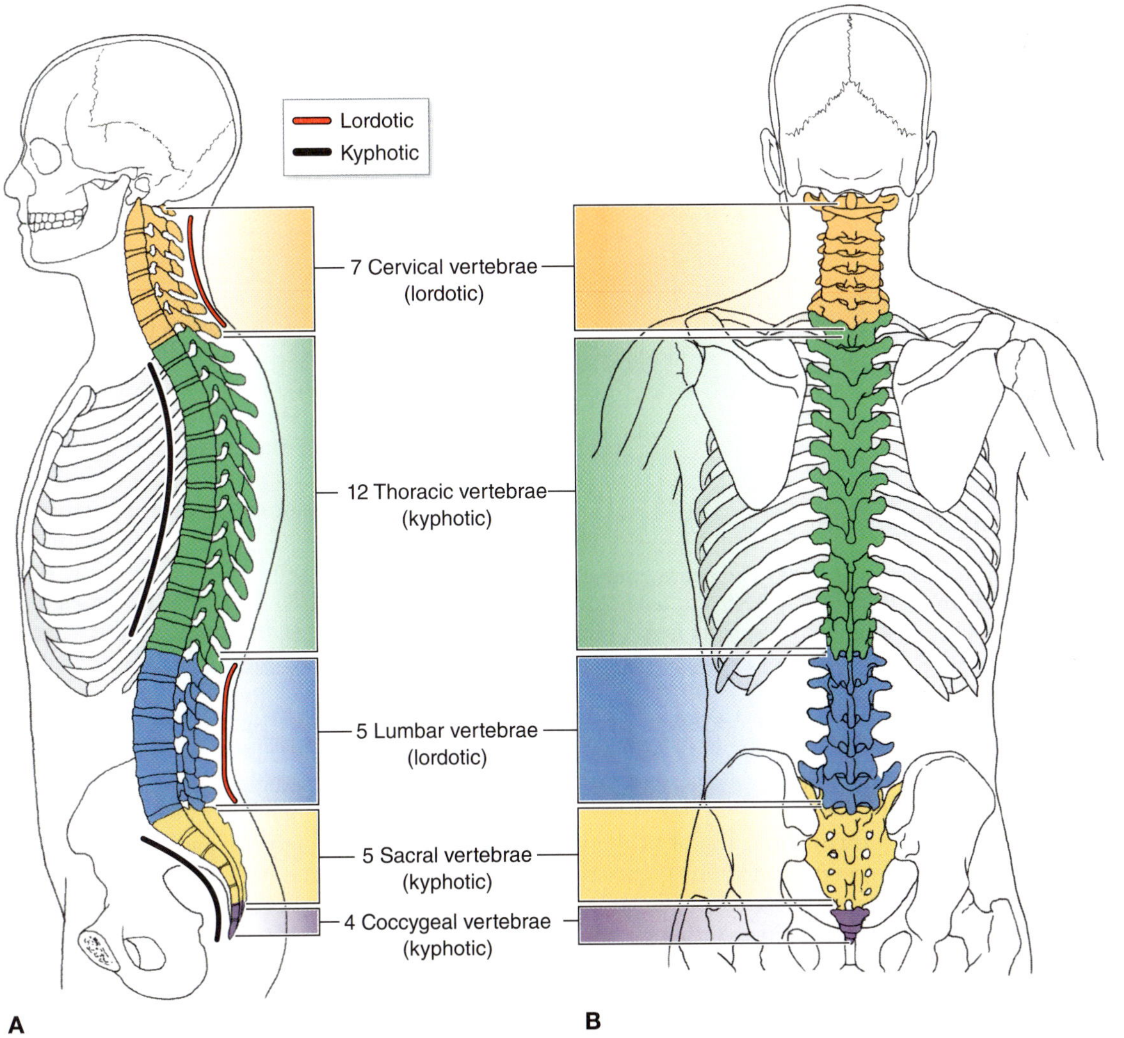

Figure 4–1 The five regions of the vertebral column include cervical, thoracic, lumbar, sacral, and coccygeal. **A.** In a side view, two lordotic curves (cervical and lumbar) and two kyphotic curves (thoracic and sacral) are evident, referencing the curves posteriorly. **B.** In a posterior view, the vertebral column bisects the trunk.

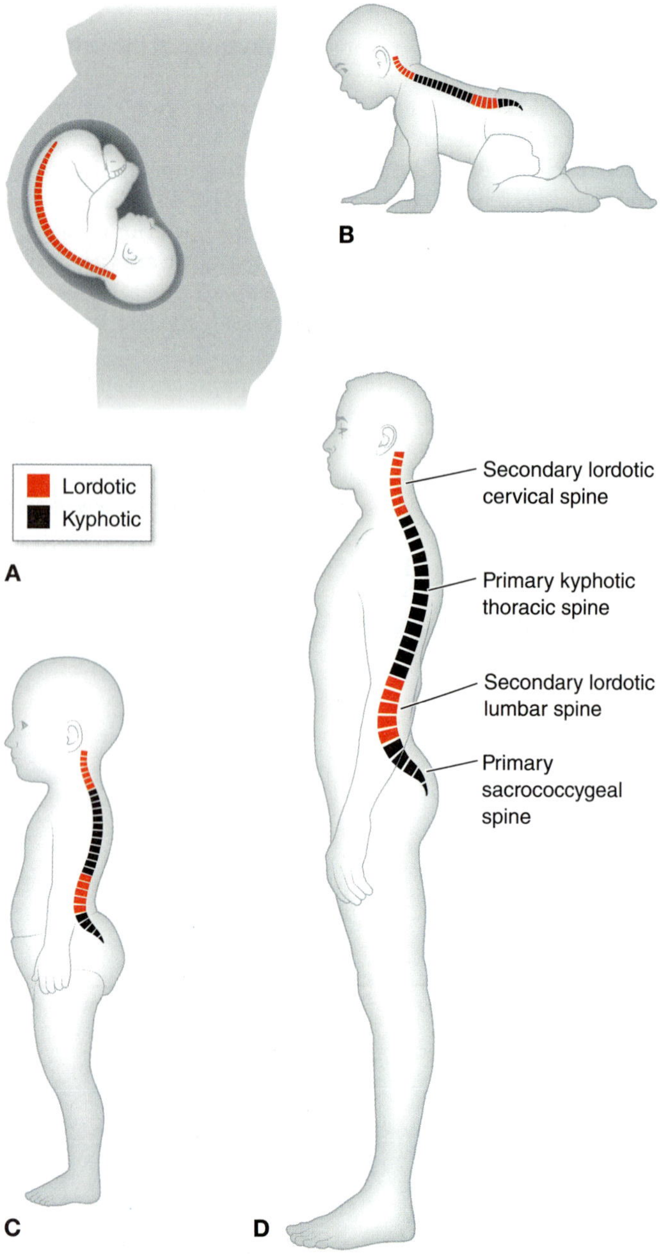

Figure 4–2 Primary and secondary curves. **A.** The entire spine is kyphotic in the fetus in utero. **B.** As the baby begins to orient its head to vertical, the secondary cervical lordosis appears first. **C.** In the toddler all four curves are evident, often with an exaggeration of the secondary lumbar lordosis. **D.** In the typical adult spine, the primary thoracic and sacrococcygeal kyphoses are evident, as are the secondary cervical and lumbar lordoses.

posterior convexity (kypohosis) throughout life are called **primary curves,** whereas the two cervical and lumbar curves that show a reversal of the original in utero posterior convexity (lordosis) are called **secondary curves.** The anteroposterior curves of the vertebral column provide a significant advantage over a straight rod because reciprocal curves can resist much higher compressive loads.[1]

When standing, the vertebral column typically functions as a closed chain, with the upright head at one end and the weight-bearing feet at the other. We can readily see how the contact of the feet to the ground "fixes" one end of the chain. The need for the head at the other end of the chain to remain vertically oriented in a somewhat stable position is less obviously "fixed." As we move, we must allow the sensory organs, particularly the eyes and ears, to be optimally positioned for function that is "fixed" with the horizontal. Each of the many separate but interdependent components of the vertebral column is designed to contribute to the overall function of the total unit, as well as to perform specific tasks.

The first section of this chapter will cover the general components of a vertebra and its articulation with its neighbor (i.e., the mobile segment), followed by regional variations and the sacroiliac joints. The second section of the chapter will cover the function of the muscles of the vertebral column and pelvis.

The Mobile Segment

It is generally held that the smallest functional unit in the spine is the **mobile segment.** A mobile segment consists of any two adjacent vertebrae, the intervening intervertebral disc (if there is one at that level), and all the soft tissues that secure them together. Vertebral movements are named by what the *cranial* vertebra and anterior aspect of the vertebra is doing, rather than what the more obvious posteriorly located spinous process is doing.

A Typical Vertebra

The structure of a typical vertebra consists of two major parts **(Fig. 4–3)**: an anterior, cylindrically shaped vertebral body **(Fig. 4–3A)** and a posterior, irregularly shaped neural arch **(Fig. 4–3B)**. The vertebral body is an important structure that can serve as an anchor for ligaments, discs, and ribs and as a source of nutrition via its marrow to the intervertebral discs. The vertebral body consists of a shell of cortical bone surrounded by a cancellous-filled cavity **(Fig. 4–4)** reinforced by trabeculae to help resist compressive (weight-bearing) loads.[2] The anterior aspect of the vertebral body has lower bone mineral density (less resistance to compression) than the posterior aspect. This may be a contributing factor to the presence of anterior compression fractures seen in those with osteoporosis.[3]

The **neural arch** can be divided into the pedicles and the posterior elements **(Fig. 4–5)**. The **pedicles** are the portion of the neural arch that lies between the articular processes and the vertebral body, connecting the posterior elements to the body **(Fig. 4-5A)**. The pedicles are short, stout pillars with thick walls and are well structured to transmit tension and bending forces from the posterior elements to the vertebral body. In general, the pedicles increase in size from the cervical to lumbar regions, which makes sense because greater forces are transmitted through the pedicles in the lumbar region. The orientation of the pedicle helps to define the size and shape of the vertebral canal through which the spinal cord or cauda equina run.

The remaining posterior elements are the laminae, the articular processes, the spinous process, and the transverse processes (Fig. 4–5A). The **laminae** serve as origination points for the rest of the posterior elements. The laminae are thin, vertically oriented pieces of bone that serve as the "closure" to the neural arch that protects the spinal cord. In addition,

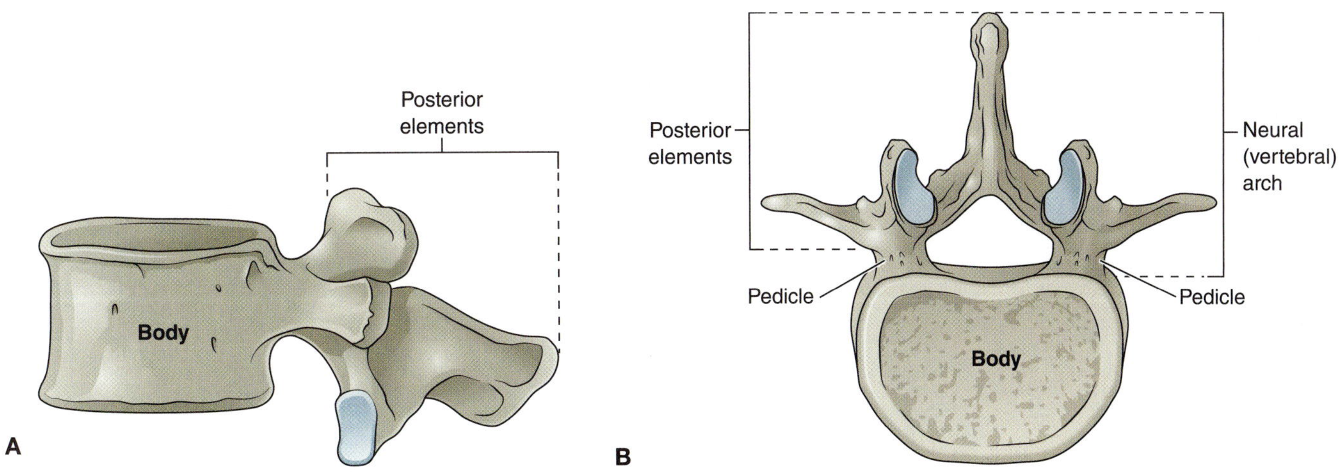

Figure 4–3 **A.** The anterior portion of a vertebra is composed of the vertebral body. **B.** The posterior portion of a vertebra is called the *vertebral* or *neural arch*. The neural arch is attached to the body via the pedicles.

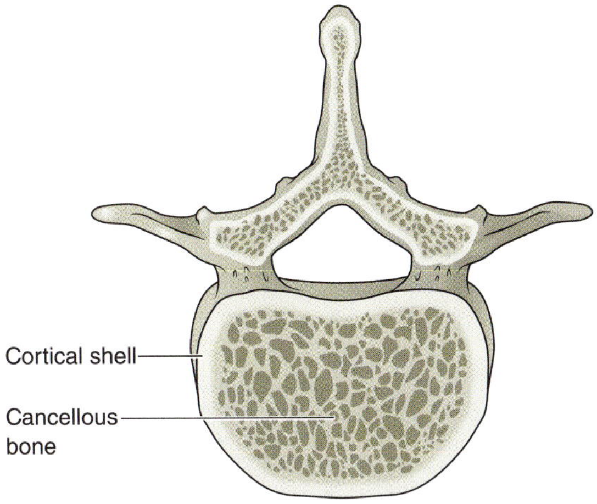

Figure 4–4 The vertebral body is comprised of a shell of cortical bone surrounding cancellous with reinforcing trabecular bone.

the laminae transmit forces from the posterior elements to the pedicles anteriorly and, via the pedicles, on to the vertebral body. This force transfer occurs through a region of the laminae called the **pars interarticularis** which, as its name suggests, is the portion of the laminae that is between the superior and inferior articular processes **(Fig. 4–5B)**.

The **articular processes** for each vertebra include two **superior** and two **inferior facets** located on the superior and inferior articular processes (Fig. 4–5B); the superior facets articulate with the inferior facets of the vertebra above while the inferior facets articulate with the superior facets of the vertebra below **(Fig. 4–5C)**. In the sagittal plane, these articular processes form a supportive column, frequently referred to as the **articular pillar.** The pars interarticularis between the articular facets (Fig. 4-5B) is subjected to bending forces that are transmitted from the more vertically oriented lamina to the horizontally oriented pedicles. The pars interarticularis is most developed in the lumbar spine, where the forces are the greatest in magnitude. Typically, an increase in cortical bone occurs to accommodate the increased forces in this region. If the cortical bone is insufficient, the pars interarticularis is susceptible to stress fractures.

Foundational Concepts 4–1
Spondylolytic Spondylolisthesis

When fractures of the pars interarticularis occur bilaterally, the result may be **spondylolytic spondylolisthesis.** In this condition, the posterior elements are separated from the remainder of the neural arch and the vertebral body. The vertebral body may then begin to slip forward on the vertebra below **(Fig. 4–6)**. This occurs most frequently at the L5–S1 mobile segment because of the angulation of the segment and the anterior shear forces that exist there.

The altered location of the slipped vertebra changes its relationship to adjacent structures and creates excessive stress on supporting ligaments and joints. Overstretched ligaments connecting the separated segments may lead to a lack of stability of the mobile segment. The forward slippage of the vertebra may cause tension or compression on the nerves of the cauda equina as well. Pain *may* arise from excessive stress on the pain-sensitive anterior and posterior longitudinal ligaments, interspinous ligament, spinal nerves, dura mater, vertebral bodies, facet joint capsules, synovial linings, or the muscles.

In the typical vertebra, the **spinous process** and two **transverse processes** are sites for muscle attachments and serve to increase the lever arm for the muscles of the vertebral column. Table 4–1 summarizes the components of a typical vertebra and Table 4–2 summarizes the regional variations in vertebral structure.

The vertebrae are subjected to a wide variety of forces; however, they have a bony architecture that suggests a generally typical loading pattern.[3] Both the vertebral bodies and the neural arch have a well-defined trabecular system that develops in response to the stresses placed on them **(Fig. 4–7)**. Specifically, the vertebrae have vertically oriented trabeculae with horizontal connections near the vertebral endplates and with denser bone areas near each pedicle's base.[3,4] Vertical systems within the vertebral bodies help support the body's weight and resist compression forces. There are also fan-shaped trabeculae introduced into the vertebral body at the area of the pedicle in response to bending and shearing forces transmitted through this region.[3]

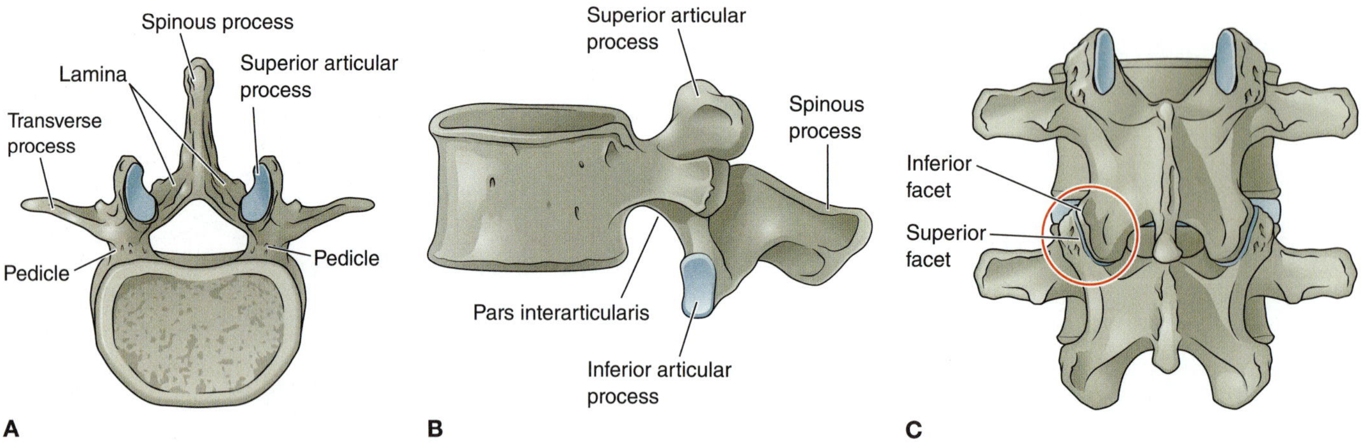

Figure 4–5 **A** and **B**. The posterior elements of a vertebra are the laminae, the articular processes, the spinous process, and the transverse processes. The pars interarticularis is the portion of each lamina that lies between the articular processes. **C.** The facets of the inferior articular processes on the vertebra above articulate with the facets of the superior articular processes on the vertebra below.

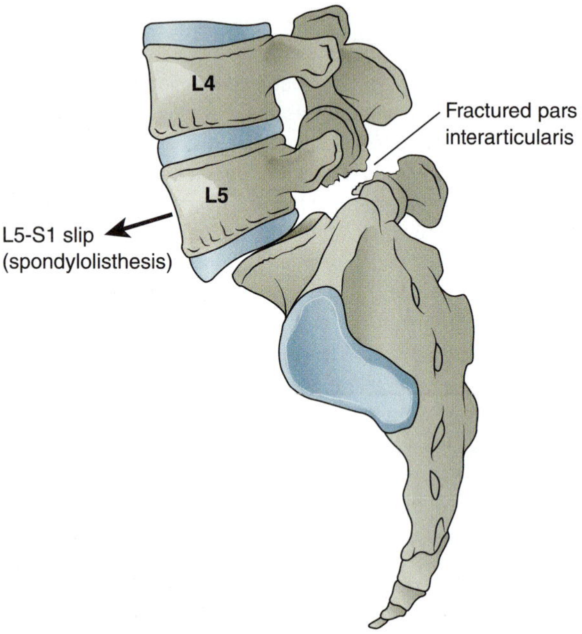

Figure 4–6 In this lateral view, a spondylolisthesis is evident, resulting from failure of the pars interarticularis. That failure allows the vertebra above to slide anteriorly on the vertebra below, most commonly occurring as a slip of L5 on S1.

Table 4–1 Components of a Typical Vertebra

	DESCRIPTION	FUNCTION
Body	Block of trabecular bone covered by a layer of cortical bone	To resist compressive loads
Arches		
Pedicle	Short, stout pillars with thick walls that connect the vertebral body to the posterior elements of the neural arch	To transmit the bending forces from the posterior elements to the vertebral body
Lamina	The vertical plate that constitutes the central portion of the arch posterior to the pedicles	To transmit the forces from the articular, transverse, and spinous processes to the pedicles
Transverse processes	Lateral projections of bone that originate from the laminae	Serve as muscle attachments and provide mechanical lever
Spinous process	A posterior projection of bone that originates from the central portion of the laminae	Serves as muscle attachment and provides mechanical lever; may also serve as a bony block to motion
Vertebral foramen	Opening bordered by the posterior vertebral body and the neural arch	Combined with all segments, forms a passage and protection for the spinal cord

Table 4–2 Regional Variations in Vertebral Structure

PART	CERVICAL VERTEBRAE	THORACIC VERTEBRAE	LUMBAR VERTEBRAE
Body	The body is small, with a transverse diameter greater than its anteroposterior diameter. The anterior surface of the body is convex; the posterior surface is flat. The superior surface of the body is saddle shaped because of the presence of uncinate processes on the lateral aspects of the superior surfaces.	The transverse and anteroposterior diameters of the bodies are similar. The anterior height is less than the posterior height. Two demifacets for articulation with the ribs are located on the posterolateral corners of the vertebral plateaus.	The body is massive, with a transverse diameter greater than the anteroposterior diameter.
Arches			
Pedicles	Project posterolaterally	Variable in shape and orientation	Short and thick
Laminae	Project posteromedially; thin and slightly curved	Short, thick, and broad	Short and broad
Superior facet facets	Face superiorly, posteriorly, and medially	Thin and flat; face posteriorly, superiorly, and laterally	Vertical and concave; face posteromedially, support mammillary processes on posterior borders
Inferior facet facets	Face inferiorly, anteriorly and laterally	Face anteriorly, inferiorly, and medially	Vertical, convex, and face anterolaterally
Transverse processes	Possess foramina for vertebral artery, vein, and venous plexus, have a gutter for the spinal nerve	Large, with thickened ends. Possess paired oval facets for articulation with the ribs. Show a caudal decrease in length.	Long, slender, and extend horizontally. Support accessory processes on the posterior inferior surfaces of the root.
Spinous processes	Short, slender, and extend horizontally. Have bifid tips.	T1–T10 slope inferiorly. T11 and T12 have a triangular shape.	Broad, thick, and extend horizontally
Vertebral foramen	Large and roughly triangular	Small and circular	Triangular; larger than the thoracic but smaller than the cervical

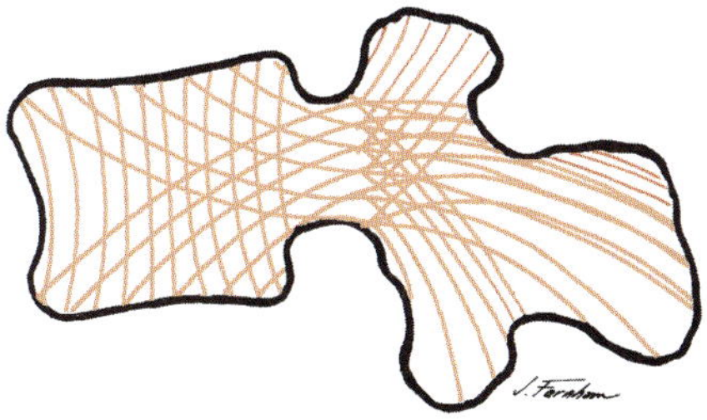

Figure 4–7 Schematic representation of the internal architecture of a lumbar vertebra (lateral view). The various trabeculae that comprise the cancellous bone are arranged along the lines of force transmission.

The Intervertebral Disc

The intervertebral disc has two principal functions: to separate two adjacent vertebral bodies, thereby increasing available motion between them, and to transmit load from one vertebral body to the next **(Fig. 4–8A)**. The size (thickness) of the intervertebral disc is related to both the amount of motion available and the magnitude of the loads that must be transmitted from one body to the next. The intervertebral discs increase in size from the cervical to the lumbar regions. The disc thicknesses vary from approximately 3 mm in the cervical region where the weight-bearing loads are the lowest, to about 9 mm in the lumbar region where the weight-bearing loads are the highest.[1] Although the discs are smallest in the cervical region and largest in the lumbar region, it is the ratio between disc thickness and vertebral body height that determines the available motion. The greater the ratio, the greater the intersegmental mobility. The ratio is *greatest* in the cervical region, followed by the lumbar region, and the ratio is *smallest* in the thoracic region. This reflects the greater functional needs for mobility in the cervical and lumbar regions and for relative stability in the thoracic region.

Most of what we know about the structure and function of the intervertebral discs has been gleaned from studies of the lumbar region. It was long thought that the discs of the cervical and thoracic regions had a structure similar to discs of the lumbar region, although this may not be the case.[5,6] This section will describe the general structure and function of the intervertebral disc. The region-specific variations will be described in the regional structure sections of the chapter.

All intervertebral discs are composed of three parts: (1) the nucleus pulposus, (2) the annulus fibrosus, and (3) the vertebral endplate **(Fig. 4–8B)**. The **nucleus pulposus** is the gelatinous mass found in the center, the **annulus fibrosus** is the fibrous outer ring, and the **vertebral endplate** is the cartilaginous layer covering the superior and inferior surfaces

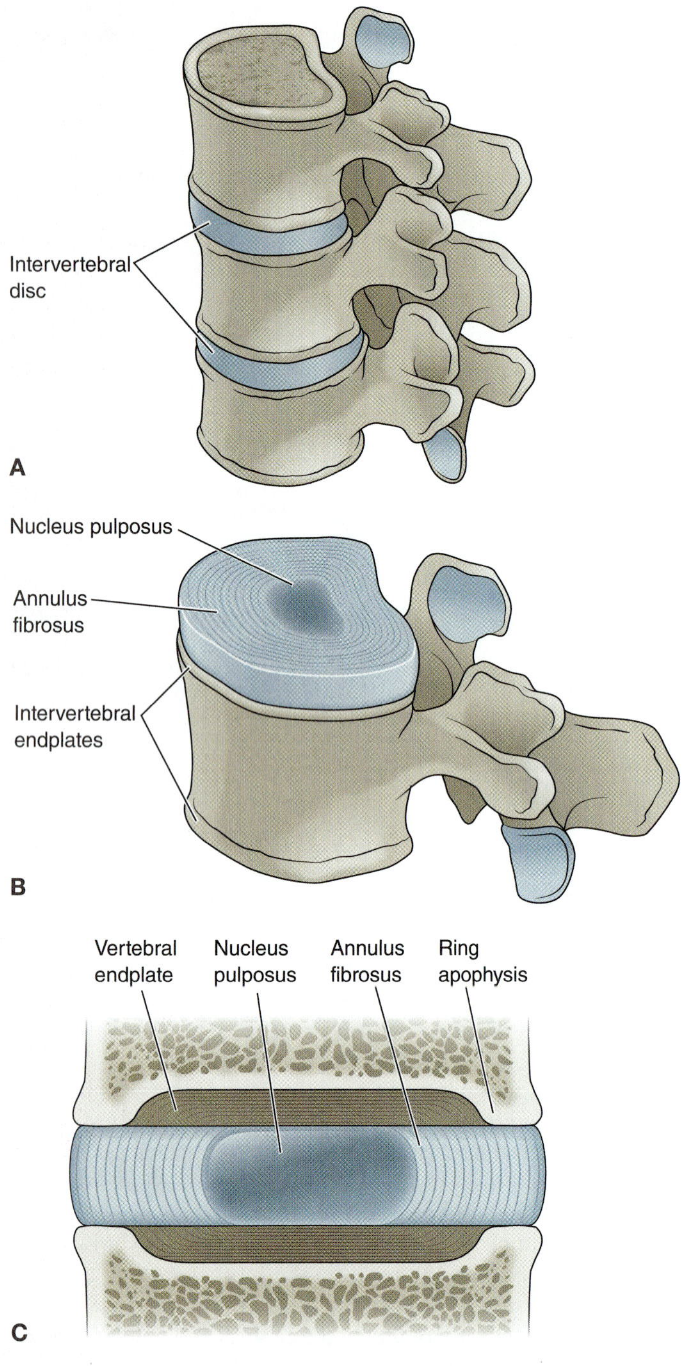

Figure 4–8 **A.** The intervertebral discs lie between each of the vertebrae. **B.** This schematic representation of a lumbar intervertebral disc shows the nucleus pulposus, the annulus fibrosus, and the vertebral endplate. **C.** On cross section, the relationship between the three components of the disc is evident, with the endplate located within the circumferential bony ring apophysis.

of the disc, separating it from the cancellous bone of the vertebral bodies above and below. All three structures are composed of water, collagen, and proteoglycans;[7] however, the relative proportions of each vary. Fluid and proteoglycan concentrations are highest in the nucleus and lowest in the outer annulus fibrosus and the outer vertebral endplate (closest to the vertebral body). Conversely, collagen concentrations are highest in the vertebral endplate and outer annulus and lowest in the nucleus pulposus. Although the center of the nucleus pulposus is clearly distinct from the annulus fibrosus and the outer rings of the annulus fibrosus are clearly distinct from the nucleus **(Fig. 4-8C)**, these structures really represent more of a continuum with no clear boundary separating the two structures where they merge. They are distinct structures only where they are farthest apart.

NUCLEUS PULPOSUS

The nucleus pulposus is approximately 80% water, depending on age and time of day.[2] Proteoglycans make up approximately 65% of the dry weight and attract water molecules because of the presence of glycosaminoglycans; hence the large water content within the extracellular matrix. Collagen fibers contribute 15% of the dry weight, and the remainder of the dry weight is composed of collagen, chondrocytes, elastin fibers, proteins, and proteolytic enzymes.[2] The nucleus pulposus has both type I and type II collagen; however, type II predominates because of its ability to resist compressive loads. Very little, if any, type I collagen is present in the center of the nucleus pulposus.[2,8] The nucleus pulposus frequently has been likened to a water balloon. When compressed, the nucleus deforms, and the increased pressure stretches the walls of the nucleus pulposus in all directions **(Fig. 4–9)**.

ANNULUS FIBROSUS

The annulus fibrosus is approximately 60% water depending on age and time of day. Proteoglycans contribute approximately 20% and collagen fibers 50% of the dry weight of the extracellular matrix of the annulus.[2] The remainder of the dry weight is made up of elastin fibers and cells such as fibroblasts and chondrocytes.[2] Again, type I and type II collagen are present in its layers; however—as for the nucleus—type I collagen predominates, particularly in the outer portions of the annulus.[2,8] This collagen makeup reflects the need for the annulus fibrosus to resist greater proportions of tensile forces. The annulus fibers are attached by Sharpey fibers to the cartilaginous endplates on the inferior and superior vertebral plateaus of adjacent vertebrae and to the bony epiphyseal ring (ring apophysis) region.

VERTEBRAL ENDPLATES

The vertebral endplates are layers of cartilage that cover the region of the vertebral bodies encircled by the ring apophysis on both the superior and inferior surfaces (see Fig. 4–8C). The endplates cover the nucleus pulposus but not the entire annulus fibrosus. The vertebral endplate is strongly attached to the annulus fibrosus but only weakly attached to the vertebral body, which is why it is considered a component of the disc.[2,8] The extracellular matrix of the vertebral endplates consist of proteoglycans, collagen, and water, as does the rest of the disc. In addition, there are cartilage cells aligned along the collagen. The cartilage of the vertebral endplates is both hyaline cartilage and fibrocartilage. Hyaline cartilage is present closest to the vertebral body and is found mainly during growth in height. Fibrocartilage is present closest to the nucleus pulposus. With increasing age, fibrocartilage becomes the major component of the vertebral endplate with little or no hyaline cartilage remaining. This presumably reflects the increasing need to tolerate higher compressive forces.

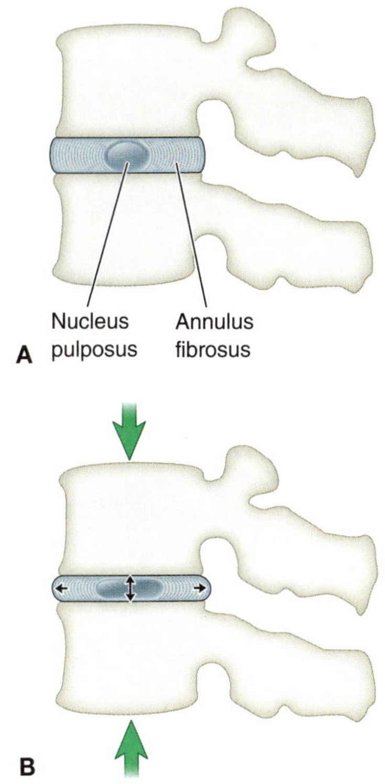

Figure 4–9 Schematic representation of compression of an intervertebral disc. Behaving somewhat like a water-filled balloon, the nucleus pulposus is contained by the annulus. **A.** In the unloaded spine, the nucleus remains spherical. **B.** Under compressive loading, the nucleus pulposus attempts to expand (becoming elliptical in shape), placing the annulus fibrosus under tension that restrains further radial expansion of the nucleus. The nuclear pressure is transmitted by the annulus fibrosus to the vertebral endplates.

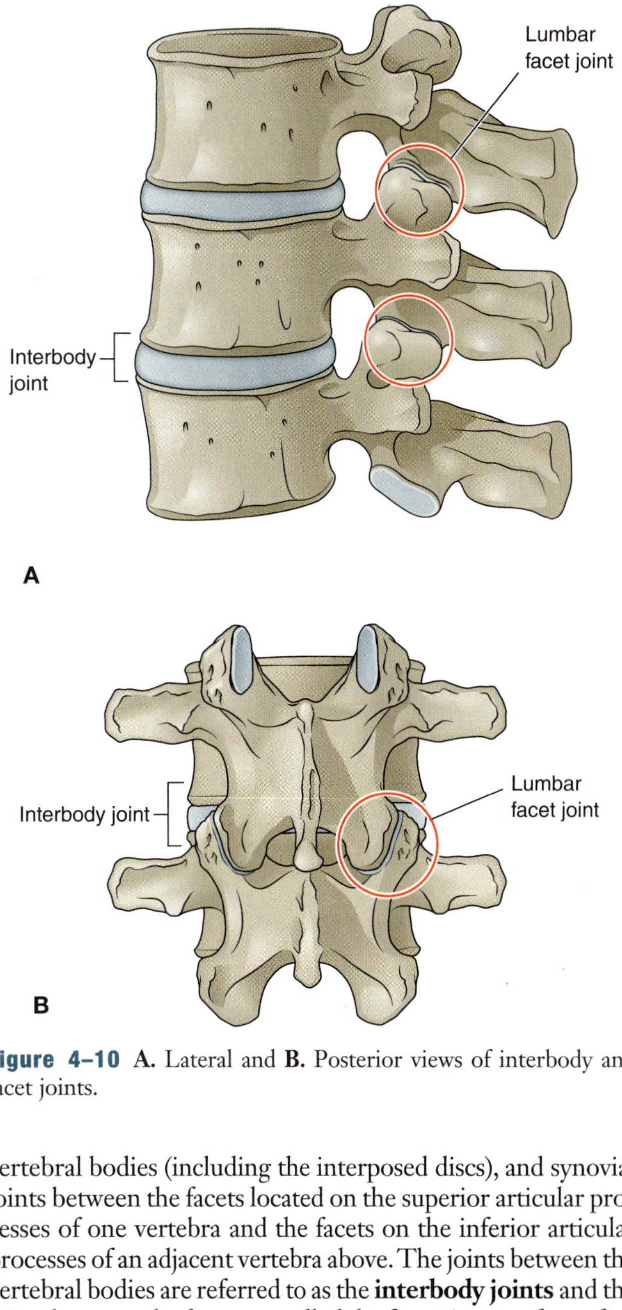

Figure 4–10 A. Lateral and **B.** Posterior views of interbody and facet joints.

INNERVATION AND NUTRITION

In healthy intervertebral discs, the annulus fibrosus is innervated in the outer one-third of the fibers, the nucleus pulposus contains no innervation, and the vertebral endplate contains peri-vascular nerve fibers.[9] Most of the nerve fibers are free nerve endings branching from the sinuvertebral nerve. As intervertebral discs degenerate, however, neural fibers increase in number and grow into previously un-innervated tissue; this is hypothesized to contribute to the pain that some individuals experience. The sinuvertebral nerve also innervates the peridiscal connective tissue and ligaments associated with the vertebral column.[2,9]

In healthy intervertebral discs, the nucleus pulposus remains avascular throughout the life span; however, the vascularization of the vertebral endplates and the outer fibers of the annulus fibrosus does change across the life span. Although they remain vascularized, the blood supply is rich in infancy and decreases with age. As with innervation, disc degeneration over time is accompanied by ingrowth of blood vessels deeper into the annulus fibrosus,[10] also hypothesized to contribute to the pain that some individuals experience.

Articulations

Two main types of articulations are found in the vertebral column: cartilaginous joints of the symphysis type between the vertebral bodies (including the interposed discs), and synovial joints between the facets located on the superior articular processes of one vertebra and the facets on the inferior articular processes of an adjacent vertebra above. The joints between the vertebral bodies are referred to as the **interbody joints** and the joints between the facets are called the **facet** (or **apophyseal** or **zygapophyseal joints**) **(Fig. 4–10)**. Synovial joints also are present where vertebrae articulate with the skull at the atlanto-occipital joints, with the pelvis at the sacroiliac joints, and where the ribs articulate with the thoracic vertebrae (see Chapter 5).

INTERBODY JOINTS

Available movements at the interbody joints include **sliding, distraction, compression,** and **tilting (Fig. 4–11)**. Sliding (translatory) motions can occur in the following directions: medial to lateral or anterior to posterior **(Fig. 4-11A** and **4-11C**, respectively). Tilt motions are rotations that can occur in the frontal, transverse, or sagittal planes **(Figs. 4-11D-F**, respectively). These motions, together with distraction and compression **(Fig. 4-11B)**, constitute six degrees of freedom.[11] The amounts of each of these motions vary by region according

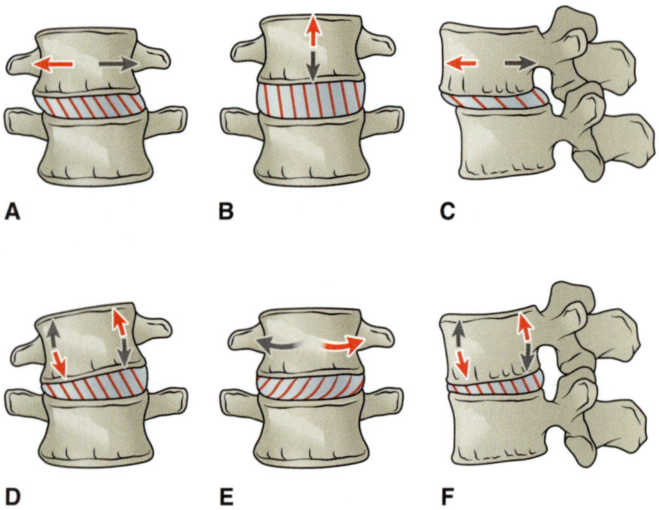

Figure 4–11 Available movements of the vertebra above on the vertebra below can take place as **A.** side-to-side sliding (translation) in the frontal plane; **B.** axial distraction and compression (superior-inferior) vertically; **C.** anteroposterior sliding (translation) in the sagittal plane; **D.** side-to-side tilting in the frontal plane around an anteroposterior axis; **E.** axial rotation in the transverse plane around a longitudinal axis; or **F.** anteroposterior tilting in the sagittal plane around a coronal axis.

to structural differences in the discs and the vertebral bodies, as well as in the ligamentous supports. In addition, the facet joints influence the total available motion of the interbody joints.

FACET JOINTS

The facet joints are composed of the articulations between the right and left inferior articulating facets of a vertebra with, respectively, the right and left superior facets of the vertebra immediately below. The facet joints are synovial joints and have regional variations in structure **(Fig. 4–12)**. Intra-articular accessory joint structures have been identified in the facet joints.[2,12,13] These accessory structures appear to be of several types, but most are classified as fibroadipose meniscoids. The structures most likely are involved in protecting articular surfaces that are exposed during flexion and extension of the vertebral column. The facet joints are innervated by the dorsal ramus of the segmental spinal nerves.[14]

Ligaments and Joint Capsules

The ligamentous system of the vertebral column is extensive and exhibits considerable regional variability. Six main ligaments are associated with the intervertebral and facet joints. These are the anterior and posterior longitudinal ligaments, the ligamentum flavum, and the interspinous, supraspinous, and intertransverse ligaments **(Fig. 4–13)**.

ANTERIOR AND POSTERIOR LONGITUDINAL LIGAMENTS

The anterior longitudinal ligament and posterior longitudinal ligament are associated with the interbody joints. The **anterior longitudinal ligament (ALL) (Figs. 4–13A and C)** runs along

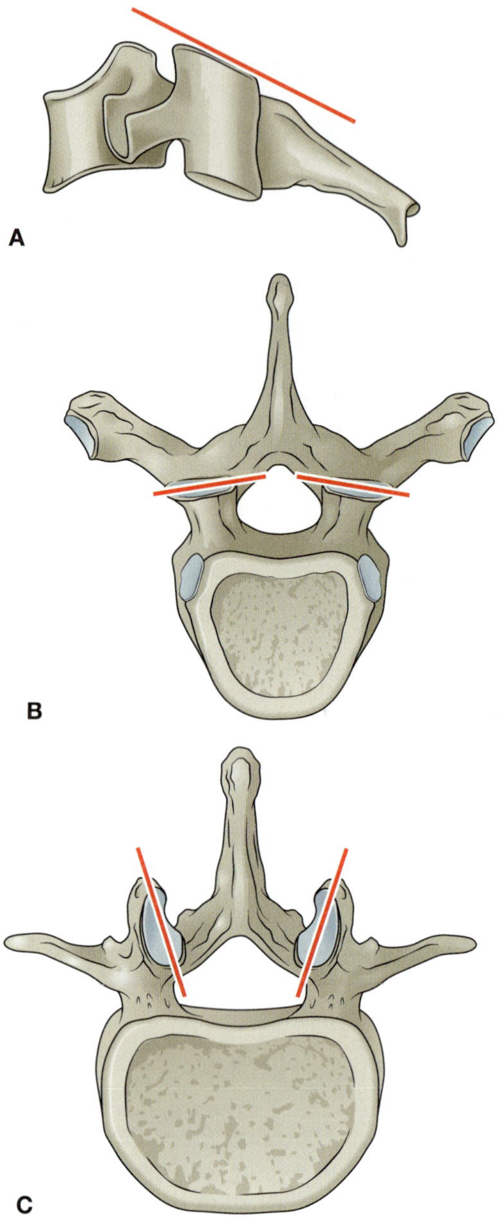

Figure 4–12 Orientation of the facet joints vary regionally. **A.** A typical cervical spine orientation (lateral view). **B.** A typical thoracic spine (superior view). **C.** A typical lumbar spine (superior view).

the anterior and lateral surfaces of the vertebral bodies from the sacrum to the second cervical vertebra. The ALL has two layers made up of thick bundles of collagen fibers; the fibers of the superficial layer are long and bridge several vertebrae, whereas the deep fibers are short and run between single pairs of vertebrae. The deep fibers blend with the fibers of the annulus fibrosus and reinforce the anterolateral portion of the intervertebral discs and the anterior interbody joints.[12] The ALL is well developed in the cervical and lumbar (lordotic) sections of the vertebral column but has little substance in the kyphotic region of thoracic spine. The tensile strength of the ALL is greatest in the lumbar region, where it is reported to be twice as strong as the region's posterior longitudinal ligament **(Fig. 4–14)**. The ALL is slack in flexion **(Fig. 4–14A)** and stretched in extension where it limits motion **(Fig. 4–14B)**.

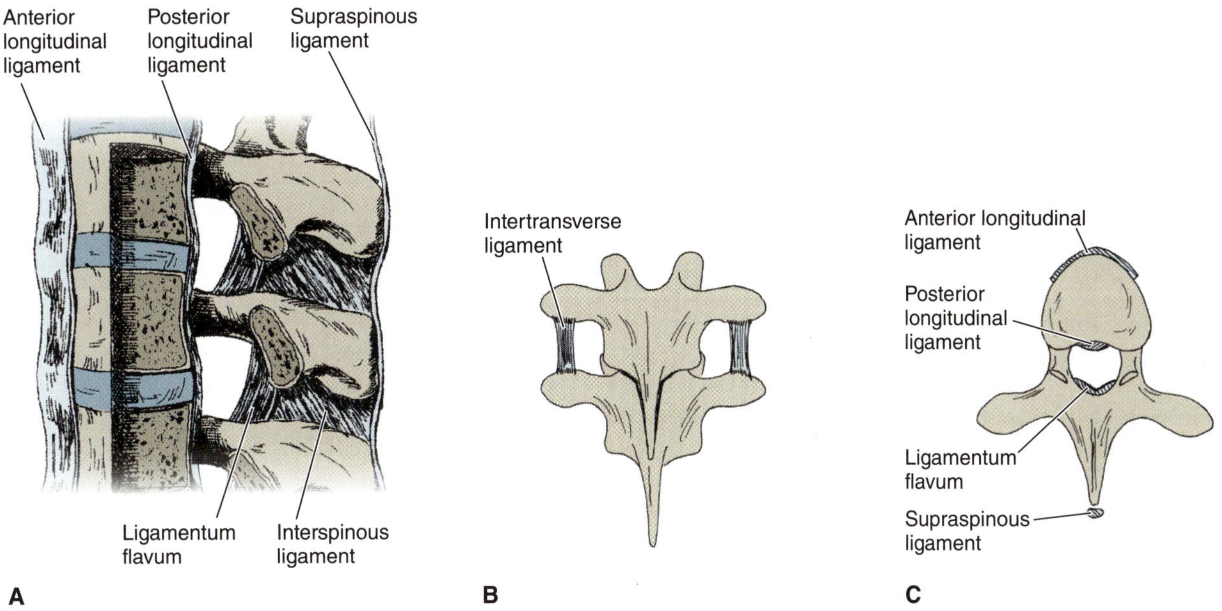

Figure 4–13 Ligamentous system of the vertebral column. **A.** The anterior and posterior longitudinal ligaments are located on the anterior and posterior aspects of the vertebral body, respectively. The ligamentum flavum runs from lamina to lamina on the posterior aspect of the vertebral canal. Portions of the bone have been removed to show the orientation of the ligament fibers. The supraspinous and interspinous ligaments run vertically along and between the spinous processes. **B.** The intertransverse ligament connects the transverse processes. **C.** The relative positions of the ligaments are shown in a superior view of the vertebra.

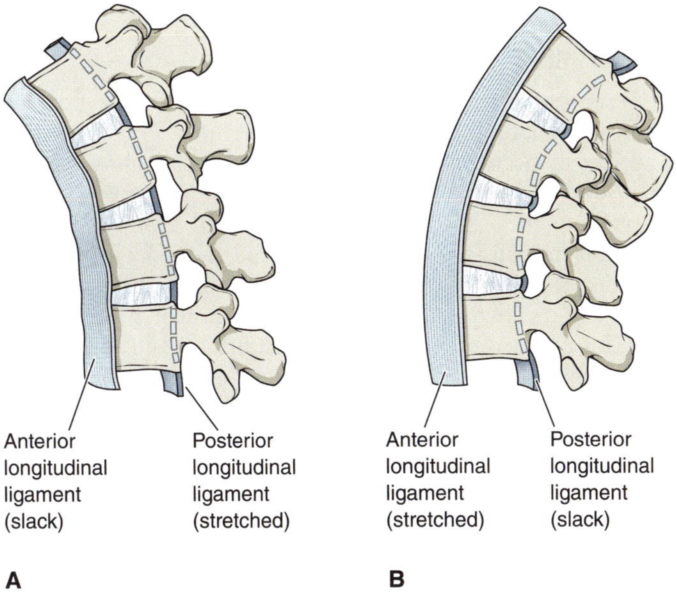

Figure 4–14 **A.** In flexion of the vertebral column, the anterior longitudinal ligament (ALL) becomes slack, whereas the posterior longitudinal ligament (PLL) is stretched. **B.** In extension of the vertebral column, the PLL is slack whereas the ALL is stretched.

It may become slackened in the neutral position of the spine when the normal height of the discs is reduced, as might occur with degenerative disc disease.

The **posterior longitudinal ligament (PLL)** (see Figs. 4–13A and 4–13C) runs along the posterior aspect of the vertebral bodies from C2 to the sacrum and forms the ventral surface of the vertebral canal. Like the ALL, the PLL also consists of a superficial and a deep layer. In the superficial layer, the fibers span several mobile segments. In the deep layer, the fibers extend only to adjacent vertebrae, interlacing with the outer layer of the annulus fibrosus and attaching to the margins of the vertebral endplates.[12] In the lumbar region, the ligament narrows to a thin ribbon that provides little support for the interbody joints. The PLL is stretched in flexion where it helps limit motion (Fig. 4–14A) and is slack in extension (Fig. 4–14B).

Foundational Concepts 4–2
Potential Role of the Posterior Longitudinal Ligament in Disc Herniation

The narrow PLL in the lumbar region does not provide much support for the intervertebral discs, which is one of the factors contributing to the higher incidence of disc herniations in a posterolateral direction in the lumbar spine than in other regions. In the lumbar spine, the posterior fibers of the annulus fibrosus are stressed most in combined flexion and rotation positions. Combined with excessive compressive loads such as occur with repetitive lifting and twisting with heavy objects, the posterior annulus can fail. The posterior annulus failure, combined with limited support from the PLL, *may* allow the nucleus pulposus to herniate in a posterolateral direction and possibly compress the exiting spinal nerve.

LIGAMENTUM FLAVUM

The **ligamentum flavum** is a thick, elastic ligament that connects lamina to lamina from C2 to the sacrum and forms the smooth posterior surface of the vertebral canal (see Figs. 4–13A and 4–13C). Some fibers extend laterally to cover the articular capsules of the facet joints. Although the highest strain in this ligament occurs during flexion when the ligament is stretched,[2] this ligament is under constant tension even when the spine is in a neutral position because of its elastic nature. This highly elastic nature serves two purposes. First, it creates a small but continuous compressive force on the discs. This increased pressure in the discs makes the discs stiffer and thus better able to provide support for the spine in the neutral position. Second, a highly elastic ligament in this location is advantageous because the ligament will not buckle on itself during movement. If the ligament were to buckle on itself, it would potentially reduce intervertebral stability in a neutral spine, and compress the spinal cord in the vertebral canal during movements into extension.

Patient Application 4–1

Joyce is a 61-year-old woman with a 10-year history of intermittent neck pain. She presents to physical therapy with familiar neck pain; however, she has new symptoms of weakness in both hands and has fallen three times in the last month. Examination confirms impaired balance and intrinsic hand muscle weakness. Compressive cervical myelopathy is suspected clinically and is confirmed by a magnetic resonance imaging (MRI) scan that also shows spondylosis, a hypertrophied ligamentum flavum, and ossified posterior longitudinal ligament.

The ligamentum flavum is subject to hypertrophy and loss of elastin due to aging, with this hypertrophy accelerated with spondylosis (degeneration) of the spine. If the ligamentum flavum is hypertrophied and less elastic, it has the potential to buckle into the spinal canal and cause compression of the spinal cord, particularly with extension motions. Because the ligamentum flavum forms the posterior surface of the spinal canal, hypertrophy can produce central spinal stenosis (narrowing of the spinal canal). The buckling potential is greatest in the presence of degenerated intervertebral discs where loss of height bring the ends of the ligament closer together, allowing the ligament to be slack at rest. Spinal stenosis associated with ligamentum flavum hypertrophy is even greater if ossification of the posterior longitudinal ligament has occurred as well. If the spinal canal space becomes small enough, myelopathy will result. If the cross-sectional area of the canal is reduced by ≥ 30%, neurological symptoms will likely be present.[15]

INTERSPINOUS LIGAMENTS

The **interspinous ligament** connects spinous processes of adjacent vertebra (see Fig. 4–13A). It is a fibrous sheet with an extracellular matrix consisting of type I collagen, proteoglycans, and profuse elastin fibers. The interspinous ligament is innervated by medial branches of the dorsal rami.[16–18] Most authors agree that the interspinous ligament resists flexion.

SUPRASPINOUS LIGAMENT

The **supraspinous ligament** is a strong, cord-like structure that connects the tips of the spinous processes (see Figs. 4–13A and 4–13C).[2,19] The supraspinous ligament, like the interspinous ligament, is stretched in flexion with its fibers resisting separation of the spinous processes. During extreme flexion, the supraspinous and interspinous ligaments are the first to fail.[20] The supraspinous ligament contains mechanoreceptors that, with stretch of the ligament, appear to play a role in the concurrent recruitment of spinal stabilizers such as the multifidus muscles.

INTERTRANSVERSE LIGAMENTS

The structure of the paired **intertransverse ligaments** is extremely variable by region. In general, the ligaments pass between transverse processes (see Fig. 4–13B) and are alternately stretched and compressed during lateral bending. The ligaments on the right side are stretched and offer resistance during lateral bending to the left, whereas the ligaments on the left side are slack and compressed during this motion. Conversely, the ligaments on the left side are stretched during lateral bending to the right and resist this motion.

FACET JOINT CAPSULES

The **facet joint capsules** assist the ligaments in limiting motion and providing stability for the vertebral column. The roles of the joint capsules also vary by region. The capsules are strongest in the transition zones where the spinal configuration changes from lordotic to kyphotic (cervicothoracic junction) or from kyphotic to lordotic (thoracolumbar junction), presumably because of the potential for excessive stress in these areas. The joint capsules, like the supraspinous and interspinous ligaments, are vulnerable in extremes of flexion, especially in the lumbar region. The facet joint capsules are richly innervated and *may* be a source of pain in cases of mechanical or inflammatory irritation.[13] Table 4–3 provides a summary of the ligaments and their functions.

Function

Kinematics

The motions available to the vertebral column are flexion/extension, lateral flexion, and axial rotation. These motions appear to occur independently of each other; however, at the level of the individual motion segment composed of two vertebrae, these motions are often coupled. **Coupling** is defined as the consistent association of one motion with another motion that will result if the axis of motion is oblique rather than in a cardinal plane. The most predominant motions that exhibit coupled behaviors are lateral flexion and rotation. It appears that pure lateral flexion and pure rotation do not occur in any region of the spine except for the atlantoaxial joint, where rotation is the primary motion as the atlas pivots around the dens of the axis in a transverse plane. Otherwise, for either lateral flexion or rotation to occur, at least some of the coupled motion must occur as well.[9,21]

Coupling patterns, as well as the types and amounts of motion that are available, are complex. The patterns differ from region to region, depending on factors that include the spinal posture and curves; the orientation of the articulating facets; the fluidity, elasticity, and thickness of the intervertebral discs; and the extensibility of the muscles, ligaments, and joint capsules.[21,22] It also appears that coupled motions vary widely among individuals and that there may be fewer patterns of coupled motions than once was believed.[23] The most consistent pattern of coupled motion occurs in the lower cervical spine, where cervical lateral flexion to one side is accompanied by cervical rotation to the same side when either lateral flexion or rotation is initiated.[24]

Motions at the interbody and facet joints are interdependent. The *amount* of motion available is determined primarily by the size of the discs, whereas the *direction* of the motion

Table 4–3 Major Ligaments of the Vertebral Column

LIGAMENTS	FUNCTION	REGION
Annulus fibrosus (outer fibers)	Resists distraction, translation, and rotation of vertebral bodies	Cervical, thoracic, and lumbar
Anterior longitudinal ligament	Limits extension and reinforces anterolateral portion of annulus fibrosus and anterior aspect of intervertebral joints	C2 to sacrum, but well developed in cervical, lower thoracic, and lumbar regions
Anterior atlantoaxial ligament (continuation of the anterior longitudinal ligament)	Limits extension	C2 to the occipital bone
Posterior longitudinal ligament	Limits forward flexion and reinforces posterior portion of the annulus fibrosus	Axis (C2) to sacrum. Broad in the cervical and thoracic regions and narrow in the lumbar region.
Tectorial membrane (continuation of the posterior longitudinal ligament)	Limits forward flexion	Axis (C2) to occipital bone
Ligamentum flavum	Limits forward flexion, particularly in the lumbar area, where it resists separation of the laminae	Axis (C2) to sacrum. Thin, broad, and long in cervical and thoracic regions and thickest in the lumbar region.
Posterior atlantoaxial ligament (continuation of the ligamentum flavum)	Limits forward flexion	Atlas (C1) and axis (C2)
Supraspinous ligaments	Limit forward flexion	Thoracic and lumbar (C7–L3 or L4). Weak in lumbar region.
Ligamentum nuchae	Limit forward flexion	Cervical region (occipital protuberance to C7)
Intertransverse ligaments	Limit forward flexion	Primarily in lumbar region, where they are well developed
Intertransverse ligaments	Limit contralateral lateral flexion	Primarily in lumbar region
Alar ligaments	Limit rotation of the head to the same side and lateral flexion to the opposite side	Atlas (C1 and C2)
Iliolumbar ligament	Resists anterior sliding of L5 and S1	Lower lumbar region
Facet joint capsules	Resist forward flexion and axial rotation	Strongest at cervicothoracic junction and in the thoracolumbar region

is determined primarily by the orientation of the facets. The intervertebral discs increase the amount of movement between two adjacent vertebrae. Without discs, the vertebrae would lie flat against each other and the movement between them would be limited to translation alone.[2] Vertebrae tilt on each other because the soft, deformable disc lies between them. Consequently, discs add substantial range of motion (ROM) to each mobile segment **(Fig. 4–15)**, with thicker discs resulting in more potential motion. The fibers of the annulus fibrosus behave as a ligamentous structure and act as restraints to motion of each mobile segment.

The motions of flexion and extension occur because of the tilting and sliding of a superior vertebra over the inferior vertebra. As the superior vertebra moves through a ROM, it follows a series of different arcs, each of which has a different instantaneous axis of rotation.[25] The nucleus pulposus acts like a pivot but, unlike a mechanical pivot, can undergo greater distortion due to its viscoelastic composition. A sliding motion occurs at the facet joints as the vertebral body tilts over the disc at the interbody joint. The differing orientation of the facet surfaces (see Fig. 4–12), determines the amount of tilting and sliding within a particular region. If the facet joints are oriented in the sagittal plane (typical lumbar orientation), the motions of flexion and extension are most facilitated **(Fig. 4–16A)**. On the other hand, if the facet surfaces are oriented in the frontal plane (given typical thoracic orientation), the predominant motion is lateral flexion **(Fig. 4–16B)**.

FLEXION

In vertebral flexion, the vertebral body above anteriorly tilts, and the inferior facets of that superior vertebra slide *upwardly* on the vertebral facets below, causing separation of the spinous processes and widening of the intervertebral foramen **(Fig. 4–17A)**. Although the amount of tilting depends partly on the size of the discs, supraspinous and interspinous ligament tension resists separation of the spinous processes and thus limits the flexion ROM. Passive tension in the facet joint capsules, ligamentum flavum, posterior longitudinal ligament, and the spinal extensors also restrains flexion. With movement into flexion, the anterior portion of the annulus fibrosus is compressed whereas the posterior portion is stretched and resists separation of the vertebral bodies, restraining motion.

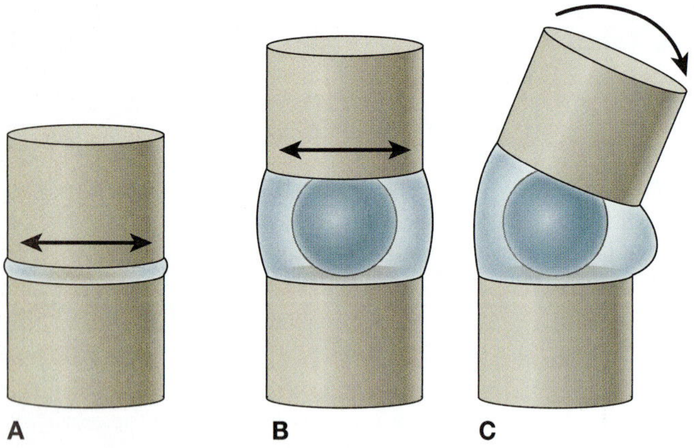

Figure 4–15 **A.** Without an intervertebral disc, only translatory motions could occur between vertebrae, limited by the interconnecting fibrous structures. **B.** The addition of an intervertebral disc separates the vertebral bodies, allowing a vertebra to both slide (translate) and tilt on the vertebra below, substantially increasing range of motion at the interbody joint.

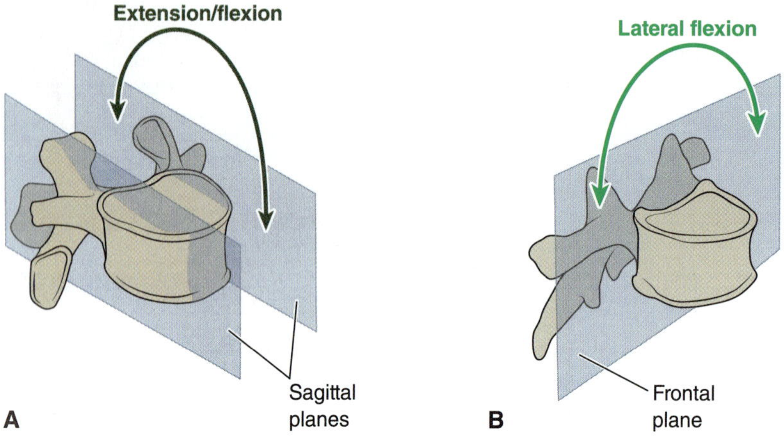

Figure 4–16 **A.** Facet surfaces oriented in the sagittal plane (seen in typical lumbar vertebra) favor the motions of flexion and extension. **B.** Facet surfaces oriented in the frontal plane (seen in typical thoracic vertebra) favor lateral flexion.

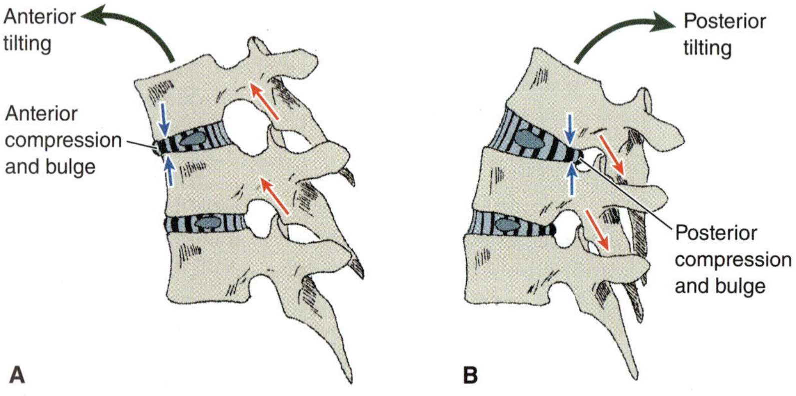

Figure 4–17 **A.** In flexion, the inferior facets of the superior vertebra slide up on the superior facets of the contiguous vertebra below, with the superior vertebral body tilting anteriorly. The anterior tilting causes compression and anterior bulging of the annulus fibrosus along with stretching of the annulus posteriorly; the intervertebral foramen widens. **B.** In extension, the inferior facets of the superior vertebra slide down on the superior facets of the vertebra below while the vertebral body tilts posteriorly. The anterior annulus fibrosus fibers are stretched, with the posterior portion of the disc compressed and bulging posteriorly; the intervertebral foramen narrows.

EXTENSION

In extension, posterior tilting and gliding of the superior vertebra on the inferior vertebra occurs, causing the spinous processes to approximate and the intervertebral foramen to narrow **(Fig. 4–17B)**. The amount of motion available in extension is limited by bony contact of the spinous processes and approximation of the facet joint surfaces, as well as tension from the anterior fibers of the annulus fibrosus, anterior longitudinal ligament, and anterior trunk muscles. The only ligament that directly limits extension is the anterior longitudinal ligament, which is likely the reason that the anterior longitudinal ligament is stronger than the posterior longitudinal ligament.

LATERAL FLEXION

In lateral flexion, the superior vertebra laterally tilts and translates over the vertebra below **(Fig. 4–18)**. The intervertebral foramen is widened contralateral to the direction of lateral flexion and narrowed on the ipsilateral side. The annulus fibrosus is compressed on the concavity of the curve and stretched on the convexity of the curve. Passive tension in the annulus fibers, intertransverse ligaments, and anterior and posterior trunk muscles on the convexity of the curve limit lateral flexion. The coupled direction of rotation that accompanies lateral flexion differs slightly from region to region because of the differing orientation of the facets.

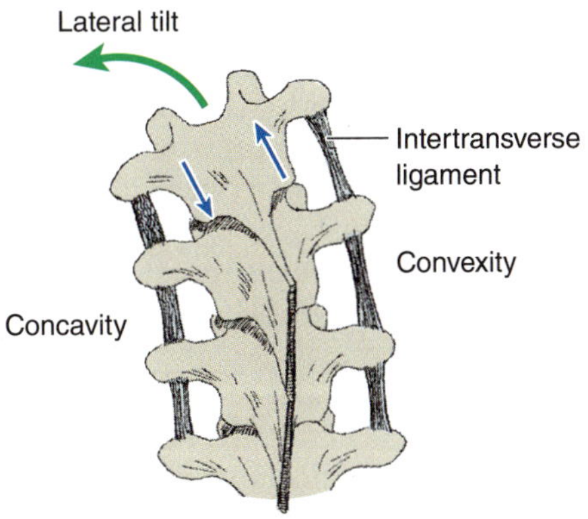

Figure 4–18 In lateral flexion to the left, the inferior facet on the concave side (the left side in the figure) slides down on the superior facet of the vertebra below, whereas the inferior facet of the superior vertebra on the convex side (on the right) slides upward. The vertebral body tilts laterally toward the concave side, widening the intervertebral foramen on the convexity and narrowing the space on the concavity. Lateral flexion is limited by tension in the intertransverse ligament on the convexity of the curve.

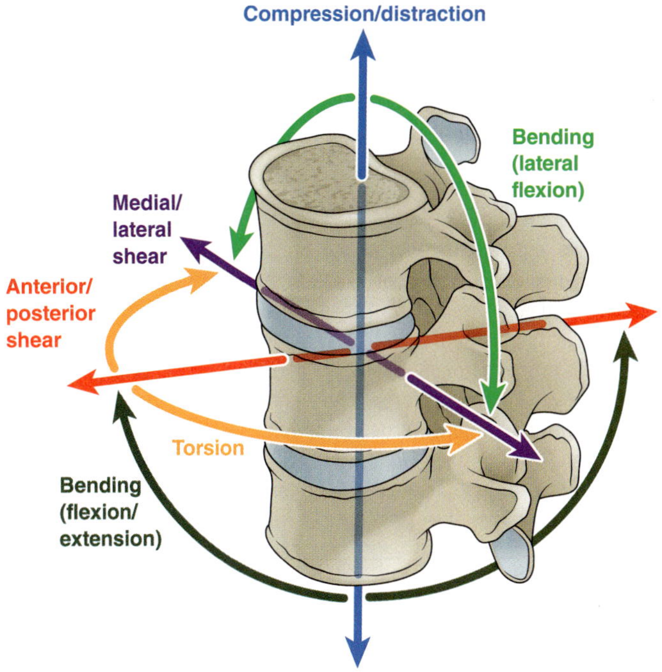

Figure 4–19 Each motion segment in the vertebral column is subjected to axial (compression/distraction), bending (flexion/extension, lateral flexion), torsional (rotation), and shear (anterior/posterior, medial/lateral) forces.

ROTATION

Rotation is available in each spinal region, but due to the drastically different shapes of the facet joints, the kinematics vary greatly by region and will be discussed by region in the following section.

Kinetics

The vertebral column is subjected to axial compression, tension (distraction), bending, torsion, and shear stress during normal functional activities as well as at rest. The column's ability to resist these loads varies among spinal regions and depends on the type, direction, duration, and rate of loading; the person's age and posture; the condition and properties of the various structural elements, and the integrity of the nervous system **(Fig. 4–19)**.

AXIAL COMPRESSION

Axial compression (force acting through the long axis of the spine at right angles to the discs) occurs due to the force of gravity, ground reaction forces, forces produced by the ligaments and muscular contractions, and any potential external load imposed on the person's body. The discs and vertebral bodies resist most of the compressive force, but the neural arches and facet joints share some of the load in certain postures and during specific motions. The compressive load is transmitted from the superior vertebral endplate, to the inferior endplate, and through the trabecular (cancellous) bone of the vertebral body and its cortical shell. The cancellous bone contributes much of the strength of a lumbar vertebra before the age of 40, and the cortical bone carries the remainder. After age 40, the cortical bone carries a greater proportion of the load, because the trabecular bone's compressive strength and stiffness decrease with decreasing bone density.[26] Depending on the posture and region of the spine, the facet joints carry from 0% to 30% of the compression load. The spinous processes also may share some of the load when the spine is in hyperextension.

The nucleus pulposus acts as a gelatinous ball that can be deformed by a compression force. The pressure created within the nucleus pulposus is greater than the force of the applied load.[27] When a weight is applied to the nucleus pulposus from above, the nucleus pulposus exhibits a swelling pressure and tries to expand outward toward the annulus fibrosus and the endplates (see Fig. 4–9). As the nucleus attempts to distribute the pressure in all directions, stress is created in the annulus fibrosus, with resulting central compressive loading on the vertebral endplates. Normally, the annulus fibrosus and the endplates provide sufficient resistance to the swelling pressure in the nucleus pulposus to reach and maintain a state of equilibrium. The pressure exerted on the endplates is transmitted to the superior and inferior vertebral bodies. The discs and trabecular bone can undergo a greater amount of deformation without failure than either the cartilaginous endplates or cortical bone when subjected to axial compression. The endplates will be the first to fail (fracture) under high compressive loading.

When the intervertebral discs are subjected to a constant load, they will exhibit creep (time-dependent deformation). This phenomenon produces typical changes in disc composition and function across each day. Under sustained compressive loading such as that incurred in the upright posture, the increase in the swelling pressure in the disc causes fluid to be expressed from the nucleus pulposus and the annulus fibrosus, reducing the height of the disc. The amount of fluid expressed from the disc depends both on the size of the load and the duration of its application. The expressed fluid is absorbed through microscopic pores in the cartilaginous endplates. When the compressive forces on the discs are reduced again, the disc imbibes fluid back from the vertebral body, regaining height.[28] The creep of the disc with compression explains why a person is slightly shorter at the end of a day of prolonged axial compression from the upright position, and slightly taller in the morning after hours of reduced compression resulting from being in a horizontal position.

Expanded Concepts 4–1

Effects of Creep Loading on the Intervertebral Discs

Adams and colleagues reported mechanical changes in the disc with creep loading that include loss of intervertebral disc height, increased bulging of the disc, and less flexibility in bending.[29] The result of these changes is that the neural arch, the ligaments, and the facet joints are subjected to greater compressive and bending forces. With prolonged compressive or excessive forces, there is a shift in load from the nucleus pulposus to the annulus fibrosus, especially at the posterior aspects of the disc. This increased load can cause buckling or prolapse of the annulus fibrosus. In addition, there is decreased exchange of fluid and a decrease in metabolism, thereby decreasing nutrition to the disc.

BENDING

Bending causes both compression and tension on the structures of the spine. In forward flexion, the anterior structures (anterior portions of the disc, anterior ligaments, and anterior muscles) are subjected to compression; the corresponding posterior structures are subjected to tension (see Fig. 4–14A). The resistance offered to the tensile forces by collagen fibers in the posterior outer annulus fibrosus, facet joint capsules, and posterior ligaments helps to limit extremes of motion and thus provides stability in flexion. Creep occurs when the vertebral column is subjected to sustained loading, such as might occur in the flexed postures commonly assumed in sitting. The resulting deformation (elongation or compression) of supporting structures such as ligaments, joint capsules, and intervertebral discs may lead to an increase in the ROM beyond otherwise normal limits. If the creep deformation of tissues occurs within the toe or elastic regions of the stress-strain curve, the structures will return to their original dimensions either immediately or within minutes or hours after cessation of the activity. If the deformation exceeds the elastic region, the vertebral structures may be injured (become plastic).

In extension, the posterior structures generally are either unloaded or subjected to compression while the anterior structures are subjected to tension (see Fig. 4–14B). In general, resistance to extension is provided by the anterior outer fibers of the annulus fibrosus, approximation (compression) of the facet joint surfaces, passive tension in the anterior longitudinal ligament, and possibly by contact of the spinous processes. In lateral bending, the ipsilateral side of the disc is compressed; that is, in right lateral bending, the right side of the disc is compressed and the outer fibers of the left side of the disc are stretched. Therefore, the contralateral fibers of the outer annulus fibrosus and the contralateral intertransverse ligament (see Fig. 4–18) help to provide stability during lateral bending by resisting extremes of motion.

TORSION

Torsional forces are created during axial rotation that occurs as a part of the coupled motions that take place in the spine. It has been suggested that the annulus fibrosus may be the most effective structure in the lumbar region for resisting torsion. However, the risk of rupture of the disc fibers is increased when there is a combination of torsion, heavy axial compression, and forward bending.[30]

When the disc is subjected to torsion, some of the annulus fibrosus fibers resist clockwise rotations whereas fibers oriented in the opposite direction resist counterclockwise rotations.

SHEAR

Shear forces occur parallel to the upper and lower surfaces of the disc and tend to cause each vertebra to slide on the one below (translation anteriorly, posteriorly, or laterally). In the lumbar spine, the facet joints resist some of the anterior shear force and the discs resist the remainder. When the load is sustained, the discs exhibit creep, and the facet joints may have to resist all the shear force. Table 4–4 summarizes vertebral function.

Table 4–4 Summary of Vertebral Function

STRUCTURE	FUNCTION
Body	Resists compressive forces. Transmits compressive forces to vertebral endplates.
Pedicles	Transmit bending forces (exerted by muscles attached to the spinous and transverse processes) to the vertebral bodies.
Laminae	Resist and transmit forces (that are transmitted from spinous and facet articular processes) to pedicles. Serve as attachment sites for muscles and ligaments.
Transverse processes	Serve as attachment sites for muscles and ligaments.
Spinous processes	Resist compression and transmit forces to laminae. Serve as attachment sites for ligaments and muscles.
Facet facets	Resist shear, compression, tensile, and torsional forces. Transmit forces to laminae.
Nucleus pulposus	Resists compression forces to vertebral endplates and translates vertical compression forces into circumferential tensile forces in annulus fibrosus.
Annulus fibrosus	Resists tensile, torsional, and shear forces.

Regional Structure and Function

The complexity of a structure that must fulfill many functions is reflected in the design of the structure's component parts, with more varied demands often requiring more complex structures. This concept is reflected in the vertebral column. Structural variations evident in the first cervical, first thoracic, fifth lumbar, and sacral vertebrae reflect adaptations necessary for joining one region of the vertebral column to adjacent regions. Differences in vertebral structure are also apparent at the cervicothoracic, thoracolumbar, and lumbosacral junctions, where there is a transition from one type of vertebral structure to another. The vertebrae located at regional junctions are called **transitional vertebrae** and usually possess characteristics common to their contiguous regions. The cephalocaudal increase in the size of the vertebral bodies reflects the increased proportion of body weight that must be supported by the lower thoracic and lumbar vertebral bodies. The sacral vertebrae fused into a solid segment reflects the need for a firm base of support for the column above. In addition to these variations, many minor alterations in structure occur throughout the column. However, only the major variations are discussed here.

Structure of the Cervical Region

The cervical portion of the vertebral column consists of seven vertebrae. Morphologically and functionally, the cervical column is divided into two distinct regions: the upper cervical spine, or craniovertebral region, and the lower cervical or subaxial cervical spine **(Fig. 4–20)**. The **craniovertebral region** includes the occipital condyles and the first two cervical vertebrae (**C1** and **C2,** or, respectively, the **atlas** and **axis**) whereas the **lower cervical spine** includes the vertebrae of **C3** to **C7** **(Fig. 4–21)**. The vertebrae from C3 to C6 display similar characteristics and therefore are the typical cervical vertebrae. The atlas, axis, and C7 exhibit unique characteristics and are considered atypical cervical vertebrae. All cervical vertebrae have the unique feature of a **transverse foramen** located on the transverse processes that serves as passage for a vertebral artery.

Craniovertebral Region

ATLAS (C1)

The atlas appears as a ring sitting between the occipital condyles and the axis (C2) **(Fig. 4–22)**. The functions of the atlas are to cradle the occiput and to transmit forces from the occiput to the cervical vertebrae below. These functions are reflected in the bony structure. The atlas is different from other vertebrae in that it has no vertebral body or spinous process and is shaped like a ring **(Fig. 4–22A)**. There are two large lateral masses on the atlas formed by the two superior and two inferior facets **(Figs. 4–22B** and **4–22C)**. These lateral masses are connected by an anterior and posterior arch that together form the ring structure and create large transverse processes for muscle attachments.[6] The transverse processes, like those elsewhere in the cervical spine, each include a transverse foramen (see Fig. 4–22A) through which a vertebral artery passes on each side. The superior facets are large, typically kidney shaped, and deeply concave to accommodate the large, convex articular surfaces of the occipital condyles. The inferior facets are slightly convex and are directed inferiorly for articulation with the superior facets of the axis (C2). There is, however, wide variation in the size and shape of these facets. The atlas also possesses a facet on the internal surface of the anterior arch for articulation with the dens **(odontoid process)** of the axis (see Fig. 4–22A).

AXIS (C2)

The primary functions of the axis are to transmit the combined load of the head and atlas to the remainder of the cervical spine and to provide rotation of the head and atlas on the axis below.[6] The axis **(Fig. 4–23)** is atypical in that the anterior portion of the body extends inferiorly and a large vertical

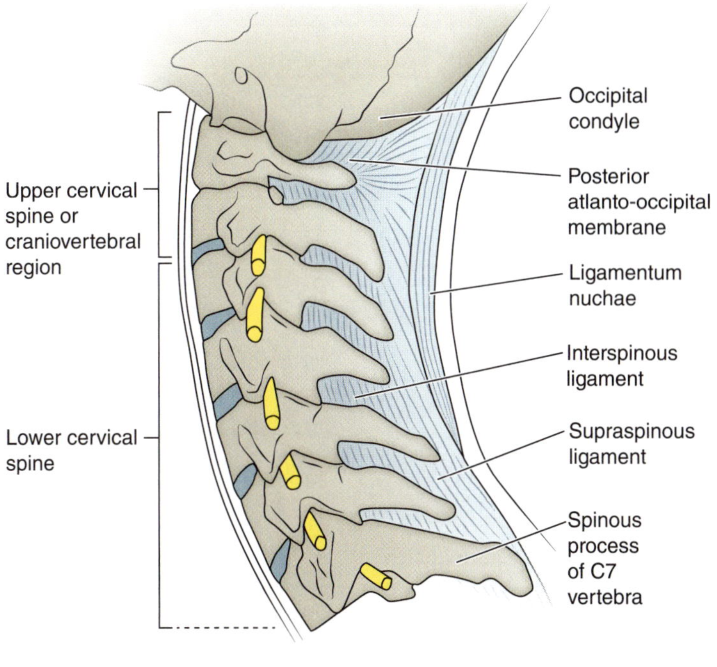

Figure 4–20 The cervical region consists of the upper cervical spine (craniovertebral region) and the lower cervical (subaxial) spine.

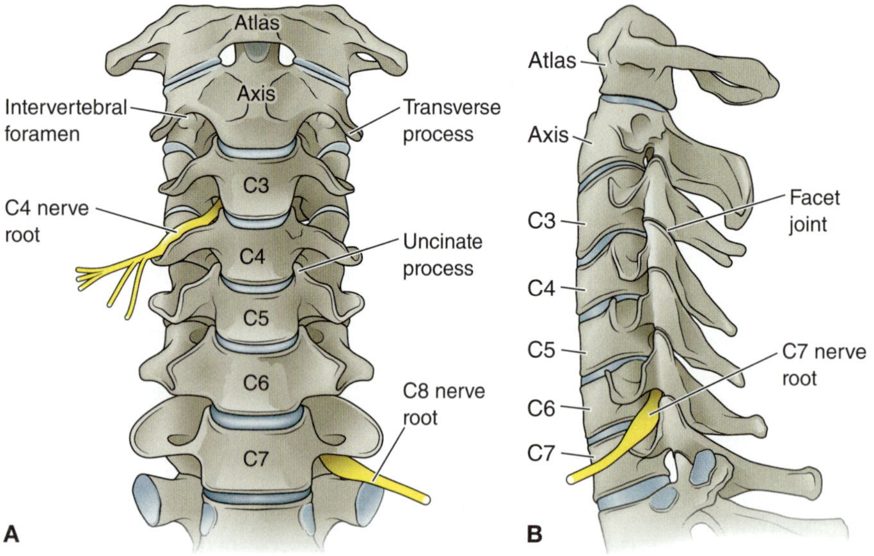

Figure 4–21 Vertebrae of the cervical spine. **A.** Lateral view. **B.** Anterior view.

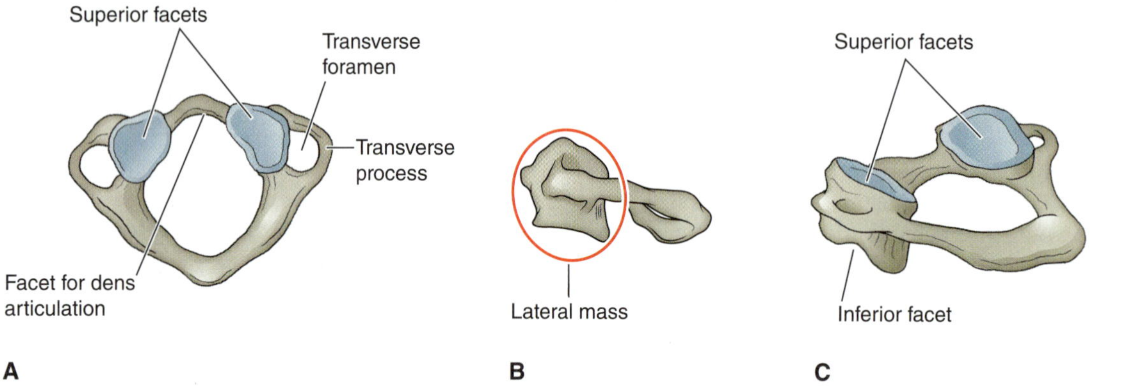

Figure 4–22 The atlas is a markedly atypical vertebra. **A.** In this superior view, it is evident that the atlas is shaped like a ring and lacks a body and a spinous process. The transverse processes each have a transverse foramen common to all cervical vertebrae. **B.** The lateral view demonstrates the lateral mass. **C.** The facets.

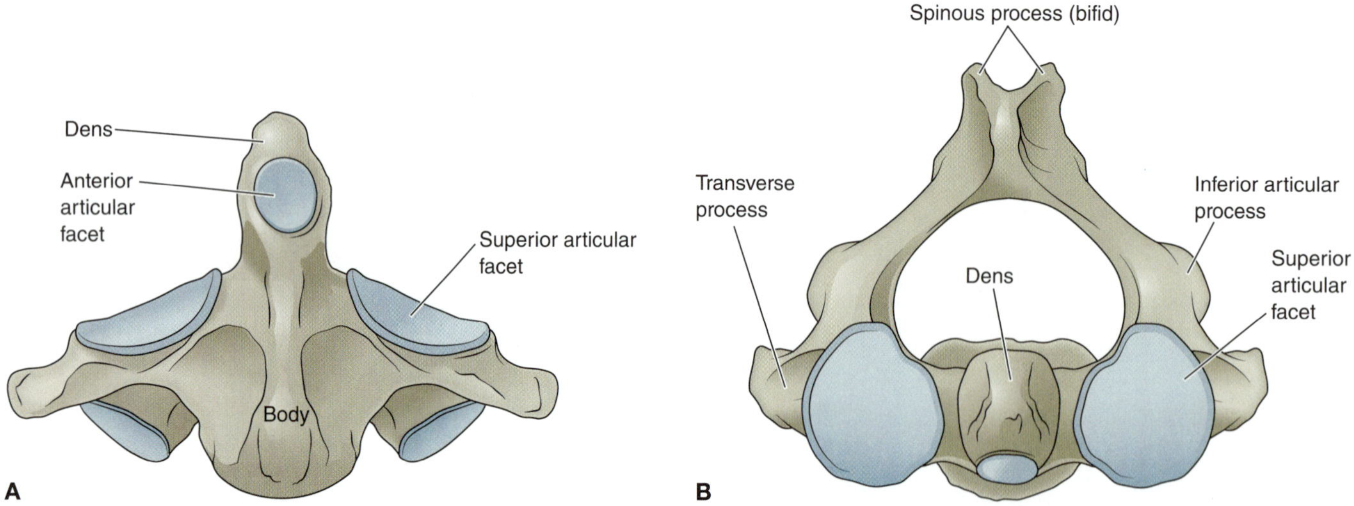

Figure 4–23 The dens (odontoid process) arises from the anterior portion of the body of the axis. The superior facets are located on either side of the dens. **A.** An anterior view shows the anterior facet on the dens for the articulation with the anterior atlas, and the inclination of the superior facets. **B.** A superior view shows the bifid spinous process and other elements of the axis.

projection called the **dens** arises from the superior surface of the body. The dens has an anterior facet for articulation with the anterior arch of the atlas (see Fig. 4–23A) and a posterior groove for articulation with the **transverse ligament.** The arch of the axis has superior and inferior facets for articulation, respectively, with atlas above and C3 below. The spinous process of the axis is large and elongated, with a bifid (split) projection (see Fig. 4–23B). The superior facets of the axis face are tilted superiorly and laterally; the inferior facets are tilted anteriorly.[31]

Articulations

The two **atlantooccipital joints** are formed by the concave superior facets of the atlas articulating with the convex occipital condyles of the skull. These joints are true synovial joints with intra-articular fibroadipose meniscoids and lie close to the horizontal plane.

There are three synovial joints that compose the **atlantoaxial joints:** There is a medial atlantoaxial joint between the dens and the anterior arch of atlas, and two lateral articulations between the superior facets of the axis and the inferior facets of the atlas **(Fig. 4–24)**. The medial joint is a synovial pivot joint in which the dens rotates within an osteoligamentous ring formed by the anterior arch of the atlas and the transverse ligament posteriorly (not shown). The two lateral joints lie in the horizontal plane and are also synovial joints. Although there is great individual variability, these joints are generally biconvex (convex in two planes).[32] Joint spaces that occur as a result of the incongruence of the biconvex structure are filled with meniscoids.

Craniovertebral Ligaments

There is a group of ligaments that are unique to the upper cervical spine. The upper cervical spine is the most mobile considering its total range of motion and has unique structures described previously. Given the increased mobility, this region is highly dependent upon ligamentous support for stability.

As shown in **Figure 4–25**, the **posterior atlantooccipital** and **posterior atlantoaxial membranes** are fibroelastic membranes that are superior (cephalad) extensions of the ligamentum flavum **(Fig. 4–25A)**. Their structure, however, varies from the ligamentum flavum in that they are less elastic and therefore restrict ROM, especially into atlantooccipital rotation.[33] The **anterior atlantooccipital** and anterior **atlantoaxial membranes** are superior extensions of the anterior longitudinal ligament **(Fig. 4–25B)**. The **tectorial membrane** is the superior extension of the posterior longitudinal ligament (PLL) in the upper two segments and is a broad, strong membrane that

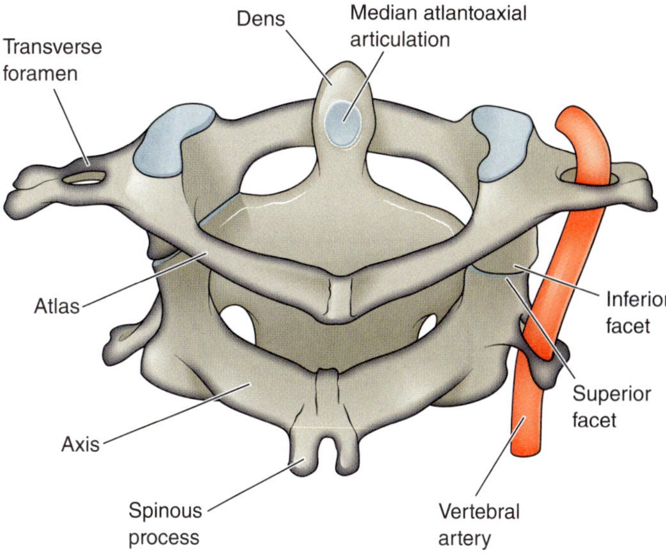

Figure 4–24 Atlantoaxial articulations. The medial atlantoaxial articulation is depicted with the posterior portion (transverse ligament) removed to show the dens and the anterior arch of the atlas. The two lateral atlantoaxial joints consisting of the superior facets of the axis and the inferior facets of the atlas lie on either side of the medial atlantoaxial joint. This view also shows the right vertebral artery as it passes through the transverse foramens.

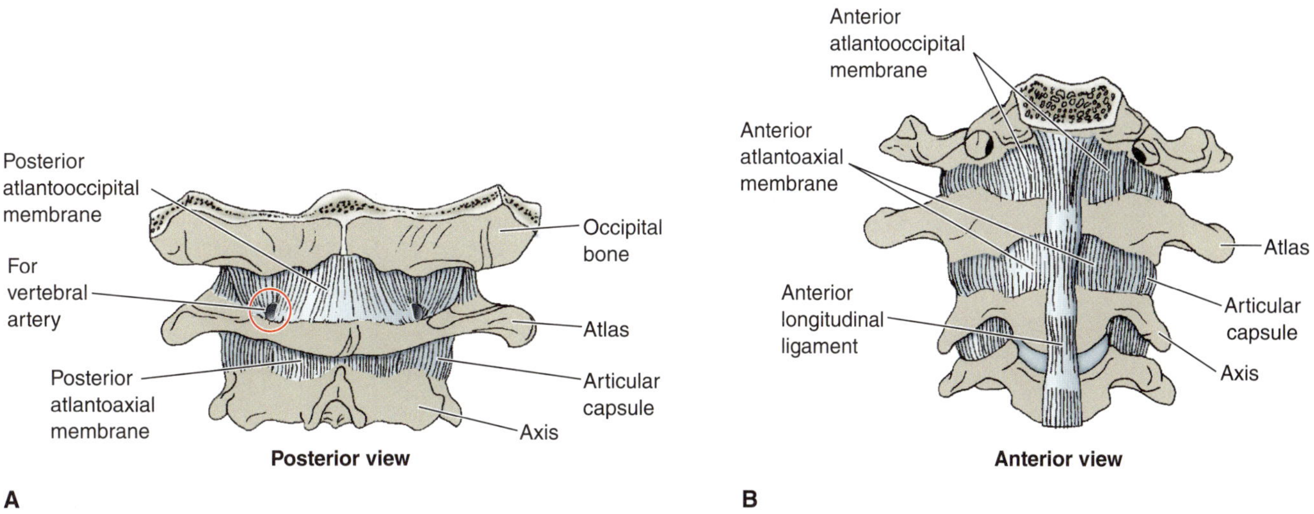

Figure 4–25 **A.** Posterior atlantooccipital and posterior atlantoaxial membranes. **B.** Anterior atlantooccipital and anterior atlantoaxial membranes.

originates from the posterior vertebral body of the axis, covers the dens and its cruciate ligament, and inserts at the basilar groove of the occiput near the anterior rim of the foramen magnum **(Fig. 4–26)**.[34] Like the PLL, the tectoral membrane lines the anterior wall of the spinal canal.

TRANSVERSE LIGAMENT

As shown in **Figure 4–27**, the **transverse ligament** stretches across the ring of the atlas and divides it into a large posterior ring for the spinal cord and a small anterior ring for the dens **(Fig. 4–27A)**. The transverse ligament has a thin layer of articular cartilage on its anterior surface where it articulates with the dens. The transverse ligament has superior fibers (known as the **apical ligament**)[19] that extend upward to attach to the occipital bone and inferior fibers extending downward to the posterior portion of the axis. The transverse ligament and its vertically oriented bands are sometimes referred to as the **cruciform** (cross-like) **ligament (Fig. 4–27B)**. The transverse portion of the ligament holds the dens against the anterior ring of the atlas and prevents anterior displacement of C1 on C2. This ligament is critical in maintaining stability at the C1–C2 segment. The transverse ligament restrains craniovertebral flexion and ensures the pivot motion of the dens during axial rotation.[34] The transverse ligament is very thick and strong; the dens often will fracture before the ligament tears with imposition of excessive forces.[19] Integrity of the transverse ligament can be compromised, however, particularly with connective tissue disorders such as rheumatoid arthritis.

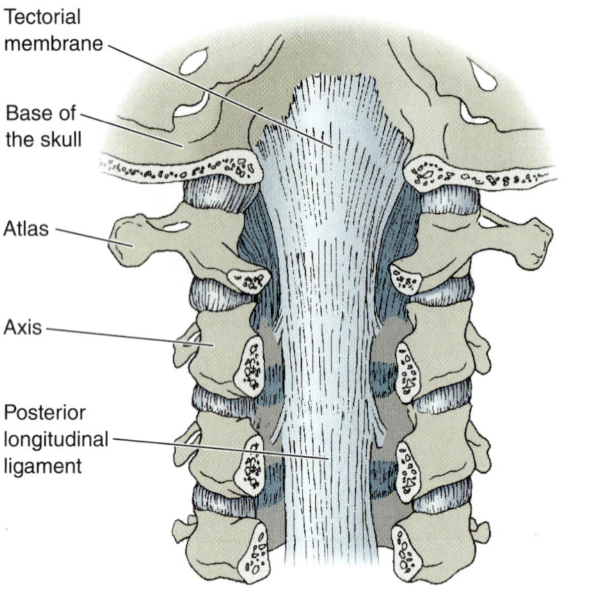

Figure 4–26 In this posterior view, the posterior vertebral arches are removed to show the tectorial membrane. The tectorial membrane is a continuation of the posterior longitudinal ligament in the craniovertebral region (occiput to axis).

ALAR LIGAMENTS

The two alar ligaments (see Figs. 4–27A and B) arise from the axis on either side of the posterior dens and extend laterally and superiorly to attach to the occipital condyles.[34,35] The ligaments consist primarily of collagen fibers. These ligaments limit craniocervical flexion. Axial rotation of the head and neck tightens both alar ligaments.[34]

The Lower Cervical Region

The lower cervical spine, also referred to as the *subaxial cervical spine*, contains the ligaments previously described for all spinal regions including the ALL, the PLL, the ligamentum flavum, and the inter-transverse ligaments. The supraspinous ligament, however, is replaced with the **ligamentum nuchae** (see Fig. 4–21). The ligamentum nuchae is a thick ligament that attaches from the external occipital protuberance and foramen magnum of the skull to the tip of C7.[18,19 36] It is a strong ligament securely attached to all cervical vertebrae and plays a primary role in resisting flexion of the head and serves as a site for muscle attachments.[37,38]

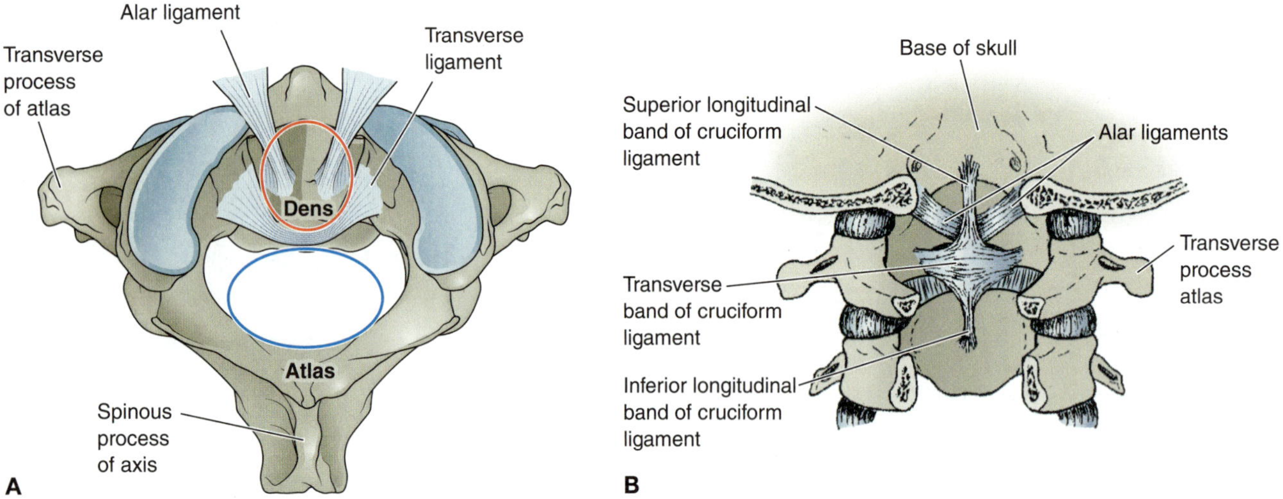

Figure 4–27 The transverse (also known as the cruciform) ligament and the alar ligaments. **A.** In a superior view, the transverse ligament divides the ring of the atlas into a smaller anterior ring and a larger posterior ring. The alar ligaments attach the axis (via the dens) to the occiput. **B.** A posterior view with the posterior portion of the vertebrae (spinous processes and portion of the arches removed) shows bands of the cruciform ligament and the attachment of the alar ligaments to the base of the skull.

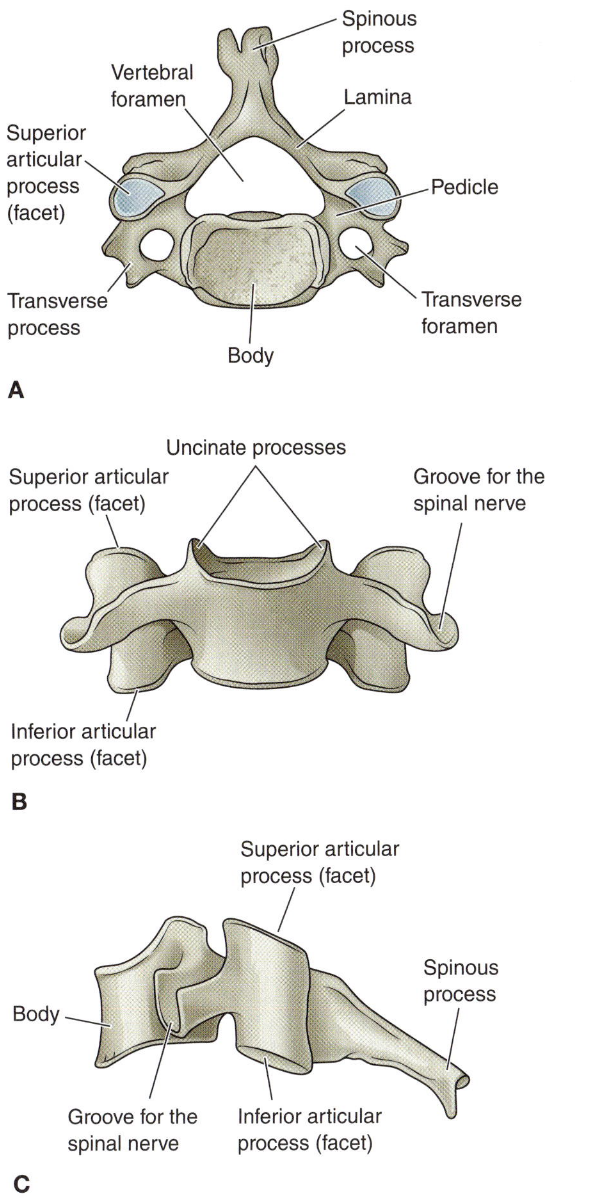

Figure 4–28 The typical cervical vertebra. **A.** The body and posterior elements of a typical cervical vertebra are evident in this superior view. **B.** In this posterior view, uncinate processes on the posterolateral superior and inferior surfaces of the body create a concavity in the frontal plane. **C.** A lateral view shows the inferior projection of the anterior body that results in a concavity of the body in the sagittal plane.

TYPICAL CERVICAL VERTEBRAE

Body

As shown in **Figure 4–28**, the body of the typical cervical vertebra is small, with a transverse diameter greater than its anteroposterior diameter and height **(Fig. 4–28A)**. The size of the body increases slightly at each level from C2 to C7. The posterolateral margins of the upper surfaces of the vertebral bodies from C3 to C7 support **uncinate processes (Fig. 4–28B)** that give the upper surfaces of these vertebrae a concave shape in the frontal plane. The uncinate processes are present prenatally, gradually enlarging between 9 to 14 years of age.[39] In addition, the anterior inferior border of the vertebral body forms a lip that hangs down toward the vertebral body below **(Fig. 4–28C)**, which produces a concave shape of the inferior surface of the vertebra in the sagittal plane.

Arches

PEDICLES. The pedicles project posterolaterally, with a thickness halfway between the superior and inferior surfaces of the vertebral body.

LAMINAE. The laminae are thin, slightly curved, and project posteromedially.

ARTICULAR PROCESSES. The cervical articular processes support paired superior and inferior facets. The superior facets are flat and oval and tilt superiorly and posteriorly; the paired inferior facets face inferiorly and anteriorly, tilting evenly between the transverse and frontal planes.

TRANSVERSE PROCESSES. Each transverse process has a transverse foramen for travel of the vertebral artery, vein, and venous plexus. Also, there is a groove for the spinal nerves that divides the cervical transverse processes into anterior and posterior tubercles (see Fig. 4–28B and C).

SPINOUS PROCESSES. The cervical spinous processes are short and slender, extend horizontally, and have a bifid tip. The length of the spinous processes decreases slightly from C2 to C3, remains constant from C3 to C5, and undergoes a significant increase at C7.

VERTEBRAL FORAMEN. The vertebral foramen is relatively large and triangular to accommodate the large proximal spinal cord.

Intervertebral Disc

The structure of the intervertebral disc in the cervical region is somewhat different from that in the lumbar region **(Fig. 4–29)**. Mercer and Bogduk state that in the cervical region the fibers of the annulus fibrosus have a crescent shape when viewed from above. The cervical discs are thick anteriorly and taper laterally as the discs approach their respective laterally located uncinate processes. The posterior fibers of the annulus fibrosus form a thinner layer with fewer concentric rings than those seen in the lumbar spine.[6,32]

Fissures in the cervical disc accompany development of the uncinate processes, becoming clefts by approximately 9 years of age **(Fig. 4–29B)**. These clefts become the joint cavity of what are termed the **uncovertebral joints** or **"joints of Luschka."**[39]

Articulations

INTERBODY JOINTS OF THE LOWER CERVICAL REGION

The interbody joints of the lower cervical region (C3 to C7) appear as saddle joints **(Fig. 4–30)**. In the sagittal plane, the inferior surface of the cranial vertebra is concave and the superior surface of the caudal vertebra is convex because of the superior uncinate processes **(Fig 4–30A)**.[7] The motions that occur in this plane are predominantly tilting motions, although translatory motions remain available.[7,32] In the frontal plane

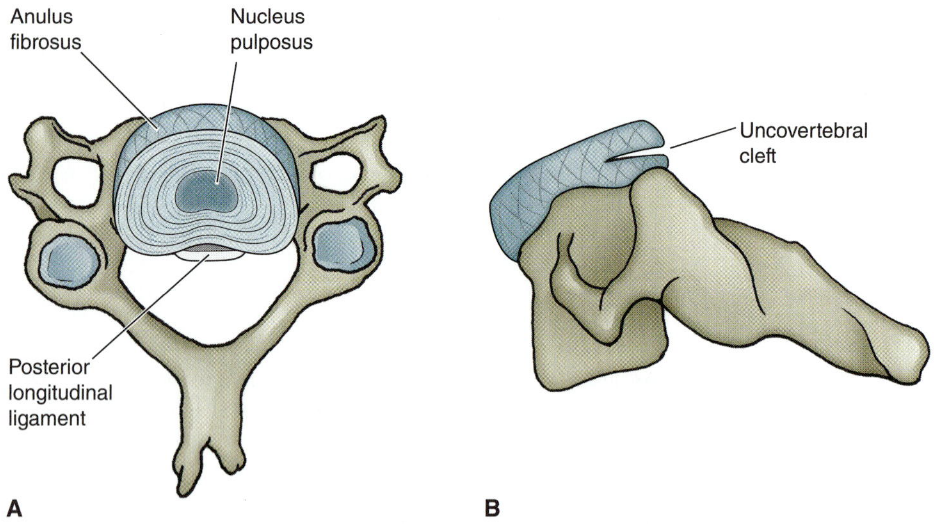

Figure 4–29 Cervical intervertebral disc. **A.** This superior view shows the crescent-shaped annulus fibrosus. **B.** The lateral view shows the uncovertebral cleft that becomes the cavity for the so-called *uncovertebral joint* or *joints of Luschka*.

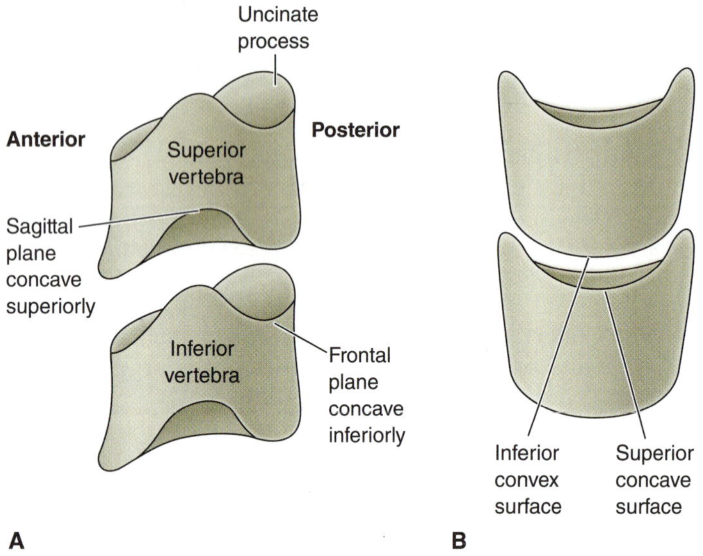

Figure 4–30 **A.** Lateral view of an interbody saddle joint in the lower cervical spine. **B.** Anterior view showing how the convex inferior surface of the superior vertebra fits into the concave superior surface of the inferior vertebra.

(Fig. 4–30B), the inferior surface of the cranial vertebra is convex and sits in the concave surface of the caudal vertebra created by the inferior uncinate processes.

FACET JOINTS

The facet joints in the lower cervical spine are true synovial joints and contain fibroadipose meniscoids.[6,7,32] The joint capsules are lax to allow a large ROM; however, the capsules will restrict motion at the end of the available ranges. The joints are generally described as oriented approximately 45° from the frontal and horizontal planes; in other words, they lie midway between the two planes (see Fig. 4–12A). However, the orientation of the joints varies widely from individual to individual, contributing to wide differences in ROM.[40]

Function of the Cervical Region

Although the cervical region demonstrates the most mobility of any of the regions of the vertebral column, stability of the cervical region—especially of the atlantooccipital and atlantoaxial joints—is essential for support of the head and protection of the brainstem, spinal cord, and vertebral arteries. The design of the atlas is such that it provides more free space for the spinal cord than does any other vertebra. The extra space helps to ensure that the spinal cord is not impinged during the large amount of motion that occurs at the atlantoaxial joint.

The differences in the two functional units of the craniocervical region and the lower cervical spine allow for different combinations of motions to occur between the head and neck in each region. Functionally, more combinations of motion facilitate optimal positioning of the sensory organs of the vestibular, visual, and auditory systems.

Kinematics

The cervical spine is designed for a relatively large amount of mobility, including flexion and extension, lateral flexion, and rotation. These motions are accompanied by translations that increase in magnitude from C2 to C7. However, the predominant translation occurs in the sagittal plane during flexion and extension.[6,7]

The atlantooccipital joints primarily allow for nodding (flexion/extension) movements between the head and the atlas, although very small amounts of lateral flexion and rotation are possible **(Fig. 4–31)**. The combined ROM for flexion/extension

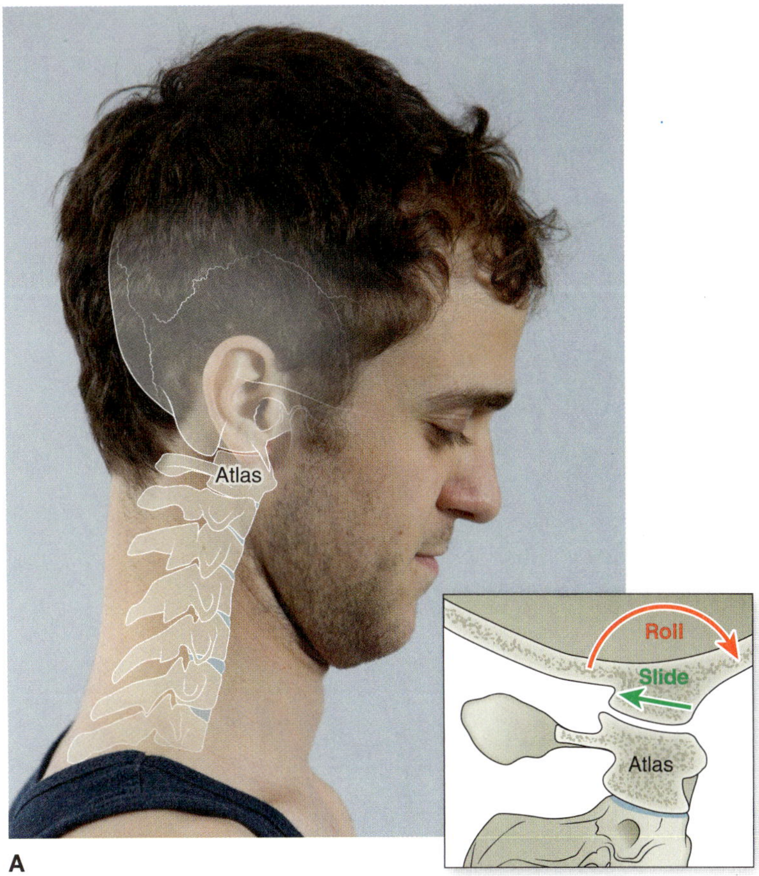

A

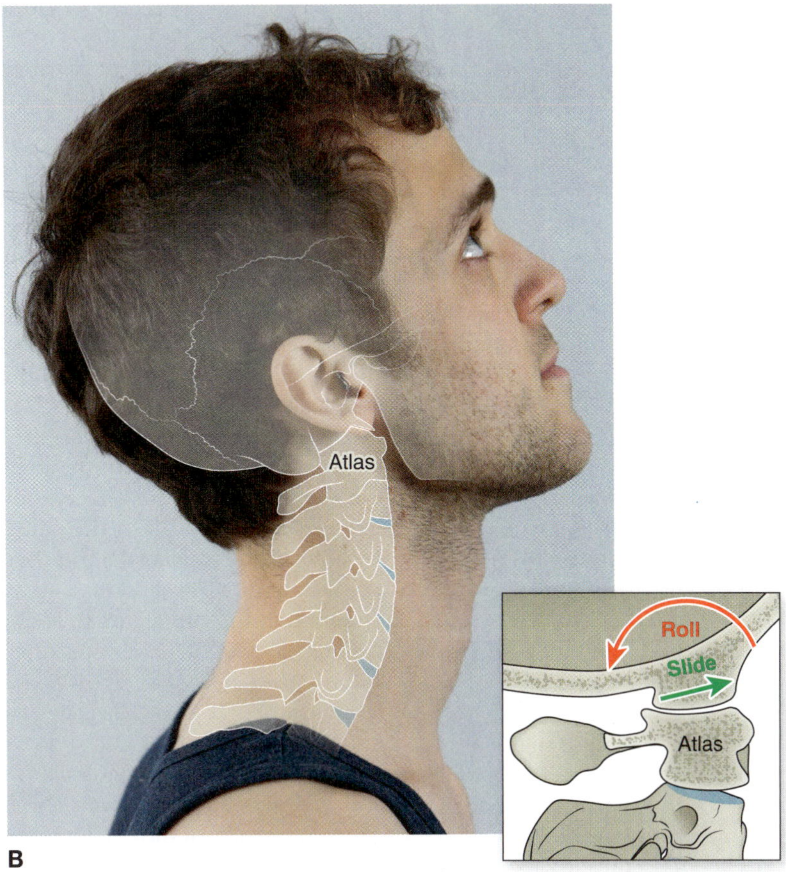

B

Figure 4–31 The primary motion available at the atlantooccipital joint is nodding (flexion/extension). **A.** In flexion, the condyles of the occiput roll forward and slide posteriorly. **B.** In extension, the condyles of the occiput roll backward and slide anteriorly.

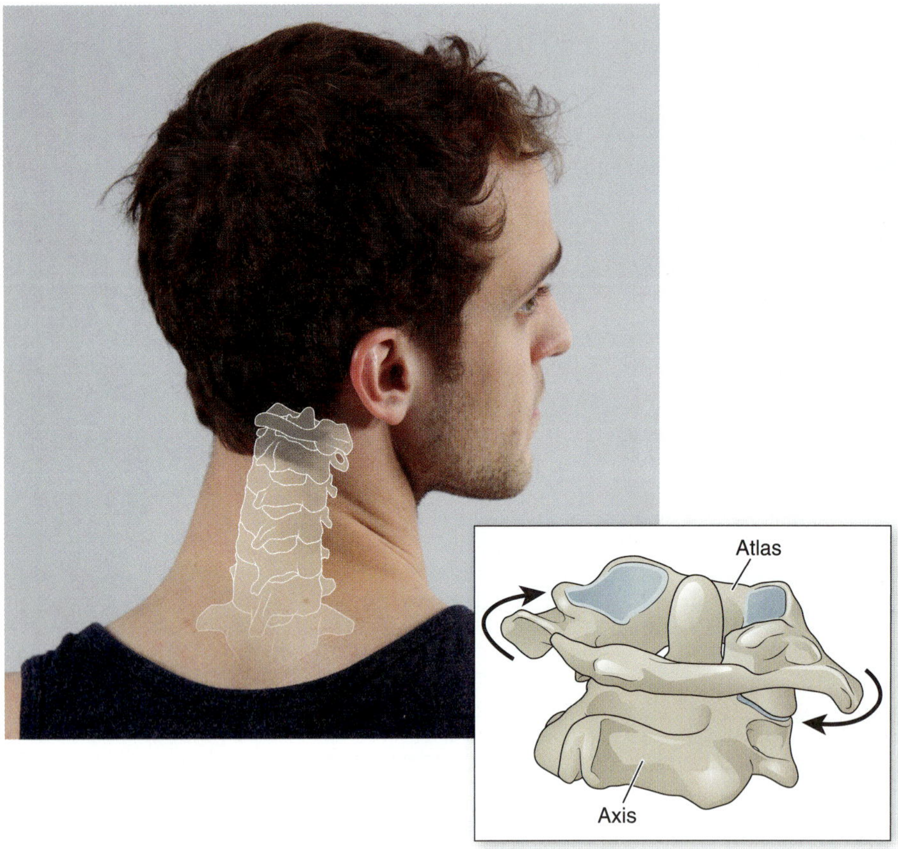

Figure 4–32 Atlantoaxial rotation takes place as motion of the occiput and atlas together on the axis below, typically resulting in 45° of rotation to either side.

is approximately 15° with approximately 3° each of lateral flexion and axial rotation.[32] In flexion, the occipital condyles roll forward and slide backward on the large superior facets of the atlas **(Fig. 4–31A)**. In extension, the occipital condyles roll backward and slide forward **(Fig. 4–31B)**. The total motion available in axial rotation and lateral flexion is extremely limited by the lack of a disc between the atlas and the occiput. Motion is also limited by the increased tension in the facet joint capsules that occurs as the occipital condyles roll up the walls of the atlantal facets contralaterally to the direction of rotation or lateral flexion.[41]

Motions at the atlantoaxial joint include rotation, lateral flexion, flexion, and extension. Approximately 60% of the total rotation of the cervical region occurs at the atlantoaxial joints[42] **(Fig. 4–32)**. The atlas pivots approximately 45° to either side for a total of about 90°.[32] The alar ligaments limit rotation at the atlantoaxial joints. The remaining 40% of total rotation available to the cervical spine is distributed evenly in the lower cervical joints.[41]

The shape of the facet and interbody joints along with the ligaments and facet joint capsules determine the motion at the lower cervical segments. The facet joint capsules are generally lax in the cervical region, contributing to the large amount of motion available here. The height of the discs, with respect to the diameter of the discs and the cervical bodies, also plays an important role in determining the amount of motion available. Generally, the height of the cervical discs is large in comparison with the anteroposterior and transverse diameters. Therefore, a large amount of flexion, extension, and lateral flexion may occur at each segment, especially in young people. Average ROMs in the cervical spine across all age groups are as follows: total flexion/extension: 126° (standard deviation [SD] = 22°), total lateral flexion: 87° (SD = 22°), and total rotation: 144° (SD = 23°), with wide variation among age groups.[43] The disc at C5–C6 is subject to a greater amount of stress than other discs because C5–C6 has the greatest range of flexion/extension and is, therefore, the area where the mechanical strain is greatest.[44]

In general, the range for flexion and extension increases from the C2–C3 mobile segment to the C5–C6 mobile segment and decreases again at the C6–C7 segment.[11] Flexion of these lower cervical segments includes anterior tilt of the superior vertebral body coupled with anterior slide at the interbody joints and upslide at the facet joints **(Fig. 4–33A)** . Extension includes posterior tilt of the cranial vertebral body coupled with posterior slide at the interbody joints and downslide at the facet joints **(Fig. 4–33B)**.

Rotation and lateral flexion are, as noted previously, coupled motions **(Fig. 4–34)**. Lateral flexion is coupled with ipsilateral rotation **(Fig. 4–34A)** and rotation is coupled with ipsilateral lateral flexion **(Fig. 4–34B)**. These motions are also a combination of vertebral tilt and slide to the ipsilateral side at the interbody joints and ipsilateral downward slide and contralateral upslide at the facet joints.[22,32] In short, these motions are coupled because of the orientation of the facet joints. Because of the oblique orientation of the facet joints (crossing cardinal planes), as rotation occurs, the ipsilateral side will experience a downward slide while the contralateral side will experience

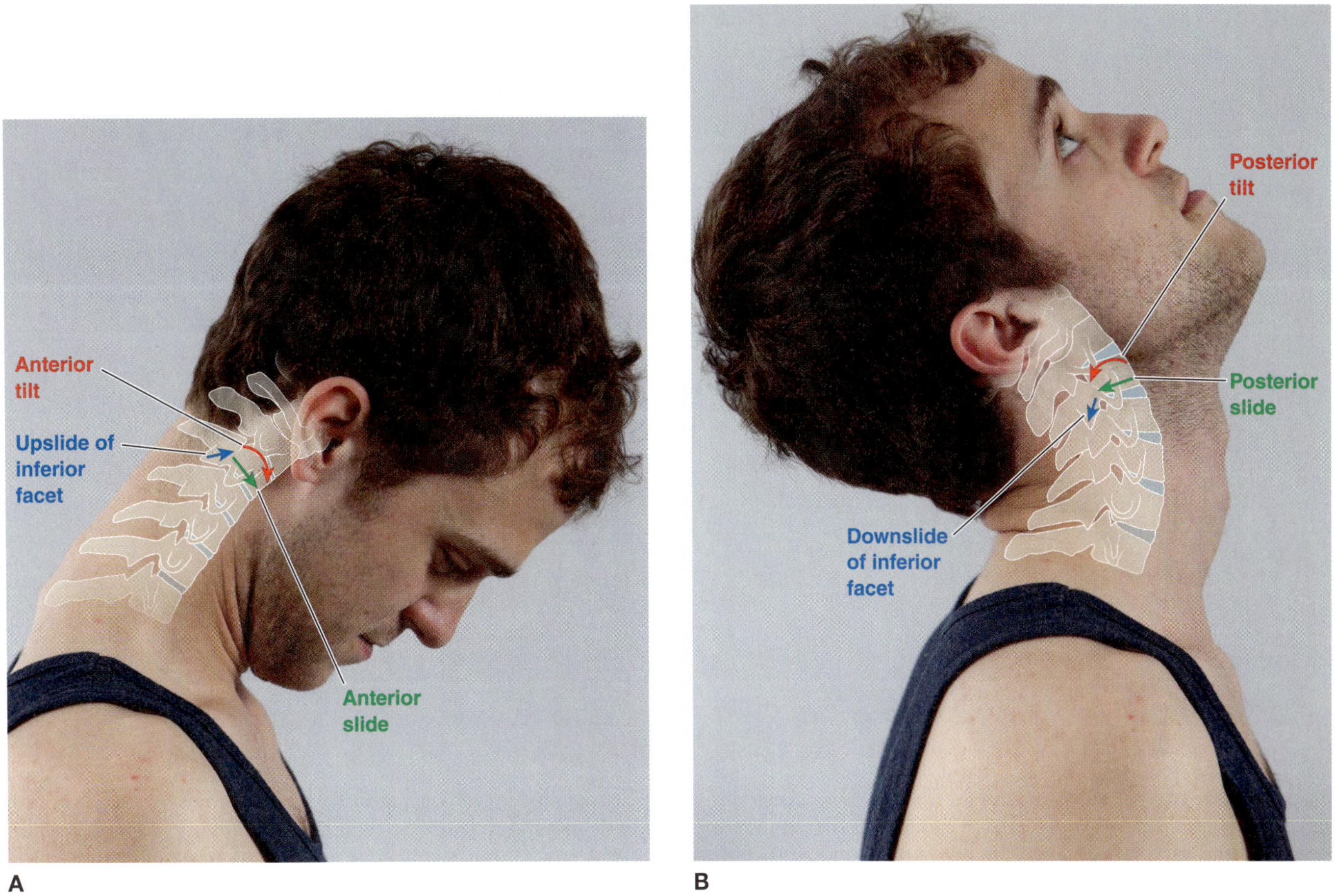

Figure 4–33 Flexion and extension of the lower cervical segments take place as movements of the cephalad vertebra (e.g., C3) on the adjacent vertebra below (e.g., C4). **A.** In flexion, the vertebral body tilts and slides anteriorly while the inferior facet slides upward on the facet below. **B.** In extension, the vertebral body tilts and slides posteriorly while the inferior facet slides downward on the facet below.

an upward slide. Thus, as rotation occurs, lateral flexion also occurs. It is clear that the role of the facet joints is to guide the motion that occurs between adjacent vertebra.

Mercer and Bogduk[6,32] suggested that the notion of lateral flexion and transverse plane rotation are an artificial construct necessary to describe motion in the cardinal planes. In their view, movement should be viewed as sliding that occurs in the plane of the facet joints.

Kinetics

The cervical region is subjected to axial compression, tension, bending, torsion, and shear stresses, as is the remainder of the spinal column; however, there are some regional differences. The cervical region differs from the thoracic and lumbar regions in that it bears less weight and is generally more mobile. The cervical spine is lordotic and therefore experiences anterior shear forces even in the ideal upright position.

No discs are present at either the atlantooccipital or atlantoaxial articulations. Therefore, the weight of the head (compressive load) must be transferred directly through the atlantooccipital joint to the articular facets of the axis. These forces are then transferred through the pedicles and laminae of the axis to the inferior surface of the body and to its two inferior articular processes. Subsequently, the forces are transferred to the adjacent disc below. The laminae of the axis are large, with the structure reflecting the functional adaptation necessary to transmit the substantial compressive loads. The trabeculae show that the laminae of both the axis and C7 are heavily loaded, while the laminae of the intervening vertebrae are not. Loads diffuse into the laminae as they are transferred from superior to inferior articular facets.[45]

The loads imposed on the cervical region vary with the position of the head and body and are minimal in a well-supported reclining body posture. In the cervical region from C3 to C7, compressive forces are transmitted by three parallel columns: a central column formed by the vertebral bodies and discs, and two posterolateral columns composed of the left and right facet joints. The posterolateral columns are often referred to as the *articular pillars*. The compressive forces are transmitted mainly by the bodies and discs, with approximately one-third transmitted by the two posterolateral columns.[31]

Foundational Concepts 4–3
Structure and Function of the Cervical Region

To summarize, the cervical region is unique in both its structure and function. The cervical vertebrae must achieve many combinations of motions to position the primary sensory organs optimally while still providing enough stability to protect the brainstem, spinal cord, and arteries that supply the brain. The sensory organs associated with vision (eyes), equilibrium (vestibular apparatus), and hearing (ears)

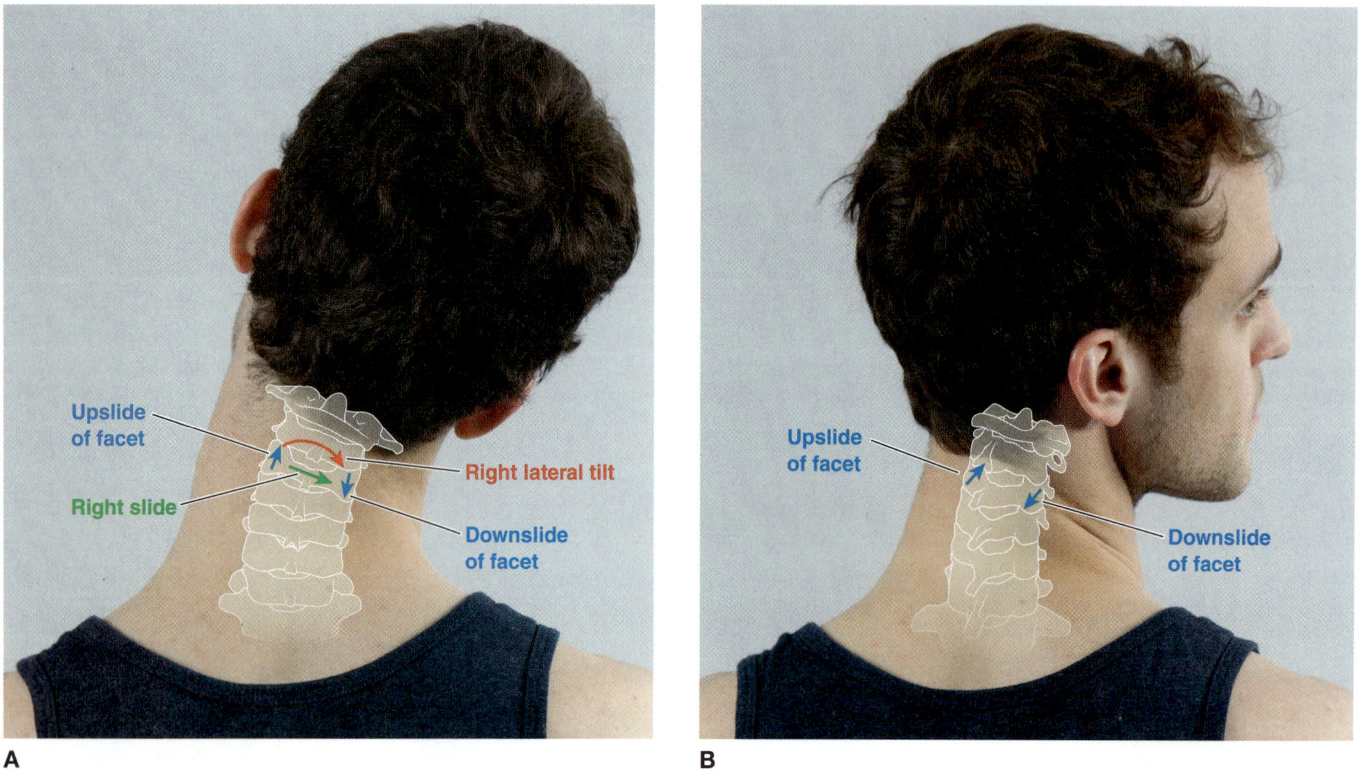

Figure 4–34 Lateral flexion and rotation of the lower cervical segments are coupled movements of the cephalad vertebra (e.g., C3) on the adjacent vertebra below (e.g., C4). **A.** In right lateral flexion, the vertebral body tilts and slides to the right while the right inferior facet slides down and the left inferior facet slides up on the facet below. The sliding of the facets produces slight rotation of the vertebral bodies to the right (ipsilaterally). **B.** In rotation to the right, the right inferior facet slides posteriorly while the left inferior facet slides anteriorly. Some right lateral tilt and slide of the vertebral body are also evident.

are all influenced by movement of the cervical spine. Ideally, these sensory organs will remain optimally oriented despite movement of our bodies. Having two distinct regions of the cervical spine (i.e., upper and lower cervical regions) that can function somewhat independently helps meet these different demands. The craniovertebral segments can move in opposite directions from the lower cervical spine as needed. Two common examples of these distinct and opposite motions within the cervical spine are found with **protraction** and **retraction** of the cervical region. Protraction involves craniovertebral extension combined with lower cervical flexion. Retraction involves craniovertebral flexion combined with lower cervical extension.

Structure of the Thoracic Region

Typical Thoracic Vertebrae

BODY

The features of a typical thoracic vertebra are shown in **Figure 4-35**. The body of a typical thoracic vertebra has equal transverse and anteroposterior diameters, which provides excellent stability. The vertebral bodies are wedge shaped, such that the posterior height is greater than the anterior height **(Fig. 4–35A)**. The most wedge-shaped vertebra, based on the peak anteroposterior height difference, occurs at T7. Anterior wedging of these vertebrae produces the normal kyphotic posture of the thoracic spine. **Demifacets** (or half facets) for articulation with the heads of the ribs are located on the posterolateral corners of the vertebral plateaus.

ARCHES

Pedicles

These generally face directly posteriorly with little to no lateral orientation, creating a smaller vertebral canal than what was observed in the cervical spine **(Fig. 4–35B)**.

Laminae

The laminae (Fig. 4-35B) are short, thick, and broad.

Facet Articular Processes

The superior facets are thin, almost flat, and face mainly posteriorly with a slight superior and lateral orientation (Fig. 4–35A). The inferior facets face primarily anteriorly, with a slight inferior and medial orientation. Consequently, the facets lie nearly in the frontal plane, with their orientation changing around T10 or T11 approximating alignment in the sagittal plane with the superior facets facing posterolaterally and the inferior facets facing anterolaterally.

Transverse Processes

The transverse processes have thickened ends that each support a large oval facet **(costotubercular facets)** for articulation with the tubercles of the ribs (Fig. 4-35A-C).

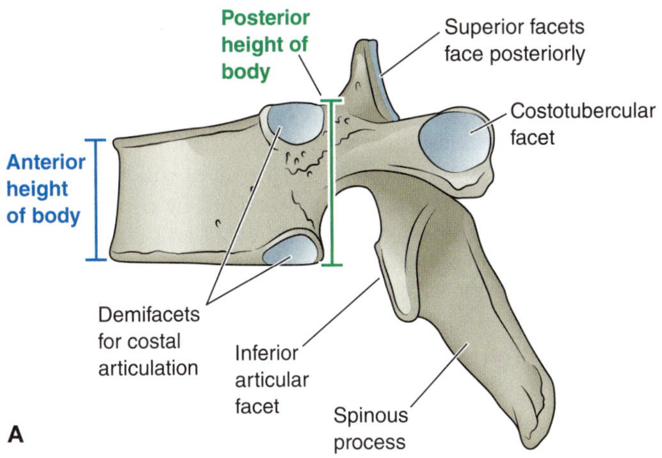

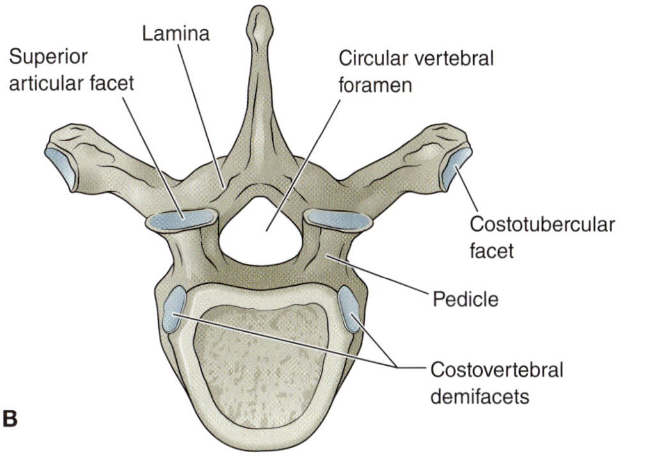

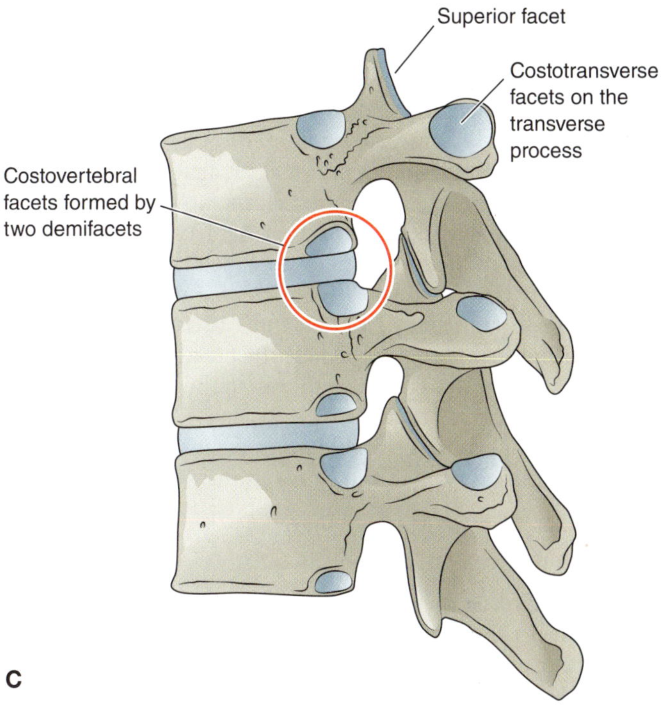

Figure 4–35 Typical thoracic vertebra. **A.** A lateral view of a thoracic vertebra shows the superior and inferior facets of the facet joints, as well as the unique demifacets for articulation with the ribs. The posterior height of the body is greater than the anterior height. **B.** A superior view of a thoracic vertebra shows the small, circular shape of the vertebral foramen, the costotubercular facets on the transverse processes for articulation with the tubercles of the ribs, and the superior costovertebral facets on the vertebral body for articulation with the heads of the ribs, and the pedicles and laminae. **C.** In this lateral view, it can be appreciated that a costovertebral facet is formed by two adjacent demifacets and the intervening disc; the overlapping of spinous processes characteristic of the thoracic region is also evident.

Spinous Processes

The spinous processes slope inferiorly and, from T5 to T8, overlap the spinous process of the vertebra below **(Fig. 4-35C)**. The spinous processes of T11 and T12 are triangular and project horizontally. For most of the thoracic spine, the tip of the spinous process lies at the level of the caudal vertebral body.

Vertebral Foramen

The vertebral foramen is small and circular (Fig. 4-35B).

Intervertebral Discs

There has been little study of the structure of the thoracic intervertebral discs; however, the structure is generally held to be like that of discs in the lumbar region, with differences only in size and shape. Thoracic intervertebral discs are thinner than those in other regions, especially those in the upper thoracic segments. Also, the ratio of disc size to vertebral body size is smallest in the thoracic region, resulting in less mobility and greater stability for this region. The endplates show a gradual increase in transverse and anteroposterior diameters from T1 to T12.

Articulations

INTERBODY JOINTS

The interbody joints of the thoracic spine involve flat vertebral surfaces that allow for translations in each direction to occur. The intervertebral discs allow for tilting of the vertebral bodies; however, relatively small disc size limits the total available motion.

FACET JOINTS

The facet joints are typical plane synovial joints with fibroadipose meniscoids present. The thoracic facet joints lie approximately 20° off the frontal plane, which allows greater ROM into lateral flexion and rotation and less ROM into flexion and extension (see Fig. 4–16B). The facet joint capsules are tighter than those of the cervical and lumbar regions, which also contributes to less available motion.

Ligaments

The ligaments associated with the thoracic region are the same as the typical vertebral ligaments described at the beginning of the chapter, with the exception that the ligamentum flavum and anterior longitudinal ligaments are thicker in the thoracic region than in the cervical region.

Atypical Thoracic Vertebrae

Most of the thoracic vertebrae adhere to the basic structural design of all vertebrae with some minor variations. The first and twelfth thoracic vertebrae are transitional vertebrae possessing characteristics of the cervical and lumbar vertebrae, respectively. The first thoracic vertebra has a typical cervical-shaped body with the transverse diameter of the body nearly twice the anteroposterior diameter. The spinous process of T1 is particularly long and prominent. The 12th thoracic vertebra has thoracic-like superior facet articular facets that face posterolaterally. The inferior facets, however, are more lumbar-like and have convex surfaces that face anterolaterally to articulate with the superior facets of the first lumbar vertebra that are vertical, concave, and oriented posteromedially. Additional differences in T1, T11, and T12 as compared with the other thoracic vertebrae include the presence of full costal facets on the vertebral bodies rather than the demifacets seen on T2-T10. This is because ribs 1, 11, and 12 articulate only with their respective vertebral bodies rather than with both the vertebral body above and below as the other ribs do.

Function of the Thoracic Region

The thoracic region is less flexible and more stable than the cervical region because of the limitations imposed by structural elements such as the rib cage,[46] spinous processes, taut facet joint capsules, a thicker ligamentum flavum, and the dimensions of the discs and the vertebral bodies. Each thoracic vertebra articulates with a set of paired ribs by way of the paired **costovertebral** and the **costotransverse joints** (Fig. 4-35). The vertebral components of the costovertebral joints are the demifacets located on most of the vertebral bodies. The vertebral components of the costotransverse joints are the oval facets on the transverse processes. These joints are discussed in detail in Chapter 5.

Kinematics

Motions across three planes occur in the thoracic region, but the range of flexion and extension is extremely limited in the upper thoracic region (T1–T6) because of the rigidity of the rib cage and the facet orientation in the frontal plane. In the lower part of the thoracic region (T9–T12), the facets lie closer to the sagittal plane, allowing an increasing amount of flexion and extension. In the upper thoracic region, lateral flexion and rotation are more available due to the facet orientation being aligned more with the frontal plane. Given facet orientation, the ROM in lateral flexion is coupled with some axial rotation. The amount of accompanying axial rotation decreases in the lower part of the thoracic region because of the changed orientation of the facets at T10 or T11. The direction of coupled rotation may vary widely among individuals.[11]

Flexion in the thoracic region is limited by tension in the posterior longitudinal ligament, the ligamentum flavum, the interspinous ligaments, and the capsules of the facet joints. Extension of the thoracic region is limited by contact of the spinous processes, laminae, and facets, as well as by tension in the anterior longitudinal ligament and abdominal muscles. Lateral flexion to either side is restricted by impact of the facets on the concavity of the lateral flexion curve and by limitations imposed by the rib cage on both sides of the lateral flexion curve. Similarly, rotation in the thoracic region also is limited by the rib cage.[46] The amount of rotation that is possible depends on the ability of the ribs to undergo distortion and the amount of motion available in the costovertebral and costotransverse joints. As a person ages, the costal cartilages of the anterior rib cage ossify and allow less rib cage distortion. This results in a reduction in the amount of thoracic rotation that is available with aging.

Kinetics

The thoracic region is subjected to increased compression forces in comparison with the cervical region because of the greater amount of body weight that needs to be supported and the region's kyphotic shape. The line of gravity of the superimposed body weight falls anterior to the thoracic spine. This produces a flexion moment on the thoracic spine that is counteracted by the posterior ligaments and the spinal extensors. The greatest flexion moment is at the peak of the kyphotic curvature due to the increased moment arm of the line of gravity.[11]

Foundational Concepts 4–4
Structure and Function of the Thoracic Region

To summarize, the primary goal of the structures of the thorax (thoracic spine and rib cage) is to protect the vital organs and the spinal cord while preserving total trunk ROM. Clinically, diminished segmental mobility of the thoracic spine occurs frequently due to prolonged sitting positions that involve a slouched posture. This may contribute to problems in adjacent spinal regions. Given that the total available motion in the thoracic segments is less than that of the cervical and lumbar regions, loss of even a small amount of thoracic motion may have a functional impact. Retaining functional mobility when there is reduced thoracic mobility may place increased mobility demands on cervical or lumbar segments. This can increase the loads on structures of those regions, contributing to neck or low back pain.

Structure of the Lumbar Region

The first four lumbar vertebrae are similar in structure to each other and share the elements common to all the vertebrae **(Fig. 4-36)**. The fifth lumbar vertebra has structural adaptations for articulation with the sacrum.

Typical Lumbar Vertebrae

BODY

The body of the typical lumbar vertebra is massive, with a transverse diameter that is greater than the anteroposterior diameter and greater than the thickness (height) of the body

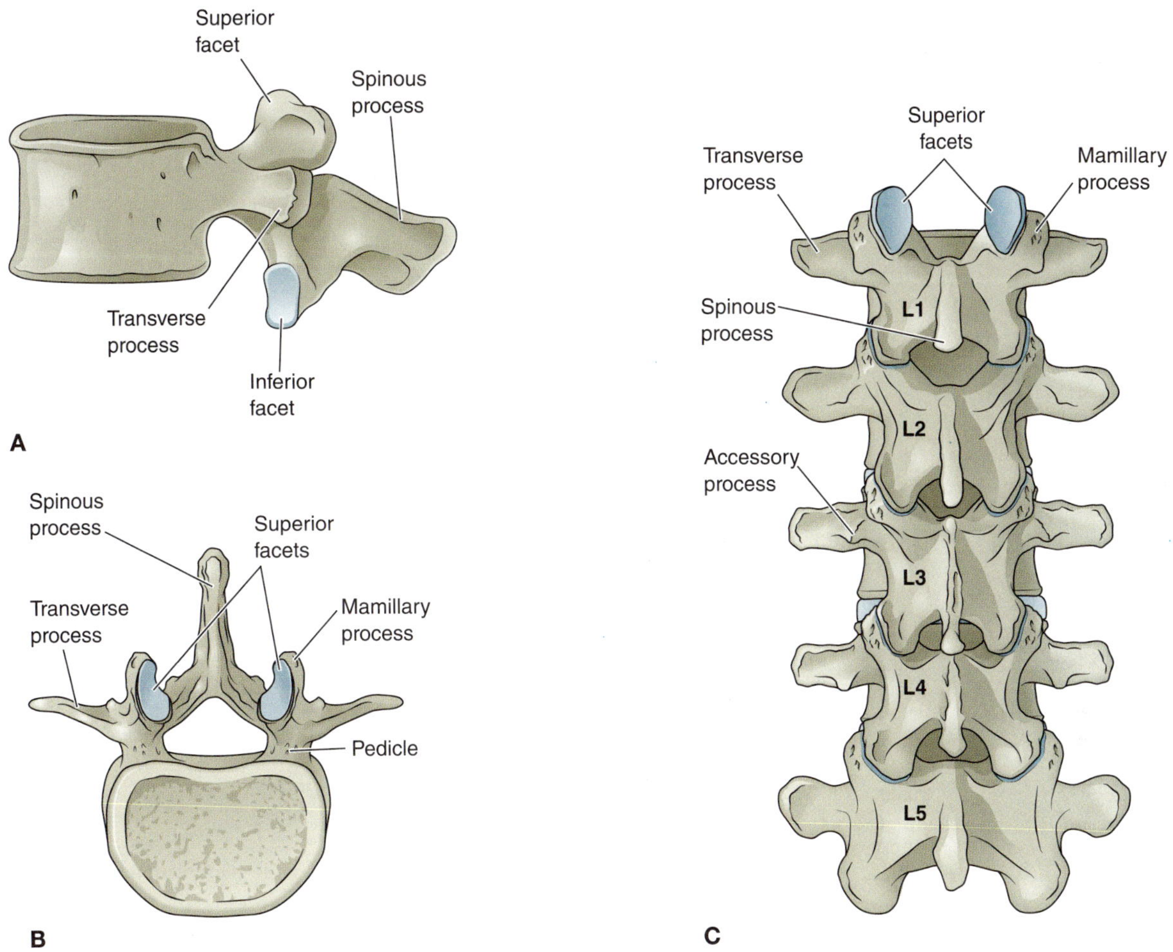

Figure 4–36 Typical lumbar vertebra. **A.** The lateral view of a typical lumbar vertebra shows the large body as well as the sagittal plane orientation of the superior and inferior facet facets. **B.** A superior view shows the triangularly shaped vertebral foramen as well as the transverse and spinous processes. The mamillary processes appear as small, smooth bumps on the posterior edges of each superior facet. **C.** A posterior view of the five lumbar vertebrae.

(Figs. 4–36A and **B)**. The size and shape reflect the need to support great compressive loads caused by body weight, ground reaction forces, and muscle contraction.

ARCHES

Pedicles

The pedicles are short and thick and project posterolaterally (Fig. 4-36B).

Laminae

The laminae posterior to the pedicle are short and broad.

Facet Articular Processes

The superior and inferior facets of lumbar vertebrae vary considerably in shape and orientation among individuals. **Mamillary processes,** unique to the lumbar vertebrae, appear as small bumps on the posterior edge of each superior facet (Fig. 4–36B). The mamillary processes serve as attachment sites for the multifidus and medial intertransverse muscles. The inferior facets are vertical and convex, oriented laterally and slightly anteriorly.

Transverse Process

The transverse processes are long and slender and extend horizontally (Fig. 4–36B).

Spinous Process

The projecting spinous process is broad, thick, and rectangular in shape, and oriented horizontally (Fig. 4–36A).

Vertebral Foramen

The vertebral foramen is triangular and larger than the thoracic vertebral foramen, but smaller than the cervical vertebral foramen (Fig. 4-36B).

Atypical Lumbar Vertebra

The fifth lumbar vertebra **(Fig. 4–37)** is a transitional vertebra and differs from the rest of the lumbar vertebrae in that it has a wedge-shaped body resulting from a greater anterior than posterior height **(Fig. 4–37A)**. The L5 spinous process is smaller than other lumbar spinous processes, with transverse processes that are large and directed superiorly and posteriorly. The inferior facets are larger and wider apart than the other

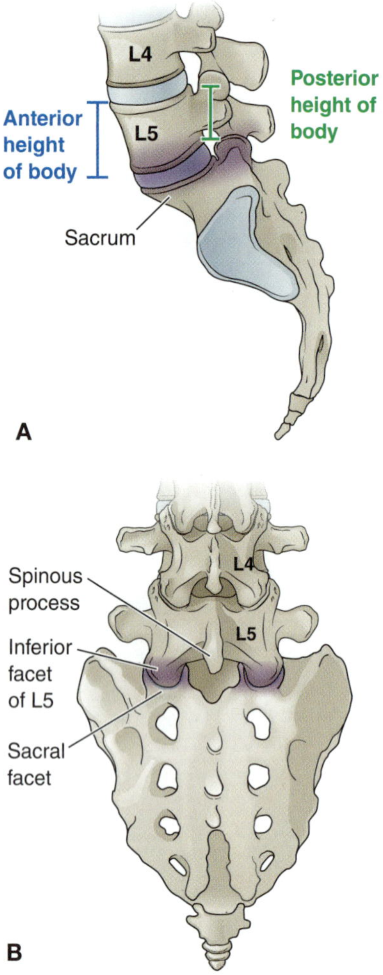

Figure 4–37 The fifth lumbar vertebra is a transitional vertebra. **A.** This lateral view demonstrates that the body of L5 is larger anteriorly than posteriorly, making it more wedge shaped than the other lumbar vertebrae; the spinous process of L5 is shorter than that of the other lumbar vertebrae. **B.** A posterior view of L5 shows that its inferior facets are oriented more anteriorly than other lumbar vertebrae in order to articulate with the posteriorly facing facets of the sacrum.

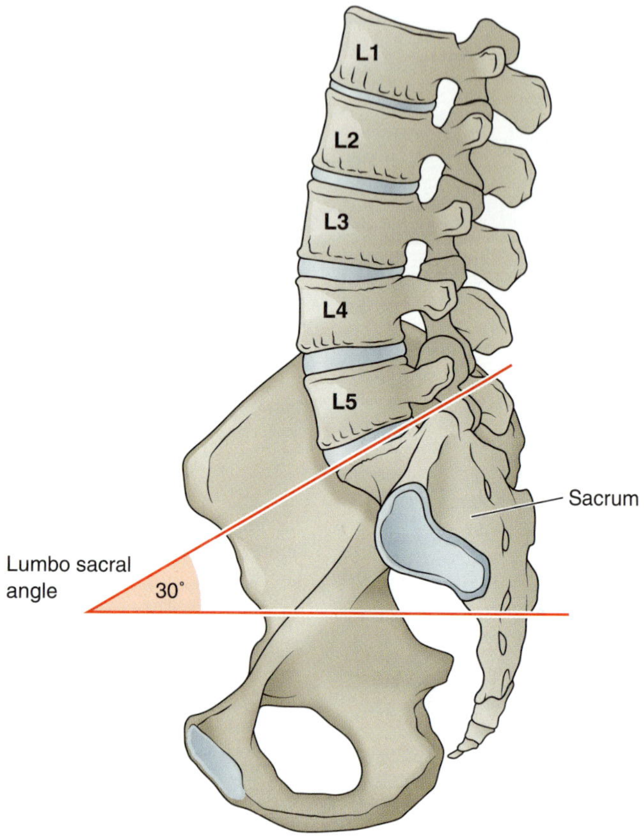

Figure 4–38 The lumbosacral angle is determined by measuring the angle formed by a line drawn parallel to the superior aspect of the sacrum and a horizontal line. The right innominate has been removed to expose the sacrum in this lateral view.

lumbar vertebrae (see Fig. 4–36C), as well as oriented more anteriorly to accommodate the large posteriorly facing sacral facets **(Fig. 4–37B)**.

The **lumbosacral articulation** (see Fig. 4–37B) is formed by the fifth lumbar vertebra and first sacral segment. The interbody articulation is sloped anteriorly and inferiorly, forming an angle with the horizontal plane called the **lumbosacral angle (Fig. 4–38)**. The size of the angle varies with the position of the pelvis and affects the superimposed lumbar curvature. An increase in this angle will result in an increase in lordosis of the lumbar curve and will increase the amount of anterior shear stress at the lumbosacral joint **(Fig. 4–39)**.

Intervertebral Discs

The lumbar discs are the largest in the body. The collagen fibers of the annulus fibrosus are arranged in sheets called **lamellae (Fig. 4–40)**. The lamellae are arranged in concentric rings that surround the nucleus. Collagen fibers in adjacent rings are oriented in opposite directions at 120° to each other.[8] The advantage of the opposing fiber orientations is that the annulus fibrosus can resist tensile forces in all directions. The shape of each disc is not purely elliptical but is concave posteriorly **(Fig. 4–41)**. This provides a greater cross-sectional area of annulus fibrosus posteriorly and thus increases the ability to resist the tension that occurs here with forward bending.

Articulations

INTERBODY JOINTS

The interbody joints of the lumbar region are capable of translations and tilts in all directions.

FACET JOINTS

The facet joints of the lumbar region, as in other regions, are true synovial joints and contain fibroadipose meniscoid structures and joint capsular ligaments. The posterior portion of the facet capsule in this region shows fibrocartilage, suggesting that this portion of the capsule is subject to compressive as well as tensile forces.[47]

In a newborn, the facet joints in the lumbar region lie predominantly in the frontal plane, as well as a lumbar kyphosis. As the child develops and assumes an upright posture, the curve of the lumbar region changes to lordosis and the orientation of the facet joints changes as well. The orientations

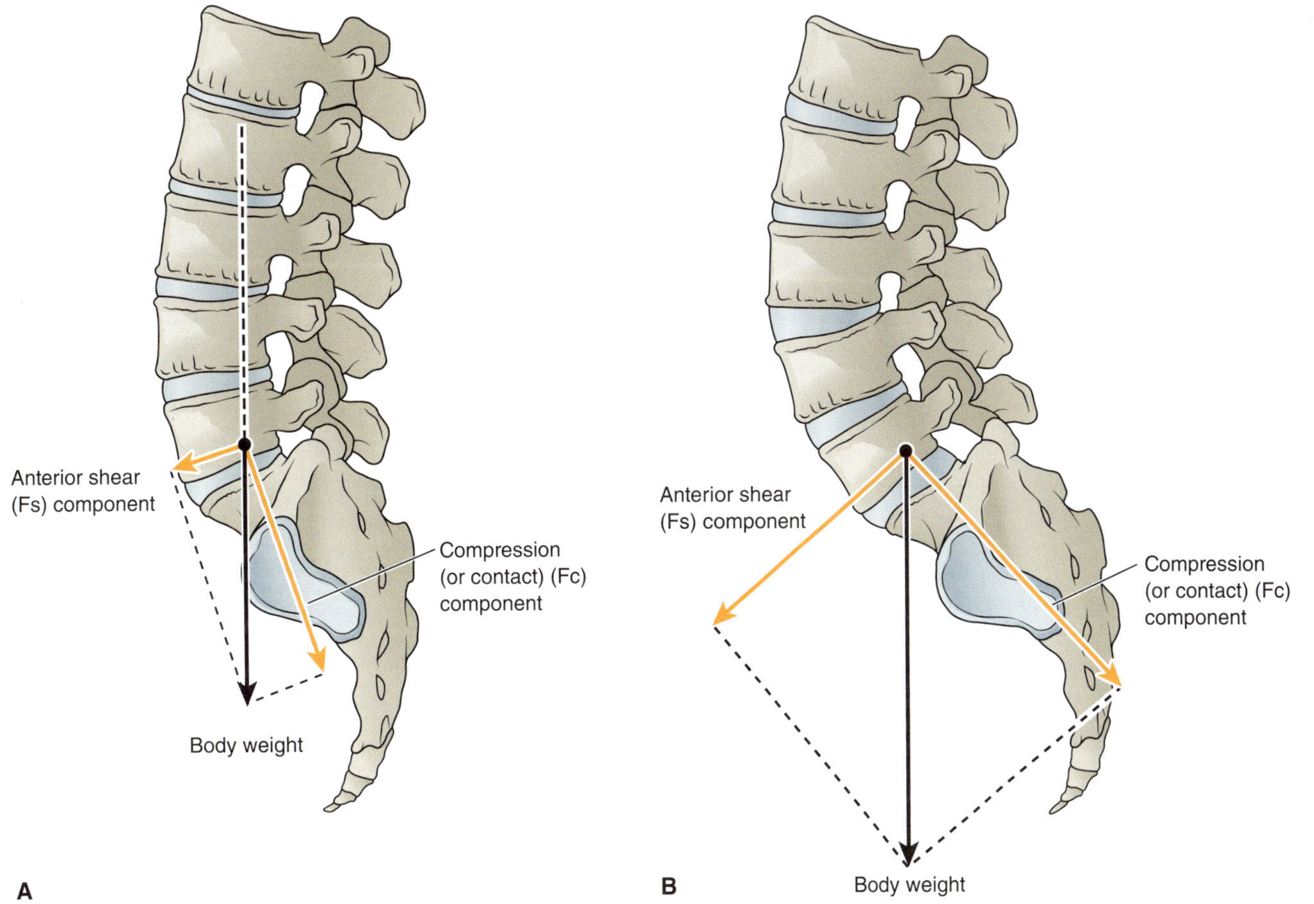

Figure 4–39 Shear stresses at the lumbosacral joint. **A.** Anterior shear typical of a lumbosacral angle of 30°. Superimposed body weight acting on L5 results in subjecting L5 to both a compressive force (Fc) and an anterior shear force (Fs) in relation to the inclined surface of S1. **B.** With an increased lumbosacral angle of 45°, the force of body weight acting on L5 results in a shear force (Fs) that is equal to the compressive force (Fc) in relation to the inclined surface of S1, increasing the tendency for L5 to slide anteriorly on the sacrum.

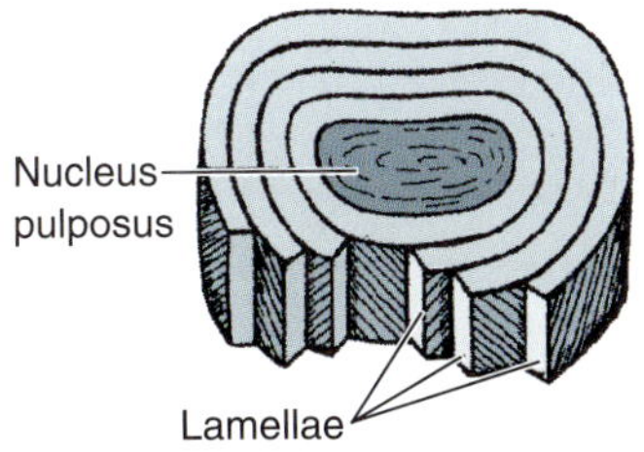

Figure 4–40 Lamellae (layers) in the annulus fibrosus of lumbar intervertebral discs shift fiber orientations from layer to layer.

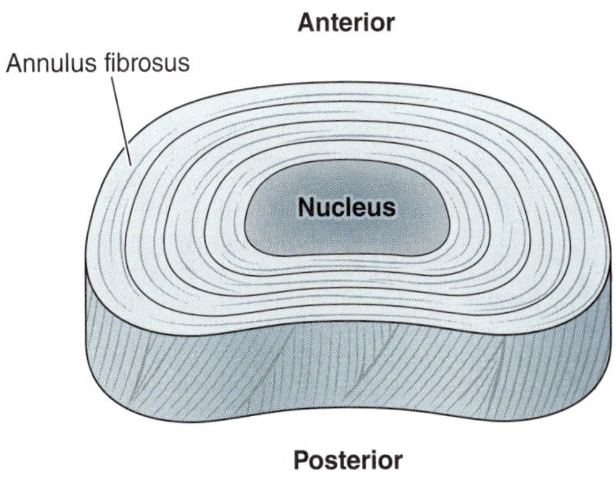

Figure 4–41 Lumbar intervertebral discs are concave posteriorly, providing a greater cross section posteriorly. This means that more annulus fibrosus is available posteriorly to resist the stretch imposed by lumbar flexion.

of the adult lumbar facet joints demonstrate great variability both between individuals and within individuals; however, the majority of the lumbar facet joints have a curved structure that is biplanar in orientation **(Fig. 4–42)**.[2,13] The anterior aspect of each facet joint remains in the frontal plane, whereas the posterior aspect is oriented close to or in the sagittal plane **(Fig. 4–42A)**. The degrees to which this happens vary. The frontal plane orientation of the anterior portion of the facets provides resistance to the anterior shear that is present in the lordotic lumbar region (see Fig. 4-39). The sagittal plane orientation of the posterior portion of the facet is evident in a posterior view of the lumbar spine **(Fig. 4–42B)**, with this orientation allowing a great range of flexion and extension motion and providing resistance to rotation.

Ligaments and Fascia

There are some regional differences in the spinal ligaments of the lumbar region. The anterior longitudinal ligament is well

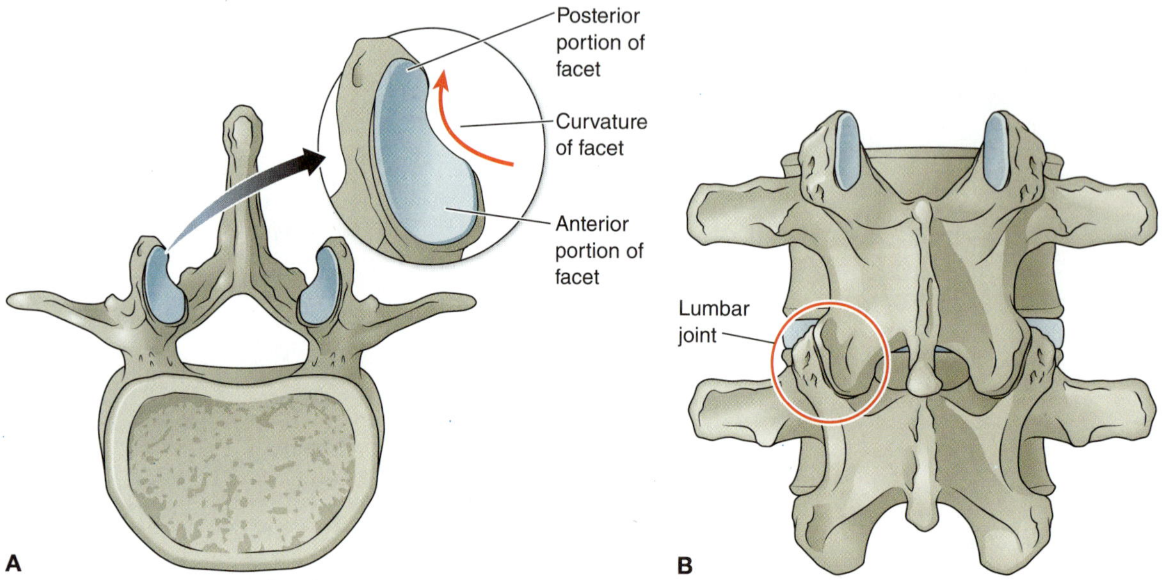

Figure 4–42 **A.** In this superior view, the biplanar curvature of the lumbar facet joints is evident. The anterior portion of the facet is oriented more in the frontal plane, whereas the posterior portion is oriented in the sagittal plan (inset). **B.** In a posterior view of the lumbar facet (circled), the shift of the posterior curvature of the facet into the sagittal plane can be appreciated.

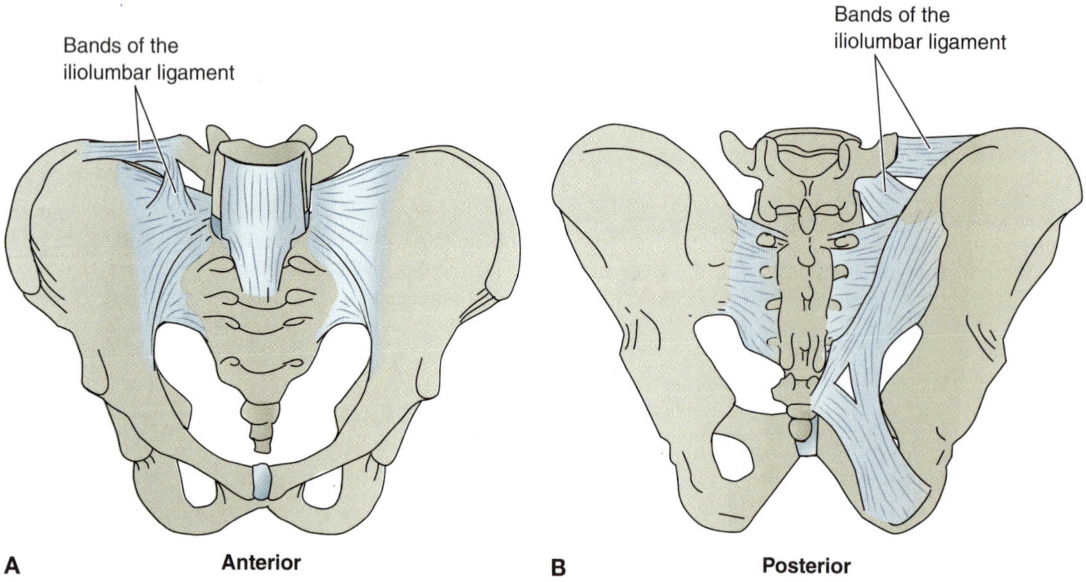

Figure 4–43 The two bands of the bilateral iliolumbar ligaments. **A.** Anterior view. **B.** Posterior view.

developed and strong, but the posterior longitudinal ligament is a thin ribbon in the lumbar region.

The supraspinous ligament is well developed only in the upper lumbar region. The middle fibers of the supraspinous ligament blend with the dorsal layer of the thoracolumbar fascia. The intertransverse ligaments are not true ligaments in the lumbar area, and are replaced by the iliolumbar ligament at L5. The ligamentum flavum is thickened here, with an indistinct interspinous ligament that blends into the ligamentum flavum.[48]

ILIOLUMBAR LIGAMENTS

The **iliolumbar ligaments** **(Fig. 4–43)** consist of two bands that run from the L5 transverse process to the iliac tuberosity with connections to the quadratus lumborum and sacroiliac ligaments.[49] The iliolumbar ligaments are very strong and play a significant role in stabilizing the fifth lumbar vertebra. These ligaments prevent anterior displacement of L5 that might result from anterior shear forces found here (see Fig. 4-39), while resisting flexion, extension, axial rotation, and lateral bending of L5 on S1. The iliolumbar ligaments are maximally loaded at the lumbosacral junction when someone is sitting in a relaxed, slouched posture. If this posture is sustained without activation of the now relaxed spinal extensor muscles, these ligaments are subject to creep and can become a source of low back pain.[50]

THORACOLUMBAR FASCIA

The thoracolumbar fascia consists of posterior, middle, and anterior layers shown in green in **Fig. 4–44**. The posterior layer is large, thick, and fibrous, arising from the spinous processes and supraspinous ligaments of the thoracic, lumbar, and

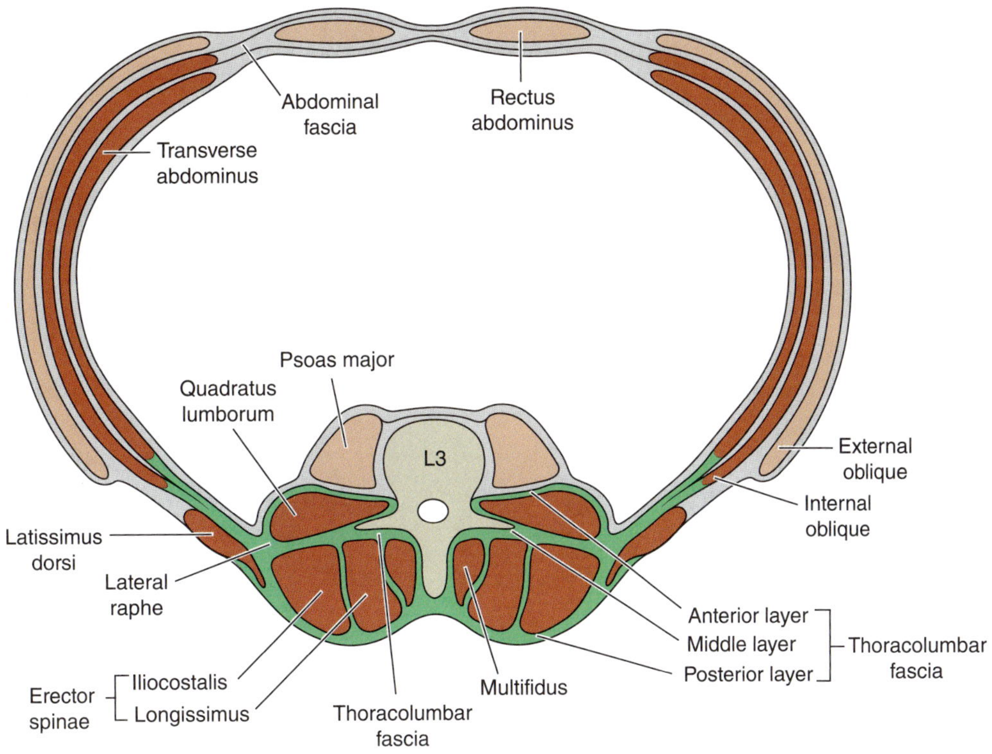

Figure 4–44 A superior view of a cross section to identify the abdominal hoop. The anterior, middle, and posterior layers of the thoracolumbar fascia (in green), along with the abdominal fascia, are the passive parts. The muscles are the active parts that pull on the fascia to tighten the hoop.

sacral spines. The posterior layer gives rise to the proximal attachment of the latissimus dorsi and is continuous with some fibers of the splenius capitis and cervicis.[51] The posterior layer travels caudally to the sacrum and ilium, and blends with the fascia of the gluteus maximus. Deep fibers of the posterior layer are continuous with the sacrotuberous ligament and are connected to the posterior superior iliac spines, iliac crests, and long posterior sacroiliac ligament.[51] The posterior layer travels laterally over the erector spinae muscles and forms the lateral raphe at the lateral aspect of the erector spinae. The internal abdominal oblique and the transversus abdominal muscles arise from the lateral raphe. The posterior layer gives rise to the middle layer as the fascia travels medially along the anterior surface of the erector spinae where it attaches to the transverse processes and intertransverse ligaments of the lumbar spine. The middle and posterior layers surround the lumbar extensor muscle group. The anterior layer of the thoracolumbar fascia is derived from the fascia of the quadratus lumborum muscle, where it joins the middle layer, inserts into the transverse processes of the lumbar spine, and blends with the intertransverse ligaments.[51]

The thoracolumbar fascia, when combined with its indirect connections to the abdominal fascia, form a hoop around the abdomen (as shown in Fig. 4–44) that adds stiffness to the lumbopelvic region.[52] Muscles that attach to the fascia can increase fascial tension when actively contracting, helping to further increase spinal stiffness and stabilize the lumbar spine. For example, contraction of the gluteus maximus and contralateral latissimus dorsi tense the superficial portions of the thoracolumbar fascia and provide a pathway for the mechanical transmission of forces between the pelvis and trunk.[51]

Function of the Lumbar Region

Kinematics

The lumbar region is capable of movement in flexion, extension, lateral flexion, and rotation. The lumbar facets favor flexion and extension because of their predominant sagittal plane orientation (Fig. 4–43B). The amount of flexion varies at each interspace, but the greatest amount of flexion takes place at the lumbosacral (L5–S1) joint. Lateral flexion and rotation are relatively more available in the upper lumbar region and progressively diminish in the lower region.

During flexion of the lumbar spine **Figure 4–45**, the body of one vertebra tilts and slides anteriorly as its inferior facets slide upward on the vertebra immediately below **(Fig. 4–45A)**. During lumbar extension, the body of a vertebra tilts and slides posteriorly as its inferior facets slide downward on the vertebra below **(Fig. 4–45B)**. During lumbar lateral flexion **Figure 4–46**, a vertebral body tilts and slides to the side of the lateral bend on the vertebra below; the inferior facet on the side of the lateral bend slides downwardly on its corresponding facet below while the contralateral inferior facet slides upwardly **(Fig. 4–46A)**. Lumbar rotation, however, has a unique motion in the lumbar region due to the shape of the facet joints. The body of a vertebra tilts and slides to the side of rotation on the vertebra below **(Fig. 4–46B)**; however, the facet

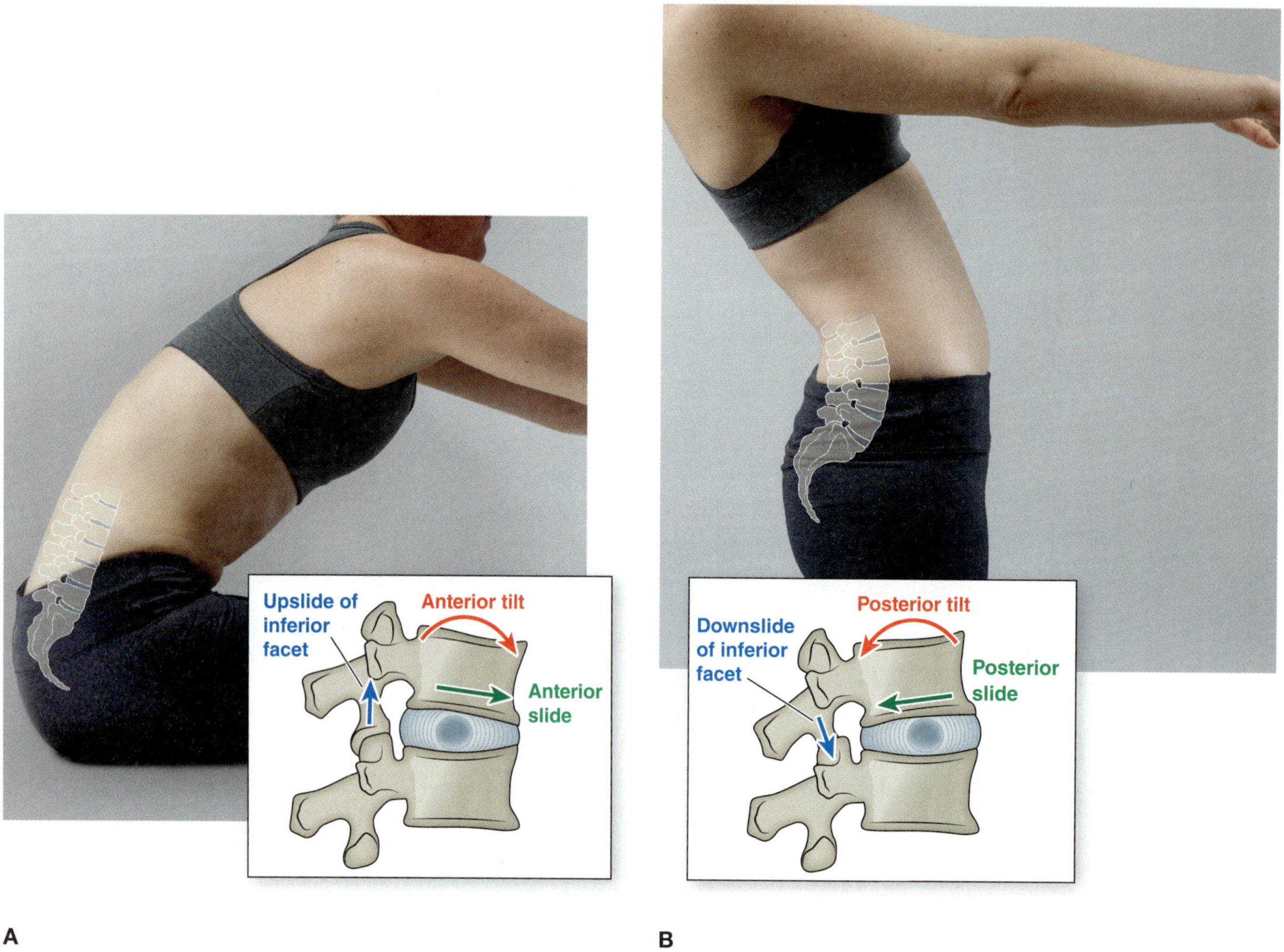

Figure 4–45 Flexion and extension of the lumbar vertebrae take place as movements of a cephalad vertebra on the contiguous vertebra below. **A.** In flexion, the vertebral body tilts and slides anteriorly while the inferior facets slide upwardly on the facets below. **B.** In extension, the vertebral body tilts and slides posteriorly while the inferior facets slide downwardly on the facets of the contiguous vertebra below.

joints of the contiguous vertebrae—given their predominant sagittal plane orientation and consequent limited ability to accept rotation—distract on the side to which the vertebra is rotating, and compress on the opposite side.

The amount of lumbar motion from a neutral lordotic position is reported to be as follows:

- Flexion: 52° (SD = 9°)
- Extension: 19° (SD = 9°)
- Lateral flexion: 30° to each side (SD = 6°)
- Rotation: 32° to each side (+/–12°)[49]

The primary restraints to motions in the lumbar region are as follows: the facet joints and capsules for axial rotation, the anterior longitudinal ligament for extension; the posterior longitudinal ligament, ligamentum flavum, and annular fibers for flexion; and the annular fibers for lateral bending.[53] In the lumbar region, coupled motions usually occur with lateral flexion and axial rotation. The pattern of coupled motion, however, appears to be inconsistent. Legaspi and Edmond performed a review of the literature to determine if a consistent pattern of coupling was demonstrated in published research. Of the 24 articles reviewed, there was little agreement about the specific characteristics of coupled motion in the lumbar spine.[23]

Lumbopelvic Rhythm

Full trunk motion, particularly in forward bending such as trying to touch your toes, is accomplished by a combination of motions at the lumbar spine and the pelvis (producing simultaneous motion at the sacroiliac and hip joints) **(Fig. 4–47)**. The ratio of contribution from different areas is identified as **lumbopelvic rhythm.** Lumbopelvic rhythm was first described by Calliet[54] as a sequential contribution from the lumbar spine first, then from the pelvis. This *sequential* pattern has since been questioned, with the lumbar and pelvic motions more likely *simultaneous*.[53,55]

Kinetics

VERTEBRAL COMPRESSION

One of the primary functions of the lumbar region is to provide support for the weight of the upper part of the body in

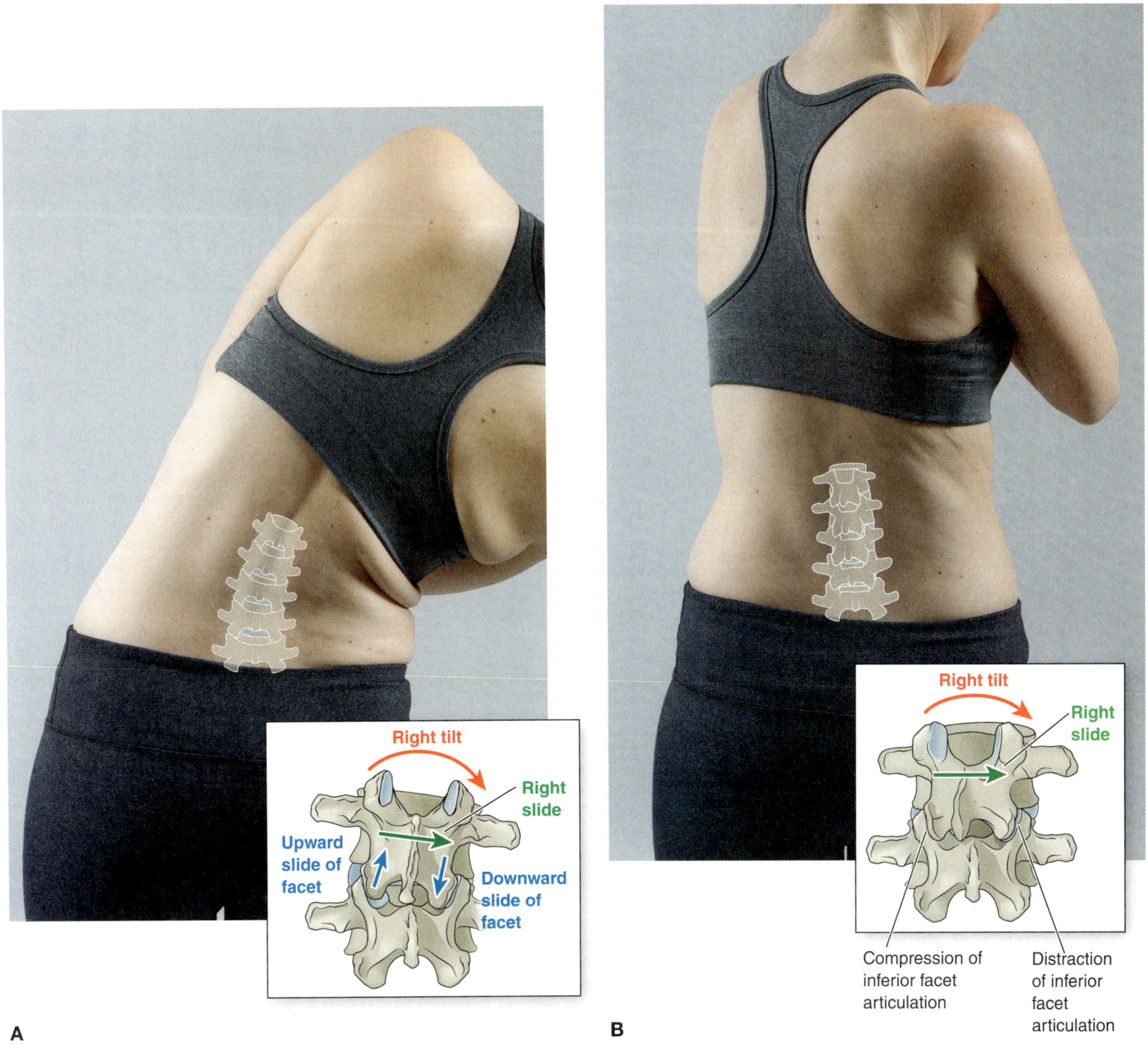

Figure 4–46 Lateral flexion and rotation of the lumbar vertebrae, although limited in range of motion, take place as movements of a cephalad vertebra on the contiguous vertebra below. **A.** In right lateral flexion, the vertebral body (and its associated posterior elements) tilts and slides to the right while the left inferior facet slides upward and the right inferior facet slides downward on the facets below. **B.** In rotation of the lumbar spine to the right, the vertebral body tilts and slides to the right while the right inferior facet joint distracts (opens) and the left inferior facet joint compresses.

static as well as dynamic situations. The increased size of the lumbar vertebral bodies and discs in comparison with their counterparts in the other spinal regions helps the lumbar structures support the cumulative superimposed weight. The lumbar region must also withstand the tremendous compressive loads produced by muscle contractions. The lumbar interbody joints bear approximately 80% of compressive forces while the lumbar facet joints bear approximately 20%. This percentage can change with altered mechanics. For example, with increased lordosis or in the presence of intervertebral disc degeneration, the facet joints will assume more of the compressive load.

Lumbosacral loads (ground reaction forces plus forces generated by erector spinae and rectus abdominis muscle groups) in the erect standing posture are about equal to one's total body weight. However, compressive loads during walking on level ground are nearly twice the body's weight.[56] Changes in the position of the body will change the location of the body's line of gravity and thus change the forces acting on the lumbar spine.

SHEAR

In the upright standing position, the lumbar segments are subjected to anterior shear forces caused by the lordotic position,

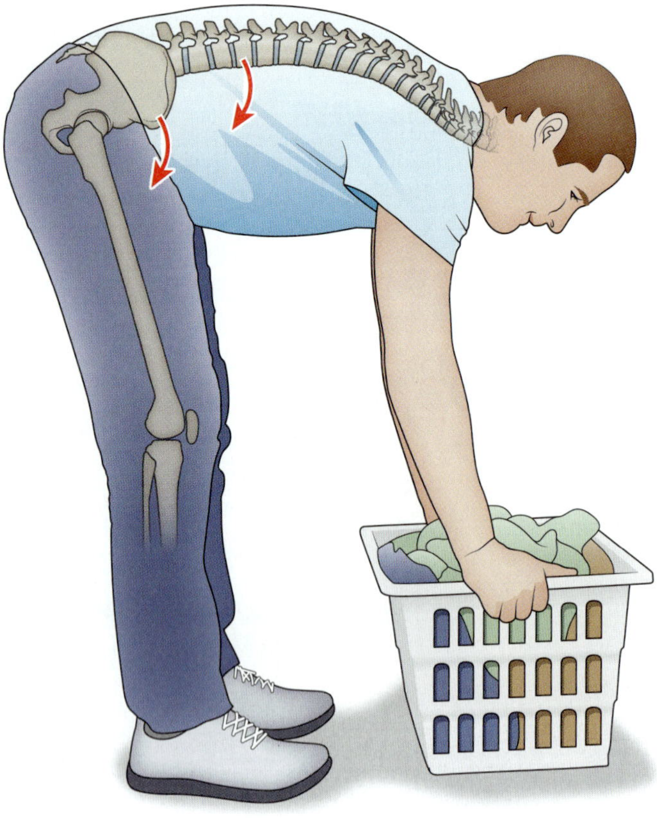

Figure 4–47 Lumbopelvic rhythm. The lumbar spine flexes (lordotic curve eliminated) and the pelvis rotates anteriorly in the sagittal plane to increase the range of forward flexion.

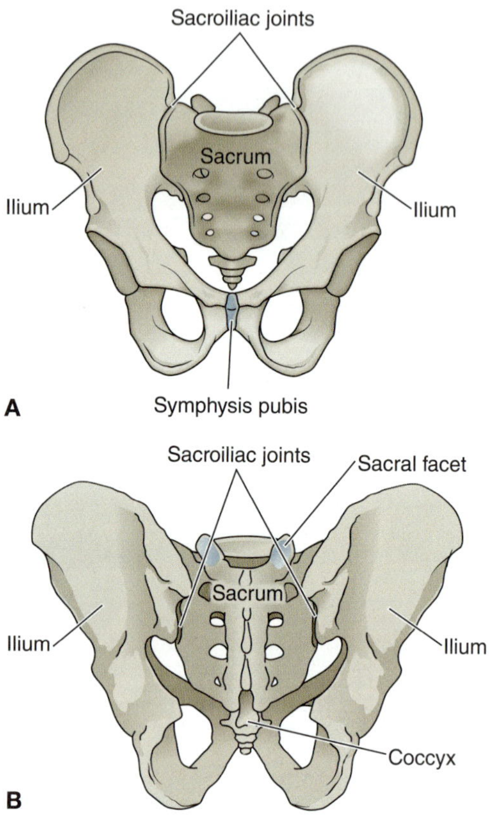

Figure 4–48 The sacroiliac joints consist of the articulations between the first three sacral segments and the two ilia of the pelvis. **A.** Anterior view. **B.** Posterior view.

body weight, and ground reaction forces (see Fig. 4–39). The anterior shear force on the vertebra is resisted by compression of its inferior facets against the superior facets of the vertebra below, as well as by the intervertebral disc, posterior ligaments, iliolumbar ligaments, and deep erector spinae muscles.

Shear loads at the L4–L5 mobile segment were examined in a variety of conditions to determine the load-bearing responses by the interbody/disc and facet joints.[53,57] With lower shear loads, the facet joints bear 65% of the load. With increasing shear loads, the disc plays a more significant role.

Expanded Concepts 4–2
Variations in Facet Joints

Structural resistance to anterior shear forces on the lumbar segments is provided by the facet joints, the facet joint capsules, the fibers of the annulus fibrosus, and at L5-S1, the iliolumbar ligaments. Individual variation in joint structure *may* be a contributing factor to pain in this region. If an individual has facet joints oriented fully in the sagittal plane, there is little to no *bony* restraint to the anterior shear forces. In such an instance, the capsuloligamentous structures will be taxed and eventually may become lengthened and irritated. Even if an individual has facet joints with a more common biplanar orientation, excessive anterior shear forces can cause damage to the stretched capsuloligamentous structures; the facet joints may undergo excessive compression and thus *may* be a source of pain. Fortunately, the body is remarkably adaptive, and the deep erector spinae muscles provide a dynamic restraint to anterior shear that will be discussed later in the chapter.

Foundational Concepts 4–5
Structure and Function of the Lumbar Region

To summarize, the primary goals of the lumbar region are to augment mobility at the hip joints to increase total mobility of the trunk, and to effectively absorb and adjust body weight forces from head, arms, and trunk above and ground reaction forces below in weight-bearing. Flexion and extension are the predominant motions available in the lumbar region, allowing us to reach our hands to the floor and overhead while also adjusting to keep the center of mass of the body over our base of support.

Structure of the Sacral Region

Five sacral vertebrae are fused to form the triangular or wedge-shaped sacrum **(Fig. 4-48A)**. The base (top) of the inverted triangle is the first sacral vertebra with two facets that face posteriorly for articulation with the inferior facets of the fifth lumbar vertebra **(Fig. 4-48B)**. The apex (bottom) of the triangle, formed by the fifth sacral vertebra, articulates with the coccyx.

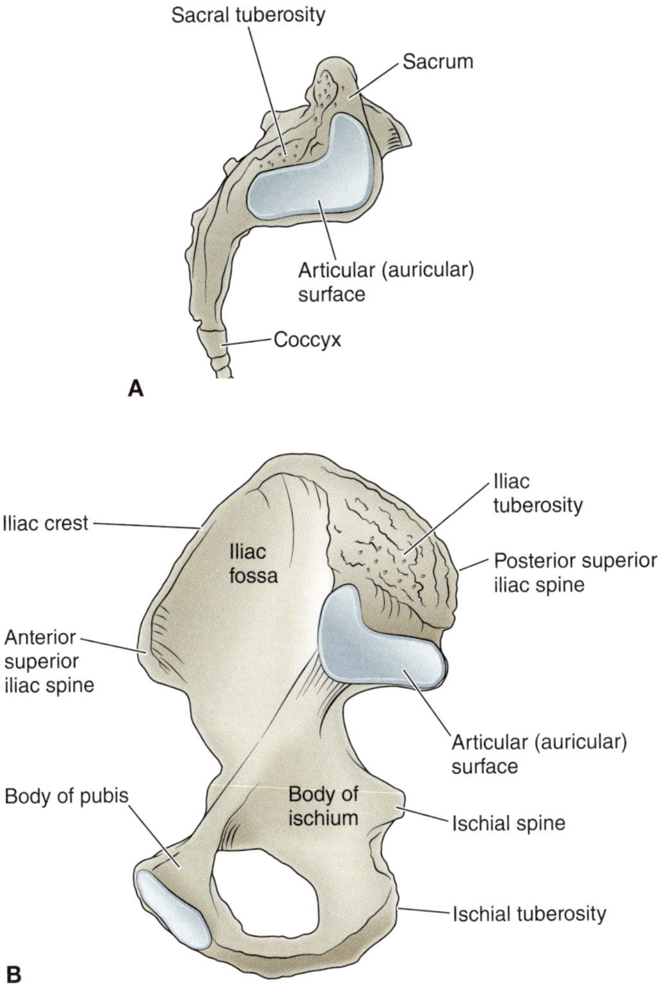

Figure 4–49 Articulating surfaces of the sacroiliac joint. **A.** Lateral view of sacrum. **B.** Medial view of the right ilium.

The two lateral parts of the sacrum, or ala, each bear an auricular (ear-shaped) surface that articulates with the corresponding iliac portion of the innominate bone **(Fig. 4–49A)**. The **innominate bone** (or innominate) refers to one side of the pelvis formed by the consolidation of the ilium, ischium, and pubis **(Fig. 4-49B)**. Each ala of the sacrum also bears the sacral tuberosity that is posterior to the auricular surface and articulates with the iliac tuberosity.

Sacroiliac Articulations

The **sacroiliac joints** are weight-bearing compound joints consisting of an anterior synovial joint between the auricular surfaces of the sacrum and ilium and a posterior syndesmosis between the tuberosities of the same bones (Fig. 4–49). The role of the sacroiliac joints appears to be to regulate the stress on the pelvic ring imparted by movement of the trunk and lower limbs, muscle contractions, the weight of the body, and ground reaction forces. The joints must allow enough movement to help dissipate forces that are ascending from the lower limb and ground and yet be stable enough to transmit the forces from the vertebral column to the lower limbs.[2]

ARTICULATING SURFACES ON THE ILIA

The auricular (ear-shaped) articulating surface on each ilium (Fig. 4–49A) is covered with hyaline cartilage less than 1 mm thick, with the cartilage containing a denser aggregate of collagen fibers than does the hyaline cartilage of the sacrum.[58,59] The articular surface of the ilium is multiplanar and curvy. The fetal and prepubertal articular faces of the ilia are flat and smooth, whereas the postpubertal surfaces develop grooves and depressions the length of the articulating surface that correspond to the grooves on the sacral articulating surfaces.[58] The tuberosities of the ilium are irregular bony surfaces located posterior and superior to the auricular surfaces. The iliac tuberosities articulate with the tuberosities of the sacrum via the sacroiliac interosseous ligaments.

ARTICULATING SURFACES ON THE SACRUM

The auricular (ear-shaped) articulating surfaces on the sacrum are located on the sides of the fused S1 to S3 vertebrae, lateral to their sacral foramina (Fig. 4–49B). These articulating surfaces, like those of the corresponding iliac surfaces, are multiplanar and curvy, showing variations over time from flat and smooth in the young to quite rough past puberty.[58] The articular surfaces are covered with hyaline cartilage that is thicker on the sacral surfaces (5 mm) than on the iliac surfaces. The tuberosities of the sacrum are, like their iliac counterparts, irregular bony surfaces posterior to the auricular surfaces that articulate with the tuberosities of the ilium via the sacroiliac interosseous ligaments.[60]

SACROILIAC LIGAMENTS

The anterior, interosseous, and long posterior sacroiliac ligaments are associated directly with the sacroiliac joints **(Fig. 4–50)**. The sacroiliac ligaments are reinforced by fibrous expansions from the quadratus lumborum, erector spinae, gluteus maximus, gluteus minimus, piriformis, and iliacus muscles, which contribute to the joints' stability. The fascial support is greater posteriorly than anteriorly because more muscles are located posteriorly. The sacroiliac ligaments are some of the strongest ligaments in the body.

The **anterior sacroiliac ligaments** are considered capsular ligaments because of their intimate connections to the anteroinferior margins of the joint capsules. These ligaments cover the anterior aspects of the sacroiliac joints and join the ilia to the sacrum **(Fig. 4–50A)**.

The **long posterior sacroiliac ligaments (Fig. 4–50B)** have superior attachments to the posterior superior iliac spines and adjacent parts of the ilium. Inferiorly, the ligaments are attached to the lateral crest of the third and fourth sacral segments. The medial fibers are connected to the deep lamina of the posterior layer of the thoracolumbar fascia and the aponeurosis of the erector spinae.[61]

The **sacrospinous ligaments** connect the ischial spines to the lateral borders of the sacrum and coccyx; the **sacrotuberous ligaments** connect the ischial tuberosities to the posterior spines at the ilia as well as the lateral sacrum and coccyx (Fig. 4–50B). The sacrospinous ligament forms the inferior

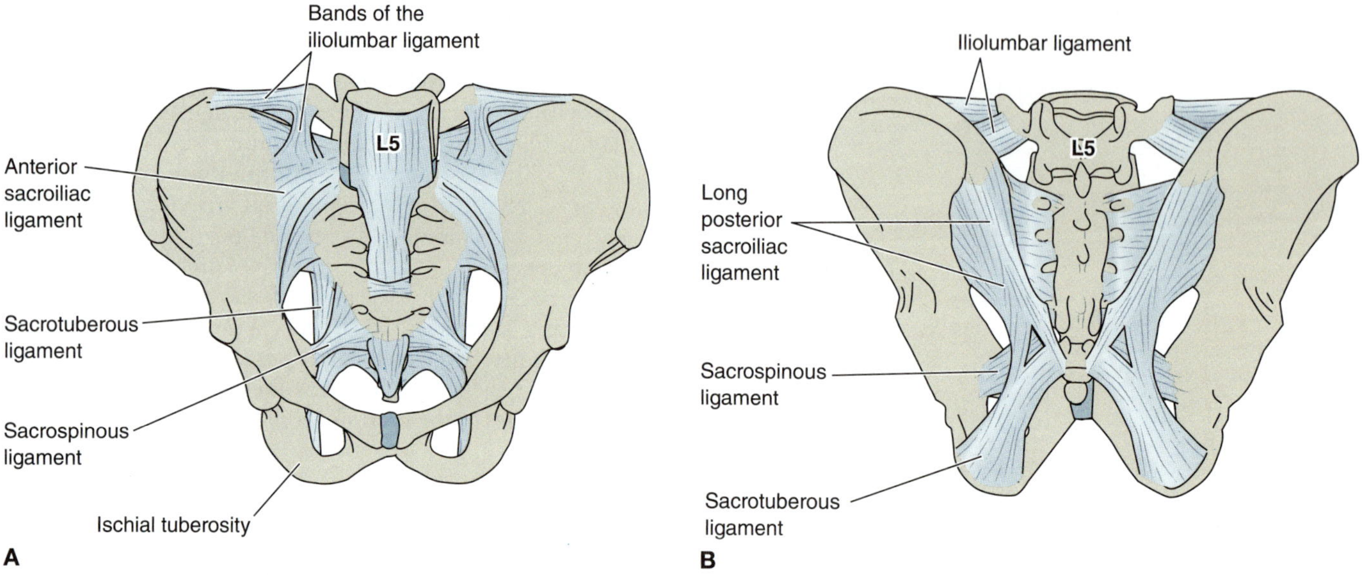

Figure 4–50 The sacroiliac ligaments. **A.** Anterior view. **B.** Posterior view.

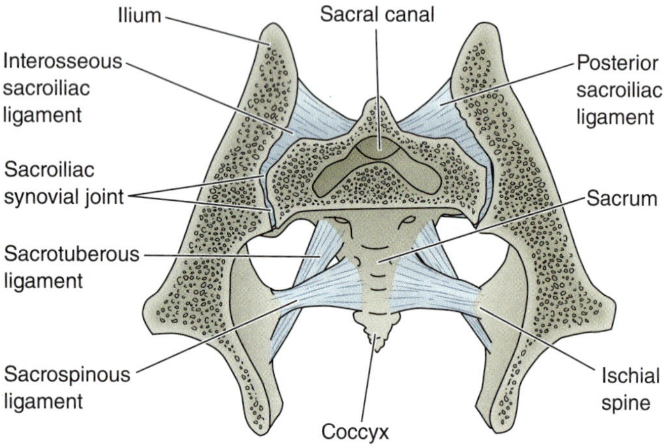

Figure 4–51 The sacroiliac ligaments in a superior view of a transverse section of the upper pelvis.

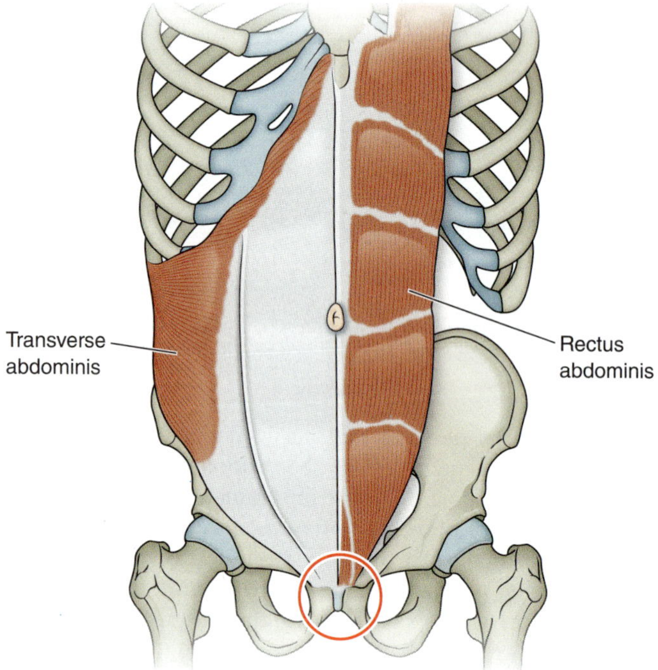

Figure 4–52 The aponeurotic expansions of several muscles cross the anterior aspect of the symphysis pubis, including those of the rectus abdominis and transverse abdominis muscles.

border of the *greater* sciatic notch, while the sacrotuberous ligament forms the inferior border of the *lesser* sciatic notch.

The **interosseous sacroiliac ligaments (Fig. 4–51)** constitute the major bonds between the sacrum and the ilia, and are considered the most important ligaments directly associated with the sacroiliac joints. These ligaments create the posteriorly located syndesmoses (fibrous union) between the tuberosities of the sacrum and ilia.

Symphysis Pubis Articulation

The symphysis pubis is a cartilaginous joint located between the two ends of the pubic bones (see Fig. 4–48). The end of each pubic bone is covered with a layer of articular cartilage, with a fibrocartilaginous disc joining the hyaline cartilage covered ends of the bones to form the joint. The three ligaments that span the symphysis pubis are the **superior pubic ligament,** the **inferior pubic ligament,** and the **posterior pubic ligament.**[1] The superior ligament is a thick and dense fibrous band that attaches to the pubic crests and tubercles and helps support the superior aspect of the joint. The inferior ligament arches from the inferior rami on one side of the joint to the inferior portion of the rami on the other side and thus reinforces the inferior aspect of the joint. The posterior ligament consists of a fibrous membrane that is continuous with the periosteum of the pubic bones.[1] The anterior portion of the joint is reinforced by aponeurotic expansions from several muscles, including the rectus abdominis and transverse abdominis **(Fig. 4–52)**.

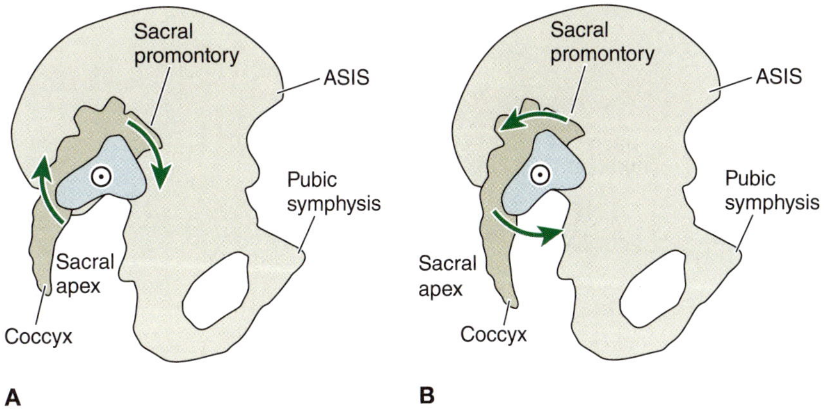

Figure 4–53 **A.** In sacral nutation, the sacral promontory moves anteriorly and inferiorly while the inferior sacrum moves posteriorly and superiorly on the innominates. **B.** With counternutation, the sacral promontory moves posteriorly and superiorly while the sacral apex moves anteriorly on the innominates.

Function of the Sacral Region

Kinematics

The kinematics of the sacroiliac joint are complex and a source of controversy as to the amount and type of motion available, as well as the axes of motion. Three-dimensional analyses of motion using mathematical and computerized modeling have been used for measuring the small amounts of motion at these joints. A recent review of biomechanical studies on sacroiliac joint motion supports what has been argued for more than a decade: The amount of rotation at the sacroiliac joints is only 1° to 3°, and the mean (average) amount of translation is less than 1 mm when testing in a variety of tasks.[60,62,63] This limited motion combined with the complex morphology of the joint brings into question the validity of clinical testing of presumably detectable sacroiliac joint motion. Although small in quantity, this motion is important for attenuating the forces transmitted via the pelvic ring to prevent sacral fracture.

Nutation is the term commonly used to refer to movement of the sacrum whereby the sacral base (S1) rotates or tips anteriorly on the innominates **(Fig. 4–53)**. During the open-chain task of forward bending from a standing position, for example, the sacrum is presumed to nutate on the two innominate bones immediately following maximal lumbar flexion and anterior rotation of the pelvis at the hip joints **(Fig. 4–53A)**. **Counternutation** refers to the opposite movement, in which the sacral base rotates or tips posteriorly on the relatively fixed innominates **(Fig. 4–53B)**. As a reminder, these motions are extremely small, with evidence showing that they cannot be palpated or measured with any clinical examination.

Motions of the sacroiliac joints have also been described as **symmetrical** or **asymmetrical.** Symmetrical motion at the sacroiliac joints occurs when both innominates move simultaneously on the relatively fixed sacrum, although again the motions are small in magnitude. In an **anterior pelvic tilt,** the innominates and sacrum move together in such a way that the anterior superior iliac spines rotate or tip anteriorly at the same time, causing relative flexion of the hips. In a **posterior pelvic tilt,** the two innominates and sacrum move together in such a way that the anterior superior iliac spines rotate or tip posteriorly at the same time, causing relative extension of the hips. During both anterior and posterior pelvic tilts, there is likely a slight movement between the innominate and the sacrum at the sacroiliac joints, but the assumption is that the innominates and sacrum are moving together as a unit.

Asymmetrical sacroiliac motion is movement of the two innominate bones in opposite directions to each other, which induces slight movements at the sacroiliac joints. Because the pelvic ring consists of the sacrum and two innominates in a closed chain, any asymmetrical motion of the innominates at the sacroiliac joints results in motion at the pubic symphysis as well. Asymmetrical motion of the two innominates at the sacroiliac joints is described as **pelvic torsion.** This type of motion is extremely small, but may occur during tasks such as ambulation, in which one hip is in a flexed position while the opposite hip is in an extended position. Although both motions are small in magnitude, the innominate on the side of the flexed hip will be torsioned in a posterior direction while the innominate on the side of the extended hip will be torsioned in an anterior direction.[64] This extremely small amount of motion cannot be palpated and is considered normal. As noted, the convention is to consider that the two innominates and the sacrum are moving together as a unit, albeit with small amounts of motion between each other.

Kinetics

Given the extremely small amount of motion between the innominates and sacrum, it is expected that the sacroiliac joints are very stable. In fact, stability of the sacroiliac joints is extremely important because these joints must support a large portion of the body weight. In normal erect posture, the weight of the head, arms, and trunk is transmitted through the fifth lumbar vertebra and lumbosacral disc to the first sacral segment. The force of the body weight creates a nutation torque on the sacrum; concomitantly, the ground reaction force creates a torque in the direction of posterior tilt of the innominates **(Fig. 4–54)**. The counter torques of nutation of the sacrum and posterior tilt of the innominates are largely offset by the ligamentous tension and fibrous expansions from adjacent muscles that reinforce the joint capsules and blend with the ligaments.

Tension developed in the sacrotuberous, sacrospinous, and anterior sacroiliac ligaments counteract the nutation torques of the sacrum. The interosseous ligaments compress the sacroiliac joint and bind the ilia to the sacrum. The long posterior sacroiliac ligament resists counter nutation of the sacrum but is relaxed in nutation.[61]

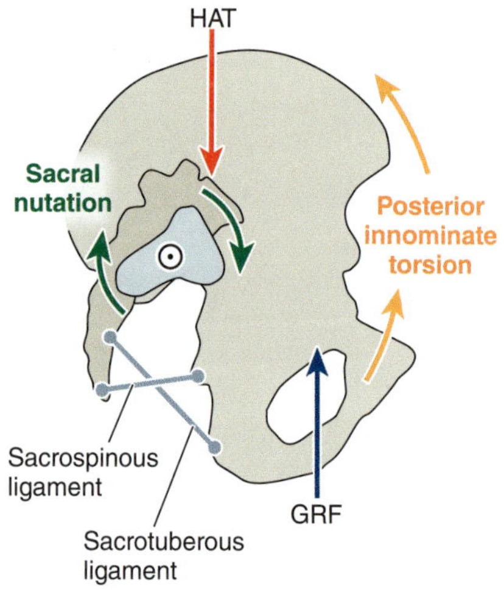

Figure 4–54 In weight-bearing, the weight of the superimposed head, arms, and trunk (HAT) creates a nutation torque of the sacrum, whereas the ground reaction force (GRF) creates a posterior torque on the innominates via the somewhat anteriorly located femoral heads and acetabula. These countertorques are offset by both muscles and ligaments, including the sacrospinous and sacrotuberous ligaments.

The complementary ridges and depressions that develop in the cartilage of the sacral and iliac surfaces also contribute to the stability of the joint. Vertical load-bearing is facilitated by the development of these ridges and depressions, but motion is limited by them.

Foundational Concepts 4–6
Structure and Function of the Pelvic Ring

To summarize, the primary function of the pelvic ring is to transmit and dissipate forces from above and below. From above, the pelvic ring receives forces from the weight of the head, arms, and trunk as well as muscle contraction and any external loads that are being carried. From below, the pelvic ring receives ground reaction forces that vary with activity. Although the sacroiliac joints and the pubic symphysis each have only very small amounts of movement, that movement is critical to allow the transmission and dissipation of all the descending and ascending forces without fracture of the pelvic ring.

Muscles of the Vertebral Column

The Craniocervical/Upper Thoracic Regions

The muscles of the craniocervical region serve two primary roles: to hold the head upright against gravity and to position the head in space to optimally position the sensory organs. The muscles of the cervicothoracic region also position the head and neck in space along with the craniocervical muscles. An additional function of the cervicothoracic muscles is to stabilize the head and neck against the pull of muscles that produce or control movements of the scapula and upper extremity while also pulling on their direct or indirect vertebral attachments. The line of gravity (LoG) of the head in an upright standing position passes anteriorly to the axes of rotation in the craniocervical region, producing a flexion moment at the joints of the region **(Fig. 4–55)**. The posterior capital extensor muscles as shown in Figure 4-55, along with the other cervical extensors and posterior ligamentous structures of this region, oppose this flexion moment. The need to position the head for the special sensory organs often includes rapid, coordinated movements, such as when a loud noise is heard and there is rapid turning of the head to locate the source of the sound.

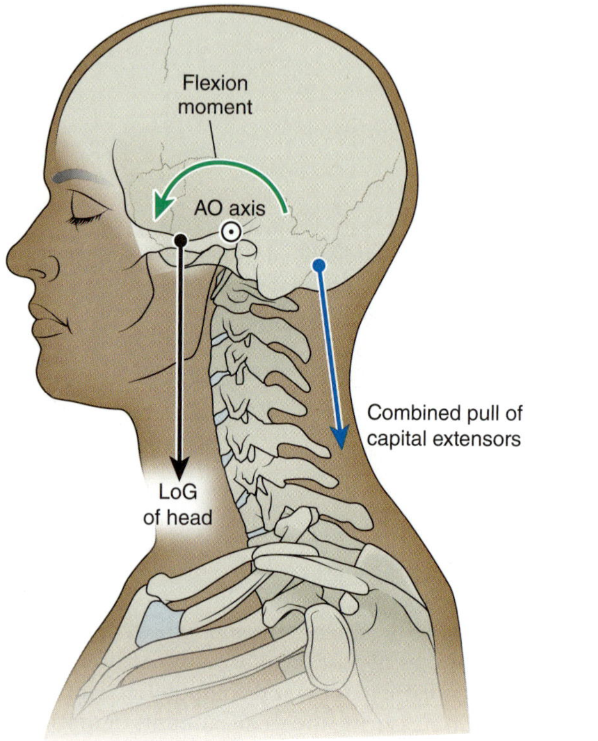

Figure 4–55 The line of gravity (LoG) of the head in the cervical region passes anteriorly to the axes of rotation of the cervical vertebrae, producing a flexion moment. There must be tension in the extensor muscles to produce a countermoment.

The muscular structure and function of the vertebral column are complex, serving the demands for what can be both subtle and large amounts of motion and yet providing sufficient stability to protect the spinal cord and allow for use of the upper extremities.

Posterior Muscles

We will examine the muscles from superficial to deep and begin with the posterior muscles **(Figs. 4–56** and **4–57)**. The **trapezius muscle** is the most superficial of the posterior muscles. It spans from the occiput to the lower thoracic spine and contains a prominent tendinous region over the cervicothoracic junction. The trapezius functions predominantly as a muscle of the shoulder region but can also produce extension of the head and neck. Acting unilaterally, the upper trapezius can produce ipsilateral lateral flexion and contralateral rotation of the head and neck.

The **levator scapula** lies deep to the trapezius. It is attached proximally to the transverse processes of the first four cervical vertebrae and distally to the vertebral border of the scapula between the root of the spine and the superior angle. This muscle has a large cross-sectional area. The levator scapula is an elevator and downward rotator of the scapula when the neck is stabilized but can produce ipsilateral lateral flexion and rotation of the cervical spine if the scapula is stabilized.

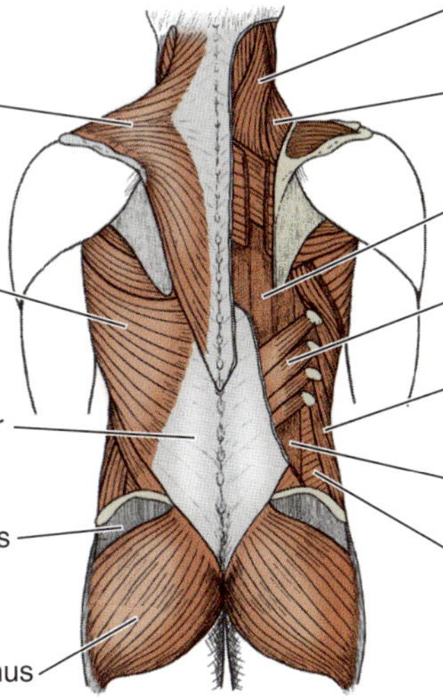

Figure 4–56 Posterior back muscles. The superficial muscles have been removed on the right side to show the erector spinae. The anterior layer of the thoracolumbar fascia is intact on the left side of the back.

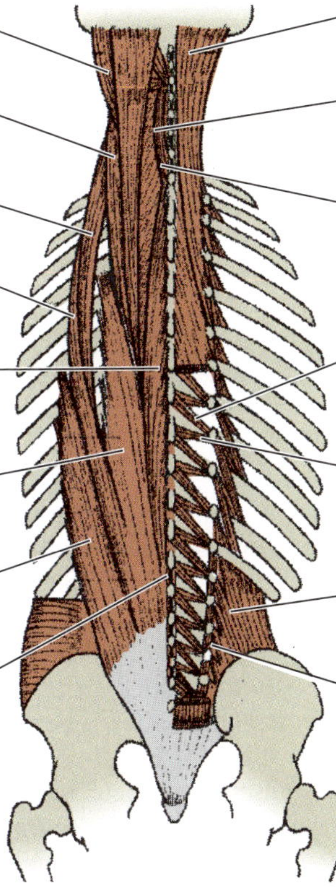

Figure 4–57 Erector spinae and deep back muscles. The erector spinae muscles have been removed from the right side of the neck to show the deeper muscles.

The cervical spine is subjected to constant anterior shear forces caused by gravity and the inclination of vertebral bodies produced by lordotic position of the spine in this region. The levator scapulae help resist these forces by producing a counteracting posterior shear force **(Fig. 4–58)**. An increase in the cervical lordosis, or a greater flexion moment as is often seen with an excessive forward head posture, will further increase the anterior shear forces on the cervical vertebrae and may cause excessive activity of the levator scapulae in resisting these more extreme anterior shear forces.

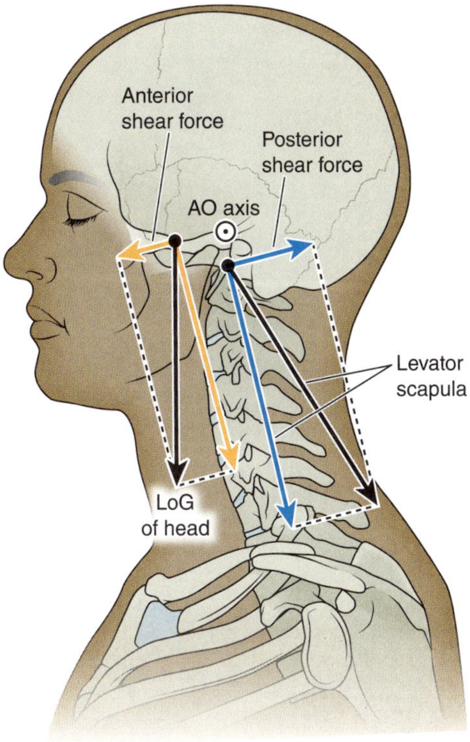

Figure 4–58 The head and cervical spine are subjected to anterior shear forces because of the lordotic curvature as well as the anteriorly located line of gravity (LoG) of the head. The levator scapulae help resist the anterior shear forces by producing posterior shear.

Patient Application 4–2

Keysha is a 23-year-old graduate student enrolled in a Doctor of Physical Therapy program. She spends approximately 15 hours per week sitting in lectures and sits to study for many additional hours. Keysha describes her seated position as slouched with a forward head (cervical protraction), thoracic flexion, lumbar flexion, and posterior pelvic tilt. She also reports that she is frequently keyboarding on her laptop both during and outside of class. Since midsemester, she has had right-sided neck pain over the insertion of the levator scapula that is now interfering with her ability to concentrate in class and type notes.

Overactivity of the levator scapulae in the presence of a forward head posture *may* be the reason that Keysha has pain and tenderness to palpation in the levator scapulae. In fact, the muscle is likely to be strained. Keysha states that she keeps trying to stretch that muscle, but the pain is only worsening. Stretching the levator scapula in the presence of forward head posture may be worsening the situation and causing further irritation because it will decrease the muscle's ability to control the anterior shear forces produced from spending so much time in this position. Reduction or elimination of the excessive anterior shear forces is necessary for adequate treatment by changing Keysha's seated position into a more retracted cervical position. In addition, the levator scapulae may need strength and endurance training.

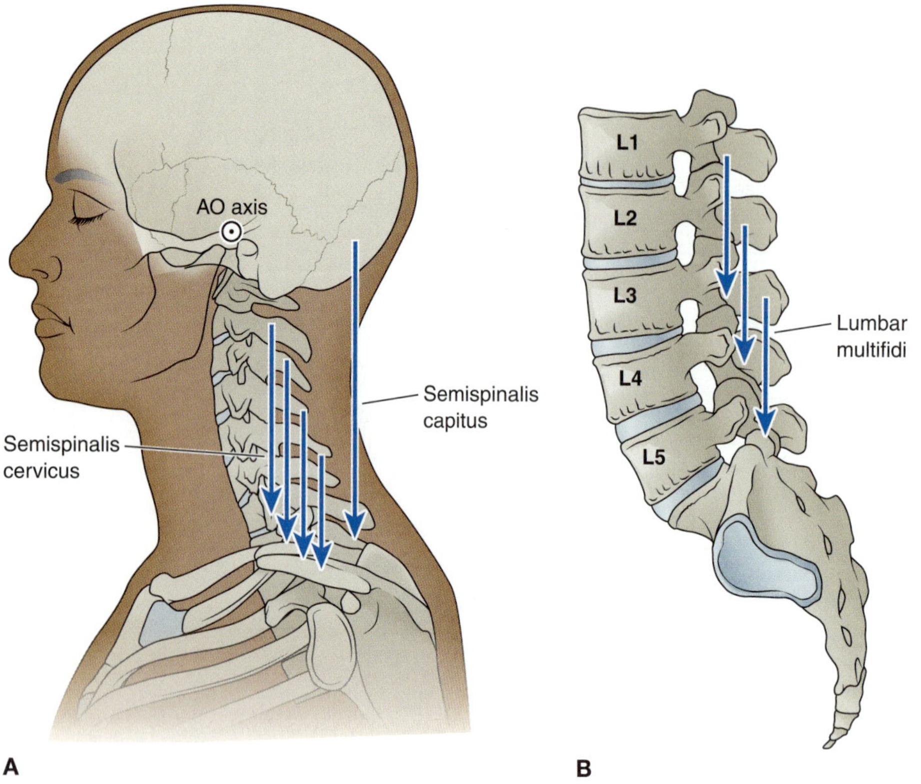

Figure 4–59 **A.** The semispinalis capitis and cervicis have optimal lines of pull to produce capital and cervical extension, respectively, which can increase the cervical lordosis. **B.** The lumbar multifidi also have a line of pull that increases lumbar extension and the lumbar lordosis. *(B from Porter JA, DeRosa C: Mechanical Neck Pain. Philadelphia, PA, Saunders/Elsevier, 1995, with permission.)*

The **splenius capitis** and **splenius cervicis muscles** lie deeper than the levator scapulae (see Fig. 4-56). The splenius muscles are large, flat muscles with proximal attachments on the superior nuchal line, mastoid processes, and transverse processes of the upper first two or three cervical vertebrae and distal attachments on the spinous processes of the seventh cervical and first three to six thoracic vertebrae. These muscles serve as prime movers of the head and neck due to their large cross-sectional area and large moment arm. These muscles produce extension of the head and neck when working bilaterally and rotation to the ipsilateral side when working unilaterally. These muscles show little electromyographic activity in normal, quiet stance.

The **semispinalis capitis** and **semispinalis cervicis muscles** are deeper than the splenius group (see Fig. 4–57). These muscles have an optimal line of pull and a large moment arm for producing extension of the head and neck. The muscles run from the occiput to the cervical spinous processes (semispinalis capitis) and from the thoracic transverse processes to the articular processes of the lower cervical spine (semispinalis cervicis). These muscles together form the cord-like bundle of muscles that can be palpated lateral to the cervical spinous processes. Their function is often likened to that of the multifidi in the lumbar region **(Fig. 4–59)**. Like the lumbar multifidi **(Fig. 4–59B)**, the semispinalis capitis and cervicis have an optimal alignment and moment arm for increasing the lordosis of the cervical spine **(Fig. 4–59A)**. It is important to note that the greater occipital nerve pierces the semispinalis capitis muscle on its way to innervate the skull. This can be a site of nerve irritation and entrapment when the semispinalis capitis is overactive or shortened, as in a forward head posture with craniocervical hyperextension; occipital region headaches can result.

The **longissimus capitis** and **longissimus cervicis** are deeper than and lateral to the semispinalis group (see Fig. 4–57). Their deep position places them close to the axis of rotation for flexion and extension, rendering them less effective as extensors because of the small moment arm, but effective compressors (stabilizers) of the cervical segments. The lateral position allows them to produce ipsilateral lateral flexion when working unilaterally. The cervical stabilization effect of the longissimus capitis and cervicis are greatest when the muscles work bilaterally.

The suboccipital extensor muscles are the deepest posterior muscles and consist of the **rectus capitis posterior major** and **minor**, and the **obliquus capitis superior** and **inferior**. These muscles run only between the occiput and C2, allowing independent movement of the craniovertebral region. Together, they produce cranial (occipital) extension. Working unilaterally, they produce ipsilateral rotation and lateral flexion of the occiput or atlas. They also serve a proprioceptive role to fine-tune the craniocervical position. The suboccipital extensor muscles have been found to have density of muscle spindles that are 15 times greater than the notably large density of the first lumbrical.[65] These muscles therefore play an important somatosensory role in the cervical spine and are involved with integrated functions of the oculomotor and vestibular systems, particularly for high-demand tasks such as head/eye coordination.

Lateral Muscles

The scalene muscles are located on the lateral aspect of the cervical spine **(Fig. 4–60)** and serve as frontal-plane stabilizers when acting as a group with the posteriorly located longissimus muscles. The **anterior scalene muscles** run

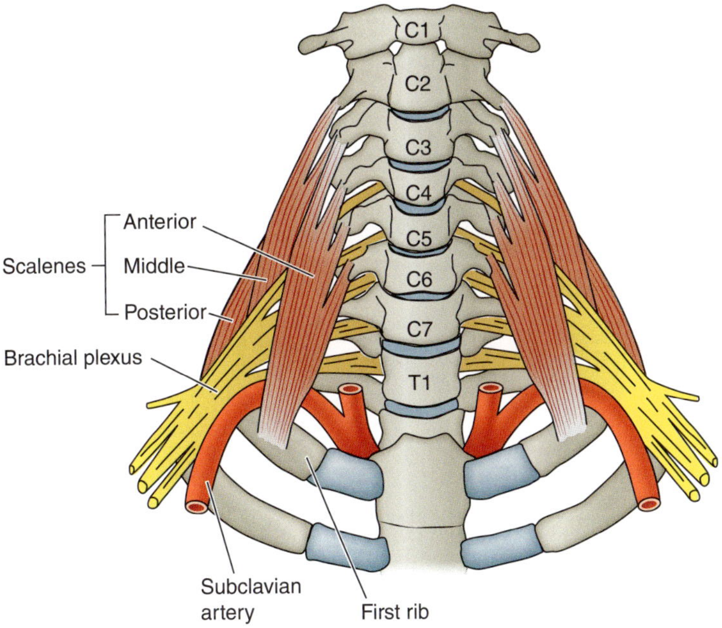

Figure 4–60 The anterior, middle, and posterior scalene. The brachial plexus and subclavian artery and vein pass between the anterior and middle scalene muscles.

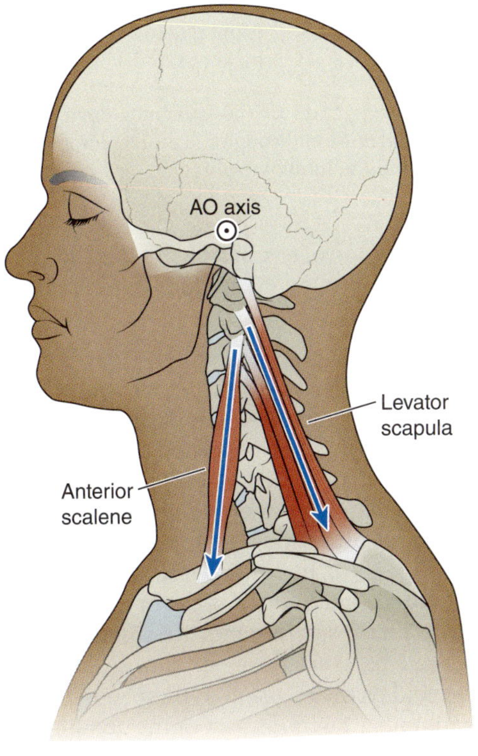

Figure 4–61 In the sagittal plane, the anterior scalene muscles work in synergy with the levator scapulae to provide balanced stabilization of the cervical spine.

from the first rib to the anterior tubercles of the transverse processes of C3 to C6. The anterior scalenes work synergistically with the levator scapulae to provide cervical stabilization **(Fig. 4–61)**. When working bilaterally, the anterior scalene will flex the cervical spine and produce an anterior shear. Unilaterally, the anterior scalene muscles will produce ipsilateral lateral flexion and rotation to the opposite side. The **middle scalene muscles** run from the first rib to the posterior tubercles of the transverse processes of C3 to C7 (see Fig. 4–60). The middle scalene muscles are placed more laterally than are the anterior scalene muscles, with lines of pull that make them excellent frontal-plane stabilizers. The **posterior scalene muscles** run from the second rib to the posterior tubercles of the transverse processes of C3 to C7 (see Fig. 4–60). The posterior scalene muscles predominantly flex the neck laterally. The scalene muscles also have a role in breathing that will be discussed in Chapter 5. The anterior and middle scalene muscles form a triangle through which the brachial plexus and the subclavian artery and vein pass (see Fig. 4–60). This can be a site for compression of the neurovascular structures by the anterior scalene muscle that can produce pain, numbness, and tingling in the arm.

The **sternocleidomastoid muscle** runs from the manubrium and medial clavicle to the mastoid process. The angle of pull of the muscle is posterior, medial, and superior. It is unique in that it lies *anterior* to the axis of rotation in the lower cervical spine but *posterior* to the atlantooccipital axis. Therefore, a bilateral contraction of the sternocleidomastoid muscles produces simultaneous flexion of the lower cervical spine and extension of the head on the neck (upper cervical spine). Acting unilaterally, the sternocleidomastoid muscle will produce ipsilateral lateral flexion and contralateral rotation of both the head and neck.

Anterior Muscles

The **longus capitis** runs from the anterior tubercles of the cervical transverse processes to the occiput. The **longus colli** runs from the thoracic vertebral bodies to the anterior tubercles of the cervical transverse processes and cranially from the anterior tubercles of the transverse processes to the atlas. These muscles lie close to the vertebral bodies and, therefore, are relatively close to the axis of rotation. Although they do have a sufficient moment arm to produce flexion, the predominant component of muscle pull produces cervical compression. The longus capitis and longus colli work synergistically with the trapezius to stabilize the head and neck so that the trapezius can act effectively on its distal attachment to produce upward rotation of the scapula[33] **(Fig. 4–62)**. Given that muscles always pull on both ends during a contraction, the trapezius would extend the lighter head and neck rather than upwardly rotate the heavier scapulohumeral complex via its attachment to the clavicle if it were not for the counterforce on the neck of the longus capitis and colli. The longus colli has a high density of muscle spindles that serve as sensory input and highlight their role in fine-tuning segmental control of the cervical region.[66]

The small **rectus capitis anterior** and **rectus capitis lateralis** run between the occiput and the atlas (C2) and are flexors of the head. Like the suboccipital extensor muscles, the small cross-sectional area and moment arms for these paired muscles likely serve a greater proprioceptive function rather than acting as prime movers of the head.

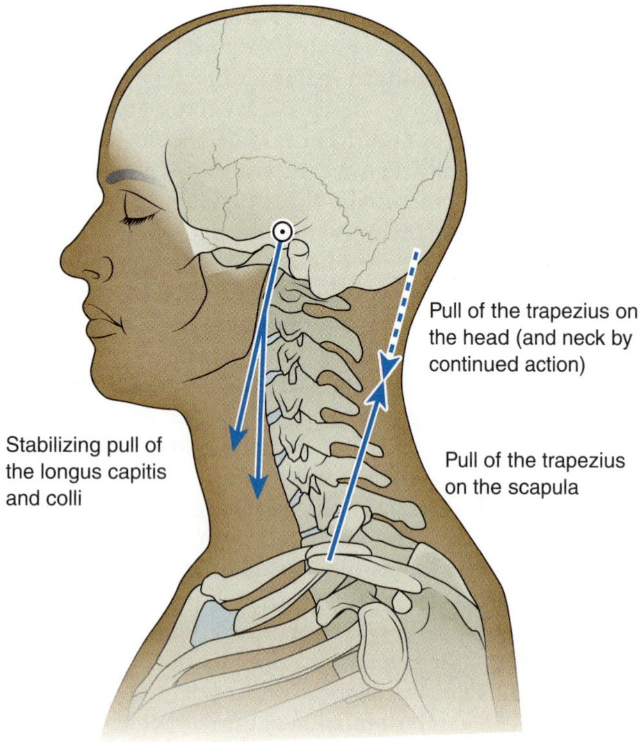

Figure 4–62 The longus capitis and longus colli work synergistically with the upper trapezius to stabilize the head so that the upper trapezius can effectively pull on the clavicle to contribute to elevation of the heavier upper extremity.

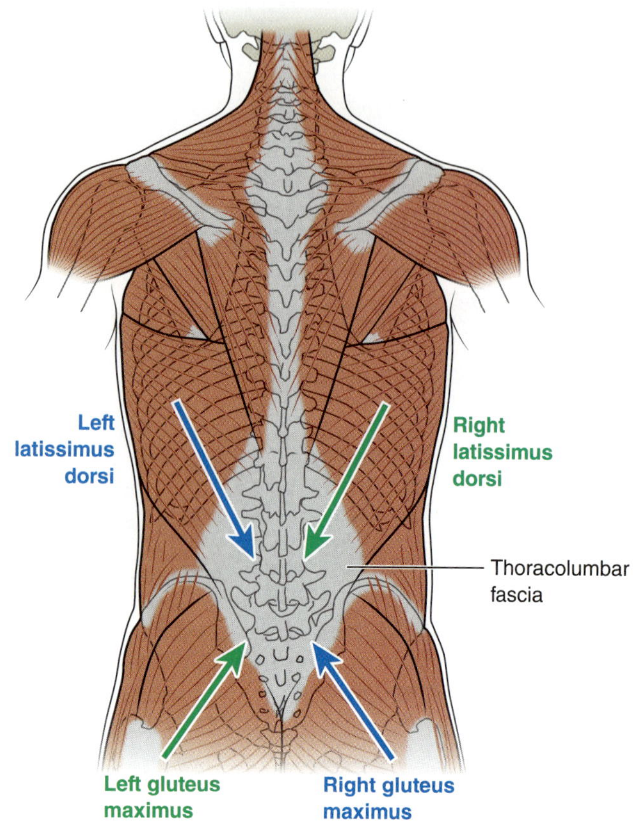

Figure 4–63 Coupled action of the latissimus dorsi and gluteus maximus muscles, and tension through the thoracolumbar fascia will compress and stabilize the lumbosacral region.

Patient Application 4–3

Casey is a 39-year-old delivery driver who was stopped at a traffic light 1 week ago when rear-ended by another car going about 20 miles per hour. Casey was wearing a seatbelt when hit. Casey is experiencing severe neck pain with activities, especially those that involve raising either arm, and is having trouble dressing, reaching overhead, and even holding the steering wheel, which is interfering with work. Radiographs were normal so it is unclear to Casey why arm elevation is causing so much pain when the arms were not injured in the accident.

Patients who have experienced a whiplash injury, as in a rear-end motor vehicle crash, often have extreme difficulty raising their arms. The longus capitis and longus colli can be overstretched and even torn in whiplash injuries without being evident on radiographs. If the longus capitis and colli are damaged, they will be unable to stabilize the head and neck against the pull of the trapezius on its proximal attachments. As a result, the trapezius moves the head and neck rather than effectively producing the upward rotation of the scapula needed to fully elevate the shoulder complex. The paradoxical action of the trapezius on the head and neck rather than on the scapula explains Casey's difficulty raising their arms.

Lower Thoracic/Lumbopelvic Regions

Muscles of the lower spine regions produce and control movement of the trunk and stabilize the trunk for motion of the lower extremities. These muscles assist in attenuating the extensive forces that affect this area and are involved with anticipatory motor control to stabilize the spine immediately before muscle activity of the extremities is initiated.

Posterior Muscles

The thoracolumbar fascia is the most superficial structure on the posterior aspect of the lower thoracic and lumbopelvic region (see Fig. 4–56) and is associated with several major muscle groups of this region. The thoracolumbar fascia blends with the latissimus dorsi, the gluteus maximus, the internal and external abdominal oblique, and the transversus abdominis (see Fig. 4–56). In addition, the fascia surrounds the erector spinae and the multifidus muscles of the lumbar region (see Fig. 4–44). These attachments are significant because tensile forces can be exerted on the thoracolumbar fascia through active and passive tension in these muscles. Tension on the thoracolumbar fascia, as part of the abdominal hoop, will produce a force that compresses the abdominal contents. Like a contraction of the abdominal muscles, the abdominal compression produced through the thoracolumbar fascia is like that of an external corset. The coupled action of the bilateral latissimus dorsi and gluteus maximus muscles together produces tension through the thoracolumbar fascia that compresses and stabilizes the lumbosacral region **(Fig. 4–63)**.[51]

Also posteriorly located, the erector spinae consist of the **longissimus** and **iliocostalis muscle groups** (Table 4–5). In general, these muscles are identified as extensors of the trunk. Bogduk[2] examined the function of the longissimus thoracis and

Table 4–5 Location and Function of the Erector Spine

NAME	LOCATION	FUNCTION
Deep Erector Spinae		
Longissimus thoracis pars lumborum (5 fascicles)	One from each lumbar TP to the PSIS	Ipsilateral lateral flexion Posterior shear: greatest at lower lumbar levels Assist with extension but close to axis of rotation; better MA at upper levels
Iliocostalis lumborum pars lumborum (4 fascicles)	One from each tip of the lumbar TP to the iliac crest	Ipsilateral lateral flexion Better rotators, due to greater MA Posterior shear, especially at lower levels Assist with extension but close to axis
Superficial Erector Spinae		
Longissimus thoracis pars thoracis (12 fascicles)	One from each thoracic TP and ribs via the ESA to L3–S3 SP	Extension of thoracic spine Extension of lumbar spine via increasing lordosis Assist with ipsilateral lateral flexion
Iliocostalis lumborum pars thoracis (7 or 8 fascicles)	One from each of the lower 7–8 ribs to PSIS and sacrum with contribution to the ESA	Extension of lumbar spine via increasing lordosis Assist with ipsilateral lateral flexion

ESA, erector spinae aponeurosis; MA, moment arm; PSIS, posterior superior sacroiliac spine; SP, posterior superior iliac spine; TP, transverse process.

the iliocostalis lumborum; he further described these muscles as each having a lumbar portion (pars lumborum) and a thoracic portion (pars thoracis). Anatomically and functionally, it is easier to group these muscles together as the superficial and deep layers. The **superficial layer** (longissimus thoracis pars thoracis and the iliocostalis lumborum pars thoracis[2]) runs from the ribs and thoracic transverse processes to form muscle bellies that are laterally located in the thoracic region. The superficial muscles have long tendons that join to form the **erector spinae aponeurosis** that inserts into the spinous processes of the lower lumbar spine, sacrum, and iliac crest **(Fig. 4–64)**. This superficial layer, with its long moment arm and excellent line of pull, produces extension of the thoracic and lumbar regions when acting bilaterally **(Fig. 4–65)**. These muscles are considered the primary extensors of the trunk. Acting unilaterally, the superficial erector spinae can laterally flex the trunk and contribute to trunk rotation. During trunk flexion from a standing position, the erector spinae are responsible for contracting eccentrically to control the motion; the gravitational moment produces forward flexion, with the amount and rate of flexion controlled by activity of the extensors and passive restraint of the erector spinae aponeurosis, the thoracolumbar fascia, and the posterior ligamentous system. The erector spinae act eccentrically until approximately two-thirds of maximal flexion, at which point these muscles become electrically silent. This is called the **flexion-relaxation phenomenon.** Flexion-relaxation is presumed to occur when the stretched passive tissues, on their own, can generate the required extension moment. However, the extensor muscles may be relaxed only in the electrical sense because they may also be generating passive force through passive stretching.[67]

The **deep layer** of the erector spinae (longissimus thoracis pars lumborum and the iliocostalis lumborum pars lumborum[2]) consists of individual fascicles with common tendinous insertions. The fascicles arise from the ilium at

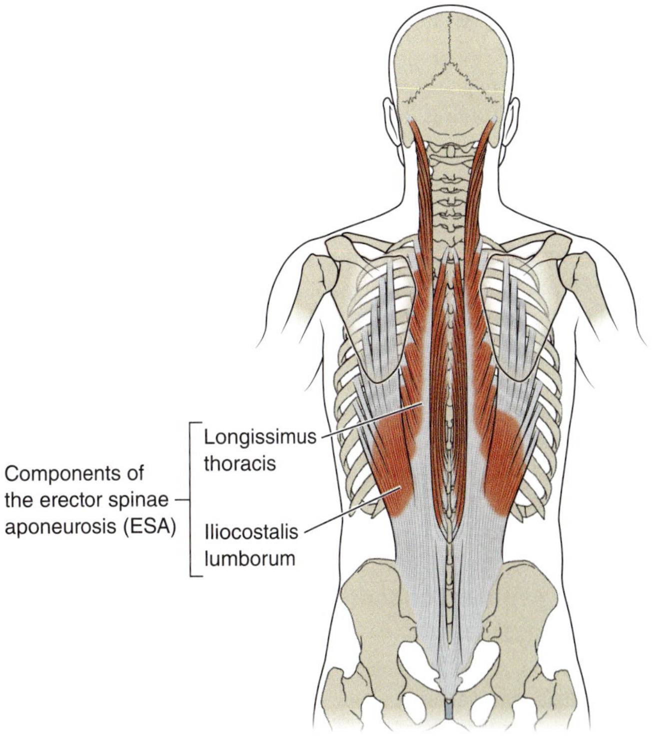

Figure 4–64 The tendons of the superficial erector spinae attach to and are part of the erector spinae aponeurosis (ESA).

the posterior superior iliac spine and iliac crest, coursing superiorly, medially, and anteriorly to insert on the lumbar transverse processes **(Fig. 4–66)**; the upper lumbar fascicles may also attach to the erector spinae aponeurosis. Porterfield and DeRosa[68] described these deep erector spinae as similar in orientation and function to the levator scapulae

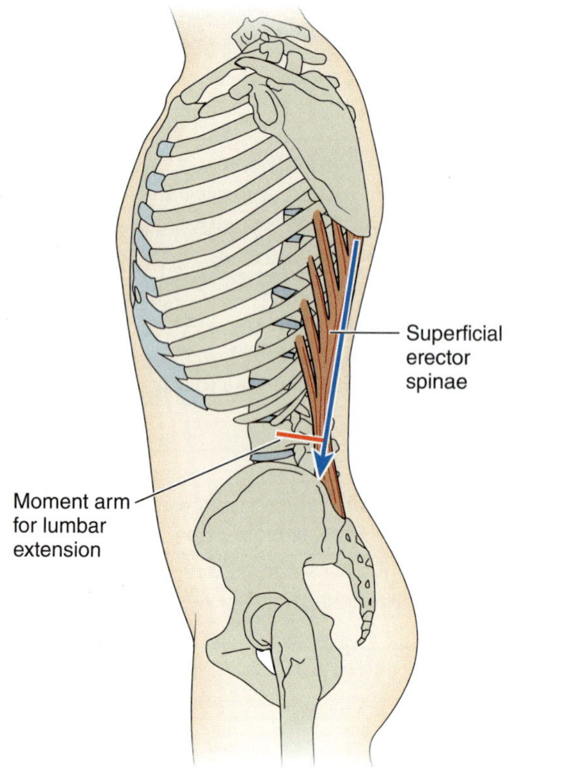

Figure 4–65 Sagittal view of the force vectors of the superficial erector spinae, demonstrating the excellent line of pull and large moment arm for thoracolumbar extension.

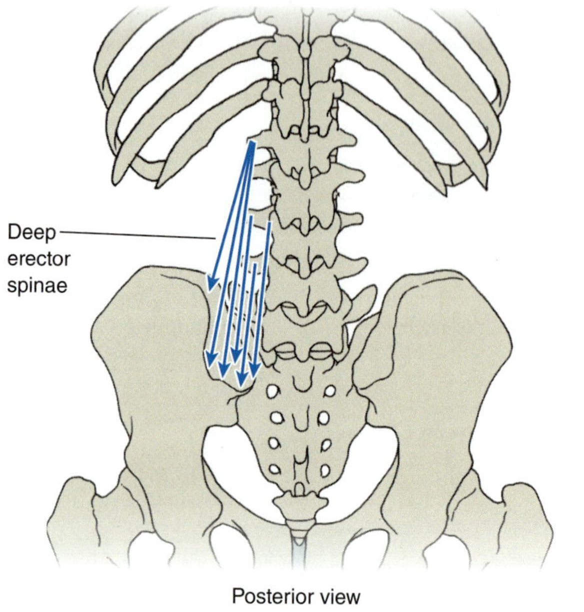

Figure 4–66 The fascicles of the deep erector spinae.

in the cervical region. Both muscle groups lie close to the flexion/extension axis without a sufficient moment arm to be prime movers for extension. The oblique orientation, however, allows the deep erector spinae muscles to exert both posterior shear and compressive forces on their vertebrae (**Fig. 4–67**). Because of their oblique line of action and ability to produce posterior shear, the deep erector spinae muscles provide an extremely important dynamic resistance to the constant anterior shear forces of the lumbar region caused by the lordotic position and the combined forces of gravity and the ground reaction. These muscles, then, have great clinical significance.

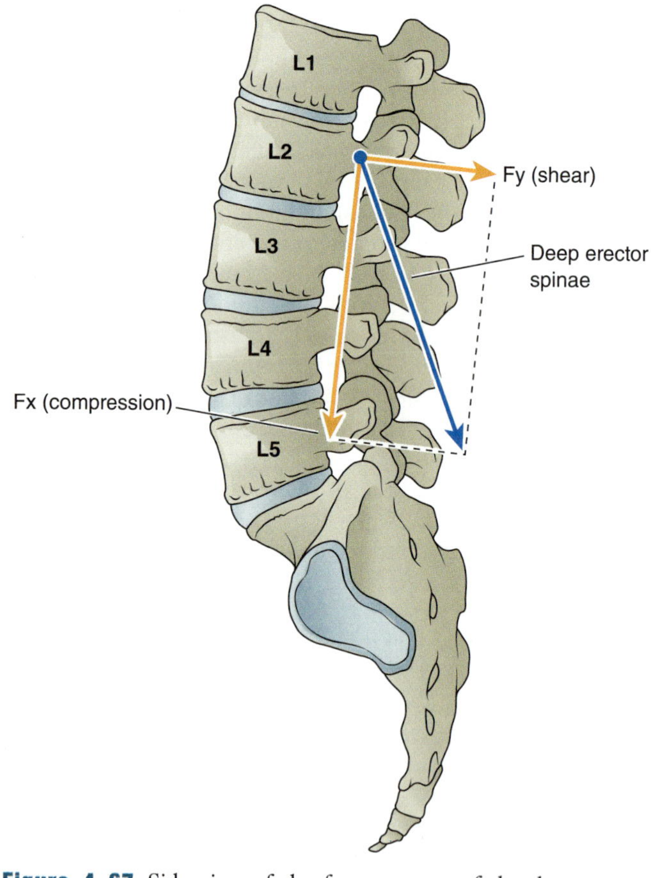

Figure 4–67 Side view of the force vectors of the deep erector spinae, demonstrating the compression (Fx) and posterior shear (Fy) components of the muscular pull.

Expanded Concepts 4–3

Negative Effects of Overstretching the Deep Erector Spinae

Like the levator scapulae in the cervical region, the deep erector spinae will become overworked, painful, and strained when counteracting excessive anterior shear forces. Overstretching the deep erector spinae muscles can remove the dynamic restraint to excessive anterior shear forces and either further load the noncontractile structures or, if the noncontractile forces have already been damaged, remove the only remaining restraint to anterior shear. In either case, stretching the deep erector spinae with exercises is likely to worsen the symptoms. It is more likely that these muscles need greater endurance and strength training.

The multifidus muscles of the spine are complex and demonstrate segmental and regional differences. The multifidus muscle group is typically considered to be part of the **transversospinales** group. However, the lumbar multifidi run from the dorsal sacrum and the ilium in the region of the posterior superior iliac spine to the spinous processes of the lumbar vertebrae and have separate fascicles.[69–71] In this region, therefore, the multifidus muscles are not characteristic of the other muscles in the transversospinales group. The lumbar multifidus muscles are a thick mass that fills the area of the sacral sulcus and are easily palpable there (unlike the other transversospinales muscles).[69,70]

The most *superficial* fibers of each fascicle of the lumbar multifidi cross as many as five segments and attach caudally to the sacrum and ilium. Their line of pull is vertically oriented, and they are distant from the flexion/extension axes of the lumbar motion segments. Therefore, the superficial fibers of the multifidi have an effective moment arm for extension, thereby increasing the lumbar lordosis (see Fig. 4–59B). The *deep* fibers of each fascicle attach from the lamina and spinous process and cross two segments to insert on the mamillary process and facet joint capsule. The deep fibers in the lumbar region have a small moment arm and, therefore, are not strong extensors. These deep fibers are ideally positioned to control segmental shear and torsion by producing compression. The role of the lumbar multifidus muscles in trunk rotation is to synergistically counteract the flexion moment of the abdominal muscles so they can produce trunk rotation. The lumbar multifidus muscles are involved in local segmental control in the lumbar region.

In the thoracic region, the multifidus muscles are like other muscles of the transversospinales group because they are more laterally oriented with an oblique line of pull. They run from all of the transverse processes of the thoracic vertebrae to the spinous processes of the more cranial vertebrae, each covering one to three segments. The thoracic multifidus muscles are activated with rotation but in a variable manner, suggesting that the thoracic multifidi, like the deep lumbar multifidi, have a role in synergistic control of motion rather than production of motion.[69]

The posteriorly located **intertransversarii** and rotatores muscles (see Fig. 4–57) are frequently described as producing lateral flexion and rotation, respectively. Because of their small cross-sectional areas and small moment arms, however, it appears likely that these muscles serve more of a proprioceptive role.

Lateral Muscles

The quadratus lumborum is deeper than the erector spinae and multifidus muscles **(Fig. 4–68)**. The quadratus lumborum, when acting bilaterally, serves as an important stabilizer and, in this role, is active in many tasks **(Fig. 4–68A)**.[17] When acting unilaterally, the quadratus lumborum can laterally flex the spine **(Fig. 4–68B)**. The *ipsilateral* quadratus lumborum can initiate lateral flexion from erect standing, but the force of gravity will continue the motion while the *contralateral* quadratus lumborum controls the movement eccentrically. The quadratus lumborum can also control rotational motion due to its attachments to the transverse processes of the lumbar vertebrae. If the pelvis is free to move, the quadratus lumborum will "hike the hip," (that is, laterally tilt the pelvis in the frontal plane) **(Fig. 4–68C)**.

Anterior Muscles

The **rectus abdominis** is the prime flexor of the trunk. It is contained within the abdominal fascia that separates the rectus abdominis into sections and attaches the rectus abdominis to the aponeurosis of the abdominal wall. The abdominal fascia also has attachment to the aponeurosis of the pectoralis major. As part of the abdominal hoop, these fascial connections are important because they transmit forces across the midline and around the trunk. Tension on this fascial system will provide stability around the trunk similar to that provided by a corset (see Fig. 4–44).

The abdominal wall consists of the **external oblique**, the **internal oblique**, and the **transversus abdominis** muscles. As described earlier in the discussion of the thoracolumbar fascia, these muscles are part of the abdominal hoop surrounding the entire abdomen circumferentially (see Fig. 4–44). The active transversus abdominis may enhance stability to the sacroiliac joints via the compressive forces resulting from the transverse orientation of the muscles to the SI joints.[72]

The **psoas major** may also be considered an anterior truck muscle. The psoas major muscle attaches to the lumbar

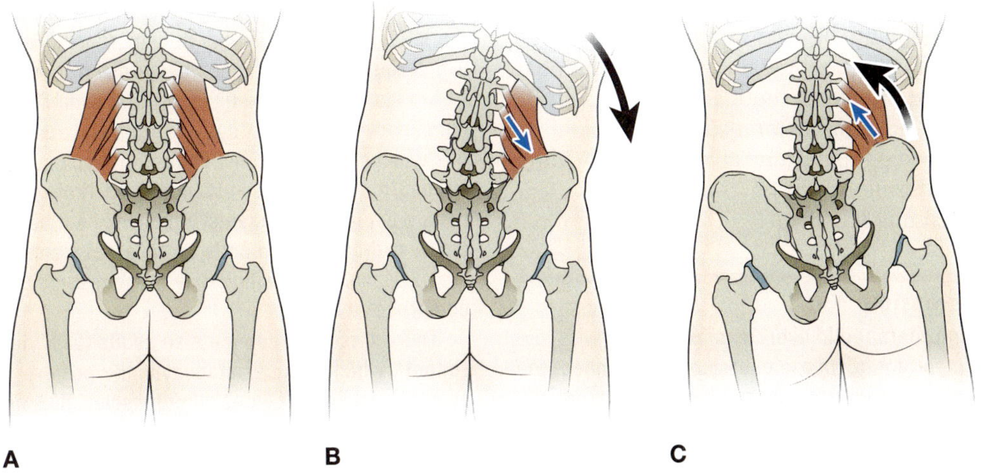

Figure 4–68 **A.** The attachments of the right and left quadratus lumborum muscles. **B.** A unilateral contraction of the right quadratus lumborum muscle when the pelvis and left leg are fixed will cause right trunk flexion. **C.** A unilateral contraction of the right quadratus lumborum muscle will lift and tilt the right side of the pelvis and "hike the hip" when the trunk is fixed and the pelvis and leg are free to move.

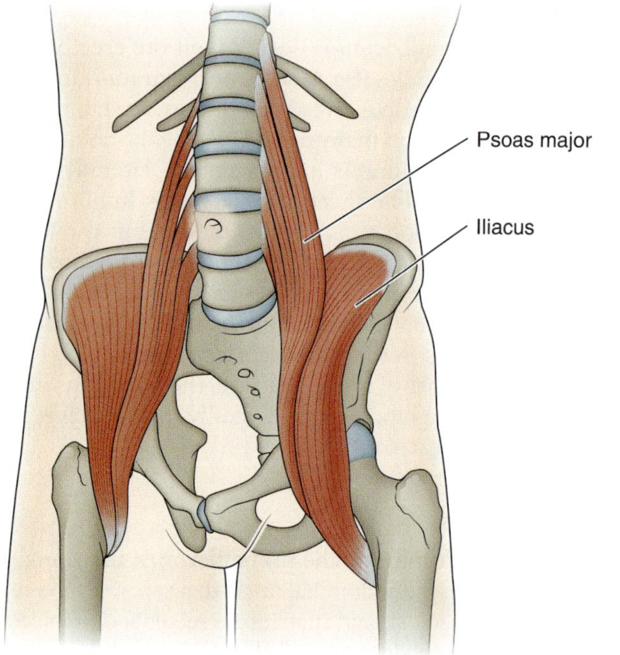

Figure 4–69 The anteriorly located psoas major and iliacus muscles are primary hip flexors. However, the iliacus simultaneously creates an anterior pull on the pelvis that would result in lumbar lordosis if not offset by the simultaneous anterior pull of the active psoas major on the lumbar vertebrae.

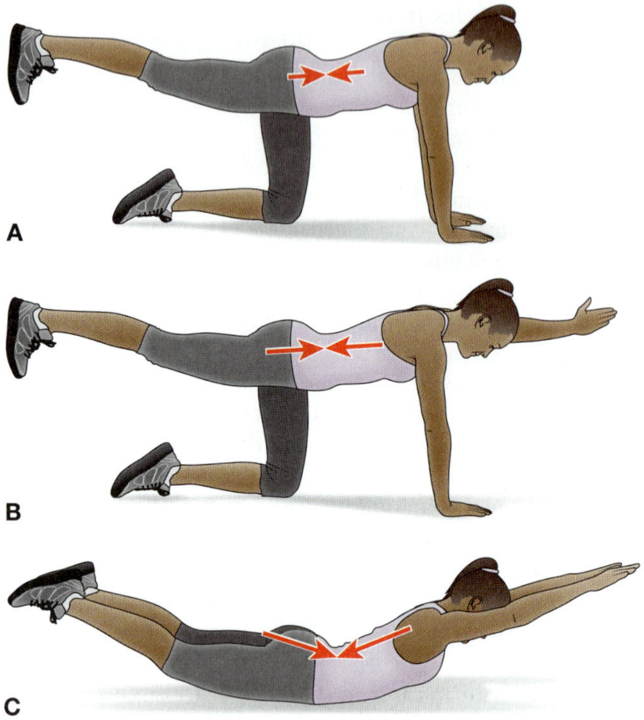

Figure 4–70 **A.** Single-leg extension in the quadruped position creates relatively low erector spinae activity and compression forces at the lumbar segments at an estimated 2,500 N. **B.** Raising the opposite leg and arm simultaneously increases demand to the lumbar erector spinae but also increases compression forces at the lumbar segments by 1,000 N. **C.** Raising all four limbs simultaneously further raises the demand for erector spinae contraction; however, this action can raise the compression at L4–L5 to an estimated 6,000 N.

transverse processes, the anterolateral vertebral bodies of T12 to L4, and the lumbar intervertebral discs and to the lesser trochanter of the femur **(Fig. 4–69)**. The psoas major courses inferiorly and laterally from its proximal attachments, with its distal tendon merging with that of the **iliacus** muscle. The primary role of the psoas major is to flex the hip. The iliacus runs from the iliac crest over the pubic ramus to the lesser trochanter with the tendon of the psoas major. When active hip flexion is initiated on a weight-bearing lower limb, the iliac muscle exerts a pull on its respective innominate that, if unopposed, would cause anterior pelvic tilt and consequent lumbar extension (lordosis) to remain upright. The psoas major, also active in non–weight-bearing hip flexion, creates an anterior pull on the lumbar vertebrae that resists the lumbar extension force created by pull of the iliacus muscle on the anterior innominate. The psoas major also provides stability to the lumbar spine during hip flexion activities by providing lumbar compression during activation. Some anterior shear is also produced when it is activated.

Clinical Application 4–1

When developing therapeutic exercises for people with low back disorders, it is important to choose exercises that connect the kinesiology and biomechanics with the chosen goal of the exercise.

For example, consider that we wish to increase strength of the deep erector spinae, including the lumbar multifidi. We may choose to use a quadruped (hands and knees) position **(Fig. 4–70)**. In **Figure 4–70A**, the person begins on hands and knees and extends one leg. The weight of the right leg creates a flexion moment at the right hip and pelvis, which will require activation of the hip extensors and erector spinae to hold their limb in the air as shown. Because both of their upper extremities are on the ground, there is some gravitational counter-torque helping to hold the trunk in neutral. With this exercise, the hip extensors are targeted more so than the erector spinae because of the counter-torque from above. The compressive forces at the lower lumbar segments are approximately 2,500 N with this exercise. In **Figure 4–70B**, the left upper extremity is now also raised, adding flexion torque to the trunk that will increase the demands on the erector spinae. The erector spinae muscle activity increases by 30%, with the compressive load across the lower lumbar segments now increasing by 1,000 N to 3,500 N.[73] When raising arms and legs bilaterally from a lying (prone) position, as in **Figure 4–70C**, the hip and trunk extensors are now raising the combined weight of the legs and arms and trunk against gravity. While this will increase the challenge to the spinal extensors for strength training, the position also produces 6,000 N of compressive force across the lower lumbar segments, which may not be tolerated. Despite the desire to increase demands on the erector spinae to meet the goal of the exercise, this position may be contra-indicated due to the large compressive loads.

This exercise sequence also sequentially decreases the base of support, which reduces stability in the posture, challenges balance, and increasingly activates other muscles. Raising one limb in quadruped also induces rotational torque to the lumbar region, which further complicates the picture. The position of the arms and legs will affect the torques produced by changing the moment arm.

This example demonstrates how an understanding of kinesiology and biomechanics is necessary to optimize exercise prescription to meet established goals.

Muscles of the Pelvic Floor

A comprehensive review of the structure and function of the pelvic floor is beyond the scope of this chapter. The role of the muscles of the pelvic floor in providing stability to the lumbopelvic ring, however, is recognized as being important to understanding biomechanics of the pelvis as well as low back pain. Dysfunction of the muscles of the pelvic floor has been identified as both a risk factor for and a result of low back pain.[74] Given the role of the pelvic floor musculature in the stability of this region, its structure and function are briefly discussed here.

Structure

The muscles of the pelvic floor are the broad muscle sheets of the **levator ani** and the **coccygeus** muscles, which together separate the pelvic cavity from the perineum **(Fig. 4–71)**. The two distinct parts of the levator ani are the **iliococcygeus** and the **pubococcygeus muscles (Fig. 4–71A)**. The pubococcygeal part of the levator ani muscle arises from the posterior aspect of the pubis and has attachments to the rectum in the anal canal, the urethra, and the walls of the vagina (in people assigned female sex at birth). The iliococcygeal portion of the levator ani arises from the obturator fascia, blends with the fibers of the anococcygeal ligament to form the median plate (raphe) of the levator ani and attaches to the last two coccygeal segments. The coccygeus muscle arises from the spine of the ischium and attaches to the coccyx and lower portion of the sacrum. The gluteal surface of the coccygeus muscle blends with the sacrospinous ligament.

Function

In addition to their roles in controlling the sphincters for micturition and defecation, the levator ani and the coccygeus muscles form a muscular (pelvic) diaphragm that supports the pelvic viscera **(Fig. 4–71B)** while also generating, maintaining, and increasing intra-abdominal pressure in functional tasks.[75,76] Increased intra-abdominal pressure created by tension in the muscles of the pelvic diaphragm increases stiffness to the lumbopelvic area, especially during co-contraction with the transverses abdominis muscle,[77] thus contributing to lumbar spine stiffness and support. In addition, the coccygeus muscle crosses the sacroiliac joint and contributes to compression of the joints in those assigned female sex at birth, which increases the stiffness of the pelvic ring.[76]

Squat Lift Versus Stoop Lift

The prevalence of back pain in workers who must do repetitive lifting tasks has led to a great deal of investigation into the safest lifting technique. Focus has primarily been on the use of a squat versus stoop lift **(Fig. 4–72)**. During a squat lift **(Fig. 4–72A)**, the spine remains as erect as possible and the trunk is brought lower to the ground primarily by hip and knee flexion. During a stoop lift **(Fig. 4–72B)**, the body is lowered primarily by thoracolumbar flexion with little to no knee flexion.

The literature remains unclear regarding whether there is biomechanical evidence to support advocating one lifting technique over another to *prevent* low back pain. It is likely that the safest posture for lifting is task specific and person specific. There are some advantages and disadvantages to each technique.[78]

Repetitive and/or heavy lifting impose large loads across the lumbar spinal segments. Biomechanical investigations have examined the kinetics across the lumbar spine and muscle activity between the two techniques, all attempting to identify the safest technique. Different positions of the body and position of the external load affect active (muscles) and passive (discs, joints, ligaments) structures differently, which alter the effects on the lumbar structures.

A squat lifting technique has some biomechanical advantages in that the spinal extensor muscles have a better length-tension to resist the flexion torque produced by the trunk and external load—and do, indeed, demonstrate more muscular activity

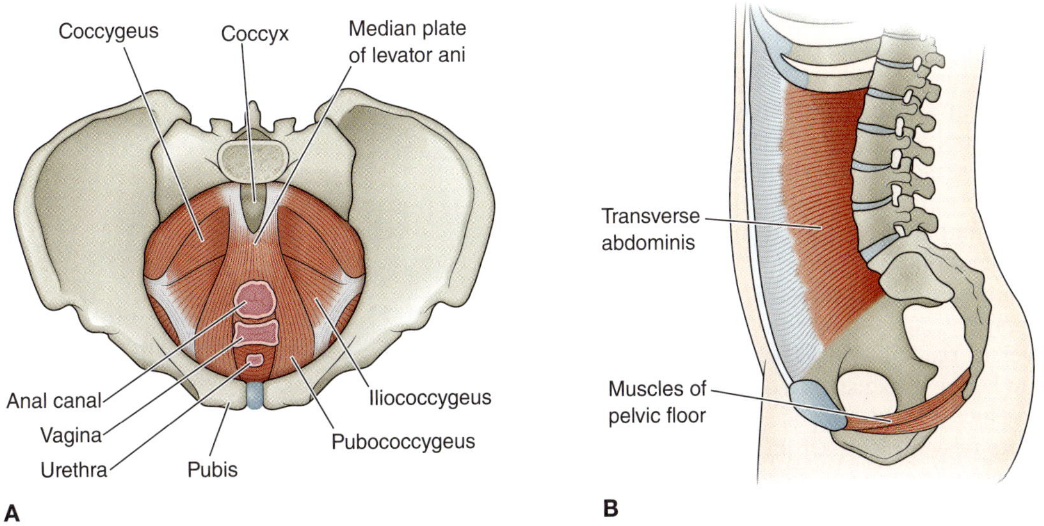

Figure 4–71 Muscles of the pelvic floor. **A.** The two components of the levator ani muscles (pubococcygeus and iliococcygeus muscles) and the coccygeus muscles form the floor of the pelvis referred to as the *pelvic diaphragm*. **B.** The pelvic diaphragm and the transverse abdominis work together actively or passively to increase support (stiffness) to the lumbopelvic region.

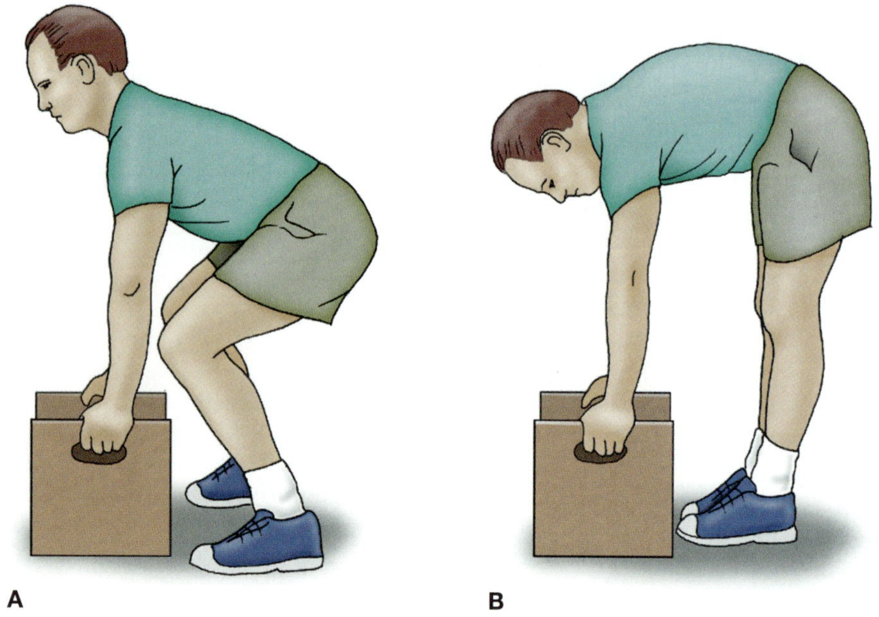

Figure 4–72 **A.** Squat lift versus **B.** Stoop lift.

in the squat than the stoop position. The squat position also has the advantage of the external load being lifted closer to the body (i.e., shorter moment arm), thereby decreasing the external flexion torque produced by the external load. In the neutral lumbar spine posture often seen in the squat lift technique, the deep layer of the erector spinae can produce a posterior shear force that helps to offset the anterior shear produced by body weight and external load.[79,80] Relatively larger shear forces are thought to be particularly damaging to disc and facet joint structures.

Stoop lifting can increase intradiscal pressures.[81,82] Similarly, shear forces on lumbar vertebrae were found to be two to four times higher for the stoop lift than for the squat lift,[43] and there is evidence that the spine is less capable of resisting shear forces than compressive forces.[80] Additionally, the deep spinal extensors can experience active insufficiency in the stoop position because attempting to shorten when fully lengthened decreases their ability to resist the anterior shear forces. Paradoxically, however, there have been findings that stoop lifting results in decreased fatigue and increased tolerance to lifting in workers. This may be explained by the decreased metabolic demands found in the stoop lift position due to increased reliance on tension in passive joint and soft-tissue structures such as the erector-spinae fascia, the thoracolumbar fascia, the facet joint capsule and ligaments. The metabolic work needed to move the load from a position lower to the ground in the squat position may also be at play.[83]

Less controversial but still critical factors in lifting in any posture appear to be the distance from the body of the object to be lifted, the velocity of the lift, and the degree of lumbar flexion. The farther away the load is from the body, the greater the gravitational moment acting on the vertebral column will be. Greater muscle activity is then required to perform the lift and, consequently, greater compressive forces are created in the discs. The higher the velocity of the lift, the greater the amount of weight that can be lifted, but the greater the load on the lumbar discs.

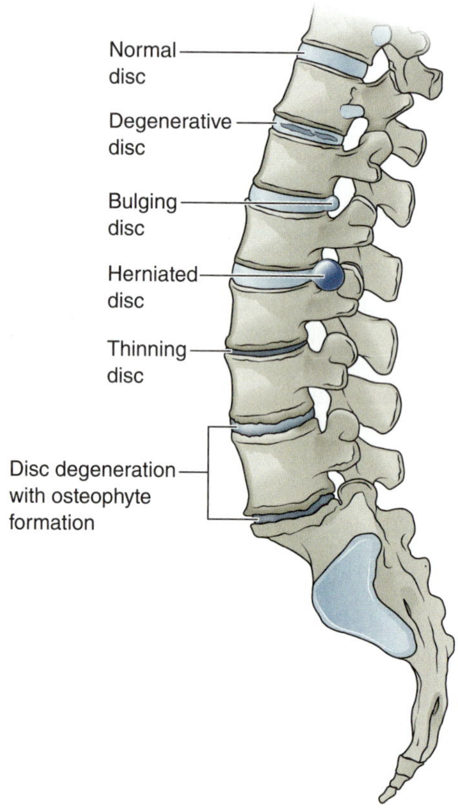

Figure 4–73 Age-related changes that can occur in the spine include disc degeneration, bulging of the annulus fibrosus with or without herniation of the nucleus pulposus, thinning of the disc, and disc degeneration with formation of osteophytes on the vertebral bodies. Disc herniation in this figure is exaggerated in magnitude for emphasis.

Effects of Aging on the Lumbar Spine

Over the life span, the vertebral column is exposed to recurrent loads that change the morphology of the column. Many of the changes described here and shown in **Figures 4–73** and **4–74**

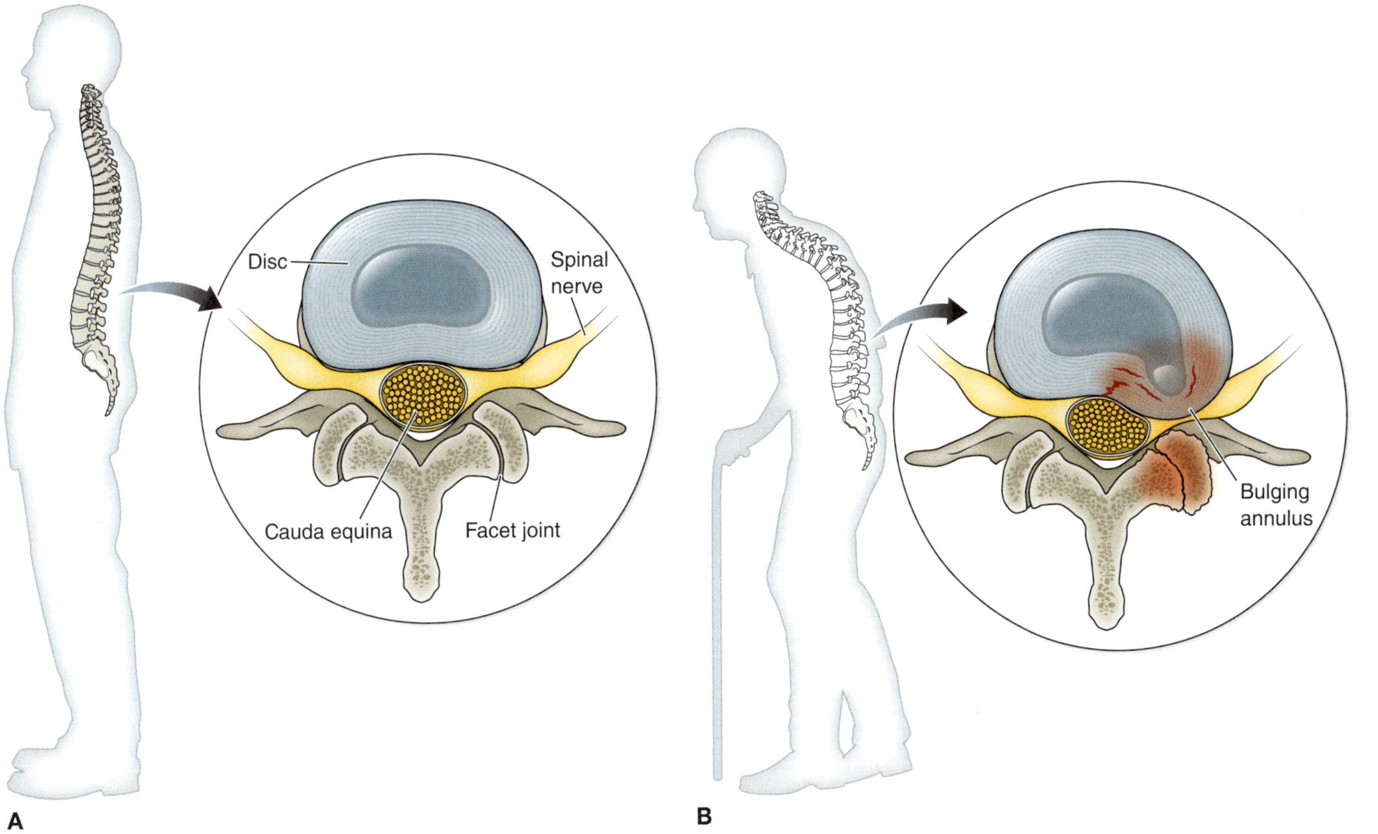

Figure 4–74 Age-related changes to the spine. **A.** In the typical adult, the annulus fibrosus maintains the central location of the nucleus pulposus. The spinal cord and spinal nerves have adequate space in, respectively, the vertebral canal and intervertebral foramen. **B.** Age-related changes to the discs, vertebral ligaments such as the ligamentum flavum, and to the facets can lead to impingement of the spinal nerve or spinal cord.

are not attributable to aging per se but are more likely to be observed in older individuals.

The vertebral bone undergoes changes in the amount and form of the trabeculae of the cancellous bone. The numbers of both horizontal and vertical trabeculae decrease with age, and the horizontal trabeculae become significantly thinner. This loss can decrease the loads that the vertebrae are able to withstand before failure.

Each of the structures of the intervertebral disc undergoes changes in the extracellular matrix that include loss in the number of proteoglycans and change in the specific type of proteoglycan, with resultant loss of water content, as well as an increase of collagen and loss of elastin. These changes in connective tissue composition result in a loss of the ability of the disc to transfer loads from one vertebra to another as the swelling ability of the nucleus decreases. The overall disc height will also decrease.

The vertebral endplate, with aging, gradually becomes more collagenous with the process of diffusion hindered.[84] Because the disc relies on the diffusion of nutrients through the vertebral endplate, nutrition of the disc becomes impaired with changes in the endplate. Eventually, the intervertebral disc can desiccate. Lamellae of the annulus separate and can result in fissures and tears that can decrease the ability of the lumbar discs to provide stiffness during movement.[85]

A disc can prolapse or protrude as a result of the pressure on the nucleus and the inability of the annulus fibrosus to restrain it. Schmorl nodes are formed when the nuclear material prolapses through the vertebral endplate and into the cancellous bone of the vertebra. This material may cause an autoimmune response when it contacts the blood supply in the cancellous bone.[84] This presentation is typically labeled *degenerative disc disease*.

With degenerative disc disease, there is a more substantial loss of disc height that can cause vertebral ligaments to reduce tension or become slack. The ligamentous prestress normally provided by the ligamentum flavum will decrease, which in turn will reduce spinal stiffness (stability). The reduction in tension in the ligamentum flavum can also result in the ligament buckling on itself with movement, potentially compressing the spinal cord. In addition, the ligamentum flavum may calcify with age, potentially leading to hypertrophic ossification that can cause compression of the spinal nerve in the vicinity of the facet joints or compress the spinal cord within the canal.[15] On occasion, blood vessels grow into the usually avascular adult discs, triggering ossification.

The facet joints also demonstrate age-related changes that may lead to eventual degeneration. With degeneration of the disc, more compressive loads are borne at the facet joints that, then, may lead to deterioration and arthritic changes. The result of these changes to the facet joints is the same as what happens to the larger synovial joints of the extremities: damage of the cartilage, including fissures and cysts, and osteophyte formation.[84] These changes can lead to localized pain or pressure on spinal nerves or the central canal or, in the cervical region, compression of the vertebral artery in the transverse foramen.

The uncovertebral joints (see Fig. 4–30), are frequent sites for age-related and degenerative changes. Osteophytes on the uncinate processes (see Fig. 4–28) occur predominantly in the lower segments, C5–C6 or C6–C7. The motion of lateral bending becomes extremely limited when these osteophytes occur.[84]

SUMMARY

In summary, it is extremely important to understand the normal structure and function, including normal variability, of the vertebral column to understand the structures at risk for injury and the best ways to treat people with dysfunction. Injury or failure occurs when the applied load is either insufficient or excessive. Repetitive strain causes injury by either the repeated application of a relatively low load or by application of a sustained load for a long duration (prolonged sitting or stooped posture).

The effects of injury, aging, disease, or developmental deficit on the vertebral column may be analyzed by considering:

- The normal function that the affected structure is designed to serve
- The stresses that are present during normal situations
- The anatomic relationship of the structure to adjacent structures
- The functional relationship of the structure to other structures

STUDY QUESTIONS

1. Describe the functional goals of each of the following regions of the spinal column: the cervical spine, the thoracic spine, the lumbar spine, and the pelvis.
2. What are the components of a typical vertebra and what are the specific functions of each?
3. How do the shapes and sizes of the components of the vertebrae differ by region and how are the changes related to the forces to which each region is subject?
4. What are the roles of the intervertebral discs? Describe how the discs fulfill these roles.
5. What are the motions that occur at the interbody joints with flexion, extension, lateral flexion, and rotation?
6. Describe the shape and orientation of the facet joints in each spinal region. What motion is most facilitated in each region based on the shape and orientation of the facets?
7. What are the motions that occur at the facet joints with flexion, extension, lateral flexion, and rotation? What is unique about the lumbar facet joint motion?
8. Describe the relative strength of the longitudinal ligaments in the lumbar region. How does this strength differ from that in the other regions? Are some structures more or less susceptible to injury in this region based on this variation?
9. Which structures are most affected if a person has a forward head posture? Describe the type and location of stresses that may occur, as well as how other structures might react to those changes in stresses.
10. Which structures are most affected if a person has an increased lumbar lordosis? Describe the type and location of stresses that may occur, as well as how other structures might react to the change in stresses.
11. Which muscles cause extension of the lumbar spine? In which position of the spine are these muscles most effective?
12. Describe what kinds of forces act on the spine during motion and at rest.
13. Explain how creep may adversely affect the stability of the vertebral column.
14. Identify the prime movers of each spinal region.
15. Identify the muscles that function specifically to control segmental motion in the cervical and lumbar spine.
16. What role has been attributed to the thoracolumbar fascia in the stability of the lumbopelvic region?
17. Describe the dynamic and static restraints to anterior shear in the lumbar and cervical regions.

REFERENCES

1. Kapandji I: The Physiology of the Joints (ed 2). Edinburgh, Scotland, E & S Livingstone, 1974
2. Bogduk N: Clinical Anatomy of the Lumbar Spine and Sacrum (ed 4). London, England, Churchill Livingstone, 2005
3. Auger JD, Frings N, Wu Y, et al: Trabecular architecture and mechanical heterogeneity effects on vertebral body strength. Curr Osteoporosis Rep 18:716-26, 2020
4. Huiskes R, Ruimerman R, van Lenthe GH, et al: Effects of mechanical forces on maintenance and adaptation of form in trabecular bone. Nature 405:704, 2000
5. Banse X, Devogelaer JP, Munting E, et al: Inhomogeneity of human vertebral cancellous bone: systematic density and structure patterns inside the vertebral body. Bone 28:563, 2001
6. Mercer SR, Bogduk N: Joints of the cervical vertebral column. J Orthop Sports Phys Ther 31:174; discussion 183, 2001
7. Singh K, Masuda K, Thonar E, An H, Cs-Szabo G: Age-related changes in the extracellular matrix of nucleus pulposis and annulus fibrosis of human intervertebral disc. Spine 34(1): 10-16, 2009
8. Lundon K, Bolton K: Structure and function of the lumbar intervertebral disk in health, aging, and pathologic conditions. J Orthop Sports Phys Ther 31:291; discussion 304, 2001
9. Groh AM, Fournier DE, Battie MC, et al: Innervation of the human intervertebral disc: a scoping review. Pain Med 22(6):1281-1304, 2021
10. Fournier DE, Kiser PK, Shoemaker JK, et al: Vascularization of the human intervertebral disc: a scoping review. JOR Spine 3:e1123, 2020
11. White A, Panjabi M: Clinical Biomechanics of the Spine (ed 2). Philadelphia, PA, Lippincott, 1990
12. Yoganandan N, Kumaresan S, Pintar FA: Biomechanics of the cervical spine part 2: cervical spine soft tissue responses and biomechanical modeling. Clin Biomech (Bristol, Avon) 16:1, 2001
13. Inami S, Kaneoka K, Hayashi K, et al: Types of synovial fold in the cervical facet joint. J Ortho Sci: Official Journal of the Japanese Orthopaedic Association 5:475, 2000
14. Kapetanakis S, Gkantsinikoudis N: Anatomy of the lumbar facet joint: a comprehensive review. Folia Morphol 80(4):799-805, 2021
15. Kim YH, Khuyagbaatar B, Kim K: Biomechanical effects of spinal cord compression due to ossification of posterior longitudinal ligament and ligamentum flavum: a finite element analysis. Med Eng Phys 35: 1266, 2013
16. Fujiwara A, Tamai K, An HS, et al: The interspinous ligament of the lumbar spine: magnetic resonance images and their clinical significance. Spine 25:358, 2000
17. McGill S: Low Back Disorders: Evidence-Based Prevention and Rehabilitation (ed 3). Champaign, IL, Human Kinetics, 2016
18. Moore K, Dalley A, Agur A: Clinically Oriented Anatomy (ed 7). Baltimore, MD, Lippincott Williams & Wilkins, 2014
19. Drake PL, Hazelwood KJ: Exposure-related health effects of silver and silver compounds: a review. Ann Occup Hyg 49:575, 2005
20. Adams MA, Hutton WC: The mechanical function of the lumbar apophyseal joints. Spine 8:327, 1983

21. Cholewicki J, Crisco JJ, Oxland TR, et al: Effects of posture and structure on three-dimensional coupled rotations in the lumbar spine: a biomechanical analysis. Spine 21:2421, 1996
22. Panjabi M, Crisco J, Vasavada A, et al: Mechanical properties of the human cervical spine as shown by three-dimensional load-displacement curves. Spine 26:2692, 2001
23. Legaspi O, Edmond SL: Does the evidence support the existence of lumbar spine coupled motion? A critical review of the literature. J Orthop Sports Phys Ther 37:169, 2007
24. Cook C, Hegedus E, Showalter C, et al: Coupling behavior of the cervical spine: a systematic review of the literature. J Manipulative Physiol Ther 29:570, 2006
25. Bogduk N, Amevo B, Pearcy M: A biological basis for instantaneous centres of rotation of the vertebral column. Proc of the Institution of Mechanical Engineers. Part H, J of Eng in Med 209:177, 1995
26. Keller T, Hansson T, Abram A, et al: Regional variations in the compressive properties of lumbar vertebral trabeculae: effects of disc degeneration. Spine 14:1012, 1989
27. Nachemson A: The lumbar spine: an orthopedic challenge. Spine 1:1, 1976
28. Twomey L, Taylor J, Oliver M: Sustained flexion loading, rapid extension loading of the lumbar spine, and the physical therapy of related injuries. Physiother Pract 4:129, 1988
29. Adams M, Dolan P, Hutton W: Diurnal changes in spinal mechanics and their clinical significance. J Bone Joint Surg Br 72:266, 1990
30. Shirazi-Adl A: Strain in fibers of a lumbar disc: analysis of the role of lifting in producing disc prolapse. Spine 14:96, 1989
31. Panjabi M, Oxland T, Takata K, et al: Articular facets of the human spine. Spine 18:1298, 1993
32. Bogduk N, Mercer S: Biomechanics of the cervical spine. I: Normal kinematics. Clin Biomech 15:633, 2000
33. Porterfield J, DeRosa C: Mechanical Neck Pain: Perspectives in Functional Anatomy. Philadelphia, PA, WB Saunders, 1995
34. Debernardi A, D'Alibert G, Talamont G, et al: The craniovertebral junction area and the role of the ligaments and membranes. Neurosurgery 68:291, 2011
35. Osmotherly PG, Rivett DA, Mercer SR: Revisiting the clinical anatomy of the alar ligaments. EurSpine J 22:60, 2013
36. Takeshita K, Peterson E, Bylski-Austrow D, et al: The nuchal ligament restrains cervical spine flexion. Spine (Phila Pa.1976) 29:E388, 2004
37. Mercer SR, Bogduk N: Clinical anatomy of ligamentum nuchae. Clin Anat 16:484, 2003
38. Johnson GM, Ahang M, Jones DG: The fine connective tissue architecture of the human ligamentum nuchae. Spine (Phila Pa.1976) 25:5, 2000
39. Hartman J: Anatomy and clinical significance of the uncinate process and uncovertebral joint: A comprehensive review. Clin Anat 27:431, 2014
40. Hsu W, Benzel EC, Chen T, et al: Axial and coronal orientation of subaxial cervical zygapophyseal joints and their effect on axial rotation and lateral bending. Spine 33:2409, 2008
41. Smith MD, Coppieters MW, Hodges PW: Postural activity of the pelvic floor muscles is delayed during rapid arm movements in women with stress urinary incontinence. Int Urogynecol J Pelvic Floor Dysfunct 18:901, 2007
42. Beyer B, Feipel V, Dugailly PM: Biomechanics of the upper cervical spine ligaments in axial rotation and flexion-extension: considerations into the clinical framework. J Craniovertebr Junction Spine 11(3):217-25, 2020
43. Takahashi I, Kikuchi S, Sato K, et al: Mechanical load of the lumbar spine during forward bending motion of the trunk—a biomechanical study. Spine 31:18, 2006
44. MacDonald D, Moseley GL, Hodges PW: Why do some patients keep hurting their back? Evidence of ongoing back muscle dysfunction during remission from recurrent back pain. Pain 142:183, 2009
45. Pal GP, Routal RV: The role of the vertebral laminae in the stability of the cervical spine. J Anat 188:485, 1996
46. Liebsch C, Wilke HJ: How does the rib cage affect the biomechanical properties of the thoracic spine? A systematic literature review. Front Bioeng Biotechnol 10:904539, 2022
47. Boszczyk BM, Boszczyk AA, Putz R, et al: An immunohistochemical study of the dorsal capsule of the lumbar and thoracic facet joints. Spine 26:E338, 2001
48. Iwanaga J, Ishak B, Saga T, et al: The lumbar ligamentum flavum does not have two layers and is confluent with the interspinous ligament: anatomical study with application to surgical and interventional pain procedures. Clin Anat 33(1):34-40, 2020
49. Hammer N, Steinke H, Böhme J, et al: Description of the iliolumbar ligament for computer-assisted reconstruction. Ann Anat–Anatomischer Anzeiger 192:162, 2010
50. Snijders CJ, Hermans PFG, Niesing R, et al: The influence of slouching and lumbar support on iliolumbar ligaments, intervertebral discs and sacroiliac joints. Clin Biomech 19:323, 2004
51. Willard FH, Vleeming A, Schuenke MD, et al: The thoracolumbar fascia: anatomy, function and clinical considerations. J Anat 221:507, 2012
52. Barker P, Guggenheimer K, Grkovic I: Effects of tensioning the lumbar fasciae on segmental stiffness during flexion and extension. Spine 31:397, 2006
53. Widmer J, Cornaz F, Scheibler G, et al: Biomechanical contribution of spinal structures to stability of the lumbar spine—novel biomechanical insights. The Spine J 20:1705-26, 2020
54. Cailliet R: Low Back Pain Syndrome (ed 5). Philadelphia, PA, FA Davis, 1995
55. Tafazzol A, Arjmand N, Shirazi-Adl A, et al: Lumbopelvic rhythm during forward and backward sagittal trunk rotations: combined in vivo measurement with inertial tracking device and biomechanical modeling. Clin Biomech 29:7, 2014
56. Khoo BC, Goh JC, Lee JM, et al: A comparison of lumbosacral loads during static and dynamic activities. Australas Phys Eng Sci Med 17:55, 1994
57. Schmidt H, Bashkuev M, Dreischarf M, et al: Computational biomechanics of a lumbar motion segment in pure and combined shear loads. J Biomech 46:2513, 2013
58. Bowen V, Cassidy JD: Macroscopic and microscopic anatomy of the sacroiliac joint from embryonic life until the eighth decade. Spine 6:620, 1981
59. Forst SL, Wheeler MT, Fortin DO, et al: The sacroiliac joint: anatomy, physiology and clinical significance. Pain Physician 9:61, 2006
60. Toyohara R, Ohashi T: A literature review of biomechanical studies on physiological and pathological sacroiliac joints: articular surface structure, joint motion, dysfunction and treatments. Clin Biomech 114:106233, 2024, doi: 10.1016/j.clinbiomech.2024.106233
61. Vleeming A, Pool-Goudzwaard A, Hammu-doghlu D, et al: The function of the long dorsal sacroiliac ligament: its implication for understanding low back pain. Spine 21:556, 1996
62. Sturesson B, Uden A, Vleeming A: A radiostereometric analysis of movements of the sacroiliac joints during the standing hip flexion test. Spine 25:364, 2000
63. Goode A, Hegedus EJ, Sizer P, et al: Three-dimensional movements of the sacroiliac joint: a systematic review of the literature and assessment of clinical utility. J Man Manip Ther 16:25, 2008
64. Cibulka MA: The Pelvis and Sacroiliac Joint: Physical Therapy Patient Management Utilizing Current Evidence in Current Concepts of Orthopaedic Physical Therapy. Lacrosse: Orthopaedic Section, American Physical Therapy Association, 2006
65. Kulkarni V, Chandy MJ, Babu KS: Quantitative study of muscle spindles in suboccipital muscles of human foetuses. Neurol India 49:355, 2001
66. Boyd-Clark LC, Briggs CA, Galea MP: Muscle spindle distribution, morphology, and density in longus colli and multifidus muscles of the cervical spine. Spine 27:694, 2002
67. McGill SM, Kippers V: Transfer of loads between lumbar tissues during the flexion-relaxation phenomenon. Spine 19:219, 1994
68. Porterfield J, DeRosa C: Mechanical Low Back Pain: Perspectives in Functional Anatomy (ed 2). Philadelphia, WB Saunders, 1998
69. Bojadsen TW, Silva ES, Rodrigues AJ, et al: Comparative study of multifidi in lumbar and thoracic spine. J Electromyogr Kinesiol: Official Journal of the International Society of Electrophysiological Kinesiology 10:143, 2000
70. Lonnemann ME, Paris SV, Gorniak GC: A morphological comparison of the human lumbar multifidus by chemical dissection. J Man Manip Ther 16:E84, 2008
71. Rosatelli AL, Ravichandiran K, Agur AM: Three-dimensional study of the musculotendinous architecture of lumbar multifidus and its functional implications. Clin Anat 21:539, 2008
72. Richardson CA, Snijders CJ, Hides JA, et al: The relation between the transversus abdominis muscles, sacroiliac joint mechanics, and low back pain. Spine 27:399, 2002
73. Callaghan JP, Gunning JL, McGill SM: The relationship between lumbar spine load and muscle activity during extensor exercises. Phys Ther 78:8, 1998
74. Smith MD, Russell A, Hodges PW: Do incontinence, breathing difficulties, and gastrointestinal symptoms increase the risk of future back pain? J Pain 10:876, 2009
75. Arab AM, Behbahani RB, Lorestani L, et al: Assessment of pelvic floor muscle function in women with and without low back pain using transabdominal ultrasound. Man Ther 15:235, 2010
76. Pool-Goudzwaard A, van Dijke GH, van Gurp M, et al: Contribution of pelvic floor muscles to stiffness of the pelvic ring. Clin Biomech 19:564, 2004

77. Sapsford RR, Hodges PW: Contraction of the pelvic floor muscles during abdominal maneuvers. Arch Phys Med Rehabil 82:1081, 2001
78. Khoddam-Khorasani P, Arjmand N, Shirazi-Adl A: Effect of changes in the lumbar posture in lifting on trunk muscle and spinal loads: a combined in vivo, musculoskeletal, and finite element model study. J Biomech 104:109728
79. El-Rich M, Shirazi-Adl A, Arjmand N: Muscle activity, internal loads, and stability of the human spine in standing postures: combined model and in vivo studies. Spine 29:2633, 2004
80. Gallagher S, Marras WS: Tolerance of the lumbar spine to shear: a review and recommended exposure limits. Clin Biomech 27:973, 2012
81. Wilke HJ, Neef P, Caimi M, et al: New in vivo measurements of pressures in the intervertebral disc in daily life. Spine 24:755, 1999
82. Nachemson A: The load on lumbar disks in different positions of the body. Clin Orthop 45:107, 1966
83. Bazrgari B, Shirazi-Adl A: Spinal stability and role of passive stiffness in dynamic squat and stoop lifts. Comput Methods Biomech Biomed Engin 10:351, 2007
84. Papadakis M, Sapkas G, Papadopoulos EC, et al: Pathophysiology and biomechanics of the aging spine. Open Orthop J 5:335-336, 2011
85. Thompson R, Pearcy M, Downing K, et al: Disc lesions and the mechanics of the intervertebral joint complex. Spine 25:3026, 2000

CHAPTER 5

The Thorax and Chest Wall

Sean Lowers, PT, DPT, CCS | Dan Cerniglia, PT, DPT

CHAPTER OUTLINE

INTRODUCTION 167
STRUCTURE AND FUNCTION OF THE THORAX 167
Structure 167
Structure of the Rib Cage 167
Articulations of the Rib Cage 168
Function 172
Kinematics of the Ribs and Manubriosternum 172
Muscles Associated With the Rib Cage 173
Coordination and Integration of Ventilatory Motions 179
LIFE SPAN AND CLINICAL CONSIDERATIONS 180
Differences Associated With the Neonate 180
Differences Associated With the Elderly 181
Pathological Changes in Structure and Function 181
SUMMARY 183
STUDY QUESTIONS 183
REFERENCES 183

Introduction

Thorax is a term that is used to describe the bones of the rib cage, the fascia and muscles that attach to the rib cage, the visceral organs within the rib cage, and even the skin that covers the rib cage. The **rib cage,** also called the *thoracic cage* or the *bony thorax*, consists of the thoracic vertebrae, the ribs, and the sternum. The rib cage provides a foundation for many of the muscle attachments of the upper extremities, head and vertebral column, and pelvis while also providing protection for the heart, lungs, and viscera. Therefore, there needs to be a certain amount of inherent stability to the thorax. The structure of the rib cage significantly increases the stability of the thoracic spine during flexion/extension, lateral bending, and rotation.[1,2] One of the important functions of the chest wall is its role in ventilation. The process of ventilation, including inhalation/exhalation (inspiration/expiration), depends on the mobility of the rib cage and the ability of the muscles of ventilation to move it.[3]

Structure and Function of the Thorax

Structure

Structure of the Rib Cage

The rib cage forms a closed chain that involves many joints and muscles. The anterior border of the rib cage is the sternum, the lateral borders are the ribs, and the posterior border is formed by the thoracic vertebrae **(Fig. 5–1)**. The superior border of the rib cage is formed by the manubrium of the sternum, the superior borders of the first costal cartilages, and the first ribs with their contiguous first thoracic vertebra. The inferior border of the rib cage is formed by the xiphoid process, the shared costal cartilages of ribs 7 through 10, the inferior portions of the 11th and 12th ribs, and the 12th thoracic vertebra (see Fig. 5–1).

The sternum is an osseous protective plate for the heart and is composed of the **manubrium, body of the sternum,** and **xiphoid process (Fig. 5–2A)**. The manubrium and the body of the sternum form a posteriorly concave angle of approximately 160° **(Fig. 5-2B)**. The xiphoid process often angles posteriorly from the distal end of the body of the sternum and therefore may be difficult to palpate.

There are 12 thoracic vertebrae to which the ribs attach, making up the posterior portion of the rib cage. The ribs articulate with a typical thoracic vertebrae at the body and transverse processes, resulting in six costal articular surfaces, four on the vertebral body (**superior** and **inferior costovertebral facets,** or **demifacets,** on each side), and one **costotransverse facet** on each of the two transverse processes **(Fig. 5–3)**. There are 12 pairs of ribs. As shown in **Figure 5–4**, the ribs are curved flat bones (Fig. 5–4A) that gradually increase in length from rib 1 to rib 7 and then decrease in length from rib 8 to rib 12. The posteriorly located head of each rib articulates with contiguous thoracic vertebral bodies, whereas the costal tubercles of ribs 1 to 10 articulate with the transverse processes of thoracic vertebrae (Fig.5–4B). Anteriorly, ribs 1 to 10 are joined either directly or indirectly to the sternum through their costal cartilages **(Fig. 5–5)**. Ribs 1 through 7 are classified as **vertebrosternal ribs** (or **"true" ribs**) because each rib articulates with both a thoracic vertebra (as previously described) and to the sternum via each rib's respective **costrochondral** and **chondrosternal** joints. Ribs 8, 9, and 10 are classified as **vertebrochondral ribs** (or **"false" ribs**). The costocartilages

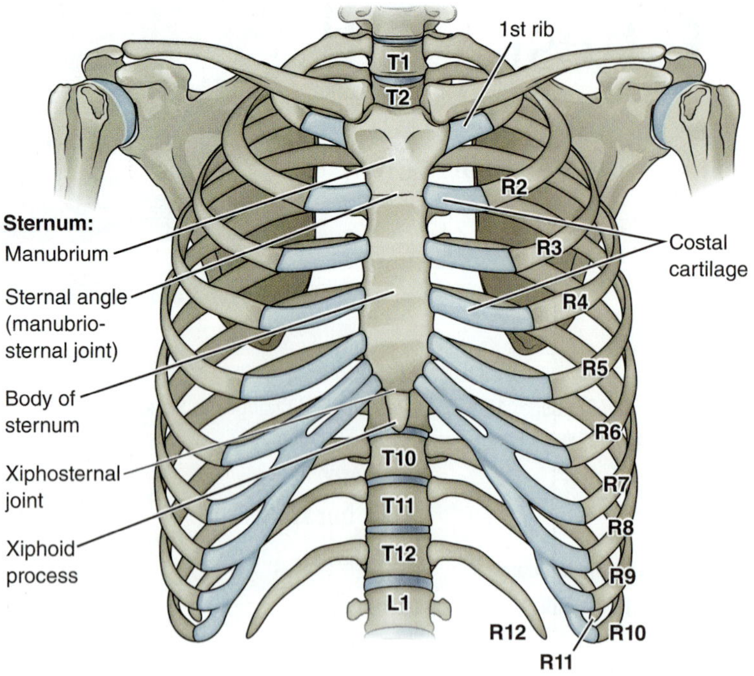

Figure 5–1 Anterior view of the thorax including its component parts: the sternum, 12 pairs of ribs (R1–R12), the costocartilages, and the thoracic vertebrae.

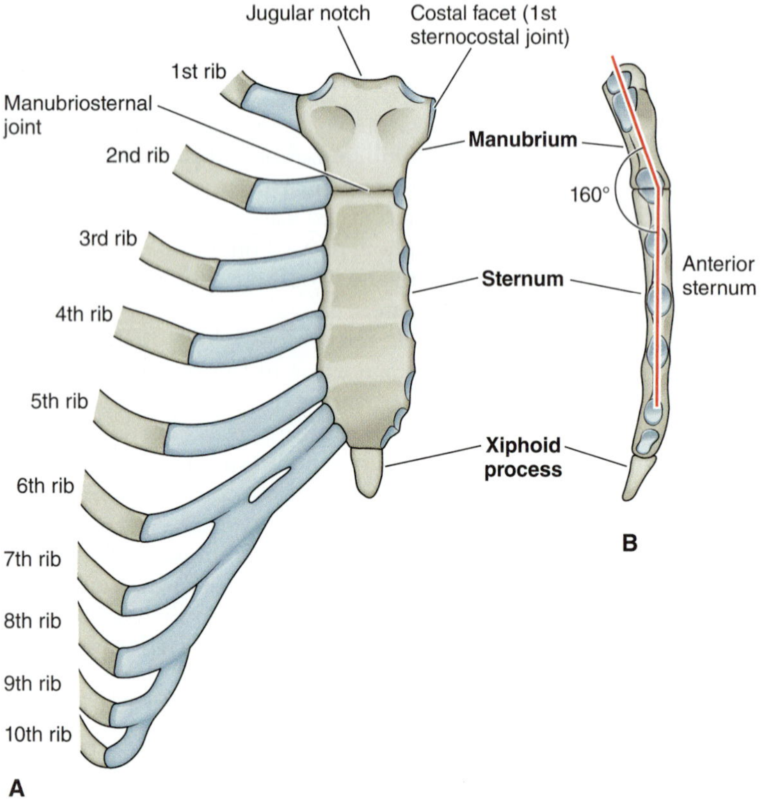

Figure 5–2 The sternum. **A.** The sternum is composed of the manubrium, the body of the sternum, and the xiphoid process. The costal notches of the sternum for the chondrosternal joints are also evident in this anterior view. **B.** Viewed laterally, the dorsal (posterior) concavity of the manubrium and sternum can be appreciated.

of these ribs articulate with the costocartilage of the rib immediately above it, indirectly articulating with the sternum via rib 7. The 11th and 12th ribs are called **vertebral ribs** (or **"floating" ribs**) because they have no attachments to the sternum.

Articulations of the Rib Cage

The articulations that join the bones of the rib cage include the **manubriosternal, xiphisternal,** costovertebral, costotransverse, costochondral, chondrosternal, and the **interchondral joints** (see Fig. 5–5).

MANUBRIOSTERNAL AND XIPHISTERNAL JOINTS

The manubrium and the body of the sternum articulate at the manubriosternal joint. This joint is also known as the *sternal angle* or the *angle of Louis* and is readily palpable as a horizontal ridge at the level of the second ribs' anterior attachments. The manubriosternal joint is a symphysis (cartilaginous) joint with an interposed fibrocartilaginous disc. Ossification of the manubriosternal joint occurs in persons older than 60 years.[4] The xiphoid process joins the inferior aspect of the sternal body at the xiphisternal joint, which is also a symphysis, and tends to ossify by 40 to 45 years of age.[4]

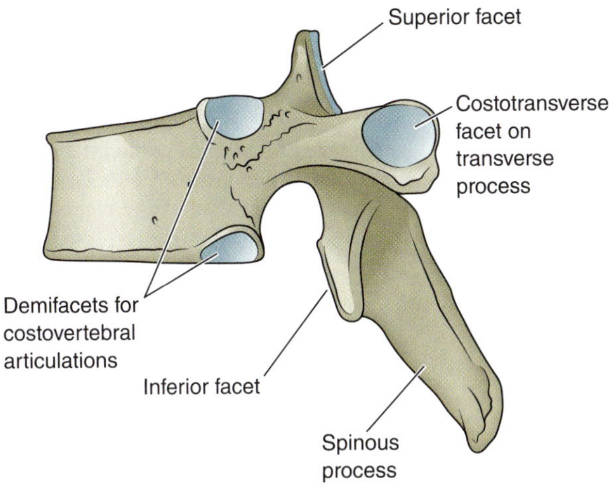

Figure 5–3 The costal facets on the typical thoracic vertebrae are found on the superior and inferior aspects of the posterior body (demifacets for the costovertebral articulations) and on the anterior transverse processes (facets for the costotransverse articulations), as shown in this lateral view.

COSTOVERTEBRAL JOINTS

The typical costovertebral joint is a synovial joint formed by the head of the rib, two adjacent vertebral bodies, and the interposed intervertebral disc (see Fig. 5–4B). Ribs 2 through 9 and their respective thoracic vertebrae (T1–T9) have typical costovertebral joints because the heads of these ribs each have two articular facets, or demifacets. The small, oval, and slightly convex demifacets of the ribs are called the *superior* and *inferior costovertebral facets* (see Fig. 5–4A). Adjacent thoracic vertebrae have facets corresponding to those on the heads of the ribs that articulate with them. The heads of ribs 2 through 9 fit snugly into the surface formed by the adjacent vertebral demifacets and the intervening disc. Each rib's superior facet articulates with the inferior facet of the vertebrae above it. Each rib's inferior facet articulates with the superior facet of its correspondingly numbered vertebrae. For example, the sixth rib's superior facet articulates with the vertebral body above (T5), and the rib's inferior facet articulates with the superior facet of the vertebral body below (T6) (see Fig. 5–4B). Ribs 1, 10, 11, and 12 are atypical ribs because they articulate with only one vertebral body and are numbered by that body. The costovertebral facets of T10 through T12 are located more posteriorly on the pedicle of the vertebra.

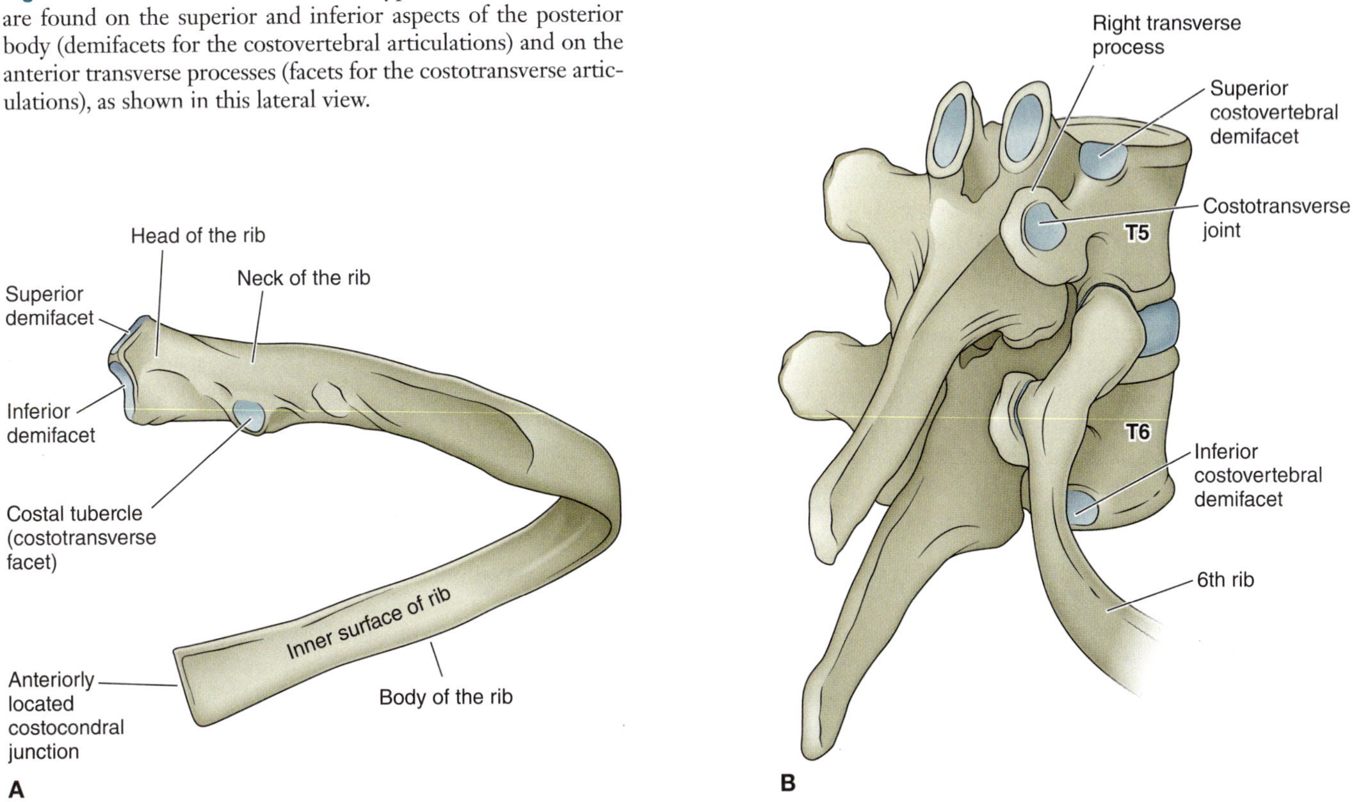

Figure 5–4 Articulation of the ribs with the vertebrae. **A.** A typical rib (ribs 2 through 9) is a curved flat bone. The posteriorly located head of this right sixth rib has superior and inferior facets (also known as *demifacets*) that articulate, respectively, with the right inferior demifacet of T5 and the right superior demifacet of the T6 vertebra to form a single costovertebral joint. **B.** The facet on the costal tubercle of the sixth rib articulates with the transverse process of T6.

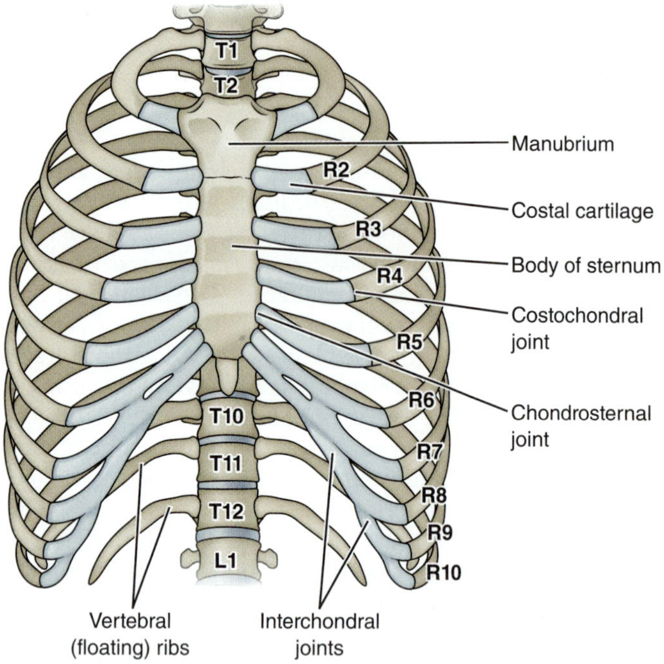

Figure 5–5 This anterior view of the rib cage shows how the ribs articulate with the costal cartilages at the costochondral joints. The costal cartilages of the first through seventh ribs articulate directly with the sternum at the chondrosternal joints. The costal cartilages of the eighth through the tenth ribs articulate indirectly with the sternum through the costal cartilages of the adjacent superior rib at the interchondral joints. Ribs 11 and 12 do not have sternal attachments.

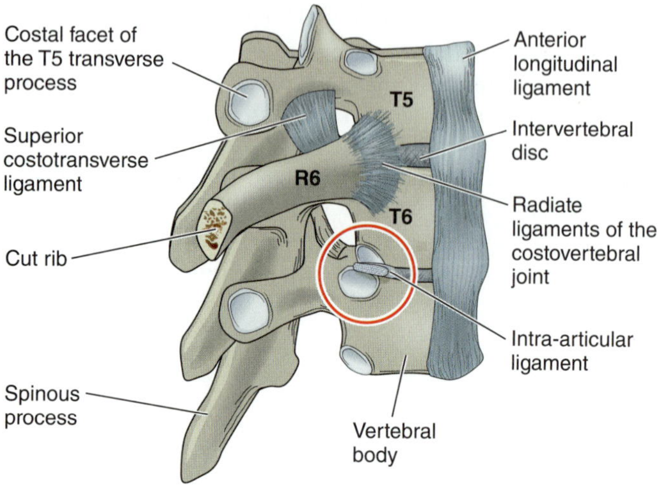

Figure 5–6 A lateral view of the costovertebral joints and ligaments. The radiate ligament reinforces the costovertebral joints. The circled costovertebral joint is shown with the radiate ligament removed to reveal the intra-articular ligament that attaches the head of the rib to the annulus fibrosus.

The typical costovertebral joint is a plane synovial joint with a fibrous capsule surrounding the entire articulation of each costovertebral joint **(Fig. 5–6)**. The joint cavity is divided into two cavities by the intracapsular **interosseous** or **intra-articular ligament.** This ligament extends from the crest of the head of the rib to attach to the anulus fibrosus of the intervertebral disc. The **radiate ligament** is also located within the capsule, with firm attachments to the anterolateral portion of the capsule.

The atypical costovertebral joints of ribs 1, 10, 11, and 12 are more mobile than the other more typical costovertebral joints because the head of these ribs articulates with only one vertebra. The interosseous ligament is absent in these joints; therefore, these each have only one cavity. The radiate ligament is present in these joints. Both rotation and gliding motions occur at each of the costovertebral joints.

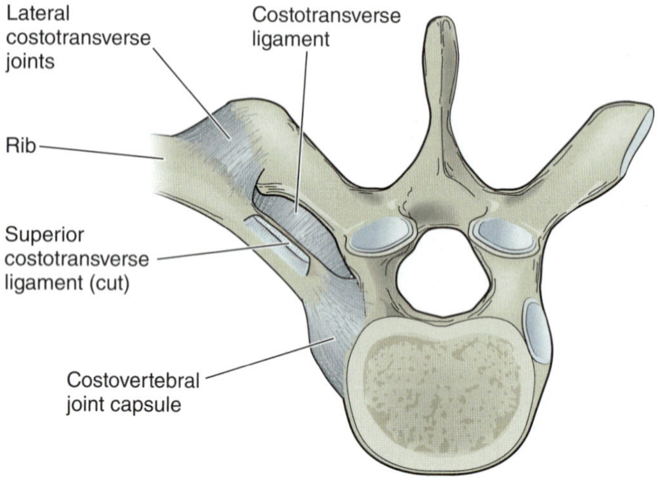

Figure 5–7 A superior view of the bilateral costovertebral and costotransverse joints shows the capsuloligamentous structures of the right side only. The vertically directed superior costotransverse ligament is shown in cross-section because it attaches to the transverse process of the vertebra immediately above.

COSTOTRANSVERSE JOINTS

The costotransverse joints are plane synovial joints formed by the articulation of the costal tubercle of the rib with a costal facet on each transverse process of the corresponding vertebra **(Fig. 5–7)**. There are 10 pairs of costotransverse joints joining vertebrae T1 through T10 with the rib of the same number. The costotransverse joints on T1 through approximately T6 (with some variations) have slightly concave costal facets on the transverse processes of the vertebrae and slightly convex costal tubercles on the corresponding ribs. This allows slight rotation movements between these segments. At the costotransverse joints of approximately T7 through T10, again with some variations, articular surfaces are flat and gliding motions predominate. The transverse processes of T11 and T12 are shorter than the other thoracic vertebrae and do not have facets for articulations with their respective ribs.

The synovial costotransverse joint is surrounded by a thin, fibrous capsule. Three major ligaments support the costotransverse joint capsule. These are the **lateral costotransverse ligament,** the **costotransverse ligament,** and the **superior costotransverse ligament** (see Fig. 5–7). The lateral costotransverse ligament is a short, stout band located between the lateral portion of the costal tubercle and the tip of the corresponding transverse process. The costotransverse ligament is composed of short fibers that run within the costotransverse foramen between the neck of the rib posteriorly and the transverse process at the same level. The superior costotransverse ligament runs from the crest of the neck of the rib to the inferior border of the cephalad transverse process.

COSTOCHONDRAL AND CHONDROSTERNAL JOINTS

The costochondral joints are formed by the articulation of the 1st through 10th ribs anterolaterally with the costal cartilages (see Fig. 5–5). The costochondral joints are cartilaginous synchondroses. The periosteum and the perichondrium are continuous, giving support to the union. The costochondral joints have no ligamentous support and begin to calcify by 35 years of age.[5]

The chondrosternal joints are formed by the articulation of the costal cartilages of ribs 1 through 7 anteriorly with the sternum. These joints also ossify with age. Rib 1 attaches to the lateral facet of the manubrium, rib 2 is attached via two demifacets at the manubriosternal junction, and ribs 3 through 7 articulate with the lateral facets of the sternal body (see Fig. 5-2A). The chondrosternal joints of ribs 1, 6, and 7 are synchondroses, while those of ribs 2 through 5 are synovial joints.

The chondrosternal joints of ribs 2 through 7 (see Fig. 5–5) have capsules that are continuous with the periosteum and support the connection of the cartilage as a whole. Ligamentous support for the capsule includes **anterior** and **posterior radiate costosternal ligaments.** The **sternocostal ligament** is an intra-articular ligament, similar to the intra-articular ligament of the costovertebral joint that divides the two demifacets of the second chondrosternal joint. The **costoxiphoid ligament** connects the anterior and posterior surfaces of the seventh costal cartilage to the front and back of the xiphoid process.

INTERCHONDRAL JOINTS

The costal cartilages of ribs 7 through 10 each articulate with the cartilage immediately above them to form interchondral joints. Thus, ribs 8 through 10 connect only indirectly to the sternum via these interchondral joints (see Fig. 5–5). The interchondral joints are synovial joints and are supported by a capsule and interchondral ligaments. The interchondral articulations, like the chondrosternal joints, tend to fuse with age.

Foundational Concepts 5–1
Summary of the Rib Cage

- Ribs 1 through 10 articulate posteriorly with the vertebral column by two synovial joints (the costovertebral and costotransverse joints) and anteriorly through the costocartilages, either directly or indirectly, to the manubriosternum. The joints of the rib cage form a closed chain in which the segments are interdependent and motion is restricted. These articulations and their associated ligaments give the thoracic cage the stability necessary to protect internal organs and yet provide enough flexibility to maximize function.
- Ribs 11 and 12 have a single costovertebral joint, no costotransverse joint, and no attachment anteriorly to the sternum. These last two ribs form an open chain so that motion of these ribs is less restricted.

Patient Application 5–1

Joanne Mann is a 14-year-old girl who has just been diagnosed with a right thoracic, left lumbar idiopathic scoliosis, a pathological lateral curvature of the spine without a known underlying cause **(Fig. 5–8A)**. As is often the case, Joanne's scoliosis is associated with substantial rotation of the thoracic vertebrae.[6] A right thoracic scoliosis is named for the side of the convexity of the vertebral curve and presents as a left lateral flexion of the thoracic spine. As in Joanne's case, an idiopathic right thoracic curvature is most often accompanied by some degree of left lumbar curvature (lateral flexion of the lumbar vertebrae to the right). Joanne's vertebral rotation, as is typically found in a right thoracic scoliosis, caused the bodies of the vertebrae to rotate to the right (spinous processes rotated to the left), and the right transverse processes of the vertebrae to rotate posteriorly, carrying the right

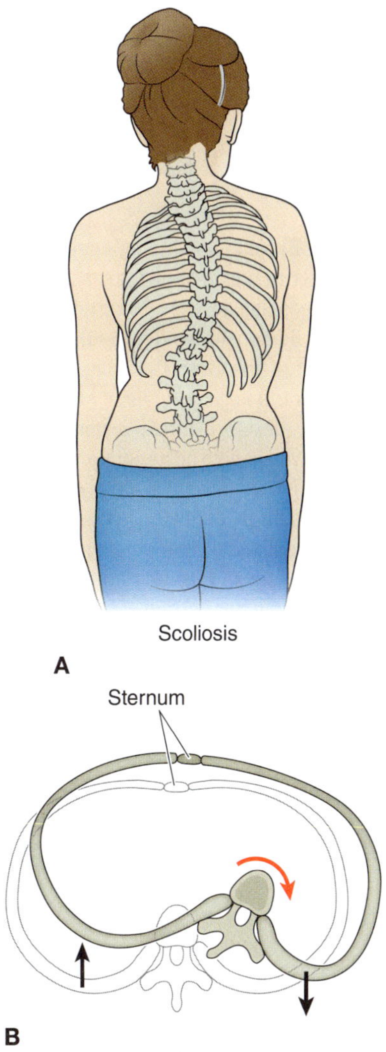

Figure 5–8 **A.** A right thoracic, left lumbar scoliosis (named for the region and side of the convexity) shows the curvature of the vertebrae and the asymmetrical spacing of the ribs (separation on the right and crowding on the left) that results from right rotation of the involved thoracic vertebrae. **B.** The bodies of the thoracic vertebrae in a right thoracic scoliosis typically rotate to the right, resulting in posterior displacement of the right transverse process and the attached right ribs, as well as anterior displacement of the opposite transverse processes and left ribs.

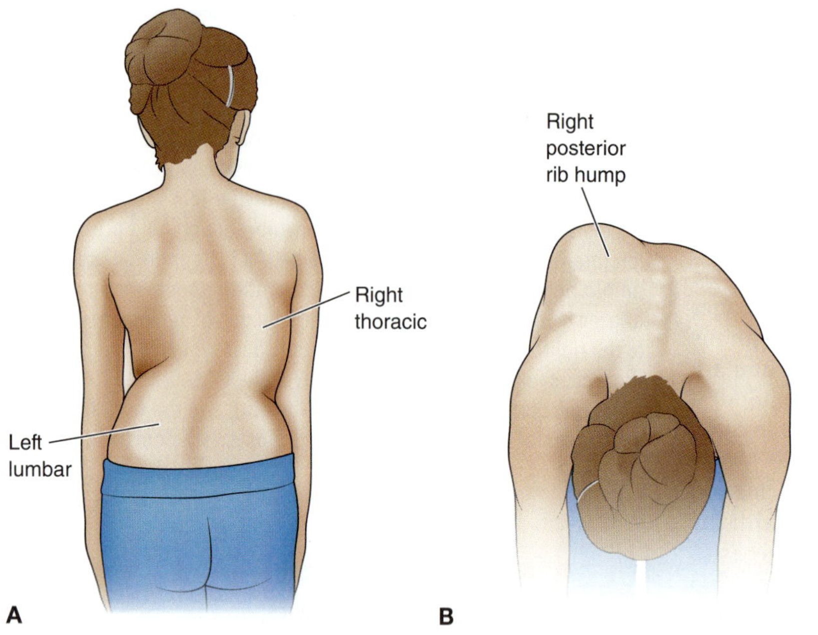

Figure 5–9 Scoliosis. **A.** From a posterior perspective in the upright position, the right thoracic and left lumbar curvature can be seen. **B.** The amount of rib rotation is often not appreciable until the subject does a forward bend.

ribs with them **(Fig. 5-8B)**. Although the amount of lateral curvature and amount of vertebral rotation are not necessarily proportional, the vertebral rotation is responsible for the classic right posterior rib hump of scoliosis that Joanne demonstrates **(Fig. 5–9)**. On the concave side of Joanne's scoliotic curve, the effects are just the opposite. The left transverse processes of the vertebrae move anteriorly, bringing the articulated ribs forward; therefore, the rib distortion that results from the vertebral rotation is evident both posteriorly and anteriorly (although less obvious anteriorly). These musculoskeletal abnormalities limit the range of motion of the rib cage. Given the limitation in rib cage range of motion and the potential distortion in the symmetry of the pleural space, Joanne will be assessed for any impairment to pulmonary function that may result from her current curvature.

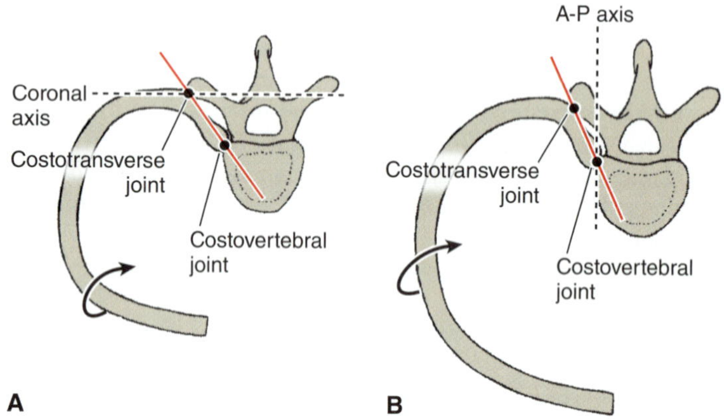

Figure 5–10 A. The common axis of motion for the upper ribs passes through the centers of the costovertebral and costotransverse joints and most closely approximates a coronal axis. **B.** The axis through the costovertebral and costotransverse joints for the lower ribs more closely approximates an A-P axis, with the costovertebral axes for transitional vertebrae 11 and 12 shifting back to approximating a coronal axis.

Function

Kinematics of the Ribs and Manubriosternum

The movements of most of the rib cage are a combination of complex geometrics that are governed by (1) the types and angles of the articulations, (2) the movement of the manubriosternum, and (3) the elasticity of the costal cartilages, given that ribs 1-10 are part of a closed chain.

The costovertebral and costotransverse joints are mechanically linked, with a single axis of motion for elevation and depression passing through the centers of both joints **(Fig. 5–10)**.[3] The length, shape, and downward angle of each rib differ; therefore, the axis of rotation for each rib is slightly different. The axes of rotation for the upper ribs most closely approximate a coronal axis **(Fig. 5–10A)**, allowing the motion of those ribs to occur predominantly in the sagittal plane. The axes of rotation for the lower ribs most closely approximate an anteroposterior (A-P) axis **(Fig. 5–10B)**, allowing the motion of those ribs to be closer to the frontal plane. The axes of rotation for ribs 11 and 12 pass through the costovertebral joint only, because ribs 11 and 12 do not articulate with their associated transverse processes. The axes of rotation for these last two ribs also approximate a coronal axis. The 12 ribs not only articulate with the vertebrae posteriorly but, for most of the ribs, with the costal cartilages anteriorly, forming a closed chain. Movement of ribs posteriorly at the vertebrae also creates movement at the anterior costochondral and chondrosternal joints.

The first ribs differ from the other ribs in that each has: an anterior articulation that is larger and thicker; a costal cartilage that is stiffer; a less mobile cartilaginous (rather than synovial) joint; and lies just inferior and posterior to its respective sternoclavicular joint. For these reasons, there is very little movement of the first rib at its attachment on the manubrium. Posteriorly, the costovertebral joint of the first rib has a single facet, which increases the mobility of that joint. Mobility of the costovertebral joints will be seen to be important in inhalation, in this instance so that the first rib can elevate.

Progressing caudally, ribs 2 through 7 increase in length and mobility. In these ribs, most of the movement occurs at the anterior aspect of the rib, given the nearly coronal axis at the vertebrae. The costocartilages rotate upward, becoming more horizontal with inhalation. The movement of the ribs pushes the sternum anteriorly and superiorly **(Fig. 5–11)**. The manubrium moves less than the body of the sternum because the shortest and least mobile first rib is attached to the manubrium. The increased movement of the body of the sternum in relation to the movement of the manubrium results in slight movement at the manubriosternal joint. The greatest effect of the motion of the upper ribs and sternum is the increase in the A-P diameter of the thorax. This combined rib and sternal motion that occurs in a predominantly sagittal plane has been termed the **"pump-handle" motion** of the thorax (Fig. 5-11).

Elevation of ribs 8 through 10 occurs about an axis of motion lying more toward the sagittal plane. The lower ribs have a more angled shape (downward obliquity increases from rib 1 to rib 10) and an indirect attachment anteriorly to the sternum **(Fig. 5–12)**. These factors allow the lower ribs more motion at the lateral aspect of the rib cage. The greatest effect of the upward rotation and elevation of the lower ribs is the increase in the frontal plane diameter of the lower thorax. This motion that occurs in a more frontal plane has been termed the **"bucket-handle" motion** of the thorax (Fig. 5–12). There is a gradual shift in the orientation of the ribs' axes of motion from cephalad to caudal; therefore, the intermediate ribs function in a transitional zone, with qualities of both pump-handle and bucket-handle types of motion.[7] The 11th and 12th ribs each have only one posterior articulation with a single vertebra and no anterior articulation to the sternum; therefore, they do not participate in the closed-chain motions of the thorax.

Patient Application 5–2

Henry Olsson is an 82-year-old man who recently had a serious fall at home. He missed the last step leading to his driveway and fell sideways into the fender of his car. He experienced immediate severe pain in his ribs and was having problems breathing. In the emergency department, Henry was told that he broke several ribs in several places, resulting in a flail chest with a pulmonary contusion **(Fig. 5–13)**. When Henry tried to take a breath in, the broken segment of ribs that was detached from the rest of the rib cage by the fractures actually went inward rather than outward as one might expect **(Fig. 5–13A)**. During typical inhalation, the ventilatory muscles pull the chest wall anteriorly and superiorly; this increase in thoracic volume causes a resultant *drop in intrapulmonary pressure* that pulls air into the lungs. Henry's flail segment, without its usual connections, was "sucked" inward by that subatmospheric pressure **(Fig. 5–13B)**. During exhalation when the rib cage ordinarily drops back down, Henry's decreased thoracic volume *increased the intrapulmonary pressure*, which forced the flail section outward **(Fig. 5–13C)**. This paradoxical motion of the flail segment was the result of the disruption of the closed chain. Henry was admitted to the hospital for management of his ventilatory dysfunction.

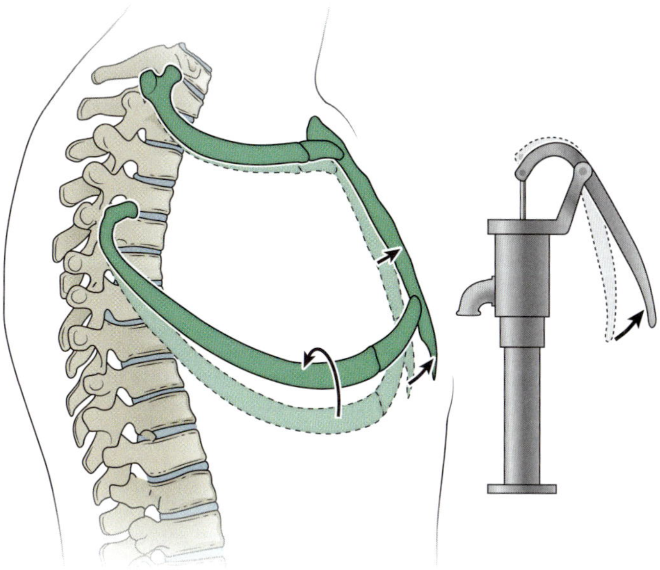

Figure 5–11 Elevation of the upper ribs at the costovertebral and costotransverse joints results in anterior and superior movement of the sternum (and accompanying torsion of the costal cartilages) as well as an increased anteroposterior diameter of the thorax. This rib motion is referred to as the "pump-handle" motion of the thorax.

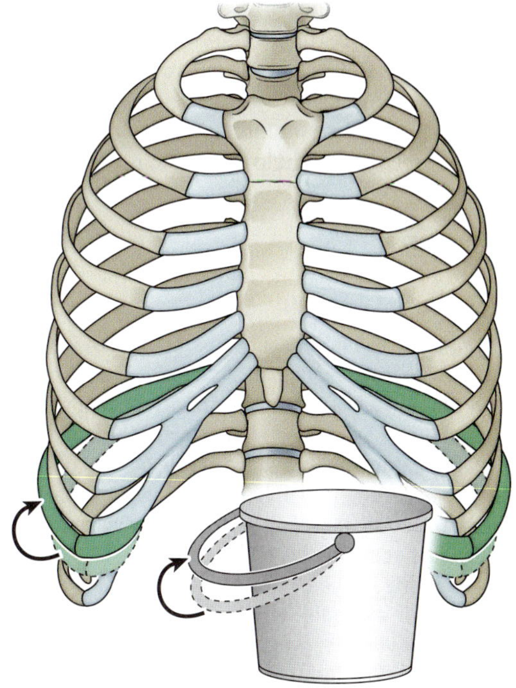

Figure 5–12 Elevation of the lower ribs at the costovertebral and costotransverse joints results in a lateral motion of the rib cage, referred to as "bucket-handle" motion of the thorax.

Muscles Associated With the Rib Cage

The muscles that act on the rib cage are generally referred to as **muscles of ventilation.** The ventilatory muscles are striated skeletal muscles that differ from other skeletal

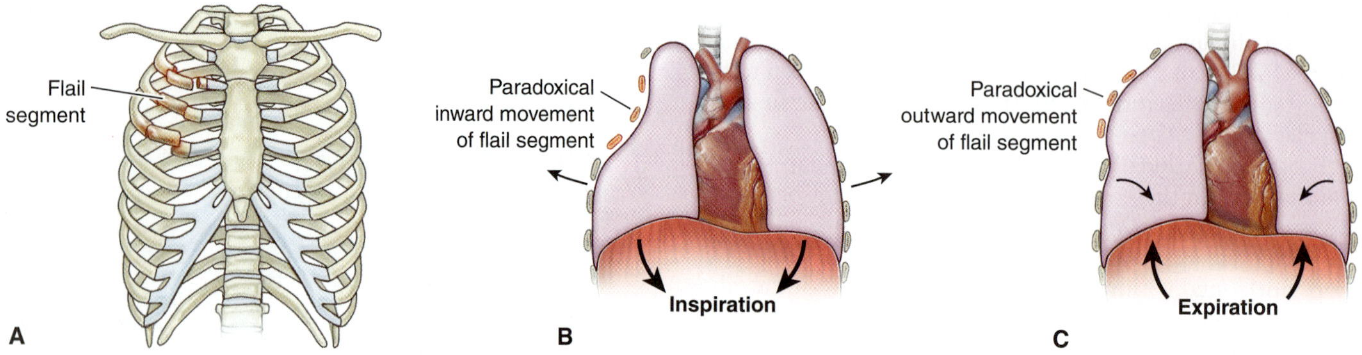

Figure 5–13 **A.** A flail chest results from the fracture of two or more ribs in two or more places. The flail segment is no longer attached to the rest of the thorax, disrupting the closed chain action of the ribs. **B.** During inspiration, the ribs are lifting up and out while the flail segment is pulled inward. **C.** During expiration, the ribs are moving down and in while the flail segment moves outward.

muscles in a number of ways: (1) they have increased fatigue resistance and greater oxidative capacity; (2) they contract rhythmically throughout life rather than episodically; (3) they work primarily against the elastic properties of the lungs and airway resistance rather than against gravitational and other external forces; (4) neurological control of these muscles is both voluntary and involuntary; and (5) the actions of these muscles are life sustaining.

Any muscle that attaches to the chest wall has the potential to contribute to ventilation. The recruitment of muscles for ventilation is related to the type of breathing being performed.[8-10] In breathing at rest, only the primary inspiratory muscles are needed for ventilation. During the active or forced breathing that occurs, for example, with increased activity or pulmonary pathologies, accessory muscles of both inhalation and exhalation are recruited to help meet the increased demand for ventilation.

Foundational Concepts 5–2
Measures of Lung Volume and Capacity

All the air that is housed in the lungs can be divided into four segments. **Tidal volume** is the amount of air that is moved in or out of the thorax during a breath while at rest. **Inspiratory reserve volume** is the amount of air that can be inhaled after a resting breath has already been inhaled. **Expiratory reserve volume** is the amount of air that can be exhaled after a resting breath has already been exhaled. Finally, **residual volume** is the amount of air that cannot be voluntarily exhaled no matter how hard someone tries.

The term **capacity** is used when two or more lung volumes are added together. For example, **vital capacity** is a combination of inspiratory reserve volume, tidal volume, and expiratory reserve volume. Vital capacity is the volume of air that can be blown out of the lungs from a full inhalation to a full exhalation. **Inspiratory capacity** is a combination of inspiratory reserve volume and tidal volume; it is the volume of air that can be breathed in from resting exhalation. **Functional residual capacity** is a combination of expiratory reserve volume and reserve volume; it is the volume of air that remains in the lungs after an exhalation at rest. Total lung capacity is a combination of all four lung volumes. Table 5–1 summarizes the definitions graphically.

Table 5–1 Lung Volumes and Lung Capacities

<table>
<tr><th>LUNG VOLUMES</th><th colspan="3">LUNG CAPACITIES</th></tr>
<tr><td>Inspiratory reserve volume (IRV)</td><td rowspan="3">Vital capacity (VC)</td><td rowspan="2">Inspiratory capacity (IC)</td><td rowspan="4">Total lung capacity (TLC)</td></tr>
<tr><td>Tidal volume (TV)</td></tr>
<tr><td>Expiratory reserve volume (ERV)</td><td rowspan="2">Functional residual capacity (FRC)</td></tr>
<tr><td>Residual volume (RV)</td><td></td></tr>
</table>

The ventilatory muscles can be classified as either **primary** or **accessory muscles of ventilation.** A muscle's action during the ventilatory cycle is neither simple nor absolute, which makes the categorizing of ventilatory muscles as either inspiratory muscles or expiratory muscles inaccurate and misleading.

PRIMARY MUSCLES OF VENTILATION

The primary muscles of ventilation are those recruited for ventilation at rest. These include the **diaphragm,** the **intercostal muscles** (particularly the **parasternal muscles** and some of the **external intercostals**), and the **scalene muscles.**[8,10] These muscles all act on the rib cage to promote inhalation. There are no primary muscles for exhalation at rest because it is a passive function.

Diaphragm

The diaphragm is the primary muscle of ventilation, accounting for approximately 70% to 80% of inhalation force during breathing at rest.[10] The diaphragm **(Fig. 5–14)** is composed of a circular set of muscle fibers that arise from the sternum, ribs, and vertebral bodies. The fibers travel cephalad (superiorly) from their origin to insert into a **central tendon.**[11] There is no bony insertion site, making the diaphragm unique. The boomerang-shaped central tendon of the diaphragm forms the top of the domes of the right and left hemidiaphragms. Functionally, the muscular portion of the diaphragm is divided

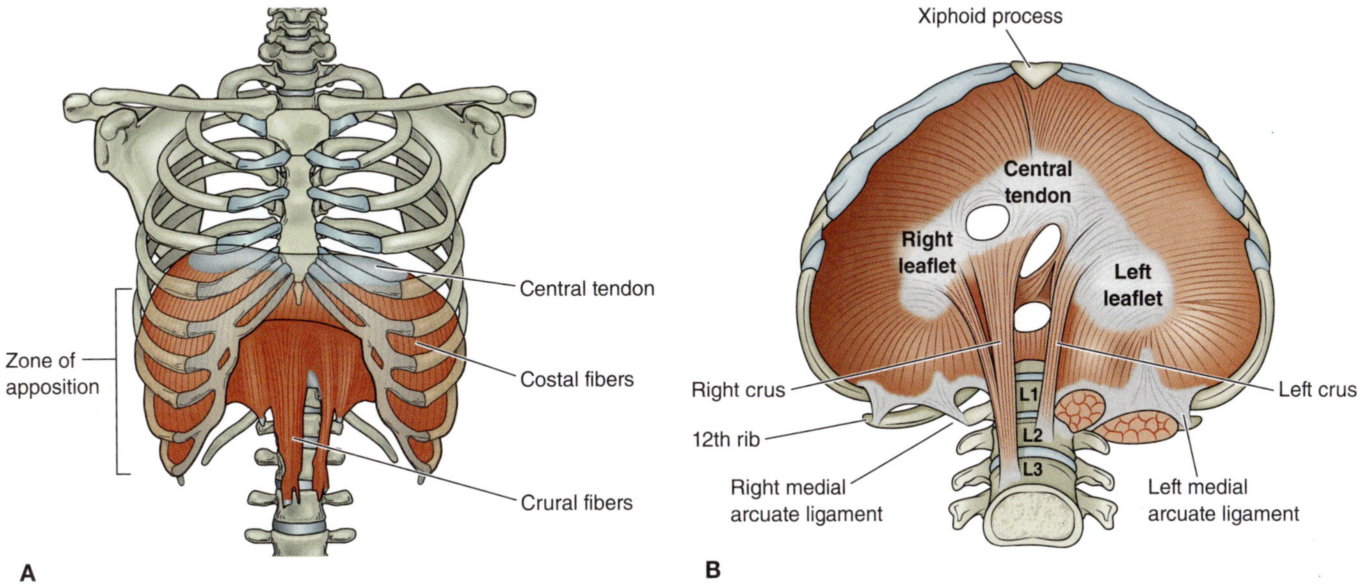

Figure 5–14 **A.** In an anterior view, the fibers of the diaphragm can be seen arising from the sternum, costocartilages, and ribs (costal fibers) and from the vertebral bodies (crural fibers). The costal fibers run vertically upward from their origin in close apposition to the rib cage and then curve and become more horizontal before inserting into the central tendon. **B.** An inferior view of the diaphragm shows the leaflets of the central tendon, the right crus, left crus, and the medial and lateral arcuate ligaments bilaterally.

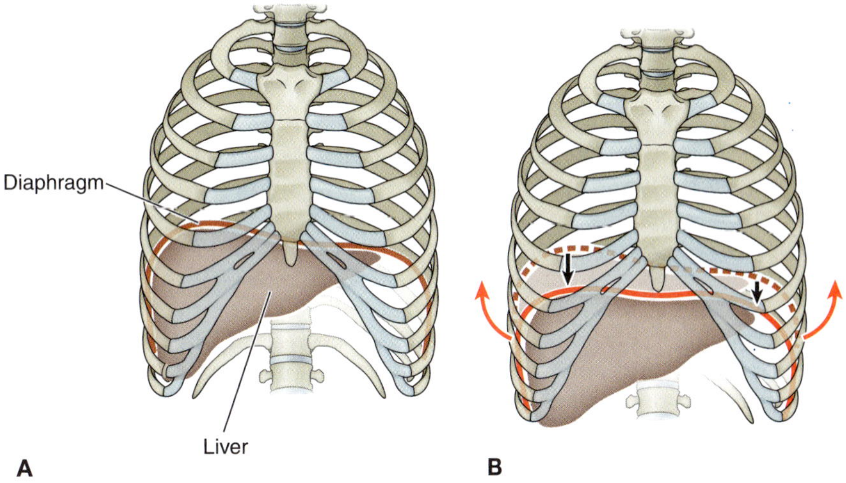

Figure 5–15 Tidal breathing. **A.** Before a new inhalation is initiated, the diaphragm is domed. **B.** During inhalation, the diaphragm contracts, the dome descends from its resting position, compressing the abdominal contents. The resulting increase in intra-abdominal pressure limits further descent of (i.e., stabilizes) the central tendon of the diaphragm so that continued contraction of the costal fibers of the diaphragm on the stabilized central tendon results in expansion (bucket-handle motion) of the lower ribs.

into posterior and anterior segments. The anterior segment, called the **costal fibers,** arises from the sternum and ribs. The posterior segment of the diaphragm, termed the **crural fibers,** arises from the vertebral bodies **(Fig. 5–14A)**.[12]

The costal fibers of the diaphragm originate from muscular slips attached to the posterior aspect of the xiphoid process, the inner surfaces of the lower six ribs, and the costal cartilages of those ribs. The costal fibers of the diaphragm run vertically from their origin, in close apposition to the rib cage, and then curve to become more horizontal before inserting into the central tendon. The vertically traveling costal fibers of the diaphragm, which lie close to the inner wall of the lower rib cage, form a functional unit called the **zone of apposition** (see Fig. 5–14A).[12]

The crural fibers of the diaphragm originate from two musculotendinous structures called the **right** and **left crus,** and from the right and left aponeurotic **medial and lateral arcuate ligaments (Fig. 5–14B)**. The musculotendinous right and left crus arise from the L1 to L3 vertebrae. These structures pass anteriorly and medially, joining together to form an arch just anterior to the aorta. The medial arcuate ligament extends from L1 or L2, covers the psoas muscles, and returns to the transverse processes of L1, L2, or L3. The lateral arcuate ligament extends from the transverse process of L1, L2, and L3, arches up and over the quadratus lumborum muscles, and returns to the caudal margin of the 12th rib.[13]

During **tidal breathing (Fig. 5–15)**, the fibers in the zone of apposition of the diaphragm contract, causing a descent

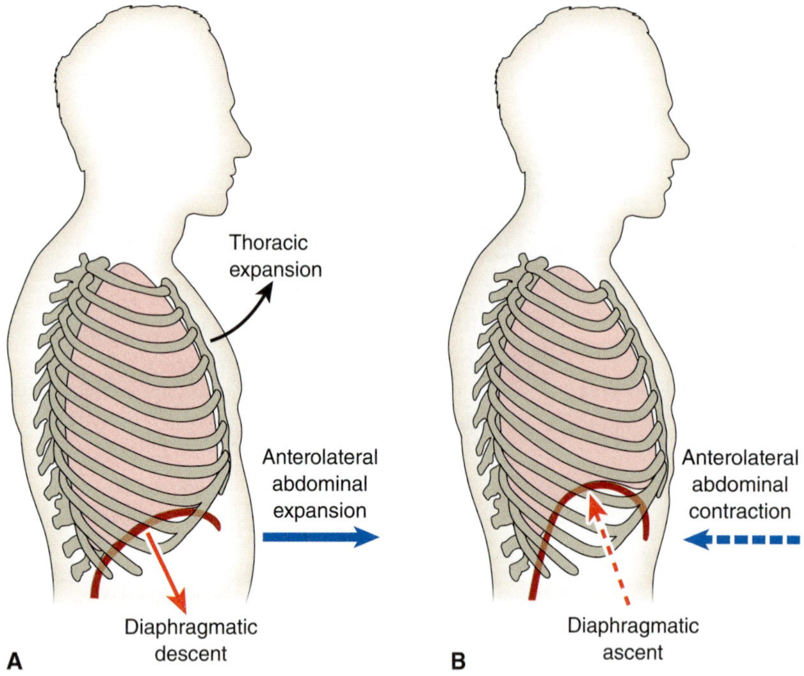

Figure 5–16 Quiet inspiration and expiration. **A.** With quiet inspiration, the typical thoracoabdominal movement is caused by contraction of the diaphragm. The diaphragm descends, increasing thoracic size and displacing the abdominal viscera anteriorly and laterally. **B.** With passive exhalation, the thorax decreases in size, and the abdominal viscera return to their resting position.

(but only a slight change in contour) of the dome of the diaphragm. As the dome descends, the abdominal contents are compressed, which increases the intra-abdominal pressure.[12] The compressed abdominal contents stabilize the central tendon of the diaphragm so that a continued contraction of the costal fibers of the diaphragm against the stabilized central tendon cause the lower ribs to lift and rotate outwardly in the bucket-handle motion (see Fig. 5–12).[14]

The crural fibers of the diaphragm have an inspiratory effect on the central tendon of the diaphragm, but, unlike the costal fibers, a less direct effect on the lower rib cage.[3,12] The action of the crural fibers of the diaphragm results in descending of the central tendon that increases intra-abdominal pressure. This increased pressure is transmitted across the apposed diaphragm to help the costal fibers of the diaphragm expand the lower rib cage.[3,12]

The thoracoabdominal movement during resting inhalation is a result of the pressures that are generated by the contraction of the diaphragm **(Fig. 5–16)**. When the diaphragm contracts and the central tendon descends, there is an increase in volume within the thorax and a resultant decreased intrapulmonary pressure that is responsible for air entering the thorax, that is, inhalation. There is also an increase in abdominal pressure, causing the abdominal contents to be displaced anteriorly and laterally **(Fig. 5–16A)**. The abdominal muscles may be active, when standing or sitting, to offer some counterbalance to this increase in abdominal pressure.[14] When active muscle contraction of the diaphragm ceases, the domes return to their higher resting position within the thorax; the thoracic volume decreases, intrapulmonary pressure increases, and, as a result, exhalation occurs. The abdominal contents return to their starting position **(Fig. 5–16B)**.

Expanded Concepts 5–1
Abdominal Compliance

Compliance (inverse of stiffness) is a measurement of the extensibility or distensibility of a structure or system. During diaphragm contraction, the abdominal cavity becomes the fulcrum for lateral expansion of the rib cage. Therefore, compliance of the abdomen is a factor in the inspiratory movement of the thorax.

$$\text{Thoracic compliance} = \Delta\,\text{volume}/\Delta\,\text{pressure}$$

Thoracic compliance = change in volume per unit of pressure

Patient Application 5–3

Hannah Rosen is a 16-year-old girl who sustained a C6 complete spinal cord injury when she dove into a pond and hit her head on a submerged tree trunk. Hannah's abdominal musculature is no longer innervated because all muscular function below the level of cervical injury was lost. Although Hannah's diaphragm is fully innervated and functioning, her pulmonary function is still impaired compared with other individuals her age.

When an individual sustains a spinal cord injury at or above the midthoracic level, loss of innervation to the intercostal and abdominal musculature affects the process of ventilation in many ways. The loss of abdominal musculature affects the function of the intact diaphragm in both inhalation and exhalation. Without intact abdominal musculature, there is increased compliance (distensibility) of the abdomen. Without the ability of the abdominal muscles to control anterior displacement of the abdominal contents, the central tendon of the diaphragm will not stabilize against the abdominal viscera, and the costal fibers of the diaphragm cannot lift the lower ribs upward and outward. The ability to inhale, as measured by vital capacity, is decreased. One strategy to help Hannah optimize her diaphragmatic function is to have her wear an elastic abdominal binder when she is sitting. The abdominal binder will replace some of the resistance to expansion that the abdominal muscles previously provided. Reducing excessive compliance facilitates improved, although not normalized, stabilization of the central tendon of the diaphragm, allowing the costal fibers to act on the lower ribs during inhalation.

Patient Application 5–4

Brittany Ludke is a 22-year-old woman in her eighth month of pregnancy. She is now noticing that she is getting a bit short of breath when she negotiates her usual two flights of stairs to her office at work. She assumed that it was due to her weight gain, but her obstetrician told her that her shortness of breath had more to do with the increased size of the fetus. The obstetrician explained that the presence of the growing baby decreased compliance of her abdomen, limiting the caudal diaphragmatic excursion in inhalation. The presence of the fetus stabilizes the diaphragm earlier in the ventilatory cycle and causes earlier lateral and upward motion of the lower rib cage during inhalation. These changes can limit Brittany's vital capacity she would usually tap into with increased exertion. The weight that Brittany gained with the baby's recent growth increased her ventilatory challenge as she ascends stairs while, at the same time, her ability to meet that challenge has been reduced.

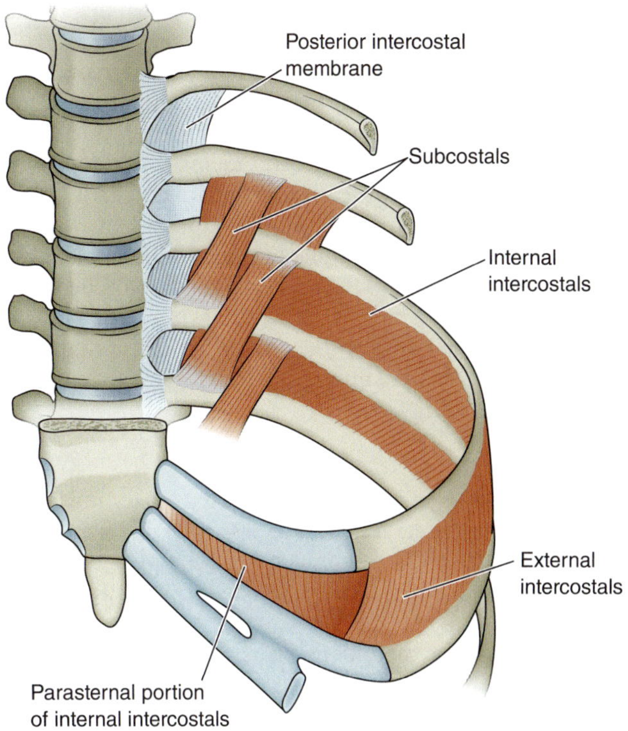

Figure 5–17 Intercostal muscles.

Intercostal Muscles

The **internal intercostal, external intercostal,** and **subcostal** muscles **(Fig. 5–17)** connect adjacent ribs to each other and are named according to their anatomic orientation and location. The internal intercostal muscles arise from the inner surfaces of ribs 1 through 11 and insert into the rib below. The fibers of the internal intercostal muscles lie deep to the external intercostal muscles and run caudally and posteriorly. The internal intercostals begin anteriorly at the chondrosternal junctions and continue posteriorly to the angles of the ribs, where they become an aponeurotic layer called the **posterior intercostal membrane.**

The external intercostal muscles originate on ribs 1 through 11 and insert into the rib below. The fibers are more superficial to the rib cage and run caudally and anteriorly at an oblique angle to the internal intercostal muscles (see Fig. 5–17).[15] The external intercostal muscles begin posteriorly at the tubercles of the ribs and extend anteriorly to the costochondral junctions, where they form the **anterior intercostal membrane.**[15]

Only the internal intercostal muscles are present anteriorly from the chondrosternal junctions to the costochondral joints. These are the segments of the internal intercostal muscles that are referred to as the **parasternal muscles** (see Fig. 5–17) and are found mainly in the first through fifth intercostal spaces.[15] There are only external intercostal muscles present posteriorly from the tubercle to the angle of the ribs. On the lateral rib cage, both internal and external intercostal muscle layers are present and may be referred to in this location as the **interosseous** or **lateral intercostal muscles.**[15]

The subcostal muscles (see Fig. 5–17) are also intercostal muscles, but they are generally found only in the posterior lower rib cage. The subcostal muscles originate at the rib angles and may span more than one intercostal space before inserting into the inner surface of a caudal rib. Their fiber directions are similar to those of the internal intercostal muscles.

The function of the intercostal muscles during ventilation is not as simple as once thought. The accepted idea that the external intercostal muscles are active during inhalation and the internal intercostal muscles are active during exhalation is not completely accurate. Both sets of intercostal muscles have been shown to be active during both phases of ventilation depending on the type of breathing and the neural recruitment of muscles.[15] Activation of the external intercostals and the parasternals (the anterior portion of the internal intercostals) has an inspiratory effect on the rib cage. The action of the parasternal muscles appears at every interspace to be a rotation of the costosternal junctions, resulting in elevation of the ribs and sternum as well as anterior movement of the sternum.[16] Another function of the parasternal muscles seems to be the stabilization of the rib cage.[17,18] This stabilizing action of the parasternal muscles opposes the decreased intrapulmonary pressure generated during diaphragmatic contraction (inhalation), preventing a paradoxical, or inward, movement of the upper chest wall during inhalation.[19]

Activity of the external intercostals, although minimal during breathing at rest, increases with increasing ventilation.[20] The external intercostals in the posterior and superior thorax have an inspiratory effect, although this inspiratory effort diminishes gradually as you move lower and anterior toward the middle of the rib cage. By the anterior lowest intercostal interspaces, the ventilatory effect of the external intercostals has changed to an expiratory effect.[16]

The internal intercostals, throughout all interspaces but especially the more caudal portions, have an expiratory effect.[16]

The function of the lateral portion of the internal and external intercostal muscles involves mainly trunk rotation.[16] The lateral intercostal muscles have a relatively small amount of activity in the ventilatory cycle in comparison with the parasternal muscles and the diaphragm.[21] The major role of the lateral intercostal muscles is in axial rotation of the thorax, with the contralateral internal and external intercostal muscles working synergistically to produce trunk rotation (e.g., right external and left internal intercostal muscles are active during trunk rotation to the left).[21]

Scalene Muscles

The scalene muscles are also considered primary muscles of ventilation at rest.[8] The scalene muscles attach to the transverse processes of C3 to C7 and descend to the upper borders of the first rib (anterior scalene and medial scalene) and second rib (posterior scalene) **(Fig. 5–18)**.

Their action lifts the first two ribs, and therefore the sternum, in the pump-handle motion of the upper rib cage (see Fig. 5–11).[22] Activity of the scalene muscles begins at the onset of inhalation and increases as inhalation gets closer to total lung capacity. The length-tension relationship of the scalene muscles allows them to generate a greater force late into the ventilatory cycle when the force from the diaphragm is decreasing. The scalene muscles also function as stabilizers of the rib cage. The scalene muscles, along with the parasternal muscles, counteract the potential paradoxical movement of the

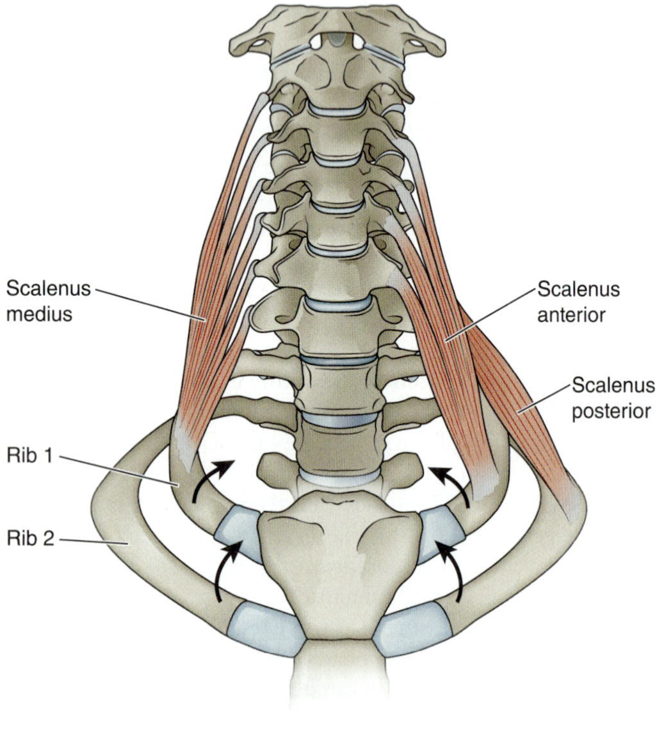

Figure 5–18 The scalenus anterior, scalenus medius, and scalenus posterior. Their action lifts the sternum and the first two ribs in the pump-handle motion.

upper chest caused by a decrease in intrapulmonary pressure created by the diaphragm's contraction.

Posteriorly, the fibers of the **levatores costae** run from the transverse processes of vertebrae C7 through T11 to the posterior external surface of the next lower rib between its tubercle and the angle and can assist with elevation of the upper ribs during inhalation.[23]

ACCESSORY MUSCLES OF VENTILATION

The muscles that attach the rib cage to the shoulder girdle, head, vertebral column, or pelvis may be classified as accessory muscles of ventilation. These muscles assist with inhalation or exhalation in situations of stress, such as increased activity or disease.

When the thorax is stabilized, the accessory muscles of ventilation move the vertebral column, arm, head, or pelvis on the trunk. During times of increased ventilatory demand, the rib cage can become the mobile segment for these muscles. The accessory muscles of inhalation, therefore, can increase the thoracic diameter by moving the rib cage upward and outward. The accessory muscles of exhalation move the diaphragm upward and the thorax downward and inward. The most commonly described accessory muscles are shown in **Figure 5–19** and are discussed in the following paragraphs.

The **sternocleidomastoid** muscle runs from the manubrium and superior medial aspect of the clavicle to the mastoid process of the temporal bone. The usual bilateral action of the sternocleidomastoid is flexion of the cervical spine. With the help of the **trapezius** muscle to stabilize the head, the bilateral action of the sternocleidomastoid muscles can pull the rib cage superiorly, expanding the upper rib cage in the pump-handle motion. The recruitment of this muscle seems to occur toward the end of maximal inhalation.[24]

The sternocostal (sternal) portion of the **pectoralis major** muscle can elevate the upper rib cage rather than act on the humerus when the humerus is stabilized. The clavicular head of the pectoralis major can be either inspiratory or expiratory in action, depending on the position of the humerus. When the arms are positioned so that the humeral attachment of the pectoralis major is below the level of the clavicle (arms below horizontal), the clavicular portion acts as an expiratory muscle by pulling the manubrium and upper ribs downward. When the humeral attachment of the pectoralis major is above the level of the clavicle (arms above horizontal), the muscle becomes an inspiratory muscle by pulling the manubrium and upper ribs up and out. The **pectoralis minor** can help elevate the third, fourth, and fifth ribs during active inhalation. The **subclavius,** a small muscle between the clavicle and the first rib, can also assist in raising the upper chest for inhalation.

The **serratus posterior superior** and **serratus posterior inferior** are located on the posterior thorax with attachments from cervical and thoracic spinous processes to the ribs (therefore they are not seen in Fig. 5–19). These muscles have been assumed to be accessory muscles of ventilation based largely on their attachments to the ribs. There is no evidence to support a ventilatory role for these muscles and they should not, at present, be considered to have a ventilatory function.[25,26]

The abdominal muscles include the **rectus abdominis, external oblique abdominis, internal oblique abdominis,** and **transversus abdominis** (deep to the other abdominals

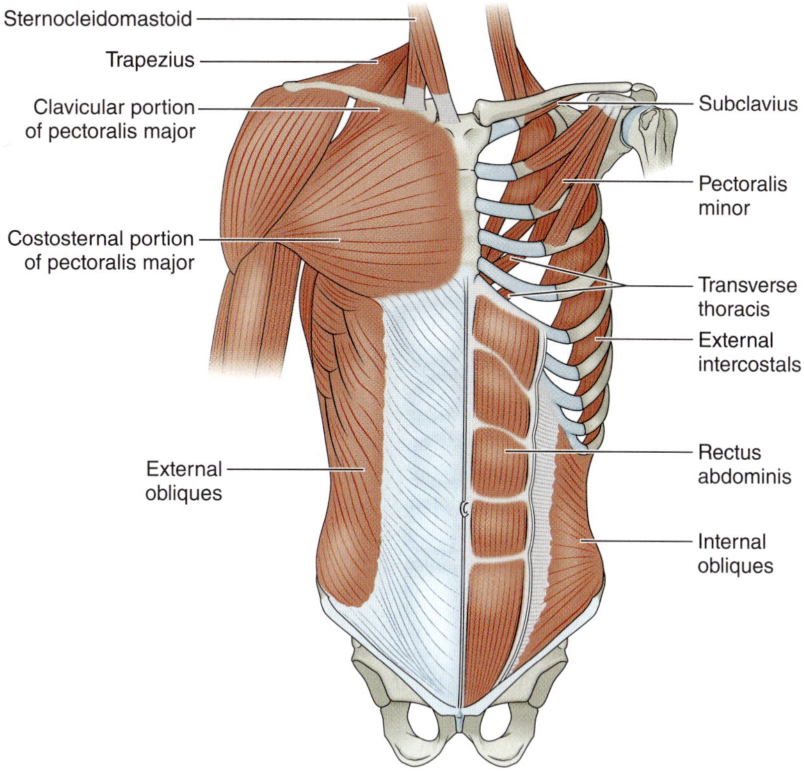

Figure 5–19 Accessory muscles of ventilation are those used during times of increased ventilatory demand. The right side of the figure shows some of the anterior superficial muscles of the thorax that can be accessory muscles of ventilation, and the left side of the thorax shows the deeper accessory muscles of ventilation.

so they are not shown in Fig. 5–19). The abdominals are also accessory muscles of ventilation as well as trunk flexors and rotators. The major function of the abdominal muscles in ventilation is to assist with forced exhalation. The muscle fibers pull the ribs and their associated costocartilage caudally, into a motion of exhalation. By increasing intra-abdominal pressure, the abdominal muscles can force the diaphragm upward into the thoracic cage, decreasing the thoracic volume, but increasing the thoracic pressure and speed of exhalation.

Although usually considered accessory muscles of exhalation, the abdominal muscles play two significant roles during inhalation. First, the increased abdominal pressure created by the lowering of the diaphragm in inhalation must be countered by tension in the abdominal musculature. Abdominal tension reduces abdominal compliance, allowing the central tendon of the diaphragm to stabilize so that the stabilized diaphragm can produce lateral chest wall expansion. Secondly, the increased intra-abdominal pressure created by active abdominal muscles during forced exhalation pushes the diaphragm cranially and exerts a passive stretch on the costal fibers of the diaphragm.[3] These changes prepare the ventilation system for the next inhalation by optimizing the length-tension relationship of the muscle fibers of the diaphragm. During periods of increased ventilatory needs, the increased muscular activity of the abdominal muscles assists in both exhalation and inhalation.[3,11]

The **transversus thoracis (triangularis sterni)** muscles comprise a flat layer of muscle that runs deep to the parasternal muscles. The transversus thoracis muscles originate from the posterior surface of the lower sternum and run cranially and laterally, inserting into the costal cartilages of ribs 3 through 7.[3] These muscles are recruited, along with the abdominal muscles, to pull the rib cage caudally. The mechanical advantage of the transverses thoracis is greater farther down the rib cage.[15] Studies have shown that these muscles are primarily expiratory muscles, especially when exhalation is active—as in talking, coughing, or laughing—or in forced exhalation into functional residual capacity.[27,28]

Gravity acts as an accessory force for ventilation in the supine position. Gravity, acting on the abdominal viscera, performs the same function as the abdominal musculature in stabilizing the central tendon of the diaphragm. In fact, in the supine position, the abdominal muscles and the trangularis sterni are silent on the electromyographic monitoring during breathing at rest.[27,28]

Coordination and Integration of Ventilatory Motions

The coordination and integration of the skeletal and muscular chest wall components during breathing are complex, given the changes in how muscles may contribute under different conditions. The recruitment of ventilatory muscles is also dependent on the activities in which a person is participating (there is a different recruitment pattern when a person is at rest than during activity), whether the body is upright against gravity or lying supine, whether the person is stationary or locomoting, and whether the person is phonating or not. Additionally, recruitment can change with disorders of the chest wall, the lung parenchyma, or the neuromuscular system.[22,23,29-31] A high and complex level of coordination is necessary for the primary and accessory muscles of ventilation to perform the necessary functions of ventilation.

Foundational Concepts 5–3
Summary of the Ventilatory Sequence During Breathing

Although the coordinated function and sequence of breathing are complex when activities are combined, the following sequence of motions and muscle actions is typical of a healthy person at rest.

- The diaphragm contracts and the central tendon moves caudally.
- The parasternal, external intercostals, and scalene muscles elevate the ribs and move the sternum anteriorly and superiorly. The muscles also stabilize the anterior upper chest wall to prevent a paradoxical inward movement caused by the decreasing intrapulmonary pressure.
- As intra-abdominal pressure increases, the abdominal contents are displaced so that the anterior epigastric abdominal wall is pushed anteriorly. Further outward motion of the abdominal wall is countered by tension in the abdominal musculature that allows the central tendon to stabilize on the abdominal viscera.
- With continued shortening of the appositional (costal) fibers of the diaphragm, the lower ribs are pulled cephalad and laterally, resulting in the bucket-handle movement of the lower ribs.
- With continued inhalation, the parasternal, scalene, and levatores costarum muscles actively rotate the upper ribs and elevate the manubriosternum, which results in an anterior (pump-handle) motion of the upper ribs and sternum.
- The lateral motion of the lower ribs and anterior motion of the upper ribs and sternum can occur simultaneously.
- Exhalation during breathing at rest is mostly passive, using the elastic recoil properties of the lungs and the cessation of inspiratory muscle contraction.

Life Span and Clinical Considerations

Differences Associated With the Neonate

The compliance, configuration, and muscle action of the chest wall change significantly from infancy to adulthood. A newborn has a cartilaginous and, therefore, extremely compliant chest wall that allows the distortion necessary for the infant's thorax to travel through the birth canal. The increased compliance of the rib cage is at the expense of thoracic stability. An infant's chest wall muscles must act as stabilizers, rather than mobilizers, of the thorax to counteract the reduced intrapulmonary pressure created by the lowered diaphragm during inhalation that would otherwise pull the ribs in. Complete ossification of the ribs does not occur for several months after birth.

The ribs in the adult thorax slope downward and the diaphragm is elliptically shaped **(Fig. 5–20A)**. The rib cage of an infant shows a more horizontal and circular alignment of the ribs **(Fig. 5–20B)**, with the angle of insertion of the costal fibers of the diaphragm also more horizontal than that of an adult. There is an increased tendency for the diaphragmatic fibers to pull the lower ribs inward, thereby decreasing ventilation efficiency and increasing distortion of the chest wall.[32] There is very little motion of the rib cage during an infant's tidal breathing.

Only 20% of the muscle fibers of the diaphragm are fatigue-resistant fibers in a healthy newborn, compared with 50% in an adult. This discrepancy predisposes infants to earlier diaphragmatic fatigue.[32] Accessory muscles of ventilation are also at a disadvantage in the infant because the inability of the infant to stabilize their upper extremities, head, and spine makes it difficult for the accessory muscles of ventilation to produce the action needed to be helpful during increased ventilatory demands.

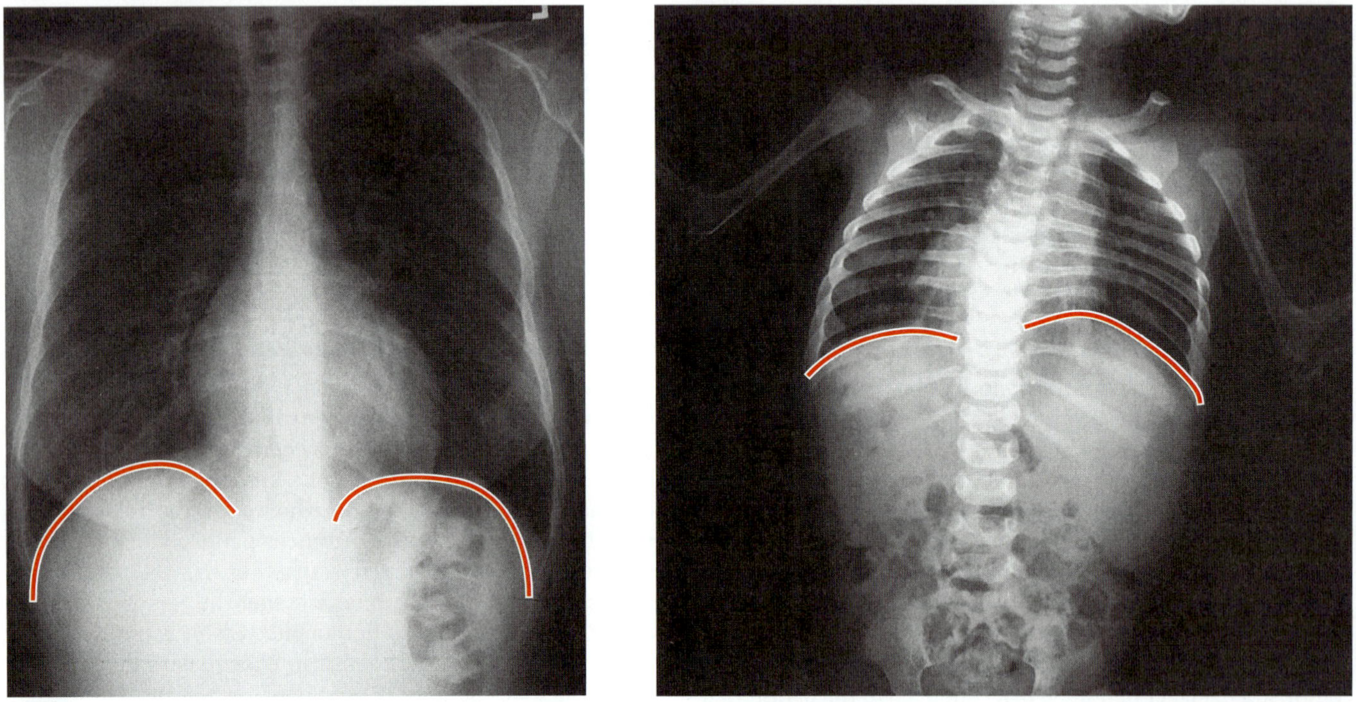

A B

Figure 5–20 **A.** In an adult, the ribs slope downward, and the diaphragm has an elliptical shape. **B.** The rib cage of an infant shows a nearly horizontal alignment of the ribs, resulting in the angle of insertion of the costal fibers of the diaphragm also more horizontal.

With increasing age, the infant's rib cage ossifies, relieving the ventilatory muscles of some of their stabilization function and allowing them to more effectively mobilize during respiration. Improving head control also allows the infant to begin to use accessory muscles for increased ventilation. As a toddler assumes independent sitting and standing, the force of gravity and postural changes allow the anterior rib cage to angle obliquely downward over time. This elongated thorax allows for a greater bucket-handle motion of the rib cage. The attachments for the muscles of ventilation move with the increasingly angled ribs, improving their action on the thorax.

Throughout childhood, the numbers of alveoli and airways continue to increase, and in early adolescence they continue to expand, as demonstrated by increases in pulmonary function test results.[33]

Differences Associated With the Elderly

Skeletal changes that occur with aging affect pulmonary function. Many of the articulations of the chest wall undergo fibrosis with advancing age.[34,35] The interchondral and costochondral joints can fibrose, and the chondrosternal joints may be obliterated. The xiphisternal and the manubriosternal junctions ossify with age. The chest wall's synovial articulations may undergo morphological changes associated with aging, including reduced mobility. The costal cartilages ossify, which interferes with their axial rotation.[14] Overall, chest wall compliance is significantly reduced (stiffness increases) with age. Reduction in diaphragm-abdomen compliance has also been reported and is at least partially related to the decreased rib cage compliance, especially in the lower ribs that are part of the zone of apposition.[36]

Aging also brings anatomical changes to the lung tissues that affect respiration. The airways narrow, the alveolar duct diameters increase, and the alveolar sacs lose surface area for gas exchange. There is a reorientation of, and a decrease in, the elastic fibers in the lung parenchyma. Overall, there is a decrease in elastic recoil and an increase in pulmonary compliance.[35] Because the resting position of the thorax depends on the balance between the elastic recoil properties of the lungs pulling the ribs inwardly and the outward pull of the ribs and costal cartilages, the reduced recoil property of the lung tissue allows the thorax to rest with an increased A-P diameter (a relatively increased inspiratory position). An increased kyphosis often observed in older individuals will further decrease the mobility not only of the thoracic spine but also of the rib cage.

Skeletal muscles of ventilation in the elderly have a documented loss of strength, fewer muscle fibers, a lower oxidative capacity, a decrease in the number or the size of type IIX (fast-twitch) fibers, and an increase in the time to peak tension.[35,36] The decrease in abdominal tension that occurs with aging allows the resting position of the diaphragm to be lower in the thorax, that is, less domed. There is an earlier recruitment pattern for accessory muscles of ventilation. For example, the transverse thoracic muscles are active during exhalation at rest in older subjects in the standing position.[26]

Overall in the elderly, there is likely to be a decreased compliance of the bony rib cage, an increased compliance of the lung tissue, and an overall decreased compliance of the ventilatory system. The result of these age-related skeletal and tissue changes is an increase in the amount of air remaining in the lungs after a typical exhalation. If the lungs retain more air at the end of exhalation (an increase in the functional residual capacity), there will be a decrease in inspiratory capacity (tidal volume plus inspiratory reserve volume) of the thorax. The decrease in the effectiveness of the ventilatory muscles means that ventilation becomes more energy-expensive with age. Functionally, the result of these multiple changes with increasing age is a decrease in the ventilatory reserve available during times of need, such as during an illness or increased activity.

Pathological Changes in Structure and Function

In this chapter, the effects of the musculoskeletal system on ventilation have been discussed. Interestingly, the opposite can also be true: Changes in the pulmonary system can affect the bony thorax. A brief discussion of this relationship is presented using **chronic obstructive pulmonary disease (COPD)** as the framework.

Patient Application 5–5

Jon Nguyen is a 58-year-old former delivery driver who smoked two to three packs of cigarettes per day for 40 years. Several years ago, Jon was diagnosed with COPD. Jon cut his smoking back to one pack per day, and he is still trying to quit smoking completely. He was forced to retire last year because his shortness of breath was limiting his ability to get in and out of his truck repeatedly throughout the day. In the past year, he has had repeated bouts of bronchitis and was admitted to the hospital a couple of times for pneumonia. Jon reports that he is now finding it more difficult to breathe even at rest and is continually fatigued. A good friend now does his food shopping for him. Pulmonary function studies show a seriously compromised ventilatory system, with impairments in ventilatory capacity and lung volume common to COPD **(Fig. 5–21)**. Jon's appearance is typical of an individual with COPD, with a barrel-shaped chest despite his slight build **(Fig. 5–22)**.

The major manifestation of COPD is damage to the airways and destruction of the alveolar walls. As tissue destruction occurs with disease, the elastic recoil property of the lung tissue diminishes. Exhalation, either passive or active, is dependent upon this elastic recoil property. In patients with COPD, exhalation becomes ineffective in removing adequate amounts of air from the thorax, leading to air trapping and hyperinflation.

The static or resting position of the thorax is a function of the balance between the elastic recoil properties of the lungs pulling inward and the typical outward spring of the rib cage. In patients with COPD, there is an imbalance in these two opposing forces that alters both lung volumes and ventilatory capacities (see Fig. 5–21). As elasticity decreases and more air remains within the lungs, an increase in the A-P diameter of the hyperinflated thorax is apparent, showing a classic barrel-shaped appearance and accompanying changes to the thorax (see Fig. 5–22).

The range of motion, or excursion, of the thorax is limited in obstructive pulmonary disease. Although the basic

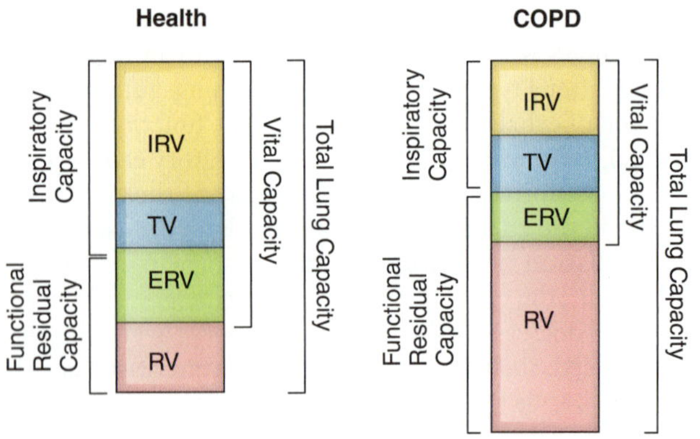

Figure 5–21 Lung volumes and capacities of a healthy person and of a patient with COPD. *COPD, chronic obstructive pulmonary disease; ERV, expiratory reserve volume; IRV, inspiratory reserve volume; RV, residual volume; TV, tidal volume.*

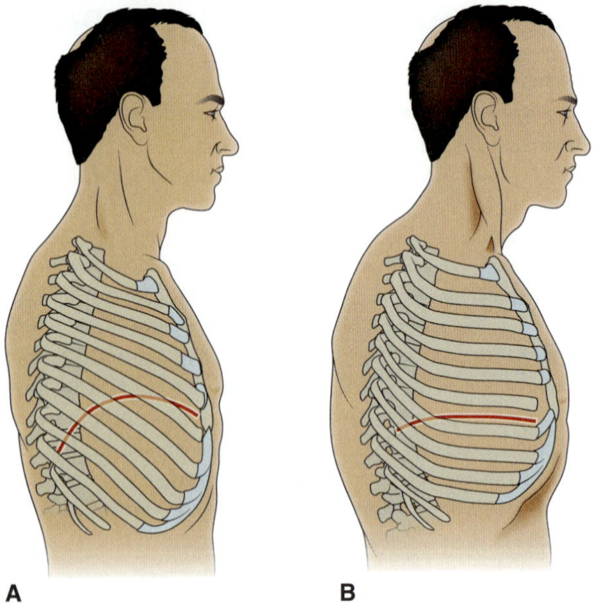

Figure 5–22 Chest changes at rest with chronic obstructive pulmonary disease (COPD). **A.** The alignment of clavicle, ribs, and diaphragm in a typical adult at rest. **B.** In individuals with COPD, the resting A-P diameter of the chest wall increases; the accompanying hyperinflation of the lungs is associated with elevation of the clavicle and sternum, more horizontally oriented ribs, a flattened diaphragm, and tension in the accessory muscles of ventilation (e.g., the sternocleidomastoid muscles).

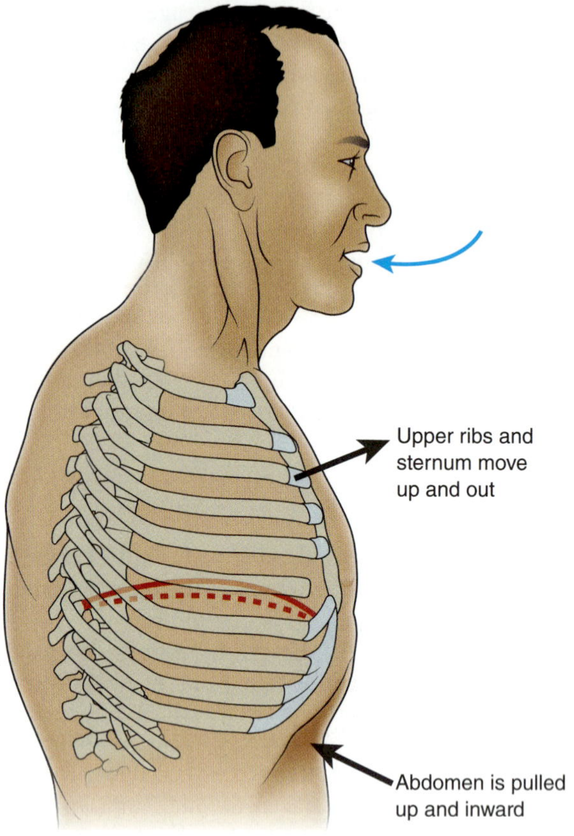

Figure 5–23 Paradoxical thoracoabdominal movement in COPD. During inspiration, the strong pull of the accessory muscles of inspiration, there is an increase in the motion of the upper chest. Rather than flattening of the diaphragm and protrusion of the abdomen usually seen with typical inspiration (see Fig. 5–16A), the expansion of the rib cage pulls the abdominal viscera and the typical flattened diaphragm of the person with COPD (dotted line) slightly upward into the thorax (solid line). With exhalation, the thorax decreases in size, and the abdominal viscera return to their resting position.

characteristic of COPD is an inability to exhale sufficiently, it is clear that inspiratory capacity is compromised as a result.

Hyperinflation affects not only the bony components of the chest wall but also the muscles of the thorax. Within the lungs, the increased residual air does not allow the diaphragm to return to its usual high domed shape and location so that there is a flattening of the diaphragm at rest. The fibers of the diaphragm remain shortened even after exhalation, decreasing the available range of contraction. The angle of pull of the flattened diaphragm fibers becomes more horizontal with a decreased zone of apposition. In severe cases of hyperinflation, the fibers of the diaphragm are aligned more horizontally than vertically. Contraction of this very flattened diaphragm will pull the lower rib cage inward and work against lung inflation.[37,38]

With the compromise of the diaphragm in COPD, the majority of inhalation is performed by other inspiratory muscles that are not as efficient as the diaphragm. The barrel-shaped and elevated thorax puts the sternocleidomastoid muscles in a shortened position, making them much less efficient. The parasternal and scalene muscles can generate a greater force as the lungs approach total lung capacity; consequently, hyperinflation has a less dramatic effect on them.

The altered muscle power during inhalation with COPD now favors movement of the upper, rather than the lower, rib cage. With a forceful contraction of the functioning inspiratory muscles of the upper rib cage in a patient with an ineffective diaphragm, the diaphragm and abdominal contents may actually be pulled upward, into the thorax.[39,40] During exhalation, the abdomen is pushed back down and out. This paradoxical thoracoabdominal breathing pattern can be seen in patients with obstructive disease who are in respiratory distress **(Fig. 5–23)**. The disadvantages of these biomechanical alterations with hyperinflation are compounded by the increased demand for ventilation in COPD. More work is required of a less effective system. The energy cost of ventilation, or the work of breathing, is markedly increased in patients with COPD.

SUMMARY

In this chapter, comprehensive coverage of the structure and function of the bony thorax and the ventilatory muscles has been provided. Chapter 7 will present additional information on the structure and function of accessory muscles of ventilation because these muscles may affect the shoulder complex.

STUDY QUESTIONS

1. Describe the articulations of the chest wall and thorax, including the costovertebral, costotransverse, costochondral, chondrosternal, and manubriosternal joints.
2. What are the different motions of the chest wall motions during breathing? Explain where these motions occur.
3. What are the roles of the diaphragm, the intercostal muscles, and the abdominal muscles during breathing at rest?
4. Describe the accessory muscles of ventilation and explain their functions.
5. Describe the inspiratory and expiratory functions of the abdominal muscles.
6. What effect does COPD have on the biomechanics of the thorax and the inspiratory muscles?
7. How does the aging process affect the structure and function of the thorax?

REFERENCES

1. Watkins Rt, Watkins R, 3rd, Williams L, et al: Stability provided by the sternum and rib cage in the thoracic spine. Spine (Phila Pa 1976) 30:1283-6, 2005
2. Horton WC, Kraiwattanapong C, Akamaru T, et al: The role of the sternum, costosternal articulations, intervertebral disc, and facets in thoracic sagittal plane biomechanics: a comparison of three different sequences of surgical release. Spine (Phila Pa 1976) 30:2014-23, 2005
3. De Troyer A, Estenne M: Functional anatomy of the respiratory muscles. Clin Chest Med 9:175-93, 1988
4. Silajiya DA, Khubchandani HT, Soni SN, et al: Radiological age estimation from sternum. National Journal of Integrated Research in Medicine 4:108, 2013
5. Levine BD, Motamedi K, Chow K, et al: CT of rib lesions. AJR Am J Roentgenol 193:5-13, 2009
6. Stehbens WE: Pathogenesis of idiopathic scoliosis revisited. Exp Mol Pathol 74:49-60, 2003
7. Wilson TA, Rehder K, Krayer S, et al: Geometry and respiratory displacement of human ribs. J Appl Physiol (1985) 62:1872-7, 1987
8. De Troyer A, Estenne M: Coordination between rib cage muscles and diaphragm during quiet breathing in humans. J Appl Physiol Respir Environ Exerc Physiol 57:899-906, 1984
9. Estenne M, Derom E, De Troyer A: Neck and abdominal muscle activity in patients with severe thoracic scoliosis. Am J Respir Crit Care Med 158:452-7, 1998
10. Tobin MJ: Respiratory muscles in disease. Clin Chest Med 9:2 63-86, 1988
11. Celli BR: Clinical and physiologic evaluation of respiratory muscle function. Clin Chest Med 10:199-214, 1989
12. De Troyer A, Sampson M, Sigrist S, et al: The diaphragm: two muscles. Science 213:237-8, 1981
13. Deviri E, Nathan H, Luchansky E: Medial and lateral arcuate ligaments of the diaphragm: attachment to the transverse process. Anat Anz 166:63-7, 1988
14. De Troyer A, Sampson M, Sigrist S, et al: Action of costal and crural parts of the diaphragm on the rib cage in dog. J Appl Physiol Respir Environ Exerc Physiol 53:30-9, 1982
15. De Troyer A, Kirkwood PA, Wilson TA: Respiratory action of the intercostal muscles. Physiol Rev 85:717-56, 2005
16. McKenzie D: To breathe or not to breathe: the respiratory muscles and COPD. J Appl Physiol (1985) 101:1279-80, 2006
17. De Troyer A, Heilporn A: Respiratory mechanics in quadriplegia: the respiratory function of the intercostal muscles. Am Rev Respir Dis 122:591-600, 1980
18. Macklem PT, Macklem DM, De Troyer A: A model of inspiratory muscle mechanics. J Appl Physiol Respir Environ Exerc Physiol 55:547-57, 1983
19. Cala SJ, Kenyon CM, Lee A, et al: Respiratory ultrasonography of human parasternal intercostal muscle in vivo. Ultrasound Med Biol 24:313-26, 1998
20. Han JN, Gayan-Ramirez G, Dekhuijzen R, et al: Respiratory function of the rib cage muscles. Eur Respir J 6:722-8, 1993
21. Whitelaw WA, Ford GT, Rimmer KP, et al: Intercostal muscles are used during rotation of the thorax in humans. J Appl Physiol (1985) 72:1940-4, 1992
22. De Troyer A: Actions of the respiratory muscles or how the chest wall moves in upright man. Bull Eur Physiopathol Respir 20:409-13, 1984
23. Goldman MD, Loh L, Sears TA: The respiratory activity of human levator costae muscles and its modification by posture. J Physiol 362:189-204, 1985
24. Raper AJ, Thompson WT, Jr., Shapiro W, et al: Scalene and sternomastoid muscle function. J Appl Physiol 21:497-502, 1966
25. Patil S: Serratus posterior muscles: anatomical properties, functional and clinical significance. International Journal of Current Research and Review 5:52-54, 2013
26. Vilensky JA, Baltes M, Weikel L, et al: Serratus posterior muscles: anatomy, clinical relevance, and function. Clin Anat 14:237-41, 2001
27. De Troyer A, Ninane V, Gilmartin JJ, et al: Triangularis sterni muscle use in supine humans. J Appl Physiol (1985) 62:919-25, 1987
28. Estenne M, Ninane V, De Troyer A: Triangularis sterni muscle use during eupnea in humans: effect of posture. Respir Physiol 74:151-62, 1988
29. De Troyer A, Kelly S, Macklem PT, et al: Mechanics of intercostal space and actions of external and internal intercostal muscles. J Clin Invest 75:850-7, 1985
30. De Troyer A, Leduc D: Role of pleural pressure in the coupling between the intercostal muscles and the ribs. J Appl Physiol (1985) 102:2332-7, 2007
31. Rimmer KP, Ford GT, Whitelaw WA: Interaction between postural and respiratory control of human intercostal muscles. J Appl Physiol (1985) 79:1556-61, 1995
32. Davis GM, Bureau MA: Pulmonary and chest wall mechanics in the control of respiration in the newborn. Clin Perinatol 14:551-79, 1987
33. Reid L: 1976 Edward B.D. Neuhauser lecture: The lung: growth and remodeling in health and disease. AJR Am J Roentgenol 129:777-88, 1977
34. Krumpe PE, Knudson RJ, Parsons G, et al: The aging respiratory system. Clin Geriatr Med 1:143-75, 1985
35. Chan ED, Welsh CH: Geriatric respiratory medicine. Chest 114:1704-33, 1998
36. Estenne M, Yernault JC, De Troyer A: Rib cage and diaphragm-abdomen compliance in humans: effects of age and posture. J Appl Physiol (1985) 59:1842-8, 1985
37. De Troyer A: Effect of hyperinflation on the diaphragm. Eur Respir J 10:708-13, 1997
38. Decramer M: Hyperinflation and respiratory muscle interaction. Eur Respir J 10:934-41, 1997
39. Aliverti A, Quaranta M, Chakrabarti B, et al: Paradoxical movement of the lower ribcage at rest and during exercise in COPD patients. Eur Respir J 33:49-60, 2009
40. Alves GS, Britto RR, Campos FC, et al: Breathing pattern and thoracoabdominal motion during exercise in chronic obstructive pulmonary disease. Braz J Med Biol Res 41:945-50, 2008

CHAPTER 6

The Temporomandibular Joint

Pamela D. Ritzline, PT, EdD | Jenna York, PT, DPT, OCS

CHAPTER OUTLINE

INTRODUCTION 186

STRUCTURE AND FUNCTION OF THE TM JOINT 186

- Structure 186
  - Articular Structures 186
  - Accessory Joint Structures 188
  - Capsule and Ligaments 189
- Function 190
  - Joint Kinematics 190
  - Muscles 193
- Relationship to the Cervical Spine and Posture 195
- Dentition 196

LIFE SPAN AND CLINICAL CONSIDERATIONS 197

- Age-Related Changes in the TM Joint 197
- Clinical Considerations 197
  - Respiratory Dysfunction and the TM Joint 197
- Inflammatory Conditions 197
  - Capsular Fibrosis 198
- Osseous Mobility Conditions 198
  - Articular Disc Displacement 198
- Degenerative Conditions 199

SUMMARY 200

STUDY QUESTIONS 200

REFERENCES 200

ANATOMY OVERVIEW

MUSCLE ACTIONS OF THE TEMPOROMANDIBULAR JOINT

TABLE KEY: Primary movers / Secondary movers

Sagittal Plane (rotation)	Elevation (closing mouth)	Depression (opening mouth)
	Temporalis (primary) Masseter (primary) Medial pterygoid (primary)	Lateral pterygoid (primary) Digastric (secondary) Stylohyoid (secondary) Mylohyoid (secondary) Geniohyoid (secondary) Omohyoid (secondary) Sternohyoid (secondary) Sternothyroid (secondary) Thyrohyoid (secondary) Platysma (secondary)
Sagittal Plane (translation)	**Protrusion**	**Retraction**
	Lateral pterygoid (primary) Masseter (secondary) Medial pterygoid (secondary)	Temporalis (primary) Masseter (secondary)

ANATOMY OVERVIEW

TEMPOROMANDIBULAR JOINT MUSCLE ATTACHMENTS		
Muscles	**Proximal Attachment**	**Distal Attachment**
Temporalis	Broad attachment to floor of temporal fossa	Narrow attachment to coronoid process and anterior border of ramus of mandible
Masseter	Quadrate muscle attaching to inferior border and medial surface of the zygomatic arch	Angle and lateral surface of ramus of mandible
Lateral pterygoid	Triangular two-headed muscle from infratemporal surface and crest of greater wing and lateral pterygoid plate of sphenoid	Superior head attaches primarily to joint capsule and articular disc of temporomandibular joint; inferior head attaches primarily to condyle of mandible
Medial pterygoid	Quadrangular two-headed muscle from medial surface of lateral pterygoid plate, palatine bone, and maxilla	Medial surface of ramus of mandible
Digastric (suprahyoid)	Inner surface of anterior body of mandible (anterior belly); mastoid process of temporal bone (posterior belly)	Hyoid bone
Stylohyoid (suprahyoid)	Styloid process of temporal bone	Hyoid bone
Mylohyoid (suprahyoid)	Medial surface of mandible	Hyoid bone
Geniohyoid (suprahyoid)	Inner surface of anterior body of mandible	Hyoid bone
Omohyoid (infrahyoid)	Superior surface of scapula	Hyoid bone
Sternohyoid (infrahyoid)	Manubrium of sternum	Hyoid bone
Sternothyroid (infrahyoid)	Posterior surface of manubrium of sternum	Thyroid cartilage
Thyrohyoid (infrahyoid)	Thyroid cartilage	Hyoid bone

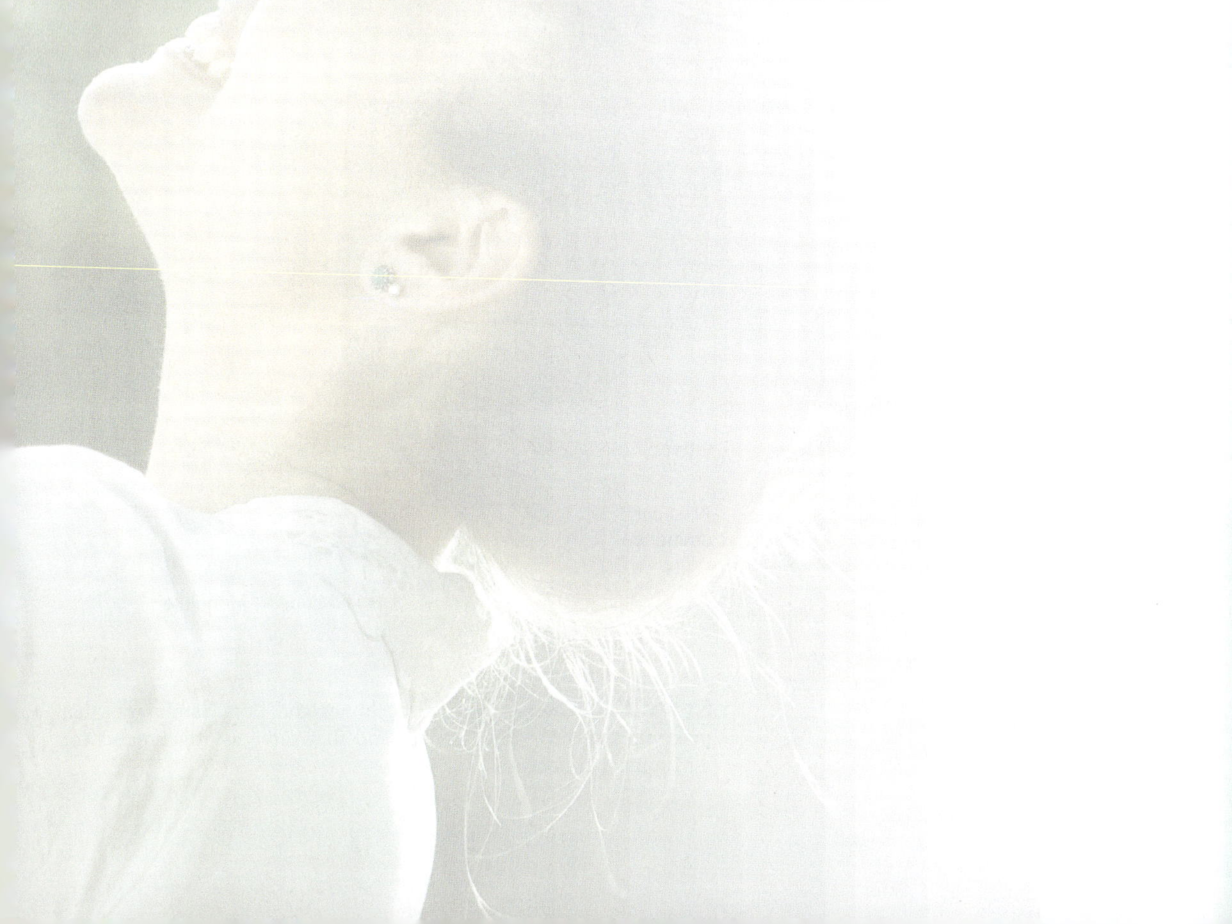

Introduction

The **temporomandibular (TM) joint** is unique in both structure and function. Structurally, the **mandible** is a horseshoe-shaped bone **(Fig. 6–1)** that articulates with the **temporal bone** at each of its posterosuperiorly located condyles and produces two distinct, but highly interdependent, articulations. Each TM joint contains a disc that separates the joint into upper and lower articulations. Functionally, mandibular movement involves concurrent movement in the four distinct joints (upper and lower articulations for the left and right TM joints), resulting in a complex structure that moves in all planes of motion to achieve typical function.

A discussion of the structure and function of the TM joint will allow the reader to appreciate and understand its unique features, its relationship with the cervical spine, and the effect of impairments and pathologies of the TM joint. Although the purpose of this chapter is to discuss the typical function and structure of the TM joint, TM disorders are a common subgroup of orofacial pain disorders. This chapter will introduce some of the common conditions that involve deviations of typical structure and function.

Structure and Function of the TM Joint

Structure

Articular Structures

Multiple bones merge to form the structure and contribute to the function of the TM joints. These bones include the mandible, **maxilla,** temporal, **zygomatic, sphenoid,** and **hyoid** bones **(Fig. 6–2)**. Although you may think of the mandible as moving on the stationary maxilla, the maxilla is not part of the TM joint. Rather, the proximal or stationary segment of the TM joint is the temporal bone. The actual articulation for the TM joint arises where the condyles of the mandible sit in the **mandibular fossa** of the temporal bone. The mandibular fossa is located between the **postglenoid tubercle** and the **articular eminence** of the temporal bone (Fig. 6–2).[1,2]

The temporal bones and the mandible form left and right TM joints that are part of a closed chain and must function together; however, each is an anatomically separate joint, and can vary from each other structurally as well as functionally. The TM joints are considered synovial joints formed by the **condyle of the mandible** as the inferior segment and the articular eminence of the temporal bone as the superior segment.[2,3] The articular eminence of the mandible contains a considerable amount of trabecular bone and serves as the primary articular surface for the mandibular condyle. Although the condyle of the mandible sits in the mandibular fossa, the bone of the fossa is thin and translucent, which would create an unlikely articular surface. Instead, the mandibular condyles articulate with the articular eminence of the temporal bone on each side. The articular eminence and the mandibular condyle are both convex structures (see Fig. 6–2), resulting in an incongruent joint.[1,2] Incongruent joints require rolling and sliding for typical range of motion (ROM) to occur.

The mandible is the largest of the facial bones and is highly mobile, arch shaped, and consists of a condyle at each posterior superior portion (see Fig. 6-1). The condyles are positioned anterior to the external auditory meatus of the

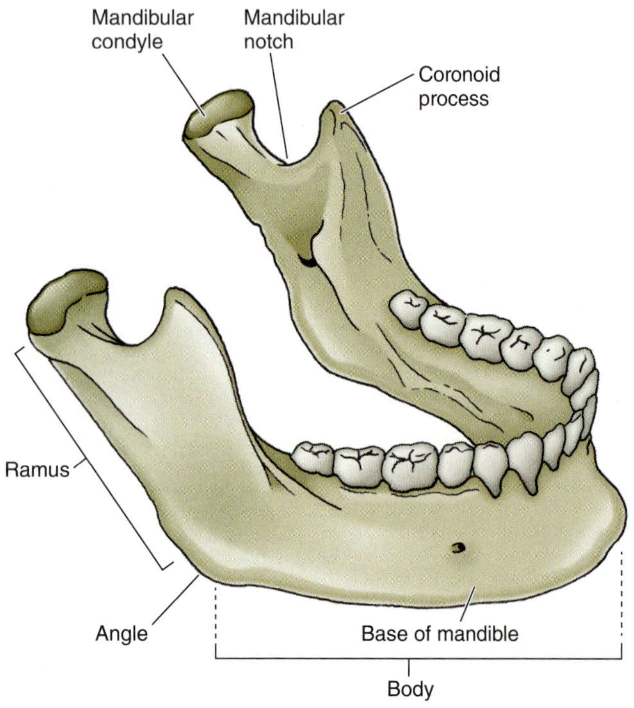

Figure 6–1 The mandible.

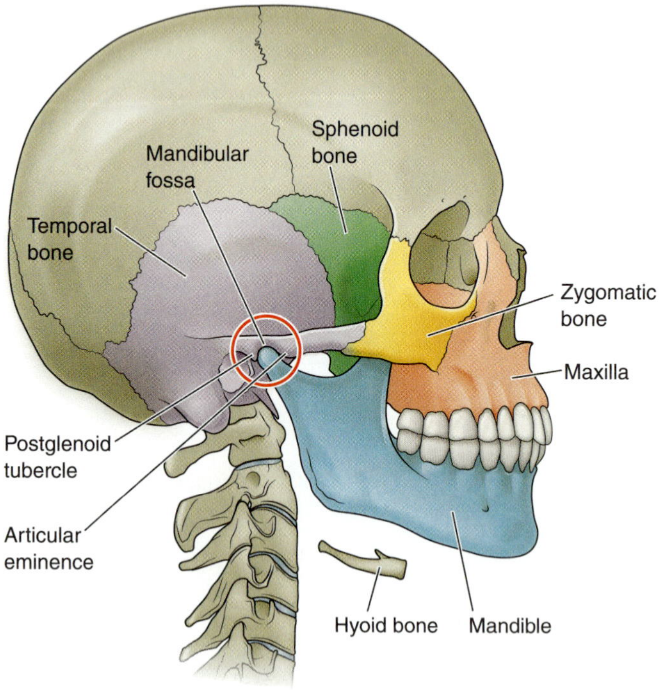

Figure 6–2 Lateral view of the bones and bony landmarks that make up the TM joint (circled) and that serve as attachments for TM joint musculature.

ear and sit within the respective mandibular fossa of each of the temporal bones. Each mandibular condyle has a medial and lateral pole **(Fig. 6–3)**, with the lateral pole being readily palpable.[4] In fact, the posterior aspect of the condyle can be palpated if a fingertip is placed into the external auditory meatus and the pad of the finger is pushed anteriorly **(Fig. 6–4)**.[5] The shape of each condyle may vary between individuals and even between sides in the same individual.[5,6] The **coronoid process** of the mandible is located anterior to the mandibular condyle and serves as an attachment for the temporalis muscle **(Fig. 6–5)**. The mandible interacts with the maxillae by way of the teeth. The importance of the articulations between the mandible and the temporal bones and maxillae will become apparent when we discuss impairments of the TM joints.

The TM joint is an atypical synovial joint because the articular surfaces are covered by fibrocartilage rather than hyaline cartilage.[3,5] The articular surfaces of both the articular eminence and the mandibular condyle are covered with dense, avascular fibrocartilage containing type I collagen fibers. As with other cartilage surfaces, these collagen fibers are aligned perpendicular to the bony surface in the deeper layers and in a parallel arrangement near the surface of the articular covering (see Chapter 2).[5,7,8] The presence of fibrocartilage rather than hyaline cartilage is significant because, unlike hyaline cartilage, fibrocartilage can repair and remodel itself.[3,5,7] Typically, fibrocartilage is present in areas that have to withstand repeated and high-level stress. The TM joints are subject to the repetitive stress of jaw motions as well as to tremendous bite forces that have been measured between 600 N and 1,200 N.[9] The TM joint surfaces are amenable to some degree of adaptation, but no clear-cut point exists between adaptive and maladaptive changes.[10] Tanaka and Koolstra[3] acknowledged that loading is necessary to stimulate the remodeling that occurs with typical functional demands to ensure homeostasis within a joint. Although no evidence exists to determine the appropriate load for the TM joint, it has been proposed that aging and some physical and mental conditions may disrupt typical load.[3]

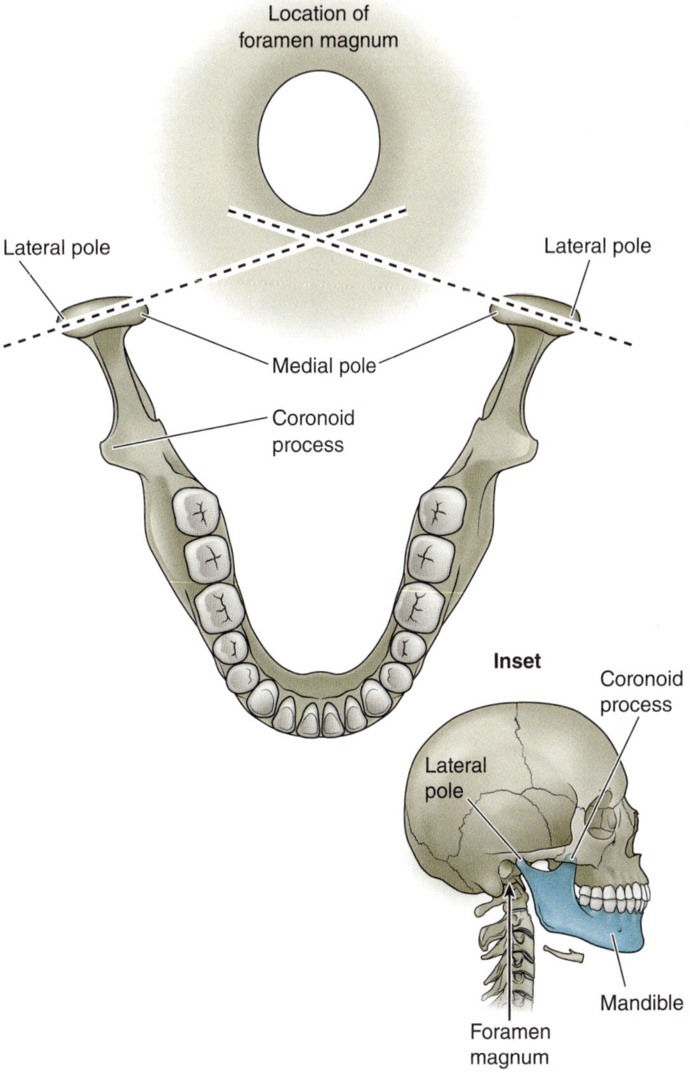

Figure 6–3 A superior view of the mandible shows the medial and lateral poles of the mandibular condyles and the coronoid processes. Mandibular rotation occurs around axes that pass through the medial and lateral poles of each condyle, with the extended lines of the axes intersecting anterior to the foramen magnum of the skull. Inset: In this right lateral view, the position of the lateral pole of the mandible anterior to the foramen magnum can be appreciated.

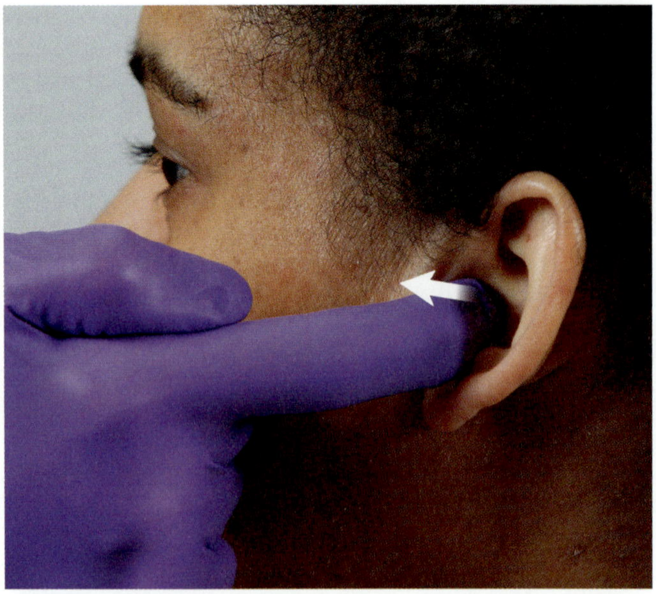

Figure 6–4 Palpation of the posterior aspect of the mandibular condyle through the external auditory meatus, pushing fingertip(s) anteriorly.

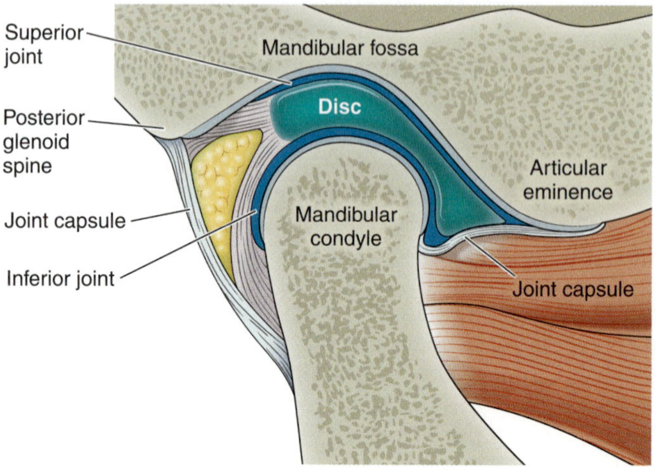

Figure 6–6 A cross-sectional lateral view of the TM joint shows the fibrocartilage-covered load-bearing surfaces on the condyle of the mandible and the articular eminence. The TM disc divides the articulation into superior and inferior joints, each with its own synovial lining. The anterior and posterior attachments of the joint capsule to the disc are shown.

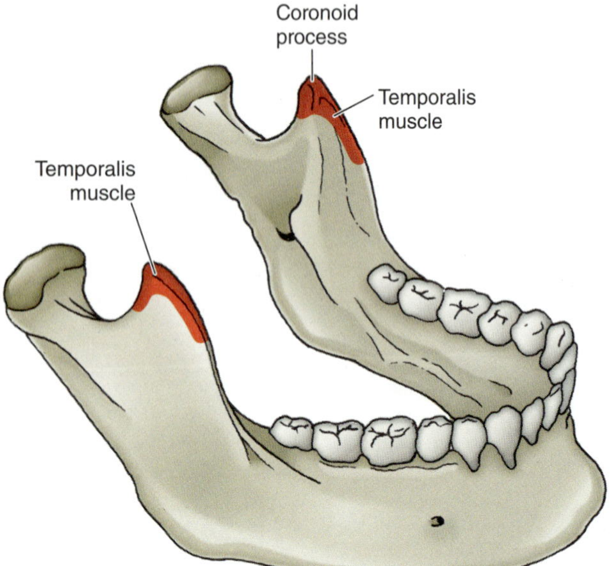

Figure 6–5 The temporalis muscle attaches to the coronoid process of the mandible.

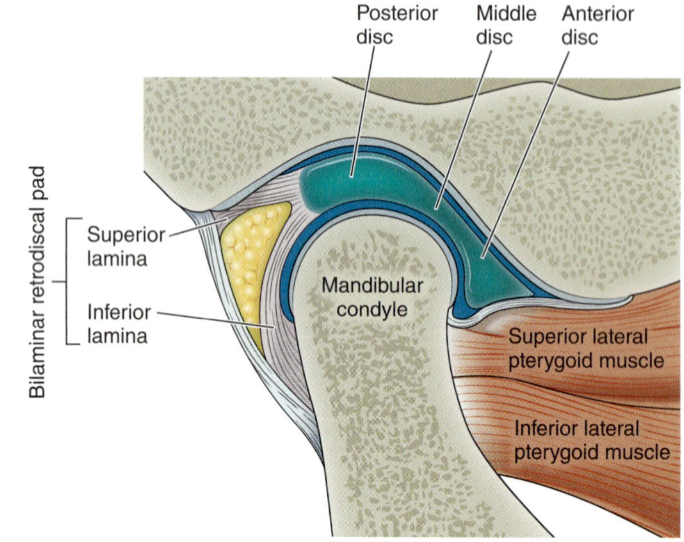

Figure 6–7 A cross-sectional lateral view of the TM joint showing the articular disc. The thickness of the disc varies within the joint, from 2 mm anteriorly to 1 mm in the center to 3 mm posteriorly.

Accessory Joint Structures

The incongruence of the TM joint is addressed by a unique **articular disc.** A disc located within each TM joint separates the articulation into distinct superior and inferior joints with slightly different functions (Fig. 6–6).[4,5,8] Thus, mandibular motion may involve the simultaneous movement of four different joints. The **inferior TM joint** is formed by the mandibular condyle and the inferior surface of the disc and functions as a simple hinge joint with one rotational degree of freedom (DOF). The **superior TM joint** is larger than the inferior joint and is formed by the articular eminence of the temporal bone and the superior surface of the disc; it functions as a plane joint.[4] The articular disc of the TM joint is biconcave; that is, the superior and inferior surfaces are both concave. Styles and Whyte describe the disc as having a "bowtie" appearance on magnetic resonance imaging (MRI), with the "knot" sitting in the center, at the thinnest portion.[11] The thickness of the articular disc varies within the joint from 2 mm anteriorly to 1 mm in the middle to 3 mm posteriorly (Fig. 6–7).[6,11,12] The purpose of the disc is to allow the convex surfaces of the articular eminence superiorly and the mandibular condyle inferiorly to remain congruent throughout the ROM of the TM joint in all planes.[6] Sicher described the TM joint as a hinge joint with movable sockets, and later investigators supported this description.[3,6,13] The articular disc, therefore, serves multiple purposes. It increases stability, minimizes loss of mobility, reduces friction, and decreases biomechanical stress on the TM joint.[5,14-16]

The disc within each TM joint has a complex set of attachments (see Fig. 6–7). On the disc's sides, the disc is firmly attached to the medial and lateral poles of the mandibular condyle, but it is not attached to the TM joint capsule medially or laterally.[6,17] These attachments allow the mandibular condyle to rotate freely on the disc in the sagittal plane. Anteriorly, the disc is attached to the joint capsule, as well as to the tendon of the **superior lateral pterygoid muscle.** These anterior attachments restrict excessive posterior slide (translation) of the disc. Posteriorly, the disc is attached to a complex structure, called the **bilaminar retrodiscal pad.** The bilaminar retrodiscal pad contains superior and inferior bands (or laminae) that attach to the posterior aspect of the disc. The superior lamina is anchored posteriorly to the tympanic plate (at the posterior mandibular fossa), while the inferior lamina is attached to the neck of the condyle.[2,4,6,8] The superior lamina consists of elastic fibers that permit the superior band to stretch, allowing the disc to translate anteriorly along the articular eminence during mandibular depression (mouth opening). The elastic properties of the superior lamina also assist in repositioning the disc posteriorly during mandibular closing. In contrast, the inferior lamina is inelastic, serving as a tether on the disc to limit excessive forward translation. It does not, however, assist with repositioning the disc during mandibular closing.[11,16] Importantly, neither of the lamina of the retrodiscal pad is under tension when the TM joint is at rest. Loose areolar connective tissue rich in arterial and neural supply is located between the two laminae[2,16] (see Fig. 6-7).

A healthy TM disc is viscoelastic and well suited for distribution of force, with the connective tissue fibers demonstrating only a small strain response even under significant stress.[18-20] The extracellular matrix of the disc consists primarily of collagen, proteoglycans (PGs), and elastin. Type I collagen is largely responsible for maintaining the disc's shape. Elastin contributes to the disc's ability to regain its form during unloading. PG composition maintains disc resiliency and resists mechanical compressive force. The biomechanical behavior of the disc may change according to changes in its composition.[19] Such changes in composition may occur as a result of aging, mechanical stress, or both.[21] Unlike the fibrocartilage on the mandibular condyles and articular eminences, the articular disc of the TM joint does not have the ability to repair and remodel itself.[19,21]

The anterior and posterior segments of the disc are vascular and innervated. The central segment of the disc is avascular and aneural.[6,20] The lack of vascularity and innervation is consistent with the fact that the middle portion of the disc is the force-accepting segment. The capsule, lateral TM ligament, and retrodiscal tissues contain mechanoreceptors and nociceptors that are responsible for proprioception and pain sensation.[4]

Capsule and Ligaments

The elasticity of the joint capsule and ligaments contributes to the available motion at the TM joint in all planes. Motion may be enhanced or restricted depending on the flexibility of these structures. Generally, the portion of the capsule superior to the disc is quite lax, whereas the portion of the capsule inferior to the disc is taut.[2,6] Consequently, the disc is more firmly attached to the condyle below and freer to move on the articular eminence above. The capsule is thin and loose in its anterior, medial, and posterior aspects, but the lateral aspect is stronger and reinforced with long fibers running from the temporal bone to the mandibular condyle.[2,17] The lack of strength of the capsule anteriorly, coupled with the incongruence of the bony articular surfaces, predisposes the joint to anterior dislocation of the mandibular condyle.[22,23] The capsule is highly vascularized and innervated, which allows it to provide a great deal of information about position and movement of the TM joint.

The primary ligaments of the TM joint are the **TM ligament**, the **stylomandibular ligament**, and the **sphenomandibular ligament** (**Fig. 6–8**). The TM ligament is strong and composed of two parts: an outer oblique element and an inner horizontal element. The outer oblique element attaches to the neck of the condyle and the articular eminence. It serves as a suspensory ligament and limits downward and posterior motion of the mandible as well as the rotation of the condyle during mandibular depression.[2,17] The inner horizontal component of the ligament is attached to the lateral pole of the condyle, the posterior portion of the disc, and the articular eminence. Its fibers are aligned horizontally to resist posterior motion of the condyle. Limiting the posterior translation of the condyle protects the retrodiscal pad.[24,25] The primary function of the TM ligament is to stabilize the lateral portion of the capsule.[2,8] Neither band of the TM ligament limits forward translation of the condyle or disc, but they do limit lateral displacement.[24-26]

The stylomandibular ligament is the weakest of the TM joint's three ligaments. It is considered a thickened part of the parotid sheath joining the styloid process to the angle of

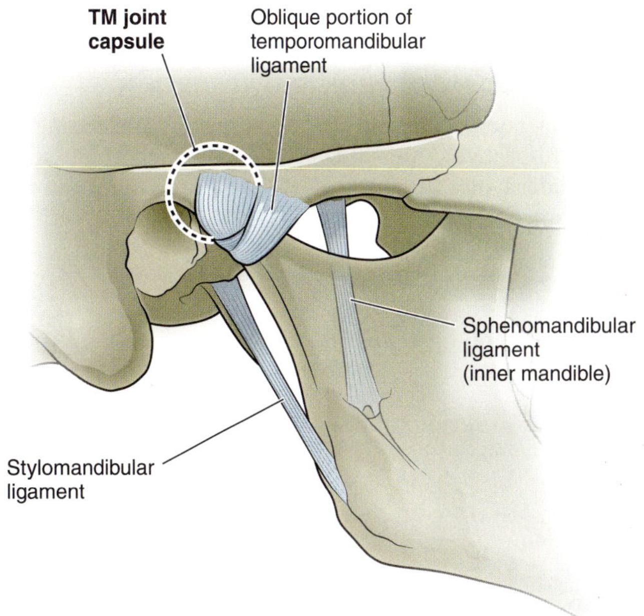

Figure 6–8 A lateral view of the TM joint capsule and ligaments.

the mandible.[2] Some investigators have identified the function of this ligament as limiting anterior translation of the mandible,[24,25,27] but others have stated that it has no known function.[23]

The sphenomandibular ligament is described as the "strong" ligament that is the "swinging hinge" from which the mandible is suspended.[2,14] Some investigators have stated that it serves to protect the mandible from excessive anterior translation.[24,25,27] Others have stated that this ligament has little or no function.[2,24,28]

Function

Joint Kinematics

The TM joint is one of the most frequently used and mobile joints in the body. It is engaged during mastication, swallowing, and speaking. Most of the time, the TM joint movements occur without resistance from chewing or contact between the upper and lower teeth.[6] However, the TM joint is designed to maintain its structure in spite of significant forces acting on it.[9] As previously noted, the articular surfaces are covered with fibrocartilage that has the ability to remodel and repair, and thus are able to tolerate repeated high-level stress. Mastication requires tremendous power, while speaking requires intricate fine motor control. The musculature controlling the TM joint is designed to accomplish each of these potentially contradictory tasks.[9,10,21] Both **osteokinematic** and **arthrokinematic** movements are required for typical function of the TM joint (see Table 6–1). Osteokinematic motions include mandibular depression (mouth opening), elevation (mouth closing), protrusion, retrusion, and left and right lateral excursions. Okeson provides a thorough overview of the detailed analysis of mandibular movements from the classic work of Posselt.[29,30] Arthrokinematic movements involve roll, anterior slide, distraction, and lateral glide.[4,8] This section describes the function of the various components of the TM joint during osteokinematic and arthrokinematic movements. For the purposes of this chapter, only movements that occur *without resistance* will be discussed.

MANDIBULAR DEPRESSION AND ELEVATION

Mandibular depression and elevation (opening and closing the mouth, respectively) are fundamental components of mastication. Under typical circumstances, the motions of mandibular depression and elevation are relatively symmetrical, with the TM joints on both sides following a similar pattern. Mandibular depression and elevation each include a combination of translatory and rotary motion (curvilinear motion), where the mandibular condyle must roll and slide **(Fig. 6–9)**.[4,8] It is generally accepted that the rolling and sliding occur concurrently, but to different extents throughout the motion.[4,8] To illustrate this, full depression and elevation are considered to occur in two phases. The initial phase of mouth opening consists primarily of rotation, in which the mandibular condyle rolls on the inferior surface of the disc in the lower TM joint **(Fig. 6–9A)**. During the second phase, there is relatively greater anterior translation than rotation, such that the mandibular condyle and disc are primarily sliding together as a condyle-disc complex along the articular eminence in the superior TM joint **(Fig. 6–9B)**.[4,5,8,14]

Normal mandibular depression ROM is 40 to 50 mm when measured between the incisal edges of the upper and lower front teeth.[5,8,14] Mastication requires approximately 18 mm of mandibular depression. The initial rolling of the mandibular condyle on the disc produces as little as 11 mm or as much as 25 mm of mandibular depression.[31] The remaining depression results primarily from anterior translation of the condyle-disc complex along the articular eminence. The shape of the condylar head and the steepness of the articular eminence positively correlate with the amount of mandibular depression, but both configurations can be asymmetrical from one TM joint to the other, thus affecting the symmetry of motion.[5,31,32] As a quick screen, the clinician may use the adult knuckles (proximal interphalangeal joints) to assess the degree of mandibular depression. Two knuckles placed between the upper and lower incisors is considered functional mandibular depression, whereas three knuckles is considered typical **(Fig. 6–10)**.[5] Gravity assists with mandibular depression, with the mandibular muscles of elevation possibly contributing eccentrically to control depression.[17]

Mandibular elevation is the reverse of mandibular depression. Arthrokinematics during the initial phase of elevation primarily involve a posterior translation of the condyle-disc complex in the superior joint. During the second phase of elevation, the mandibular condyles roll on the disc in the inferior joint to complete mouth closing.[4,8]

Active and passive control of the articular disc during mandibular depression and elevation is attributed to the disc's connections **(Fig. 6–11)**. Passive control occurs through the capsuloligamentous attachments of the disc to the condyle.

Table 6-1 Kinematics of the Temporomandibular Joint[8]

OSTEOKINEMATIC MOTION	NORMAL RANGE OF MOTION	ARTHROKINEMATIC MOTION
Depression	Normal: 40 mm–50 mm Functional: 18 mm–20 mm	Phase I: 11 mm–25 mm opening • Posterior roll* Phase II: 25 mm–50 mm opening • Anterior slide of disc and condyle along the articular eminence
Protrusion	Lower incisors anterior to upper incisors	Anterior slide of disc and condyle along the articular eminence
Lateral excursion	8 mm–11 mm	Ipsilateral: condyle spins on disc Contralateral: anterior slide of disc and condyle along the articular eminence

*In this case, the roll is named according to the direction the mandibular ramus rotates.[8]

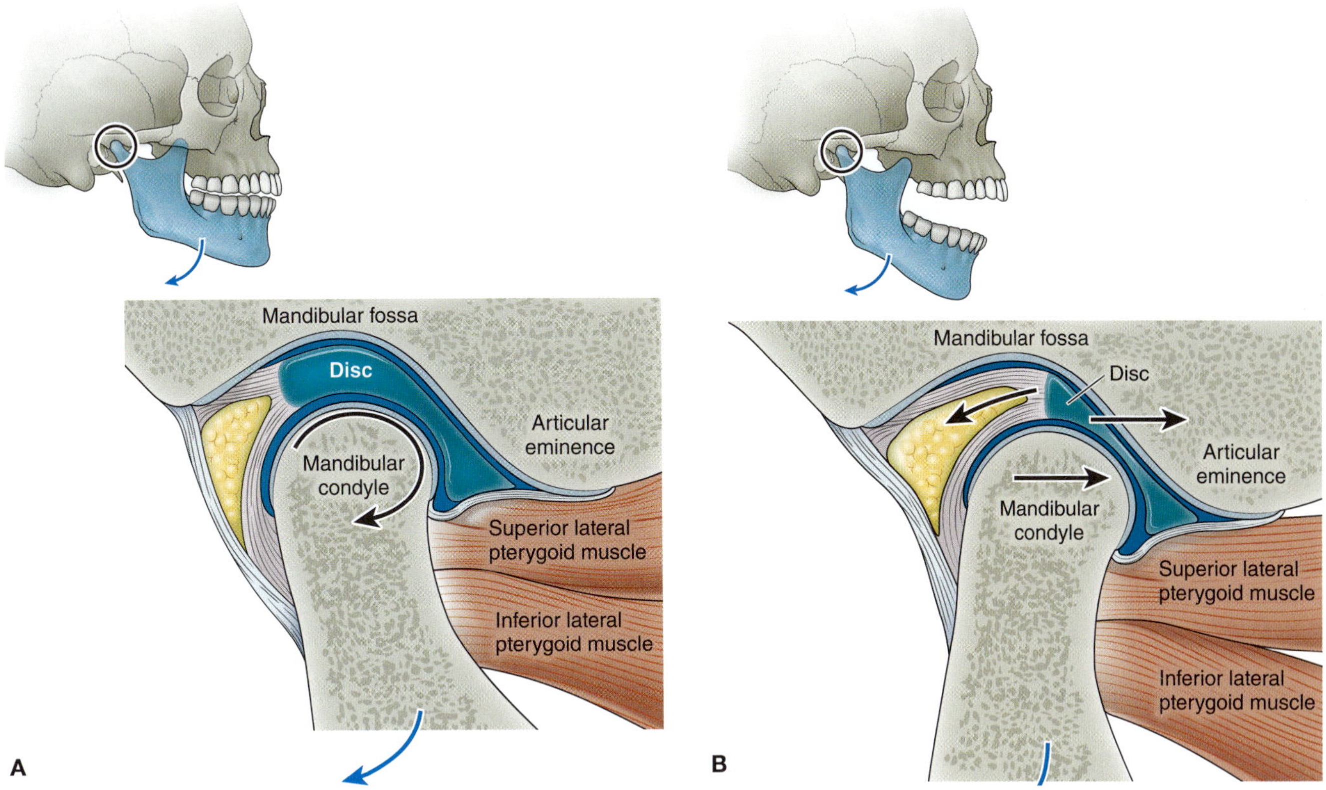

Figure 6–9 **A.** When the mouth begins to open, the motion at the TM joint may be limited to a roll of the condyle on the disc (clockwise rotation in this view). **B.** Anterior slide (translation) of the condyle and disc together on the articular eminence occur either after or simultaneously with sliding in the later stages of mouth opening. The inelastic inferior lamina limits the amount of anterior translation, whereas the elastic properties of the superior lamina control anterior translation.

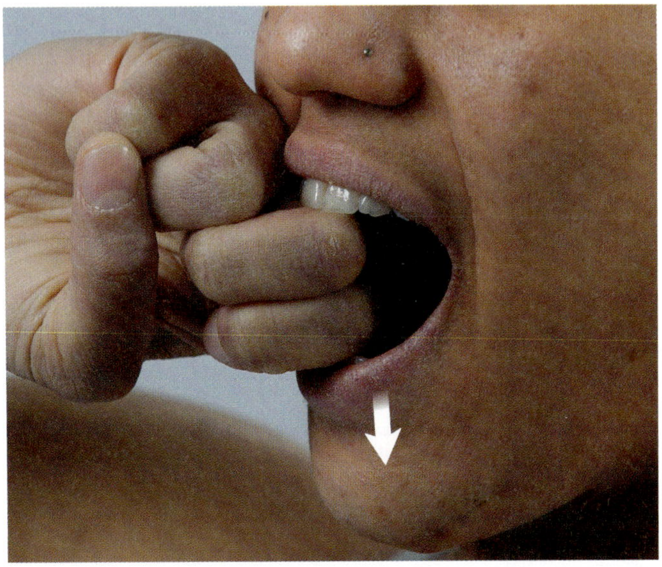

Figure 6–10 Mandibular depression (mouth opening) is considered *functional* if the proximal interphalangeal joints of two fingers can be inserted between the teeth, and *normal* if the joints of three fingers can be inserted.

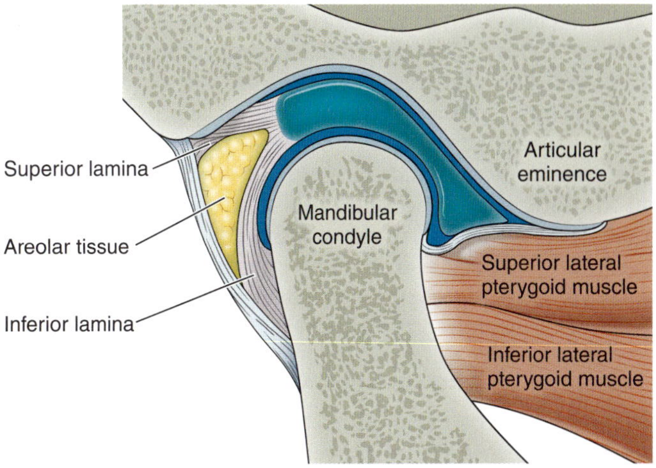

Figure 6–11 The TM disc attaches posteriorly to the joint capsule and to the superior and inferior laminae (segments of the bilaminar retrodiscal pad). Anteriorly, the disc attaches to the joint capsule and to the lateral pterygoid muscle.

The lateral pterygoid muscle attaches to the anterior portion of the disc, producing active control,[31] although this attachment may not be consistently present.[33] During mandibular depression, the medial and lateral attachments securing the disc to the condyle effectively restrict the motion between the disc and condyle to that of rolling (see Fig. 6–9A). As the condyle translates anteriorly during depression (see Fig. 6–9B), the biconcave shape of the disc causes it to travel anteriorly with the condyle without the need for active or passive assistance. The inelastic inferior retrodiscal lamina limits anterior translation of the disc. The superior portion of the lateral pterygoid muscle

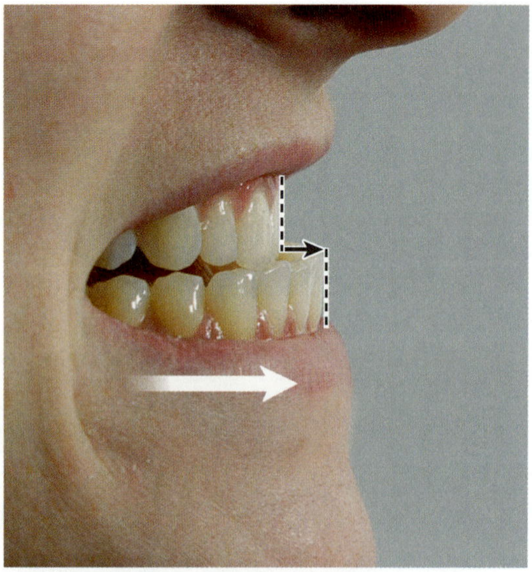

Figure 6–12 With maximum mandibular protrusion, the lower teeth should be in front of the upper teeth.

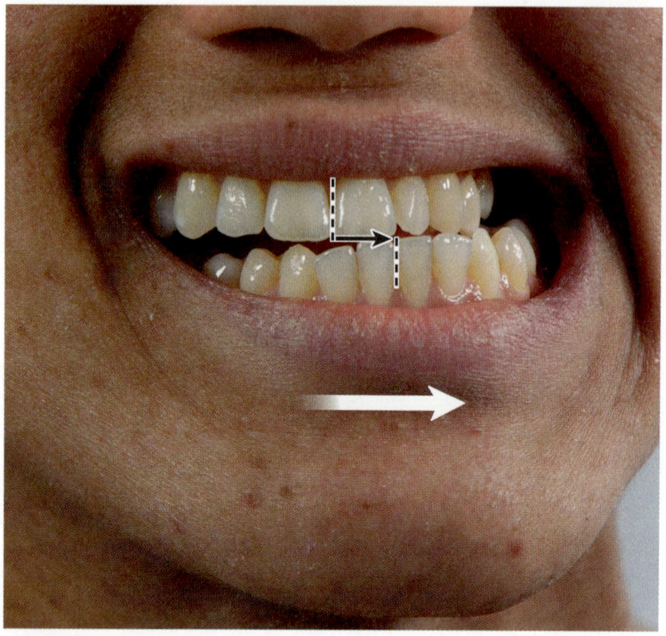

Figure 6–13 With normal lateral deviation of the mandible to the right, for example, the midline of the lower teeth should move from the midline of the upper teeth (dashed lines) by the full width of the right upper central incisor.

attaches to the disc and appears to be positioned to assist with anterior translation; however, no muscle activity is noted in the lateral pterygoid muscle during mandibular depression.[5,34]

During mandibular elevation (mouth closing), the elastic properties of the stretched superior retrodiscal lamina applies a posteriorly directed force on the disc. In addition, the superior portion of the lateral pterygoid appears to eccentrically control the posterior movement of the disc, while maintaining the disc in an anterior position until the mandibular condyle completes its rolling phase in its return to a typical resting position.[14,15,19,34] Abe and colleagues suggested that the sphenomandibular ligament also assists this restraining action[35] (see Fig. 6-8).

Other muscles (to be further explored later in this chapter) may also assist with controlling the disc position during active movement. These include the masseter muscle, which attaches to the anterolateral portion of the disc and may counteract the slight medial pull of the anteromedially directed lateral pterygoid.[6,34] The masseter, temporalis, and medial pterygoid muscles work together to provide a constant pressure and prevent dislocation of the disc.[34]

MANDIBULAR PROTRUSION AND RETRUSION

Mandibular protrusion and retrusion (forward thrust and retraction of the mandible) occur in the superior TM joints. Working bilaterally, the condyle-disc complex translates (slides) in an anterior (and slightly inferior) direction, following the downward slope of the articular eminence during protrusion, and returning along a posterior (and somewhat superior) path during retrusion.[4,8] Rolling of the condyles does not occur during protrusion and retrusion. These motions occur when the teeth are separated. In protrusion, the lower teeth ideally should surpass the upper teeth by several millimeters **(Fig. 6–12)**; however, protrusion is considered adequate when the upper and lower front incisal edges touch.[5] Rather than having a functional purpose in isolation, protrusion is an important component necessary for maximal mandibular depression. Similarly, retrusion is an important component of mandibular elevation from a maximally depressed position.[4,8]

During protrusion, the posterior attachments of the disc (the bilaminar retrodiscal tissue) stretch 6 to 9 mm to allow completion of the motion.[14,27] The degree of retrusion is limited by tension in the TM ligament as well as by compression of the posterior soft tissues in the retrodiscal area between the condyle and the posterior glenoid spine. An estimated 3 mm of translation occurs during retrusion; however, this motion is rarely measured clinically.[14]

MANDIBULAR LATERAL EXCURSION

Lateral excursion of the TM joint involves moving the mandible to the left and to the right. The degree of lateral excursion considered typical for an adult is 8 to 11 mm.[4,5,8] One functional screen to estimate whether this motion is typical is to observe whether the mandible can move the full width of one of the **central incisors** in each direction **(Fig. 6–13)**.[5] Active lateral excursion is described as *contralateral* or *ipsilateral* relative to the primary muscle action. To accomplish lateral excursion, the ipsilateral mandibular condyle spins around a vertical axis within the mandibular fossa, while the contralateral mandibular condyle translates anteriorly along the articular eminence **(Fig. 6–14)**. A slight degree of spin and lateral slide of the contralateral mandibular condyle is necessary to achieve maximal lateral excursion.[5]

Another typically asymmetrical movement of the TM joint involves the spin of one condyle around an anteroposterior axis while the other condyle depresses (slides downward).[14] This movement results in a frontal plane motion of the mandible, with the chin moving downward and deviating from the midline toward the condyle that is spinning. These motions are generally combined into one complex motion used for chewing and grinding food.

Deviations and **deflections** may be noted during osteokinematic movements of the mandible **(Fig 6–15)**. Deviations and deflections may result from left vs. right asymmetries in the mandibular condyle head shape. If no other signs or symptoms accompany these asymmetries, then deviation or deflection is considered inconsequential. However, as will be discussed later in this chapter, deviations and deflections may indicate a pathology.[5]

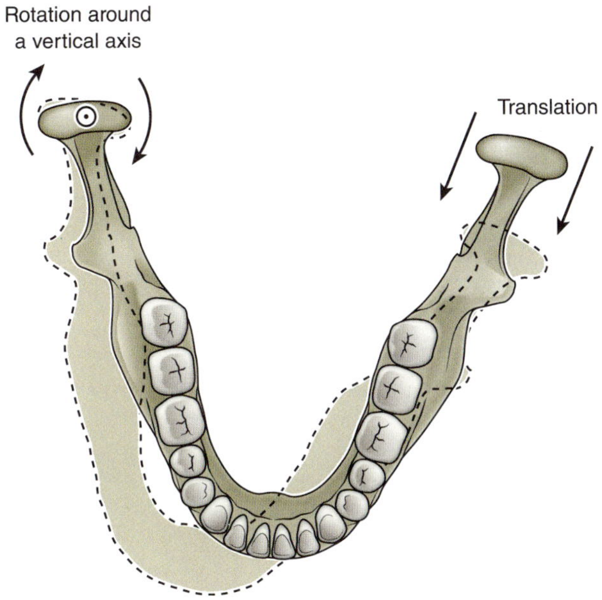

Figure 6–14 In this superior view of the mandible, lateral deviation of the mandible (chin) to the right occurs effectively as a rotation (spin) of the right condyle around a vertical axis, and the left condyle translates anteriorly.

Muscles

As an overview, mastication involves depression, elevation, and lateral excursion of the mandible. The muscles of mastication include the medial and lateral pterygoids, masseter, and temporalis, along with other accessory muscles. Specifically, the lateral pterygoid, stylohyoid, mylohyoid, and geniohyoid muscles, with assistance from the digastric muscle, depress the mandible, whereas the temporalis, medial pterygoid, and masseter muscles elevate the mandible. Contralateral contraction of the inferior belly of the lateral pterygoid is responsible for lateral excursion of the mandible.[6] The information in the next section provides details specific to the muscles of mastication.

PRIMARY MUSCLES

The muscles acting on the TM joint are divided into primary and secondary muscle groups **(Fig. 6–16)**. The primary muscles include the temporalis, masseter, lateral pterygoid, and medial pterygoid[3]

The temporalis is a flat, fan-shaped muscle that is wide at the proximal portion and narrow at the inferior portion **(Fig. 6–16A)**. The superior fibers attach to the cranium, and the inferior fibers attach to the coronoid process and the medial surface of the ramus of the mandible. The temporalis fills the concavity of the temporal fossa and can be palpated easily over the temporal bone.[2,4] The masseter is a thick, powerful muscle with its superior attachments on the zygomatic bone and its inferior attachment on the external surface of the ramus of the mandible **(Fig. 6–16B)**. This muscle can be palpated easily superior to the angle of the mandible.[2] Okeson noted that the temporalis and masseter are responsible for elevating the mandible. Additionally, the temporalis assists with retrusion whereas the masseter contributes to protrusion.[29] Van der Bilt and colleagues noted that the bilateral masseters and

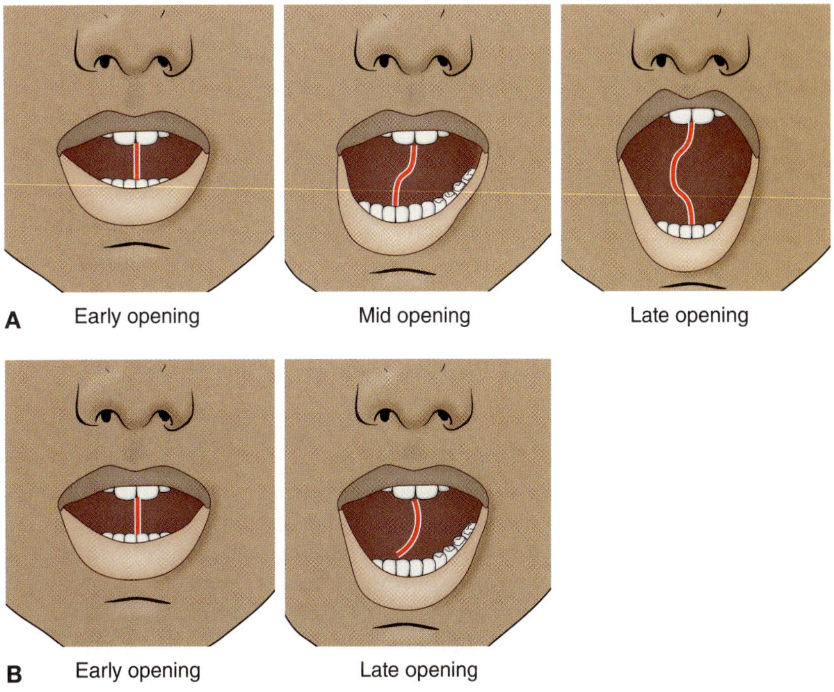

Figure 6–15 **A.** A mandibular *deviation* to the right is a motion where the mandible moves away from midline during depression and returns to midline at the end range. **B.** A mandibular *deflection* to the right is a motion where the mandible moves away from midline during depression and does **not** return to midline at the end range.

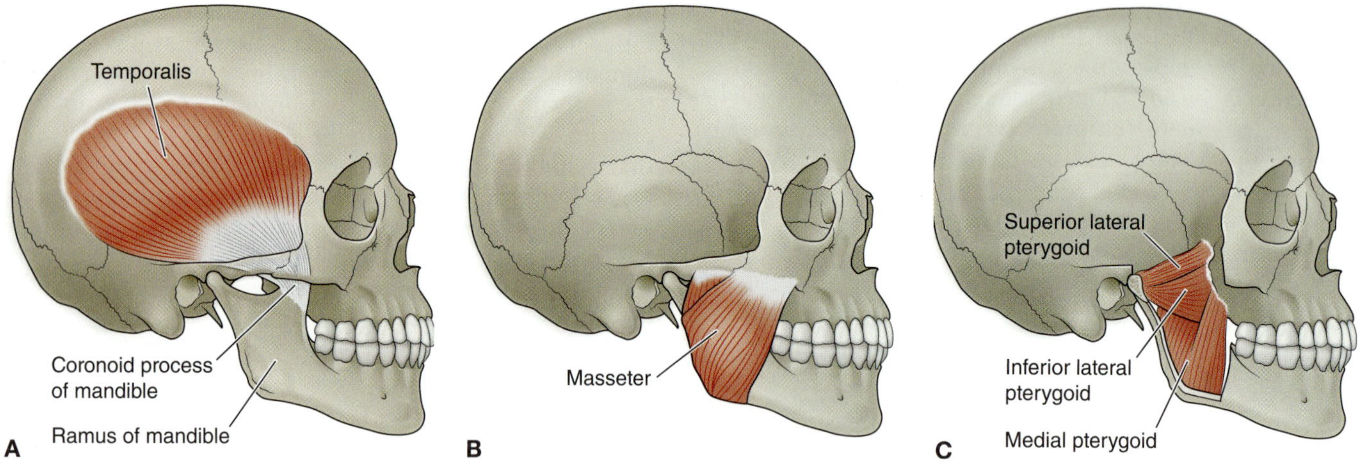

Figure 6–16 Primary TM joint muscles. **A.** The temporalis muscle attaches to the medial aspect of the coronoid process and ramus of the mandible. **B.** The masseter muscle attaches to the external surface of the ramus of the mandible. **C.** The superior and inferior lateral pterygoid and medial pterygoid muscles lie inside the mandible (shown cut away here), attaching to the neck of the mandible, disc, and TM joint capsule.

anterior temporalis muscles were 30% more active during bilateral maximum voluntary bite force than during unilateral bite force.[10] Furthermore, during unilateral clenching, these investigators reported symmetrical muscle activity of the bilateral masseters but noted significantly greater activity in the anterior fibers of the ipsilateral temporalis than in the contralateral temporalis muscles.[10]

The lateral pterygoid, as already noted, consists of superior and inferior segments **(Fig. 6–16C)** that travel in a horizontal direction and combine posteriorly to attach to the neck of the mandible, the articular disc, and the joint capsule (see Fig. 6–11).[2] The literature is contradictory as to whether this muscle can be palpated. The lateral pterygoid muscles are thought to assist with mandibular depression.[1,17,36] Okeson noted that the superior fibers stabilize the condyle and disc during mandibular loading, whereas the inferior fibers protrude the mandible and contribute to lateral movements and mandibular depression.[29,34]

The medial pterygoid parallels the masseter in line of force and size. The superior fibers attach to the medial surface of the lateral pterygoid plate on the sphenoid bone, and the inferior attachment is on the internal surface of the ramus near the angle of the mandible (Fig. 6–16C).[2] The medial pterygoid muscles elevate the mandible and contribute to protrusion.[29] Although we may be unable to palpate the lateral pterygoid muscle, an intraoral palpation of the medial pterygoid is possible.

SECONDARY MUSCLES

The secondary muscles are smaller than the primary muscles and consist of the **suprahyoid** and **infrahyoid groups** **(Fig. 6–17)**. The digastric, geniohyoid, mylohyoid, and stylohyoid muscles compose the suprahyoid group. The infrahyoid group includes the **omohyoid, sternohyoid, sternothyroid,** and **thyrohyoid** muscles.[4,8] The suprahyoid muscles assist with mandibular depression, whereas the infrahyoid muscles are responsible for stabilizing the hyoid bone. Both the suprahyoid and infrahyoid muscle groups are involved in speech, tongue movements, and swallowing. The suprahyoid muscles attach between the base of the cranium, the hyoid, and the mandible. The superior fibers of the infrahyoid muscles attach to the hyoid and the inferior fibers attach to the thyroid cartilage, sternum, and scapula.

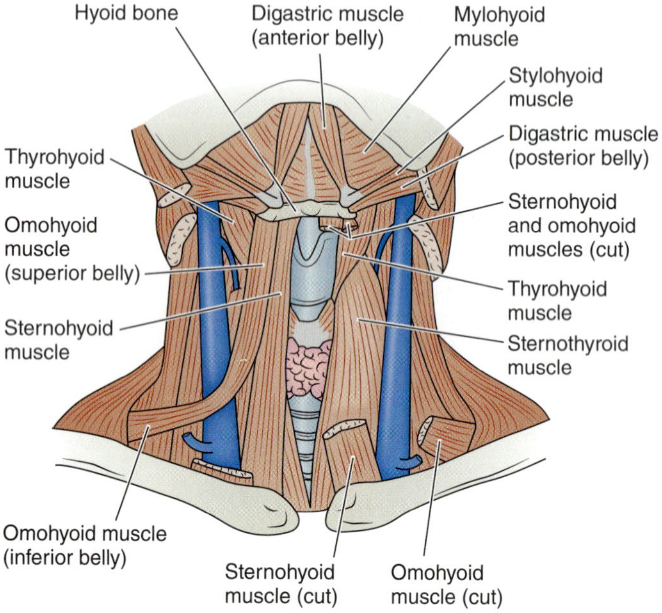

Figure 6–17 The suprahyoid and infrahyoid muscle groups shown from an anterior view of the neck.

The posterior fibers of the digastric muscle attach to the mastoid notch and the anterior fibers attach to the inferior mandible; the tendon joining the anterior and posterior segments is connected to the hyoid bone in the neck by a fibrous loop **(Fig. 6–18)**. The digastric muscle is predominantly responsible

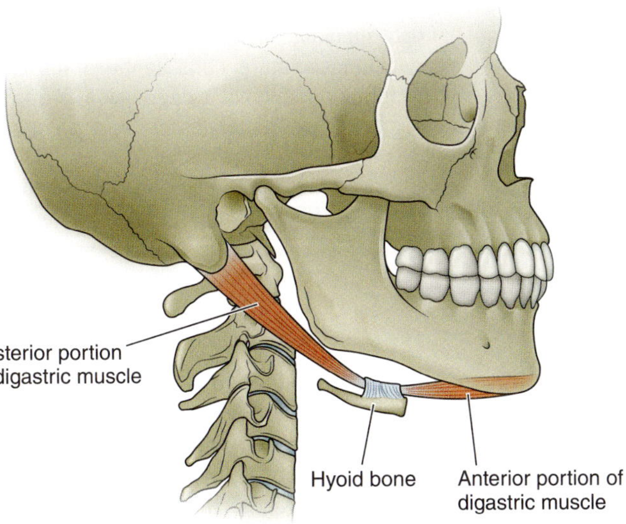

Figure 6–18 The posterior portion of the digastric muscle arises from the mastoid notch and the anterior portion arises from the inferior mandible. The tendon that joins the anterior and posterior portions is connected by a fibrous loop to the hyoid bone in the neck.

for mandibular depression, but also plays a role in elevating the hyoid bone.[29] The hyoid bone must be stabilized for the digastric muscle to depress the mandible. This stabilization is provided by the infrahyoid muscles.[4]

The muscles associated with the TM joint are directly innervated by the cranial nerves or cranial nerve branches. The neurological evidence indicates TM joint conditions may present similarly to trigeminal neuralgia or an ear pathology, possibly resulting in inaccurate diagnoses. Loughner and colleagues suggest that pain felt in the ear may be referred from the TM joint as a result of injury or inflammation.[28]

COORDINATED MUSCLE ACTIONS

Mandibular depression occurs from the concentric action of the bilateral digastric muscles in conjunction with the inferior portion of the lateral pterygoid muscles, coupled with passive contributions from gravity when the head is upright. Mandibular elevation results from the collective concentric action of the bilateral masseter, temporalis, and medial pterygoid muscles. The bilateral superior lateral pterygoid muscles eccentrically control the TM discs as the mandibular condyles relocate into the mandibular fossa during mandibular elevation.[4,33]

The other mandibular motions of protrusion, retrusion, and lateral deviation are produced by the same muscles that elevate and depress the mandible, but in different sequences. Mandibular protrusion is produced by the bilateral action of the masseter, medial pterygoid, and lateral pterygoid muscles.[5,33] Retrusion is generated through the bilateral action of the posterior fibers of the temporalis muscles, with assistance from the anterior portion of the digastric muscle.[33] Lateral deviation of the mandible is produced by the unilateral action of a selected set of these muscles. The medial and lateral pterygoid muscles each deviate the mandible to the opposite side.[33] The temporalis muscle can deviate the mandible to the same side. Although the temporalis and lateral pterygoid muscles on the left appear to create opposite motions of the mandible, concomitant contractions of the right lateral pterygoid and left temporalis muscles function as a force couple. The lateral pterygoid muscle is attached to the medial pole of the condyle and pulls the condyle forward. The temporalis muscle on the ipsilateral side is attached to the coronoid process and pulls it posteriorly. Together, these muscles effectively spin the left condyle to create deviation of the mandible to the left.[4,8] Because the temporalis muscle is also an elevator of the mandible, this combination of muscular activity is particularly useful in chewing.

Patient Application 6–1

Jill Smith is a 48-year-old insurance actuarial who is a parent to three young children. She is complaining of jaw pain with mouth opening, as well as intermittent headaches and ear pain. Jill's medical history is unremarkable, except for a history of serious hay fever present since childhood. After questions about a history of trauma, she recalled a biking accident when she was 12 years old where she flew forward off the seat of her bike, hitting her chin hard enough on the handlebars that she had to have a couple of stitches.

Upon examination, Jill demonstrates decreased active ROM with mandibular depression, protrusion, and left lateral excursion. Passive mobility of the right TM joint is limited in distraction and anterior translation, as well as lateral slide. Her mandible deflects to the right with mandibular depression. Palpation of the mandibular condyles reveals a larger space on the left than the right during active mandibular depression and protrusion. These findings indicate that the right mandibular condyle and disc are not translating as far anteriorly as are the left mandibular condyle and disc. The asymmetry may be due either to hypomobility on the right or to hypermobility on the left, but the differential (asymmetrical) activity or stretch on muscles and capsuloligamentous structures may be the source of Jill's jaw pain.

Relationship to the Cervical Spine and Posture

The cervical spine and TM joint are intimately connected. A biomechanical relationship exists between the position of the head, the cervical spine, and the dentofacial structures.[32,37] The proximal and distal attachments of the primary and secondary TM muscles have both direct and indirect connections to the cervical spine, throat, clavicle, and scapula, which implies that dysfunction in these areas (e.g., postural deviations) can affect the TM joint, or vice versa. Head and neck position may affect active or passive tension in the cervical muscles, which may in turn influence the position or movement of the mandible.[37-39] A desirable posture should minimize the forces required of the cervical spine extensors as well as the other cervical muscles to support the weight of the head. Over time, deviations from this expected posture can lead to adaptive shortening or lengthening of the muscles around the head, cervical spine, and upper quarter (including all structures including and superior to the scapulae). Deviations in posture may alter ROM, muscular forces, and joint morphology. Many of the symptoms associated with TM joint dysfunction are similar to the symptoms associated with primary cervical spine impairment. Therefore, the cervical spine and upper quarter should be thoroughly examined when clients present with TM joint complaints.[37,38]

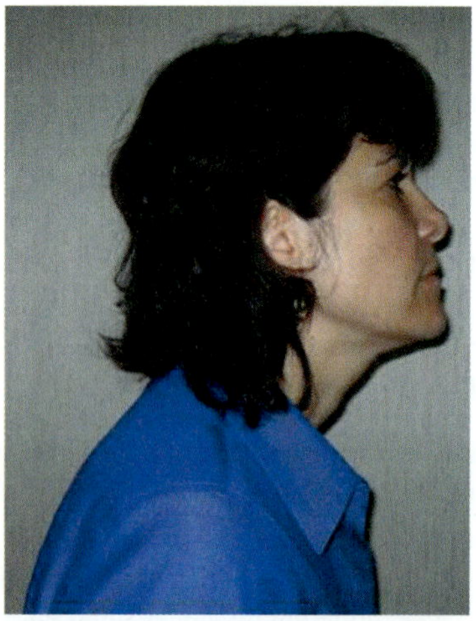

Figure 6–19 Poor cervical posture, such as forward head as shown here, may increase the physical demands on the craniocervical structures, contributing to TM joint dysfunction.

Expanded Concepts 6–1
TM/Cervical Joint Interrelationships

Pain often occurs concurrently in the head, neck, and jaw. The mechanical changes that occur with forward head posture are postulated to stimulate nociceptors and contribute to altered kinematics.[40-44] However, investigation into the relationship between forward head posture and pain is ongoing.[45-47] Forward head posture consists of flexion of the lower cervical and upper thoracic spine with concurrent extension of the occiput and the upper cervical spine to achieve a level head position **(Fig. 6–19)**. In a forward head position, the upper cervical extensors are maintained in a shortened position and may adaptively shorten over time, whereas the deep anterior cervical muscles are in an elongated position and may develop stretch weakness.[41] For example, with the occiput extended on the atlas, there may be adaptive shortening of the suboccipital tissues, the upper fibers of the upper trapezius, and the semispinalis capitis and splenius capitis muscles, while the posterior belly of the digastric muscles and the stylohyoid muscles may adaptively lengthen. The forces necessary to maintain the head against gravity with altered cervical posture and forward head can result in muscle imbalances and altered movement patterns. Such alterations may lessen the capacity of particular structures to adaptively respond to physical stresses.

Shortening of the suboccipital tissues may contribute to headaches that originate from the suboccipital area, limit active ROM of the upper cervical spine, and contribute to TM joint dysfunction. Furthermore, pain in the TM region may be referred from the cervical region.[44,48] For example, individuals with TM dysfunction report higher perceptions of pain with palpation of the cervical muscles.[49] Thus, the cervical region should be assessed thoroughly to appropriately evaluate dysfunction in the TM joint complex.[48]

Patient Application 6–2

In addition to Jill Smith's TM joint asymmetry, Jill's postural exam shows a forward head (see Fig. 6–19) with rounded shoulders, winging scapulae, increased thoracic kyphosis, increased lumbar lordosis, genu recurvatum, and overpronated feet. The noted posture and elevation of her right shoulder may imply tightness of some of the suboccipital and cervical musculature, consistent with her limited active ROM when performing mandibular depression, protrusion, and left lateral excursion. Jill reports tenderness with palpation of the muscles at the base of her head, the right side of her face, and under her chin. Tenderness and muscle guarding may be related to the stresses placed on the tissues from improper positioning.[44]

Dentition

Occlusion (contact of the upper and lower teeth) is intimately involved in the function of the TM joint because, in part, chewing is one of its functions. Although the teeth are only estimated to be in contact for approximately 15 minutes each day, the presence and position of the teeth are critical to typical TM joint function. Contact of the upper and lower teeth necessarily limits motion of the TM joint during empty mouth (non-chewing) movements. The complexities of the TM joint and the interrelated issues with the teeth underscore the necessity for comprehensive management of TM joint disorders. Normal adult dentition includes 32 teeth divided into four quadrants. The only teeth we will refer to by name are the upper and lower central incisors. These are the two central teeth of the maxilla and the two central teeth of the mandible.[9,50] When the central incisors are in firm approximation, the position is called **maximal intercuspation** or the **occlusal position.**[51] This position is not the typical resting position of the mandible. Rather, there is typically 1.5 mm to 5 mm of **"freeway space"** between the upper and lower incisors.[52] By maintaining this freeway space, the intra-articular pressure within the TM joint is decreased, the stress on the articular structures is reduced, and the tissues of the area are able to rest and repair.[9]

The American Academy of Orofacial Pain and others have identified occlusion as a causative factor in TM disorders.[40] However, the related literature has been contradictory and inconclusive. Lack of uniformity in research methods and techniques has been suggested as the source of these discrepancies. Peck noted that malocclusion is not necessarily a predictor of TM disorders because individuals with and without TM disorders demonstrate similar occlusal patterns.[9] He agreed, however, that altered articular patterns of the TM joint could occur as the result of occlusal changes. Clinicians should be aware that dental occlusion and TM disorders are more than a biomechanical concern. Just like with all other body regions, the biobehavioral aspect must be included in treating patients with TM disorders.[9]

Sonnesen and colleagues studied a sample of 96 children with severe malocclusion prior to orthodontic intervention.[39] These investigators identified a direct correlation between the occurrence of muscle tenderness in the masticatory muscles and a long-face craniofacial morphology. They provided two possible explanations: (1) The muscle tenderness could be the result of functional overloading of weak mandibular elevator muscles, or (2) the muscle tenderness may lead to temporary hypofunction of the masticatory muscles, resulting in decreased bite force. Additionally, the investigators confirmed an association between posture and TM dysfunction in the studied sample. Clicking (joint noise), locking of the mandible, and asymmetric mandibular depression were noted in children with a marked forward inclination of the cervical column and an increased craniocervical angle.[38,39]

Life Span and Clinical Considerations

TM joint dysfunction is a vague term that encompasses numerous clinical problems involving the masticatory system. Mechanical stress is the most critical factor in the multifactorial etiology.[20,39] Dysfunction of either the muscles or the joint structure is generally at fault. Most clients with TM dysfunction do not fit into a specific diagnostic classification category, which creates a clinical challenge.[53] Additionally, only 20% to 30% of individuals with internal derangement of the TM joint develop symptomatic joints, with symptoms progressing or resolving spontaneously.[11,17] One group of investigators identified the most common signs of TM dysfunction in children with headaches (from most to least frequent) as joint pain, muscular pain, joint noise, and mandibular deviation.[54] Pathomechanics of the TM joint may result from postural deviations, an isolated traumatic event such as a fall, cervical whiplash, or chronic inflammation of the TM joint resulting from indirect trauma. Although treatment of TM dysfunction is beyond the scope of this text, collaboration between dentists, orofacial pain specialists, physical therapists, and counselors provides the best functional outcomes.[38]

Determining whether a client has TM dysfunction requires an evidence-based diagnostic approach. This process should include a thorough clinical assessment performed by a TM clinician, classification of patients according to the *Research Diagnostic Criteria for TM Disorders*,[53] and MRI as the diagnostic gold standard. Because of the complexity associated with TM joint dysfunction, clinicians should seek advanced education before attempting to manage this patient clientele. Common etiologies of TM joint dysfunction include aging, inflammatory conditions, capsular fibrosis, osseous mobility, articular disc displacement, and degenerative conditions.

Age-Related Changes in the TM Joint

The aging process affects the joints of the human body, and the TM joint is no exception. However, degenerative changes are not always the result of typical aging and may occur instead from a preexisting dysfunction. Furthermore, degenerative changes do not necessarily indicate disability. Rowe and Kahn described successful aging as "multidimensional, encompassing the avoidance of disease and disability, the maintenance of high physical and cognitive function, and sustained engagement in social and productive activities."[55] With progression through life, the body's tissues become less supple, less elastic, and less able to withstand maximal forces. Pathology or biomechanical dysfunction will not necessarily result from these changes.[55] Alexiou and colleagues conducted a retrospective study of data from 71 individuals aged 20 to 75, each with characteristics of degenerative arthritis on diagnostic imaging.[56] They noted evidence of flattening, resorption, or sclerosis in the condylar head of the mandible in 56%, 43%, and 25% of the patients, respectively. They concluded that osteoarthritis of the TM joint is an age-related degenerative disease in patients over the age of 40.[56] Nannmark and colleagues examined cadaver mandibular condyles from 37 TM joints of people ages 55 to 99.[57] Structural changes were identified in 38% of the mandibular condyles examined, but no signs of inflammatory cell infiltration were found, suggesting that the observed changes were the result of biomechanical stresses rather than inflammation. Additionally, they noted that 22 (59%) of the articular discs had perforations, roughness, or were thinned. Only 3 (8%) of the discs were in an anterior position and each was perforated. The investigators concluded that TM osteoarthritis may be expected in 14% to 40% of adults, with increased frequency with age in both men and women.[57]

Clinical Considerations

Internal derangement is the abnormal position and function of the disc and articulating surfaces with the TM joint.[17] De Leeuw and colleagues performed radiography and MRI studies of 46 former patients 30 years after the diagnosis of osteoarthritis and internal derangement of the TM joint.[58] Compared to a group of 22 age-matched controls without known TM joint dysfunction, it was noted that radiographic changes were more common and severe in the former patient group. MRIs revealed a higher percentage of osteoarthritis and internal derangement in the TM joints on the side of diagnosed dysfunction, as well as in the contralateral TM joints. However, degenerative changes in the contralateral TM joints were largely asymptomatic, with only 25% of the subjects reporting any symptoms; none of this latter group had pursued intervention. MRIs of the study's control group showed only infrequent evidence of osteoarthritis and internal derangement.[58]

These studies suggest that TM joint degeneration does not necessarily occur with aging and that degenerative changes evident on radiograph or MRI are not necessarily associated with symptoms or dysfunction.[57,58]

Respiratory Dysfunction and the TM Joint

Children with chronic respiratory allergies may develop TM joint dysfunction as a result of altered growth and developmental patterns.[38] For example, a child with allergies who has difficulty breathing through the nose may assume a forward head position to increase the diameter of the upper respiratory tract and improve ventilation.[38,59] This posture, however, also changes the dynamics of the TM joint. As an additional example, blocked nasal passages impede inhalation and promote the use of accessory muscles of ventilation (scalene and sternocleidomastoid muscles) to assist with breathing. Such excessive use of accessory muscles may lead to a forward head posture.[60] Over time, this forward head posture may contribute to a cycle of increased musculoskeletal dysfunction,[61] including repeated episodes of TM inflammation that can result in fibrosis of the TM joint capsule.

Inflammatory Conditions

Inflammatory conditions of the TM joint include **capsulitis** and **synovitis.** Capsulitis involves inflammation of the joint capsule, and synovitis is characterized by fluctuating edema caused by effusion within the synovial membrane of the TM joint. Rheumatoid arthritis (RA) is the most common cause of synovial membrane inflammation, but gout, psoriatic arthritis, ankylosing spondylitis, systemic lupus erythematosus, juvenile chronic arthritis, and calcium pyrophosphate dehydrate deposition may also contribute to inflammation of the synovia.[17] Individuals with inflammatory conditions such as RA experience pain and inflammation within the joint complex, which may result in diminished mandibular depression.[6] Eventually, unresolved inflammation can lead to adhesions that restrict the movement of the disc and mechanically limit the function of the TM joint.[11] Although a discussion of rheumatoid arthritis is beyond the scope of this text, clinicians should be aware that RA often affects the TM joint.[62]

Capsular Fibrosis

Chronic inflammation of the TM joint capsule stimulates overproduction of fibrous connective tissue that can create **capsular fibrosis** of the TM joint complex.[5] The resultant fibrosis causes progressive damage and loss of tissue function.[5] A thorough client history is the key to identifying this condition. The clinician should listen for reports of repeated episodes of capsulitis. Circumstances leading to chronic capsulitis with progression to capsular fibrosis may include prolonged periods of immobilization, direct or indirect trauma, or arthritis.[5] Physical examination will reveal limited or altered osteokinematic motions, suggestive of a decrease in translatory motion on the involved side. Active motion of the TM joint capsule will typically elicit pain.[5]

Patient Application 6–3

Jill Smith's musculoskeletal complaints and limited active ROM of the mandible may be attributed to capsular fibrosis, as well as to her faulty posture. Most likely she has had repeated episodes of acute capsulitis of the right TM joint, with her initial episode following her childhood bicycle accident. The trauma to her face from hitting her chin on the handlebars of her bicycle likely caused compression forces to both TM areas, resulting in an inflammatory process with edema and pain. Her faulty posture may have developed as a result of her long-standing allergies and is exacerbated by her job that requires extended time in front of a computer screen in an ergonomically poor workspace. The stress of being a working mother may have exacerbated the inflammation without the opportunity for resolution, leading to a chronic and progressive capsular fibrosis of the TM joint.[32]

Osseous Mobility Conditions

Osseous mobility disorders of the TM joint complex include **joint hypermobility** and **dislocation.** Many similarities are noted in the client history and clinical findings for these two conditions. Hypermobility, or excessive motion, of the TM joint is a common phenomenon found in both symptomatic and asymptomatic populations. Joint hypermobility is a result of laxity of the joint capsules, tendons, and ligaments.[5,63] Joint hypermobility may occur as a generalized connective tissue disorder that involves all joints of the body, including the TM joints.[36,64] Individuals seen clinically for TM joint hypermobility typically report that the jaw "goes out of place," produces noises, or "catches" when the mouth is in the fully opened position. Physical examination of clients with TM joint hypermobility may reveal a larger indentation posterior to the lateral pole of the mandibular condyle. Joint noises (i.e., clicks) may occur at the end of mandibular depression and at the beginning of mandibular elevation. These noises may be audible to the person; however, the clinician often can palpate the clicking or crepitus associated with these noises. Unilateral hypermobility of one TM joint results in the deflection of the mandible toward the contralateral side during mandibular depression. In addition, the presence of excessive laxity may contribute to mandibular depression that exceeds 40 mm.[5] Yang and colleagues examined MRIs of 98 patients diagnosed with TM joint hypermobility during jaw opening.[36] They found pathological changes (hypertrophy, atrophy, or contracture) in 77% of the lateral pterygoid muscles, with changes more common in the superior portion of the muscle. Further, more symptoms were reported by individuals with anterior disc displacement with reduction (disc returns to resting position) compared to people with typical mobility or with disc displacement without reduction (sustained malposition of the disc).[36]

Many aspects of the client history and physical examination of individuals with dislocation of the TM joint are similar to those of individuals with hypermobility. However, with unilateral TM joint dislocation, full mandibular depression results in deflection (lateral deviation) of the mandible to the uninvolved side and an inability to close the mouth. The individual may experience pain with this condition. With dislocation, both the mandibular condyle and the disc have translated anteriorly beyond the articular crest of the tubercle of the temporal bone, thus "sticking" in the extreme end-range position.[5,11] Dislocation of the TM joint is usually temporary and resolves with manual joint mobilization.

Articular Disc Displacement

Articular disc displacement occurs when the articular disc anteriorly translates excessively to a point beyond the articular eminence.[5,65] Two conditions can result: disc displacement with reduction and disc displacement without reduction.[5,36,65] Without intervention, disc displacement with reduction often advances to disc displacement without reduction.[5,11,36,65] Disc displacement is an internal derangement that may be identified by diagnostic imaging or during a physical examination.[11] MRI is the imaging modality of choice to identify disc displacement.[17]

Individuals exhibiting disc displacement *with reduction* experience "joint noise" at two intervals: during mandibular depression and during mandibular elevation. The joint noise is referred to as a **reciprocal click** and is the gold standard necessary to diagnose disc displacement with reduction.[5,11,66] At rest, the articular disc sits anterior to the mandibular condyle; therefore, the mandibular condyle is in contact with the retrodiscal tissue rather than with the disc. During mandibular depression, the condyle translates anteriorly and captures the inferior surface of the disc to obtain a more congruent relationship with the disc. If the condylar translation is excessive and the condyle slips under the disc, an audible click is often present. Once the condyle-disc relationship is restored, typical motion continues through full mandibular depression. As the mandible elevates to close the mouth, the condyle translates posteriorly and slips back out from under the disc, while the disc remains in its displaced anterior position. Thus, elevation produces a second audible click. The second click signifies that the condyle and disc have lost the typical condyle-disc relationship. When the click occurs early in opening and late in closing, the amount of anterior displacement of the disc is relatively limited. The later the click occurs in the opening phase, the more severe the disc dislocation.[5,66]

Individuals exhibiting disc displacement *with* reduction may continue in this state or progress rapidly, within months, to an acute condition of disc displacement *without* reduction. Over time, the posterior attachments to the anteriorly displaced disc can become overstretched and unable to relocate the disc during mandibular depression, which results in the loss of the reciprocal clicks.[5,11,66] On MRI, Yang and colleagues discovered a strong correlation between abnormalities of the lateral pterygoid muscles and TM joints with disc displacements both with and without reduction of the disc.[36] The abnormalities of the lateral pterygoid muscle included hypertrophy, contracture, and atrophy of the superior and inferior bellies of the lateral pterygoid muscles of the involved TM joint. Recall that the lateral pterygoid muscle attaches to the anterior portion of the disc (see Fig. 6–11) and is typically active with mandibular elevation, presumably to eccentrically control the disc's return to its resting position. Hypertrophy of this muscle indicates overactivity that may lead to excessive or sustained anterior positioning of the articular disc.[36]

Whether acute or chronic, disc displacement without reduction indicates that the disc does not relocate onto the mandibular condyle. Thus, clients with acute disc displacement without reduction demonstrate limited mandibular motion because the disc creates a mechanical obstruction to condylar motion, rather than facilitating condylar translation. Individuals with disc displacement without reduction typically describe an inability to fully depress the mandible, as well as difficulty performing functional movements involving the jaw, such as chewing, talking, or yawning.

Degenerative Conditions

Morales and Cornelius conducted imaging studies of the TM joint using MRI.[12] The authors noted that degenerative joint changes were one of the most common pathologies affecting the TM joint, second only to internal derangement.[12]

Two degenerative conditions may affect the TM joint: osteoarthritis and rheumatoid arthritis, with rheumatoid arthritis discussed previously. It is estimated that 80% to 90% of the population older than 60 years have some symptoms of osteoarthritis in the TM joint.[36] Osteoarthritis usually occurs unilaterally (unlike rheumatoid arthritis, which usually presents bilaterally). Although multifactorial in nature, one common cause of osteoarthritis is repeated minor trauma to the joint, particularly trauma that creates an impact between the articular surfaces.[11,67] The radiographic features of degenerative changes in the TM joint, similar to those elsewhere in the body, include joint space narrowing, erosion, osteophyte formation, sclerosis, and remodeling.[11] Loss of posterior teeth may also contribute to degenerative changes because the occlusion of the remaining teeth can alter the forces that occur between the TM joint forces.[5]

Foundational Concepts 6–1
Signs and Symptoms of TM Joint Dysfunction

Clinical manifestations of TM joint dysfunction can vary widely, depending on the extent of the condition and the presence of complicating factors. Signs and symptoms may include the following:

- Pain in the area of the jaw
- Edema around the mandibular condyle
- Increased or decreased active or passive ROM
- Popping or clicking noises
- Difficulty with functional activities (e.g., eating, talking) or parafunctional activities (e.g., clenching, nail biting, pencil chewing) of the mandible
- Catching or locking of the jaw
- Forward head posture

Patient Application 6–4

Jill Smith's symptoms may be attributed to trauma to the TM joint, poor cervical posture (e.g., forward head position), or some combination of these sources. Factors such as stress from work or family life also may play a role in her clinical presentation. Although the research literature does not explicitly draw a direct link between the cited sources, research does suggest that such biomechanical variables may play a role in a patient's pain presentation. Therefore, clinical interventions are aimed at improving the structural balance and alignment of the head, neck, and thorax **(Fig. 6–20)**. These are important augmentations to any direct intervention at the TM joint. Task modification in her work environment and stress management strategies may be therapeutic adjuncts.

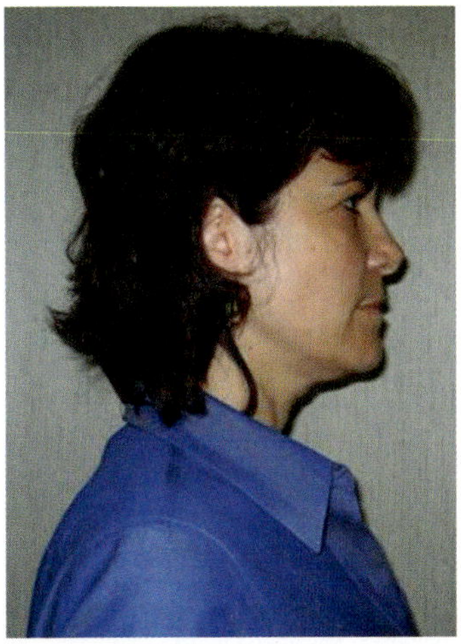

Figure 6–20 Corrected cervical posture restores the muscles of the cervical spine and TM joint to a more balanced length-tension relationship.

SUMMARY

- The TM joints are unique both structurally and functionally. The magnitude and frequency of mandibular movement, the daily resistance encountered during mastication, the physical stress imposed by sustained sitting and standing postures, and the chronic adaptation of muscles around the TM joint complex make this joint particularly vulnerable to problems.
- The influence of the cervical spine and posture upon the TM joint must always be recognized. The typical changes associated with aging must be considered as well.
- Intervention for clients with TM disorders presents many clinical challenges, and practitioners with interest in this clientele should seek advanced education beyond entry level in this specialty area.

As we proceed in subsequent chapters to examine the joint complexes of the appendicular skeleton, evidence will indicate that each joint complex has its own unique features. We will not see again, however, the complexity of intra-articular and discal motions that can be observed at the TM joints.

STUDY QUESTIONS

1. Describe the articulating surfaces of the TM joint.
2. Although the TM joint is classified as a synovial joint, its articular surfaces are covered with fibrocartilage rather than hyaline cartilage. Discuss the significance of this difference.
3. What is the importance of the differing thicknesses and vascularity of the disc?
4. How do the superior and inferior laminae of the retrodiscal area differ?
5. Describe the motions in the upper and lower joints within the TM joint during mouth opening and closing.
6. What limits posterior motion of the condyle? How is the motion limited?
7. What are the consequences of a left TM joint that does not anteriorly slide?
8. What are the consequences of a right disc that cannot move freely on the mandibular condyle?
9. Describe the control of the disc when moving from an open mouth position to a closed mouth position.
10. What is the potential effect of cervical spine posture on the function of the TM joint complex?
11. Discuss the effects of aging on the TM joint.
12. Compare and contrast the functional presentations of hypo- and hypermobile TM joint complexes.

REFERENCES

1. Matsumoto M, Matsumoto W, Bolognese A: Study of the signs and symptoms of temporomandibular dysfunction in in dividuals with normal occlusion and malocclusion. Cranio 20:274-81, 2002
2. Standring S: Gray's Anatomy: The Anatomical Basis of Clinical Practice (ed 42). New York, NY, Elsevier Health Sciences, 2020
3. Tanaka E, Koolstra JH: Biomechanics of the temporomandibular joint. J Dent Res 87:989-91, 2008
4. Helland MM: Anatomy and function of the temporomandibular joint. J Orthop Sports Phys Ther 1:145-52, 1980
5. Kraus S: Temporomandibular joint, in Saunders H, Saunders R (eds): Evaluation, Treatment, and Prevention of Musculoskeletal Disorders (ed 4). Bloomington, MN, Educational Opportunities, 2004
6. Bag AK, Gaddikeri S, Singhal A, et al: Imaging of the temporomandibular joint: an update. World J Radiol 6:567-82, 2014
7. Mueller MJ, Maluf KS: Tissue adaptation to physical stress: a proposed "physical stress theory" to guide physical therapist practice, education, and research. Phys Ther 82:383-403, 2002
8. Shaffer SM, Brismée J, Sizer PS, et al: Temporomandibular disorders. Part 1: anatomy and examination/diagnosis. J Man Manip Ther 22:2-12, 2014
9. Peck CC: Biomechanics of occlusion—implications for oral rehabilitation. J Oral Rehabil 43:205-14, 2016
10. van der Bilt A, Tekamp A, Glas H, et al: Bite force and electromyograpy during maximum unilateral and bilateral clenching. Eur J Oral Sci 116:217-22, 2008
11. Styles C, Whyte A: MRI in the assessment of internal derangement and pain within the temporomandibular joint: a pictorial essay. Br J Oral Maxillofac 40:220-8, 2002
12. Morales H, Cornelius R: Imaging approach to temporomandibular joint disorders. Clin Neuroradiol 26:5-22, 2016
13. Sicher H: Functional anatomy of the temporomandibular joint, in Sarnat B (ed): The temporomandibular joint (ed 2). Springfield, IL, Charles C Thomas, 1964
14. Hertling D, Kessler R: Management of common musculoskeletal disorders: physical therapy principles and methods (ed 4). Philadelphia, PA, Lippincott-Raven, 2006
15. Koolstra JH, Tanaka E: Tensile stress patterns predicted in the articular disc of the human temporomandibular joint. J Anat 215:411-16, 2009
16. Magee D: Orthopedic physical assessment (ed 5). Philadelphia, PA, WB Saunders, 2008
17. Sommer OJ, Aigner F, Rudisch A, et al: Cross-sectional and functional imaging of the temporomandibular joint: radiology, pathology, and basic biomechanics of the jaw. Radiographics 23:e14, 2003
18. Hattori-Hara E, Mitsui SN, Mori H, et al: The influence of unilateral disc displacement on stress in the contralateral joint with a normally positioned disc in a human temporomandibular joint: an analytic approach using the finite element method. J Cranio-Maxillo-Facial Surg: 42:2018-24, 2014
19. Tanaka E, Kawai N, Hanaoka K, et al: Shear properties of the temporomandibular joint disc in relation to compressive and shear strain. J Dent Res 83:476-9, 2004
20. Tanaka E, Shibaguchi T, Tanaka M, et al: Viscoelastic properties of the human temporomandibular joint disc in patients with internal derangement. J Oral Maxillofac Surg 58:997-1002, 2000
21. Willard VP, Arzi B, Athanasiou KA: The attachments of the temporomandibular joint disc: a biochemical and histological investigation. Archives of Oral Biology 57:599-606, 2012
22. Horton LM, John RM, Karibe H, et al: Jaw disorders in the pediatric population. J Am Assoc Nurse Pract 28:294-303, 2016
23. Sicher H: Functional anatomy of the temporomandibular articulation. Aust J Dent 55:73-85, 1951
24. Cuccia AM, Caradonna C, Caradonna D: Manual therapy of the mandibular accessory ligaments for the management of temporomandibular joint disorders. J Am Osteopath Assoc 111:102-12, 2011
25. Sencimen M, Yalçin B, Doğan N, et al: Anatomical and functional aspects of ligaments between the malleus and the temporomandibular joint. Int J Oral Maxillofac Surg, 37:943-7, 2008
26. Curtis N: Craniofacial biomechanics: an overview of recent multibody modelling studies. J Anat 218:16-25, 2011
27. Alomar X, Medrano J, Cabratosa J, et al: Anatomy of the temporomandibular joint. Seminars in Ultrasound, CT, and MR 28:170-83, 2007
28. Loughner BA, Gremillion HA, Mahan PE, et al: The medial capsule of the human temporomandibular joint. J Oral Maxillofac Surg 55:363-9; discussion 369-70, 1997
29. Okeson JP: Management of temporomandibular disorders and occlusion (ed 7). St. Louis, MO, Mosby, 2013
30. Posselt U: Movement areas of the mandible. J Prosthet Dent 7:375-85, 1957
31. van der El A: The Temporomandibular Joint, Orthopaedic Manual Therapy Diagnosis: Spine and Temporomandibular Joints. Boston, MA, Jones & Bartlett Learning, 2010
32. Rocabado M: Craniovertebral-craniomandibular disorders in headache patients. Vancouver, Canada, Physiotherapy, pp S1-S2
33. Dutton M: The Temporomandibular Joint, Manual Therapy of the Spine: An Integrated Approach. New York, NY, McGraw-Hill, 2002
34. Okeson JP: Joint intracapsular disorders: diagnostic and nonsurgical management considerations. Dent Clin N Am 51:85-103, vi, 2007

35. Abe S, Ouchi Y, Ide Y, et al: Perspectives on the role of the lateral pterygoid muscle and the sphenomandibular ligament in temporomandibular joint function. Cranio 15:203-7, 1997
36. Yang X, Pemu H, Pyhtinen J, et al: MRI findings concerning the lateral pterygoid muscle in patients with symptomatic TMJ hypermobility. Cranio 19:260-8, 2001
37. Armijo-Olivo S, Jara X, Castillo N, et al: A comparison of the head and cervical posture between the self-balanced position and the Frankfurt method. J Oral Rehab 33:194-201, 2006
38. Solow B, Sandham A: Cranio-cervical posture: A factor in the development and function of the dentofacial structures. Eur J Orthod 24:447-56, 2002
39. Sonnesen L, Bakke M, Solow B: Temporomandibular disorders in relation to craniofacial dimensions, head posture and bite force in children selected for orthodontic treatment. Eur J Orthod 23:179-92, 2001
40. Almăşan O, Kui A, Duncea I, et al: Temporomandibular joint disk displacements in class II malocclusion and cervical spine alterations: Systematic review and report of a hypodivergent case with MRI bone and soft tissue changes. Life (Basel, Switzerland) 12:908, 2022
41. Kendall FP, McCreary EK, Provance PG, et al: Muscles: Testing and Function With Posture and Pain (ed 5). Baltimore, MD, Lippincott Williams & Wilkins, 2005
42. La Touche R, París-Alemany A, Von Piekartz H, et al: The influence of cranio-cervical posture on maximal mouth opening and pressure pain threshold in patients with myofascial temporomandibular pain disorders. Clin J Pain 27:48-55, 2011
43. Sambataro S, Cervino G, Bocchieri S, et al: TMJ dysfunctions systemic implications and postural assessments: a review of recent literature. J Funct Morphol Kinesiol 4:58, 2019
44. Saunders H, Saunders R: Evaluation, Treatment and Prevention of Musculoskeletal Disorders (ed 4). Chaska, MN, The Saunders Group, 2004
45. Kim D, Kim C, Son S: Neck pain in adults with forward head posture: effects of craniovertebral angle and cervical range of motion. Osong Public Health Res Perspect 9:309-13, 2018
46. Mahmoud NF, Hassan KA, Abdelmajeed SF, et al: The relationship between forward head posture and neck pain: a systematic review and meta-analysis. Curr Rev Musculoskelet Med 12:562-77, 2019
47. Sarig Bahat H, Levy A, Yona T: The association between forward head posture and non-specific neck pain: a cross-sectional study. Physiother Theory Pract 39:1736-45, 2023
48. Ali HM: Diagnostic criteria for temporomandibular joint disorders: a physiotherapist's perspective. Physiother 88:421-6, 2002
49. Andrade AV, Gomes PF, Teixeira-Salmela LF: Cervical spine alignment and hyoid bone positioning with temporomandibular disorders. J Oral Rehab 34:767-72, 2007
50. Brand R, Isselhard D: Anatomy of Orofacial Structures (ed 7). St. Louis, MO, CV Mosby, 2013
51. Lila-Krasniqi ZD, Shala K, Pustina-Krasniqi T, et al: Differences between centric relation and maximum intercuspation as possible cause for development of temporomandibular disorder analyzed with T-scan III. Eur J Dent 9:573-9, 2015
52. Suvinen TI, Kemppainen P: Review of clinical EMG studies related to muscle and occlusal factors in healthy and TMD subjects. J Oral Rehabil 34:631-44, 2007
53. Manfredini D, Chiappe G, Bosco M: Research diagnostic criteria for temporomandibular disorders (RDC/TMD) axis I diagnoses in an Italian patient population. J Oral Rehabil 33:551-8, 2006
54. de Paiva Bertoli FM, Antoniuk SA, Bruck I, et al: Evaluation of the signs and symptoms of temporomandibular disorders in children with headaches. Arquivos De Neuro-Psiquiatria 65:251-5, 2007
55. Rowe JW, Kahn RL: Successful aging and disease prevention. Adv Ren Replace Ther 7:70-77, 2000
56. Alexiou KE, Stamatakis HC, Tsiklakis K: Evaluation of the severity of temporomandibular joint osteoarthritic changes related to age using cone beam computed tomography. Dentomaxillofac Radiol 38:141-7, 2009
57. Nannmark U, Sennerby L, Haraldson T: Macroscopic, microscopic and radiologic assessment of the condylar part of the TMJ in elderly subjects: an autopsy study. Swed Dent J 14:163-9, 1990
58. de Leeuw R, Boering G, Kuijl B, et al: Hard and soft tissue imaging of the temporomandibular joint 30 years after diagnosis of osteoarthrosis and internal derangement. J Oral Maxiofac Surg 54:1270-80; discussion 1280-81, 1996
59. Muto T, Takeda S, Kanazawa M, et al: The effect of head posture on the pharyngeal airway space (PAS). Int J Oral Maxillofac Surg 31:579-83, 2002
60. Ribeiro EC, Marchiori SC, Silva AT: Electromyographic muscle EMG activity in mouth and nasal breathing children. Cranio 22:145-50, 2004
61. Han J, Park S, Kim Y, et al: Effects of forward head posture on forced vital capacity and respiratory muscles activity. J Phys Ther Sci 28:128-31, 2016
62. Kretapirom K, Okochi K, Nakamura S, et al: MRI characteristics of rheumatoid arthritis in the temporomandibular joint. Dentomaxillofac Radiol 42:31627230, 2013
63. Goodman CC, Fuller KS: Pathology: Implications for the Physical Therapist (ed 4). Philadelphia, PA, WB Saunders, 2014
64. Winocur E, Gavish A, Halachmi M, et al: Generalized joint laxity and its relation with oral habits and temporomandibular disorders in adolescent girls. J Oral Rehabil 27:614-22, 2000
65. Yang X, Pernu H, Pyhtinen J, et al: MR abnormalities of the lateral pterygoid muscle in patients with nonreducing disk displacement of the TMJ. Cranio 20:209-21, 2002
66. Okeson JP, Leeuw R: Differential diagnosis of temporomandibular disorders and other orofacial pain disorders. Dent Clin N Am, 55: 105-20, 2011
67. Wang XD, Zhang JN, Gan YH, et al: Current understanding of pathogenesis and treatment of TMJ osteoarthritis. J Dental Research 94:666-73, 2015

SECTION 3

Upper Extremity Joint Complexes

CHAPTER 7 **The Shoulder Complex** 204

CHAPTER 8 **The Elbow Complex** 242

CHAPTER 9 **The Wrist and Hand Complex** 269

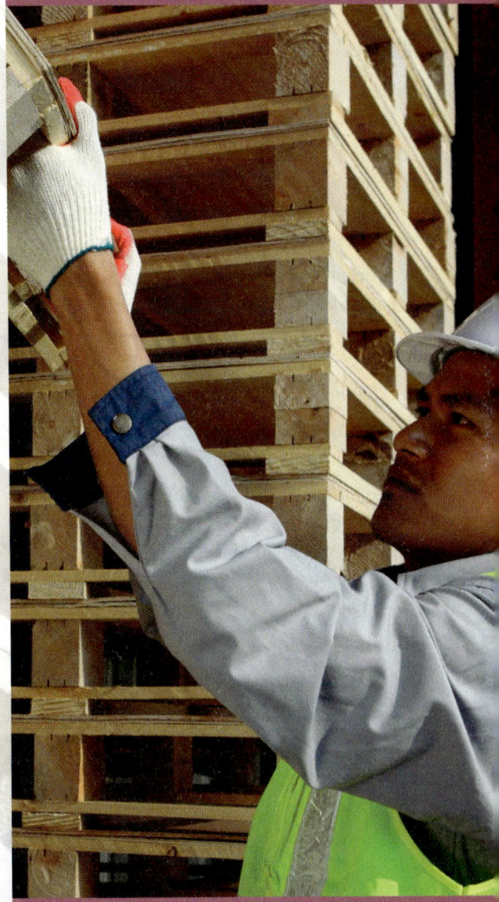

CHAPTER 7

The Shoulder Complex

Paula M. Ludewig, PT, PhD, FAPTA | John Borstad, PT, PhD

CHAPTER OUTLINE

INTRODUCTION 207
SHOULDER COMPLEX JOINTS AND STRUCTURES 207
Sternoclavicular Joint Structure 207
Sternoclavicular Articulation 208
Sternoclavicular Accessory Joint Structures 208
Sternoclavicular Capsule and Ligaments 208
Acromioclavicular Joint Structure 209
Acromioclavicular Articulation 209
Acromioclavicular Accessory Joint Structures 209
Acromioclavicular Capsule and Ligaments 209
Scapulothoracic Joint Structure 210
Scapulothoracic Articulation 210
Glenohumeral Joint Structure 211
Proximal Articular Surface 212
Distal Articular Surface 212
Glenohumeral Accessory Structures 213
Glenohumeral Capsule and Ligaments 213
Coracoacromial Arch and Bursae 215
SHOULDER JOINT FUNCTION 216
Sternoclavicular Motion 216
Elevation and Depression 217
Protraction and Retraction 217
Anterior and Posterior Rotation 217
Sternoclavicular Stability 217
Acromioclavicular Kinematics 218
Internal and External Rotation 218
Anterior and Posterior Tilting 218
Upward and Downward Rotation 218
Acromioclavicular Stability 219
Scapulothoracic Kinematics 220
Upward and Downward Rotation 220
Elevation and Depression 221
Protraction and Retraction 221
Internal and External Rotation 221
Anterior and Posterior Tilting 222
Scapulothoracic Stability 223
Glenohumeral Kinematics 223
Flexion and Extension 223
Medial and Lateral Rotation 223
Abduction and Adduction 224
Intra-Articular Glenohumeral Motion 224
Static Glenohumeral Joint Stability in the Dependent Arm 225
Dynamic Glenohumeral Joint Stabilization 225
The Deltoid and Glenohumeral Stabilization 225
The Rotator Cuff and Glenohumeral Stabilization 226
The Supraspinatus and Glenohumeral Stabilization 227
The Long Head of the Biceps Brachii and Glenohumeral Stabilization 227
Costs of Dynamic Stabilization of the Glenohumeral Joint 228
INTEGRATED FUNCTION OF THE SHOULDER COMPLEX 229
Integrated Joint Function 229
Scapulothoracic and Glenohumeral Function 229
Sternoclavicular and Acromioclavicular Function 230
Scapula Motion and Muscle Function 232
Integrated Shoulder Muscle Function: Elevation 233
Deltoid 233
Supraspinatus 234
Infraspinatus, Teres Minor, and Subscapularis 235
Trapezius and Serratus Anterior 235
Rhomboids 236
Integrated Shoulder Muscle Function: Depression 236
Latissimus Dorsi and Pectoralis 236
Teres Major and Rhomboids 237
LIFE SPAN AND CLINICAL CONSIDERATIONS 238
Life Span Considerations 238
Structural Dysfunction 238
SUMMARY 239
STUDY QUESTIONS 239
REFERENCES 239

ANATOMY OVERVIEW

MUSCLE ACTIONS OF THE GLENOHUMERAL JOINT

TABLE KEY: Primary movers *Secondary movers*

Sagittal Plane	Flexion	Extension
	Deltoid (anterior) Pectoralis major (clavicular head) *Biceps brachii* *Coracobrachialis*	Deltoid (posterior) Latissimus dorsi *Triceps brachii (long head)* *Pectoralis major (sternal head)* *Teres major*
Frontal Plane	**Abduction**	**Adduction**
	Supraspinatus Deltoid (middle)	Pectoralis major Latissimus dorsi Teres major *Coracobrachialis*
Transverse Plane	**Medial Rotation**	**Lateral Rotation**
	Pectoralis major Subscapularis Teres major *Latissimus dorsi* *Deltoid (anterior)*	Infraspinatus Teres minor *Deltoid (posterior)*

MUSCLE ACTIONS OF THE SCAPULOTHORACIC JOINT

TABLE KEY: Primary movers *Secondary movers*

Protraction	Retraction
Serratus anterior Pectoralis major *Pectoralis minor*	Middle trapezius Rhomboids *Lower trapezius*
Elevation	**Depression**
Upper trapezius *Levator scapulae* *Rhomboids*	Lower trapezius *Latissimus dorsi* *Pectoralis minor*
Upward Rotation	**Downward Rotation**
Serratus anterior Upper trapezius *Lower trapezius*	Rhomboids Latissimus dorsi *Levator scapulae* *Pectoralis minor*

SHOULDER MUSCLE ATTACHMENTS

Muscle	Proximal Attachment	Distal Attachment
Pectoralis major	Clavicular head: Anterior surface of medial half of clavicle Sternocostal head: Anterior surface of sternum, superior six costal cartilages, aponeurosis of external oblique muscle	Lateral lip of intertubercular (bicipital) groove and crest of greater tubercle of humerus
Pectoralis minor	3rd–5th ribs near their costal cartilages	Medial border and superior surface of coracoid process of scapula
Serratus anterior	External surfaces of lateral parts of 1st–8th ribs	Anterior surface of medial border of scapula
Trapezius	Medial third of superior nuchal line, external occipital protuberance, nuchal ligament, spinous processes of C7–T12 vertebrae	Lateral third of clavicle, acromion, and spine of scapula
Latissimus dorsi	Spinous processes of inferior 6 thoracic vertebrae, thoracolumbar fascia, iliac crest, and inferior 3 or 4 ribs	Floor of intertubercular sulcus of humerus
Levator scapulae	Transverse processes of C1–C4 vertebrae	Superior aspect of medial border of the scapula
Rhomboid minor	Nuchal ligament; spinous processes of C7 and T1 vertebrae	Smooth triangular area at medial end of scapular spine
Rhomboid major	Spinous processes of T2–T5 vertebrae	Medial border of scapula from level of spine to inferior angle
Deltoid	Lateral 1/3 of clavicle; acromion and spine of scapula	Deltoid tuberosity of humerus
Supraspinatus	Supraspinous fossa of scapula	Superior facet of greater tubercle of humerus
Infraspinatus	Infraspinous fossa of scapula	Middle facet of greater tubercle of humerus
Teres minor	Middle aspect of lateral border of scapula	Inferior facet of greater tubercle of humerus
Teres major	Posterior surface of inferior angle of scapula	Medial lip of intertubercular (bicipital) groove of humerus
Subscapularis	Subscapular fossa (most of anterior surface of scapula)	Lesser tubercle of humerus
Biceps brachii	Short head: Tip of coracoid process of scapula Long head: Supraglenoid tubercle of scapula	Tuberosity of radius
Coracobrachialis	Tip of coracoid process of scapula	Middle third of medial surface of humerus
Triceps brachii	Long head: Infraglenoid tubercle of scapula	Proximal end of olecranon of ulna

Introduction

The shoulder complex—composed of the clavicle, scapula, and humerus—is an intricately designed combination of three joints that links the upper extremity to the thorax. The articular structures of the shoulder complex are designed primarily for mobility, allowing us to move and position the hand through a wide range of space. The **glenohumeral (GH) joint,** which links the humerus and scapula, has greater mobility than any other joint in the body. Although the components of the shoulder complex constitute half the mass of the entire upper limb, they are connected to the axial skeleton by a single joint, the **sternoclavicular (SC) joint.**[1] As a result, muscle forces serve as a primary mechanism for securing the shoulder girdle to the thorax and providing a stable base of support for upper extremity movements.

The contradictory requirements on the shoulder complex for both mobility and stability are met through active forces, or **dynamic stabilization,** a concept for which the shoulder complex is considered a classic example. In essence, dynamic stability exists when a moving segment or set of segments is not limited very much by passive forces such as articular surface configuration, capsule, or ligaments, but instead relies heavily on active forces or dynamic muscular control. Dynamic stabilization results in a wide range of mobility for the shoulder complex and provides adequate stability when the complex is functioning in a typical manner. However, the competing mobility and stability demands on the shoulder girdle, coupled with the intricate structural and functional design mediating the compromise between structure and function, make the shoulder complex highly susceptible to dysfunction and instability.

The osseous segments of the shoulder complex are the clavicle, scapula, and humerus **(Fig. 7–1)**. These three segments are joined by three interdependent linkages: the SC joint, the **acromioclavicular (AC) joint,** and the glenohumeral joint **(Fig. 7-1A)**. The articulation between the scapula and the thorax **(Fig. 7-1B)** is often described as the **scapulothoracic (ST) "joint,"** although it does not have the characteristics of a fibrous, cartilaginous, or synovial joint. Instead, scapula motion on the thorax is a function of SC, AC, or combined SC and AC joint motions. The scapulothoracic joint is frequently described as a "functional joint." An additional region of the shoulder complex is the **subacromial** (or **suprahumeral**) space. This space is between the head of the humerus and the coracoacromial arch. We will refer to this region as the **subacromial space** and consider it a component of the glenohumeral joint rather than a separate joint.

The joints that compose the shoulder complex can, in combination with trunk motion, contribute as much as 180° of elevation to the upper extremity, although typical range of motion (ROM) for most individuals is closer to 150° to 160°. **Elevation** of the upper extremity refers to the combination of scapular, clavicular, and humeral motion that occurs when the arm is raised either *across the body*, *forward*, or *to the side*, including sagittal plane flexion, frontal plane abduction, and all the motions in between. Motion of the scapula on the thorax typically contributes about one-third of the total shoulder complex motion necessary for arm elevation, whereas the glenohumeral joint contributes about two-thirds of the total motion. Although the integrated function of all three joints is of primary interest, each of the articulations and components of the shoulder complex must be examined individually before their integrated dynamic function can be appreciated.

Shoulder Complex Joints and Structures

Sternoclavicular Joint Structure

The SC joint is the only structural attachment between the axial skeleton and the shoulder and upper extremity. The SC

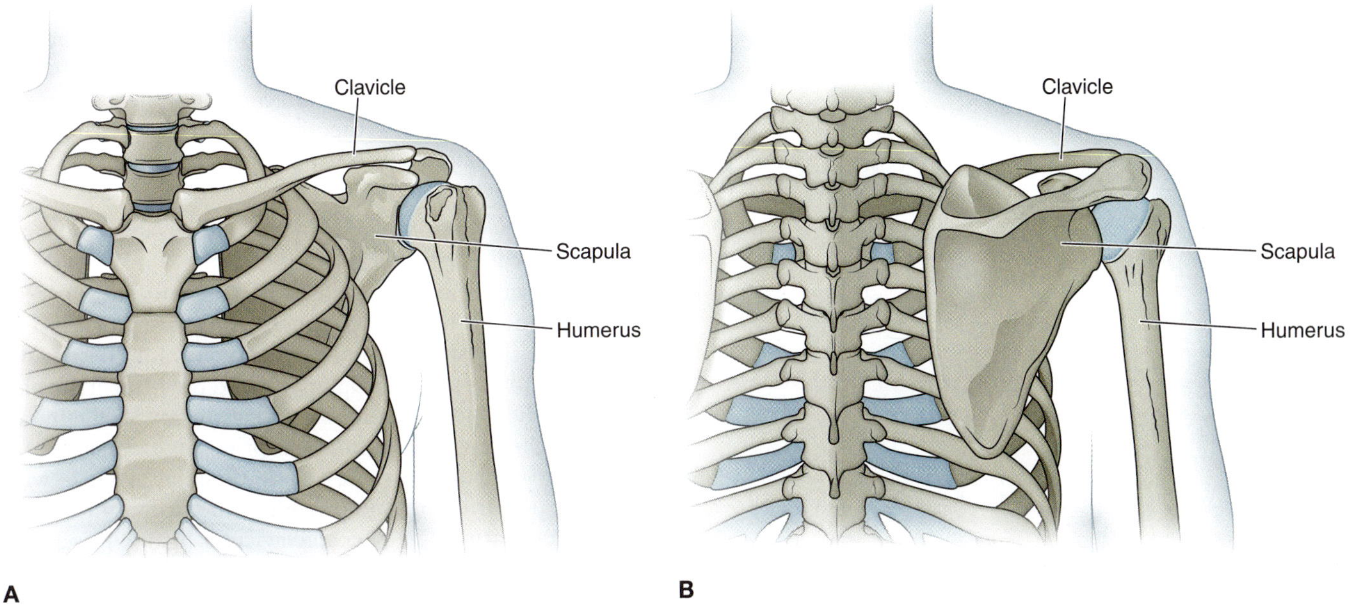

Figure 7–1 A. Anterior view of the three components of the shoulder complex: the humerus, the scapula, and the clavicle. **B.** Posterior view of the three components.

joint is classified as a synovial joint with three rotary and three translatory degrees of freedom.

Sternoclavicular Articulation

The SC articulation **(Fig. 7–2)** consists of two shallow, saddle-shaped surfaces between the medial clavicle and the manubrium, but is often considered a plane (rather than saddle) synovial joint because of the subtlety of the saddle configuration and minimal joint congruency. The smaller articular surface of the medial clavicle is located anteroinferiorly where it articulates with the cartilage of the 1st rib, whereas the larger articular surface of the medial clavicle covers nearly the width of the manubrial facet on the sternum.[2] The superior and posterior portions of the medial clavicle do not contact the sternum but serve as attachments for the accessory joint structures: the **SC joint disc,** the **joint capsule**, and the interclavicular ligament. Movements of the clavicle relative to the manubrium result in contact area changes between the clavicle, the SC joint disc, and the costal cartilage.

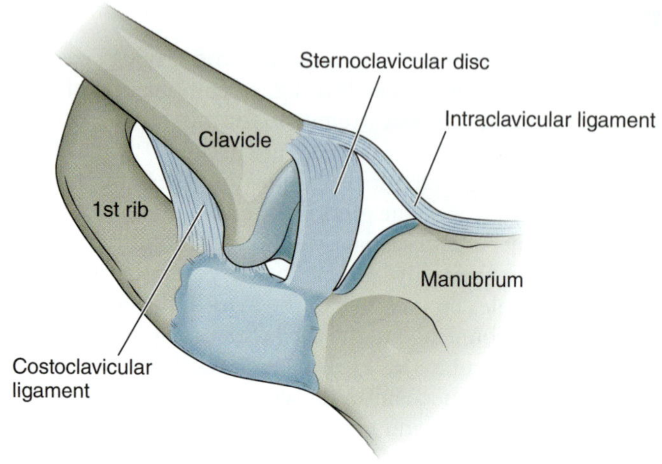

Figure 7–3 The SC disc is contained within the SC joint capsule (removed), and transects the joint into two separate joint cavities (shown with the clavicle pulled away slightly to facilitate visualization).

Sternoclavicular Accessory Joint Structures

The SC joint has a fibrocartilage disc that increases congruence between the articulating surfaces and dissipates joint loads. The upper portion of the disc is attached to the posterosuperior clavicle and the lower portion is attached to the manubrium and first costal cartilage, as well as to the anterior and posterior portions of the fibrous SC capsule.[3] As shown in **Figure 7–3**, the disc transects the SC joint space diagonally, dividing the joint into two separate cavities.[1] The disc improves SC stability by increasing joint congruence and by absorbing forces transmitted along the clavicle from its lateral end to the SC joint.

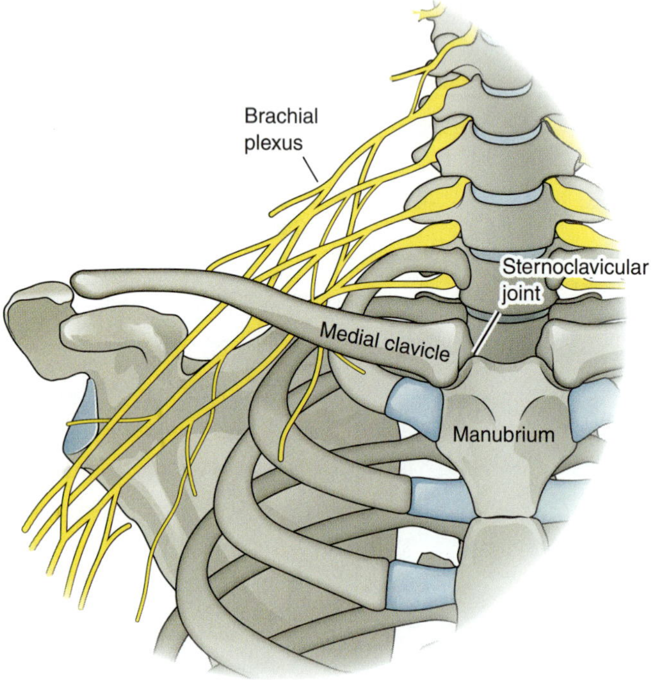

Figure 7–2 The SC joint is the articulation of the reciprocally convex and concave (saddle-shaped) surfaces of the medial clavicle with the manubrium of the sternum and the first costal cartilage; it is considered either a saddle or a plane synovial joint.

In Figure 7–3, note that the diagonal attachments of the SC disc will limit medial translation of the clavicle, which might otherwise cause the medial articular surface of the clavicle to override the shallow manubrial facet. The substantial area of disc contact with the medial clavicle also helps dissipate medially directed forces from the clavicle, protecting the small manubrial facet from high concentrations of pressure. Although one might think that medially directed forces on the clavicle are infrequent, we shall see that this is not the case when we examine the function of the AC joint, the upper trapezius muscle, and the coracoclavicular ligament.

During arm and shoulder motion, the disc acts like a pivot point for the medial end of the clavicle, but its role is different depending on the motion. With **clavicular elevation** and **depression,** the medial articular surface of the clavicle rolls and slides on the relatively stationary disc, with the upper attachment of the disc serving as a pivot point. With **clavicular protraction** and **retraction,** the SC disc and medial articular surface of the clavicle roll and slide *together* on the manubrial facet, with the lower attachment of the disc serving as a pivot point.[1] The disc, therefore, is considered part of the manubrium during elevation and depression and part of the clavicle during protraction and retraction.

Sternoclavicular Capsule and Ligaments

The SC joint is surrounded by a fairly strong fibrous capsule but depends on three ligament complexes for most of its support: the **anterior** and **posterior SC ligaments,** the bilaminar **costoclavicular ligament,** and the **interclavicular ligament (Fig. 7–4)**. The anterior and posterior SC ligaments reinforce the capsule and function primarily to check anterior and posterior translation of the medial clavicle, with the thick posterior capsule providing the primary restraint to both translations.[4] The costoclavicular ligament is a very strong ligament between the clavicle and first rib that has two segments, or *laminae.* Both laminae limit lateral clavicle elevation and may contribute to roll and slide kinematics of the medial clavicle on the disc.[5] The costoclavicular ligament

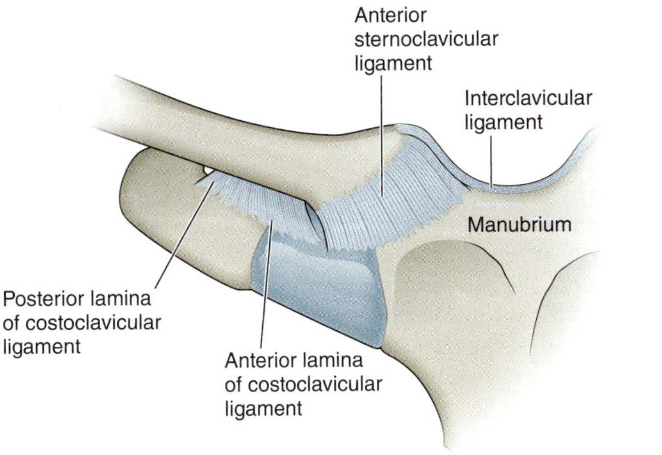

Figure 7–4 The SC joint ligaments. The axes for SC joint motion appear to occur at the location of the costoclavicular ligament.

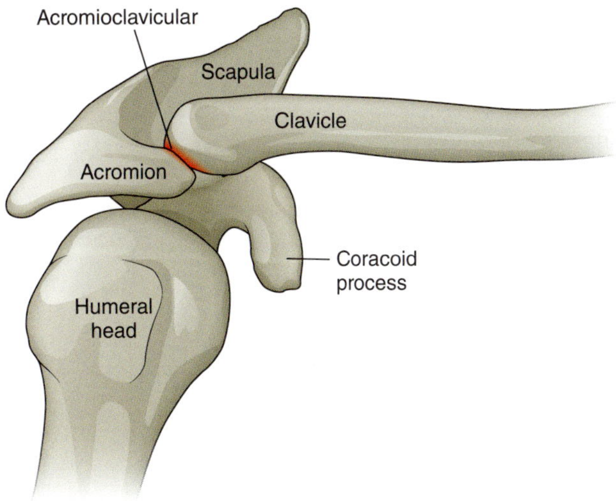

Figure 7–5 The AC joint is the articulation of the lateral clavicle with the acromion on the scapula, forming an incongruent plane synovial joint.

also absorbs and transmits the superiorly directed forces applied to the clavicle by the pull of the sternocleidomastoid and sternohyoid muscles, whereas the posterior lamina will resist medial translation of the clavicle. The interclavicular ligament limits excessive depression of the lateral clavicle and superior sliding of the medial clavicle on the manubrium.[6,7] The limitation of clavicular depression by the interclavicular ligament is critical to protecting structures such as the brachial plexus and subclavian artery, which pass under the clavicle and over the first rib (see Fig. 7–2).

Acromioclavicular Joint Structure

The AC joint attaches the scapula to the lateral clavicle. It is generally described as a plane synovial joint with three rotational and three translational degrees of freedom. The primary function of the AC joint is to allow the scapula to rotate in three dimensions during arm movement. This function satisfies three objectives: increasing upper extremity motion; positioning the glenoid beneath the humeral head; and helping to maximize scapula contact with the thorax. The AC joint also helps to transmit forces from the upper extremity to the clavicle.

Acromioclavicular Articulation

The AC joint is the articulation between the lateral end of the clavicle and a small facet on the acromion of the scapula **(Fig. 7–5)**. The articular facets are considered to be incongruent and vary in configuration from flat to concave-convex.[8] The vertical orientation of the articulating surfaces may make the joint susceptible to the degenerative effects of shear forces.[9]

Acromioclavicular Accessory Joint Structures

In early childhood, the AC joint is a fibrocartilaginous union between the clavicle and acromion. With upper extremity use over time, a joint space develops that may leave a "meniscal homologue" within the joint.[10] This fibrocartilage remnant, or disc, may vary in size between individuals, within an individual as they age, and between the shoulders of the same individual.

Acromioclavicular Capsule and Ligaments

The capsule of the AC joint is weak and maintains integrity of the joint with support from the **superior** and **inferior AC ligaments** and the **coracoclavicular ligaments (Fig. 7–6)**. The AC ligaments assist the capsule in approximating the articular surfaces; the superior AC ligament is the main restraint to movement caused by anterior and posterior forces applied to the lateral clavicle.[11,12] The fibers of the superior AC ligament are reinforced by aponeurotic fibers of the **trapezius** and **deltoid muscles,** making the superior ligament stronger than the inferior capsule and ligament.

The coracoclavicular ligament, although not directly attaching at the AC joint, firmly unites the clavicle and scapula to provide most of the joint's superior, inferior, and rotational stability.[12] This ligament is divided into a medial **conoid ligament** and a lateral **trapezoid ligament** (Fig. 7–6). The conoid ligament is more triangular and vertically oriented, whereas the trapezoid ligament is quadrilateral in shape and oriented nearly horizontal.[8] The two portions are separated by adipose tissue and a large bursa.[6] Both ligaments attach to the undersurface of the clavicle and their influence on shoulder biomechanics will be described in the section on Integrated Function of the Shoulder Complex. Although the AC capsule and ligaments can resist small rotary and translatory forces at the AC joint, restraint of larger translations and rotations is credited to the coracoclavicular ligament.

The conoid portion of the coracoclavicular ligament provides the primary restraint to inferior translation of the acromion relative to the lateral clavicle.[12] The trapezoid portion of the ligament provides more restraint to posterior translations of the lateral clavicle relative to the acromion.[13,14] Both portions of the ligament limit upward rotation of the scapula at the AC joint. When medially directed forces on the humerus are transferred to the glenoid fossa of the scapula, medial displacement of the scapula on the clavicle is prevented by the coracoclavicular ligament complex, particularly the horizontal trapezoid portion. Such medial forces are transferred by the ligament to the clavicle and then to the strong SC joint **(Fig. 7–7)**. In addition, one of the most critical functions of the coracoclavicular ligament relative to shoulder function is to couple posterior clavicle rotation and scapula upward rotation during arm elevation.

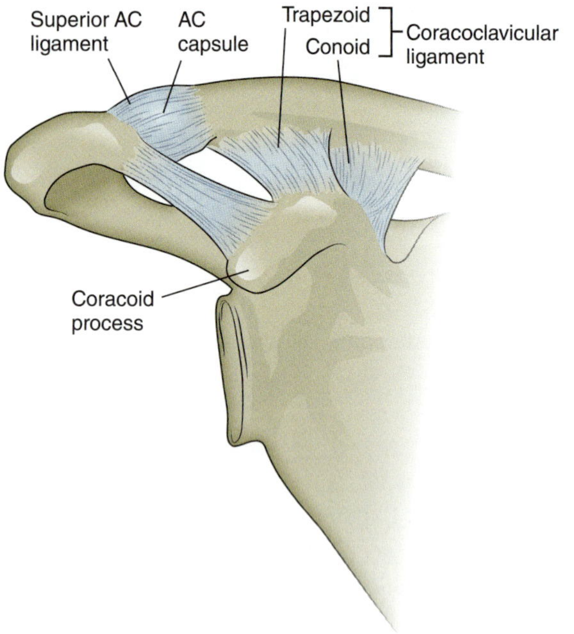

Figure 7–6 The AC joint capsule and ligaments, including the coracoclavicular ligament with its conoid and trapezoid portions.

Scapulothoracic Joint Structure

Scapulothoracic Articulation

The scapulothoracic "joint" is formed by the articulation of the anterior surface of the scapula with the thorax. It is not a true anatomical joint because it is not a union of bony segments joined by fibrous, cartilaginous, or synovial tissues. By contrast, the articulation of the scapula with the thorax depends on the integrity of the anatomical AC and SC joints. The SC and AC joints are interdependent with scapulothoracic motion because the scapula is attached by its acromion process to the lateral end of the clavicle through the AC joint; the clavicle, in turn, is attached to the axial skeleton at the SC joint. Any movement of the scapula on the thorax must therefore result in movement at the AC joint, the SC joint, or both. This makes the functional scapulothoracic joint part of a true closed chain with the AC joint, SC joint, and the thorax. Observation and measurement of individual SC and AC joint motions are considerably more difficult than observing or measuring motions of the scapula on the thorax. Consequently, scapulothoracic position and motions are described and measured far more frequently than are the SC and AC joint motions upon which scapulothoracic motions are dependent.

At rest, the scapula sits on the posterior thorax approximately 5 cm from the midline between the second through seventh ribs **Figure 7–8**. The resting position of the scapula on the thorax is upwardly rotated 5° to 10° from vertical, with upward rotation described as the angular deviation of a "longitudinal" reference line positioned perpendicular to a line running from the root of the scapular spine to the AC

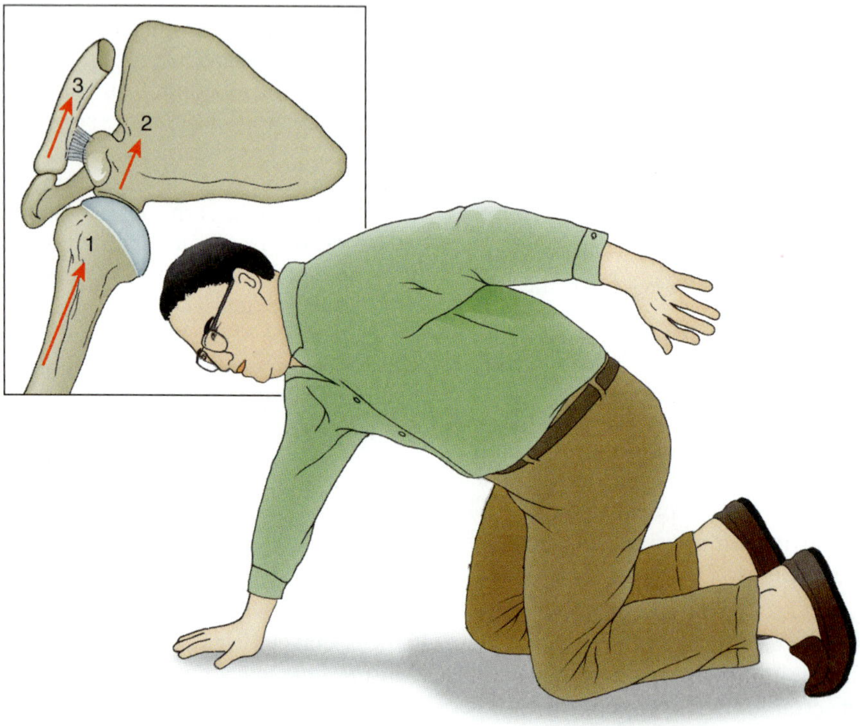

Figure 7–7 When a person bears weight (or falls) on an arm, a medially directed force up the humerus (1) is transferred to the glenoid fossa of the scapula (2) then to the clavicle via the coracoclavicular ligament (3) and finally ending at the stable SC joint.

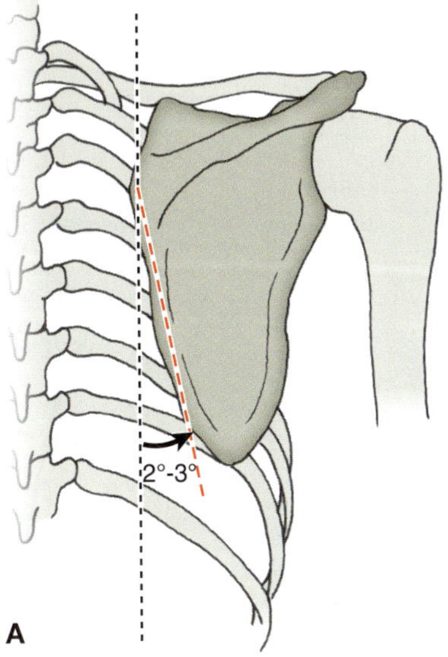

A

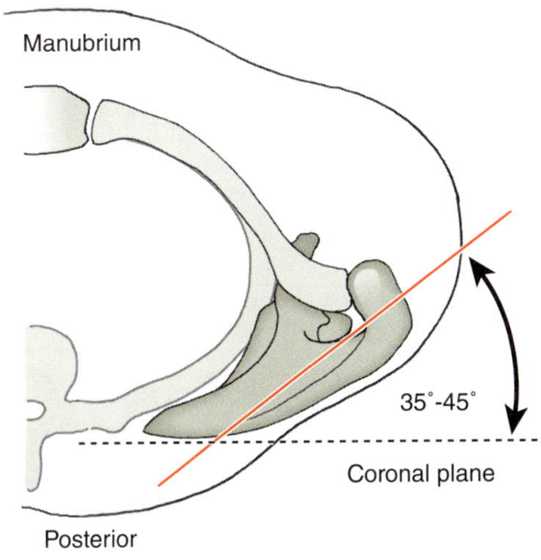

B

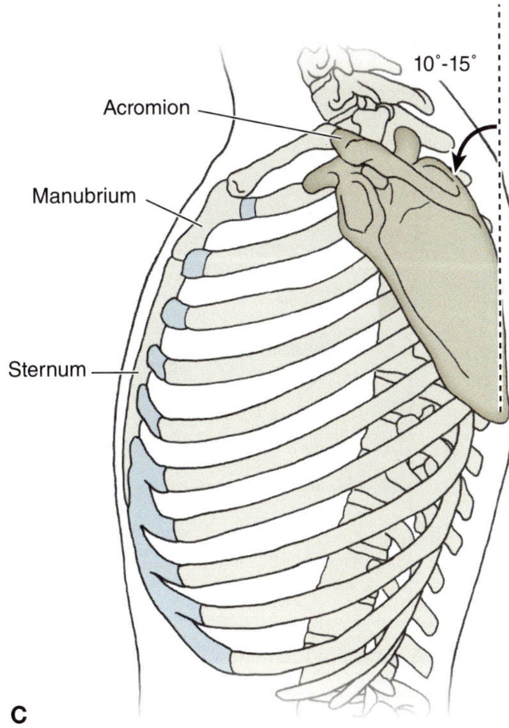

C

Figure 7–8 The resting position of the scapula on the thorax. **A.** This posterior view shows the scapula resting between the 2nd and 7th ribs, with the axis of the vertebral border of the scapula upwardly rotated 2° to 3° from vertical. **B.** This superior view shows the scapula resting in an internally rotated position 35° to 45° anterior to the coronal plane. **C.** This side view shows that the scapula at rest is anterior tilted approximately 10° to 15° to the vertical plane.

joint. If instead, the vertebral (medial) border of the scapula is used as the reference "longitudinal" line, the magnitude of upward rotation at rest is usually described as 2° to 3° from vertical **(Fig. 7–8A)**.[17] The resting scapula is also internally rotated 35° to 45° from the coronal plane **(Fig. 7–8B)**, and is tilted anteriorly approximately 10° to 15° from vertical **(Fig. 7–8C)**.[15,16] Although these typical values for the resting scapula are cited, substantial individual variability exists in scapular rest position, even among healthy subjects.[18]

Glenohumeral Joint Structure

The glenohumeral joint is a ball-and-socket synovial joint with three rotary and three translatory degrees of freedom. It has a capsule as well as several associated ligaments and bursae. The articulation is composed of the large head of the humerus and the smaller glenoid fossa **(Fig. 7–9)**. Because the glenoid fossa of the scapula is the proximal segment of the glenohumeral joint, any motions of the scapula will influence glenohumeral joint function. The glenohumeral joint sacrifices articular congruency to increase the mobility of the upper extremity, allowing flexible positioning of the hand. As such, the reduced stability results in increased susceptibility to degenerative changes, instability, and derangement.

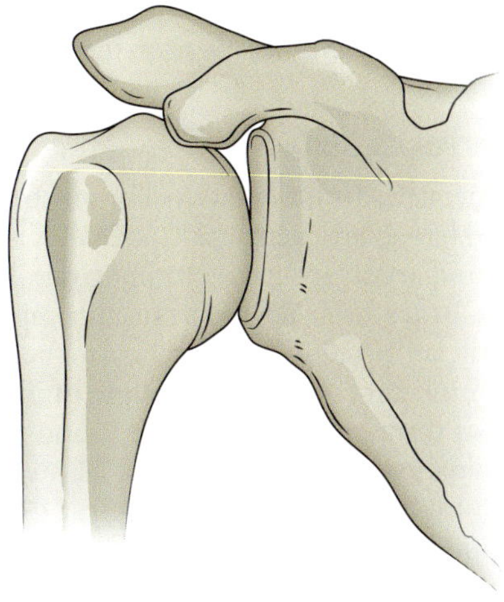

Figure 7–9 The glenohumeral joint.

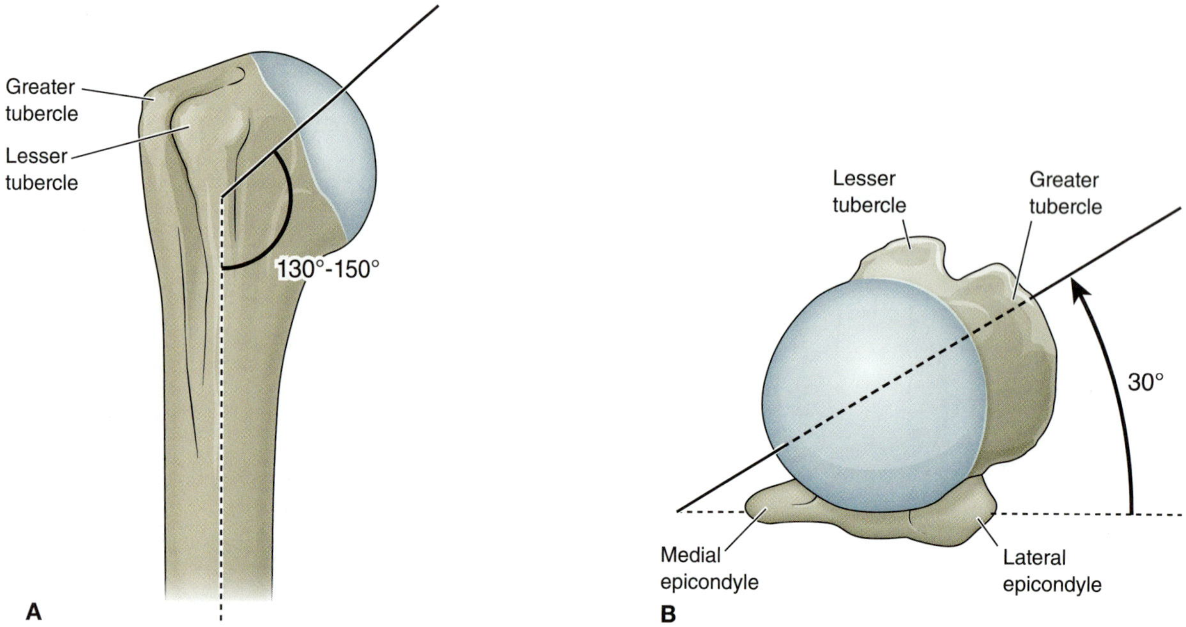

Figure 7–10 **A.** Angle of Inclination: The typical angle between the humeral head and the shaft varies between 130° and 150°. **B.** Angle of Torsion: Viewing the humeral head from above and looking down the shaft, the humeral head is typically angled posteriorly approximately 30° with regard to an axis through the humeral condyles (angle of torsion).

Proximal Articular Surface

The glenoid fossa of the scapula serves as the proximal articular surface for the glenohumeral joint. The orientation of the shallow concavity of the glenoid fossa in relation to the thorax varies with the resting position of the scapula on the thorax and with motion at the SC and AC joints. In addition, the orientation of the glenoid fossa may vary with the form of the scapula itself. The glenoid fossa may be tilted slightly upward or downward when the arm is at the side, although representations most commonly show a slight upward tilt.[18-20] Similarly, the fossa does not always lie in a plane perpendicular to the plane of the scapula; it may be anteverted or retroverted up to 10°, with 6° to 7° of retroversion most typical.[20] With anteversion, the glenoid fossa faces slightly anterior in relation to the plane or body of the scapula, and with retroversion it faces slightly posterior.

Distal Articular Surface

The humeral head is the distal articular surface of the glenohumeral joint and has an articular surface area that is larger than that of the glenoid articular surface, forming one-third to one-half of a sphere. In anatomic position, the humeral head faces medially, superiorly, and posteriorly with regard to the shaft of the humerus and the humeral condyles. The **angle of inclination** is formed by an axis through the humeral head and neck in relation to a longitudinal axis through the shaft of the humerus and is typically between 130° to 150° in the frontal plane **(Fig. 7–10A)**. The **angle of torsion** is formed by an axis through the humeral head and neck in relation to an axis through the humeral condyles. This transverse plane angle varies but is approximately 30° posterior **(Fig. 7–10B)**. This posterior orientation of the humeral head with regard to the humeral condyles is also called **posterior torsion, retrotorsion,** or **retroversion** of the humerus. When the arms hang dependently (passively) at the side, the two articular surfaces of the glenohumeral joint have little contact; the inferior surface of the humeral head rests on only a small inferior portion of the glenoid fossa (see Fig. 7–9).[21,22]

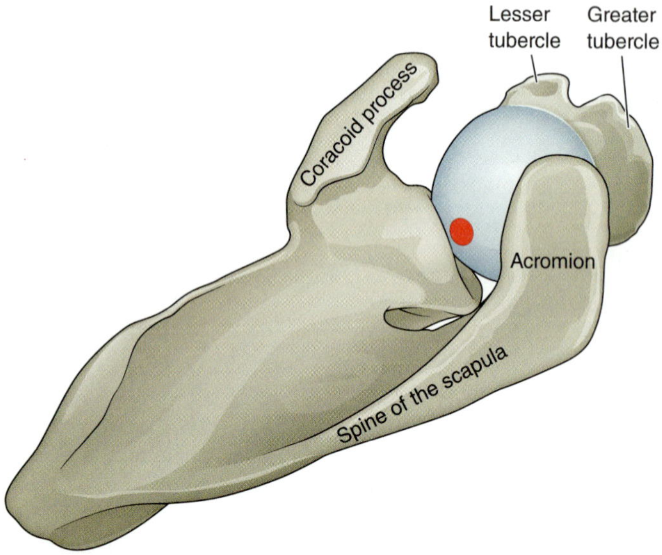

Figure 7–11 In a superior view of the scapula and humerus, the slightly retroverted angle of humeral torsion effectively centers the humeral head on the somewhat anteriorly-facing glenoid fossa of the internally rotated scapula, a typical position when the scapula is at rest and the humerus is in neutral position.

Foundational Concepts 7–1
Humeral Retroversion

Because of the internally rotated resting position of the scapula on the thorax (see Fig. 7–8B), typical retroversion of the humeral head increases congruence of the glenohumeral joint by orienting the humeral head toward the articular surface of the glenoid fossa **(Fig. 7–11)**. A humerus with an *increased* humeral retroversion angle results in the

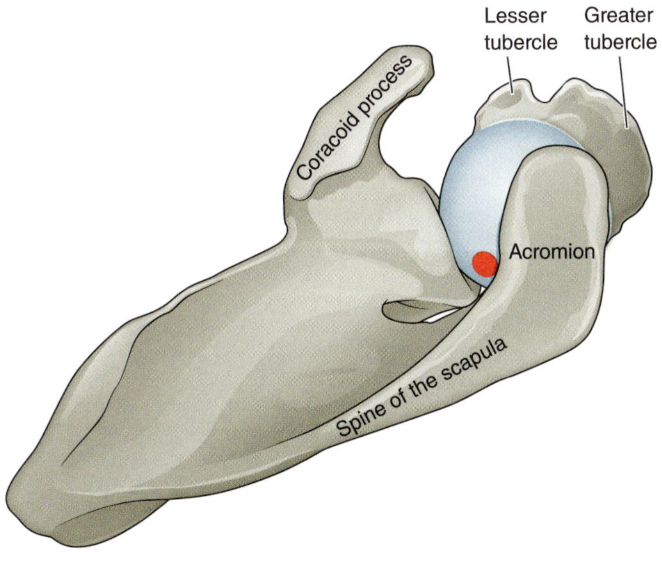

Figure 7–12 Excessive retroversion of the humerus places the humeral head more posteriorly on the glenoid fossa of the scapula when the scapula is at rest and the humerus is in neutral position.

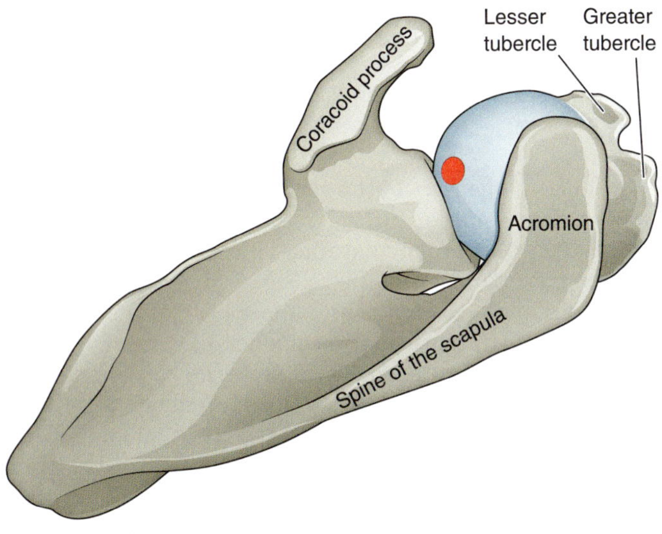

Figure 7–13 Retroversion that is reduced or actually anteverted places the humeral head more anteriorly on the glenoid fossa of the scapula when the scapula is at rest and the humerus is in neutral position.

humeral head sitting more posteriorly on the glenoid surface when the humeral condyles are aligned in the coronal plane (anatomic neutral) **(Fig. 7–12)**. Importantly, this increased humeral retroversion may result in increased range of lateral rotation of the humerus and reduced range of medial rotation. Increased glenohumeral lateral rotation and decreased glenohumeral medial rotation have been demonstrated in the dominant arm of throwing athletes, and evidence suggests that increased humeral retroversion may be one contributing mechanism for this ROM adaptation.[23,24] Although not as common, *decreased* humeral retroversion (or actual anteversion) may increase medial rotation ROM and decrease lateral rotation ROM **(Fig 7–13)**.

Glenohumeral Accessory Structures

The total available articular surface of the glenoid fossa is enhanced by the **glenoid labrum.** This accessory structure

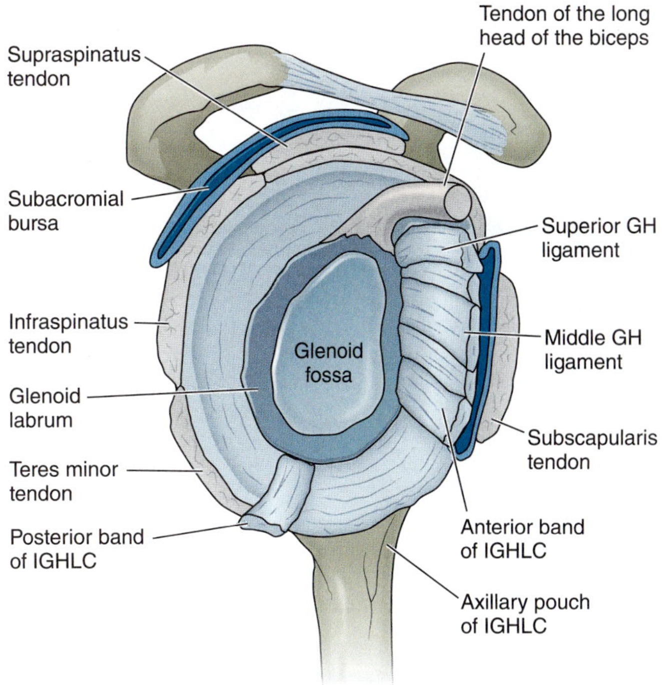

Figure 7–14 Looking directly into the glenoid fossa (with the humerus removed), it can be appreciated that the glenoid labrum increases the articular area of the glenoid fossa, as well as serving as the attachment for the glenohumeral (GH) capsule, the capsular ligaments, and the inferior glenohumeral ligament complex (IGHLC).

surrounds and is attached to the periphery of the glenoid fossa **(Fig. 7–14** and **Fig. 7–15)**, enhancing the depth or concavity of the fossa by approximately 50%.[25,26] The labrum also functions to restrict humeral head translations, protect the bony edges of the glenoid fossa, minimize GH joint friction, and dissipate joint contact forces.[27] The glenoid labrum serves as the attachment site for the glenohumeral ligaments and the tendon of the **long head of the biceps brachii** (see Fig. 7–14).[28]

Glenohumeral Capsule and Ligaments

The glenohumeral joint is surrounded by a large, loose capsule that, when the arm is dependent at the side, is taut superiorly and slack anteriorly and inferiorly (see Fig. 7–15). The capsule tightens when the humerus is abducted and laterally rotated, making this the close-packed position for the glenohumeral joint.[29] The capsular surface area is twice that of the humeral head, and more than 2.5 cm of distraction of the head from the glenoid fossa is possible in the loose-packed position.[8] The relative laxity of the glenohumeral capsule is necessary for the large excursions of the joint but provides little stability without the reinforcement of ligaments and muscles. The capsule is reinforced by the **superior, middle,** and **inferior glenohumeral ligaments** and by the **coracohumeral ligament (Fig. 7–16)**. The superior, middle, and inferior glenohumeral ligaments are thickened regions within the capsule tissue itself. In addition to these passive capsular reinforcements, the **rotator cuff muscles** and their tendons provide dynamic reinforcement to the capsule through their anatomic proximity to the joint and because the tendons of the cuff muscles insert directly

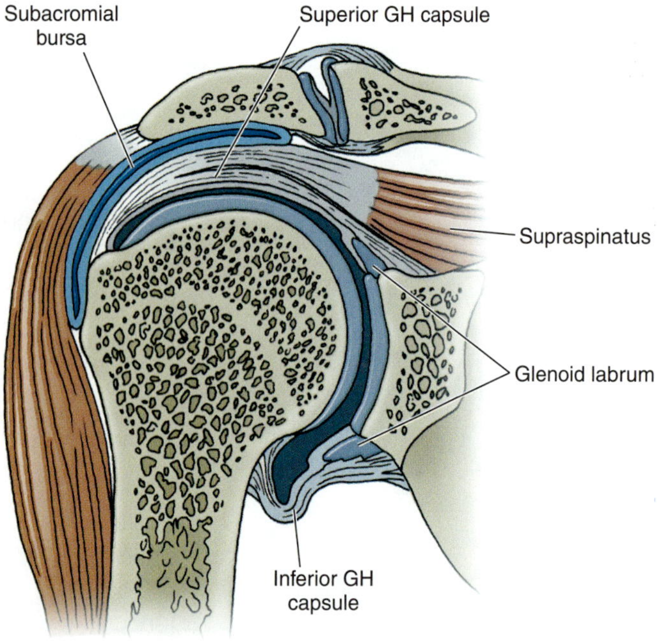

Figure 7–15 When the arm is at rest at the side, the superior glenohumeral (GH) capsule is taut, whereas the inferior capsule is slack.

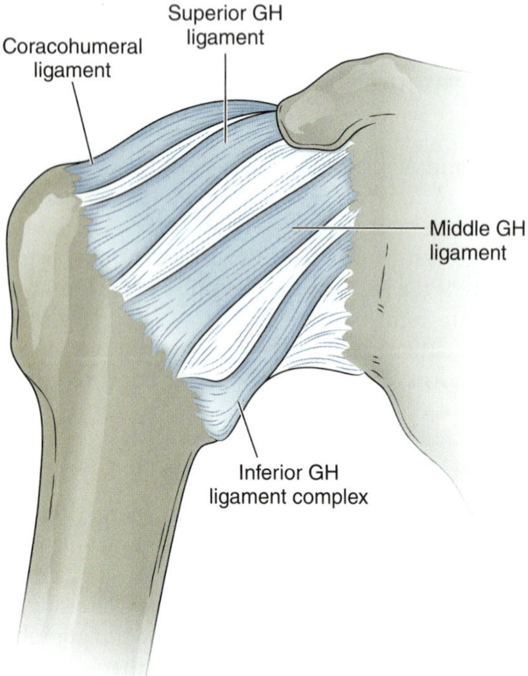

Figure 7–16 The ligamentous reinforcements to the glenohumeral (GH) capsule include the superior, middle, and inferior glenohumeral ligaments, along with the coracohumeral ligament.

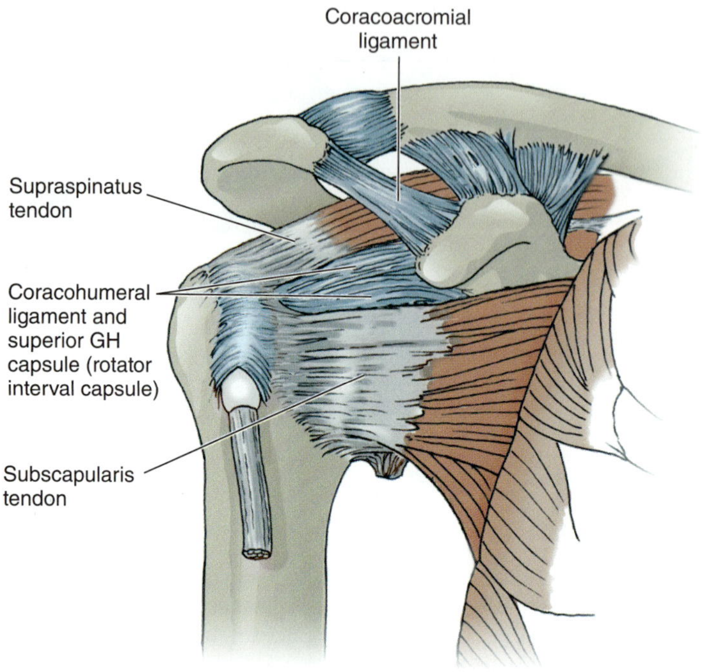

Figure 7–17 The rotator interval capsule is made up of the superior glenohumeral (GH) capsule, superior glenohumeral ligament, and coracohumeral ligament. Together, these structures bridge the gap between the supraspinatus and subscapularis muscle tendons and form the rotator interval capsule.

onto the glenohumeral capsule. The effects of the cuff muscles (**supraspinatus, infraspinatus, subscapularis**, and **teres minor**) on the GH joint will be discussed in detail further in this chapter. Even with ligamentous and musculotendinous reinforcements, the glenohumeral joint is vulnerable to dislocations, particularly in the anterior direction. The superior, middle, and inferior glenohumeral ligaments (Fig. 7-16) vary considerably in size, extent, and attachment sites between individuals.[30] Figure 7–14 shows these three ligaments as they appear on the interior surface of the joint capsule, as well as the tendons of the four rotator cuff muscles.

The superior glenohumeral ligament passes from the superior glenoid labrum to the upper neck of the humerus deep to the extracapsular coracohumeral ligament. The superior glenohumeral ligament, the superior capsule, and the coracohumeral ligament are interconnected structures that bridge the space between the supraspinatus and subscapularis muscle tendons and form the **rotator interval capsule (RIC)** (see **Fig. 7–17**).[31] The middle glenohumeral ligament runs obliquely from the superior anterior labrum to the anterior aspect of the proximal humerus below the superior glenohumeral ligament attachment (see Figs. 7–14 and 7–16). This ligament may be absent in up to 30% of individuals.[30] The inferior glenohumeral ligament is described as having three components and thus has been termed the **inferior GH ligament complex (IGHLC)**.[32] The three components of the IGHLC are the anterior and posterior ligament bands and the axillary pouch in between (see Fig. 7–14). The IGHLC shows position-dependent variability in function, as well as variations in viscoelastic behavior.[25,33]

Study of the movement restraint provided by the glenohumeral ligaments indicates that each ligament contributes differently to glenohumeral stability **(Fig. 7–18)**. The superior glenohumeral ligament and its associated rotator interval capsule structures contribute to anterior and inferior joint stability mostly by limiting anterior and inferior translations of the humeral head when the arm is at the side (0° abduction) (see **Fig. 7–18A**). The middle glenohumeral ligament contributes primarily to anterior joint stability by limiting anterior humeral translation with the arm at the side and up to 60° of abduction

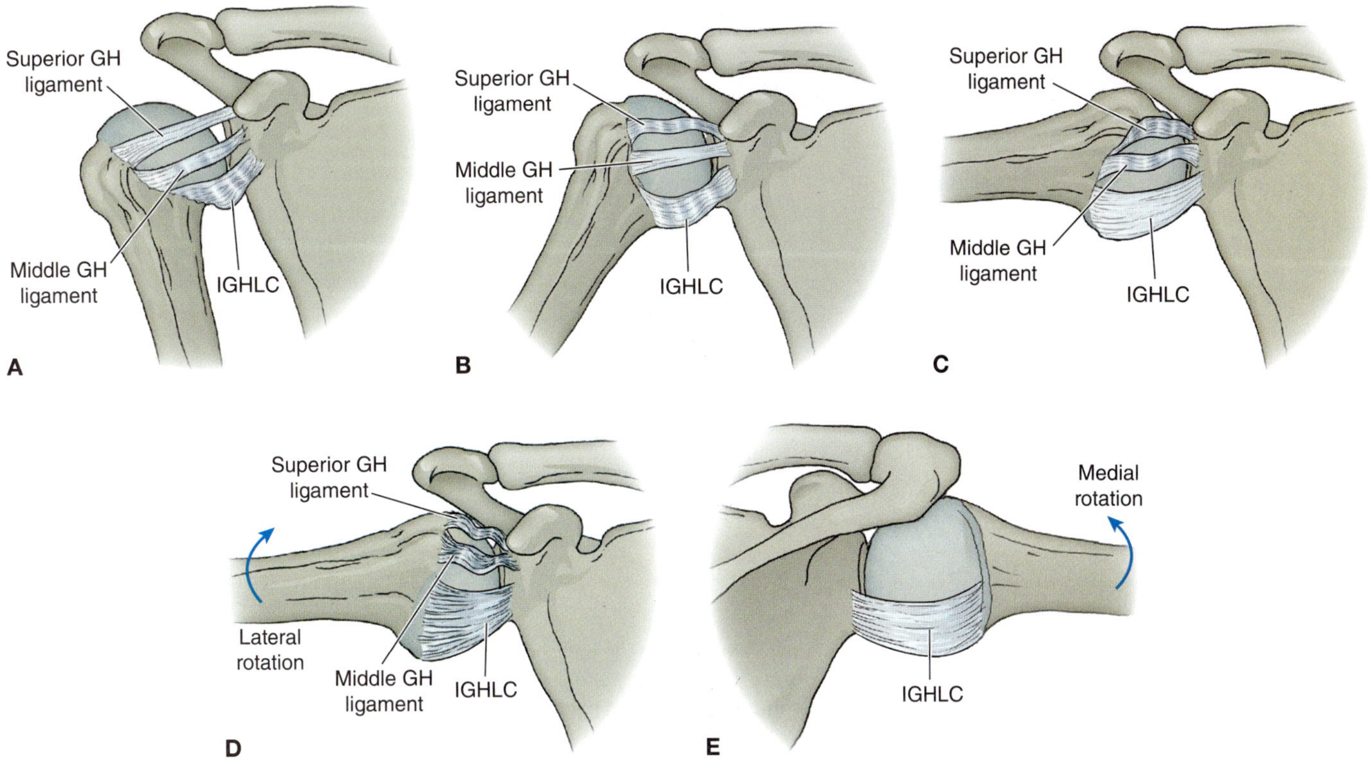

Figure 7–18 The glenohumeral (GH) ligaments and inferior glenohumeral ligament complex (IGHLC) shown in **A.** an anterior view slightly adducted from neutral; **B.** at 45° humeral abduction and neutral rotation; **C.** at 90° humeral abduction and neutral rotation; and **D.** at 90° humeral abduction and external rotation. **E.** In a posterior view, the IGHLC is shown at 90° humeral abduction and medial rotation.

(see **Fig. 7–18B**).[34] With abduction beyond 45° or with combined abduction and rotation (see **Fig. 7–18C**), the IGHLC plays the major role of joint stabilization.[25,32,33,35,36] With abduction, the axillary (inferior capsule) slack is taken up, and the IGHLC resists inferior humeral head translation. If lateral rotation is added to the abducted humerus (see **Fig. 7–18D**), the anterior band of the IGHLC fans out anteriorly to provide anterior joint stability and resistance to anterior and inferior humeral head translation. When the abducted humerus is medially rotated (see **Fig. 7–18E**), the posterior band of the IGHLC fans out posteriorly and provides posterior joint stability and resistance to posterior and inferior humeral head translation.[37] In all positions of humeral abduction, lateral or medial rotation of the humerus tightens the capsule and glenohumeral ligaments and increases glenohumeral joint stabilization.[38]

The coracohumeral ligament (see Figs. 7–16 and 7–17) originates from the base of the coracoid process and has two bands. The first band inserts into the edge of the supraspinatus tendon and onto the greater tubercle, joining the superior glenohumeral ligament. The second band inserts into the subscapularis and lesser tubercle.[31,39] The two bands contribute to the tunnel through which the tendon of the long head of the biceps brachii passes.[40] As part of the rotator interval capsule, the coracohumeral ligament limits inferior translation of the humeral head in the dependent arm position. In addition, the coracohumeral ligament resists humeral lateral rotation with the arm *adducted*. The ligament may also assist in preventing superior translation of the humerus, especially when the dynamic stabilizing force of the rotator cuff muscles is impaired.[39]

Coracoacromial Arch and Bursae

The **coracoacromial** (or **suprahumeral**) **arch** is formed by the coracoid process, the acromial undersurface, the **coracoacromial ligament,** and the inferior surface of the AC joint **(Fig. 7–19)**. The coracoacromial arch forms an osteoligamentous roof over the humeral head; the region between the arch and the humeral head is called the *subacromial space*. The subacromial bursa, the rotator cuff tendons, and a portion of the tendon of the long head of the biceps brachii lie within the subacromial space and are protected superiorly from direct trauma by the coracoacromial arch. Such trauma could occur through simple daily tasks such as carrying a heavy bag over the shoulder. The arch also acts as a physical barrier to superior translatory forces acting on the humeral head, preventing it from dislocating superiorly. Although beneficial to joint stability, upward translation of the humeral head toward the undersurface of the arch can simultaneously cause painful impingement or mechanical abrasion of the interposed structures within the subacromial space. The supraspinatus tendon is particularly vulnerable because of its location beneath the potentially impinging structures of the acromion, coracoacromial ligament, and distal clavicle (see Fig. 7–19).

Several bursae are associated with the shoulder complex in general and with the glenohumeral joint specifically, reflecting adaptation to frictional forces between anatomic structures. Although all bursae at the shoulder contribute to function, the most important are the subacromial and subdeltoid bursae. These bursae separate the supraspinatus tendon and head of the humerus from the acromion, coracoid process, coracoacromial

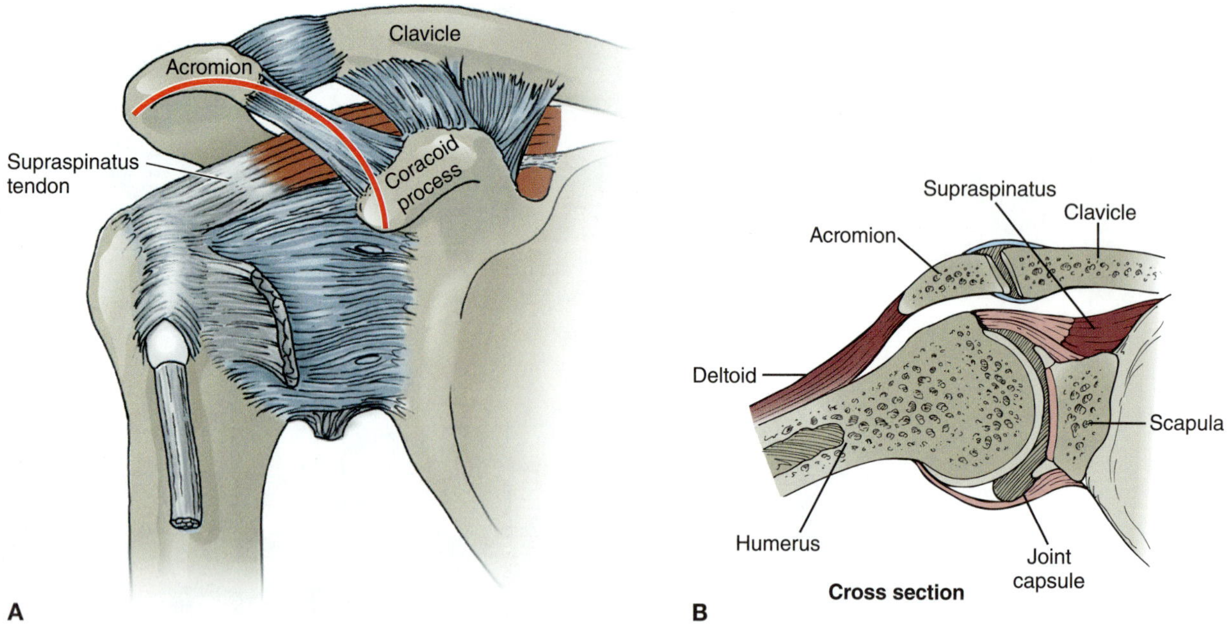

Figure 7–19 The coracoacromial (suprahumeral) arch is formed by the coracoid process anteriorly, the acromion and AC joint posteriorly, and the coracoacromial ligament superiorly. **A.** Together, these structures form an osteoligamentous roof over the humeral head. **B.** As the humerus abducts to 90°, the supraspinatus is pulled medially, which somewhat vacates the subacromial space.

ligament, and deltoid muscle. These bursae may be separate entities but are commonly continuous with each other and are collectively known as the **subacromial bursa** (see Fig. 7–15). The subacromial bursa reduces friction to permit smooth sliding between the humerus and supraspinatus tendon, as well as the surrounding structures. Subacromial bursitis is a common finding on imaging, often assumed to be secondary to inflammation or degeneration of the supraspinatus tendon.[10] In the absence of inflammation, bursae are merely layers of synovial tissue in contact with each other with a very thin layer of fluid in between. However, when inflamed, the subacromial bursa may decrease the subacromial space available for rotator cuff tendon clearance.

The subacromial space, also referred to as the **suprahumeral space** or **supraspinatus outlet**, has been quantified by measuring the superior-to-inferior **acromiohumeral interval** (vertical distance between the acromion and humeral head) on radiographs. This interval averages 10 mm in healthy subjects with the arm resting at the side and decreases to about 5 mm during elevation of the arm.[41,42] As the acromiohumeral interval decreases, it must accommodate the soft tissue structures within it, as well as the humeral articular cartilage and the capsuloligamentous structures. For this reason, even during typical motion into humeral elevation, there is some contact (small impingement) of the musculotendinous rotator cuff with the coracoacromial arch above it.[41] However, three-dimensional (3D) imaging has determined that anatomic approximation of the supraspinatus tendon with the acromion typically occurs at humeral elevation angles below 60°, whereas the smallest acromiohumeral interval is between the acromion and the greater tuberosity of the humerus at approximately 90° of elevation.[43,44] By 90°, however, the supraspinatus tendon has rotated medially past the undersurface of the acromion. Subsequently, typical decreases in the acromiohumeral distance during arm elevation may not affect the rotator cuff for most people at elevation angles higher than 60° because the tendon is no longer between the two bony prominences (see **Fig 7–19B**).[45]

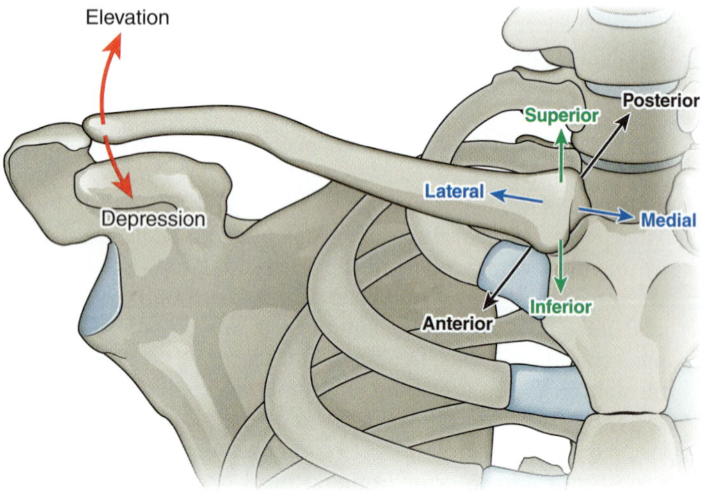

Figure 7–20 Elevation and depression of the clavicle are named by what is happening to the *lateral* end of the clavicle during rotation at the SC joint around an anteroposterior (A-P) axis. Translatory motions of the *medial* end of the clavicle may occur in a medial/lateral, superior/inferior, or anterior/posterior direction.

Shoulder Joint Function

Sternoclavicular Motion

The three rotational degrees of freedom at the SC joint are most commonly described as elevation/depression, protraction/retraction, and **anterior/posterior rotation** of the clavicle. Elevation/depression **(Fig. 7–20)** and protraction/retraction **(Fig. 7–21)** are named according to the movement

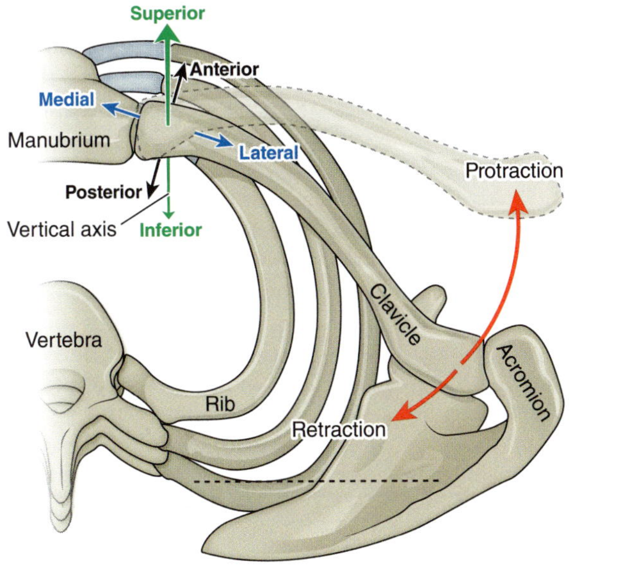

Figure 7–21 Protraction and retraction of the clavicle are named by what is happening to the *lateral* end of the clavicle during rotation at the SC joint around a vertical axis (superior view). Translatory motions of the medial clavicle may occur in a medial/lateral, superior/inferior, or anterior/posterior direction.

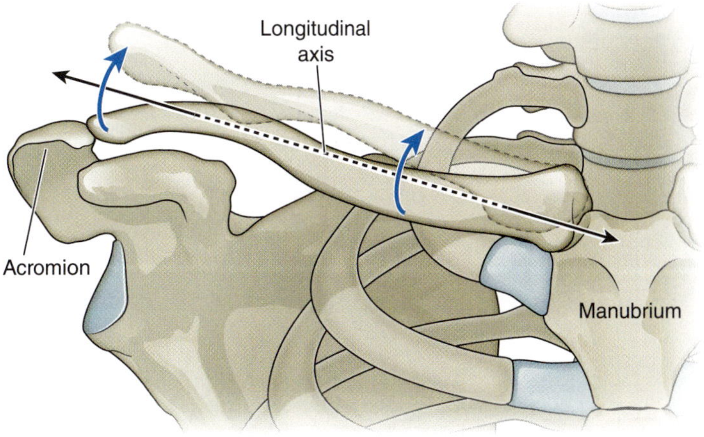

Figure 7–22 Clavicular rotation at the SC joint occurs as a spin of the entire clavicle around a long axis that has a medial/lateral orientation. As the clavicle posteriorly rotates, the lateral end of the clavicle flips up because of its s-shape. Anterior rotation is predominantly a return to resting position.

of the *lateral* end of the clavicle. Anterior/posterior rotations are long-axis rolling motions of the entire clavicle **(Fig. 7–22)** and are named for motion of a point located on the anterior clavicle. Three degrees of translatory motion at the SC joint can also occur, although clavicle translations are very small in magnitude in a healthy joint. Translations of the medial clavicle on the sternum are usually defined as occurring in anterior/posterior, medial/lateral, and superior/inferior directions (see Figs. 7–20 and 7–21).

Elevation and Depression

The clavicular motions of elevation and depression occur around an approximately anteroposterior (A-P) axis (see Fig. 7–20) between the somewhat convex clavicular surface and the concave surface formed by the sternum and first costal cartilage. The SC joint axis is described as lying at the costoclavicular ligament located lateral to the anatomic joint. The location of this *functional* axis relatively far from the joint reflects the large intra-articular motion of the medial clavicle. With clavicle elevation, the lateral end of the clavicle moves upward as its medial articular surface rolls superiorly and slides inferiorly on the sternum and first rib. During depression, the lateral clavicle moves downward as its medial articular surface rolls inferiorly and slides superiorly. The range of clavicular elevation has been reported as up to 48°, whereas passive depression from neutral is limited to less than 15°.[46] The full available range of clavicle elevation is generally not used during functional arm elevation.[47,48]

Protraction and Retraction

Protraction and retraction of the clavicle occur at the SC joint around an approximately vertical axis that also appears to be located at the costoclavicular ligament (see Fig. 7–21). With protraction, the lateral end of the clavicle moves anteriorly in the transverse plane, while with retraction the lateral clavicle moves posteriorly. The configuration of joint surfaces in this plane is the opposite of that for elevation/depression, with a concave medial end of the clavicle meeting a sternum surface that is convex. During protraction, the medial clavicle is expected to roll and slide anteriorly on the sternum and first costal cartilage with the opposite joint kinematics occurring during retraction. Approximately 15° to 20° of protraction and 30° of retraction are available.[16,46,48,49]

Anterior and Posterior Rotation

Anterior/posterior (or long axis) rotation of the clavicle (see Fig. 7–22) occurs as a spin of the saddle-shaped surfaces of the medial clavicle on the manubriocostal facet and the SC disc. Unlike many joints, which can rotate in either direction from their resting position, the clavicle rotates primarily *posteriorly* from neutral, bringing the inferior surface of the clavicle to face anteriorly. This motion has alternatively been referred to as "backward" or "upward" rotation.[1] From its posteriorly rotated position, the clavicle can rotate anteriorly to return to neutral. Available anterior rotation beyond neutral is limited to less than 10°.[1] The range of available clavicular posterior rotation may be as much as 50°.[46] The axis of rotation runs longitudinally through the clavicle, intersecting the SC and AC joints (see Fig. 7–22).

Sternoclavicular Stability

The bony morphology, capsule, ligaments, and disc of the SC joint combine to create an articulation that contributes to the substantial mobility of the arm while remaining a stable link to the axial skeleton. Although the SC joint is considered incongruent, it does not typically undergo the degree of degenerative change common to the other joints of the shoulder complex.[9,10] Strong force-dissipating structures such as the SC disc and the costoclavicular ligament (see Fig. 7–3) minimize articular stresses and limit intra-articular motion that could lead to subluxation or dislocation. Reported dislocations of

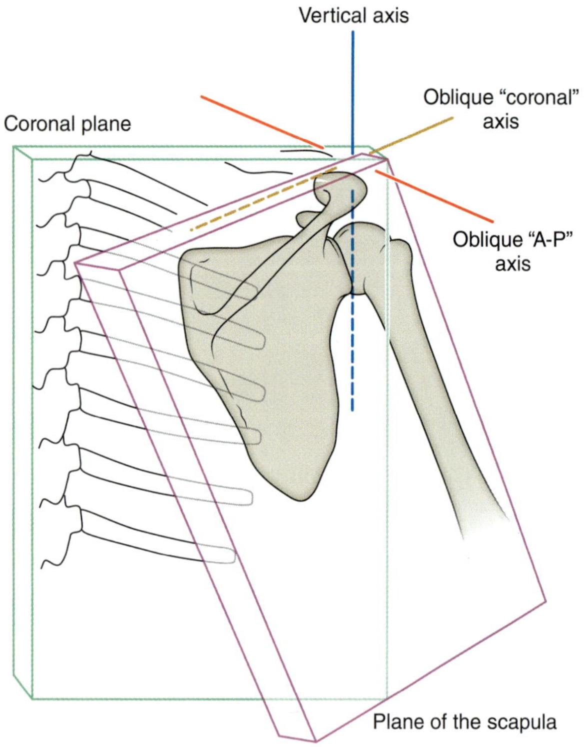

Figure 7–23 The AC rotary axes of motion are oriented in relation to the plane of the scapula rather than in relation to the cardinal planes, resulting in coronal and anteroposterior (A-P) axes that are oblique to their cardinal orientation.

the SC joint represent only 1% of joint dislocations in the body and only 3% of shoulder girdle dislocations, although subluxations may be more frequent.[50]

Acromioclavicular Kinematics

The small articular facets of the AC joint vary widely across individuals and afford limited motion, leading to difficulty in clearly determining axes of motion and joint movements. The primary rotations at the AC joint are **internal/external rotation, anterior/posterior tilting,** and **upward/downward rotation.** These motions occur around axes that are oriented relative to the **plane of the scapula** rather than to the cardinal planes. The plane of the scapula is where the scapula sits on the thorax at rest, 30° to 45° in front of the coronal plane (see Fig. 7–9A). Although internal/external rotation of the scapula at the AC joint occurs around a nearly vertical axis, anterior/posterior tilting occurs around an oblique "coronal" axis, while upward/downward rotation occurs around an oblique "A-P" axis **(Fig. 7–23)**. Acromioclavicular joint motion also influences, and is influenced by, long-axis rotation of the clavicle. In addition, small-magnitude translations at the AC joint can occur. Acromioclavicular translations are usually described as anterior/posterior, medial/lateral, and superior/inferior.

Internal and External Rotation

Internal/external rotation of the scapula relative to the clavicle occurs around an approximately vertical axis through the AC joint **(Fig. 7–24)**. Internal and external rotation at the AC joint can be visualized best as orienting the glenoid fossa of the scapula anteromedially and posterolaterally, respectively **(Fig. 7–24A)**. These motions occur in part to maintain contact of the scapula with the horizontal curvature of the thorax as the clavicle protracts and retracts, maintaining apposition by internally and externally rotating the scapula as it slides around the thorax **(Fig. 7–24B)**. These motions also "aim" the glenoid fossa toward the plane of humeral elevation, which is an important function for maintaining congruency and stability between the humeral head and scapula, and for maximizing the function of glenohumeral muscles, capsule, and ligaments. The available ROM at the AC joint is difficult to measure. A range of 30° for combined internal and external rotation ROM in cadaveric AC joints separated from the thorax has been described.[1] Smaller values (20° to 35°) have been reported in vivo during arm motions, although up to 60° may be possible with full-range motions reaching forward and across the body.[16,46,48,49]

Anterior and Posterior Tilting

Anterior/posterior tilting of the scapula relative to the clavicle occurs around an oblique "coronal" axis through the joint **(Fig. 7–25)**. Anterior tilting results in the acromion moving forward and the inferior angle of the scapula moving backward (see **Fig. 7–25A**). During posterior tilting, the acromion moves backward and the inferior angle moves forward. Scapular tilting, like scapula internal/external rotation, occurs to maintain the contact of the scapula with the contour of the thorax and to orient the glenoid fossa relative to the humeral head. As the scapula moves upward or downward on the rib cage in elevation or depression, tilting may occur to maximize contact between the anterior scapula and the curvature of the ribs (see **Fig. 7–25B**). However, the scapula does not always follow the curvature of the thorax precisely. For example, during typical flexion or abduction of the arm, the scapula posteriorly tilts on the thorax as the scapula is upwardly rotating. Available passive motion into anterior/posterior tilting at the AC joint is 60° in cadaveric AC joint specimens separated from the thorax.[1] The magnitude of anterior/posterior tilting during in vivo arm elevation is approximately 20°, although up to 40° or more may be possible in the full range from maximum flexion to extension.[16,51]

Upward and Downward Rotation

Upward/downward rotation of the scapula relative to the clavicle occurs about an oblique "A-P" axis that is roughly perpendicular to the plane of the scapula, passing midway between the joint surfaces **(Fig. 7–26)**. Upward rotation tilts the glenoid fossa upward and moves the inferior angle laterally, while downward rotation does the opposite. The amount of available passive motion into upward/downward rotation occurring directly at the AC joint is limited by the coracoclavicular ligament. For isolated upward rotation at the AC joint, the coracoid process and superior border of the scapula need to move downward (inferiorly) relative to the clavicle, a motion that is restricted by tension in the coracoclavicular ligaments (see Fig. 7–17). The amount of available upward rotation is also dependent in part on rotation of the clavicle around its long axis. Because of the attachment of the coracoclavicular ligaments to the undersurface and posterior edge of the clavicle, posterior rotation of the clavicle releases tension on

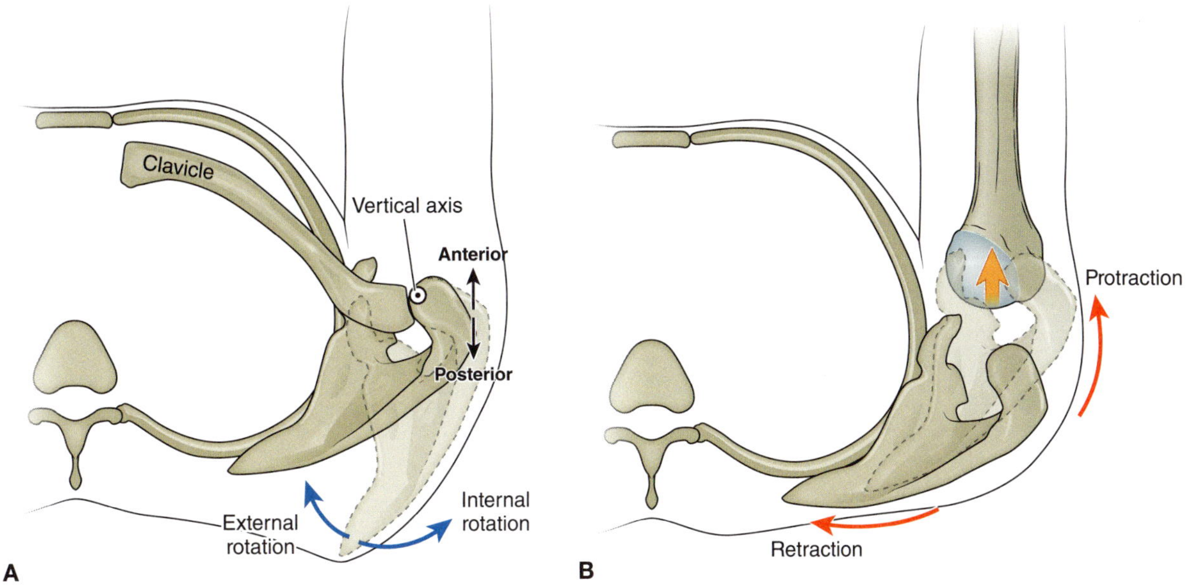

Figure 7–24 **A.** A superior view of scapular internal and external rotation at the AC joint. Although the rotational arrows are drawn at the vertebral border, the motions are named with reference to the orientation of the glenoid fossa of the scapula. The acromion also has small amounts of anterior and posterior translatory motions. **B.** Protraction and retraction of the scapula require internal and external rotation at the AC joint for the scapula to maintain maximal contact with the convex thorax and orient the glenoid fossa with the plane of elevation (e.g., anteriorly with flexion of the arm).

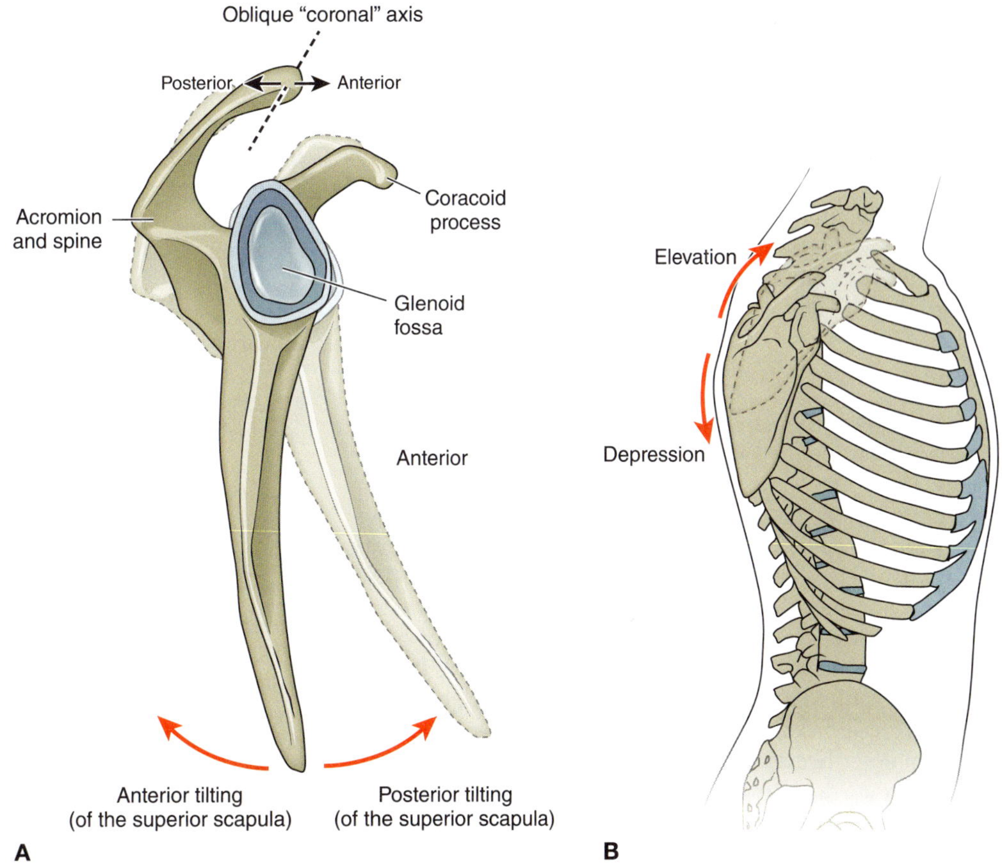

Figure 7–25 **A.** A lateral view of scapular anterior and posterior tilting at the AC joint. Although the directional arrows are drawn at the inferior angle, the motions are named with reference to the *superior* aspect of the scapula (e.g., acromion). The acromion also has small amounts of anterior and posterior translatory motions. **B.** Elevation and depression of the scapula can include AC anterior and posterior tilting, respectively, for the scapula to approximate the convexity of the thorax.

the coracoclavicular ligaments, thereby no longer restricting further AC joint upward rotation.[47] Conway describes 30° of upward rotation and 17° of downward rotation actively at the AC joint in vivo.[46] Others have described 15° to 16° of upward rotation occurring during active humeral abduction.[16,51]

Acromioclavicular Stability

Unlike the SC joint, the AC joint is not very stable, making it susceptible to both trauma and degenerative changes. Trauma to the AC joint most often occurs in the first three decades of life, during either contact sports or a fall on the shoulder

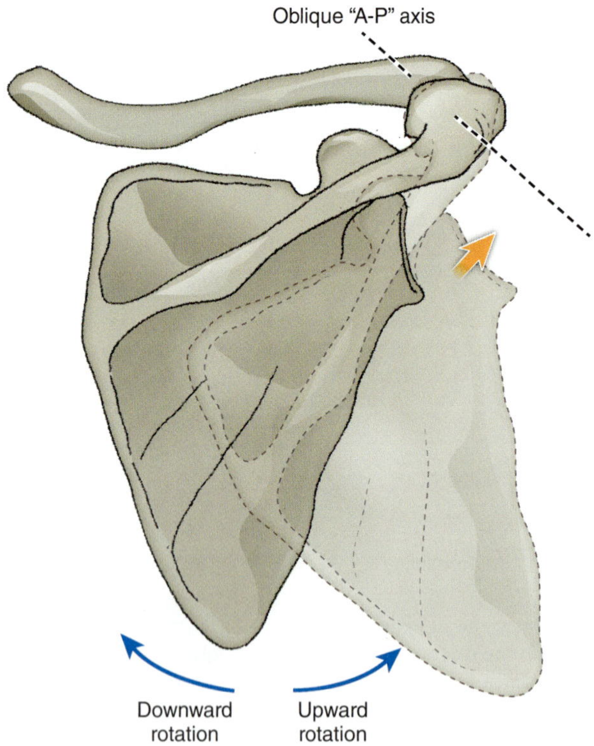

Figure 7–26 Upward/downward rotation of the scapula at the AC joint occurs around an approximately A-P (perpendicular to the plane of the scapula) axis. Although the directional arrows are drawn at the inferior angle, the motions are named with the glenoid fossa of the scapula as the reference, with the glenoid facing upwardly in upward rotation.

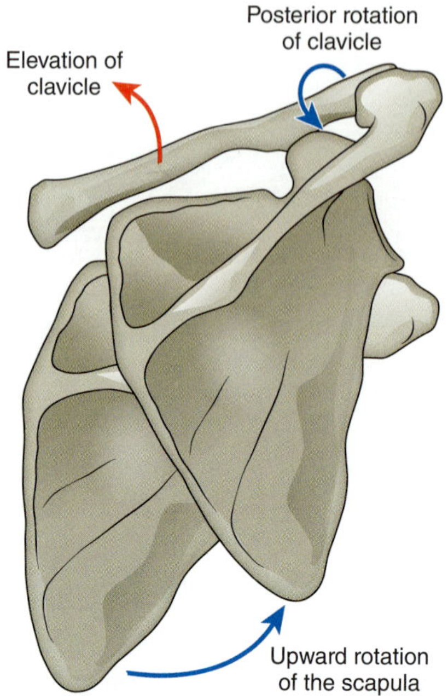

Figure 7–27 Full upward rotation of the scapula is produced in part by scapular elevation at the SC joint, and more so by clavicular posterior rotation at both the SC and AC joints, and upward rotation at the AC joint.

with the arm adducted. Trauma most often is the result of high inferior forces on the acromion, resulting in AC joint disruption that can range from sprains and subluxations to dislocations.

Scapulothoracic Kinematics

The motions of the functional scapulothoracic joint include three rotations that are similarly named as those that occur at the AC joint. These are upward/downward rotation, internal/external rotation, and anterior/posterior tilting. Scapulothoracic motions take place between the scapula and the thorax rather than between the scapula's acromion and the clavicle as at the AC joint. Scapulothoracic movements involve SC joint motions, AC joint motions, or a combination of both. The scapula on the thorax is also often described as having translatory motions of scapulothoracic **elevation/depression** and **protraction/retraction.** These scapulothoracic motions are often described as if they occur independently. However, the linkage of the scapula to the AC and SC joints actually prevents scapulothoracic motions from occurring in isolation or as true translatory motions.

Upward and Downward Rotation

Upward rotation of the scapula on the thorax **(Fig. 7–27)** is the principal motion of the scapula observed during active elevation of the arm and plays a significant role in increasing the arm's range of elevation overhead. Approximately 50° to 60° of upward rotation of the scapula on the thorax is typically available. Because scapulothoracic motions are combined joint motions, differing proportions of upward/downward rotation of the scapula on the thorax are contributed by clavicular posterior/anterior rotation and elevation/depression at the SC joint, and by upward/downward rotation of the scapula at the AC joint.[52]

Because the axes of the SC and scapulothoracic joints for upward/downward rotation are not parallel to each other, the relationships between SC and AC joint motions and scapulothoracic motion may be challenging to visualize. However, considering the orientation of the SC and scapulothoracic joint axes in two hypothetical configurations may assist in visualizing these relationships **(Fig. 7–28)**. First, assume the long axis of the clavicle at rest was *parallel* to the plane of the scapula yielding an AC joint internal rotation of 0° (see **Fig. 7–28A**); scapulothoracic upward rotation would directly couple with *clavicular elevation at the SC joint.* In other words, SC elevation (rise of the lateral end of the clavicle) would result in scapulothoracic upward rotation, and vice versa. Second, assume the long axis of the clavicle at rest was *perpendicular* to the plane of the scapula such that there is 90° of internal rotation at the AC joint (see **Fig. 7–28B**); scapulothoracic upward rotation would directly couple with *posterior rotation of the clavicle at the SC joint.* The typical angle of AC joint internal rotation at rest actually is approximately 60° **(Fig. 7–28C)**, thus about two-thirds of a 90° AC joint internal rotation position.[16,52] Consequently, two-thirds of the motion of scapulothoracic upward rotation couples with (results from) *clavicular posterior rotation at the SC joint;* one-third of scapulothoracic upward rotation couples with (results from) *clavicular elevation at the SC joint.*[52]

Expanded Concepts 7–1
Terminology

Upward and downward rotation of the scapula are defined by upward and downward movement of the glenoid fossa, respectively. However, the inferior angle of the scapula may also be used as the referent, with upward and downward rotation described as movement of the inferior angle away from the vertebral column (upward rotation) or movement of the inferior angle toward the vertebral column (downward rotation). Some also refer to upward/downward rotation of the scapula (regardless of reference point on the scapula) as *abduction/adduction* or *lateral/medial rotation,* respectively.[1,53]

Elevation and Depression

Scapulothoracic elevation and depression can be performed by shrugging the shoulder up and depressing the shoulder downward, respectively. Elevation and depression of the scapula on the thorax are sometimes described as translatory motions in which the scapula moves upward (cephalad) or downward (caudal) along the rib cage from its resting position. Scapular elevation, however, actually occurs as elevation of the clavicle around an A-P axis at the SC joint **(Fig. 7–29)** and may include subtle adjustments in anterior/posterior tilting and internal/external rotation at the AC joint to keep the scapula in contact with the thorax.

Protraction and Retraction

Protraction and retraction of the scapula on the thorax are often described as translatory motions of the scapula away from and toward the vertebral column, respectively. These theoretical translatory motions have also been termed *scapular abduction* and *adduction*. However, if protraction or abduction of the scapula on the thorax occurred as a pure translatory movement, the scapula would move directly away from the vertebral column, and the glenoid fossa would face laterally. Only the vertebral border of the scapula would remain in contact with the rib cage. Full scapular protraction actually results in the glenoid fossa facing anteriorly, with the scapula in contact with the rib cage. The scapula protracts and retracts on the thorax through protraction and retraction of the clavicle at the SC joint (vertical axis) and follows the contour of the ribs by rotating internally and externally at the AC joint **(Fig. 7–30)**.

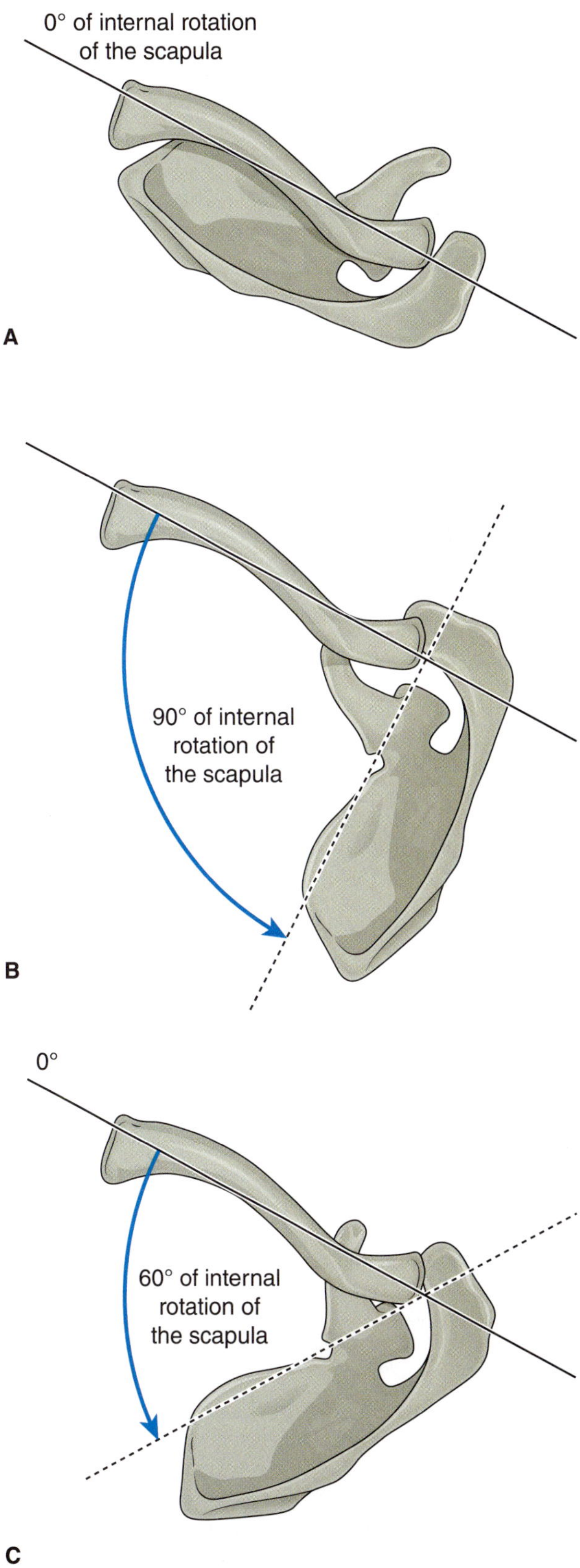

Figure 7–28 Coupling of scapular motion on the thorax and rotation of the clavicle at the SC joint. **A.** Theoretical AC joint internal rotation of 0° (clavicular long axis and scapular plane are parallel) would result in direct coupling of scapular upward rotation with clavicular elevation at the SC joint. **B.** Theoretical AC joint internal rotation of 90° would result in direct coupling of scapular upward rotation with clavicular posterior rotation at the SC joint. **C.** A typical AC joint internal rotation of approximately 60° (or approximately two-thirds of the way toward 90°) means that two-thirds of the upward rotation of the scapula on the thorax is linked with posterior rotation motion of the clavicle, whereas one-third of the scapular rotation on the thorax is linked to clavicular elevation at the SC joint.

Internal and External Rotation

The scapulothoracic motions of internal and external rotation are less obvious on physical observation but are critical to movement of the scapula along the curved rib

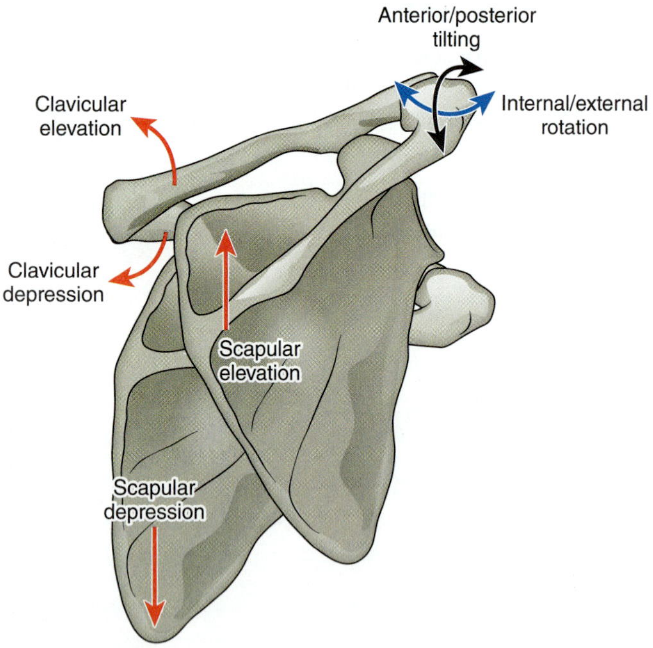

Figure 7–29 Elevation and depression of the scapula on the thorax are produced by elevation/depression of the clavicle at the SC joint, accompanied by rotations (anterior/posterior tilting and internal/external rotation) at the AC joint.

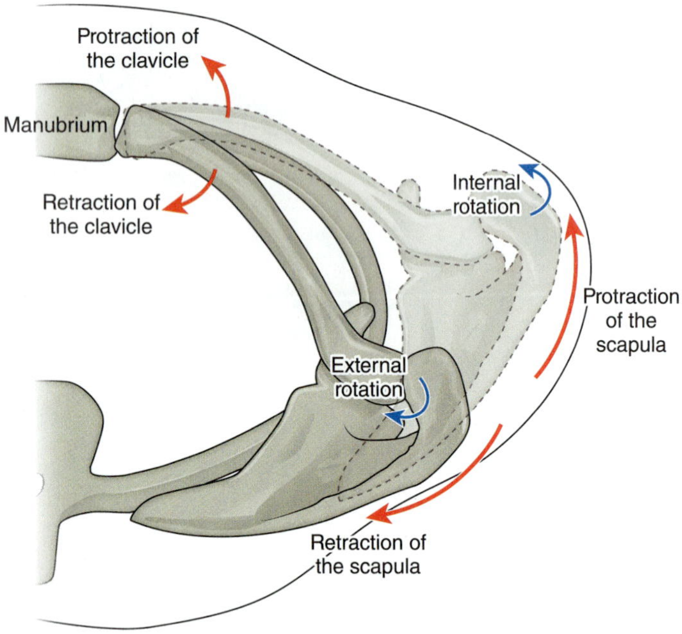

Figure 7–30 Protraction and retraction of the scapula are produced by protraction/retraction of the clavicle at the SC joint, accompanied by rotations at the AC joint, especially internal/external rotation to maintain the scapula on the curved thorax.

cage. Internal/external rotation of the scapula on the thorax typically accompany protraction/retraction of the clavicle at the SC joint (see Fig. 7–30). Approximately 15° to 16° of internal rotation occurs at the AC joint during typical elevation of the arm.[16,51] A larger amount of internal rotation of the scapula on the thorax that is isolated to (or occurs excessively at) the AC joint results in prominence of the

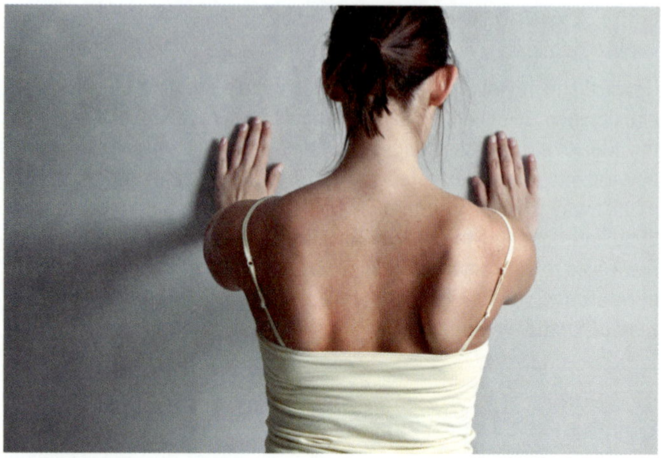

Figure 7–31 Scapular winging. With attempted protraction of the scapula (or elevation of the arms), excessive internal rotation of the scapulae at the AC joint causes prominence of the medial border of the scapula.

medial vertebral border of the scapula as a result of loss of contact with the thorax. This excessive internal rotation is often referred to clinically as **scapular winging (Fig. 7–31)**. Excessive internal rotation may be indicative of pathology or poor neuromuscular control of the scapulothoracic muscles (particularly but not exclusively the **serratus anterior muscle**).

Anterior and Posterior Tilting

As is true for internal/external rotation, scapulothoracic anterior/posterior tilting is typically not very obvious on clinical observation and yet is critical to maintaining contact of the scapula against the curvature of the rib cage. Anterior/posterior tilting of the scapula on the thorax occurs predominately at the AC joint around an oblique coronal axis that lies in the plane of the scapula.[16] Because of the differing SC and AC axis alignment described earlier (see Fig. 7–28), scapulothoracic anterior/posterior tilting and elevation/depression of the clavicle at the SC joint can also couple.[52] If the clavicle was perpendicular to the axis for AC internal rotation (see Fig 7–28B), anterior tilting of the scapula on the thorax would couple with or result from clavicle elevation , and vice versa. Given the approximately 60° typical internal rotation angle of the AC joint (see Fig. 7–28C), two-thirds of the magnitude of anterior tilting of the scapula on the thorax will couple with or result from clavicle elevation. Anterior tilting beyond resting values will result in prominence of the inferior angle of the scapula **(Fig. 7–32)**. An excessive anteriorly tilted scapula may occur with poor neuromuscular control or abnormal posture. Scapulothoracic posterior tilting can occur directly through posterior tilting at the AC joint or it can be coupled with posterior rotation of the clavicle at the SC joint. If the clavicle were aligned parallel to the plane of the scapula at a 0° AC internal rotation angle (see Fig. 7–29A), posterior tilting of the scapula on the thorax would couple with clavicle posterior rotation. Given the approximately 60° typical internal rotation angle of the AC joint, only one-third of the magnitude of posterior tilting of the scapula on the thorax will result from clavicle posterior rotation.

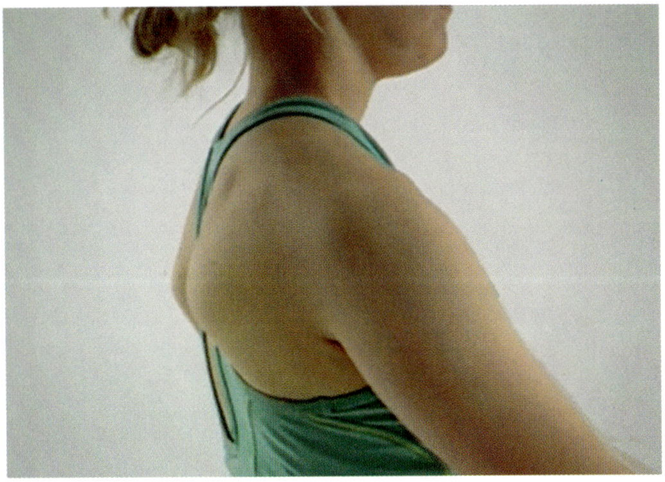

Figure 7–32 This scapula is anteriorly tilted with attempted flexion of the arm, causing the inferior angle of the scapula to lift off the thorax and become visually prominent. The condition typically occurs if the anterior deltoid and coracobrachialis are inadequately opposed by the serratus anterior, also referred to as "reverse action" as the deltoid and coracobrachialis move their unstabilized (now more mobile) proximal attachments.

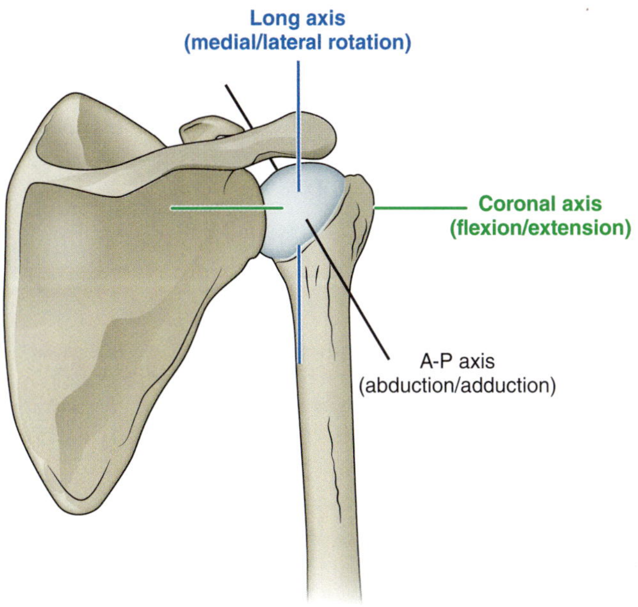

Figure 7–33 Glenohumeral rotations. Flexion/extension occur around a coronal axis (green); abduction/adduction occur around an A-P axis (black); and medial/lateral rotation occur around a long axis (blue).

Scapulothoracic Stability

Stability of the scapula on the thorax is provided by the structures that maintain integrity of the linked AC and SC joints. The muscles that attach to both the thorax and scapula maintain contact between these surfaces while producing the movements of the scapula. In addition, stabilization is provided by the scapulothoracic musculature, which pulls or compresses the scapula to the thorax.[53]

The ultimate functions of scapular motion are to orient the glenoid fossa for optimal contact with the humeral head, to add range to elevation of the arm, and to provide a stable base for the controlled motions between the humeral head and glenoid fossa. The scapula, with its associated muscles and linkages, performs these mobility and stability functions so well in healthy shoulder function that it serves as a premier example of dynamic stabilization in the human body.

Patient Application 7–1
Anterior-Lateral Shoulder Pain

Denzel Harris is a 57-year-old dentist who reports shoulder pain localized at the proximal lateral humerus. This location is consistent with pain originating from the rotator cuff tendons, the long head of the biceps tendon, or the subacromial bursa. His pain may be related to a rotator cuff or biceps tendinopathy, or possible shoulder subacromial mechanical impingement due to repetitive work at low angles of humeral elevation. Repetitive mechanical impingement can create tendinopathy and progress to partial- and full-thickness rotator cuff tears.[54] In addition, he reports pain when sleeping on his right side. This is a common complaint of persons with pain originating from the subacromial space because additional compression of the subacromial tissues is experienced while lying on the affected side.

Glenohumeral Kinematics

The glenohumeral joint is usually described as having three rotational degrees of freedom: **flexion/extension, abduction/adduction,** and **medial/lateral rotation** **(Fig. 7-33)**. The range of each of these motions occurring solely at the glenohumeral joint varies considerably.

Flexion and Extension

Flexion and extension occur about a coronal axis passing through the center of the humeral head. The glenohumeral joint is often considered to have 120° of flexion and about 50° of extension.[55] However, more recent work measuring 3D glenohumeral motion reported peak humeral flexion of only 97° in relation to the scapula in a small sample of subjects averaging 50 years of age.[56] This lesser value of glenohumeral motion is also supported by studies in young, healthy subjects.[16] The higher values classically attributed to glenohumeral flexion may not have fully isolated glenohumeral motion from possible accompanying trunk and scapular motion.

Medial and Lateral Rotation

Medial and lateral rotation occur about a long axis parallel to the shaft of the humerus and passing though the center of the humeral head. The range of medial/lateral rotation of the humerus varies with position. With the arm at the side, medial and lateral rotation may be limited. Abducting the humerus to 90° frees the arc of rotation, with glenohumeral values of 130° or greater.[55] The restricted arc of medial/lateral rotation when the arm is at the side may be related to different alignment of the greater and lesser tubercles, which creates a mechanical block, or to different areas of capsular or muscular tightness when the arm is adducted versus abducted.

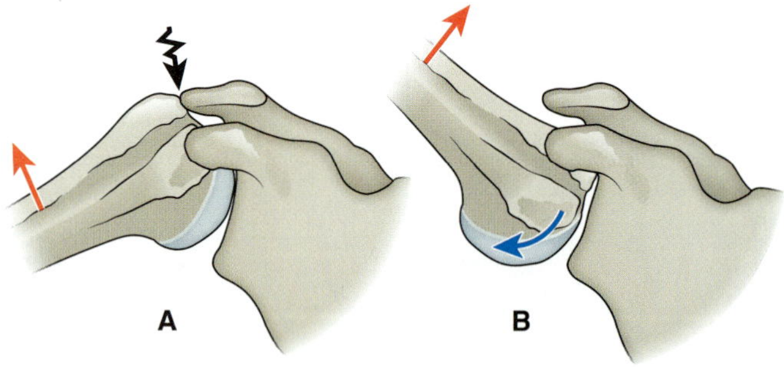

Figure 7–34 **A.** Without downward sliding of the articular surface of the humeral head, the humeral head will roll up the glenoid fossa and impinge upon the coracoacromial arch. **B.** With downward sliding of the humeral head's articular surface as the humeral abducts, a full ROM can occur.

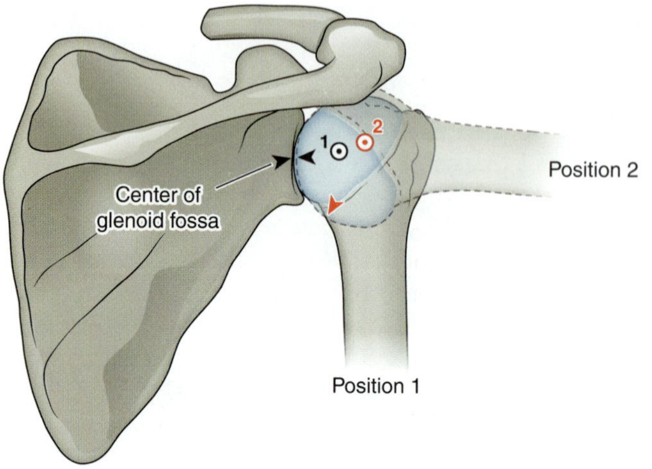

Figure 7–35 Slight superior translation of the center of the humeral head (from position 1 to position 2) may still occur during humeral abduction despite inferior sliding of the head's articular surface.

Abduction and Adduction

Abduction/adduction of the glenohumeral joint occurs around an A-P axis passing through the humeral head center. The maximum range of abduction at the glenohumeral joint is the topic of much disagreement. There is general consensus, however, that the range of abduction of the humerus in the frontal plane (whether the abduction is active or passive) will be diminished if the humerus is maintained in neutral or medial rotation through the motion. The restriction to abduction in medial or neutral rotation is commonly attributed to impingement of the greater tubercle on the coracoacromial arch. When the humerus is laterally rotated 35° to 40°, the greater tubercle will pass under or behind the arch so that abduction can continue through greater range.[57,58]

The ROMs for abduction of the glenohumeral joint (if impact of the greater tubercle is avoided) are reported to be anywhere from 90° to 120°.[1,10,56,59,60] Early study found active abduction to be limited to 90° when the scapula does not participate in the motion, but that 120° of motion was available passively.[47] Further increasing the variability between investigations, some studies examined the range of abduction in the traditional frontal plane, whereas others have investigated elevation in the plane of the scapula (30° to 45° anterior to the frontal plane as shown in Fig. 7-8A). The available passive range for abduction in the scapular plane may be slightly greater than for abduction in the frontal plane.[58] When the humerus is elevated in the plane of the scapula (referred to as *abduction in the plane of the scapula*, *scapular abduction*, or **scaption** in clinical jargon), there is presumably less restriction to motion because the capsule is less twisted than when the humerus is brought farther back into the frontal plane. During active arm elevations in all planes of elevation, availability of glenohumeral lateral rotation has been demonstrated.[16,61]

Intra-Articular Glenohumeral Motion

Full ROM of the glenohumeral joint is, to a reasonable degree, a function of the intra-articular movement of the incongruent articular surfaces. The convex humeral head is a substantially larger surface and may have a different radius of curvature than the shallow concave fossa. Given this incongruence, rotations of the joint around its three axes do not occur as pure spin but have changing centers of rotation and shifting contact patterns within the joint. There is a somewhat surprising lack of consensus on the extent and direction of movement of the humeral head on the fossa.[25] However, elevation of the humerus requires that the articular surface of the humeral head slide inferiorly (caudally) in a direction opposite to movement of the shaft of the humerus. Failure of the humeral articular surface to slide downward in abduction of the humerus would cause purely superior (cephalad) rolling of the humeral head surface on the fossa **(Fig. 7–34A)**. The large humeral head would soon run out of glenoid surface, and the head of the humerus would impinge upon the overhanging coracoacromial arch. If, as it should, the articular surface of the head of the humerus slides inferiorly while the head rolls up the fossa, full ROM can be achieved (see **Fig. 7–34B**).

There is consensus that inferior sliding of the humeral head's articular surface is necessary to offset upward rolling of the humeral head. However, the humeral head as a whole (referencing its center of rotation) is often reported to still move somewhat superiorly (translate upwardly) on the glenoid fossa in spite of the articular surface downward sliding **(Fig. 7–35)**, although the magnitude of superior versus inferior humeral head center translation differs among investigators.[25,58,62-65] The humeral articular surface may also slide anteriorly or posteriorly and medially or laterally on the glenoid fossa. The humeral head's center is believed to move slightly superior (1–2 mm of translation) until about 60° of active elevation motion.[19,62-64] With further elevation, the humeral head's center is believed to remain relatively stable and centered on the glenoid fossa.

A lack of consensus exists regarding the anterior and posterior translations of the humeral head's center. Slight anterior positioning and translation (1–2 mm) has been reported during active elevation, including in abduction and scapular plane abduction.[63,65] Other investigators have reported slight anterior or posterior translations early in the range and opposite translations later in the range of active elevation, including during flexion.[62,64-66] All studies of active translations show smaller magnitudes of slide (less than 5 mm) during active motions than is available in a passive laxity examination, in which translations up to 20 mm have been reported.[67] These data support the premise that rotator cuff forces help to stabilize and center the humeral head on the glenoid fossa during active motion. Most investigators also agree that many variables determine the patterns of movement of the humeral head on the glenoid fossa, including articular geometry, capsuloligamentous influences, influences of arm position, and muscle forces.

Much of the confusion surrounding reported motions of the humeral head on the glenoid fossa may be attributed to the differences in the point on the humerus that is being followed (combinations of rolling and sliding versus translations), as well as to the small magnitudes of these motions and the limitations of currently available measurement systems.

Expanded Concepts 7–2

The Role of the Capsule

The glenohumeral capsule and its associated glenohumeral ligaments (see Fig. 7–16) provide stability to the glenohumeral joint by limiting anterior, inferior, or posterior humeral head translation on the glenoid fossa. The stabilizing function of these structures is minimal at less than 90° of humeral elevation when only the superior segment of the capsule is under any significant tension. At these lower elevation angles, the rotator cuff muscles and tendons actively stabilize the glenohumeral joint based on their angle of pull as they cross the joint. Toward the end range of humeral motions, however, the capsule becomes tight passively, and this tension restricts glenohumeral translation. At end ranges, this tension begins to produce rather than restrict humeral head center translations.[68] With asymmetrical tightening of the capsule, this forced translation occurs in a direction away from the tight and toward the looser capsular tissue.[68] For example, with increasing medial rotation, the posterior capsule becomes tight and produces anterior translation of the humeral head center that is not restricted by the relatively slack anterior capsule. A tight posterior capsule is, therefore, one potential mechanism for shoulder mechanical impingement, because it may produce increased anterior humeral head translation and reduce the subacromial space.[62]

Static Glenohumeral Joint Stability in the Dependent Arm

With the arm relaxed and unsupported at one's side, gravity imparts a caudally directed translatory force on the humerus. Glenohumeral joint bony geometry, particularly the nearly vertical orientation of the glenoid fossa, cannot fully resist this caudal force. To maintain equilibrium, a cranially directed force (or force with a cranially directed component) is needed to maintain stability. Because the muscles of the shoulder complex are electrically silent in the relaxed, unloaded limb,[18,29] forces generated by passive structures provide the cranially directed force needed to maintain glenohumeral joint stability. The rotator interval capsule tissues (superior capsule, superior glenohumeral joint ligament, and coracohumeral ligament) have the orientation and tensile properties to generate the force vector needed to compress the humeral head into the fossa and prevent caudal humeral translation **(Fig. 7–36)**.[31,33,36]

In addition to passive tension from the rotator interval capsule, two other mechanisms help provide static stability to the glenohumeral joint in the dependent arm. In a healthy

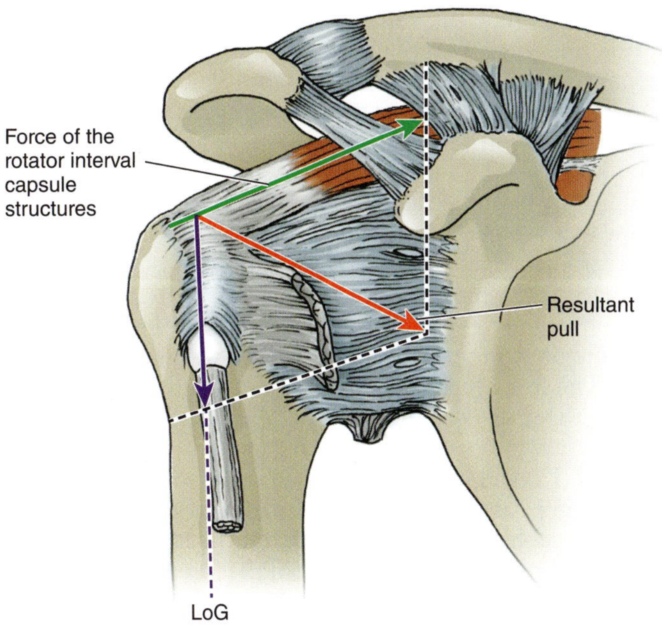

Figure 7–36 Mechanism for stabilization of the dependent arm. With the arm relaxed at the side, the downward pull of gravity on the arm (the LoG extended upward from the center of gravity of the upper extremity) is opposed by the passive tension in the rotator interval capsule. The resultant of these forces stabilizes the humeral head on the glenoid fossa.

glenohumeral joint, the capsule is airtight and there is negative intra-articular pressure that creates a relative vacuum that helps resist the inferior humeral translation caused by the force of gravity.[33] Loss of intra-articular pressure, produced by venting the capsule or tears in the glenoid labrum, results in large increases in inferior humeral translations.[69,70] The degree of glenoid inclination also influences glenohumeral joint stability with the arm in the dependent position.[35] A slight upward tilt of the glenoid fossa, either anatomically in the structure of the scapula or through scapular upward rotation at rest, creates bony resistance against humeral inferior translation.

When passive forces alone are inadequate for glenohumeral joint stabilization, as may occur in the heavily loaded arm, the supraspinatus provides active assistance through its attachments to the rotator interval capsule.[18,39] In fact, the role of the supraspinatus may be more critical than its activity indicates as measured by electromyography (EMG) because paralysis or dysfunction in the supraspinatus may lead to inferior subluxation of the glenohumeral joint over time. Without the reinforcing passive tension of the intact supraspinatus muscle, the sustained load on the connective tissue structures of the rotator interval capsule apparently causes these structures to gradually stretch (become plastic), resulting in a loss of joint stability. Inferior glenohumeral subluxation is commonly encountered in patients with diminished rotator cuff function caused by stroke or other brain injuries.

Dynamic Glenohumeral Joint Stabilization

The Deltoid and Glenohumeral Stabilization

It is generally accepted that the middle deltoid muscle is the prime mover (along with the supraspinatus) for glenohumeral abduction, while the anterior and posterior deltoid are the prime movers for glenohumeral flexion and extension, respectively. All three elevation activities share biomechanical similarities; the deltoid segment or segments that participate in elevation will vary by role and function.[71,72] Importantly, deltoid activation during elevation activities also generates potentially harmful translatory motions at the glenohumeral joint that require joint stabilization forces. Examination of the resultant line of action of the deltoid muscle in abduction can be used to highlight the stabilization needs of the glenohumeral joint in elevation activities. **Figure 7–37** shows the line of action of the deltoid muscle with the arm at the side. The force vectors of the three segments of the deltoid acting together coincide with the fibers of the middle deltoid. When the muscle force vector (FD) is resolved into its parallel (Fx) and perpendicular (Fy) components in relation to the long axis of the humerus, the parallel component (Fx) directed cephalad (superiorly) is by far the larger of the two components. That is, the majority of the force of contraction of the deltoid from this initial position causes the humerus and its humeral head to translate superiorly. With the arm at the side, only a small moment arm (and small Fy component) exists to directly contribute to humeral abduction.

At the majority of joints in the body, the force component parallel to the long bone is larger and has a stabilizing effect because it contributes to joint compression. At the glenohumeral joint, however, when the arm is at the side, the nearly vertical glenoid fossa is almost parallel with the shaft of the humerus. Consequently, a force (Fx) applied parallel to the long axis of the humerus creates a substantial shear force at the joint (approximately parallel to the contacting articular surfaces) rather than a stabilizing (compressive) force. An unopposed deltoid contraction generates a large superior humerus translation effect because of the greater superiorly directed force component, and a small rotation effect because of the much smaller Fy component vector and short moment arm. To prevent the humerus from translating superiorly and impacting the coracoacromial arch, and to improve the mechanical advantage for rotation, a set of forces complementary to the deltoid are needed. These forces are actively generated by the rotator cuff muscles.

The Rotator Cuff and Glenohumeral Stabilization

The supraspinatus, infraspinatus, teres minor, and subscapularis muscles and tendons comprise the rotator cuff. These muscles are considered to be part of a "cuff" because the inserting tendons of each muscle of the cuff blend with and reinforce the glenohumeral capsule both anteriorly (subscapularis) and posteriorly (supraspinatus, infraspinatus, and teres minor). Each of the rotator cuff muscles has lines of action that significantly contribute to the dynamic stabilization of the glenohumeral joint.

The force of the infraspinatus, teres minor, or subscapularis muscles taken together (as well as individually) resolves into components such that the perpendicular force component (Fy) causes at least some rotation of the humerus, given its orientation to the axis of rotation, and also (unusual for a muscular Fy component) compresses the humeral head into the glenoid fossa **(Fig. 7–38)**. Because of the nearly vertical orientation of the glenoid fossa, this compression force is critical to stabilizing the glenohumeral joint by countering the downward directed force of gravity on the humerus. This example also illustrates how muscle forces produce not only movement through joint rotations but also produce functionally relevant translatory forces.

In addition to glenohumeral joint compression forces, the infraspinatus, teres minor, and subscapularis muscles also generate an inferior translatory force that opposes the deltoid muscle contraction (see Fig. 7-38). The sum of these three rotator cuff muscles together with the subscapularis combine to produce an inferior force component vector that limits the superior humeral head translatory effect created

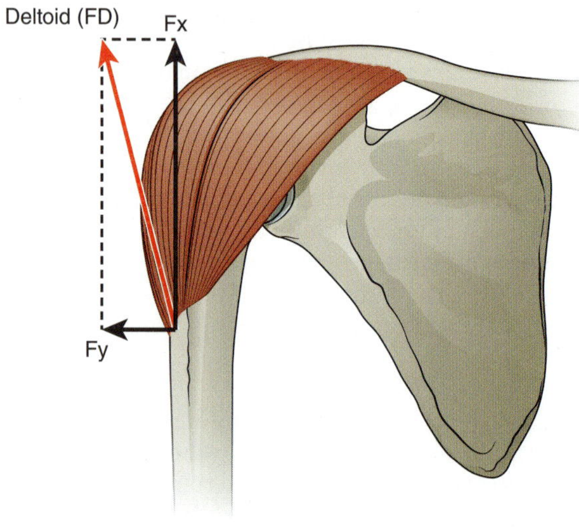

Figure 7–37 The action line of all three segments of the deltoid follows the line of pull of the middle deltoid. The resultant pull of the three deltoid segments (FD) resolves into a very large upward translatory component (Fx) and a small rotary component (Fy) so that an isolated contraction of the deltoid would cause the deltoid to produce more superior translation than rotation of the humerus.

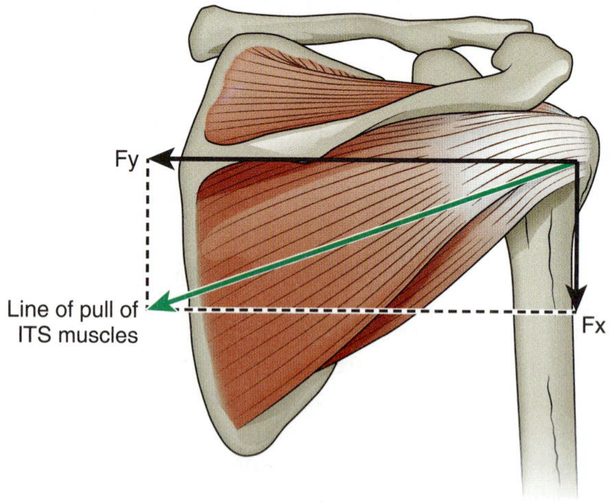

Figure 7–38 The combined action line of the infraspinatus, teres minor, and the anteriorly located subscapularis (ITS) muscles of the rotator cuff has a large Fy component that, atypically, compresses the humeral head into the glenoid fossa, and a downwardly directed Fx component.

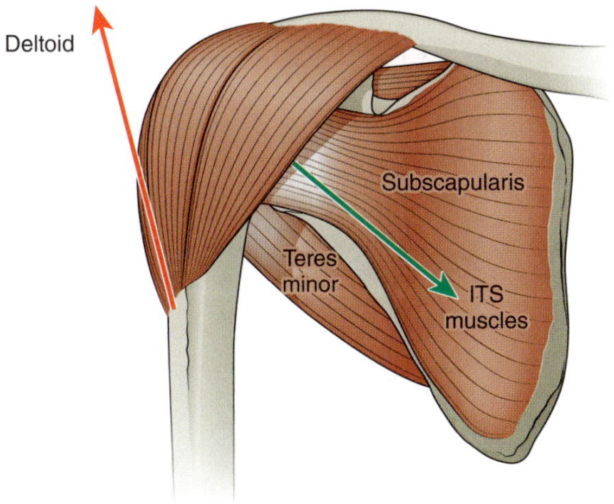

Figure 7–39 The line of pull of the deltoid muscle and the combined pulls of the posteriorly located infraspinatus and teres minor, along with the anteriorly located subscapularis (ITS muscles), approximate a force couple with nearly parallel lines of pull that produce almost perfect rotation of the humeral head around a stable A-P axis with minimal translation of the humeral head.

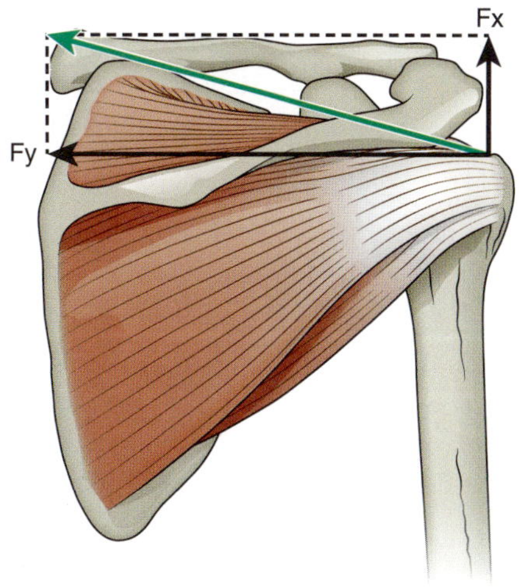

Figure 7–40 The supraspinatus, like the other muscles of the rotator cuff, has a large Fy component that compresses the head of the humerus but, unlike the other muscles of the rotator cuff, has a *superiorly* (rather than inferiorly) directed Fx component. The line of action of the supraspinatus lies far enough from the joint axis that it can abduct the humerus independently without the deltoid muscle.

by the deltoid. Cadaver experiments demonstrated that arm abduction without the forces generated by the infraspinatus, teres minor, and subscapularis results in substantial superiorly directed shifts in humerus position on the glenoid fossa.[73]

Acting together, the rotator cuff muscles compress the glenohumeral joint and limit superior humerus translations. However, when activated individually, each muscle has the potential to create other glenohumeral motions. As glenohumeral lateral rotators, the teres minor and infraspinatus create lateral rotation during humerus elevation to help clear the greater tubercle from beneath the acromion. The subscapularis, a medial rotator, does not actively prevent lateral rotation from happening, but works synergistically with the lateral rotators to help center the humeral head in the anterior/posterior direction, a function that has been referred to as "steering."[74]

The action of the deltoid and the combined actions of the infraspinatus, teres minor, and subscapularis muscles approximate a force couple **(Fig. 7–39)**. The nearly equal and opposite superior (deltoid) and inferior (rotator cuff) forces acting on the humerus create an *almost* perfect rotation of the humeral head around a relatively stable axis of rotation with minimal translation.

The Supraspinatus and Glenohumeral Stabilization

Although the supraspinatus muscle is part of the rotator cuff, its line of action has a slightly superior (cephalad) translatory component **(Fig. 7–40)**, rather than the inferior (caudal) component of the other cuff muscles (see Fig. 7–38). Given its line of pull, the supraspinatus cannot contribute to offsetting the upward translatory action of the deltoid.[75] The supraspinatus is still an effective stabilizer of the glenohumeral joint, however, because of its contribution to joint compression. The more superior location of the supraspinatus results in a line of action that lies farther from the glenohumeral joint axis than the action lines of the other rotator cuff muscles, establishing a moment arm that is capable of *independently* producing a full or nearly full range of glenohumeral joint abduction while simultaneously stabilizing the joint.[29] Gravity acts as a stabilizing synergist to the supraspinatus by offsetting the small upward translatory pull of the muscle.

Expanded Concepts 7–3
The Supraspinatus as an Independent Abductor

The supraspinatus can, at least theoretically, independently produce abduction of the arm through most or all of its range, whereas the deltoid cannot. The resultant of the force vectors of an active supraspinatus contraction and gravity is essentially identical to the resultant vector in Figure 7–36 because the line of action of the supraspinatus is the same as that of the rotator interval capsule with which it blends. With a concentric contraction of the supraspinatus, the proportionally small superiorly directed translatory force is offset by the inferiorly directed force of gravity, which results in translatory equilibrium but effective rotation. The resultant of the gravitational and supraspinatus force vectors contributes to an inferior sliding of the humeral head articular surface during abduction of the arm, allowing full articulation of the joint surfaces and preventing unwanted superior displacement. The supraspinatus can also contribute small amounts of either medial or lateral rotation torque, depending on the position of the arm, although its moment arm for long axis rotation is very small.[76]

The Long Head of the Biceps Brachii and Glenohumeral Stabilization

The long head of the biceps brachii runs superiorly along the anterior shaft of the humerus through the bicipital groove between the greater and lesser tubercles to attach to the supraglenoid tubercle and superior labrum **(Fig. 7–41)**. Within the bicipital groove, the biceps tendon is enveloped by a tendon sheath and tethered there by the **transverse humeral ligament** that runs between the greater and lesser tubercles (see **Fig. 7–41A**). The long head tendon enters the glenohumeral

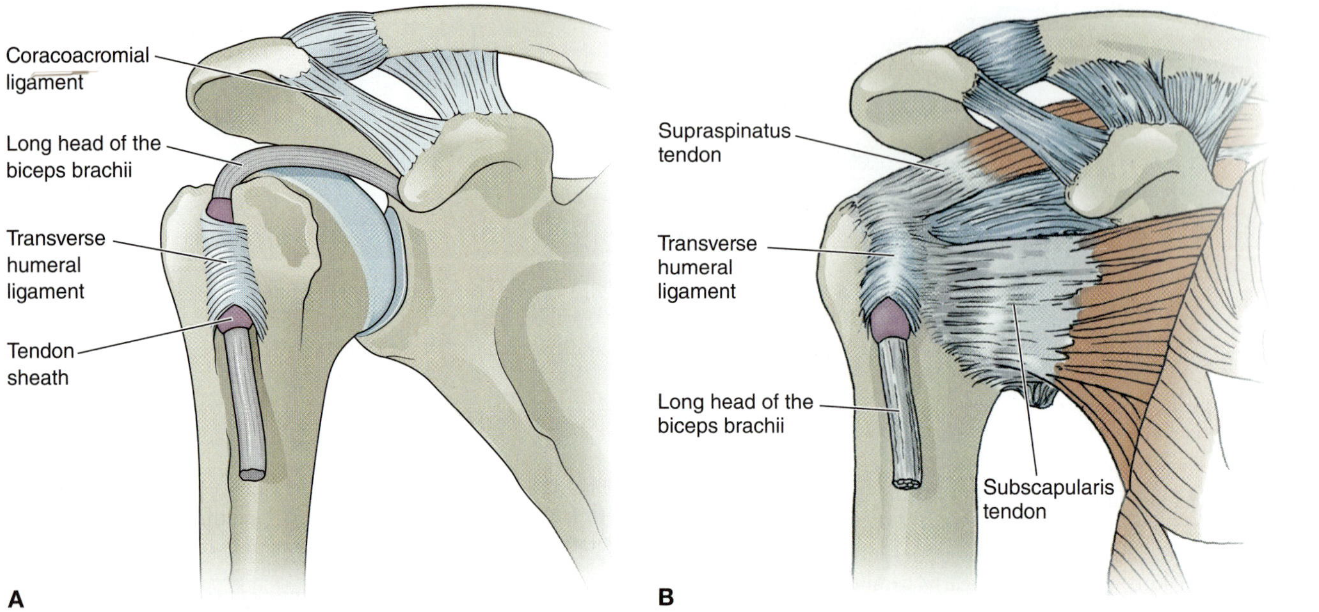

Figure 7–41 The long head of the biceps brachii. **A.** The tendon passes through a fibro-osseous tunnel formed by the bicipital groove and the transverse humeral ligament, protected from frictional forces by a tendon sheath. **B.** The tendon enters the glenohumeral joint capsule (but not its synovial lining) through an opening between the supraspinatus and subscapularis tendons.

joint capsule through an opening between the supraspinatus and subscapularis tendons (see **Fig. 7–41B**), where it penetrates the capsule but not the synovium.

The long head of the biceps brachii, because of its position at the superior capsule and its connections to structures of the rotator interval capsule, is sometimes considered part of the reinforcing cuff of the glenohumeral joint.[39] Activity of the biceps' long head can contribute to glenohumeral joint flexion and, if the humerus is laterally rotated, contribute to abduction.[47] Although elbow and shoulder position modify its function, the long head appears to contribute to glenohumeral stabilization by centering the humeral head in the fossa and by reducing vertical (superior and inferior) and anterior translations.[77-80] Pagnani and colleagues hypothesized that the long head may produce its effect by tightening the relatively loose superior labrum and transmitting increased tension to the superior and middle glenohumeral ligaments.[80] This idea follows from their observation that lesions of the anterosuperior labrum did not affect stability of the glenohumeral joint unless the attachment of the long head of the biceps brachii was also disrupted.[81] The overall contribution of the long head to glenohumeral stabilization is supported by the observation that the tendon sometimes hypertrophies with rotator cuff tears.[80]

Foundational Concepts 7–2
Dynamic Stabilization of the Glenohumeral Joint

Dynamic stabilization at any point in the glenohumeral range is a function of (1) the force of the prime mover or movers; (2) the force of gravity; (3) the force of the muscular stabilizers; (4) articular surface geometry; (5) passive capsuloligamentous forces; and (6) the joint reaction force, because compression of the humeral head into the glenoid fossa is opposed by an equal force from the glenoid fossa in the opposite direction (joint reaction force).[47] Due to muscular compression forces, joint reaction forces can reach magnitudes of 9 to 10 times the weight of the upper extremity as the arm is elevated.[26,47] When the medially directed resultant muscular forces have slightly superior or inferior components, shear forces will occur. The greatest shear forces during humeral elevation typically occur between 30° and 60° of elevation.[26]

Costs of Dynamic Stabilization of the Glenohumeral Joint

When all stabilization forces and factors are intact and properly functioning, the head of the humerus rotates the arm into flexion or abduction around a relatively stable axis with minimal translation. Over time, however, even typical stresses related to dynamic stabilization may lead to degenerative changes or dysfunction at the glenohumeral joint. Any disruption in the synergistic action of the dynamic stabilization factors may accelerate degenerative changes in or around the joint.

The supraspinatus muscle is a particularly key structure in dynamic stabilization. The supraspinatus is either passively stretched or actively contracting when the arm is at the side (depending on load); it also contributes to humeral elevation throughout the glenohumeral ROM. Consequently, the tendon is under tension most of a person's waking hours and is vulnerable to tensile overload and chronic overuse. Mechanical compression and impingement of the stressed supraspinatus tendon may occur on either the superior or inferior surface of the tendon for a variety of reasons. Compression may increase when the subacromial space is reduced by osteoligamentous factors, when there is increased superior or anterior translation of the humeral head center, when the scapula does not posteriorly tilt or upwardly rotate adequately during humeral elevation, or when occupational factors require heavy lifting or sustained overhead arm postures. Mechanical "impingement" of the undersurface of the supraspinatus on the glenoid can also occur at higher humeral elevation angles.[82] The supraspinatus tendon is the most vulnerable of the rotator cuff muscles, although overuse and potential impingement issues also affect the other cuff muscles. Both symptomatic and asymptomatic partial- or full-thickness rotator cuff tears are present in many people over the age of 60, with the supraspinatus likely to show lesions earlier than other cuff tendons.[83] Rotator cuff tendinopathy or tears typically produce pain between 60° and 120° of humeral elevation in relation to the trunk, a ROM described as the **painful arc.** Within this arc of motion, the tendons of the rotator cuff were previously described as passing beneath the coracoacromial arch in a cadaveric investigation.[41] However, as noted earlier, more recent investigation of active motion in human subjects revealed that, in continuing beyond 60° of abduction of the arm from the side, the supraspinatus tendon has rotated past the overlying acromion in most cases.[43] Subsequently, the source of the pain in a painful arc of motion may be related to factors other than supraspinatus compression, such as the need to produce high active forces against gravity.

Patient Application 7–2
Glenohumeral Joint Instability

Megan Schultz is a 17-year-old girl who reports symptoms of pain, weakness, and a feeling of "giving out" during some reaching activities. She is unable to lie on her shoulder when sleeping because of this same "giving out" sensation. Holding the position of 90° abduction and 90° external rotation is uncomfortable for her. These symptoms are consistent with loss of static stabilization of the GH joint, which is often related to hypermobility or laxity of the anterior capsule and glenohumeral ligaments. In such cases, the dynamic stabilizers—primarily the rotator cuff—must be relied on to support the joint and maintain the humeral head position on the glenoid. These patients often note increased symptoms at the end of the day or after repetitive use of the upper extremity, presumably from fatigue of the dynamic stabilizers.

Integrated Function of the Shoulder Complex

Integrated Joint Function

The shoulder complex joints, muscles, tendons, and ligaments act in a coordinated manner to produce the smoothest and greatest ROM possible to the upper limb. Motion at the glenohumeral joint alone would not account for the full range of elevation (abduction or flexion) available to the humerus; the remainder of the range is realized by scapula motion on the thorax (the functional scapulothoracic joint) through motions at the anatomical SC and AC joints. The ability to move the arm from its position parallel to the thorax (0°) is known as **scapulohumeral motion**, and is attributable to the combination of anatomical SC, AC, and glenohumeral joint motions. Multi-joint scapulohumeral motion (1) distributes the motion between the contributing joints, permitting a large ROM with less reduction in stability than would occur if the same range occurred at one joint; (2) maintains the glenoid fossa in an optimal position in relation to the head of the humerus, increasing joint congruency while decreasing

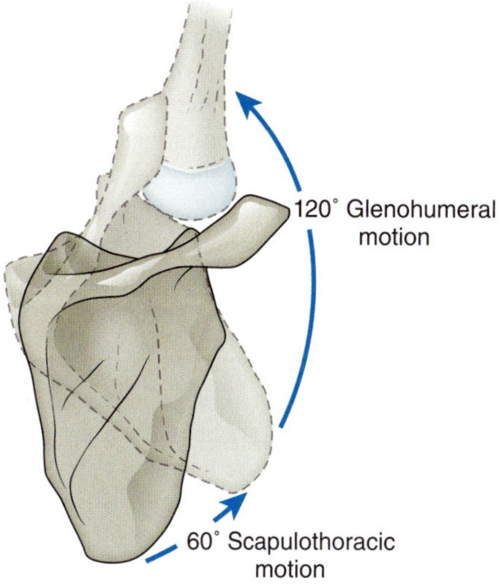

Figure 7–42 When it is assumed that the total range of elevation is 180°, it is common to attribute 120° of the ROM to the humerus at the glenohumeral joint and 60° to the scapula on the thorax—with the two segments moving *synchronously* rather than sequentially.

shear forces; and (3) permits muscles acting on the humerus to maintain a good length-tension relationship that minimizes or prevents active insufficiency of the deltoid.

Scapulothoracic and Glenohumeral Function

Scapula motion on the thorax contributes to elevation (flexion and abduction) of the humerus by upwardly rotating the glenoid fossa 50° to 60° from its resting position.[16,48] If the humerus were immobile at the glenohumeral joint, the scapula alone theoretically would result in as much as 60° of humeral elevation (relative to the thorax). The humerus and its glenohumeral joint, of course, are not immobile but can move independently on the glenoid fossa, contributing 100° to 120° to flexion and 90° to 120° to abduction. The combination of scapular and humeral movement results in a maximum range of elevation of 150° to 180° **(Fig. 7–42)**.[56,84] During arm elevation, an *overall* ratio of 2° of glenohumeral to 1° of scapulothoracic motion is commonly described, and this combined motion is commonly referred to as **scapulohumeral rhythm.** According to the two-to-one ratio framework, flexion or abduction of 90° in relation to the thorax would be accomplished through approximately 60° of glenohumeral and 30° of scapulothoracic motion.

The two-to-one ratio of glenohumeral to scapulothoracic contribution to arm elevation is an oversimplification, with substantial variability in scapular and humeral contributions at different points in the ROM and among individuals. However, the ratio is still a useful conceptualization of a typical motion pattern.

Expanded Concepts 7–4
Variations in Scapulohumeral "Rhythm"

Inman and coworkers reported that during the initial 60° of flexion or the initial 30° of abduction of the humerus, an inconsistent amount and type of scapular motion occurred in relation to glenohumeral motion.[47] The scapula has been described as seeking a position of stability in relation to the humerus during this period.[47,72,85] In this early phase, motion occurs primarily at the glenohumeral joint, although stressing the arm may increase the scapular contribution.[69] A number of studies have investigated the scapulohumeral "rhythm," with ratios reported varying between 1.25:1 and 2.69:1.[19,59,60,74,85,86] Ratios are often described as nonlinear, indicating changing ratios during different portions of the ROM for elevation of the arm. The rhythm varies among individuals and may vary with external constraints.[86] Synchronous upward rotation of the scapula with glenohumeral elevation is certainly an important concept. However, the utility of the term *rhythm* seems limited because there does not appear to be a definitive scapulohumeral "rhythm."

The scapula contributes to arm elevation not only by upwardly rotating on the thorax but also through the scapulothoracic motions of anterior/posterior tilting and internal/external rotation. While the exact magnitudes of these scapular motions vary across studies, the general patterns are relatively consistent. As the arm is elevated into flexion, scapular plane abduction (scaption) or abduction in the frontal plane, the scapula posteriorly tilts on the thorax.[15-17,48,53] As the arm moves from the side to 150° of elevation, the magnitude of posterior tilting is about 20° to 30°.[16,48] This posterior tilting allows the inferior angle of the scapula to move anteriorly and stay in contact with the thorax as it slides upward and around the rib cage. Posterior tilting of the scapula also has the effect of bringing the anterior acromion superior and back. This may serve to minimize reduction in the subacromial space as the humerus elevates.

Internal/external rotation of the scapula is more variable within and between people during arm elevation.[15,16,48] In general, the scapula is externally rotating on the thorax at the end ranges of elevation.[15,16,48,53] However, slight internal rotation of the scapula on the thorax occurs early in the ROM for flexion. Prevention of excess internal rotation of the scapula is important for keeping the scapula, particularly the medial border, in contact with the thorax as the scapula upwardly rotates during arm elevation. In flexion, the scapula initially protracts and internally rotates to orient the glenoid fossa closer to the coronal plane.[16,48] Structural limitations or the inability of muscles to appropriately stabilize the scapula may result in anterior tilting, internal rotation, and downward rotation of the scapula with attempted flexion of the arm, through reverse action of the deltoid **(Fig. 7–43)**.

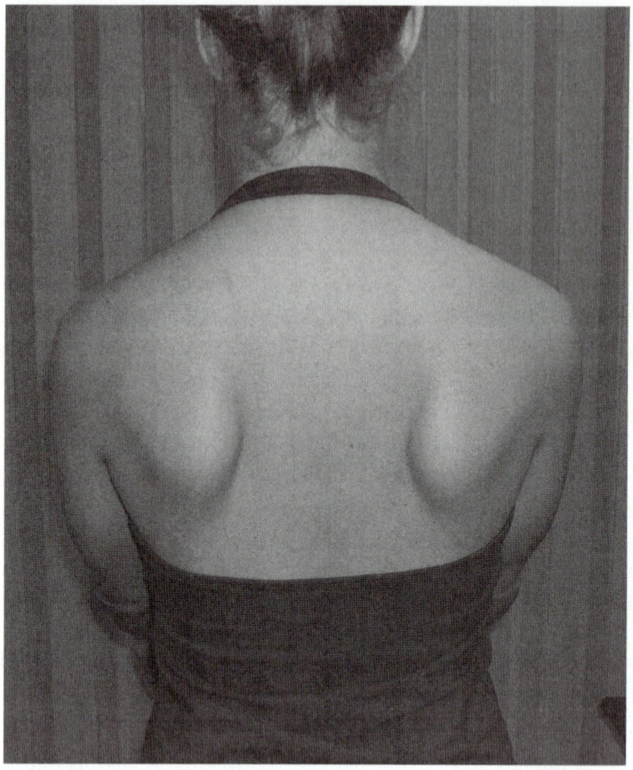

Figure 7–43 Structural limitations or the inability of muscles to appropriately stabilize the scapula may result in anterior tilting, internal rotation, and downward rotation of the scapula during arm elevation, lifting the inferior and medial angles of the scapula off the thorax.

Sternoclavicular and Acromioclavicular Function

Arm elevation in any plane involves motion of the SC and AC joints to produce scapulothoracic motion. Given the complexity of the linkages, there is limited description in the literature on the relative contributions of the SC and AC joints to the potential 60° arc of upward rotation of the scapula on the thorax. However, recent investigations report consistent average values for SC and AC joint motions during active elevation despite varying measurement methods.[16,48,51]

During arm flexion or abduction, the initiation of scapulothoracic upward rotation appears to couple with clavicular posterior rotation and elevation at the SC joint **(Fig. 7–44)**. The coupling is based on the nonparallel clavicular-scapular axis relationships previously described (see Fig. 7–28).[72] This scapular upward rotation occurs around an oblique A-P axis, passing through the costoclavicular ligament (SC joint axis of motion), and projecting backward through the root of the scapular spine (axis of scapulothoracic motion). As arm elevation progresses, the scapulothoracic axis for upward rotation gradually shifts laterally, reaching the AC joint at the end of the ROM **(Fig. 7–45)**.[72] This major shift in

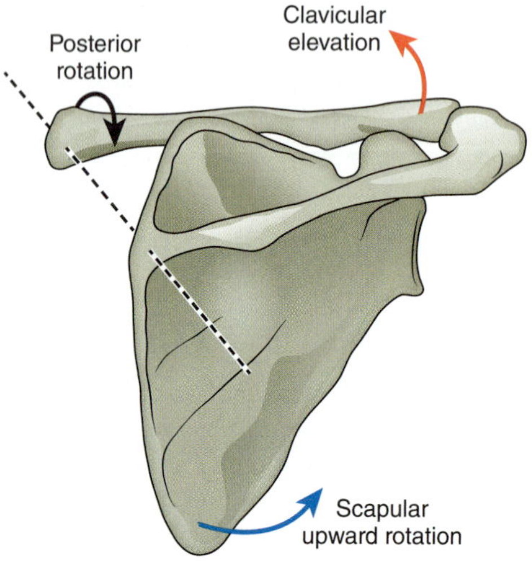

Figure 7–44 The scapulothoracic upward rotation contribution to arm elevation begins as posterior rotation and elevation at the SC joint around an axis that appears to pass posteriorly from the costoclavicular ligament to the root of the spine of the scapula.

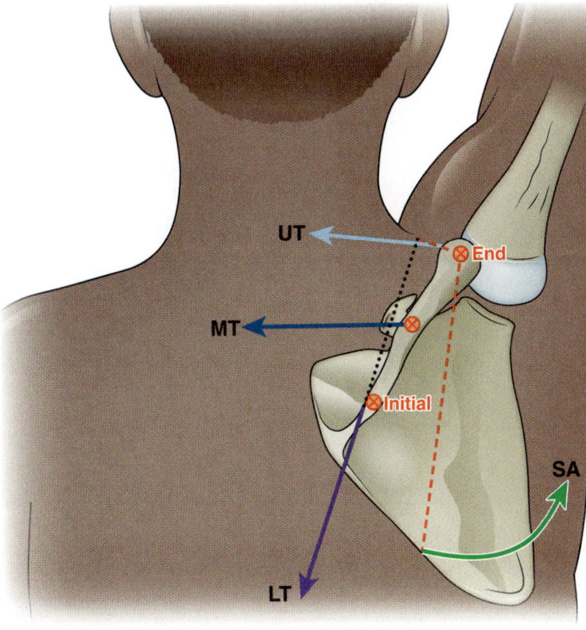

Figure 7–45 The axis of scapular upward rotation (red circles) progresses laterally from its initial position near the root of the scapular spine to its final location near the AC joint at the end of arm elevation. The action lines of the middle trapezius (MT), lower trapezius (LT), and serratus anterior (SA) muscles produce scapulothoracic upward rotation through their scapular attachments, while the upper trapezius (UT) contributes by elevating the clavicle. The red dashed lines show the moment arms of the lower trapezius (its vector extended by the black dotted line) and serratus anterior with respect to the axis of rotation at the end of the motion, with the moment arm of the serratus being much longer.

the axis of rotation happens because scapulothoracic motion can occur only through a combination of motions at the SC and AC joints. When the axis of scapular upward rotation is near the root of the scapular spine, scapulothoracic motion is primarily a function of SC joint motion. When the axis of scapular upward rotation is at the AC joint, AC joint motions predominate. When the axis of scapular upward rotation is in an intermediate position, both the SC and AC joints contribute to scapulothoracic motion (see Fig. 7–45).

Current 3D descriptions of clavicular motion show about 10° or less of clavicular elevation during arm elevation.[16,51] In addition, as described previously (see Fig. 7–29), approximately one-third of this elevation (about 3°) will couple with scapular upward rotation.[52] For upward rotation of the scapula to occur at the AC joint, described in 3D studies as 15°–20° of scapular upward rotation at the AC joint, AC motion constraints imposed by the coracoclavicular ligament must be overcome.[16,51] Tension in the coracoclavicular ligament (especially the conoid portion) increases as the coracoid process moves downward with muscle forces attempting to upwardly rotate the scapula at the AC joint. The tightened conoid ligament pulls its posteroinferior clavicular attachment forward and down as the coracoid process drops, causing clavicle posterior rotation. Posterior rotation of the clavicle around its longitudinal axis results in additional scapulothoracic upward rotation (see Figs. 7–22 and 7–27). Thus, scapulothoracic upward rotation at the AC joint occurs through coupling with clavicle posterior SC joint rotation and through reduced tension in the coracoclavicular ligament.[52] The magnitude of posterior rotation of the clavicle ranges from 30° to 50°, with about two-thirds of this motion coupled with scapulothoracic upward rotation.[16,47] Consequently, SC and AC joint rotations work synchronously and cumulatively to contribute to overall scapular upward rotation on the thorax during arm elevation.

Throughout arm elevation (flexion, scapular plane abduction, or frontal plane abduction), the clavicle also retracts at the SC joint, typically 20° to 30°, which couples with external rotation of the scapula on the thorax.[16,48,51] Because of the approximately vertical orientation of both the SC and scapulothoracic axes for protraction, SC retraction and protraction will directly result from—or couple with—scapulothoracic external and internal rotation, respectively. This coupling only exists if there is no motion at the AC joint, however. Instead, during functional arm elevation movements, the scapula is *internally* rotating 10° to 15° at the AC joint,[16,48] while the clavicle retracts at the SC joint. Internal/external rotation at the AC joint occurs about an approximately vertical axis as well, and thus is parallel to the scapulothoracic internal/external rotation axis. As a result, the AC joint *internal rotation* offsets a large portion of the scapulothoracic *external rotation* that would otherwise occur from SC joint retraction during arm elevation.

The magnitudes of AC joint internal rotation with arm elevation will differ with variations in scapular resting position, rib cage configuration, and muscle dynamics. However, the component motions of the SC (retraction) and AC (internal rotation) joints are similar regardless of whether the arm elevation motion is performed in the sagittal, scapular, or frontal planes. In other words, with arm elevation in each of these planes, it is expected that the SC joint will always retract, and the AC joint will always internally rotate in a typically functioning shoulder.[16]

The plane of arm elevation will also result in different starting positions of the SC and AC joints. With flexion of the arm, the clavicle and scapula begin in less retraction and more internal rotation, respectively, to bring the glenoid fossa forward and in line with the elevating humeral head.[16] During abduction of the arm, the clavicle and scapula begin in more retraction and less internal rotation, respectively, to bring the glenoid fossa more lateral for closer alignment with the humeral head during the motion.

The final component motion of the scapula on the thorax during arm elevation in all planes is posterior tilting. Although about one-third of SC posterior rotation of the clavicle will couple with scapulothoracic *posterior tilting*, two-thirds of SC elevation (about 6°) will couple with scapulothoracic *anterior tilting* during the same range of arm elevation.[52] As a reminder, this is because the AC joint internal rotation angle is about two-thirds of the way to a 90° alignment between the clavicular long axis and the scapular plane. In a 90° alignment, clavicular elevation would produce scapulothoracic anterior tilting. As a result, the clavicular elevation and posterior rotation at the SC joint offset one another with regard to scapulothoracic tilting at the AC joint, and minimal scapulothoracic posterior tilting is produced at the SC joint during typical arm elevation. The predominance of scapulothoracic posterior tilting during elevation of the arm occurs with AC joint posterior tilting, which averages 20° or more.[16,51]

Expanded Concepts 7–5
Thoracic Spine Motion

In addition to the motions that occur at the shoulder complex joints during arm elevation, there is also concurrent motion of the thoracic spine. With unilateral arm elevation, the lower thoracic spine side-bends contralaterally, whereas the upper thoracic spine undergoes contralateral axial rotation.[87] During bilateral arm elevation, there is extension of both the lower and upper thoracic regions.[87] Mobility of the thoracic spine region should also be considered when assessing shoulder complex function because decreased or increased thoracic motion has the potential to influence shoulder kinematics.

Scapula Motion and Muscle Function

There is agreement that the motions of the scapula are primarily produced by a balance of the forces between the trapezius and serratus anterior muscles through their attachments on the clavicle and the scapula. The upper portion of the trapezius muscle is attached to the lateral clavicle and is positioned to contribute directly to the initial elevation of the clavicle as well as to the SC joint retraction that occurs during typical arm elevation.[88] The serratus anterior muscle makes its contribution to the combined clavicular and scapular motion through its action on the scapula. When the location of the axis for scapulothoracic upward rotation is at or approaching its final position near the AC joint, the lower trapezius may contribute to upward rotation, although the lower serratus anterior muscle has a much greater moment arm (see Fig. 7–45).

There are substantial implications for muscle function during scapulothoracic upward rotation due to the large shift in the scapulothoracic axis of rotation. The upward rotation torque capabilities of the lower trapezius increase with increasing range of elevation as the scapular axis for upward rotation shifts laterally,[88] whereas the serratus anterior muscle maintains a large moment arm for scapulothoracic upward rotation throughout the entire range of elevation.

Despite a line of action and moment arm that are less effective for producing scapulothoracic upward rotation, the trapezius is clearly active during arm elevation and plays a role in the balance of forces that move and control the scapula on the thorax.[47] If the serratus anterior muscle acted in isolation, the lateral line of action would result in substantial scapular lateral translation (protraction) and less effective upward rotation, as is seen with accessory nerve damage affecting the trapezius **(Fig. 7–46)**. The medial translatory action of the trapezius muscle is necessary to offset the lateral translatory action of the serratus and results in more effective upward rotation by the serratus.

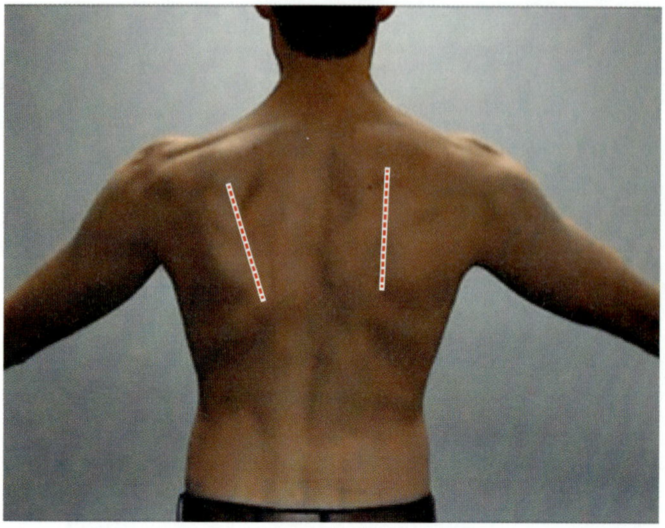

Figure 7–46 Individual with *left* spinal accessory nerve palsy, with partial paralysis of the ipsilateral trapezius, particularly the middle and lower trapezius. Note visible atrophy of all aspects of the affected trapezius as well as reduced scapular upward rotation and increased lateral translation of the root of the scapular spine on the left side during abduction. The unopposed action of the serratus anterior results in excessive lateral translation and, consequently, less effective scapular upward rotation.

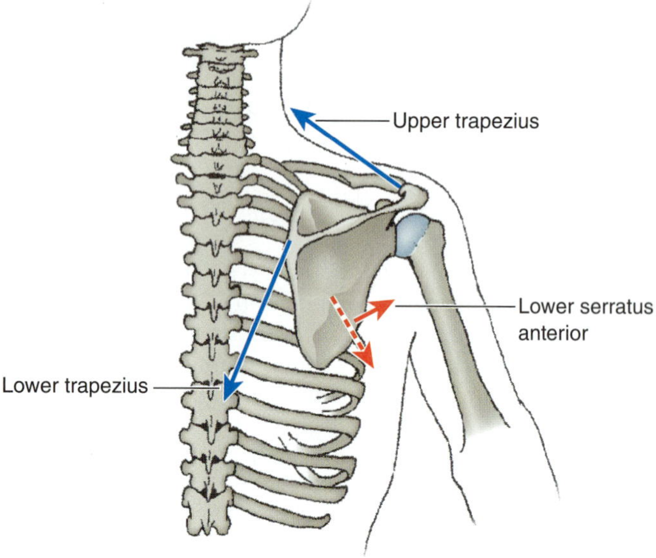

Figure 7–47 Classically described action lines for the upward rotators of the scapula that *may* overestimate the ability of the trapezius to upwardly rotate the scapula.

Foundational Concepts 7–3
Trapezius Function Reconsidered

Johnson and colleagues identified how the lines of action for the trapezius muscle were based on actual muscle fiber orientation that differed from the traditional descriptions and depictions of muscle line of action in older textbooks.[88] Historically, the upper trapezius has been shown with a superior and medial line of action on the scapula and the lower trapezius with an inferior medial line of action **(Fig. 7–47)**. Johnson and colleagues suggested, on the basis of cadaveric dissection, that the upper trapezius fibers act minimally on the scapula and more through elevation and retraction of the clavicle, thus only minimally contributing directly to upward rotation of the scapula on the thorax.[88] Johnson and colleagues also suggested, on the basis of actual fiber orientation and cross-sectional area, that the lower trapezius action line should be directed more medially and less inferiorly than traditionally depicted.[88] Consequently, the lower trapezius (see Fig. 7–45) would have an even smaller moment arm to contribute to scapular upward rotation on the thorax than has been classically described. These descriptions are consistent with Dvir and Berme's model of shoulder function, which identifies the lower serratus anterior muscle as the prime mover of the scapula and the trapezius as the prime stabilizer.[72]

The contribution of scapulothoracic muscles to producing and controlling scapulothoracic anterior/posterior tilting and internal/external rotation is not well described in the literature. The middle and lower serratus anterior muscles, with their insertions into the medial border and inferior angle of the scapula, play a primary role in stabilizing the scapula against the thorax through lines of action that produce AC joint external rotation.[89] During scapula protraction, external rotation at the AC joint keeps the medial border against the thorax. In fact, paralysis of the serratus anterior muscle classically presents with scapular "winging" (see Fig. 7–31), a motion deviation that includes internal rotation and anterior tilting of the scapula produced by the remaining muscles without the stabilizing external rotation and posterior tilting influence of the middle and lower serratus. The lower serratus anterior muscle also has a large moment arm to produce posterior tilting of the scapula. The middle and lower trapezius can also contribute to external rotation torques of the scapula at the AC joint, and the upper trapezius contributes to clavicular retraction torque at the SC joint.[88,89]

Integrated Shoulder Muscle Function: Elevation

Elevation and depression are the two primary patterns of shoulder complex function. Elevation activities are those that require muscles to overcome or control the weight of the limb and its load. The completion of typical elevation depends on not only the freedom of movement and integrity of the SC, AC, and glenohumeral joints, but also the appropriate strength and function of the muscles producing and controlling movement. A closer look at the activity of these muscles should enhance an understanding of typical function, as well as contribute to an understanding of the deficits seen in pathological situations.

Deltoid

The deltoid is at resting length (optimal length-tension) when the arm is at the side. When at resting length, the deltoid's angle of pull results in a predominance of superior translatory pull on the humerus with an active contraction (see Fig. 7–37). With an appropriate synergistic inferior pull from the infraspinatus, teres minor, and subscapularis muscles, the rotary component of the deltoid muscle is an effective primary mover for elevation. The anterior deltoid is the prime mover for flexion but also assists with abduction.[90,91] During abduction in the plane of the scapula, the anterior and middle deltoid segments are optimally aligned to produce elevation of the humerus.[24] The line of action of the posterior deltoid has too small a moment arm (and too small a rotary component) to contribute effectively to frontal plane abduction. As such, minimal EMG activity is noted in the posterior deltoid during abduction, and it serves primarily as a joint compressor and in motions such as horizontal abduction and extension.[21,71]

As the humerus elevates, the superior translatory component of the deltoid diminishes as its resultant force vector shifts increasingly toward the glenoid fossa. At the same time, the rotary component of the deltoid force must counteract the increasing torque of gravity as the arm moves toward horizontal. Analysis of EMG shows gradually increasing activity in the deltoid, peaking between 90° to 120° of humeral abduction with a plateau or drop off for the remainder of the motion.[74,91] At higher elevation angles, the shortening deltoid is not able to produce as much active tension, and passive tension is diminished. As a result, a greater number of motor units must be recruited to maintain force output. The multipennate structure and considerable cross-sectional area of the deltoid help compensate for its relatively small moment arm, low mechanical advantage, and less than optimal length-tension relationship as elevation progresses.

Clinical Application 7–1
Shoulder Flexion Exercises: Variations

Clinicians often use arm elevation resistance exercises to strengthen the muscles used for functional tasks that require reaching overhead. Clinicians can modify a variety of factors during these exercises in order to meet therapeutic goals. For example, shoulder flexion performed in a supine position challenges the shoulder flexor muscles differently than does shoulder flexion performed in sitting or standing positions. In the supine position, the external extension moment arm (gravity acting on the upper extremity) is longest at the beginning of the exercise when the patient's arm is at their side **(Fig. 7–48)**. The long moment arm results in the greatest amount of extension torque as the exercise is initiated, which in turn requires the greatest amount of anterior deltoid concentric force to be generated. As the glenohumeral joint further flexes in this supine position, the external moment arm decreases, reducing the extension torque that must be overcome by the shoulder flexors. Importantly, when the shoulder flexes beyond a vertical position (roughly beyond 90° of flexion ROM), gravity begins generating an external *flexion* torque requiring the activation of the extensor muscles acting eccentrically to control the flexion torque imposed by gravity. In contrast, the same motion performed in an upright position requires the shoulder flexors to be active concentrically throughout the full ROM. In addition, the longest external moment arm and greatest external extension torque now occurs when the arm is horizontal (roughly 90°), which in turn requires the highest muscle force. In summary, one can challenge the shoulder flexors differently by how the patient is oriented to gravity. In supine, the flexors are most active early and are no longer the agonist beyond 90°, while in a standing position the flexor muscles are active throughout the full range and are most active at 90°.

For the patient with a painful arc near 90°, the supine position may allow pain-free exercises. Therapists can further manipulate patient orientation to gravity to progress the demand on the shoulder muscles by using increasingly inclined positions for flexion exercises.

Maintaining an advantageous deltoid muscle length-tension relationship is strongly dependent on simultaneous scapular movement. When the scapula is restricted and cannot upwardly rotate, the loss of tension in the deltoid with increased shortening has been reported to result in a reduced range of active glenohumeral abduction (whether the supraspinatus is available for assistance or not).[47] If the scapular upward rotators (serratus anterior and trapezius

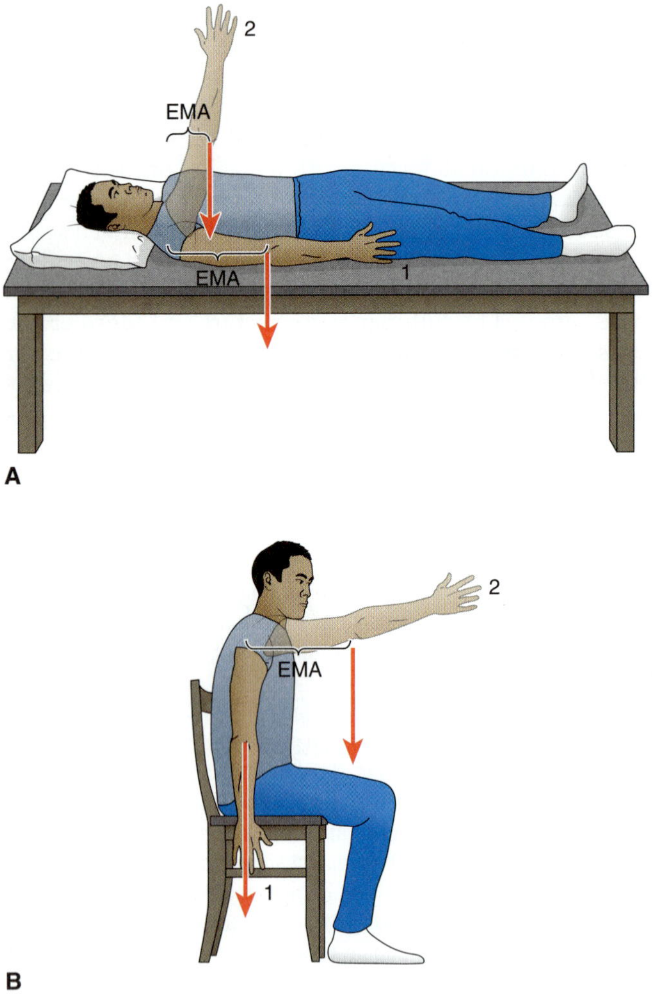

Figure 7–48 As shoulder flexion exercises are performed in different positions, the demands on the flexor muscles change as the moment arm (MA) of the external force (EF) of gravity changes. **A.** When performed in a supine position, there is greater muscle force required at the initiation of flexion (position 1) due to the large gravitational moment arm; as the arm is raised toward position 2, the MA of the EF gradually *decreases* so less muscle force is needed to continue active flexion. **B.** In contrast, when sitting, the muscle force requirement is smallest at the initiation of movement (position 1), but greatest when the arm is around 90°(position 2) where the moment arm of EF (gravity) in sitting is greatest.

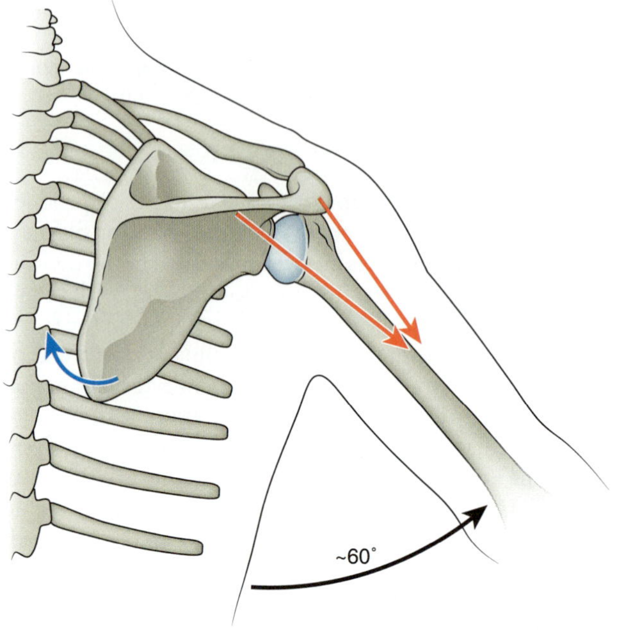

Figure 7–49 Without the upward rotatory effect of the trapezius and serratus anterior, activity of the middle and posterior deltoid during attempted abduction will downwardly rotate the lighter scapula while attempting to abduct the heavier arm. The net effect of abduction of the GH joint on the downwardly rotated scapula will be to achieve only 60°to 75° of active abduction of the *arm from the side* (shown as 60° here).

muscles) are absent, the middle and posterior fibers of the active deltoid (originating on the acromion and spine of the scapula) will not move the heavier arm but will, instead, move the lighter scapula; that is, without the stabilizing force of the scapula upward rotators, the middle and posterior deltoid will downwardly rotate the lighter scapula **(Fig. 7–49)** (typically referred to as reverse action). Although the deltoid can still produce glenohumeral motion with restricted or limited scapula motion, the glenohumeral motion may occur on a downwardly rotated scapula. Depending on the plane of elevation and amount of loss of scapulothoracic muscle force production, deltoid reverse action can also produce undesired scapular anterior tilt and increased scapular internal rotation. The net effect of attempted abduction by the deltoid when there is trapezius and serratus anterior muscle paralyses is that the arm will rise from the side only about 60° to 75° (Fig. 7–49).[92]

Effective deltoid function also depends on intact rotator cuff muscles. With complete derangement of the cuff, a contraction of the deltoid results in a shrug of the shoulder (clavicular elevation at the SC joint and upward translation of the humerus) rather than in abduction of the humerus from the side **(Fig. 7–50)**. Isolated electrical stimulation of the axillary nerve (innervating the deltoid and teres minor muscles alone) produces approximately 40° of abduction.[93] Partial tears in or partial paralysis of the cuff will weaken the effective elevation produced by the deltoid, even though deltoid activation may increase.[94]

Supraspinatus

The supraspinatus muscle is considered a humerus abductor that functions in all planes of arm elevation. The pattern of activity of the supraspinatus is essentially the same as that found in the deltoid.[47] The moment arm of the supraspinatus is fairly constant throughout elevation ROM and is larger than that of the deltoid for the first 60° of shoulder abduction.[21] When the deltoid is paralyzed, the supraspinatus alone can bring the arm through most, if not all, of the glenohumeral range but torque will be reduced.

The secondary functions of the supraspinatus are to compress the glenohumeral joint, to act as a "steerer" for the humeral head, and to assist in maintaining the stability of the dependent arm. With isolated and complete paralysis of

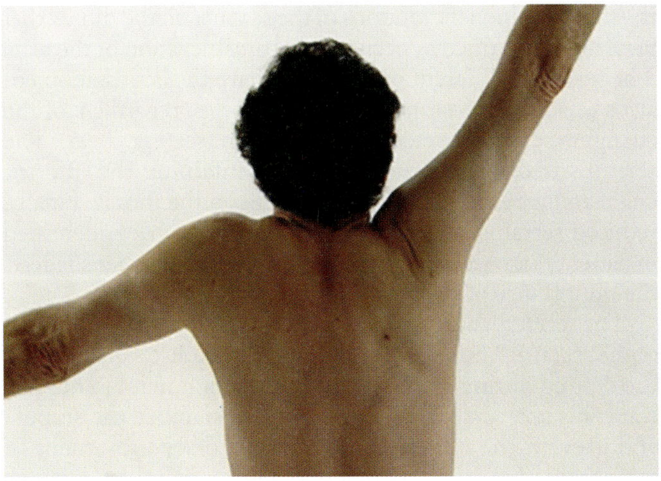

Figure 7–50 Patient attempting to elevate both arms. On the left, there is excess clavicle elevation (shoulder shrugging) produced by increased upper trapezius and deltoid activation. This muscle force imbalance often contributes to excess superior humeral translation, and inadequate scapular upward rotation as noted in this patient. This movement pattern in varying degrees may be a result of a massive rotator cuff tear, extreme shoulder stiffness with adhesive capsulitis, severely reduced glenohumeral mobility with osteoarthritis, or force production deficits of the inferior force-producing components of the rotator cuff or the serratus anterior.

the supraspinatus muscle, or an isolated supraspinatus tear, some loss of abduction force is evident, but most of its functions can be performed by remaining musculature. Isolated paralysis of the supraspinatus is unusual, however, because its innervation is the same as the infraspinatus and related to that of the teres minor muscle. Often, tears of the rotator cuff muscles do not remain isolated to the supraspinatus but extend to the infraspinatus or subscapularis, producing a more extensive deficit than is seen with loss of the supraspinatus alone.

Infraspinatus, Teres Minor, and Subscapularis

When Inman and coworkers assessed the combined actions of the infraspinatus, teres minor, and subscapularis muscles, EMG activity indicated a nearly linear rise in action potentials from 0° to 115° elevation.[47] Muscle activity then dropped slightly between 115° and 180°. These patterns are generally consistent with that reported by a more recent study in abduction.[91] Total muscle activity during flexion was slightly greater than that observed in abduction.[47] As noted earlier, the medial rotary function of the subscapularis muscle diminishes with abduction, serving instead to steer the head of the humerus horizontally while continuing to work with the other cuff muscles to compress and stabilize the glenohumeral joint.[74,90]

Trapezius and Serratus Anterior

The upper trapezius, along with the levator scapula muscle, supports the shoulder girdle against the downward pull of gravity. Although support of the scapula in the dependent limb is nearly passive in many individuals, loading the limb will produce activity in the upper trapezius and levator scapula muscles.[29,47] As previously discussed, the trapezius and lower serratus anterior muscles work synergistically to produce upward rotation of the scapula on the thorax. When activity of the upper and lower trapezius and serratus anterior muscles was monitored by EMG during humeral elevation, the curves were similar and complementary. Activity in the trapezius peaks above 90° in abduction, with less activity in flexion. The serratus anterior muscle shows an increase in action potentials above 90° in flexion, with less activity in abduction.[47,91] The middle trapezius muscle is also active during elevation (especially abduction) and may contribute to scapula upward rotation early in the range; however, it is likely to be more important in contributing to medial stabilization against the lateral pull of the serratus anterior.

Expanded Concepts 7–6
EMG and Muscle Function

EMG activity must be interpreted as only an indirect representation of muscle force production. If the length of the muscle is not held constant, an increase in EMG activity may not be indicative of increased force production; rather, increased muscle activity may be compensating for a muscle's loss of tension with active shortening (from decreasing length-tension relationship), as is proposed to be the rationale for increased end-range activity of many muscles. Such higher activity levels are commonly seen in muscles at the end range despite the necessity for peak torque production near the midrange of motion where gravitational resistance torques are often greatest. In addition, for increased EMG activity to relate to increased muscle force, the velocity of contraction and type of contraction (concentric, eccentric, isometric) must not change across comparison conditions. Finally, moment arms may change during movement, which will modify the force output requirements of muscle and result in an altered EMG signal.

The EMG activity of a muscle during a specific motion does not define the function of the muscle. Often, muscles are active as synergists offsetting unwanted translatory or rotary effects of a prime mover. For example, if a muscle is active during scapular upward rotation, it may be active to stabilize against excessive upward rotation rather than to produce upward rotation. This was discussed previously with trapezius function to offset lateral scapular motion from the pull of the serratus anterior; it will also be discussed as it occurs with rhomboid function during arm elevation.

The force and alignment of the trapezius seem more critical to scapulothoracic motion in active arm abduction than it is in active flexion. When the trapezius is intact and the serratus anterior muscle is paralyzed, full active abduction of the arm can occur, although it is weakened, whereas flexion is more difficult. With EMG analysis, the trapezius has been found to be more active in abduction than in flexion.[89] This may be related to the increased need for scapulothoracic and AC joint internal rotation noted in flexion as compared with abduction.[16] Without the trapezius (with or without the serratus anterior muscle), the scapula rests in a downwardly rotated position as a result of the unopposed effect of gravity on the clavicle and scapula (Fig. 7–51). In addition, with full paralysis of the trapezius, full abduction may not be possible even with a fully intact serratus anterior.

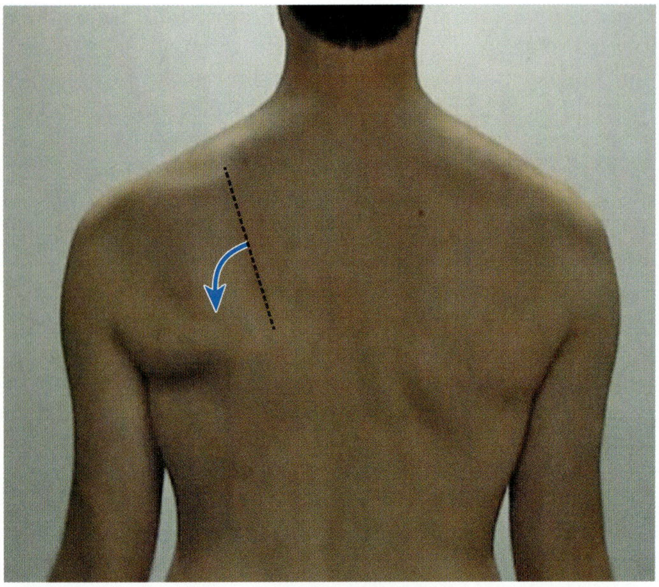

Figure 7–51 Weakness or paralysis of the left trapezius. With trapezius weakness or paralysis, the scapula rests in a downwardly rotated position on the thorax because the pull of gravity on the shoulder girdle is largely unopposed by remaining musculature.

Patient Application 7–3

Upper Trapezius Overuse

Excess activation of the upper trapezius has been identified in some patients with shoulder pain,[15] causing an imbalance of forces between the trapezius and serratus. The result can be an accompanying shoulder shrug type of motion (excess clavicle elevation) during arm elevation and less efficient upward rotation of the scapula on the thorax, although typically less pronounced than that seen with a massive rotator cuff tear or other severe conditions (see Fig. 7–50). Because of the coupling of clavicle elevation to scapular anterior tilt, excess upper trapezius activation may also result in reduction of the typical scapular posterior tilt that should occur during arm elevation. Prolonged overuse of the upper trapezius can result in muscle fatigue and pain in this muscle. Patients who report pain over the upper trapezius region should be evaluated for an upper trapezius overuse pattern with arm elevation.

Just as the trapezius is more active in abduction, the serratus anterior muscle seems to be better aligned and the more critical of the two muscles in producing scapular upward rotation during flexion of the arm. If the trapezius muscle is paralyzed but the serratus anterior muscle is intact, there is a loss of force of shoulder flexion but a fairly typical range of active flexion can still take place. If the serratus anterior muscle is paralyzed (even in the presence of a functioning trapezius), flexion will be diminished in strength and limited in range. When the scapular retraction component of the trapezius is not opposed by the serratus anterior muscle as it usually is, the trapezius is less effective in upwardly rotating the scapula—a necessary component for full flexion.

The role of the serratus anterior muscle in typical shoulder function appears to be essential in many aspects. The serratus anterior is the only muscle capable of producing simultaneous scapular upward rotation, posterior tilting, and external rotation, the three component motions of the scapula on the thorax that have been identified as occurring during elevation of the arm. The serratus's different portions also have the largest moment arms of any of the scapulothoracic muscles, regardless of the changing scapulothoracic axis of rotation (see Fig. 7–45). The serratus is the primary stabilizer maintaining the inferior angle and medial border of the scapula on the thorax. Finally, reduced serratus anterior muscle activity has been identified in patients with shoulder impingement, which further suggests the importance of this muscle to typical shoulder function.[15]

The serratus anterior is the prime mover for upward rotation of the scapula. The serratus and trapezius are also synergists for the deltoid during abduction at the glenohumeral joint. The trapezius and serratus anterior muscles stabilize the scapula and prevent the undesired downward rotary movement of the scapula by the middle and posterior deltoid segments, each of which are attached to the scapula (see Fig. 7–49). The trapezius and serratus anterior muscles maintain an optimal length-tension relationship with the deltoid and permit the deltoid to carry its heavier distal lever through its full ROM. Thus, the role of the scapular forces of the trapezius and the serratus anterior muscles is both agonistic to scapular movement and synergistic with glenohumeral movement.

Rhomboids

The **rhomboid major** and **minor** muscles are active in elevation of the arm, especially in abduction.[91] These muscles serve a critical function as stabilizing synergists to the muscles that upwardly rotate the scapula. If the rhomboids, which are downward rotators of the scapula, are active during upward rotation of the scapula, these muscles must be working eccentrically to control the change in position of the scapula produced by the trapezius and the serratus anterior muscles.[95] Paralysis of these muscles causes disruption of the typical scapulohumeral rhythm and may result in diminished ROM. Like the middle and lower trapezius, the rhomboid muscles act primarily to offset the lateral translation component of the serratus anterior muscle and help prevent excess internal rotation of the scapula at the AC joint by stabilizing the medial or vertebral border of the scapula against the thorax.

Integrated Shoulder Muscle Function: Depression

Shoulder **depression** is the second of the two primary patterns of shoulder complex function. Depression involves the *forceful* downward movement of the arm against resistance. When the arm is weight-bearing on the forearms or hands or holding on to an object overhead (e.g., a pull-up bar), shoulder depression is a motion of the trunk upward beneath the relatively fixed arms. During shoulder depression, the scapula tends to rotate downward, tilt anteriorly and adduct, but a consistent pattern or ratio of scapula to humeral movement has not been described.

Latissimus Dorsi and Pectoralis

Through its attachment to both the scapula and humerus, **latissimus dorsi** activation will adduct and depress the scapula, as well as raise the trunk relative to the scapula and humerus when the arm is weight-bearing or fixed. The latissimus dorsi is a critical muscle when a cane, crutches, or walker is needed to assist with gait. When the hands are bearing weight through one of these assistive devices, latissimus dorsi activation lifts the pelvis unilaterally or bilaterally (along with one or both lower extremities) beneath the fixed scapula to allow forward progression of the leg(s).

The **sternal portion** of the **pectoralis major** is also an important shoulder complex depressor. The action of the pectoralis major parallels that of the latissimus dorsi muscle, with the pectoralis major located anterior to the glenohumeral joint rather than posterior **(Fig. 7–52)**. During upper-extremity weight-bearing, the pectoralis major and the latissimus dorsi muscles combine to depress the shoulder complex while synergistically offsetting anterior/posterior translation of the humerus and protraction/retraction of the shoulder. The **pectoralis minor** muscle assists the latissimus dorsi and pectoralis major (see Fig. 7–52) by directly depressing the scapula through its attachment on the coracoid process. The pectoralis minor is also oriented to internally rotate, downwardly rotate, and anteriorly tilt the scapula so that the length of this muscle may influence full scapula movement during arm elevation.[96] The pectoralis minor is considerably active during weight-bearing activities that involve scapula internal rotation.[97]

Teres Major and Rhomboids

The **teres major** and rhomboid muscles are strongly synergistic during adduction and depression of the humerus. Teres major activation is high during resisted humeral adduction and extension, but these functions depend on stability of the muscle's proximal attachment on the scapula. Without this scapular stability, teres major force would move the lighter scapula toward the heavier humerus (in another example of reverse action) rather than move the humerus on the scapula. The rhomboids, through their attachment on the scapula medial border and their oblique orientation, provide this proximal segment stabilization **(Fig. 7–53)**. The scapular downward rotation torque of the rhomboid muscles offsets the undesired upward rotary torque of the teres major muscle, allowing the teres major to move the heavier humerus. The rhomboids are assisted in this stabilization function by the anteriorly located pectoralis minor muscle.

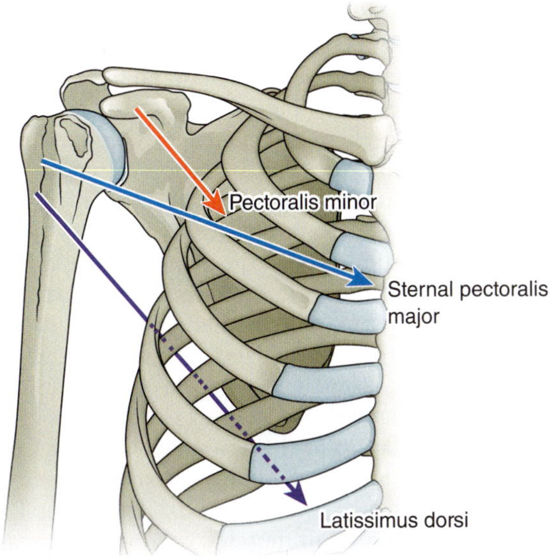

Figure 7–52 Muscles of depression. The anteriorly located sternal portion of the pectoralis major and pectoralis minor works with the large posteriorly located latissimus dorsi to forcefully depress the shoulder girdle.

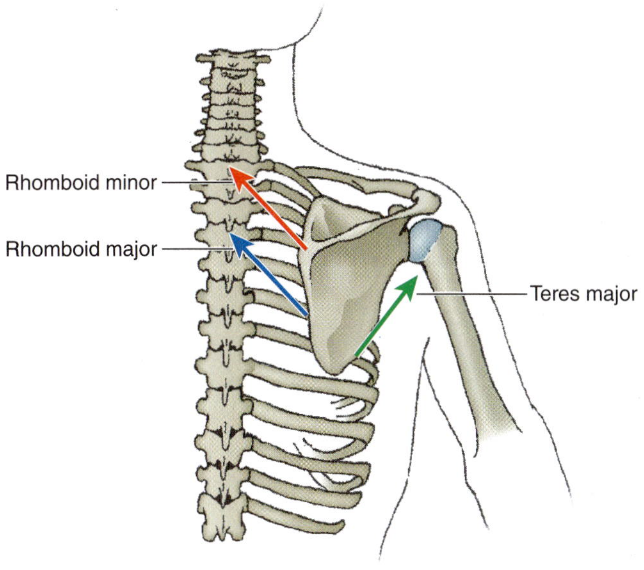

Figure 7–53 For the teres major muscle to extend the heavier humerus rather than upwardly rotate the lighter scapula, the synergy of the rhomboid muscles is necessary to stabilize the scapula.

Patient Application 7–4
Postural Faults

Louis Haddad is a 17-year-old boy who has recently taken up free weights in an attempt to correct his bad posture but is now having shoulder pain when he reaches over shoulder level. He presents with a forward (rounded) shoulder posture that may be contributing to his symptoms. This posture is often related to medial rotation of the humerus and, indirectly, clavicular protraction due to pectoralis major tightness, and to scapular downward rotation, internal rotation, and anterior tilting from pectoralis minor tightness.[96] These motions are all antagonistic to the motions of the scapula and humerus that must occur during typical arm elevation. Because of the attachment of the pectoralis minor muscle to the coracoid process and rib cage (see Fig. 7–52), decreased extensibility (passive lengthening) or hypertonicity during arm elevation could cause the muscle to limit scapular upward rotation, posterior tilting, and external rotation.[96] Decreased extensibility in the pectoralis major could limit the ability to laterally rotate the humerus and retract the clavicle during arm elevation. A subtle but potentially important effect may also be to increase the risk of mechanical impingement of the subacromial bursa, the rotator cuff tendons, and long head of the biceps brachii in elevation of the arm. The risk may be increased by a decreased subacromial space because of the inability of the scapula to posteriorly tilt and externally rotate to move the acromion away from the humeral head during elevation. A reduction in scapular upward rotation may also result in an offsetting hypermobility of the glenohumeral joint, increasing the likelihood that the humerus will impinge on the coracoacromial arch. Furthermore, a restriction in lateral rotation of the humerus from pectoral major tightness may not allow the greater tubercle to adequately clear the acromion.

Life Span and Clinical Considerations

Life Span Considerations

As might be expected, aging and the cumulative effects of joint loading may have negative effects on the shoulder complex. However, the relatively minimal weight-bearing function of the upper extremity results in less severe degenerative changes than those recognized in the large lower extremity joints. Degenerative changes to the shoulder complex joints and structures usually begin around the fourth decade of life and occur most often at the AC joint and lateral clavicle. These changes include osteophytes, sclerosis, and joint narrowing or degeneration.[98,99] Acromial osteophytes are more frequently seen with aging, whereas glenohumeral degenerative changes become more frequent after age 60.[100,101] The more frequent degenerative changes at the AC joint suggest that this articulation is subject to high stresses over the life span. Bone mineral density of the proximal humerus also declines with age.[102]

Gross shoulder motion gradually declines with age, with decreasing shoulder flexion and abduction after the fifth decade of life, and small decreases in lateral rotation ROM that are correlated with age.[103-105] Kinematic studies report less glenohumeral joint lateral rotation and scapulothoracic internal rotation during functional tasks in older individuals, whereas children have demonstrated decreased scapulothoracic posterior tilt during arm elevation compared with healthy adults.[106,107] Age-related declines in isometric strength are seen in both men and women, with greater decreases in rotational strength noted in men only after age 60.[104,108] Despite age-related strength and range declines, corresponding decreases in function were not present when measured using both functional tasks and standardized outcome measures.[104]

Degenerative changes in the AC joint may result in pain in the same area of the shoulder as pain from supraspinatus or rotator cuff lesions. Pain due to AC degeneration is reported to be found more typically when the arm is raised to end range or when the arm is adducted across the body, compressing the AC joint surfaces.[109] The long head of the biceps brachii similarly can produce pain in the anterosuperior shoulder. Because the long head of the biceps tendon also passes directly beneath the impinging structures of the coracoacromial arch, it is subject to some of the same degenerative changes and the same trauma seen in the tendons of the rotator cuff. Whether the biceps is actively contributing to elevation of the arm, to joint stabilization, or is passive, the tendon of the biceps must be able to slide within the bicipital groove and under the transverse humeral ligament as the humerus moves. If the bicipital tendon sheath is worn or inflamed, or if the tendon is hypertrophied (as often seen with rotator cuff tears), the sliding mechanism may be interrupted and pain may occur. A tear in the transverse humeral ligament may result in the tendon of the long head popping in and out of the bicipital groove with rotation of the humerus, a potentially wearing and painful microtrauma.

Patient Application 7–5
AC Joint Degeneration

Mary Czerny is a 71-year-old woman who presents with shoulder pain located at the AC joint, which may be related to AC joint degeneration. The AC joint frequently shows evidence of degeneration after the sixth decade of life, which may be a source of pain, crepitus, and movement faults. When pain is noted at the end of arm elevation, it may be indicative of AC joint pathology or degeneration.

Structural Dysfunction

Completion of the range of elevation of the arm depends on the ability of the glenohumeral, SC, and AC joints to each make the needed contribution. Disruption of movement in any of the participating joints can result in a loss of ROM. Once restrictions to function are introduced, the concept of scapulohumeral rhythm is altered; that is, a reduction in glenohumeral joint range may *not* result in a proportional decrease in scapulothoracic range. The ratio of movement is no longer consistent because the body will likely recruit remaining motion at other joints.[110] Although it is not necessarily predictable, the restriction of motion at any one joint in the shoulder complex may result in the development of some hypermobility (and reduced stability) in remaining articulations.

Foundational Concepts 7–4
Glenohumeral Joint Hypomobility

If motion at the glenohumeral joint is restricted by pain or disease, the total ROM available to the humerus will be reduced. Whatever portion of the motion remains at the glenohumeral joint will still be accompanied by scapulothoracic motion. A restriction of the humerus, limiting glenohumeral joint abduction to approximately 60°, theoretically can combine with up to 60° of scapulothoracic motion to provide a total available range of 120° as the arm is raised from the side. Recent research has also provided evidence of increased scapulothoracic upward rotation, or scapular "substitution" in cases where glenohumeral mobility is reduced, such as with glenohumeral osteoarthritis or adhesive capsulitis.[110]

Mechanical deviations in glenohumeral stabilization factors may result in injury to other structures of the joint other than the rotator cuff, and lead to subluxation or dislocation of the glenohumeral joint. The glenohumeral joint is the most frequently dislocated of all the joints in the body. Capsuloligamentous and muscle reinforcement to the glenohumeral joint are weakest inferiorly, but it is most common for the glenohumeral joint to dislocate anteriorly—or anteriorly and inferiorly—because of the type of forces to which it is exposed. Although the subscapularis and the glenohumeral ligaments reinforce the capsule anteriorly, a force applied to an abducted, laterally rotated arm can force the humeral head beyond the limits of the anterior glenoid and its labrum. Some individuals may be predisposed to glenohumeral subluxation or dislocation based on these structural deviations: (1) anterior tilt of the glenoid fossa in relation to the scapular plane, resulting in less of a mechanical limitation of the glenoid fossa to anterior translation; (2) excessive retroversion of the humeral head; or (3) weakened rotator cuff muscles.[82] Conversely, scapular internal rotation may result in less anterior humeral head translation and greater tension in the anterior capsule.[111]

The most common diagnosis for shoulder pain and dysfunction is shoulder "impingement." This is typically divided into entrapment of the rotator cuff tendons beneath the coracoacromial arch (referred to as *subacromial impingement*) or entrapment between the humeral head and glenoid (referred to as *internal impingement*).[82] However, it is becoming increasingly recognized that the impingement diagnosis is overly broad and may include a wide variety of tissue pathologies and movement deviations.[112]

Two other common clinical presentations are shoulder instabilities and stiffness. Instabilities or hypermobilities of the shoulder joints are not surprising, as noted earlier, given the large ROM necessary for typical function of the shoulder joint. Stiffness (hypomobility) is most commonly seen with adhesive capsulitis or "frozen shoulder," where the large redundancy of the glenohumeral joint capsule can become adhered to itself or to the humerus, substantially limiting ROM. Glenohumeral hypomobility can also occur with osteoarthritis or rheumatoid arthritis. Continued enhancement of our understanding of joint structure and function will be integral to continuing to advance the most useful diagnostic classifications for shoulder pain and dysfunction, including diagnoses based on the movement system. Diagnostic classification provides a necessary foundation for targeted and effective preventive and rehabilitative strategies.

SUMMARY

- In this chapter, we laid the foundation for understanding more distal upper extremity joint function by exploring the intricate dynamic stabilization of the shoulder complex. The more distal joints of the upper extremity depend on the dual mobility/stability roles of the shoulder complex.
- Whereas function in the hand, for instance, can continue on a limited basis with loss of shoulder mobility, loss of shoulder stability can render the remaining function in the hand unusable, with the hand unable to reach a necessary positional workspace. In the next chapter, we will explore the elbow as the intermediary between the shoulder and the hand.

STUDY QUESTIONS

1. Describe the motions of the SC joint for elevation/depression, protraction/retraction, and axial rotation.
2. Describe the roles of the costoclavicular and interclavicular ligaments at the SC joint.
3. Discuss the relevance of the SC disc to SC joint congruency, joint motion, and joint function.
4. Describe the scapular movements that take place at the AC joint.
5. Discuss the relevance of the coracoclavicular ligament to AC joint function.
6. Discuss the anatomical configuration of the humerus and the glenoid fossa as they relate to glenohumeral joint stability. What role do the glenoid labrum and joint capsule play in joint stability?
7. What is the most frequent direction of glenohumeral dislocation? Why?
8. Compare the relative stability and tendency toward degenerative changes in the glenohumeral, AC, and SC joints.
9. What are the advantages of the coracoacromial arch? What are the disadvantages?
10. What intra-articular motions must occur at the glenohumeral joint for full abduction to occur? What is the typical ROM?
11. What muscle is the prime mover in shoulder glenohumeral flexion and abduction? What synergy is necessary for typical function of this muscle? Why?
12. Why is the supraspinatus able to abduct the shoulder without additional muscular synergy?
13. What accounts for the static stabilization of the glenohumeral joint when the arm is at the side? What happens if the hanging (dependent) limb is excessively loaded?
14. Identify factors that contribute to dynamic stabilization of the glenohumeral joint in either flexion or abduction.
15. What is the total ROM available to the humerus in elevation? How is this full range achieved?
16. What muscles are necessary to produce the typical scapular and humeral movements in elevation of the arm?
17. If the scapulothoracic joint were fused in neutral position, what active range of elevation would still be available to the upper extremity?
18. What are the consequences of a rupture of the coracoclavicular ligaments?
19. If the glenohumeral joint were immobilized by osteoarthritis, what range of elevation would be available to the upper extremity?
20. If isolated paralysis of the supraspinatus were to occur, what would be the likely functional deficit?
21. If the muscles of the rotator cuff are paralyzed, what is the effect when abduction of the arm is attempted?
22. When there is paralysis of the trapezius and the serratus anterior muscles, what is the functional deficit when abduction of the arm is attempted?
23. If the deltoid alone is paralyzed, what happens with attempted abduction of the arm? What occurs with attempted flexion of the arm?
24. What is the role of the rhomboids in elevation of the arm?
25. What differences do you see in attempted abduction if the trapezius alone is paralyzed, compared with the differences you see if the serratus anterior muscles are paralyzed?
26. What muscular synergy does the teres major muscle require to perform its function?
27. Describe why electromyographic activity of the deltoid in typical abduction typically shows a rise in activity beyond the ROM (90°) where the greatest gravitational torque resists its function.
28. Which of the joints of the shoulder complex is most likely to undergo degenerative changes over time? Which joint is least likely to undergo these changes?

REFERENCES

1. Dempster WT: Mechanisms of shoulder movement. Arch Phys Med Rehabil 46:49-70, 1965
2. van Tongel A, MacDonald P, Leiter J, et al: A cadaveric study of the structural anatomy of the sternoclavicular joint. Clin Anat 25:903-10, 2012
3. Brossmann J, Stabler A, Preidler KW, et al: Sternoclavicular joint: MR imaging—anatomic correlation. Radiology 198:193-8, 1996
4. Spencer EE, Kuhn JE, Huston LJ, et al: Ligamentous restraints to anterior and posterior translation of the sternoclavicular joint. J Shoulder Elbow Surg 11:43-7, 2002
5. Pronk GM, van der Helm FC, Rozendaal LA: Interaction between the joints in the shoulder mechanism: The function of the costoclavicular, conoid and trapezoid ligaments. Proc Inst Mech Eng H 207:219-29, 1993

6. Sarrafian SK: Gross and functional anatomy of the shoulder. Clin Orthop Relat Res:11-9, 1983
7. Tubbs RS, Loukas M, Slappey JB, et al: Surgical and clinical anatomy of the interclavicular ligament. Surg Radiol Anat 29:357-60, 2007
8. Standring S: Gray's Anatomy: The Anatomical Basis of Clinical Practice (ed 42). New York, NY, Elsevier Health Sciences, 2020
9. Depalma A: Degenerative Changes in Sternoclavicular and Acromioclavicular Joints in Various Decades. Springfield, IL, Charles C. Thomas, 1957
10. Cailliet R: Shoulder Pain (ed 2). Philadelphia, PA, F.A. Davis, 1991
11. Dawson PA, Adamson GJ, Pink MM, et al: Relative contribution of acromioclavicular joint capsule and coracoclavicular ligaments to acromioclavicular stability. J Shoulder Elbow Surg 18:237-44, 2009
12. Debski RE, Parsons IM, 3rd, Fenwick J, et al: Ligament mechanics during three degree-of-freedom motion at the acromioclavicular joint. Ann Biomed Eng 28:612-8, 2000
13. Debski RE, Parsons IMt, Woo SL, et al: Effect of capsular injury on acromioclavicular joint mechanics. J Bone Joint Surg Am 83:1344-51, 2001
14. Lee KW, Debski RE, Chen CH, et al: Functional evaluation of the ligaments at the acromioclavicular joint during anteroposterior and superoinferior translation. Am J Sports Med 25:858-62, 1997
15. Ludewig PM, Cook TM: Alterations in shoulder kinematics and associated muscle activity in people with symptoms of shoulder impingement. Phys Ther 80:276-91, 2000
16. Ludewig PM, Phadke V, Braman JP, et al: Motion of the shoulder complex during multiplanar humeral elevation. J Bone Joint Surg Am 91:378-89, 2009
17. Ludewig PM, Cook TM, Nawoczenski DA: Three-dimensional scapular orientation and muscle activity at selected positions of humeral elevation. J Orthop Sports Phys Ther 24:57-65, 1996
18. Basmajian JV, Bazant FJ: Factors preventing downward dislocation of the adducted shoulder joint: an electromyographic and morphological study. J Bone Joint Surg Am 41-A:1182-6, 1959
19. Poppen NK, Walker PS: Normal and abnormal motion of the shoulder. J Bone Joint Surg Am 58:195-201, 1976
20. Saha AK: Dynamic stability of the glenohumeral joint. Acta Orthop Scand 42:491-505, 1971
21. Poppen NK, Walker PS: Forces at the glenohumeral joint in abduction. Clin Orthop Relat Res:165-70, 1978
22. Walker PS, Poppen NK: Biomechanics of the shoulder joint during abduction in the plane of the scapula [proceedings]. Bull Hosp Joint Dis 38:107-11, 1977
23. Crockett HC, Gross LB, Wilk KE, et al: Osseous adaptation and range of motion at the glenohumeral joint in professional baseball pitchers. Am J Sports Med 30:20-6, 2002
24. Reagan KM, Meister K, Horodyski MB, et al: Humeral retroversion and its relationship to glenohumeral rotation in the shoulder of college baseball players. Am J Sports Med 30:354-60, 2002
25. Bigliani LU, Kelkar R, Flatow EL, et al: Glenohumeral stability: biome- properties of passive and active stabilizers. Clin Orthop Relat Res:13-30, 1996
26. Howell SM, Galinat BJ: The glenoid-labral socket: a constrained articular surface. Clin Orthop Relat Res:122-5, 1989
27. Hill AM, Hoerning EJ, Brook K, et al: Collagenous microstructure of the glenoid labrum and biceps anchor. J Anat 212:853-62, 2008
28. Beltran J, Bencardino J, Padron M, et al: The middle glenohumeral ligament: normal anatomy, variants and pathology. Skeletal Radiol 31:253-62, 2002
29. MacConaill M, Basmajian J: Muscles and Movement: A Basis for Human Kinesiology. Baltimore, MD, Williams & Wilkins, 1969
30. Ide J, Maeda S, Takagi K: Normal variations of the glenohumeral ligament complex: an anatomic study for arthroscopic Bankart repair. Arthroscopy 20:164-8, 2004
31. Harryman DT, 2nd, Sidles JA, Harris SL, et al: The role of the rotator interval capsule in passive motion and stability of the shoulder. J Bone Joint Surg Am 74:53-66, 1992
32. O'Brien SJ, Neves MC, Arnoczky SP, et al: The anatomy and histology of the inferior glenohumeral ligament complex of the shoulder. Am J Sports Med 18:449-56, 1990
33. Warner JJ, Deng XH, Warren RF, et al: Static capsuloligamentous restraints to superior-inferior translation of the glenohumeral joint. Am J Sports Med 20:675-85, 1992
34. Burkart AC, Debski RE: Anatomy and function of the glenohumeral ligaments in anterior shoulder instability. Clin Orthop Relat Res:32-9, 2002
35. Itoi E, Motzkin NE, Morrey BF, et al: Scapular inclination and inferior stability of the shoulder. J Shoulder Elbow Surg 1:131-9, 1992
36. O'Connell PW, Nuber GW, Mileski RA, et al: The contribution of the glenohumeral ligaments to anterior stability of the shoulder joint. Am J Sports Med 18:579-84, 1990
37. Halder AM, Itoi E, An KN: Anatomy and biomechanics of the shoulder. Orthop Clin North Am 31:159-76, 2000
38. Gohlke F, Essigkrug B, Schmitz F: The pattern of the collagen fiber bundles of the capsule of the glenohumeral joint. J Shoulder Elbow Surg 3:111-28, 1994
39. Soslowsky LJ, Carpenter JE, Bucchieri JS, et al: Biomechanics of the rotator cuff. Orthop Clin North Am 28:17-30, 1997
40. Ferrari DA: Capsular ligaments of the shoulder: anatomical and functional study of the anterior superior capsule. Am J Sports Med 18:20-4, 1990
41. Flatow EL, Soslowsky LJ, Ticker JB, et al: Excursion of the rotator cuff under the acromion: patterns of subacromial contact. Am J Sports Med 22:779-88, 1994
42. Petersson CJ, Redlund-Johnell I: The subacromial space in normal shoulder radiographs. Acta Orthop Scand 55:57-8, 1984
43. Bey MJ, Brock SK, Beierwaltes WN, et al: In vivo measurement of subacromial space width during shoulder elevation: technique and preliminary results in patients following unilateral rotator cuff repair. Clin Biomech (Bristol) 22:767-73, 2007
44. Giphart JE, van der Meijden OA, Millett PJ: The effects of arm elevation on the 3-dimensional acromiohumeral distance: a biplane fluoroscopy study with normative data. J Shoulder Elbow Surg 21:1593-600, 2012
45. Lawrence RL, Schlangen DM, Schneider KA, et al: Effect of glenohumeral elevation on subacromial supraspinatus compression risk during simulated reaching. J Orthop Res 35:2329-37, 2017
46. Conway AM: Movements at the sternoclavicular and acromioclavicular joints. Phys Ther Rev (1948) 41:421-32, 1961
47. Inman VT, Saunders JB, Abbott LC: Observations of the function of the shoulder joint. 1944. Clin Orthop Relat Res:3-12, 1996
48. McClure PW, Michener LA, Sennett BJ, et al: Direct 3-dimensional measurement of scapular kinematics during dynamic movements in vivo. J Shoulder Elbow Surg 10:269-77, 2001
49. Fung M, Kato S, Barrance PJ, et al: Scapular and clavicular kinematics during humeral elevation: a study with cadavers. J Shoulder Elbow Surg 10:278-85, 2001
50. Wirth MA, Rockwood CA, Jr: Acute and chronic traumatic injuries of the sternoclavicular joint. J Am Acad Orthop Surg 4:268-78, 1996
51. Sahara W, Sugamoto K, Murai M, et al: Three-dimensional clavicular and acromioclavicular rotations during arm abduction using vertically open MRI. J Orthop Res 25:1243-9, 2007
52. Teece RM, Lunden JB, Lloyd AS, et al: Three-dimensional acromioclavicular joint motions during elevation of the arm. J Orthop Sports Phys Ther 38:181-90, 2008
53. van der Helm FC, Pronk GM: Three-dimensional recording and description of motions of the shoulder mechanism. J Biomech Eng 117:27-40, 1995
54. Zuckerman JD, Kummer FJ, Cuomo F, et al: The influence of coracoacromial arch anatomy on rotator cuff tears. J Shoulder Elbow Surg 1:4-14, 1992
55. Norkin CC, White DJ: Measurement of Joint Motion: A Guide to Goniometry. Philadelphia, PA, FA Davis, 2009
56. Rundquist PJ, Anderson DD, Guanche CA, et al: Shoulder kinematics in subjects with frozen shoulder. Arch Phys Med Rehabil 84:1473-9, 2003
57. An KN, Browne AO, Korinek S, et al: Three-dimensional kinematics of glenohumeral elevation. J Orthop Res 9:143-9, 1991
58. Soslowsky LJ, Flatow EL, Bigliani LU, et al: Quantitation of in situ contact areas at the glenohumeral joint: a biomechanical study. J Orthop Res 10:524-34, 1992
59. Doody SG, Freedman L, Waterland JC: Shoulder movements during abduction in the scapular plane. Arch Phys Med Rehabil 51:595-604, 1970
60. Freedman L, Munro RR: Abduction of the arm in the scapular plane: scapular and glenohumeral movements. A roentgenographic study. J Bone Joint Surg Am 48:1503-10, 1966
61. Aliaj K, Foreman KB, Chalmers PN, et al: Beyond Euler/Cardan analysis: true glenohumeral axial rotation during arm elevation and rotation. Gait Posture 88:28-36, 2021
62. Ludewig PM, Cook TM: Translations of the humerus in persons with shoulder impingement symptoms. J Orthop Sports Phys Ther 32: 248-59, 2002
63. Graichen H, Stammberger T, Bonel H, et al: Glenohumeral translation during active and passive elevation of the shoulder—A 3D open-MRI study. J Biomech 33:609-13, 2000
64. Kelkar R, Flatow EL, Bigliani LU, et al: A stereophotogrammetric method to determine the kinematics of the glenohumeral joint. Adv Bioeng ASME 19:143-6, 1992
65. Lawrence RL, Braman JP, Staker JL, et al: Comparison of 3-dimensional shoulder complex kinematics in individuals with and without shoulder pain, part 2: glenohumeral joint. J Orthop Sports Phys Ther 44:646-55, B1-3, 2014

66. Sahara W, Sugamoto K, Murai M, et al: The three-dimensional motions of glenohumeral joint under semi-loaded condition during arm abduction using vertically open MRI. Clin Biomech (Bristol) 22:304-12, 2007
67. Harryman DT, 2nd, Sidles JA, Harris SL, et al: Laxity of the normal glenohumeral joint: a quantitative in vivo assessment. J Shoulder Elbow Surg 1:66-76, 1992
68. Harryman DT, 2nd, Sidles JA, Clark JM, et al: Translation of the humeral head on the glenoid with passive glenohumeral motion. J Bone Joint Surg Am 72:1334-43, 1990
69. Gibb TD, Sidles JA, Harryman DT, 2nd, et al: The effect of capsular venting on glenohumeral laxity. Clin Orthop Relat Res:120-7, 1991
70. Habermeyer P, Schuller U, Wiedemann E: The intra-articular pressure of the shoulder: an experimental study on the role of the glenoid labrum in stabilizing the joint. Arthroscopy 8:166-72, 1992
71. De Duca CJ, Forrest WJ: Force analysis of individual muscles acting simultaneously on the shoulder joint during isometric abduction. J Biomech 6:385-93, 1973
72. Dvir Z, Berme N: The shoulder complex in elevation of the arm: a mechanism approach. J Biomech 11:219-25, 1978
73. Sharkey NA, Marder RA: The rotator cuff opposes superior translation of the humeral head. Am J Sports Med 23:270-5, 1995
74. Saha A: Theory of Shoulder Mechanism: Descriptive and Applied. Springfield, IL, Charles C. Thomas, 1961
75. Wuelker N, Plitz W, Roetman B, et al: Function of the supraspinatus muscle: abduction of the humerus studied in cadavers. Acta Orthop Scand 65:442-6, 1994
76. Ihashi K, Matsushita N, Yagi R, et al: Rotational action of the supraspinatus muscle on the shoulder joint. J Electromyogr Kinesiol 8:337-46, 1998
77. Itoi E, Hsu HC, An KN: Biomechanical investigation of the glenohumeral joint. J Shoulder Elbow Surg 5:407-24, 1996
78. Itoi E, Kuechle DK, Newman SR, et al: Stabilising function of the biceps in stable and unstable shoulders. J Bone Joint Surg Br 75:546-50, 1993
79. Malicky DM, Soslowsky LJ, Blasier RB, et al: Anterior glenohumeral stabilization factors: progressive effects in a biomechanical model. J Orthop Res 14:282-8, 1996
80. Pagnani MJ, Deng XH, Warren RF, et al: Role of the long head of the biceps brachii in glenohumeral stability: a biomechanical study in cadavera. J Shoulder Elbow Surg 5:255-62, 1996
81. Pagnani MJ, Deng XH, Warren RF, et al: Effect of lesions of the superior portion of the glenoid labrum on glenohumeral translation. J Bone Joint Surg Am 77:1003-10, 1995
82. Edelson G, Teitz C: Internal impingement in the shoulder. J Shoulder Elbow Surg 9:308-15, 2000
83. Gschwend N, Ivosevic-Radovanovic D, Patte D: Rotator cuff tear—relationship between clinical and anatomopathological findings. Arch Orthop Trauma Surg (1978) 107:7-15, 1988
84. Barnes CJ, Van Steyn SJ, Fischer RA: The effects of age, sex, and shoulder dominance on range of motion of the shoulder. J Shoulder Elbow Surg 10:242-6, 2001
85. Braman JP, Engel SC, Laprade RF, et al: In vivo assessment of scapulohumeral rhythm during unconstrained overhead reaching in asymptomatic subjects. J Shoulder Elbow Surg 18:960-7, 2009
86. McQuade KJ, Smidt GL: Dynamic scapulohumeral rhythm: the effects of external resistance during elevation of the arm in the scapular plane. J Orthop Sports Phys Ther 27:125-33, 1998
87. Crosbie J, Kilbreath SL, Hollmann L, et al: Scapulohumeral rhythm and associated spinal motion. Clin Biomech (Bristol) 23:184-92, 2008
88. Johnson G, Bogduk N, Nowitzke A, et al: Anatomy and actions of the trapezius muscle. Clin Biomech (Bristol) 9:44-50, 1994
89. Phadke V, Camargo P, Ludewig P: Scapular and rotator cuff muscle activity during arm elevation: a review of normal function and alterations with shoulder impingement. Rev Bras Fisioter 13:1-9, 2009
90. Otis JC, Jiang CC, Wickiewicz TL, et al: Changes in the moment arms of the rotator cuff and deltoid muscles with abduction and rotation. J Bone Joint Surg Am 76:667-76, 1994
91. Wickham J, Pizzari T, Stansfeld K, et al: Quantifying 'normal' shoulder muscle activity during abduction. J Electromyogr Kinesiol 20:212-22, 2010
92. Houglum PA, Bertoti DB: Brunnstrom's Clinical Kinesiology (ed 6). Philadelphia, PA, FA Davis, 2012
93. Celli L, Balli A, de Luise G, et al: Some new aspects of the functional anatomy of the shoulder. Ital J Orthop Traumatol 11:83-91, 1985
94. McCully SP, Suprak DN, Kosek P, et al: Suprascapular nerve block results in a compensatory increase in deltoid muscle activity. J Biomech 40:1839-46, 2007
95. Reed D, Halaki M, Ginn K: The rotator cuff muscles are activated at low levels during shoulder adduction: an experimental study. J Physiother 56:259-64, 2010
96. Borstad JD, Ludewig PM: The effect of long versus short pectoralis minor resting length on scapular kinematics in healthy individuals. J Orthop Sports Phys Ther 35:227-38, 2005
97. Castelein B, Cagnie B, Parlevliet T, et al: Serratus anterior or pectoralis minor: which muscle has the upper hand during protraction exercises? Man Ther 22:158-64, 2016
98. Bonsell S, Pearsall AW, Heitman RJ, et al: The relationship of age, gender, and degenerative changes observed on radiographs of the shoulder in asymptomatic individuals. J Bone Joint Surg Br 82:1135-9, 2000
99. Edelson JG: Patterns of degenerative change in the acromioclavicular joint. J Bone Joint Surg Br 78:242-3, 1996
100. Mahakkanukrauh P, Surin P: Prevalence of osteophytes associated with the acromion and acromioclavicular joint. Clin Anat 16:506-10, 2003
101. Petersson CJ: Degeneration of the acromioclavicular joint: a morphological study. Acta Orthop Scand 54:434-8, 1983
102. Mantila Roosa SM, Hurd AL, Xu H, et al: Age-related changes in proximal humerus bone health in healthy, white males. Osteoporos Int 23:2775-83, 2012
103. Gill H, Gustafsson L, Hawcroft L, et al: Shoulder joint range of motion in healthy adults aged 20 to 49 years. British J Occup Ther 69: 556-61, 2006
104. Roy JS, Macdermid JC, Boyd KU, et al: Rotational strength, range of motion, and function in people with unaffected shoulders from various stages of life. Sports Med Arthrosc Rehabil Ther Technol 1:4, 2009
105. Soucie JM, Wang C, Forsyth A, et al: Range of motion measurements: reference values and a database for comparison studies. Haemophilia 17:500-7, 2011
106. Habechian FA, Fornasari GG, Sacramento LS, et al: Differences in scapular kinematics and scapulohumeral rhythm during elevation and lowering of the arm between typical children and healthy adults. J Electromyogr Kinesiol 24:78-83, 2014
107. Rundquist PJ, Bratton J, Fasano E, et al: A comparison of 3-d shoulder kinematics to perform ADLs between older and younger adults. Phys Occup Ther Geriatr 29:300-10, 2011
108. Hughes RE, Johnson ME, O'Driscoll SW, et al: Age-related changes in normal isometric shoulder strength. Am J Sports Med 27:651-7, 1999
109. Kessel L, Watson M: The painful arc syndrome: clinical classification as a guide to management. J Bone Joint Surg Br 59:166-72, 1977
110. Fayad F, Roby-Brami A, Yazbeck C, et al: Three-dimensional scapular kinematics and scapulohumeral rhythm in patients with glenohumeral osteoarthritis or frozen shoulder. J Biomech 41:326-32, 2008
111. Weiser WM, Lee TQ, McMaster WC, et al: Effects of simulated scapular protraction on anterior glenohumeral stability. Am J Sports Med 27:801-5, 1999
112. Braman JP, Zhao KD, Lawrence RL, et al: Shoulder impingement revisited: evolution of diagnostic understanding in orthopedic surgery and physical therapy. Med Biol Eng Comput 52:211-9, 2014

CHAPTER 8

The Elbow Complex

Jane Fedorczyk, PT, PhD, CHT, FAPTA

CHAPTER OUTLINE

INTRODUCTION 244
STRUCTURE AND FUNCTION OF THE HUMEROULNAR AND HUMERORADIAL ARTICULATIONS 244
Structure 244
Proximal Joint Surfaces 244
Distal Joint Surfaces 244
Joint Articulations 244
Joint Capsule 246
Ligaments 247
Muscles 249
Function 250
Axis of Motion 250
Mobility/Stability 251
Muscle Action 253
STRUCTURE AND FUNCTION OF THE PROXIMAL AND DISTAL RADIOULNAR ARTICULATIONS 254
Structure 254
Proximal (Superior) Radioulnar Joint 254
Distal (Inferior) Radioulnar Joint 255
Ligaments 255
Muscles 256
Function 257
Radioulnar Axis and Radioulnar Motions 257
Radioulnar ROM 258
Muscle Action 258
Stability 258
MOBILITY AND STABILITY OF THE ELBOW COMPLEX 260
Functional Activities 260
Relationship to the Hand and Wrist 260
LIFE SPAN AND CLINICAL CONSIDERATIONS 260
Effects of Age 261
Injury 261
Compression Injuries 261
Distraction Injuries 263
Varus/Valgus Injuries (Thrower's Elbow) 263
Peripheral Nerve Injuries 264
SUMMARY 265
STUDY QUESTIONS 266
REFERENCES 266

ANATOMY OVERVIEW

MUSCLE ATTACHMENTS OF THE ELBOW JOINT		
TABLE KEY: Primary movers, Secondary movers		
Sagittal Plane (Humeroulnar and Humeroradial Joints)	**Flexion**	**Extension**
	Biceps brachii (primary) Brachialis (primary) Brachioradialis (secondary) Pronator teres (secondary)	Triceps brachii (primary) Anconeus (primary)
Transverse Plane (Radioulnar Joints)	**Supination**	**Pronation**
	Biceps brachii (primary) Supinator (primary)	Pronator teres (primary) Pronator quadratus (primary)

ANATOMY OVERVIEW

ELBOW MUSCLE ATTACHMENTS		
Muscles	**Proximal Attachment**	**Distal Attachment**
Biceps brachii	Short head: Tip of coracoid process of scapula Long head: Supraglenoid tubercle of scapula	Tuberosity of radius and fascia of forearm via bicipital aponeurosis
Brachialis	Distal half of anterior surface of humerus	Coronoid process and tuberosity ulna
Brachioradialis	Proximal 2/3 of lateral supracondylar ridge of humerus	Lateral surface of distal end of radial styloid process
Pronator teres	Ulnar head: Coronoid process Humeral head: Medial epicondyle of humerus	Middle convexity of lateral surface of radius
Triceps brachii	Long head: Infraglenoid tubercle of scapula Lateral head: Posterior surface of humerus, superior to radial groove Medial head: Posterior surface of humerus, inferior to radial groove	Proximal end of olecranon of ulna
Anconeus	Lateral epicondyle of humerus	Lateral surface of olecranon and superior part of posterior surface of ulna

Introduction

Elbow movement is the essential linkage between the hand and the shoulder for positioning the hand to interact with the environment.[1,2] The joints and muscles bend and straighten the upper limb to position the hand for reaching and grasping, and rotation of the forearm refines the position of the hand and wrist. Loss of motion at the elbow greatly affects functional use of the upper extremity and can significantly limit a person's ability to participate in both activities of daily living (ADLs) and in recreational and occupational activities. In conjunction with providing mobility for the hand, elbow structures also provide stability when performing functional tasks in both the open chain and closed chain. Many of the 15 muscles that cross the elbow complex also act at the wrist or shoulder, thereby linking the elbow with function of the joints both proximal and distal to the elbow.[2]

The elbow complex includes three joints: **humeroulnar**, **humeroradial**, and the **proximal radioulnar joints**.[2] These joints are distinct, highly congruent articulations enclosed in a single joint capsule. The capsule is known for its unpredictable inflammatory reaction with even minor injury and is prone to contracture with prolonged immobilization.[3,4]

The humeroulnar and humeroradial joints may be considered as a single compound joint that functions as a modified or loose hinge joint with one degree of freedom, permitting the motions of flexion and extension in the sagittal plane around a coronal axis. A small amount of axial rotation and side-to-side motion (abduction/adduction) of the ulna occurs during flexion and extension, which is why the elbow is a modified or loose hinge joint rather than a pure hinge joint.[5] Two ligament complexes and five muscles are directly associated with the compound elbow joint. Three of the muscles are flexors that cross the anterior aspect of the joint. The other two muscles are extensors that cross the posterior aspect of the joint.

The proximal radioulnar joint at the elbow is linked functionally to the **distal radioulnar joint** of the wrist to act together to produce forearm rotation with one degree of freedom of motion. The radioulnar joints are both uniaxial (pivot) synovial joints and permit rotation (supination and pronation) occurring in the transverse plane around a longitudinal axis through the forearm.[5] Six ligaments and four muscles are associated with the radioulnar joints. Two muscles produce supination and two produce pronation.

The remaining content of this chapter will expand on this introduction and will explore in more depth the structure and function of the elbow complex to provide a better understanding of and appreciation for the interaction of the joint structures that provide stability and mobility in multiplanes. We will also develop an understanding of how the elbow is a vital link in the entire upper extremity chain, rendering it vulnerable to traumatic and repetitive injury.

Structure and Function of the Humeroulnar and Humeroradial Articulations

Structure

Proximal Joint Surfaces

The articulating surfaces on the anterior aspect of the distal humerus are the hourglass-shaped trochlea and the spherical capitulum **(Fig. 8–1)**. These structures are situated between the medial and lateral epicondyles of the humerus. The **trochlea** forms the proximal portion of the medially located *humeroulnar* articulation and is set at an angle on the medial aspect of the distal humerus, lying slightly anterior to the humeral shaft. The **trochlear groove** spirals obliquely around the trochlea and divides the trochlea into medial and lateral portions.

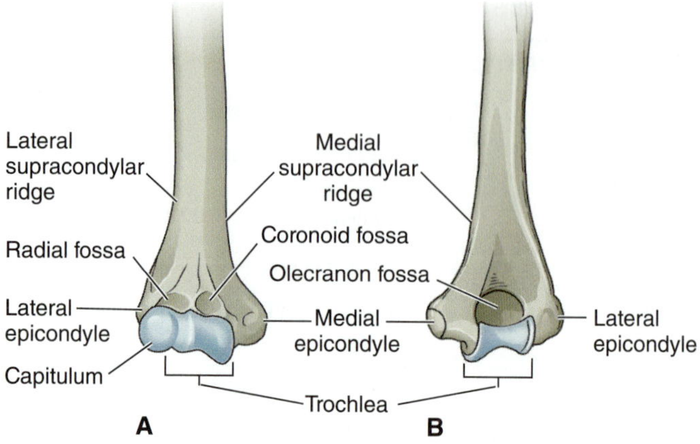

Figure 8–1 Proximal articular surfaces of the right elbow joint. **A.** Articulating surfaces (trochlea and capitulum) on the anterior aspect of the right distal humerus. **B.** The olecranon fossa on the posterior aspect of the right distal humerus.

The depression on the anterior distal humerus is the **coronoid fossa,** designed to receive the coronoid process of the ulna at full elbow flexion range of motion (ROM). The **capitulum** is the proximal portion of the *humeroradial* articulation and is located on the lateral distal humerus. The capitulum, like the trochlea, lies anterior to the shaft of the humerus. The **radial fossa** just above the capitulum is designed to receive the head of the radius in full elbow flexion. Posteriorly, the concavity of the **olecranon fossa** can be seen, designed to receive the olecranon process of the ulna at the end of the elbow extension ROM (see **Fig. 8–1B**).

Distal Joint Surfaces

The proximal joint surfaces of the ulna and radius articulate, respectively, with the trochlea and capitulum of the humerus **(Fig. 8–2)**. The ulnar articulating surface of the humeroulnar joint is a deep, semicircular concavity called the **trochlear notch (Fig. 8–3)**.[6] The proximal portion of the notch is divided into two unequal parts by the **trochlear ridge** that corresponds to the trochlear groove on the humerus. The **coronoid process** of the ulna forms the distal end of the notch, whereas the **olecranon process** forms the proximal end of the notch. There is a facet on the ulna lateral to the coronoid process, the **radial notch,** where the head of the radius articulates (see **Fig. 8-3A** and **B**). The distal articulating surface of the humeroradial joint is composed of the **head of the radius (Fig. 8–4)**. The radial head has a slightly cup-shaped concave surface called the **fovea** that is surrounded by a rim.

Joint Articulations

Motion at the humeroulnar joint occurs primarily as a sliding motion between the trochlear notch of the ulna and the trochlea

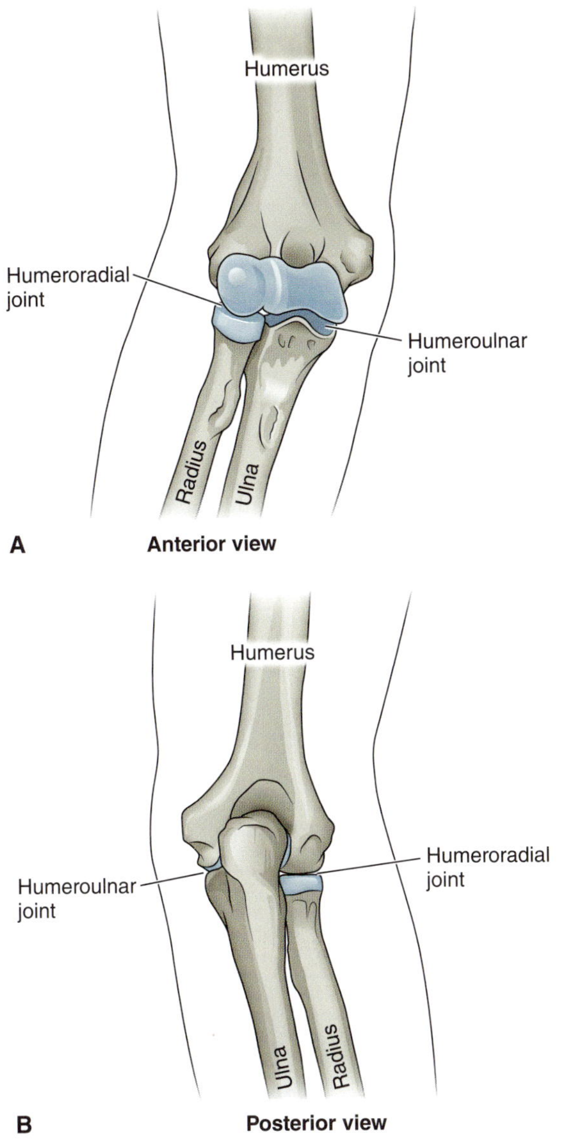

Figure 8–2 Right elbow articulations. **A.** An anterior view of the right elbow showing the proximal articulating surfaces of the ulna and radius that are part of the humeroulnar and humeroradial joints. **B.** A posterior view of the right elbow showing the posterior aspects of the proximal ulna and radius that form the humeroulnar and humeroradial joints.

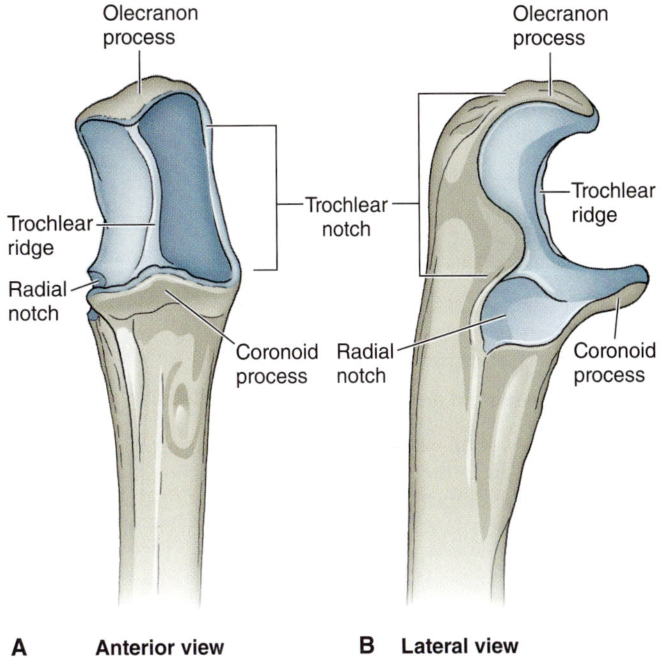

Figure 8–3 Trochear notch of the ulna. **A.** Anterior view of the right ulna's trochlear notch and ridge. **B.** Lateral view of the right trochlear notch and ridge, formed in part by the coronoid process anteriorly and the olecranon process posteriorly.

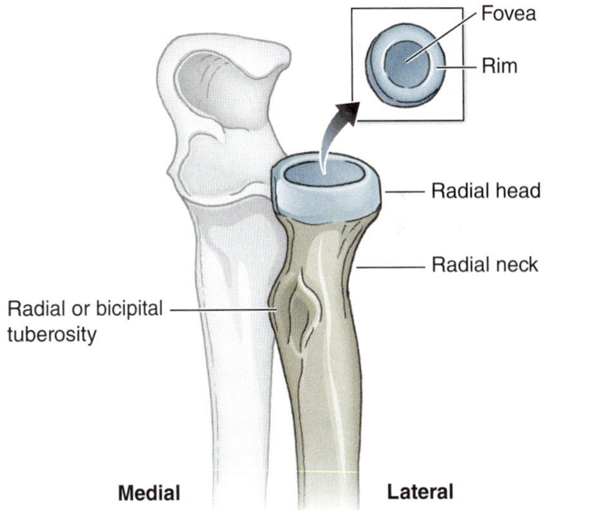

Figure 8–4 The radial head on the proximal radius with its articular surface formed by its fovea and rim.

of the humerus **(Fig. 8–5)**. In flexion, the trochlear notch of the ulna slides along the trochlea until the coronoid process of the ulna enters the coronoid fossa approaching the end-range of flexion (see **Fig. 8–5A**).[6] In extension, sliding between the surfaces continues until the olecranon process enters and impacts the olecranon fossa (see **Fig. 8–5B**).

Although the opposing articulating surfaces of the trochlea and trochlear notch appear to be completely congruent, experiments with cadaveric specimens have shown that the articulating surface of the trochlea does not contact the deepest portion of the trochlear notch unless the joint is heavily loaded **(Fig. 8–6)**.[6-9] In cadaveric specimens, Eckstein and colleagues found that small loads of 25 N (simulating resisted elbow extension) resulted in no contact between the trochlea and the depths of the trochlear notch between 30° and 120° of flexion (see **Fig. 8–6A**).[8] However, contact did occur when the load was raised to 500 N (see **Fig. 8–6B**).

Articulation between the radial head and the capitulum at the humeroradial joint involves sliding the shallow concave radial head over the convex surface of the capitulum **(Fig. 8–7)**. The humeral capitulum is slightly smaller than the corresponding radial fovea, so the joint surfaces are somewhat incongruent.[10] In full flexion, the rim of the radial head slides into the radial fossa at the end of the flexion range (see **Fig. 8–7A**).[11] In full extension, no contact occurs between the articulating radial head and capitulum (see **Fig. 8–7B**).

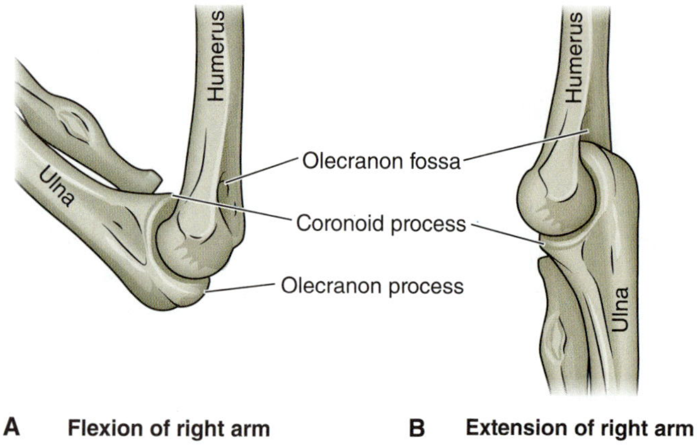

Figure 8–5 **A.** With elbow flexion, the coronoid process enters the coronoid fossa. **B.** As the elbow reaches full extension, the olecranon process enters and impacts the olecranon fossa.

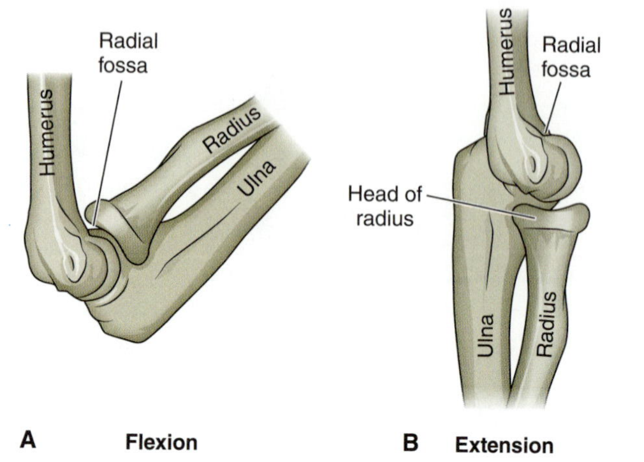

Figure 8–7 **A.** Toward end-range of elbow flexion, the rim of the radius slides in the radial fossa on the humerus. **B.** In full elbow extension, there is no contact between the capitulum and the radial head.

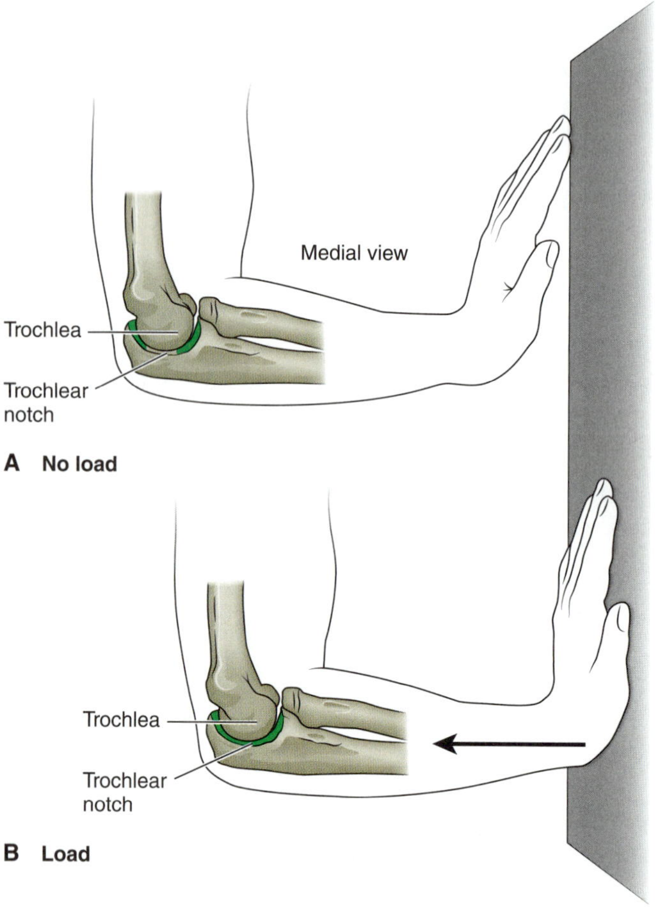

Figure 8–6 Left elbow joint. **A.** No contact occurs between the trochlea and deepest portion of the trochlear notch from 30° to 120° of flexion in an unloaded condition. **B.** Contact areas of the humeroulnar joint expand when a load is applied.

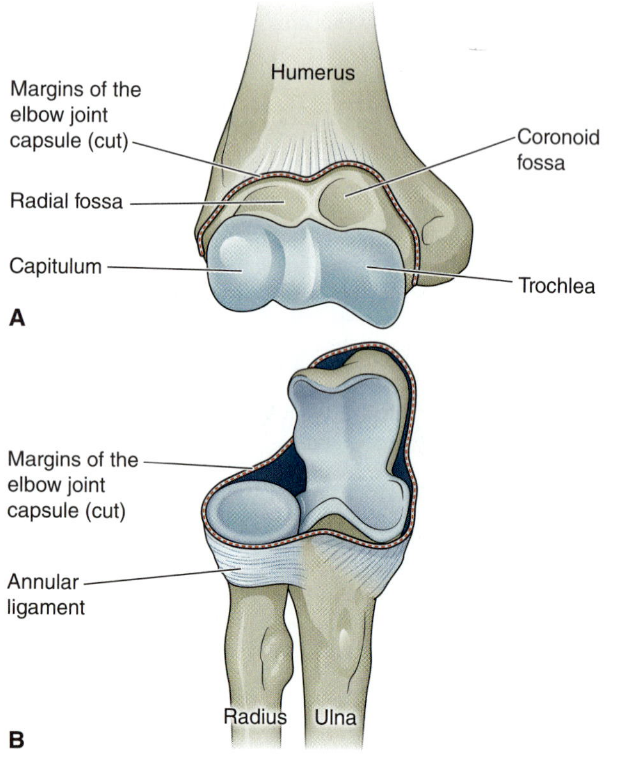

Figure 8–8 The margins (dashed lines in red) of the excised elbow joint capsule encompass three joints: the humeroradial, the humeroulnar, and the proximal radioulnar articulations.

Joint Capsule

The humeroulnar, humeroradial, and proximal radioulnar joints are enclosed in a single joint capsule. The proximal humeral attachment of the capsule is just above the coronoid and radial fossae **(Figure 8–8A)**. The capsule is distally attached to the ulna along the margin of the coronoid process and blends with the proximal border of the annular ligament **(Fig. 8-8B)**. Medially and laterally, the capsule is continuous with the collateral ligaments.[6] Posteriorly, the capsule is attached to the humerus along the upper edge of the olecranon fossa and to the back of the medial epcondyle.[6] The capsule passes just below the annular ligament to attach to the posterior and inferior margins of the neck of the radius.[6]

The capsule is fairly large, loose, and weak anteriorly and posteriorly. Fat pads are located between the capsule and the

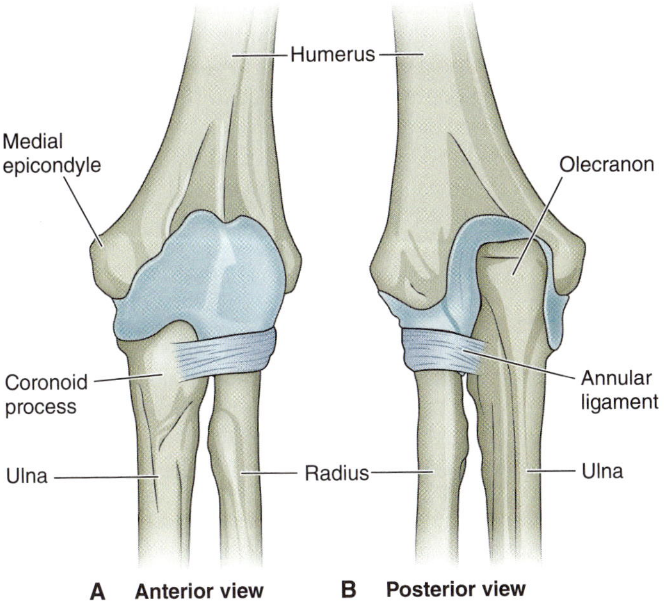

Figure 8–9 Synovium of the elbow joint. **A.** anterior view and **B.** posterior view.

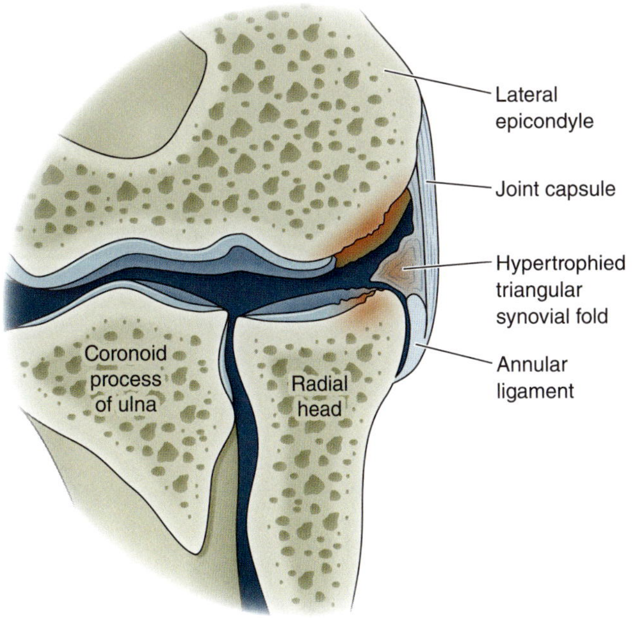

Figure 8–10 In this cross section of the elbow articulation, hypertrophy of the radial portion of a synovial fold can lead to entrapment in the humeroradial joint and potentially be a cause of lateral elbow pain and inflammatory or degenerative changes.

synovial membrane adjacent to the olecranon, coronoid, and radial fossae.[6] Laterally and medially, the capsule is reinforced by the collateral ligaments.

The synovial membrane that lines the capsule encompasses the three articular surfaces and associated fossae (**Fig. 8-9**). A triangular synovial fold between the proximal radius and ulna partially divides the elbow joint into two joints.[3] The synovium has folds that permit the large elbow ROM. Duparc and colleagues found that synovial folds varied from 1 to 4 mm in thickness and from 9 to 51 mm in length, and contained fat pads and nerve fibers.[12]

Expanded Concepts 8–1

Hypertrophied Synovial Folds

Hypertrophied triangular synovial folds have been identified as a source of pain in cases of lateral epicondylalgia (pain in the region of the lateral epicondyle).[12,13] Lateral elbow pain may arise from an irritation of the nerve fibers in a hypertrophied triangular synovial fold located between the radial head and ulna (inside the annular ligament) or at the junction of the annular ligament and joint capsule (**Fig. 8–10**).

Patient Application 8–1

Bill Garcia is a 40-year-old man who reports to physical therapy with an insidious onset of right lateral elbow pain approximately 2 months ago. Pain is worsened with repetitive elbow motion especially terminal extension, prolonged computer work, and doing push-ups. Key objective findings are as follows:

- No pain with palpation on or near the lateral epicondyle or common extensor tendon
- Pain with palpation along the humeroradial joint line, especially posteriorly
- Pain with active wrist extension, active elbow extension, and compression of the humeroradial joint (weight-bearing with push-ups)
- Significant reduction of pain with distraction of humeroradial joint
- Occasionally experiences a clicking or snapping sensation with active elbow movements

Bill's presentation is a classic case of synovial fold syndrome of the elbow (also called *posterolateral plica syndrome*). Hypertrophied triangular synovial folds have been identified as a source of persistent lateral elbow pain in the region of the lateral epicondyle, which mimics tennis elbow.[12,13] Lateral elbow pain may arise from an irritation of the nerve fibers in a hypertrophied triangular synovial fold located between the radial head and ulna (inside the annular ligament) or at the junction of the annular ligament and joint capsule (see Fig. 8–10).

The compression of Bill's humeroradial joint while performing push-ups into full elbow extension, and prolonged computer work with his wrist in extension was enough to create inflammation of the synovial tissue that extended into the joint space. If not thoroughly examined, this presentation can be easily mistaken for a lateral elbow tendinopathy (tennis elbow), which would require a very different treatment approach.

Ligaments

Typical of most hinge joints in the body, the elbow has collateral ligaments. Collateral ligaments are located on the medial and lateral sides of hinge joints to provide medial/lateral stability and to keep joint surfaces in apposition. The two main ligaments associated with the elbow joints are the medial (ulnar) and lateral (radial) collateral ligaments (**Fig. 8–11**).

MEDIAL (ULNAR) COLLATERAL LIGAMENT

The **medial collateral ligament,** often referred to as the **ulnar collateral ligament,** consists of anterior, posterior, and transverse bundles (see **Fig. 8-11A**).[14–18] The proximal attachment of the ligament is described as a round area on the

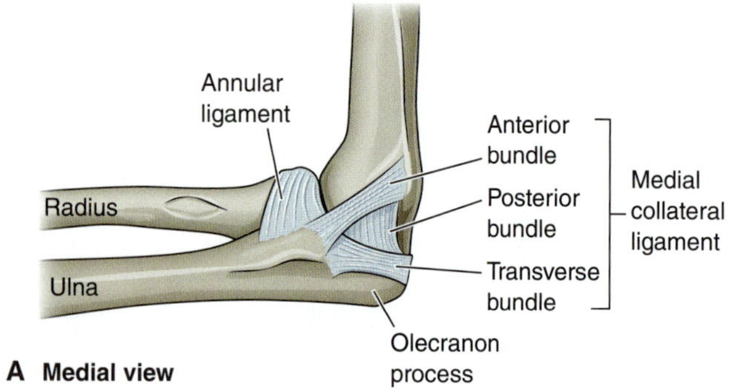

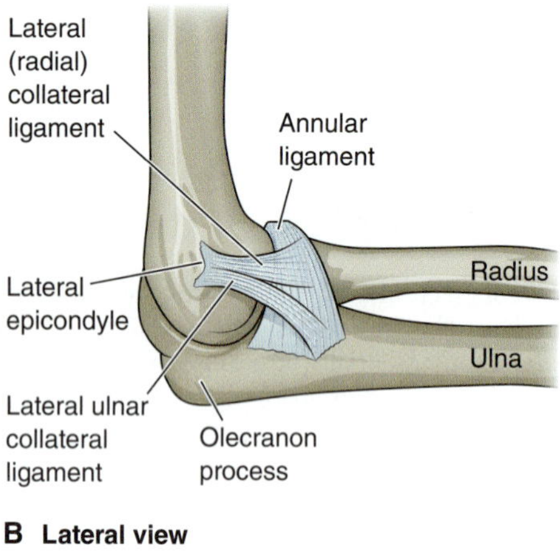

Figure 8–11 **A.** Three parts of the medial (ulnar) collateral ligament are shown on the medial aspect of the right elbow with the joint capsule removed so the ligaments stand out. **B.** The lateral collateral ligament complex includes the lateral (radial) collateral ligament, lateral ulnar collateral ligament, and annular ligament.

flat portion of the anterior and inferior aspect of the medial humeral epicondyle.[16,19] Milz and colleagues determined that the proximal attachment of the medial collateral ligament was essentially fused with the common flexor tendon as well as with part of the humeral articular cartilage where the ligament wraps around the articular cartilage of the edge of the trochlea.[19]

The distal attachment of the medial collateral ligament on the coronoid process of the ulna is broad proximally and tapers distally, with fibers of the ligament crossing the coronoid process and inserting further distally on the proximal and medial ulna.[20] This type of spread-out insertion is also a mechanism for distribution of stress.[21] Mechanoreceptors (Golgi organs, Ruffini terminals, Pacini corpuscles, and free nerve endings) are densely distributed near the ligament's humeral and ulnar attachments.[22]

The anterior bundle of the medial collateral ligament is the primary ligamentous restraint to valgus stress from 20° to 120° of elbow flexion.[23-25] Callaway and colleagues described the anterior bundle as a combination of bands that tighten in a reciprocal manner as the elbow flexes and extends.[15] The anterior capsule and radial head also make contributions to medial joint stability, but these structures fail to provide stability against valgus stress when the anterior bundle is cut.[26]

The posterior bundle of the medial collateral ligament is not as distinct as the anterior bundle, and its fibers may blend with the fibers from the medial portion of the joint capsule. The posterior bundle limits elbow extension but plays a less significant role than the anterior bundle in providing valgus stability for the elbow.[23-25] The transverse bundle of the medial collateral ligament extends between the olecranon and coronoid processes of the ulna. This portion of the ligament appears to contribute little to valgus stability, but it may help to keep the joint surfaces in approximation.

Foundational Concepts 8–1
Functional Summary for Medial (Ulnar) Collateral Ligament

1. Stabilizes against valgus torques at the medial elbow[15,23-28]
2. Limits extension at the end of the elbow extension ROM[17,20]
3. Guides joint motion throughout flexion ROM[17]
4. Provides some resistance to longitudinal distraction of joint surfaces.

LATERAL COLLATERAL LIGAMENTOUS COMPLEX

The **lateral collateral ligament complex** includes the **lateral (radial) collateral ligament,** the **lateral ulnar collateral ligament,**[29,30] and the **annular ligament** (see **Fig. 8–11B**).[30] The lateral radial collateral ligament is a fan-shaped structure that extends from the inferior aspect of the lateral epicondyle of the humerus to merge with the annular ligament that encircles the head of the *radius*. Fibrous tissue extending from the lateral humeral epicondyle to the lateral aspect of the *ulna* and the annular ligament is referred to as the lateral ulnar collateral ligament.[20] This ligament adheres closely to the supinator, extensor, and anconeus muscles, which lie just posterior to the lateral collateral ligament complex.[31]

In a study of cadaveric specimens, Wavreille and colleagues determined that the positions of the forearm and elbow affect the length of the lateral collateral ligaments and, therefore, may affect the posterolateral stability of the elbow.[32] For example, when the forearm was in neutral pronation/supination, the lateral collateral ligament was longest between 0° and 30° and at 90° of elbow flexion. When the forearm was in full pronation, the results differed. In contrast to the effects of forearm rotation on the lateral collateral ligament, forearm rotation had little effect on the length of the lateral ulnar collateral ligament.[32]

The lateral radial collateral ligament provides reinforcement for the humeroradial articulation,[33] offers some protection against varus stress in some positions of the elbow, and assists in providing resistance to longitudinal distraction of the humeroradial joint surfaces.[33] Some fibers of the lateral radial collateral ligament remain taut throughout the flexion ROM, thus able to resist varus stresses fairly consistently.[20] Elbows with a torn lateral collateral ligament are most unstable when moving the elbow into extension with the forearm in supination, and is often injured as a result of an elbow dislocation.[34,35]

Olsen and colleagues concluded that the lateral radial collateral ligament is the primary soft tissue restraint on the lateral side of the elbow, with the lateral ulnar collateral ligament and the annular ligament serving as secondary restraints to combined forced varus and supination stresses and forced valgus stress.[36] Others found that the lateral ulnar collateral ligament has the potential for assisting the lateral radial collateral ligament in resisting varus stress and in providing lateral support to the elbow joint.[31,36,37]

Foundational Concepts 8–2
Functional Summary for Lateral Collateral Ligament Complex

1. Stabilizes the elbow against varus torque[29,30,33,35,36]
2. Stabilizes against combined varus and supination torques[29,30,35,36]
3. Reinforces the humeroradial joint and helps provide some resistance to longitudinal distraction of the articulating surfaces[33]
4. Stabilizes the radial head, thus providing a stable base for rotation[38]
5. Maintains posterolateral rotatory stability[30,31,34,35,39,40]
6. Prevents subluxation of the humeroulnar joint by securing the ulna to the humerus[35]
7. Prevents the radial head from rotating off the capitulum when valgus force is applied during extension from the fully flexed position with the forearm in supination[34,35]

Patient Application 8–2

Joshua Rodes, a 27-year-old man, reports to physical therapy with reports of pain and weakness in his right upper extremity, particularly with using it during activities such as pulling weeds and lifting weights. He feels that his elbow is "unstable" when placing a dinner plate of food on a table. In fact, he has felt his elbow "shift" a couple times during these activities. During his history, Joshua explained how he fell on an outstretched hand while playing soccer 4 months ago, an injury termed a FOOSH (**f**all **o**n **o**ut**s**tretched **h**and). This fall resulted in immediate pain and his elbow "looking funny." Joshua attempted to straighten his elbow, resulting in a "clunk," with his elbow returned back to a normal appearance. He did not seek further medical intervention and managed with rest and ice. Upon testing, Joshua presented with positive findings of lateral ligament complex laxity and elbow instability and was referred for further confirmation with imaging and surgical consultation.

Isolated tears of the lateral collateral ligament are uncommon, but chronic insufficiency may lead to symptomatic posterolateral joint subluxation.[40] Complete disruption of the lateral collateral ligament complex is most often seen in fracture dislocations and fractures involving the coronoid or radial head.[41] A patient presenting with lateral elbow pain with painful clicking or locking of the elbow may have posterolateral instability, which would require further examination and stress radiographs.[34]

Muscles

Nine muscles cross the anterior aspect of the elbow joint, but only three of these muscles (the **brachialis, biceps brachii,** and **brachioradialis**) have primary functions at the elbow joint. Of the other six, the **supinator** and **pronator teres** muscles have major functions at the radioulnar joints, while the **flexor carpi radialis, flexor carpi ulnaris, flexor digitorum superficialis,** and **palmaris longus** muscles are weak elbow flexors with primary functions at the wrist, hand, and fingers **(Fig. 8–12)**.

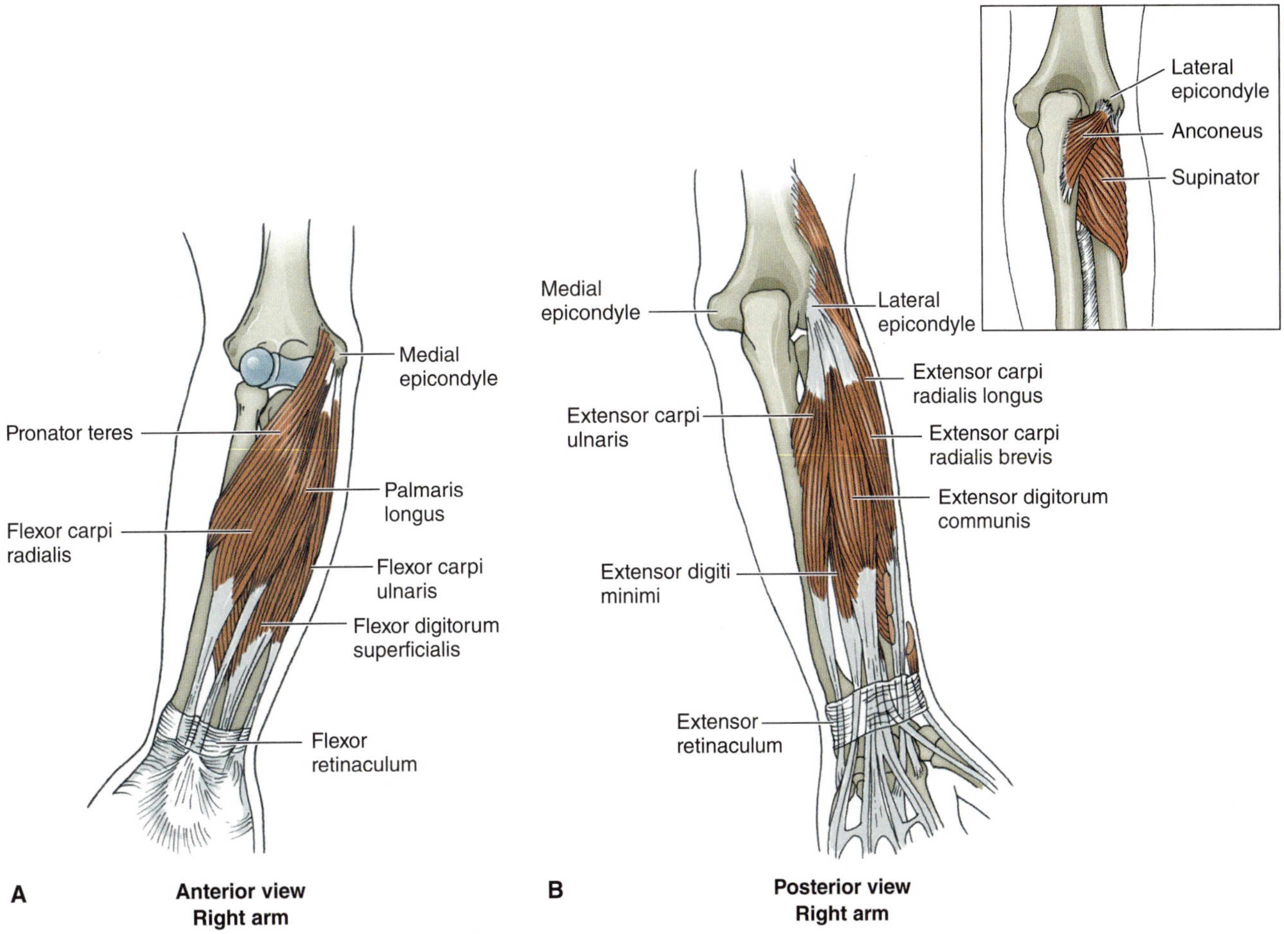

Figure 8–12 Secondary muscles of the elbow joint. **A.** Proximal attachments of secondary elbow flexor muscles on the medial epicondyle of the humerus. **B.** Proximal attachments of secondary elbow extensor muscles on the lateral epicondyle of the humerus.

The major flexors of the elbow are the brachialis, the biceps brachii, and the brachioradialis. The biceps brachii cross and acts on the elbow and proximal radioulnar joints, and have a common attachment to the proximal radius; the long head also acts on the glenohumeral joint as discussed in the previous chapter. The brachioradialis crosses and acts on the elbow and proximal radioulnar joints, while the brachialis crosses and acts only on the elbow joint. The two extensors of the elbow joint are the **triceps brachii** and the **anconeus** muscles. The triceps brachii has long, medial, and lateral heads, all of which cross and act on the elbow joint, with only the long head also crossing the shoulder. The anconeus is a small triangular muscle that only crosses and acts on the elbow joint.[6] A number of muscles with primary actions at the wrist and fingers insert into the lateral humeral epicondyle, along with the anconeus, by way of a common extensor tendon. Because these muscles cross the elbow, they can potentially act on the elbow, but their effect is predominantly compressive (stabilization). These muscles include the **extensor carpi radialis longus, extensor carpi radialis brevis, extensor digitorum communis, extensor carpi ulnaris,** and **extensor digiti minimi** (see **Fig. 8–12B**).[6]

Expanded Concepts 8–2
Muscles and Tendons of the Elbow Complex

The extensor carpi radialis longus and brevis, and the extensor digitorum communis are active during gripping, hammering, and sawing tasks. The repetitive pull of these muscles on the lateral epicondyle during forceful, repetitive activities could injure the muscle tissue or their attachment via the common extensor tendon. Pathology at the enthesis of the common tendon (enthesopathy) is commonly seen in tennis elbow.[42] If a patient reports numerous episodes of elbow pain over several years, one may suspect a chronic condition that results from degenerative changes affecting the tendon.

Over the past two decades, the clinical terminology has changed from *tendinitis* or *epicondylitis* to **tendinopathy**, a nonrupture injury in the tendon or peritendon aggravated by repetitive mechanical loading.[43] Lateral elbow tendinopathy involves degenerative changes to the extensor carpi radialis brevis primarily, but the extensor digitorum communis and extensor carpi radialis longus may also be involved. This is the most common tendinopathy of the elbow.[44]

The basis for the shift in terminology is that pain and impaired muscle function may be related to a spectrum of changes to the structure and histology of the tendon as well as the presence of chemical mediators of pain and inflammation.[44] Failure of the tendon to repair itself may contribute to the observed tissue changes.[45] The extensor carpi radialis brevis is vulnerable to shearing forces against the capitulum during elbow motion[46] and the relatively limited blood supply may also affect the potential for injury and limit healing.[47,48]

Imaging studies such as magnetic resonance imaging (MRI) and ultrasound have been used in cases of lateral elbow tendinopathy that have failed to respond to therapeutic interventions commonly offered in physical therapy. However, the diagnostic value of these modalities to determine a plan of care based on identified tissue changes of the tendon has not been validated.[44]

Function

Axis of Motion

Traditionally, the axis for flexion and extension has been described as a relatively fixed line that passes horizontally through the center of the trochlea and capitulum and bisects the longitudinal axis of the shaft of the humerus **(Fig. 8–13)**.[49,50] However, some studies have found that the axis is not as fixed as previously thought.[51-53]

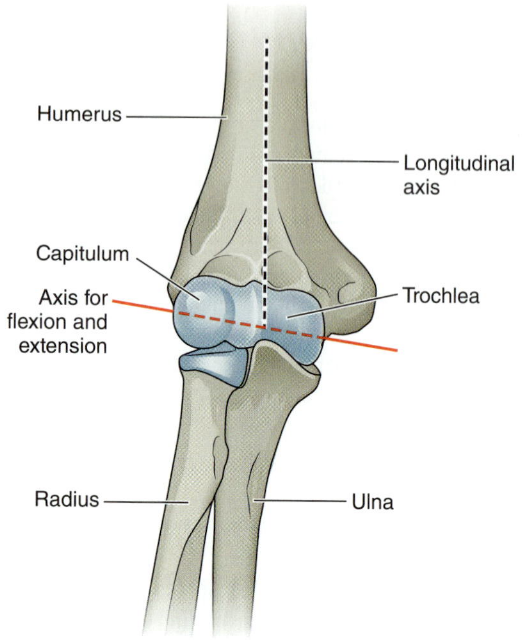

Figure 8–13 The axis of motion for elbow flexion/extension is centered in the middle of the trochlea on a line that intersects the longitudinal (anatomic) axis of the humerus.

An exact determination of the axis of motion at the elbow is important because of the need to position elbow braces and prostheses (following amputation) in such a way that they correctly mimic elbow joint motion. Variations found in the inclination of the instantaneous axis support the hypothesis that activity of the various muscles may influence the pattern of motion during active flexion/extension and that differences in contours of the joint surfaces may explain interindividual differences. Ericson and coworkers found that the orientation of the instantaneous axes varied as much as 14° between subjects (more in the frontal plane than in the transverse plane).[51] However, the inclination of the average axis across subjects in the transverse plane differed little from a line through the centers of the trochlea and capitulum. Bottlang and colleagues similarly found in their research that all instantaneous axes of rotation nearly intersected on the medial facet of the trochlea.[53]

CARRYING ANGLE OF THE ELBOW

When the upper extremity is in the anatomic position (shoulder in lateral rotation, elbow in extension, and forearm fully supinated), the long axes of the humerus and forearm form an acute angle laterally at the elbow **(Fig. 8–14)**. The angulation occurs because the medial aspect of the trochlea extends more distally than does the lateral aspect, with the capitulum slightly above the trochlea (see Fig. 8–13). This angulation is called the **carrying angle** and is typically around 15° (see **Fig 8–14A**) but may vary among individuals. When this carrying angle exceeds 15° to 20°, the condition is referred to as **cubitus valgus** (see **Fig. 8–14B**), whereas a reduced (< 5°) or reversed carrying angle is referred to as **cubitus varus** (see **Fig. 8–14C**).

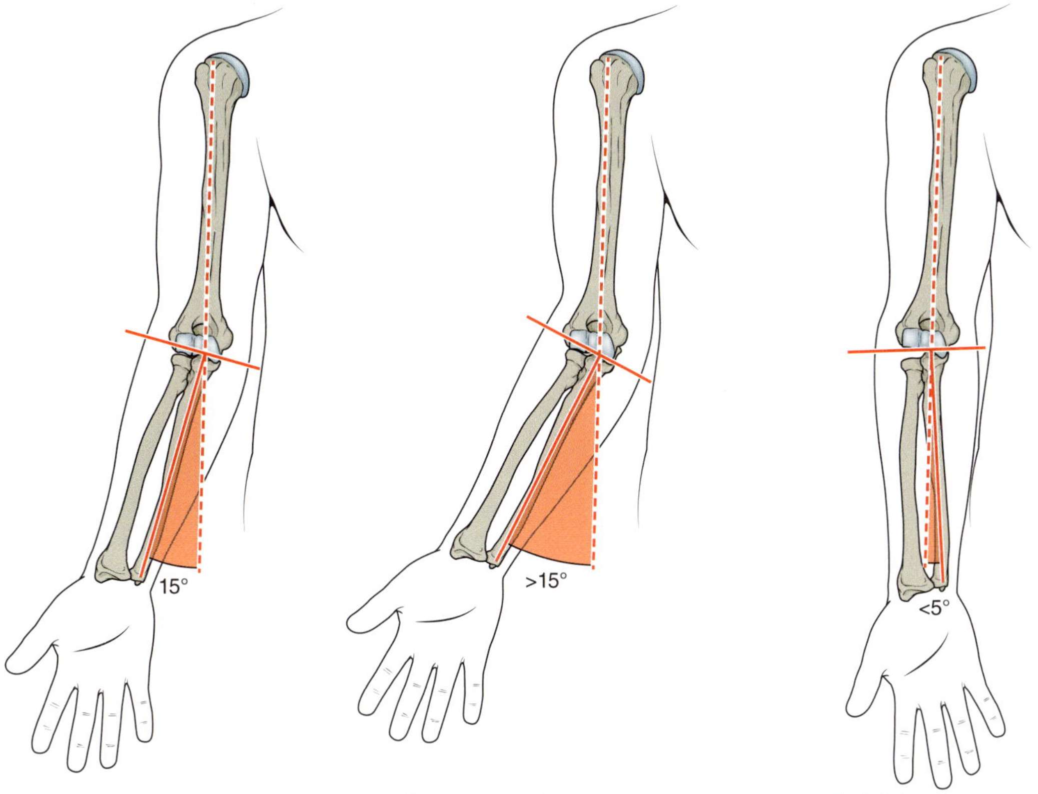

Figure 8–14 Carrying angle at the elbow. **A.** The forearm typically lies slightly lateral to the humerus when the elbow is fully extended in the anatomic position; this angulation is referred to as the *carrying angle of the elbow.* **B.** When the carrying angle is excessive (>15°), the angulation is referred to as *cubitus valgus.* **C.** When the carrying angle at the elbow is reduced (<5°) or even reversed, it is referred to as *cubitus varus.*

A "gunstock" deformity is an excessive cubitus varus that likely developed from a complex fracture.[54]

Khare and colleagues found that in the first year of life, there is no difference in the carrying angle between males and females.[55] However, in children greater than 1 year old, the carrying angle is larger in females than in males when matched for age.[55-58]

Although there is a normal angulation between the humerus and the forearm in elbow extension, the obliquity of the elbow axis results in a change in the relationship of the forearm and humerus with elbow flexion **(Fig. 8–15)**. With a typical inclination of the elbow joint axis, the ulna is guided progressively medially from extension to flexion so that in full flexion, the forearm comes to rest in the same plane as the humerus (see **Fig. 8–15A**).[11] With an increase in the angulation of the elbow joint axis (cubitus valgus), the forearm may come to rest medial to the humerus in full flexion, or may come to rest lateral to the humerus with more extreme degrees of cubitus varus[11,49] (see **Fig. 8–15B**).

Mobility/Stability

Several factors determine the amount of motion that is available at the elbow joint. These factors include the type of motion (active or passive), the position of the radioulnar joints (pronation/supination), body mass index (BMI), and the position of the shoulder. The range of active flexion at the elbow is usually less than the range of passive flexion because the muscle bulk of the contracting flexors on the anterior surface of the humerus may interfere with the approximation of the forearm with the humerus. The active ROM for elbow flexion with the forearm supinated is typically considered to be from about 135° to 145°, whereas the range for passive flexion is between 150° and 160°.[11] The position of the forearm at the radioulnar joints also affects the flexion ROM. When the forearm is either in pronation or in neutral supination/pronation, the ROM is less than it is when the forearm is supinated. A high body-mass index (BMI) may also limit the elbow ROM.[59]

The position of the shoulder may affect the elbow's ROM because of the influence of the two- or multijoint biceps brachii and triceps brachii. If a full ROM is attempted at the shoulder and the elbow simultaneously, these muscles may become actively or passively insufficient.

Foundational Concepts 8–3
Effects of Two-Joint Muscles on Elbow ROM and Function

Multijoint muscles do not have sufficient length (or ability to generate active tension) to allow (or complete) full ROM simultaneously at all joints crossed. In **Figure 8–16**, the woman is attempting to complete elbow flexion as she performs a pull-up to the bar. With simultaneous shoulder and elbow flexion, the long head of the two-joint triceps is lengthened over both joints, whereas the three-joint biceps is shortened

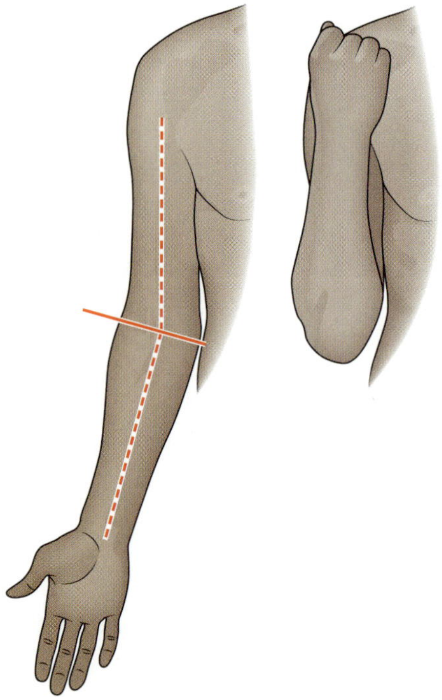

A

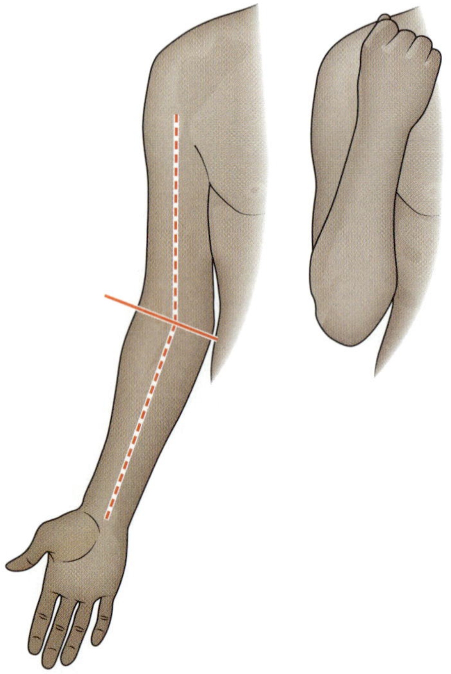

B

Figure 8–15 Forearm angulation. **A.** In the most common inclination of the elbow joint axis (15°), the ulna is guided progressively medially from extension to flexion by the angled trochlea so that, in full flexion, the forearm comes to rest in the same plane as the humerus. **B.** When the inclination of the elbow joint axis is increased (e.g., 20°), the forearm comes to rest medially to the humerus in passive flexion.

across the flexed shoulder, flexed elbow, and supinated forearm. The ability of the biceps to actively complete the elbow flexion ROM is limited by poor active tension generation (active insufficiency) in this fully shortened position, whereas the lengthened triceps is simultaneously providing passive resistance to further elbow flexion.

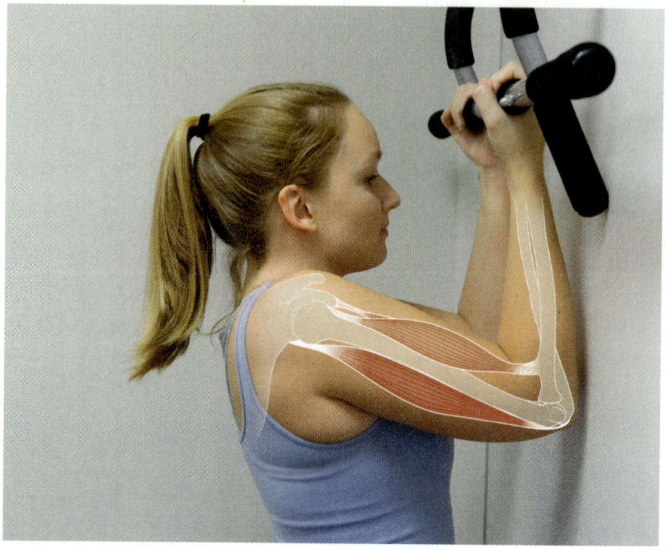

Figure 8–16 Pull-up. In a pull-up exercise, the long head of the biceps brachii is attempting to shorten over the flexed shoulder while both heads are attempting to shorten over the flexed elbow and supinated forearm. The muscle may not be able to shorten sufficiently or create enough tension to complete the available ROM at all three joints. At the same time, the long head of the triceps brachii is being stretched over the shoulder and the elbow, potentially providing passive resistance that the biceps must overcome.

The elbow joint has inherent articular stability at the extremes of extension and flexion.[24,25,33] In full extension, the humeroulnar joint is in a close-packed position. Bony contact of the olecranon process in the olecranon fossa limits the end of the extension range (see Fig.8–5B), and the configuration of the joint structures helps provide valgus and varus stability. The bony components provide 50% of the resistance to varus stress in full extension, and the lateral collateral complex and joint capsule provide the other 50% of the resistance.[33] The anterior portion of the joint capsule provides the majority of the resistance to anterior displacement of the distal humerus out of the trochlear notch, with the medial and lateral collateral ligaments contribute only slightly.[24]

Approximation of the coronoid process with the coronoid fossa and the rim of the radial head in the radial fossa limit elbow flexion (see Fig. 8-5A). At 90° of flexion, the anterior part of the medial collateral ligament provides the primary resistance to both distraction and valgus stress. If the anterior portion of the medial collateral ligament becomes lax through overstretching, medial instability will result when the elbow is in flexed positions. Most of the resistance to varus stress when the elbow is flexed to 90° is provided by the osseous structures of the joint, with only a slight amount provided by the lateral collateral ligament and the joint capsule. Active and passive tension in the muscles that cross the elbow, as is true of most muscles, contributes to stabilization of the joint through compression. Co-contractions of the flexor and extensor muscles at the elbow provide a stable base for forceful motions of the wrist and fingers because several of the muscles that cross the wrist and fingers also cross the elbow joint.

Swelling or pain may limit the range of elbow motion. McGuigan and Bookout investigated the effects of intra-articular fluid on ROM. They found that the flexion arc of motion decreased 2.1° for every milliliter of injected fluid.[60]

Muscle Action

FLEXORS

The brachialis is considered a mobility muscle because its insertion is close to the elbow joint axis, an attachment that favors production of a large arc of motion at the distal segment. The muscle has the potential to generate substantial tension due to its physiological cross-sectional area.[2] The moment arm of the brachialis is greatest at slightly more than 100° of elbow flexion.[61] Because the brachialis attachments are on the humerus and the ulna, it is unaffected by changes in shoulder or forearm position. According to electromyography studies, the brachialis muscle works in flexion of the elbow with and without resistance and during both slow and fast motions.[62]

The biceps brachii, like the brachialis, is considered a mobility muscle because of its insertion close to the elbow joint axis that favors a large arch of distal movement. The long head of the biceps brachii has the largest volume among the elbow flexors, but the muscle has a relatively small physiological cross-sectional area.[2] The moment arm of the biceps is greatest between 80° and 100° of elbow flexion **(Fig. 8–17)**. This gives the biceps a strong torque generation potential in this range (see **Fig. 8–17A**).[61] The moment arm of the biceps is small as the elbow approaches full extension, with most of the muscle force applied parallel to and toward the joint (translatory compression) (see **Fig. 8–17B**). Therefore, the biceps muscle is less effective as an elbow flexor when the elbow is fully extended than when the elbow is flexed to 100°. When the elbow is flexed beyond 100°, the translatory component of the muscle force is directed away from the elbow joint and therefore acts as a distracting or dislocating force as discussed in Chapter 1 (see Fig. 1–36D).

The biceps brachii is active during unresisted elbow flexion if the forearm is supinated or in neutral pronation/supination, but tends *not* to be active in unresisted elbow flexion when the forearm is pronated. When the magnitude of the resistance increases much beyond limb weight, the biceps is active in all positions of the forearm.[63]

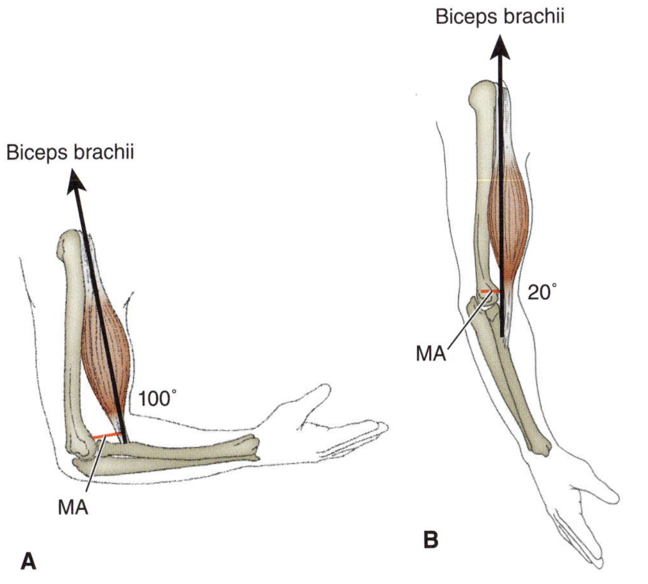

Figure 8–17 **A.** Moment arm (MA) of the biceps brachii is maximal at 100° of elbow flexion. **B.** As the elbow approaches full extension, the moment arm (MA) of the biceps is relatively small, and most of the muscle force contributes to joint compression.

The brachioradialis is inserted at a distance from the joint axis, with the largest component of muscle force being translation toward the joint surfaces and, hence, toward compression and stabilization. The brachioradialis has a relatively small mean physiological cross-sectional area (1.2 cm), but a relatively large moment arm in comparison with other elbow flexors given its superficial location, with the peak moment arm for the brachioradialis occurring between 100° and 120° of elbow flexion.[61] The brachioradialis shows no electrical activity during eccentric elbow flexor activity when the motion is performed slowly with the forearm supinated, or during slow, unresisted, concentric elbow flexion.[64] When the speed of the motion is increased, or when a load is applied with the radioulnar joint at neutral or full pronation, the brachioradialis shows moderate activity.[62,65]

The pronator teres and other muscles that cross the elbow joint (palmaris longus, flexor digitorum superficialis, flexor carpi radialis, and flexor carpi ulnaris) are weak elbow flexors with primary actions at the radioulnar and wrist joints.[6]

EXTENSORS

The effectiveness of the three heads of the triceps brachii as an elbow extensor is unaffected by changes in position of the forearm because the triceps attaches to the ulna (does not cross the radioulnar joint). Because the long head crosses both the shoulder and the elbow, the long head's ability to produce elbow extension force diminishes with simultaneous shoulder hyperextension due to encroaching active insufficiency. The one-joint medial head of the triceps brachii is active in unresisted active elbow extension; all three heads are active when heavy resistance is given to extension, or when quick extension of the elbow is attempted even in a gravity-assisted position (as in hammering).[62] Although maximum isometric torque has been observed at 90° of elbow flexion, the total amount of extensor torque generated at 90° varies with the position of the shoulder and the body.[66-68]

The variations in the ability of the triceps brachii to produce effective elbow extension force is most often represented by the function of the muscles during a push-up exercise **(Fig. 8–18)**. In a push-up, the triceps are active eccentrically to control the elbow flexion produced by the body weight as the body is lowered to the ground (see **Fig. 8–18A**). To raise the body back up, the triceps are active concentrically to extend the elbow against the resistance of the body weight (see **Fig. 8–18B**). Throughout the push-up exercise, the relative ability of the long head of the triceps to generate force is maintained. This is because elbow extension (pushing up phase) is accompanied by shoulder flexion; the shortening at the elbow is offset by the long head of the triceps lengthening at the shoulder. Similarly, in the lowering phase, elbow flexion lengthens the active long head while the muscle is shortening over the extending shoulder. The combination of stretch and shortening in the active muscles helps minimize active insufficiency.

Zhang and Nuber[69] found that in voluntary isometric extension, the uniarticular lateral and medial heads of the triceps provide 70% to 90% of the total elbow extension torque. The small anconeus muscle contributes about 15%, whereas the biarticular long head of the triceps contributes

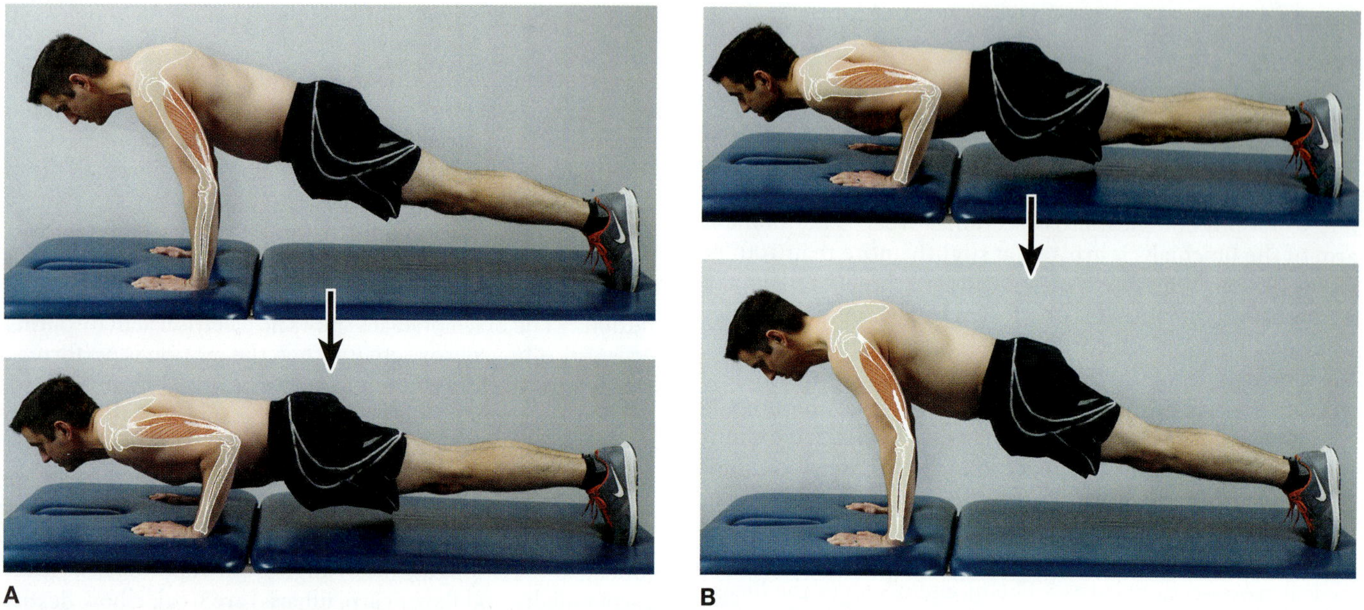

Figure 8–18 Triceps brachii activity during a push-up. **A.** The triceps work eccentrically to control the elbow flexion produced by the body weight during the lowering phase of a push-up. **B.** As the elbows extend against the resistance of body weight, the triceps work concentrically to return to the start position in the push-up.

even less. This seems to follow the premise that the central nervous system *tends to* recruit one-joint muscles before two- and multijoint muscles.

The triceps may be active during activities requiring stabilization of the elbow. For example, the triceps acts as a synergist to the biceps when the biceps is performing isolated forearm supination, counterbalancing the unwanted elbow flexion force of the biceps brachii. The anconeus assists in elbow extension and arguably acts as a stabilizer during many activities.[70] Prodoehl and colleagues demonstrated that muscle activation patterns change with the force requirements of the task and the amount of available muscle force.[71]

Structure and Function of the Proximal and Distal Radioulnar Articulations

Structure

Proximal (Superior) Radioulnar Joint

The articulating surfaces of the proximal radioulnar joint include the radial notch of the ulna, the annular ligament, rim and fovea of the head of the radius **(Fig. 8–19)**, and the humeral capitulum. The concave **radial notch** of the ulna is located on the lateral aspect of the proximal ulna directly below the trochlear notch. The nearly circular annular ligament is attached to the anterior and posterior edges of the notch. The rim and fovea of the radial head are hyaline cartilage–covered, as is the inner aspect of the annular ligament, and the radial notch; together, these create a fibro-osseous ring within which the head of the radius rotates (see **Fig. 8–19A**). The capitulum and the proximal surface of the head of the radius (the fovea) are part of both the proximal radioulnar joint as well as part of the previously discussed humeroradial (elbow) articulation[6] (see **Fig. 8–19B**).

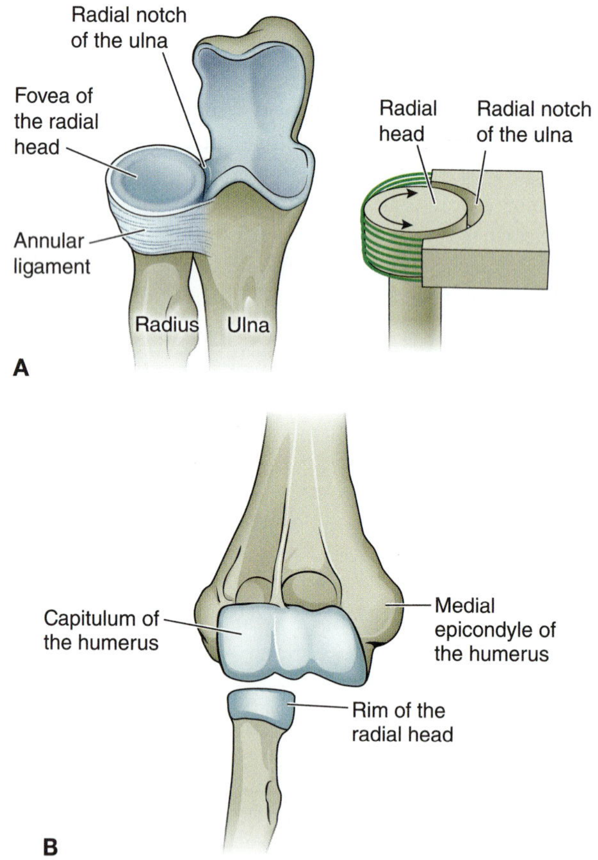

Figure 8–19 The proximal radioulnar joint. **A.** One part of the proximal radioulnar joint is formed by the fibro-osseous ring of the annular ligament and radial notch of the ulna within which the radial head rotates. **B.** The joint also includes the articulation of the fovea (see **A.**) of the radial head with the capitulum of the distal humerus.

Distal (Inferior) Radioulnar Joint

The articulating surfaces of the distal radioulnar joint include the **ulnar notch** of the radius, the **radioulnar articular disc**, and the **head of the ulna** (**Fig. 8–20**). The **ulnar notch** of the radius is located at the distal end of the radius. The curvature of the concave ulnar notch is larger than that of the small ulnar head. The **radioulnar disc** is commonly referred to as either the **triangular fibrocartilage (TFC)** because of its triangular shape, or as a part of the **triangular fibrocartilage complex (TFCC)** because of its extensive fibrous and ligamentous connections to the structures of the wrist.[6]

The base of the triangular fibrocartilage is attached to the distal edge of the ulnar notch of the radius (see Fig. 8-20). The apex of the triangular fibrocartilage has one attachment to the fovea on the ulnar head and another to the base of the ulnar styloid process.[72] The triangular fibrocartilage has numerous attachments, leading to the common designation as the triangular fibrocartilage complex. The TFCC has been described as resembling a shelf whose medial border is embedded in a wedge of vascular connective tissue containing fine ligamentous bands that join the triangular fibrocartilage to the ulna and articular capsule.[73] Medially, the triangular fibrocartilage is continuous with the fibers of the ulnar collateral ligament that arises from the sides of the styloid process.[72] The margins of the triangular fibrocartilage are thickened, being thinner centrally, and are either formed by, or are integral parts of, the **dorsal and palmar radioulnar ligaments** (see **Fig 8–20B**).[74-76] The ligaments are firmly attached to the radius; the ulnar attachments are somewhat less firmly attached.[72] In cadaveric specimens, Chidgey and colleagues found that the central portion of the fibrocartilage was avascular in most specimens, in contrast to the peripheral area of the triangular fibrocartilage.[76] Clinically, the disc vascularity has led to the recommendation that peripheral tears of the triangular fibrocartilage can be made in the more commonly vascularized zone, whereas tears in the central and more commonly avascular region are simply debrided.[77] Ohmori and Azuma found free nerve endings in the ulnar side of the triangular fibrocartilage, particularly around the periphery. The authors suggested that, in view of their findings, the disc may be a source of wrist pain.[78]

The triangular fibrocartilage and its associated complex physically divides the distal radioulnar joint from the radiocarpal joint, each of which is anatomically distinct with its own joint capsule (**Fig. 8–21**). Consequently, the triangular fibrocartilage has two articulating surfaces. The proximal (superior) surface of the triangular fibrocartilage is part of the distal radioulnar joint, while the disc's distal (inferior) surface is part of the radiocarpal joint.[72] Both the proximal and distal surfaces of the triangular fibrocartilage are concave to accommodate the convexity of the ulnar head superiorly and the convexity of the carpal bones distally.[72] The peripheral portions of both the proximal and distal triangular fibrocartilage surfaces are covered by synovium lining their respective joint capsules.[75]

Ligaments

There are a number of ligaments that contribute to stability of the proximal and distal radioulnar joints. Because the proximal and distal joints are mechanically linked, all radioulnar ligaments provide at least indirect support to both joints, although some are clearly associated with one joint more than the other. The three ligaments associated specifically with the proximal radioulnar joint are the **annular** and **quadrate ligaments** and the oblique cord (**Fig. 8–22**). The annular ligament, as previously discussed, is a strong band that forms a ring that encircles the radial head and forms part of the articular surface of the proximal radioulnar joint (see Fig. 8–19A). The proximal border of the annular ligament blends with the elbow joint capsule, and the lateral aspect is reinforced by fibers

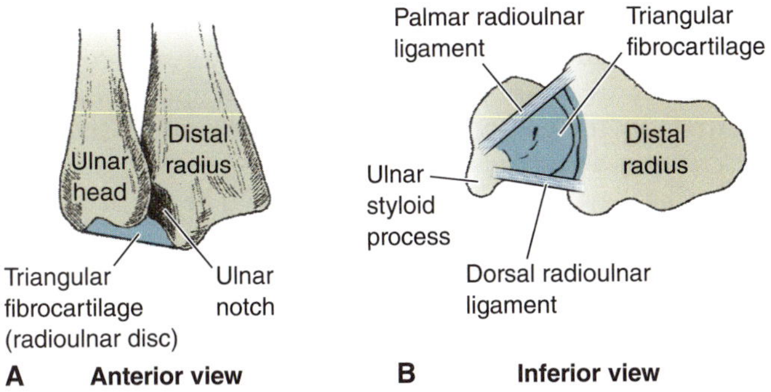

Figure 8–20 The distal radioulnar joint. **A.** An anterior view of the distal radioulnar joint shows the triangular fibrocartilage (radioulnar disc) in its normal position in a supinated forearm. **B.** An inferior view of the distal radius and ulna shows how the triangular fibrocartilage (not actually transparent) covers the inferior aspect of the distal ulna. The palmar and dorsal radioulnar ligaments contribute to stability of the radioulnar articulation and the triangular fibrocartilage, all being part of the triangular fibrocartilage complex (TFCC).

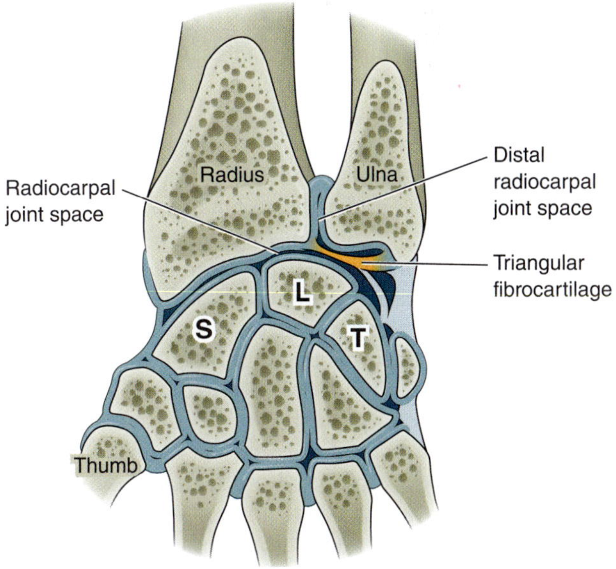

Figure 8–21 Triangular fibrocartilage. A cross section through the right distal forearm and hand allows one to see that the triangular fibrocartilage divides, and serves as a physical barrier between, the distal radioulnar synovial joint and the radiocarpal synovial joint. The triangular fibrocartilage, therefore, is part of both the distal radioulnar and the radiocarpal articular surfaces. S, scaphoid; L, lunate; T, triquetrum.

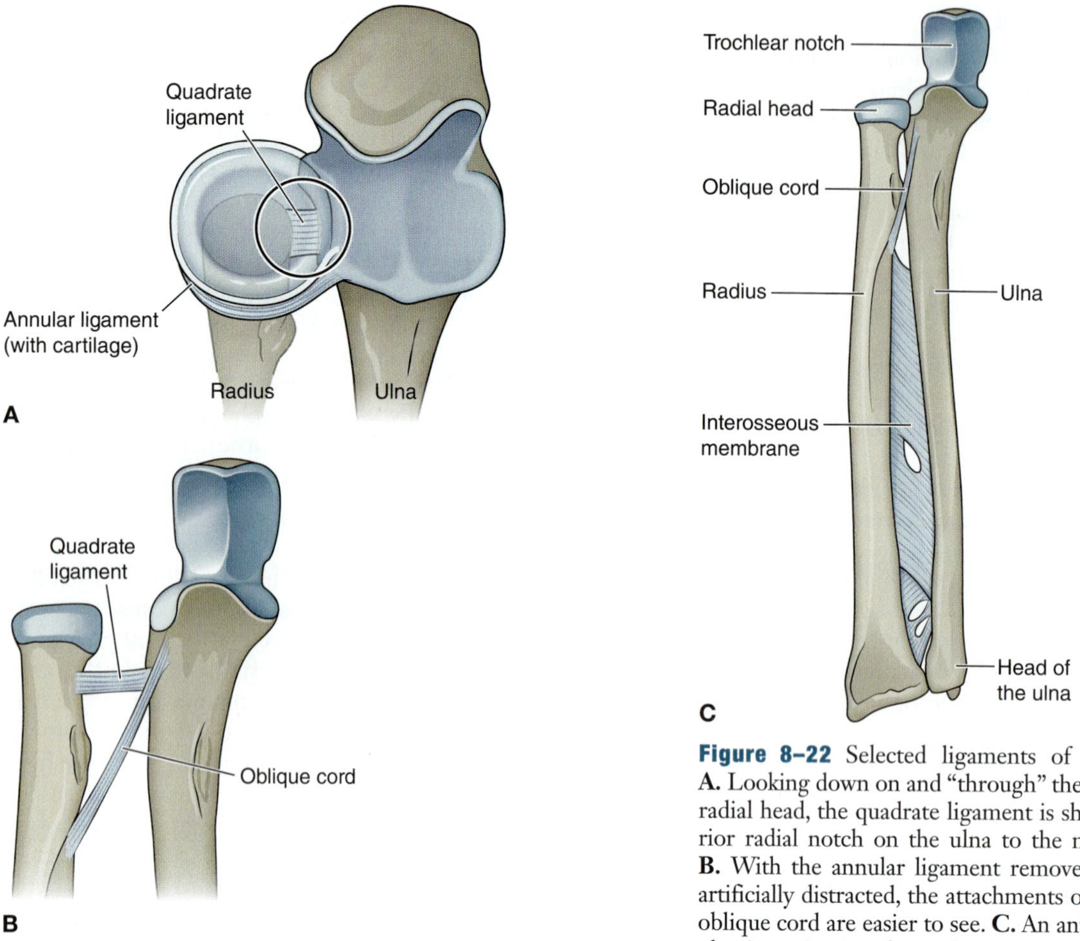

Figure 8–22 Selected ligaments of the right radioulnar joint **A.** Looking down on and "through" the artificially semi-transparent radial head, the quadrate ligament is shown running from the inferior radial notch on the ulna to the medial radius below its rim. **B.** With the annular ligament removed and the radius and ulnar artificially distracted, the attachments of the quadrate ligament and oblique cord are easier to see. **C.** An anterior view of the radius and ulna in supination shows the interosseous membrane.

from the elbow's lateral collateral ligament. The quadrate ligament extends from the inferior edge of the ulna's radial notch to insert in the neck of the radius (see **Fig. 8–22A** and **B**). The quadrate ligament reinforces the inferior aspect of the joint capsule and helps maintain the radial head against the radial notch. The quadrate ligament also limits the spin of the radial head in supination and pronation because it is attached to the radius just below the rim of the radial head. The proximally located **oblique cord** (see Fig. 8-22B and C) is a flat fascial band on the ventral (anterior) forearm that attaches to the anterolateral aspect of the coronoid process of the ulna and just below the bicipital tuberosity on the radius.[79] The fibers of the oblique cord are at right angles to the fibers of the interosseous membrane (see **Fig. 8-22C**). The functional significance of the oblique cord is not clear, but it may assist in preventing separation of the radius and ulna.

The **dorsal** and **palmar radioulnar ligaments** provide direct support to the distal radioulnar joint. The dorsal and palmar ligaments are formed by longitudinally oriented collagen fiber bundles originating from the dorsal and palmar aspects of the ulnar notch of the radius. As shown previously, the two ligaments extend along the margins of the triangular fibrocartilage to insert on the ulnar fovea and base of the ulnar styloid process (see Fig. 8–20B).[75]

The **interosseous membrane** lies between the radius and ulna, providing stabilization at both the proximal and distal radioulnar joints (see Fig. 8–22C).[79,80] It is a complex structure consisting of a central band, a thin membranous portion, and a dorsal oblique cord. The key central band is described as being strong and thick, consisting of bundles of fibers that run obliquely from the radius to the ulna.[79,81,82] When the tensile strength of the central band was compared with that of the patellar tendon, investigators found that the ultimate tensile strength of the central band was 84% of the strength of the patellar tendon.[83] Nakamura and associates found that the central band remained taut throughout forearm rotation, apparently to keep the radius and ulna in apposition.[84] In contrast to the central band, the membranous portion is described as a soft and thin structure that lies adjacent to the central band both proximally and distally.[79] The dorsal oblique cord (not be confused with the oblique cord of the proximal radioulnar joint) has fibers that have a direction opposite to those of the central band, so assists with approximation of the radius and ulna against additional forces.[79]

The triangular fibrocartilage and distal radioulnar joint capsule also provide stability for the distal radioulnar joint by binding the distal radius and ulna together. The distal radioulnar joint capsule can be a source of limitation of motion when it is invaded by scar tissue after wrist injuries.[82]

Muscles

The primary muscles associated with the radioulnar joints are the pronator teres, **pronator quadratus**, biceps brachii, and supinator **(Fig. 8–23)**. The two pronators are the pronator

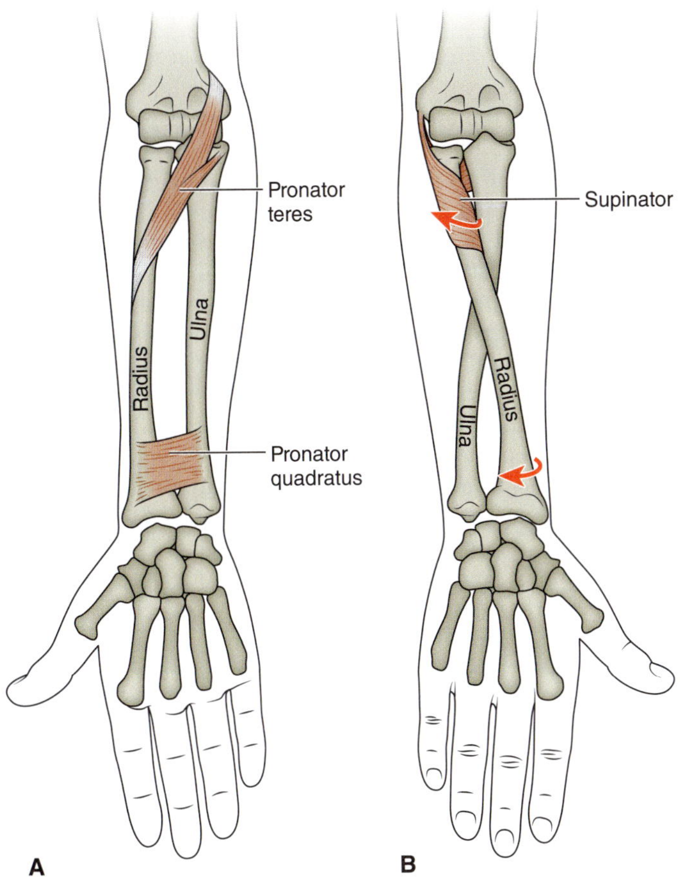

Figure 8–23 Primary pronator and supinator muscles of the radioulnar joints. **A.** An anterior view of the right forearm shows the pronator teres and pronator quadratus muscles on the *supinated* forearm. When these muscles shorten, the radius will cross over the ulna into pronation. **B.** In radioulnar *pronation*, the supinator is coiled around the radius. When the supinator shortens, it will uncoil and pull the radius back into supination.

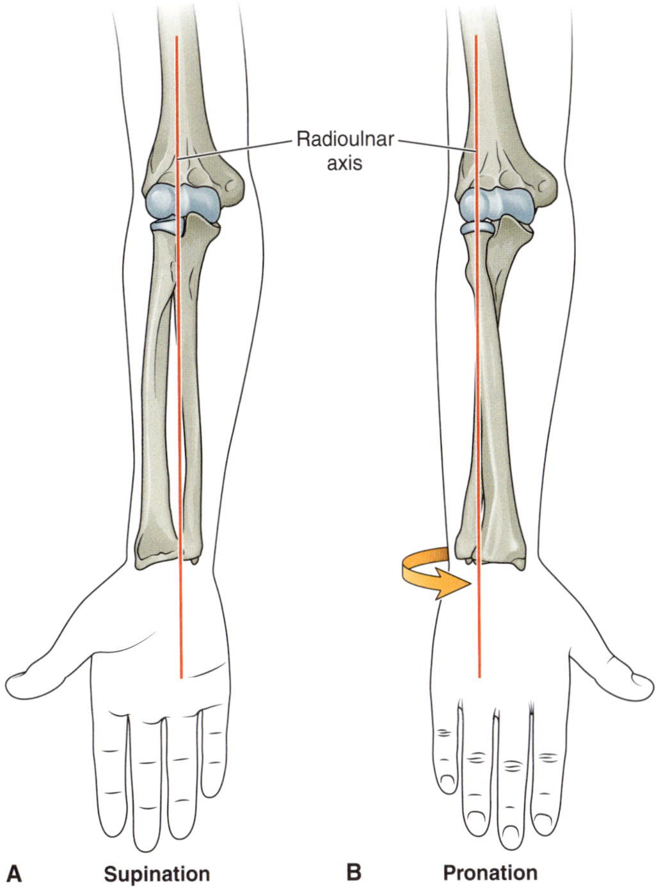

Figure 8–24 Mechanical linkage of the proximal and distal radioulnar joints **A.** The radius and ulna are parallel to each other in the supinated position of the forearm, with the single longitudinal axis passing through the proximal and distal radioulnar joints. **B.** During pronation, the radius rotates within the annular ring proximally and pivots around the triangular fibrocartilage distally, with the radius crossing over the relatively stable ulna as the radius rotates around the longitudinal joint axis.

teres and the pronator quadratus (see **Fig. 8–23A**). The pronator teres has two heads: a humeral head and an ulnar head. Both heads attach distally to the surface of the lateral side of the middle of the radius. The anteriorly located **pronator quadratus** has both deep and superficial portions, both located at the distal end of the forearm with attachments to the ulna and the radius.[85]

The biceps brachii, as was noted in the discussion of muscles acting on the elbow joint, is a radioulnar supinator as well as an elbow flexor. The short, broad **supinator** muscle is a one-joint radioulnar supinator. In pronation, the supinator wraps around the radius, uncoiling and spinning the radius when the supinator actively shortens (see **Fig. 8–23B**).

Function

Radioulnar Axis and Radioulnar Motions

The proximal and distal radioulnar joints are mechanically linked by a single longitudinal axis that extends from the center of the radial head proximally to the center of the ulnar head distally **(Fig. 8–24)**.[72] Because the linked proximal and distal radioulnar joints have a common axis, motion must occur simultaneously at both joints.

In supination, the radius and ulna lie parallel to one another (see **Fig. 8–24A**), whereas the radius crosses over the ulna in pronation (see **Fig. 8–24B**). Proximally, the head of the radius spins within the osteoligamentous ring formed by the radial notch and the annular ligament, with the fovea of the radial head simultaneously spinning on the capitulum of the humerus. Distally, the concave surface of the ulnar notch on the radius slides around the ulnar head, accompanied by the triangular fibrocartilage that sweeps beneath the ulnar head as it pivots around its attachment to the ulnar styloid.

Although the predominant motion at the radioulnar joints is motion of the radius, there is some motion of the distal ulna as well, but of less magnitude.[86] The ulnar head moves distally and dorsally in pronation, while moving proximally and medially in supination. Therefore, at the distal radioulnar joint, the ulnar head sits on the dorsal lip of the ulnar notch of the radius in pronation while it sits on the palmar aspect of the ulnar notch in full supination.[74] Contact between the head of the ulna and the ulnar notch of the radius is minimal at these end ranges, and maximal when the forearm is midway between supination and pronation.[87]

Radioulnar ROM

A total ROM of 150° has been ascribed to the radioulnar joints.[88,89] However, Shaaban and colleagues found supination and pronation ROM to vary based on the elbow position.[87] Controlling for all humeral motion, these investigators found a significant increase in supination with the elbow fully flexed and, conversely, greater pronation with the elbow extended.[87] From a function standpoint, it is advantageous to have more supination when putting the hand to the mouth to eat, generally accompanied by elbow flexion.[72] Pronation in all elbow positions is limited by bony approximation of the radius and ulna and by tension in the dorsal radioulnar ligament and the posterior fibers of the medial collateral ligament of the elbow.[87] Supination is limited by passive tension in the palmar radioulnar ligament and the oblique cord. The quadrate ligament that attaches to the radius immediately below the radial head limits spin of the radial head in both pronation and supination. The annular ligament does not limit motion because the radial head rotates within the annular ring but does help maintain stability of the proximal radioulnar joint by holding the radius in close approximation to the radial notch.

Clinical Application 8-1
Measuring Forearm ROM

In the clinic, the ROM of pronation and supination is assessed with the elbow held against the side of the trunk in 90° of flexion **(Fig. 8–25)**. This position stabilizes the humerus so that humeral medial/lateral rotation aren't affecting the measurement of radioulnar pronation/supination. For example, if an examiner erroneously tested pronation with the elbow in extension and the shoulder in 90° of flexion (arm held straight out in front of the body), then apparent pronation would actually include quite a bit of glenohumeral medial rotation. Likewise, in this erroneously tested position, an assessment of supination would also include considerable glenohumeral lateral rotation. Maintaining a consistent standardized position is important for test-retest reliability and ensures that clinicians are measuring and recording motion at the joint of interest.

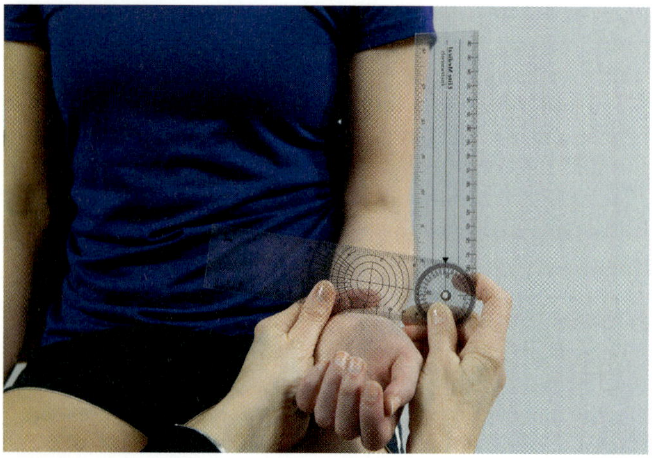

Figure 8–25 Clinical measurement of radioulnar motion. Measurement of the end range of supination with a goniometer. The subject's left elbow is flexed to 90° and the elbow is held close to the trunk. The same position is used for measuring the end range of pronation.

Muscle Action

The pronator teres has its major action at the radioulnar joints, but the long head also crosses the elbow joint. Lying very close to the elbow joint axis, the pronator teres plays only a slight role in elbow flexion but can contribute to stabilization of the proximal radioulnar and humeroradial joints. The pronator quadratus, a one-joint muscle, is unaffected by changing positions at the elbow. The pronator quadratus is active in unresisted and resisted pronation and in both slow and fast pronation. The pronator quadratus is thought to act as a dynamic stabilizer to maintain compression of the distal radioulnar joint.[85]

In a mechanical study on cadavers, the pronators were found to be most efficient around the neutral position of the forearm when the elbow was flexed to 90°, with pronation torque of the pronator teres and pronator quadratus maximal at midrange with a decline at the extremes of pronation and supination.[90,91]

The supinator muscle, as a one-joint muscle, may act alone during unresisted slow supination for all positions of the elbow or forearm. It can also act alone during unresisted fast supination when the elbow is extended. However, activity of the biceps brachii is always evident when supination is performed against resistance, or during fast supination when the elbow is flexed to 90°. Supination torque values were greatest when the forearm was partially pronated.[92,93]

The brachioradialis also plays a role in supination and pronation. Naito and colleagues demonstrated in unimpaired subjects that the brachioradialis showed high levels of activity during rapid alternating supination/pronation motions with the elbow held at 90° of flexion, with higher levels of activity noted when the forearm was pronated.[65] Bremer suggested that the brachioradialis acts as a pronator in supination and as a supinator while the forearm is in pronation.[91]

Stability

Muscular support of the distal radioulnar joint is attributed to the pronator quadratus [85,94,95] and the extensor carpi ulnaris tendon.[72,82] The deep head of the pronator quadratus is active throughout supination and pronation, and therefore is thought to provide dynamic stabilization for the distal radioulnar joint.[96] Activity in the extensor carpi ulnaris muscle **(Fig. 8–26)** exerts an anteriorly directed force on the dorsal aspect of the ulnar head as the tendon is stretched over the ulnar head during supination. Tension in the tendon helps to maintain the position of the ulnar head during both supination and pronation.[72]

The extensor carpi radialis brevis, like the extensor carpi ulnaris, appears to provide support for the radioulnar joints, as evidenced by the magnitude of motor unit activity during radioulnar motion and its activity during forceful pronation.[92]

Patient Application 8-3

Belinda Chambliss, a 47-year-old woman who is a textile worker, reports left lateral elbow pain for the past 2 months with no history of trauma. Her job consists of sitting at a sewing machine for half her workday, with the remainder spent folding, packing, and lifting boxes of clothes. She does not report any change in her daily activity

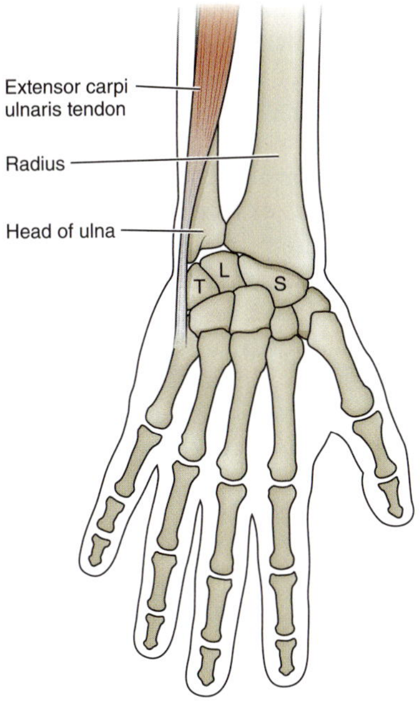

Figure 8–26 Extensor carpi ulnaris. This dorsal (posterior) view of the right forearm and hand shows the extensor carpi ulnaris tendon as it passes distally through the notch in the ulnar head to its attachments on the base of the fifth metacarpal. The distal tendon can stabilize the head of the ulna during pronation and supination. T, triquetrum; L, lunate; S, scaphoid.

over the past couple of months. She has had a history of neck pain but indicated that it is not bothering her at this time. Key objective findings are as follows:

- Pain with palpation to the common extensor tendon
- Elbow pain with resisted wrist extension
- Preference for sitting in a slumped manner with forward head and rounded shoulders
- Limited cervical ROM with extension, right rotation, and right side-bending
- Pain provoked along the right upper trapezius with cervical provocation tests
- Slight decrease in elbow pain with cervical distraction

This is a very common presentation of elbow pain seen in many outpatient physical therapy clinics. It is not uncommon to find poor postural habits and cervical dysfunction in combination with repetitive upper extremity activity that results in complaints of elbow pain of insidious onset.

O'Sullivan and Gallwey found a direct link between gripping during forearm rotations and high muscular activity in the extensor carpi radialis brevis.[92] Research has also shown a poor prognosis in cases of lateral elbow tendinopathy (tennis elbow) associated with manual job employment with a high level of physical strain at work and a high level of pain at baseline.[97] Treatment focused on patient education and ergonomic instruction combined with specific treatment to the spine and elbow will give the therapist and patient the best chance for success. If only localized treatment to the elbow is implemented, results can vary.

Passive support of the distal radioulnar joint is provided by the dorsal and palmar radioulnar ligaments, the interosseous membrane, and the triangular fibrocartilage. The dorsal radioulnar ligament becomes taut in pronation, whereas the palmar radioulnar ligament becomes taut in supination.[72,95,98] The radioulnar ligaments have limited cross-sectional areas and low structural stiffness, but they are able to prevent separation of the radius from the ulna during loading and may also contribute to force transmission from the radius to the ulna through the distal radioulnar joint. However, these ligaments do not augment longitudinal stability, allowing approximately 5 mm of play between the radius and ulna before providing resistance to further distraction.[74] The interosseous membrane and triangular fibrocartilage provides stability for the distal joint by binding the radius and ulna together. However, they also provide important *longitudinal stabilization*, preventing translatory motion (shifting) between the radius and ulna.[81,82]

The interosseous membrane protects the *proximal* radioulnar joint and head of the radius by transferring some of the longitudinal loads across the wrist and distal radius to the proximal ulna.[99] At the wrist, the base of the radius is substantially larger than the small head of the ulna, with more of the radiocarpal compression (as in weightbearing on the hand) creating a superiorly directed force on the radius, with the smaller ulna also somewhat protected by the soft tissues of the triangular fibrocartilage complex (see Fig. 8–20B). If not attenuated, the force imposed on the distal radius would potentially cause large compressive stress at the small *proximal* articulation between the radial head and the capitulum (rather than the much larger and more congruent proximal articulation between the ulna and trochlea. When bearing weight on the wrist and hand, the direction of the central fibers of the interosseous membrane limits the proximal shift of the radius on the ulna **(Fig. 8–27)**, and shifting a proportion of the force imposed on the distal radius to the ulna.

DeFrate and colleagues determined that the average proportion of total compressive load transmission through the radius and ulna differed with forearm position. In supination, load distribution was 68% in the distal radius and 32% in the distal ulna; proximally, the proportions shifted to 51% in the proximal radius and 49% in the proximal ulna.[100] The axial force transmitted through the radius was found to be least in full supination and greater as the forearm moved toward pronation; the ulnar load—as one might expect—was just the opposite.[101] Markolf and associates also studied load-sharing between the radius and ulna, noting a shift in load with the elbow in varus, valgus, and neutral positions.[102] When the elbow was in a relative varus position (no contact between the radial head and capitulum), force was transmitted from the distal radius through the interosseous membrane to the proximal ulna. When the elbow was in a relative valgus position (increasing the contact between the radial head and the capitulum), the force was transmitted through the radius.[102]

The triangular fibrocartilage acts as a cushion as compressive forces are transmitted from the carpals to the ulna, and acts as a stabilizer of the ulnar side of the carpals.[72,103] Also, like the interosseous membrane, the triangular fibrocartilage assists in the transmission of compressive forces from the radius to the ulna.[102,104] Using a distractive force to simulate the effects of the separation of articulating surfaces that accompanies a power grip, investigators concluded that, although strain distribution was dependent on forearm position, the triangular fibrocartilage regularly bears both compressive and tensile strains.[88,105,106]

A summary of ligamentous and muscular support for both radioulnar joints is presented in Table 8–1.

Mobility and Stability of the Elbow Complex

Functional Activities

The joints and muscles of the elbow complex (including the proximal radioulnar joint and its linked distal radioulnar joint) are used in almost all ADLs, such as dressing, eating, carrying, keyboarding, and lifting. They are also used in tasks such as splitting firewood and hammering nails, and in sports such as tennis, golf, basketball, and baseball. Most of the ADLs require combinations of motion at the elbow and radioulnar joints. Morrey and associates measured elbow and forearm motion in 33 healthy subjects during 15 activities. The authors concluded that a total arc of 100° of elbow flexion (between 30° and 130°) and 100° of forearm rotation (50° supination and 50° pronation) were sufficient to accomplish simple tasks such as eating, drinking, brushing hair, brushing teeth, and dressing[107] **(Fig. 8–28)**. Other researchers found similar findings for elbow flexion and forearm rotation.[108,109] A more recent paper has noted that full elbow flexion and full pronation are required for tasks such as use of a mobile phone or keyboarding.[1] Therefore, mobility of the complex is necessary for normal functioning in most activities.

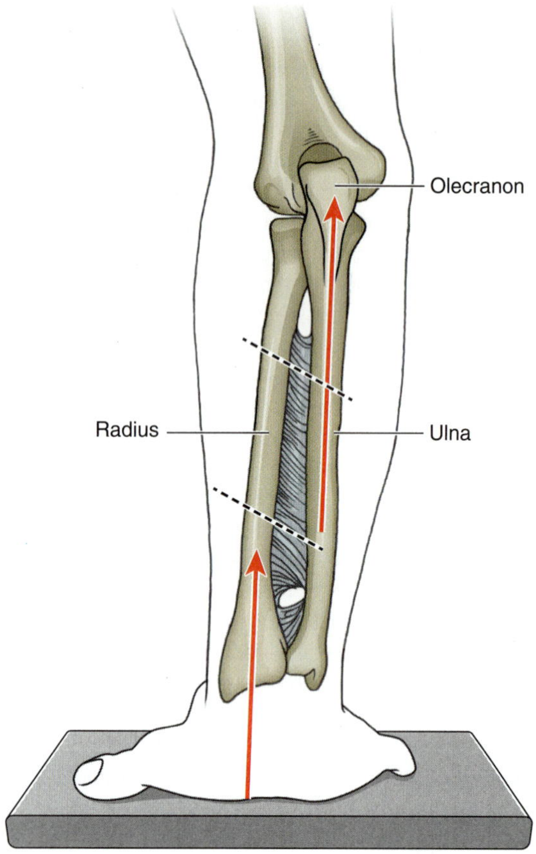

Figure 8–27 Interosseous membrane in force transmission. In bearing weight on the right hand (posterior view), the greater proportion of the ground reaction force is borne by the large base of the radius. As the interosseous membrane tightens, superiorly directed motion of the radius is checked and transferred to the ulna and, from there, to the larger humeroulnar surfaces proximally.

Relationship to the Hand and Wrist

The design of the radioulnar joints enhances the mobility of the hand. In primitive mammalian species, the ulna was a major weight-bearing structure and was connected directly to the carpals through a dense immobile syndesmosis.[110] The complete separation of the ulna from the carpals by the articular disc and formation of synovial joints are features that permit pronation and supination to occur in every position of the hand in relation to the forearm.

The hand and wrist muscles, as noted earlier, attach proximally to the humerus and cross the elbow joint. This creates a close structural and functional relationships between the elbow and wrist/hand complexes. Anatomically, the hand and wrist muscles help reinforce the elbow joint capsule and contribute to stability of the elbow complex. Evidence suggests that the flexor carpi ulnaris, flexor digitorum superficialis, and flexor carpi radialis function as dynamic stabilizers, with the flexor carpi ulnaris being the primary stabilizer for elbow valgus stability and reinforcement of the medial collateral ligament of the elbow; wrist/hand extensor muscle activity actually increased the valgus strain on the medial collateral ligament.[111,112]

Life Span and Clinical Considerations

Like other joints in the body, the joints and muscles of the elbow complex may be subject to the effects of age, injury, and immobilization. Knowledge of these effects will significantly improve a clinician's ability to evaluate and treat elbow problems in patients of all ages.

Table 8–1 Ligamentous and Muscular Contributions to Stability at the Proximal and Distal Radioulnar Joints

JOINT	LIGAMENTOUS	MUSCULAR
Proximal radioulnar joint	Annular and quadrate ligaments Oblique cord (limits supination) Interosseous membrane	Passive tension in the biceps brachii in the fully extended elbow position Pronator teres (helps maintain contact of radial head and capitulum) Anconeus
Distal radioulnar joint	Interosseous membrane Dorsal radioulnar ligament (limits pronation) Palmar radioulnar ligament (limits supination) Triangular fibrocartilage complex Joint capsule	Pronator quadratus Extensor carpi ulnaris Pronator teres

Effects of Age

As can be seen in the sampling of experimental findings presented in Table 8–2, the decrease in muscle strength that accompanies increasing age appears to be affected by the type of muscle action involved (eccentric vs. concentric), the muscle group involved, and gender, along with other factors such as level of physical activity.[113-117] Pennation angles and fascicle lengths tend to become smaller as we get older, which may account for as much of 50% of the loss of muscle function. Fortunately, resistance training may be able to increase fascicle length and increase the number of sarcomeres.[118]

Numerous studies across young to old age groups have demonstrated a decline in torque generation and shortening velocity of elbow flexor and extensor muscle with age, with some observing that declines were most notable after 50-60 years of age. [120,122-125]

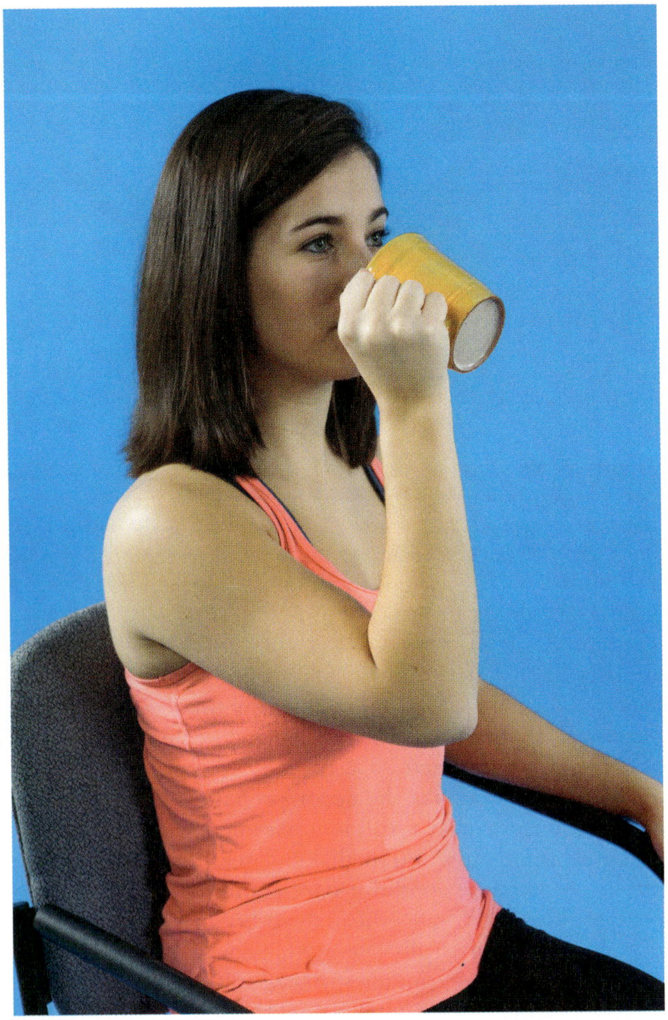

Figure 8–28 Functional ROM. Common activities in healthy subjects (such as drinking from a mug) can be accomplished with an arc of elbow flexion from 30° to 130°, and a radioulnar range between 50° supination and 50° pronation.[107]

Injury

Injuries to the elbow are common and recovery is dependent on restoring ROM, preventing instability, and decreasing/resolving pain. An understanding of the mechanisms of elbow injuries and their relation to elbow joint structures is necessary for determining the effects of the injuries on joint function.

Compression Injuries

Longitudinal compression forces across the elbow joint are absorbed mainly by bony contact; therefore, excessive compression forces at the elbow often result in bony failure. Falling on a pronated hand when the elbow is in a close-packed (extended) position may result in the transmission of forces through the distal radius and ulna to the elbow, leading to fractures of one or both bones depending on the direction of forces, or dislocation of the radial head **(Fig. 8–29)**. If the forces are transmitted through the radius, as may happen with a concomitant valgus stress, a fracture of the radial head may result from impact of the radial head on the capitulum. A fracture of the radial head can be accompanied by a tear of the central band of the interosseous membrane given that one of the functions of the interosseous membrane is to limit compressive forces at the radial head. The central band of the interosseous membrane has little physiological ability to heal, so such a tear may result in longitudinal instability of the radioulnar joints if the injuries are not addressed surgically.[126] If the force from the fall is transmitted to the ulna, a fracture of either the coronoid or olecranon processes may occur from the impact of the ulna on the humerus. If

Table 8–2 Effects of Aging on Elbow Muscles

HUGHES et al[119]	LYNCH et al[120]	GALLAGHER et al[121]	RUNNELS et al[122]
n = 68 women	n = 339 women	n = 60 men	n = 75
n = 52 men	n = 364 men		
Age 1st eval, 47–78 yr	Age 19–93 yr	Age 20–60 yr	Age 20–83 yr
Age 2nd eval, 56–88 yr			
Isokinetic strength in the elbow flexors and extensors declined by 2% per decade for women and 12% per decade for men.	Muscle quality (peak torque per unit of muscle mass) for concentric peak torque showed a 28% decrease in men and a 20% decrease in women. Eccentric peak torque showed a 25% decline in men, but the decline was not significant in women.	Active elbow flexion/extension peak torque, power, and angle of peak torque production measured bilaterally and showed highly significant differences between young and old. However, no age-related differences occurred in supination and pronation.	Isokinetic elbow flexor and extensor peak torque was less in men 60 to 83 years than in men 20 to 59 years. Maximal isometric force production also declined at age 60.

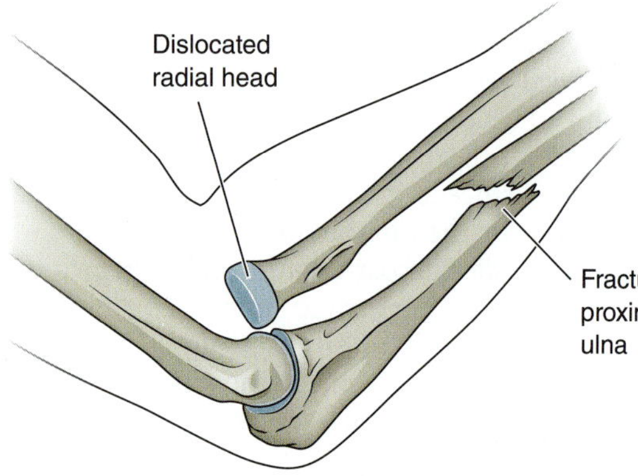

Figure 8–29 A fall on an outstretched hand with the elbow in extension (close-packed position) and the forearm pronated will result in the transmission of forces through the radius, the ulna, or both. When the force is sufficient, a common pattern is a fracture of the proximal ulna and anterior dislocation of the radial head.

neither the radius nor the ulna absorbs the excessive force by fracturing, then the force may be transmitted to the distal humerus. Elbow and forearm fractures account for about 5% of all fractures of the body and 30% of upper extremity fractures.[127] The incidence of fracture is relatively equal for the radius, ulna, and distal humerus. High-energy fractures to two or more of the bones with dislocations are more common with high-velocity injuries, such as what might occur in sports or motor vehicle crashes. The most common low-energy fracture (a fall on the hand from standing upright) occurs at the radial head.[128]

Clinical Application 8-2
Elbow Stability Throughout the ROM

The articular surfaces of the elbow joint, especially the humeroulnar joint, are highly congruent. This articular congruency is greatest when the elbow is in full flexion. As the elbow joint extends, it becomes less stable until it is "locked" in full extension with the olecranon process snug in the olecranon fossa of the posterior distal humerus. This bony congruency of the elbow in both full flexion and full extension is why the elbow is considered one of the most stable joints in the upper extremity. The ligaments and muscles provide static and dynamic stability to supplement the bony congruency. Following traumatic injury (e.g., dislocation or surgical repair) of the elbow, the elbow is typically fixed in 90° of flexion. However, fixing the joint in any one position for an extended period, upon release, is likely to show joint stiffness. Therefore, early sagittal plane ROM exercises are indicated to reduce joint stiffness, but they are performed within a limited arc or full arc to protect the healing structures. These ROM exercises are done with the patient in the supine position with the shoulder at 90° of flexion to support compression at the elbow joint. If the lateral collateral ligaments are healing, flexion and extension are performed with the forearm in full pronation. If the medial collateral ligaments are healing, flexion and extension are performed with the forearm in supination, and if both medial and lateral collateral ligament complexes are healing, flexion and extension are performed with the forearm placed in neutral.

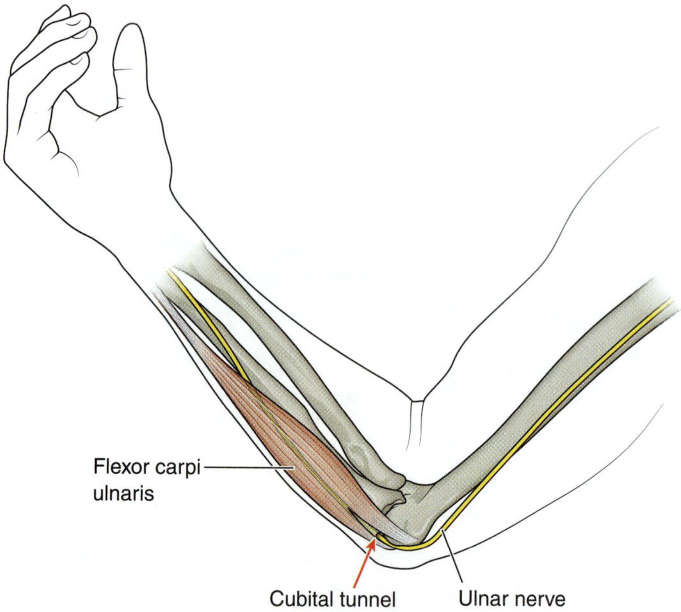

Figure 8–30 Ulnar nerve in the right cubital tunnel. The ulnar nerve passes through the cubital tunnel formed by the two heads of the flexor carpi ulnaris muscle. A contraction of the flexor carpi ulnaris muscle can cause compression of the ulnar nerve between the two heads of the muscle, which are located on either side of the ulnar nerve at the elbow.

Muscle contractions also may cause high-compression forces at the elbow. For example, during the acceleration and deceleration phases of baseball pitching, the compression forces at the elbow can reach 90% of body weight.[129] Repetitive forceful contractions of the flexor/pronator muscle group of the medial elbow may result in ulnar nerve irritation, medial elbow tendinopathy, and medial collateral ligament tears or attenuation. These conditions are commonly referred to as *thrower's elbow*.[14,130] In overhead throwers, pronator/supinator muscle groups are usually hypertrophied. Consequently, with repetitive throwing, the ulnar nerve may be compressed as it passes through the cubital tunnel between the medial epicondyle of the humerus and olecranon process of the ulna **(Fig. 8–30)**.[131] Nerve compression may be worsened with increasing elbow flexion because both the cubital tunnel and ulnar nerve cross sections decrease with increased flexion.[132]

Patient Application 8–4

Margaret Blevins is a 46-year-old nurse who slipped backward on a wet floor and attempted to cushion the fall with her right hand extended behind her. She immediately noted pain in her right wrist and elbow, but she did not report the injury until the end of her shift. She was seen by an occupational health nurse practitioner who referred her to physical therapy the next day with a diagnosis of an elbow contusion (bruise). Upon examination in physical therapy, the patient reported right lateral elbow pain and was holding her right elbow in a flexed position. She was found to have noticeable swelling at the joint line and tenderness at the joint with palpation. Patients will typically attempt to reduce this joint pain by assuming a position of about 80° of flexion, considered to be the elbow position at which the least amount of tension is present in the joint capsule.[132] Therefore, it is a position of relative comfort for patients with intra-articular swelling. The patient in this case was referred for imaging that revealed an intra-articular radial head fracture. The patient was subsequently placed in an immobilizer to allow the radial head fracture to heal.

Distraction Injuries

Both ligaments and muscles at the elbow provide resistance to longitudinal tensile (distraction) forces placed on the forearm. A tensile force of sufficient magnitude exerted on an extended forearm may cause the radius to be pulled inferiorly out of the annular ligament leading to a distraction injury or subluxation of the radial head. This injury is most likely to occur in children younger than 5 years, affecting females more than males.[133,134] The predominance in young children is attributed to the laxity or elasticity of the annular ligament common in childhood. Lifting or swinging a small child up into the air by one or both hands or yanking a child's arm by the hand, especially when the tug isn't anticipated by the child, are the usual causative mechanisms, with the injury referred to as **nursemaid's elbow** or *pulled elbow* **(Fig. 8–31)**.[133,134]

Varus/Valgus Injuries (Thrower's Elbow)

Valgus and varus stresses at the elbow occur in many activities. When such stresses occur, one side of the joint is subjected to distraction forces whereas the other side is subjected to compression forces. In the more commonly occurring valgus stress at the elbow, the radial head and capitulum are compressed while the proximal ulna and trochlea are distracted **(Fig. 8–32)**. With repeated valgus stresses, the medial collateral ligament may become overstretched or torn, which then allows greater distraction medially and results in even greater compression between the radial head and capitulum. The opposite circumstances will occur with the less common varus stresses at the elbow.

During the backswing or "cocking" phase of pitching a baseball **(Fig. 8–33)**, the stress on the medial collateral ligament is repetitive, leading to ligamentous laxity and inability of the ligament to reinforce the medial aspect of the joint.[110] The resulting medial laxity may cause an increase in the normal carrying angle and excessive compression between the radial head and capitulum.[135] If the abnormal compression forces are prolonged, these forces may interfere with the blood supply of the humeroradial joint cartilage and result in **avascular necrosis** of the capitulum.[110]

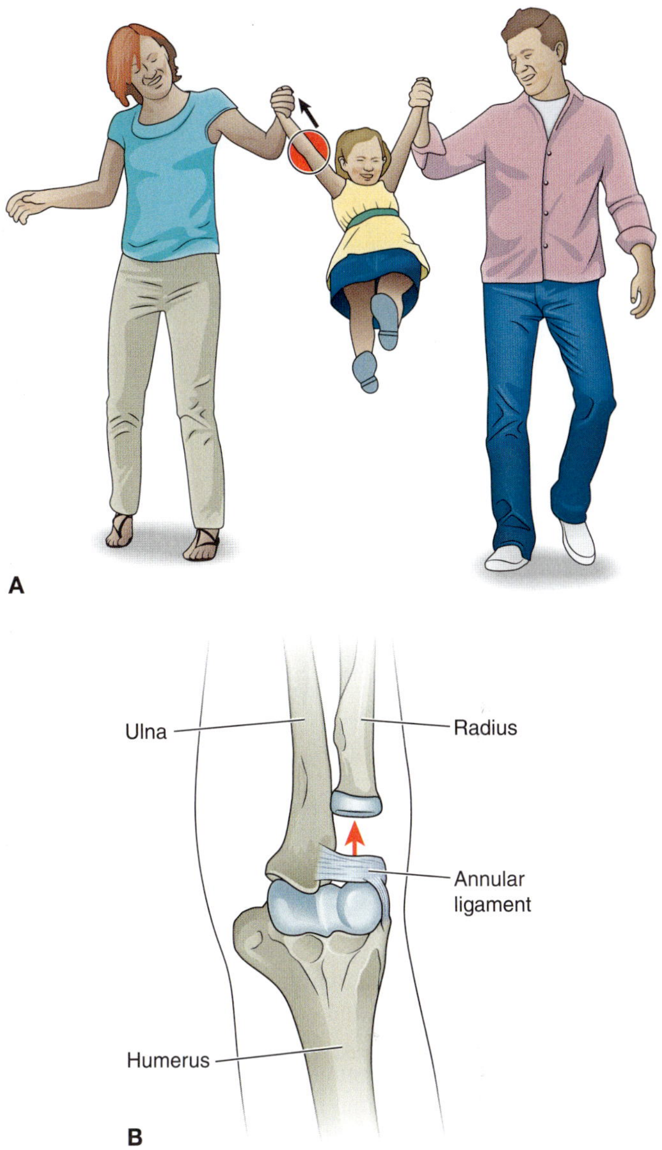

Figure 8–31 Nursemaid's elbow. **A.** An upward longitudinal force on the child's hands can create distraction at the humeroradial joint. **B.** The right radial head can slip out of the annular ligament, especially if the child is relaxed and the active muscle forces crossing the elbow are not producing an offsetting joint compression.

Patient Application 8–5

Steve Cho is a 13-year-old boy who joined two baseball teams during the summer to practice his pitching on a more frequent basis. Three weeks into the summer season, Steve noticed medial elbow soreness in his throwing arm after pitching and that his pitching velocity and control were declining. When the elbow became painful with casual throwing of the ball, his parents sought medical advice. Palpation along the medial collateral ligament of the elbow was painful. Excessive laxity was found with a valgus stress applied to the elbow in comparison with his nonthrowing arm; the valgus stress reproduced the sharp pain that he was experiencing during pitching. It was determined that Steve had sprained (developed microtears in) his medial collateral ligament, so he was pulled out of the pitching rotation until complete healing occurred.

This scenario is very common as evidenced by the substantial increase in the number of youth baseball players seeking medical attention for elbow injuries, specifically medial collateral ligament sprains and tears.[136] This has led to recommendations and guidelines for youth baseball pitchers regarding pitch count limits and rest recommendations.[137]

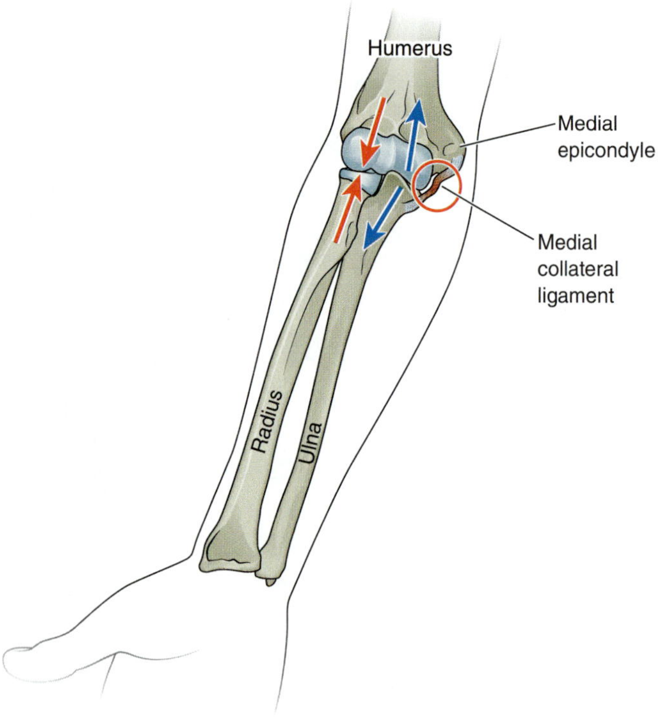

Figure 8–32 Valgus injuries. The application of a valgus stress across the elbow joint produces compression at the humeroradial joint and distraction at the humeroulnar joint. With repeated valgus stress, the medial collateral ligament that ordinarily checks joint distraction may become stretched and inflamed.

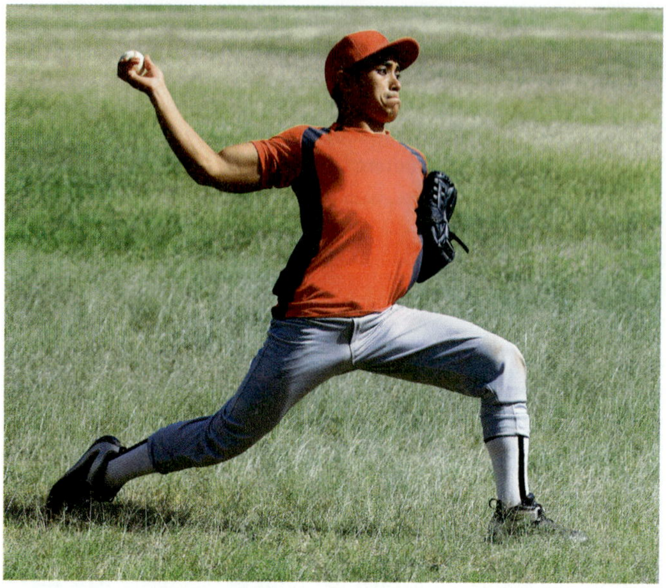

Figure 8–33 During the cocking phase of a baseball pitch, the valgus stress on the elbow is high. Repetitive valgus stresses to the elbow of a pitcher may lead to laxity or inflammation of the medial collateral ligament and elbow joint instability. *(sonofpioneer/iStock/Thinkstock)*

Garrison and colleagues examined baseball players who were diagnosed with a medial collateral ligament tear and compared these players with age- and position-matched healthy control players.[138,139] Their studies suggest that alterations in motion, strength, or proximal motor control are associated with medial collateral ligament injury, most likely due to an increased valgus stress at the elbow.

Peripheral Nerve Injuries

The elbow has amongst the highest incidences of peripheral nerve injuries in the body.[140] Factors such as superficial positioning of nerves, unique anatomic structures, trauma (fractures/dislocations), and common repetitive stress to the elbow make the nerves susceptible to injury. Classic examples of peripheral entrapments around the elbow are associated with repetitive or excessive valgus stress to the ulnar nerve with throwing, or a compressive stress to the median nerve from repetitive gripping or forceful repeated pronation, such as when using a screwdriver.[136,141,142] Even simple activities such as resting an elbow on the armrest or back of a chair for a prolonged period of time can result in localized nerve ischemia to the ulnar or radial nerves, respectively.

Patient Application 8–6

Nijee Warfield, a 21-year-old college student, visited the emergency department with reports of wrist weakness and forearm pain upon waking, but without a contributory history. The patient was referred to the physical therapist for consultation and key objective findings were as follows:

- Localized tenderness with palpation to the radial tunnel on the dorsal aspect of his forearm
- Only trace ability to activate his wrist extensors
- Negative cervical provocation

Upon further inquiry, Nijee admitted to waking up in an "awkward" position in which his head was resting on his forearm without a pillow. He was diagnosed with radial nerve entrapment, also known as "Saturday night palsy," and was discharged home with a splint and instructions for self-management.[143]

Neuropathies are traditionally diagnosed on the basis of the findings from the clinical history, physical examination, and electrodiagnostic study.[144] Other pathologies, such as tendinopathies, collateral ligament pathology, and arthritic changes, can mimic peripheral neuropathies around the elbow and must be ruled out during the examination process.

A "double crush" syndrome refers to multiple sites of compression along the course of a peripheral nerve. Individually, each mechanical stress is not enough to produce symptoms, but collectively can result in clinical findings. A thorough examination throughout the length of the nerve, from cervical spine to terminal nerve ending, is needed to appropriately diagnose these neuropathies.[145] It is generally considered that the ulnar nerve is most susceptible to injury at the elbow. Refer to Table 8–3 for a list of common elbow entrapments and mechanical causes.

Table 8–3 Common Sites of Peripheral Nerve Injuries of the Elbow

NERVE	LOCATION(S) OF ENTRAPMENT	MECHANISM OF INJURY	SYMPTOMS
Ulnar	Cubital tunnel (cubital tunnel syndrome)	• Prolonged compression (resting medial elbow on armrest or table • Traction (excessive valgus stress during throwing) • Overuse (repeated/prolonged flexion, sleeping in the fetal position) • Medial epicondyle fracture (direct trauma or prolonged flexion in brace)	• Aching/pain along the medial elbow • Motor and sensory changes in the ulnar nerve distribution of forearm and hand that may affect grasp and prehension
Median	Proximal entrapment (biceps aponeurosis or pronator teres)	Compression injury due to forceful contraction of biceps such as in weight-lifting or rowing Compression injury (pronator syndrome) due to repetitive pronation or traction injury from repetitive supination associated with hypertrophy of the pronator muscle bellies	Proximal anterior forearm ache/pain and sensory changes in the median nerve distribution without nocturnal pain of the wrist common to carpal tunnel syndrome Motor changes rare
	Median nerve in forearm	Related to ulna and/or radius fractures throughout length of bones due to compression or traction forces	Motor changes to hand intrinsics to thumb or lumbricals affecting prehension Sensory loss in median nerve distribution of hand
	Anterior interosseous nerve (proximal edge of flexor digitorum superficialis)	Direct compression or traction with fracture Iatrogenic injection (needlestick) with IV or blood collection in cubital fossa	Dull ache in proximal to mid anterior forearm Weakness of the flexor pollicis longus and/or index flexor digitorum profundus; inability to make OK sign with thumb and index finger
Radial	Radial tunnel syndrome—posterior interosseous branch (supinator muscle, arcade of Frohse)	• Forceful repetitive forearm pronation/supination (manual stirring action of viscous substance) • Direct compression or traction associated with fall or fractures to radius and distal 1/3 of humerus • Direct pressure to proximal posterior forearm	• Proximal dorsal forearm pain distal to the lateral epicondyle including the dorsum of wrist • Motor changes–weakness for digit extensors
	High radial nerve–(Saturday night palsy)	• Prolonged position of the upper extremity away from the trunk (traction) such as the back of a chair or arm position to clear the trunk for surgery	• Arm and forearm pain • Motor changes–weakness may include triceps, wrist and digit extensors, supinator

Sources: Data from Latinovic R, Gulliford MC, Hughes RA: Incidence of common compressive neuropathies in primary care. J Neurol Neurosurg Psychiatry 77:263-5, 2006; Andreisek G, Crook DW, Burg D, et al: Peripheral neuropathies of the median, radial, and ulnar nerves: MR imaging features. Radiographics 26:1267-87, 2006; Miller TT, Reinus WR: Nerve entrapment syndromes of the elbow, forearm, and wrist. AJR Am J Roentgenol 195:585-94, 2010

SUMMARY

- The interrelationship between the elbow complex and the wrist and hand complex makes normal functioning of the elbow vitally important. If elbow function is impaired, function of the hand or joints, such as the shoulder and trunk, may be impaired as well. For example, if the elbow cannot be flexed, it is impossible for the hand to bring food to the mouth. Alternatively, if the shoulder is limited in motion, then injury related to increased valgus stress at the elbow may result.
- Because many important vascular and neural structures that supply the hand are closely associated with the elbow, it is important to prevent excessive stress and to protect the elbow from injury. If the radial nerve is injured at the level of the epicondyle, the wrist extensors, supinator, and thumb and finger extensors will be affected. If the median nerve is injured at the level of the elbow, the pronators, flexor carpi radialis, finger flexors, thenar muscles, and lumbricals will be affected. In the following chapter, we will discuss the specific functions of the hand muscles and will be better able to appreciate the significance of injury to some of the muscles associated with the elbow complex.
- Some of the interrelationships between the structure and function of the elbow, shoulder, wrist, and hand have been introduced in this chapter. Muscles that have their primary

actions at the wrist and hand also cross the elbow and contribute to its stability and function, whereas the stability and ROM at the shoulder and elbow help to enhance the function of the wrist and hand.

- Compensations at the elbow complex often are necessary when the ROM is limited at the shoulder or wrist. New relationships for the joints and muscles of the upper extremity will be introduced in the detailed study of the wrist and hand that follows in the next chapter.

STUDY QUESTIONS

1. Name and locate all of the articulating surfaces of the joints of the elbow complex and describe the method of articulation at each joint, including axes of motion and degrees of freedom.
2. Describe the articulation at the humeroradial joint between the radial head, capitulum, and annular ligament in supination and pronation, with the elbow flexed and extended.
3. Explain the stabilizing function of the brachioradialis by diagramming the translatory and rotatory components for this muscle at different elbow joint angles.
4. Explain why active elbow flexion is more limited than passive flexion. Which structures limit extension?
5. Describe the "carrying angle" of the elbow and explain why it is present.
6. Which structures limit supination and pronation?
7. If slow pronation of the forearm is attempted without resistance, which muscle(s) will be used?
8. How does the structure and function of the annular ligament differ from that of the other elbow joint ligaments?
9. Describe the activity of the biceps brachii during the entirety of a chin-up exercise and the activity of the triceps during the entirety of a push-up exercise.
10. Describe a common mechanism of injury in what is commonly called *tennis elbow*.
11. Provide a rationale for evaluating joints proximal to the elbow when treating lateral epicondylalgia.
12. Explain why the term *tendinopathy* may be a more appropriate diagnostic term than *epicondylitis* for tennis elbow.
13. Compare the medial and lateral collateral ligaments based on structure and function.
14. Compare the biceps brachii and the brachialis based on structure and function.
15. Explain the function of the interosseous membrane.
16. What ligaments provide primary support to the distal radioulnar joint?
17. In what position(s) of the shoulder, elbow, and forearm might you expect the biceps brachii to be passively insufficient? What is the consequence of that passive insufficiency?
18. What is the role of the triangular fibrocartilage at the distal radioulnar joint?

REFERENCES

1. Sardelli M, Tashjian RZ, MacWilliams BA: Functional elbow range of motion for contemporary tasks. J Bone Joint Surg Am 93:471-7, 2011
2. An KN, Hui FC, Morrey BF, et al: Muscles across the elbow joint: a biomechanical analysis. J Biomech 14:659-69, 1981
3. Reichel LM, Morales OA: Gross anatomy of the elbow capsule: a cadaveric study. J Hand Surg Am 38:110-6, 2013
4. Morrey BF: Posttraumatic stiffness: distraction arthroplasty. Orthopedics 15:863-9, 1992
5. Lockard M: Clinical biomechanics of the elbow. J Hand Ther 19:72-80, 2006
6. Standring S: Gray's Anatomy: The Anatomical Basis of Clinical Practice (ed 42). New York, NY, Elsevier Health Sciences, 2020
7. Eckstein F, Lohe F, Muller-Gerbl M, et al: Stress distribution in the trochlear notch: a model of bicentric load transmission through joints. J Bone Joint Surg Br 76:647-53, 1994
8. Eckstein F, Lohe F, Hillebrand S, et al: Morphomechanics of the humero-ulnar joint: I. Joint space width and contact areas as a function of load and flexion angle. Anat Rec 243:318-26, 1995
9. Eckstein F, Merz B, Muller-Gerbl M, et al: Morphomechanics of the humero-ulnar joint: II. Concave incongruity determines the distribution of load and subchondral mineralization. Anat Rec 243:327-35, 1995
10. Milz S, Eckstein F, Putz R: Thickness distribution of the subchondral mineralization zone of the trochlear notch and its correlation with the cartilage thickness: an expression of functional adaptation to mechanical stress acting on the humeroulnar joint? Anat Rec 248:189-97, 1997
11. Putz R, Milz S, Maier M, et al: Functional morphology of the elbow joint. Orthopade 32:684-90, 2003
12. Duparc F, Putz R, Michot C, et al: The synovial fold of the humeroradial joint: anatomical and histological features, and clinical relevance in lateral epicondylalgia of the elbow. Surg Radiol Anat 24:302-7, 2002
13. Cerezal L, Rodriguez-Sammartino M, Canga A, et al: Elbow synovial fold syndrome. AJR Am J Roentgenol 201:W88-96, 2013
14. Cain EL, Jr, Dugas JR, Wolf RS, et al: Elbow injuries in throwing athletes: a current concepts review. Am J Sports Med 31:621-35, 2003
15. Callaway GH, Field LD, Deng XH, et al: Biomechanical evaluation of the medial collateral ligament of the elbow. J Bone Joint Surg Am 79:1223-31, 1997
16. Dugas JR, Ostrander RV, Cain EL, et al: Anatomy of the anterior bundle of the ulnar collateral ligament. J Shoulder Elbow Surg 16:657-60, 2007
17. Fuss FK: The ulnar collateral ligament of the human elbow joint. Anatomy, function and biomechanics. J Anat 175:203-12, 1991
18. Jones KJ, Osbahr DC, Schrumpf MA, et al: Ulnar collateral ligament reconstruction in throwing athletes: a review of current concepts. AAOS exhibit selection. J Bone Joint Surg Am 94:e49, 2012
19. Milz S, Tischer T, Buettner A, et al: Molecular composition and pathology of entheses on the medial and lateral epicondyles of the humerus: a structural basis for epicondylitis. Ann Rheum Dis 63:1015-21, 2004
20. Regan WD, Korinek SL, Morrey BF, et al: Biomechanical study of ligaments around the elbow joint. Clin Orthop Relat Res:170-9, 1991
21. Benjamin M, Toumi H, Ralphs JR, et al: Where tendons and ligaments meet bone: attachment sites ('entheses') in relation to exercise and/or mechanical load. J Anat 208:471-90, 2006
22. Petrie S, Collins JG, Solomonow M, et al: Mechanoreceptors in the human elbow ligaments. J Hand Surg Am 23:512-8, 1998
23. Sojbjerg JO, Ovesen J, Nielsen S: Experimental elbow instability after transection of the medial collateral ligament. Clin Orthop Relat Res: 186-90, 1987
24. Ahmad CS, ElAttrache NS: Elbow valgus instability in the throwing athlete. J Am Acad Orthop Surg 14:693-700, 2006
25. Hassan SE, Parks BG, Douoguih WA, et al: Effect of distal ulnar collateral ligament tear pattern on contact forces and valgus stability in the posteromedial compartment of the elbow. Am J Sports Med 43:447-52, 2015
26. Gurbuz H, Kutoglu T, Mesut R, et al: Anatomical dimensions of anterior bundle of ulnar collateral ligament and its role in elbow stability. Folia Med (Plovdiv) 47:47-52, 2005
27. Safran MR, McGarry MH, Shin S, et al: Effects of elbow flexion and forearm rotation on valgus laxity of the elbow. J Bone Joint Surg Am 87:2065-74, 2005
28. Chantelot C, Wavreille G, Dos Remedios C, et al: Intra-articular compressive stress of the elbow joint in extension: an experimental study using Fuji films. Surg Radiol Anat 30:103-11, 2008
29. Reichel LM, Milam GS, Sitton SE, et al: Elbow lateral collateral ligament injuries. J Hand Surg Am 38:184-201; quiz 201, 2013
30. Seki A, Olsen BS, Jensen SL, et al: Functional anatomy of the lateral collateral ligament complex of the elbow: configuration of Y and its role. J Shoulder Elbow Surg 11:53-9, 2002
31. Imatani J, Ogura T, Morito Y, et al: Anatomic and histologic studies of lateral collateral ligament complex of the elbow joint. J Shoulder Elbow Surg 8:625-7, 1999
32. Wavreille G, Seraphin J, Chantelot C, et al: Ligament fibre recruitment of the elbow joint during gravity-loaded passive motion: an experimental study. Clin Biomech (Bristol) 23:193-202, 2008

33. Morrey BF, An KN: Articular and ligamentous contributions to the stability of the elbow joint. Am J Sports Med 11:315-9, 1983
34. Karbach LE, Elfar J: Elbow instability: anatomy, biomechanics, diagnostic maneuvers, and testing. J Hand Surg Am 42:118-26, 2017
35. O'Driscoll SW: Elbow instability. Acta Orthop Belg 65:404-15, 1999
36. Olsen BS, Sojbjerg JO, Nielsen KK, et al: Posterolateral elbow joint instability: the basic kinematics. J Shoulder Elbow Surg 7:19-29, 1998
37. Kim PT, Isogai S, Murakami G, et al: The lateral collateral ligament complex and related muscles act as a dynamic stabilizer as well as a static supporting structure at the elbow joint: an anatomical and experimental study. Okajimas Folia Anat Jpn 79:55-61, 2002
38. Olsen BS, Sojbjerg JO, Dalstra M, et al: Kinematics of the lateral ligamentous constraints of the elbow joint. J Shoulder Elbow Surg 5:333-41, 1996
39. Dunning CE, Zarzour ZD, Patterson SD, et al: Ligamentous stabilizers against posterolateral rotatory instability of the elbow. J Bone Joint Surg Am 83:1823-8, 2001
40. Ball CM, Galatz LM, Yamaguchi K: Elbow instability: treatment strategies and emerging concepts. Instr Course Lect 51:53-61, 2002
41. McKee MD, Schemitsch EH, Sala MJ, et al: The pathoanatomy of lateral ligamentous disruption in complex elbow instability. J Shoulder Elbow Surg 12:391-6, 2003
42. Benjamin M, Kumai T, Milz S, et al: The skeletal attachment of tendons—tendon "entheses." Comp Biochem Physiol A Mol Integr Physiol 133:931-45, 2002
43. Fredberg U, Stengaard-Pedersen K: Chronic tendinopathy tissue pathology, pain mechanisms, and etiology with a special focus on inflammation. Scand J Med Sci Sports 18:3-15, 2008
44. Lucado AM, Day JM, Vincent JI, et al: Lateral elbow pain and muscle function impairments. J Orthop Sports Phys Ther 52:CPG1-CPG111, 2022
45. Faro F, Wolf JM: Lateral epicondylitis: review and current concepts. J Hand Surg Am 32:1271-9, 2007
46. Bunata RE, Brown DS, Capelo R: Anatomic factors related to the cause of tennis elbow. J Bone Joint Surg Am 89:1955-63, 2007
47. Bales CP, Placzek JD, Malone KJ, et al: Microvascular supply of the lateral epicondyle and common extensor origin. J Shoulder Elbow Surg 16:497-501, 2007
48. Schneeberger AG, Masquelet AC: Arterial vascularization of the proximal extensor carpi radialis brevis tendon. Clin Orthop Relat Res:239-44, 2002
49. Youm Y, Dryer RF, Thambyrajah K, et al: Biomechanical analyses of forearm pronation-supination and elbow flexion-extension. J Biomech 12:245-55, 1979
50. Deland JT, Garg A, Walker PS: Biomechanical basis for elbow hinge-distractor design. Clin Orthop Relat Res:303-12, 1987
51. Ericson A, Arndt A, Stark A, et al: Variation in the position and orientation of the elbow flexion axis. J Bone Joint Surg Br 85:538-44, 2003
52. Duck TR, Dunning CE, King GJ, et al: Variability and repeatability of the flexion axis at the ulnohumeral joint. J Orthop Res 21:399-404, 2003
53. Bottlang M, Madey SM, Steyers CM, et al: Assessment of elbow joint kinematics in passive motion by electromagnetic motion tracking. J Orthop Res 18:195-202, 2000
54. Randsborg PH: Elbow fractures in children remain a challenge: commentary on an article by Noora Vallila, MD, et al.: "Pediatric distal humeral fractures and complications of treatment in Finland: a review of compensation claims from 1990 through 2010." J Bone Joint Surg Am 97:e34, 2015
55. Khare GN, Goel SC, Saraf SK, et al: New observations on carrying angle. Indian J Med Sci 53:61-7, 1999
56. Golden DW, Jhee JT, Gilpin SP, et al: Elbow range of motion and clinical carrying angle in a healthy pediatric population. J Pediatr Orthop B 16:144-9, 2007
57. Golden DW, Wojcicki JM, Jhee JT, et al: Body mass index and elbow range of motion in a healthy pediatric population: a possible mechanism of overweight in children. J Pediatr Gastroenterol Nutr 46:196-201, 2008
58. Balasubramanian P, Madhuri V, Muliyil J: Carrying angle in children: a normative study. J Pediatr Orthop B 15:37-40, 2006
59. Zwerus EL, Willigenburg NW, Scholtes VA, et al: Normative values and affecting factors for the elbow range of motion. Shoulder Elbow 11:215-24, 2019
60. McGuigan FX, Bookout CB: Intra-articular fluid volume and restricted motion in the elbow. J Shoulder Elbow Surg 12:462-5, 2003
61. Murray WM, Delp SL, Buchanan TS: Variation of muscle moment arms with elbow and forearm position. J Biomech 28:513-25, 1995
62. Murray WM, Buchanan TS, Delp SL: The isometric functional capacity of muscles that cross the elbow. J Biomech 33:943-52, 2000
63. Kasprisin JE, Grabiner MD: Joint angle-dependence of elbow flexor activation levels during isometric and isokinetic maximum voluntary contractions. Clin Biomech (Bristol) 15:743-9, 2000
64. Nakazawa K, Kawakami Y, Fukunaga T, et al: Differences in activation patterns in elbow flexor muscles during isometric, concentric and eccentric contractions. Eur J Appl Physiol Occup Physiol 66:214-20, 1993
65. Naito A, Sun YJ, Yajima M, et al: Electromyographic study of the elbow flexors and extensors in a motion of forearm pronation/supination while maintaining elbow flexion in humans. Tohoku J Exp Med 186:267-77, 1998
66. Provins KA, Salter N: Maximum torque exerted about the elbow joint. J Appl Physiol 7:393-8, 1955
67. Currier DP: Maximal isometric tension of the elbow extensors at varied positions. I. Assessment by cable tensiometer. Phys Ther 52:1043-9, 1972
68. Bohannon RW: Shoulder position influences elbow extension force in healthy individuals. J Orthop Sports Phys Ther 12:111-4, 1990
69. Zhang LQ, Nuber GW: Moment distribution among human elbow extensor muscles during isometric and submaximal extension. J Biomech 33:145-54, 2000
70. Molinier F, Laffosse JM, Bouali O, et al: The anconeus, an active lateral ligament of the elbow: new anatomical arguments. Surg Radiol Anat 33:617-21, 2011
71. Prodoehl J, Gottlieb GL, Corcos DM: The neural control of single degree-of-freedom elbow movements: effect of starting joint position. Exp Brain Res 153:7-15, 2003
72. Lees VC: Functional anatomy of the distal radioulnar joint in health and disease. Ann R Coll Surg Engl 95:163-70, 2013
73. Mohiuddin A, Janjua MZ: Form and function of radioulnar articular disc. Hand 14:61-6, 1982
74. Linscheid RL: Biomechanics of the distal radioulnar joint. Clin Orthop Relat Res:46-55, 1992
75. Mikic ZD: Detailed anatomy of the articular disc of the distal radioulnar joint. Clin Orthop Relat Res:123-32, 1989
76. Chidgey LK, Dell PC, Bittar ES, et al: Histologic anatomy of the triangular fibrocartilage. J Hand Surg Am 16:1084-100, 1991
77. Sachar K: Ulnar-sided wrist pain: evaluation and treatment of triangular fibrocartilage complex tears, ulnocarpal impaction syndrome, and lunotriquetral ligament tears. J Hand Surg Am 37:1489-500, 2012
78. Ohmori M, Azuma H: Morphology and distribution of nerve endings in the human triangular fibrocartilage complex. J Hand Surg Br 23:522-5, 1998
79. Noda K, Goto A, Murase T, et al: Interosseous membrane of the forearm: an anatomical study of ligament attachment locations. J Hand Surg Am 34:415-22, 2009
80. Moritomo H: The distal interosseous membrane: current concepts in wrist anatomy and biomechanics. J Hand Surg Am 37:1501-7, 2012
81. Pfaeffle HJ, Fischer KJ, Manson TT, et al: Role of the forearm interosseous ligament: is it more than just longitudinal load transfer? J Hand Surg Am 25:683-8, 2000
82. Skahen JR, 3rd, Palmer AK, Werner FW, et al: The interosseous membrane of the forearm: anatomy and function. J Hand Surg Am 22:981-5, 1997
83. Pfaeffle HJ, Tomaino MM, Grewal R, et al: Tensile properties of the interosseous membrane of the human forearm. J Orthop Res 14:842-5, 1996
84. Nakamura T, Yabe Y, Horiuchi Y, et al: Normal kinematics of the interosseous membrane during forearm pronation-supination—a three-dimensional MRI study. Hand Surg 5:1-10, 2000
85. Johnson RK, Shrewsbury MM: The pronator quadratus in motions and in stabilization of the radius and ulna at the distal radioulnar joint. J Hand Surg Am 1:205-9, 1976
86. Palmer AK, Werner FW: Biomechanics of the distal radioulnar joint. Clin Orthop Relat Res:26-35, 1984
87. Shaaban H, Giakas G, Bolton M, et al: Contact area inside the distal radioulnar joint: effect of axial loading and position of the forearm. Clin Biomech (Bristol) 22:313-8, 2007
88. Palmer AK: The distal radioulnar joint. Orthop Clin North Am 15:321-35, 1984
89. Shaaban H, Pereira C, Williams R, et al: The effect of elbow position on the range of supination and pronation of the forearm. J Hand Surg Eur Vol 33:3-8, 2008
90. Haugstvedt JR, Berger RA, Berglund LJ: A mechanical study of the moment—forces of the supinators and pronators of the forearm. Acta Orthop Scand 72:629-34, 2001
91. Bremer AK, Sennwald GR, Favre P, et al: Moment arms of forearm rotators. Clin Biomech (Bristol) 21:683-91, 2006
92. O'Sullivan LW, Gallwey TJ: Upper-limb surface electromyography at maximum supination and pronation torques: the effect of elbow and forearm angle. J Electromyogr Kinesiol 12:275-85, 2002
93. Gordon KD, Pardo RD, Johnson JA, et al: Electromyographic activity and strength during maximum isometric pronation and supination efforts in healthy adults. J Orthop Res 22:208-13, 2004
94. Stuart PR: Pronator quadratus revisited. J Hand Surg Br 21:714-22, 1996

95. Van der Heijden EP, Hillen B: A two-dimensional kinematic analysis of the distal radioulnar joint. J Hand Surg Br 21:824-9, 1996
96. Askew LJ, An KN, Morrey BF, et al: Isometric elbow strength in normal individuals. Clin Orthop Relat Res:261-6, 1987
97. Haahr JP, Andersen JH: Prognostic factors in lateral epicondylitis: a randomized trial with one-year follow-up in 266 new cases treated with minimal occupational intervention or the usual approach in general practice. Rheumatology (Oxford) 42:1216-25, 2003
98. af Ekenstam F: Anatomy of the distal radioulnar joint. Clin Orthop Relat Res:14-8, 1992
99. Birkbeck DP, Failla JM, Hoshaw SJ, et al: The interosseous membrane affects load distribution in the forearm. J Hand Surg Am 22:975-80, 1997
100. DeFrate LE, Li G, Zayontz SJ, et al: A minimally invasive method for the determination of force in the interosseous ligament. Clin Biomech (Bristol) 16:895-900, 2001
101. Shaaban H, Giakas G, Bolton M, et al: The load-bearing characteristics of the forearm: pattern of axial and bending force transmitted through ulna and radius. J Hand Surg Br 31:274-9, 2006
102. Markolf KL, Lamey D, Yang S, et al: Radioulnar load-sharing in the forearm: a study in cadavera. J Bone Joint Surg Am 80:879-88, 1998
103. Schuind F, An KN, Berglund L, et al: The distal radioulnar ligaments: a biomechanical study. J Hand Surg Am 16:1106-14, 1991
104. Bade H, Koebke J, Schluter M: Morphology of the articular surfaces of the distal radio-ulnar joint. Anat Rec 246:410-4, 1996
105. Adams BD, Holley KA: Strains in the articular disk of the triangular fibrocartilage complex: a biomechanical study. J Hand Surg Am 18:919-25, 1993
106. Schmidt HM: The anatomy of the ulnocarpal complex. Orthopade 33:628-37, 2004
107. Morrey BF, Askew LJ, Chao EY: A biomechanical study of normal functional elbow motion. J Bone Joint Surg Am 63:872-7, 1981
108. Magermans DJ, Chadwick EK, Veeger HE, et al: Requirements for upper extremity motions during activities of daily living. Clin Biomech (Bristol) 20:591-9, 2005
109. Safaee-Rad R, Shwedyk E, Quanbury AO, et al: Normal functional range of motion of upper limb joints during performance of three feeding activities. Arch Phys Med Rehabil 71:505-9, 1990
110. Drobner WS, Hausman MR: The distal radioulnar joint. Hand Clin 8:631-44, 1992
111. Davidson PA, Pink M, Perry J, et al: Functional anatomy of the flexor pronator muscle group in relation to the medial collateral ligament of the elbow. Am J Sports Med 23:245-50, 1995
112. Lin F, Kohli N, Perlmutter S, et al: Muscle contribution to elbow joint valgus stability. J Shoulder Elbow Surg 16:795-802, 2007
113. Cheng JC, Wing-Man K, Shen WY, et al: A new look at the sequential development of elbow-ossification centers in children. J Pediatr Orthop 18:161-7, 1998
114. Patel B, Reed M, Patel S: Gender-specific pattern differences of the ossification centers in the pediatric elbow. Pediatr Radiol 39:226-31, 2009
115. Leahy I, Schorpion M, Ganley T: Common medial elbow injuries in the adolescent athlete. J Hand Ther 28:201-10; quiz 211, 2015
116. Wood LE, Dixon S, Grant C, et al: Isokinetic elbow torque development in children. Int J Sports Med 29:466-70, 2008
117. Deighan M, De Ste Croix M, Grant C, et al: Measurement of maximal muscle cross-sectional area of the elbow extensors and flexors in children, teenagers and adults. J Sports Sci 24:543-6, 2006
118. Tonson A, Ratel S, Le Fur Y, et al: Effect of maturation on the relationship between muscle size and force production. Med Sci Sports Exerc 40:918-25, 2008
119. Hughes VA, Frontera WR, Wood M, et al: Longitudinal muscle strength changes in older adults: influence of muscle mass, physical activity, and health. J Gerontol A Biol Sci Med Sci 56:B209-17, 2001
120. Lynch NA, Metter EJ, Lindle RS, et al: Muscle quality. I. Age-associated differences between arm and leg muscle groups. J Appl Physiol (1985) 86:188-94, 1999
121. Gallagher MA, Cuomo F, Polonsky L, et al: Effects of age, testing speed, and arm dominance on isokinetic strength of the elbow. J Shoulder Elbow Surg 6:340-6, 1997
122. Runnels ED, Bemben DA, Anderson MA, et al: Influence of age on isometric, isotonic, and isokinetic force production characteristics in men. J Geriatr Phys Ther 28:74-84, 2005
123. John EB, Liu W, Gregory RW: Biomechanics of muscular effort: age-related changes. Med Sci Sports Exerc 41:418-25, 2009
124. Valour D, Pousson M: Compliance changes of the series elastic component of elbow flexor muscles with age in humans. Pflugers Arch 445:721-7, 2003
125. Toji H, Kaneko M: Effects of aging on force, velocity, and power in the elbow flexors of males. J Physiol Anthropol 26:587-92, 2007
126. Murray PM: Diagnosis and treatment of longitudinal instability of the forearm. Tech Hand Up Extrem Surg 9:29-34, 2005
127. Ennis O, Miller D, Kelly CP: (v) Fractures of the adult elbow. Curr Orthop 22:111-31, 2008
128. Duckworth AD, Clement ND, Jenkins PJ, et al: The epidemiology of radial head and neck fractures. J Hand Surg Am 37:112-9, 2012
129. Werner SL, Fleisig GS, Dillman CJ, et al: Biomechanics of the elbow during baseball pitching. J Orthop Sports Phys Ther 17:274-8, 1993
130. Patel RM, Lynch TS, Amin NH, et al: The thrower's elbow. Orthop Clin North Am 45:355-76, 2014
131. Dowdle SB, Chalmers PN: Management of the ulnar nerve in throwing athletes. Curr Rev Musculoskelet Med 13:449-56, 2020
132. Green JR, Jr, Rayan GM: The cubital tunnel: anatomic, histologic, and biomechanical study. J Shoulder Elbow Surg 8:466-70, 1999
133. Mohd Miswan MF, Othman MS, Muhamad Effendi F, et al: Pulled/nursemaid's elbow. Malays Fam Physician 12:26-28, 2017
134. Vitello S, Dvorkin R, Sattler S, et al: Epidemiology of nursemaid's elbow. West J Emerg Med 15:554-7, 2014
135. Anand P, Parks BG, Hassan SE, et al: Impact of ulnar collateral ligament tear on posteromedial elbow biomechanics. Orthopedics 38:e547-51, 2015
136. Gregory B, Nyland J: Medial elbow injury in young throwing athletes. Muscles Ligaments Tendons J 3:91-100, 2013
137. https://www.mlb.com/pitch-smart/pitching-guidelines, accessed November 11, 2025.
138. Garrison JC, Cole MA, Conway JE, et al: Shoulder range of motion deficits in baseball players with an ulnar collateral ligament tear. Am J Sports Med 40:2597-603, 2012
139. Garrison JC, Johnston C, Conway JE: Baseball players with ulnar collateral ligament tears demonstrate decreased rotator cuff strength compared to healthy controls. Int J Sports Phys Ther 10:476-81, 2015
140. Latinovic R, Gulliford MC, Hughes RA: Incidence of common compressive neuropathies in primary care. J Neurol Neurosurg Psychiatry 77:263-5, 2006
141. Wei SH, Jong YJ, Chang YJ: Ulnar nerve conduction velocity in injured baseball pitchers. Arch Phys Med Rehabil 86:21-5; quiz 180, 2005
142. Lee MJ, LaStayo PC: Pronator syndrome and other nerve compressions that mimic carpal tunnel syndrome. J Orthop Sports Phys Ther 34:601-9, 2004
143. Spinner RJ, Poliakoff MB, Tiel RL: The origin of "Saturday night palsy"? Neurosurgery 51:737-41; discussion 741, 2002
144. Kim SJ, Hong SH, Jun WS, et al: MR imaging mapping of skeletal muscle denervation in entrapment and compressive neuropathies. Radiographics 31:319-32, 2011
145. Kane PM, Daniels AH, Akelman E: Double crush syndrome. J Am Acad Orthop Surg 23:558-62, 2015

CHAPTER 9

The Wrist and Hand Complex

Mia Erickson, PT, EdD, CHT

CHAPTER OUTLINE

INTRODUCTION 272
STRUCTURE AND FUNCTION OF THE WRIST JOINT 272
- **Joints of the Wrist** 273
  - Structure of the Radiocarpal Joint 273
  - Structure of the Midcarpal Joint 274
- **Ligaments of the Wrist** 275
  - Dorsal Wrist Ligaments 275
  - Volar Wrist Ligaments 276
  - Intrinsic Wrist Ligaments 277
- **Muscle Function** 277
  - Dorsal Wrist Muscles — Extensors 277
  - Volar Wrist Muscles — Flexors 280
- **Wrist Kinematics** 281
  - Flexion/Extension 281
  - Radial/Ulnar Deviation 283
- **Wrist Kinetics** 284

STRUCTURE AND FUNCTION OF THE HAND COMPLEX 284
- **Digits 2–5** 284
  - Carpometacarpal Joints 2–5 284
  - Metacarpophalangeal Joints 2–5 285
  - Interphalangeal Joints 2–5 288
- **Muscles of the Digits** 289
  - Extrinsic Flexors for Digits 2–5 289
  - Extrinsic Extensors for Digits 2–5 292
  - Intrinsic Finger Muscles for Digits 2–5 292
  - Extensor Mechanism for Digits 2–5 294
- **The Thumb** 297
  - Joints of the Thumb 297
  - Thumb Muscles 299

PREHENSION 300
- **Power Grip** 301
  - Cylindrical Grip 301
  - Spherical Grip 301
  - Hook Grip 302
- **Lateral Prehension** 302
- **Precision Grip** 302
  - Precision Handling 302
  - Pulp Pinch 303
  - Tip Pinch 303

FUNCTIONAL POSITION OF THE WRIST AND HAND 304
SUMMARY 304
STUDY QUESTIONS 304
REFERENCES 305

ANATOMY OVERVIEW

MUSCLE ACTIONS OF THE WRIST AND FINGERS (DIGITS 2–5)			
TABLE KEY: Primary movers Secondary movers			
Sagittal Plane	**Joint**	**Flexion**	**Extension**
	Radiocarpal Midcarpal Carpometacarpal	Flexor carpi radialis Flexor carpi ulnaris Palmaris longus Flexor digitorum superficialis Flexor digitorum profundus Flexor pollicis longus Abductor pollicis longus Opponens Digiti Minimi	Extensor carpi radialis brevis Extensor carpi radialis longus Extensor carpi ulnaris (when the forearm is supinated) Extensor digitorum communis Extensor indicis Extensor digiti minimi Extensor pollicis longus Extensor pollicis brevis
	Metacarpophalangeal	Interossei (palmar and dorsal) Lumbricals Flexor digitorum superficialis Flexor digitorum profundus Flexor digiti minimi	Extensor digitorum communis Extensor indicis Extensor digiti minimi
	Proximal interphalangeal	Flexor digitorum superficialis Flexor digitorum profundus	Lumbricals Extensor digitorum communis Extensor indicis Extensor digiti minimi
	Distal interphalangeal	Flexor digitorum profundus	Lumbricals Extensor digitorum communis Extensor indicis Extensor digiti minimi
Frontal Plane		**Radial Deviation/Abduction**	**Ulnar Deviation/Adduction**
	Radiocarpal Midcarpal Carpometacarpal	Extensor carpi radialis longus Extensor carpi radialis brevis Flexor carpi radialis Extensor indicis Flexor pollicis longus Abductor pollicis longus Extensor pollicis longus Extensor pollicis brevis	Extensor carpi ulnaris (when in pronated position) Flexor carpi ulnaris
	Metacarpophalangeal	Dorsal interossei Abductor digiti minimi	Palmar interossei

ANATOMY OVERVIEW

Muscles	Proximal Attachment	Distal Attachment
Flexor carpi radialis (FCR)	Medial epicondyle of humerus (common flexor origin)	Base of 2nd and 3rd metacarpals
Palmaris longus	Medial epicondyle of humerus (common flexor origin)	Distal half of flexor retinaculum and apex of palmar aponeurosis
Flexor carpi ulnaris (FCU)	Radial head: Medial epicondyle of humerus (common flexor origin) Ulnar head: Olecranon and posterior border of ulna (via aponeurosis)	Pisiform, hook of hamate, base of 5th metacarpal
Extensor carpi radialis longus (ECRL)	Lateral supracondylar ridge of humerus	Dorsal aspect of base of 2nd metacarpal
Extensor carpi radialis brevis (ECRB)	Lateral epicondyle of humerus (common extensor origin)	Dorsal aspect of base of 3rd metacarpal

Muscles	Proximal Attachment	Distal Attachment
Extensor carpi ulnaris (ECU)	Lateral epicondyle of humerus; posterior border of ulna via a shared aponeurosis	Dorsal aspect of base of 5th metacarpal
Flexor digitorum superficialis (FDS)	Humeroulnar head: Medial epicondyle of humerus, ulnar collateral ligament, and coronoid process of ulna Radial head: Superior half of anterior border of radius	Bodies of middle phalanges of medial four digits
Flexor digitorum profundus (FDP)	Proximal 3/4 of medial and anterior surfaces of ulna and interosseous membrane	Bases of distal phalanges of medial four digits
Extensor digitorum communis (ED or EDC)	Lateral epicondyle of humerus (common extensor origin)	Extensor expansions of 2nd–5th digits
Extensor indicis (EI)	Posterior surface of distal 1/3 of ulna and interosseous membrane	Extensor expansion of 2nd digit
Extensor digiti minimi (EDM)	Lateral epicondyle of humerus (common extensor origin)	Extensor expansion of 5th digit
Abductor pollicis longus (APL)	Posterior surface of proximal half of ulna, radius, and interosseous membrane	Lateral aspect of base of 1st metacarpal
Extensor pollicis longus (EPL)	Posterior surface of middle 1/3 of ulna and interosseous membrane	Dorsal aspect of base of distal phalanx of thumb
Extensor pollicis brevis (EPB)	Posterior surface of distal 1/3 of radius and interosseous membrane	Dorsal aspect of base of proximal phalanx of thumb
Flexor pollicis longus (FPL)	Anterior surface of radius	Base of distal phalanx of thumb
Flexor pollicis brevis (FPB)	Flexor retinaculum and tubercles of scaphoid and trapezium	Lateral side of base of proximal phalanx of thumb
Adductor pollicis (AP)	Oblique head: Bases of 2nd and 3rd metacarpals, capitate, and adjacent carpals Transverse head: Anterior surface of shaft of 3rd metacarpal	Medial side of base of proximal phalanx of thumb
Abductor pollicis brevis (APB)	Flexor retinaculum and tubercles of scaphoid and trapezium	Lateral side of base of proximal phalanx of thumb
Opponens pollicis (OP)	Flexor retinaculum and tubercles of scaphoid and trapezium	Lateral side of 1st metacarpal
Abductor digiti minimi (ADM)	Pisiform	Medial side of base of proximal phalanx of 5th digit
Flexor digiti minimi (FDM)	Hook of hamate and flexor retinaculum	Medial side of base of proximal phalanx of 5th digit
Opponens digiti minimi (ODM)	Hook of hamate and flexor retinaculum	Medial border of 5th metacarpal
Lumbricals, 1st and 2nd	Lateral two tendons of FDP (as unipennate muscles)	Lateral sides of extensor expansions of 2nd–3rd digits
Lumbricals, 3rd and 4th	Medial three tendons of flexor digitorum profundus (as bipennate muscles)	Lateral sides of extensor expansions of 4th–5th digits
Dorsal interossei, 1st–4th	Adjacent sides of two metacarpals (as bipennate muscles)	Bases of proximal phalanges; extensor expansions of 2nd–4th digits
Palmar interossei, 1st–3rd	Palmar surfaces of 2nd, 4th, and 5th metacarpals (as unipennate muscles)	Bases of proximal phalanges; extensor expansions of 2nd, 4th, and 5th digits

Introduction

The human wrist and hand are topics of universal interest. They are integral parts of the upper kinematic chain. Joints proximal to the wrist serve to expand hand placement in space and increase the degrees of freedom available to the hand. The shoulder serves as a mobile base of support; the elbow allows the hand to approach or extend away from the body; and the forearm and wrist refine the approach of the hand to its target. Any loss of function in the upper limb, regardless of the segment, ultimately translates into diminished function of its distal joints.

This chapter will explore the wrist and hand, starting with joint structure. Specific anatomic structures will be highlighted, including the bones, joints that are formed by their interconnections, and soft tissue structures that support these articulations—including the capsule and ligaments. The osteo- and arthrokinematics will highlight how these structures move, followed by a discussion of how the various muscles in the area interact to enable functional use. Finally, the chapter concludes with a discussion of how all these elements integrate to provide a well-adapted tool that allows for interaction with the environment.

Structure and Function of the Wrist Joint

The wrist **(carpus)** consists of eight carpal bones aligned in proximal and distal rows **(Fig. 9–1)**. From lateral (radial) to medial (ulnar), the proximal row includes the **scaphoid**, **lunate**, and **triquetrum**. The **pisiform** is also associated with the proximal row although it is a sesamoid bone encased within the flexor carpi ulnaris tendon. From lateral to medial, the distal row includes the **trapezium**, **trapezoid**, **capitate**, and **hamate**. The proximal and distal rows are interposed between the forearm and the metacarpals (see Fig. 9-1), and are collectively referred to as the **wrist joint**[1]. The compound wrist joint is considered to function as a biaxial, synovial joint **(Fig. 9–2)**. It is traditionally classified as having two degrees of freedom, **flexion/extension** (see **Fig. 9–2A**) around a coronal axis and **radial deviation/ ulnar deviation** around an anterior-posterior (A-P) axis (see **Fig. 9–2B**).

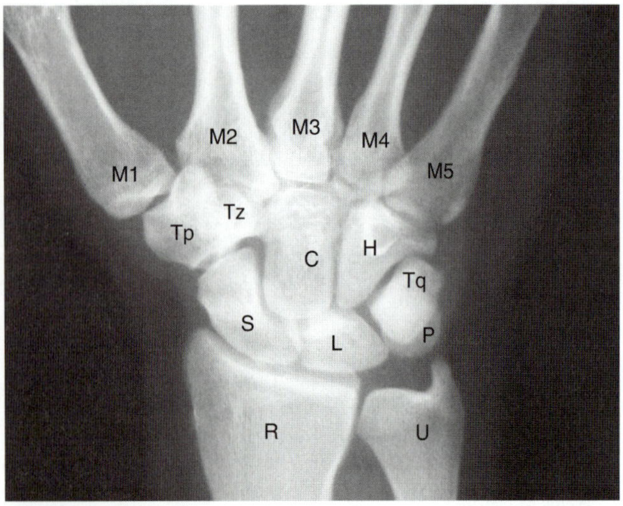

Figure 9–1 Wrist complex as shown on radiograph with metacarpals (M) 1 through 5, and the scaphoid (S), lunate (L), triquetrum (Tq), pisiform (P), trapezium (Tp), trapezoid (Tz), capitate (C), and the hamate (H).

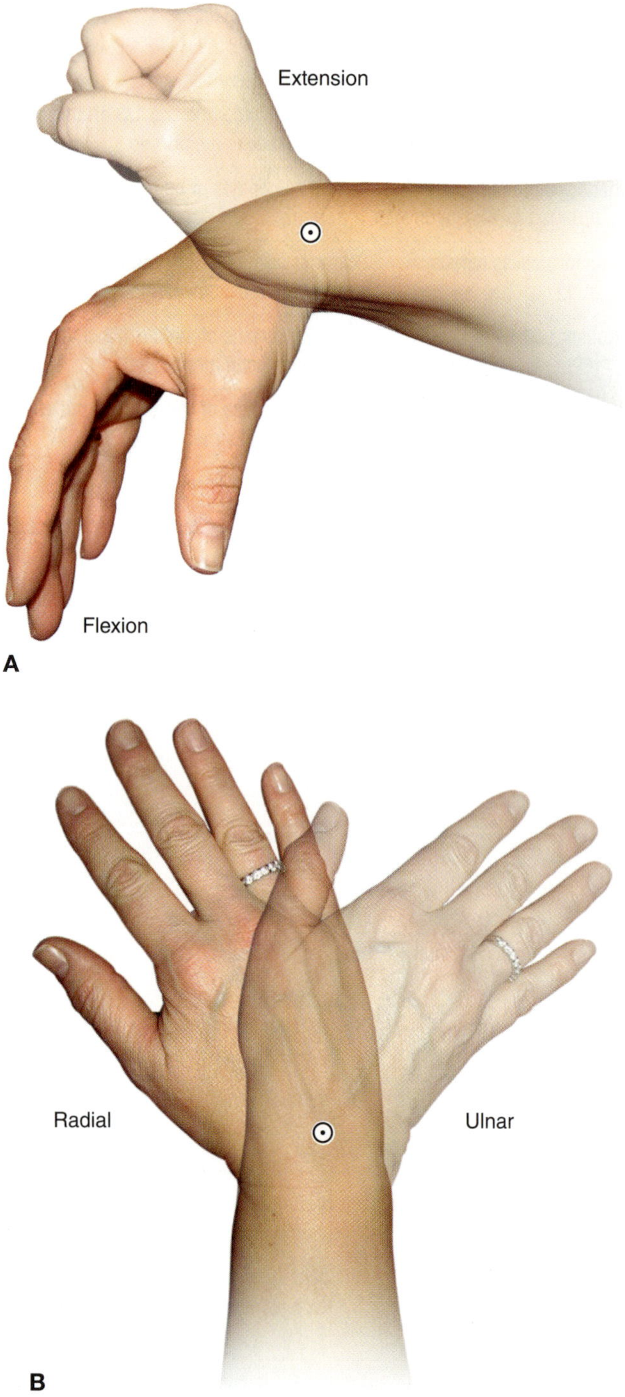

Figure 9–2 A. Wrist flexion/extension around a coronal axis; **B.** radial deviation and ulnar deviation around an anterior/ posterior axis.

Foundational Concepts 9–1
Nomenclature

As is true of many other joints of the body, there are variations in nomenclature for the wrist and hand. Flexion/extension of the wrist may also be termed volar **(palmar) flexion/dorsiflexion**, respectively. Radial/ulnar deviation of the wrist may also be called *abduction/adduction*, respectively. When referring to joints and structures in the wrist/hand anteriorly, the terms *volar* and *palmar* are used virtually interchangeably, whereas reference to the posterior aspect of the hand is more consistently referred to as the dorsum. The terms **medial** and **lateral** may be used in lieu of **ulnar** and **radial**. We will use *flexion/extension* and *radial/ulnar deviation* for the wrist motions, although frontal plane motions of the fingers are referred to most commonly as *abduction/adduction*—a convention that we will follow. The terms **volar** and **palmar** will be used interchangeably to accurately represent terms found in the cited literature.

Joints of the Wrist

Structure of the Radiocarpal Joint

The **radiocarpal joint** is composed proximally of the combination of the distal radius and the **radioulnar disc** of the **triangular fibrocartilage complex,** and distally with the proximal row of carpals **(Fig. 9–3)**. The distal radius has a biconcave curvature that is long and shallow from medial to lateral (in the frontal plane) and shorter and sharper anterior to posterior (in the sagittal plane). The **lateral radial facet,** also known as the *radial* or *scaphoid fossa*, articulates with the convex, proximal pole of the scaphoid, whereas the **medial radial facet,** also known as the *lunate fossa*, articulates with the convex surface of the lunate. The concave articular disk articulates predominantly with the convex, proximal aspect of the triquetrum, although it also has some contact with the lunate in the neutral wrist position.

The radioulnar disc (previously discussed as part of the distal radioulnar joint) is made of fibrocartilage and has a limited blood supply, especially in the central and radial portions.[2] The radioulnar disc is part of the triangular fibrocartilage complex (**TFCC**) that also includes: (1) the posterior (dorsal) and anterior (volar) distal radioulnar joint ligaments, and (2) the ulnolunate and ulnotriquetral ligaments—all named for their respective attachments; (3) the subsheath of the extensor carpi ulnaris tendon; and (4) a meniscal homologue. The extensor carpi ulnaris tendon sheath consists of collagen fibers that run from the tendon to the triquetrum and ulnar styloid process, a projection off the distal ulna.[2] The meniscal homologue is made of both loose and tight collagen fibers with variable attachments between the radioulnar disc, triquetrum, wrist joint capsule, fifth metacarpal base, hamate, and the ulnar styloid process. The triangular fibrocartilage complex and the various fibrous attachments provide the primary support for the distal radioulnar joint **(Fig. 9–4)**.[3] Overall, the triangular fibrocartilage complex should be considered to function at the wrist as an extension of the distal radius, just as it does at the distal radioulnar joint.

The scaphoid is the largest carpal bone. It has a convex proximal pole that articulates with the radial fossa and a distal pole that articulates with the trapezium. The tubercle of the scaphoid is on the anterior aspect and is an important bony landmark used for palpation in a clinical examination. The narrow area between the poles is the *scaphoid waist*. The proximal aspect of the lunate is convex and articulates with the concave lunate fossa of the distal radius. The concave

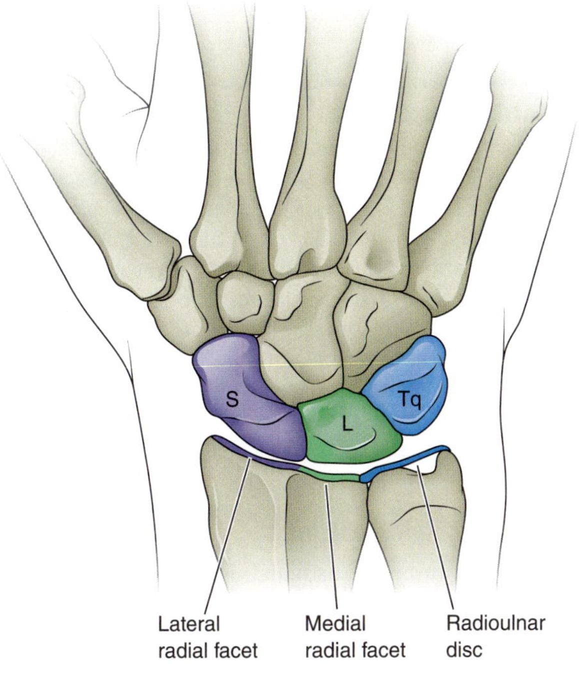

Figure 9–3 The compound radiocarpal joint formed by the articulation of the distal scaphoid (S) with the proximal lateral facet of the radius; the distal lunate (L) with the proximal medial facet of the radius; and the distal triquetrum (Tq) with the triangular fibrocartilage complex (radioulnar disc).

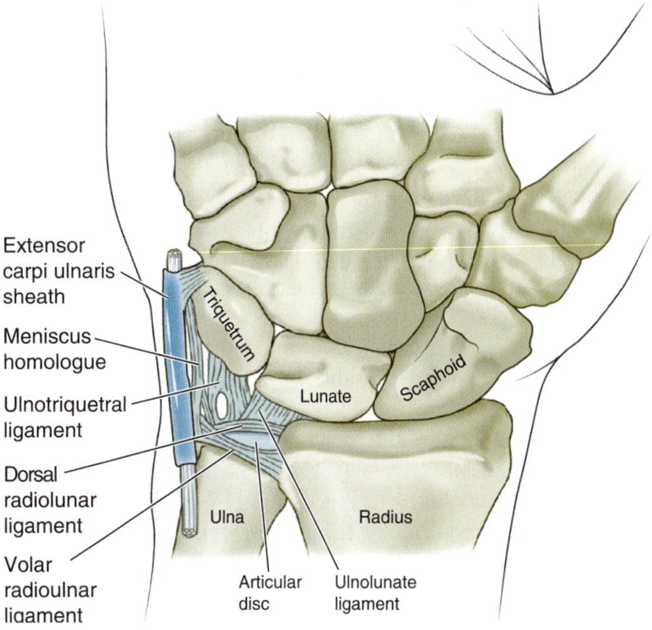

Figure 9–4 The triangular fibrocartilage complex, including the radioulnar disc with its various fibrous attachments, provides support to the wrist and distal radioulnar joint.

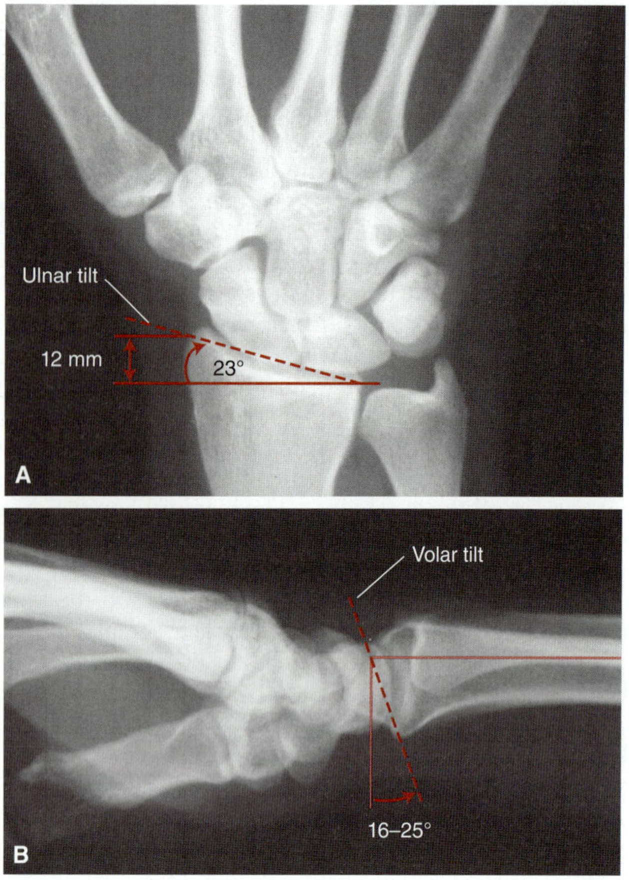

Figure 9–5 **A.** The typical angle of inclination of the radius in the frontal plane results because the distal radius is longer on the radial side than on the ulnar side. **B.** A typical volar, or palmar tilt resulting from a radius that is longer posteriorly than anteriorly.

surface of the lunate articulates with the capitate and hamate to form the "central column" of the wrist.[4,5] The triquetrum is irregularly shaped. Its proximal tubercle is covered in cartilage where it is in contact with the radioulnar disc; the anterior surface of the triquetrum is flat so that it can articulate with the pisiform.[1]

The proximal, convex surfaces of the scaphoid, lunate, and triquetrum—taken together—are sharper than the articular surface of the distal radius and radioulnar disc in both the sagittal and frontal planes, making the radiocarpal joint somewhat incongruent. The overall contact between the scaphoid and lunate with the distal radius and radioulnar disc is never more than about 20% of the available articular surface throughout the entire range of motion (ROM).[1]

In the frontal plane, the radiocarpal joint surface is oblique and angled medially **(Fig. 9–5)**. This is known as the *radial inclination angle*, or ulnar tilt. It is formed by the intersection of a line drawn perpendicular to the long axis of the radius and a line drawn across the radial articular surface (see **Fig. 9–5A**). Normal radial inclination values range from 15° to 25° (see Fig. 9-5A).[6] This inclination occurs because the radial length (height) is about 12 mm greater on the lateral side than on the medial side.[7] In the sagittal plane, the distal aspect of the radius and its articular surface are tilted in an anterior direction. This is known as *volar*, or *palmar tilt*, and typical values range from 16° to 25° (see **Fig. 9–5B**).[7] The posterior aspect of the distal radius is slightly longer than the anterior aspect because of this volar tilt.[7] The volar and ulnar tilt of the distal radius joint surface result in a greater range of radiocarpal joint flexion than extension and in greater radiocarpal joint ulnar deviation than radial deviation, respectively.[8]

The relationship between the length of the ulna and the length of the radius at the wrist is known as **ulnar variance.** In a typical wrist, the distal radius and ulna should be aligned on the same level for the articulation with the lunate.[6] **Negative ulnar variance** is described as a short ulna in comparison with the distal articular surface of the radius, whereas **positive ulnar variance** occurs when the distal ulna is long in relation to the distal radius **(Fig. 9–6)**. Both have important clinical implications. With positive ulnar variance, there is a potential for impingement of the triangular fibrocartilage complex interposed between the distal ulna and the triquetrum.[9] Consequently, the presence of a positive ulnar variance has been associated with triangular fibrocartilage complex thinning.[10] Positive ulnar variance can be congenital or result from an injury such as a distal radius fracture that healed in a shortened position. Pain is commonly present at end range of pronation and ulnar deviation because these motions increase the likelihood of impinging the ulnar structures. Surgical intervention may include a joint-levelling procedure, such as ulnar shortening, to unload the ulnar side of the wrist.[11] In contrast, negative ulnar variance can result in abnormal force distribution across the radiocarpal joint.[12] **Avascular necrosis** of the lunate, or **Kienböck's disease** **(Fig. 9–7)**, has been associated with negative ulnar variance.[13] Like positive ulnar variance, negative variance can also be congenital or arise from an injury.

Patient Application 9–1

Gail Antanasi is a 26-year-old woman who sustained a right distal radius fracture **(Fig. 9–8)** after a **f**all **o**n an **o**ut**s**tretched **h**and (known by the acronym **FOOSH**). A posteroanterior radiograph demonstrated a reduction in length of the radius and a reduction in the typical ulnar tilt (see **Fig. 9–8A**). The volar tilt of the distal radius is now dorsally angulated as can be seen in the postreduction lateral radiograph (see **Fig. 9–8B**). These changes would be likely to result in a loss of ROM and the likelihood of future radioulnar joint degeneration. Correcting the relative lengths of the radius and ulna would most likely require open reduction and internal fixation (ORIF) with plate and screws.

Structure of the Midcarpal Joint

The **midcarpal joint** is the articulation between the scaphoid, lunate, and triquetrum proximally and the distal carpal row **(Fig. 9–9)**. The midcarpal joint does not form a single uninterrupted articular surface as does the radiocarpal joint. It is anatomically separate from the radiocarpal joint and has a fibrous capsule and synovial lining that is continuous with each intercarpal articulation and may be continuous with some of the carpometacarpal joints.[14] The midcarpal joint surfaces

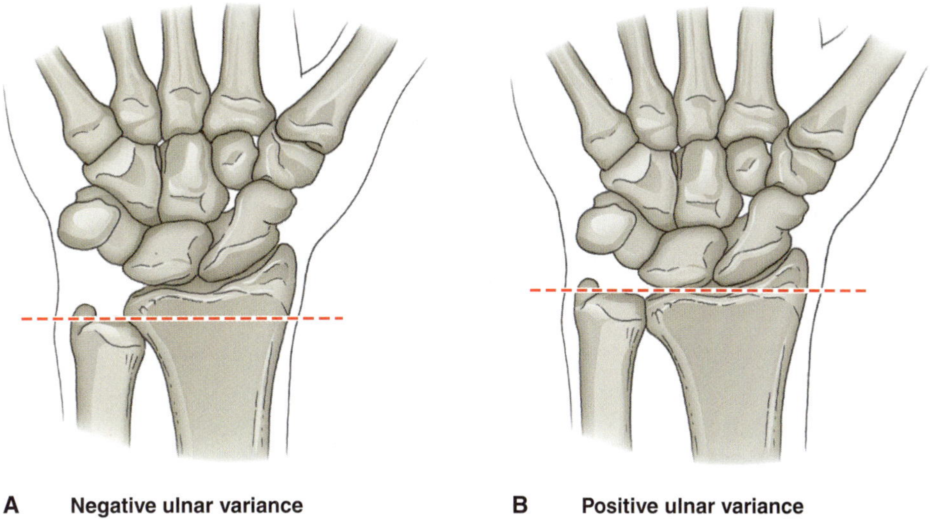

Figure 9–6 Ulnar variance. **A.** Negative. **B.** Positive.

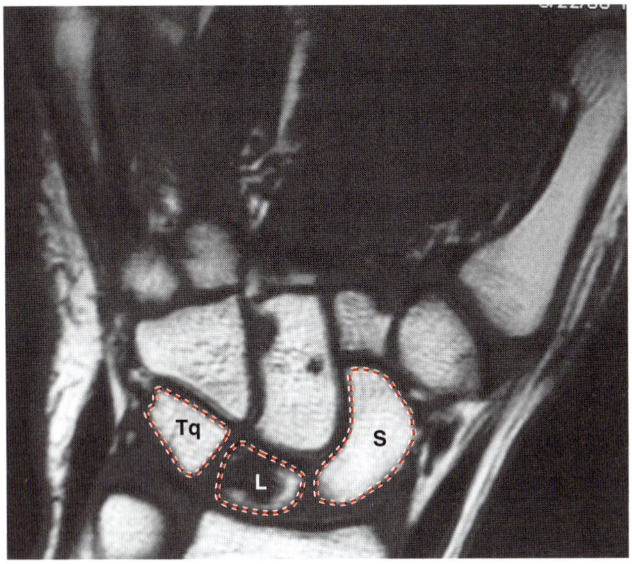

Figure 9–7 In this magnetic resonance image of the wrist, the dark area seen on the lunate demonstrates avascular necrosis, known as Kienböck's disease, and has been associated with negative ulnar variance. L, lunate; S, scaphoid; Tq, triquetrum.

are complex. The distal pole of the scaphoid is convex and articulates with the concave trapezium and trapezoid at the **scaphotrapeziotrapezoid joint**, a common site for degenerative changes. The concave distal lunate articulates with the convex proximal aspect of the capitate. The **triquetrohamate joint** has both convex and concave regions.[1] The hamate has an important bony prominence on its volar aspect called the **hook of hamate.** It serves as an important site for ligament attachment and is vulnerable to fracture.

The distal carpal row is tightly positioned against the metacarpal bases, and collectively form a dorsal convexity known as the **proximal transverse (carpal) arch**[15] **(Fig. 9–10)**. This arch persists even when the hand is fully opened and is created by the curved shape of the carpals and the ligaments that maintain their position in the wrist. The carpal bones form the floor of the carpal tunnel.

Ligaments of the Wrist

There is considerable variability in names, anatomic descriptions, and ascribed functions of wrist ligaments from investigator to investigator.[16] Although there may not be universal agreement on the structure and function of individual ligaments, there is consensus that the carpal ligaments are responsible for articular stability and for guiding and checking motion between and among the carpals.[17] The ligaments of the wrist are typically classified as either extrinsic or intrinsic ligaments. The **extrinsic ligaments** attach to the radius or ulna and one or more carpal bones; **intrinsic ligaments** form connections between the carpal bones and are also known as *intercarpal,* or *interosseous ligaments.*[18] The intrinsic ligaments connect bones of the proximal or distal carpal rows, or they span the midcarpal joint (*midcarpal ligaments*).[19] Unlike the extrinsic ligaments, the intrinsic ligaments lie within the synovial lining and, therefore, must rely on synovial fluid for nutrition rather than from contiguous vascularized tissues.[20]

Dorsal Wrist Ligaments

The dorsal wrist ligaments are thin and somewhat loose, allowing full wrist flexion while stabilizing the carpus. Dorsally, the major extrinsic wrist ligament is the **dorsal radiocarpal ligament (Fig. 9–11)**. It originates from posteriorly located Lister's tubercle of the distal radius and spans distally and obliquely toward the medial aspect of the wrist to insert on the triquetrum. Along the way, it attaches to the lunate.[1] Another important dorsal wrist ligament is an intrinsic, midcarpal ligament called the **dorsal intercarpal ligament** (see Fig. 9–11). It spans from the triquetrum to the scaphoid and has attachments to the lunate and variable attachments to the trapezium[18] and second metacarpal.[21] Together, the dorsal radiocarpal and dorsal intercarpal ligaments form a horizontal "V" with the apex at the triquetrum.

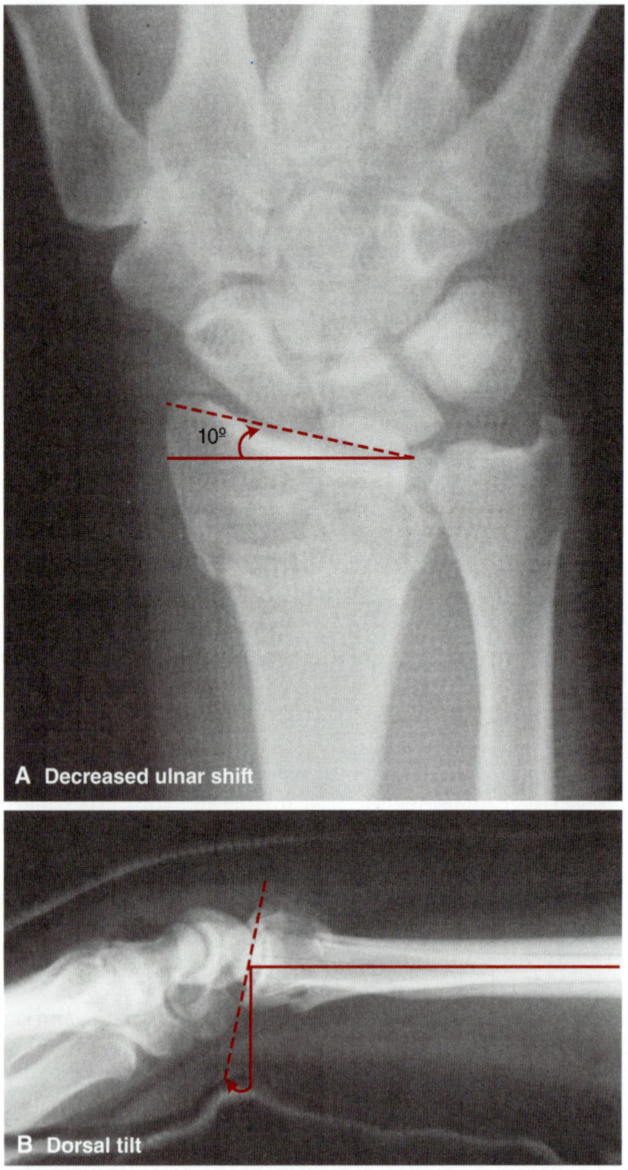

Figure 9–8 **A.** A radial fracture from a **f**all **o**n an **o**utstretched **h**and (FOOSH) resulting in diminished ulnar angulation and length of the distal radius (ulnar positive variance). **B.** Relative shortening of the radius also results in a reversal of the typical volar inclination of the radius.

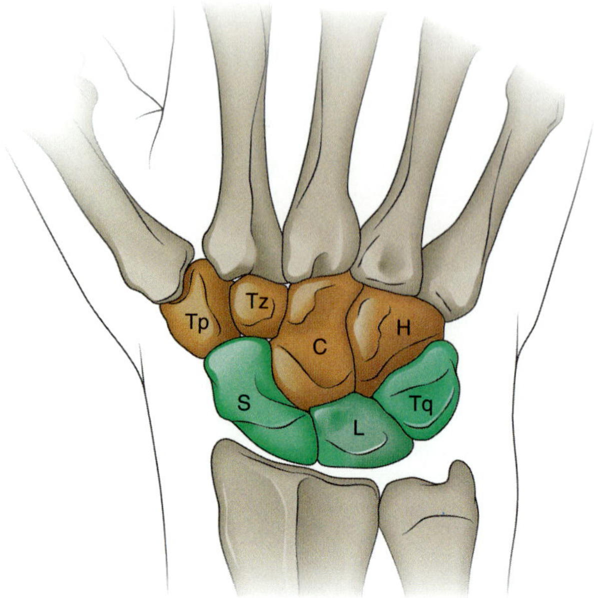

Figure 9–9 Midcarpal joint is formed proximally by the scaphoid (S), lunate (L), and triquetrum (Tq), and distally by the trapezium (Tp), trapezoid (Tz), capitate (C), and hamate (H).

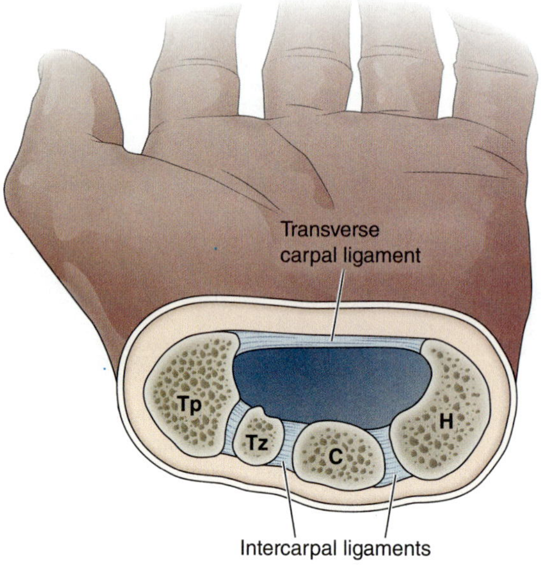

Figure 9–10 The proximal transverse arch, or carpal arch, forms the tunnel through which the median nerve and long finger flexors travel. The transverse carpal ligament and intercarpal ligaments assist in maintaining this concavity. C, capitate; H, hamate; Tp, trapezium; Tz, trapezoid.

Volar Wrist Ligaments

The volar ligaments are more numerous, thicker, and stronger than those on the dorsal surface, and effectively limit wrist extension. They are also more prone to injury.[21] The volar extrinsic ligaments attach to either the radius or ulna and insert onto the carpus **(Fig. 9–12)**. Those on the lateral aspect of the wrist include the following[21]:

1. The **radioscaphocapitate ligament** spans from the volar radial styloid to the capitate with a variable attachment on the scaphoid.[18]
2. The **radiolunotriquetral ligament** is comprised of the short and long radiolunate ligaments. The *long radiolunate ligament* attaches between the radial styloid and the lunate and triquetrum, while the *short radiolunate ligament* attaches to the bones for which it is named.[18]
3. The **radioscapholunate ligament** is not a true ligament, together with the short radiolunate ligament providing a conduit for neurovascular structures.[19]
4. The **radial collateral ligament** runs between the radial styloid and scaphoid.

Volar ligaments arising from the medial aspect of the wrist (see Fig. 9–12) include the **ulnolunate** and **ulnotriquetral**

ligaments. These run between the anteriorly located distal radioulnar ligament and the lunate and triquetrum, respectively. The **ulnocapitate ligament** originates from the ulnar fovea and inserts onto the capitate.[19] Along with the **ulnar collateral ligament**, the ulnolunate and ulnotriquetral ligaments are part of the triangular fibrocartilaginous complex. Neither the ulnar collateral nor the radial collateral ligament play a large role in wrist stability.[21]

Intrinsic Wrist Ligaments

Two short intrinsic ligaments join the scaphoid to the lunate, and the lunate to the triquetrum. Named by their attachments, these are the **scapholunate** and **lunotriquetral ligaments** (see Fig 9–12). These ligaments are covered with cartilage proximally, joining the three proximal carpals to make up the continuous distal articulating surface of the radiocarpal joint.[22] These two ligaments have received particular attention for their role in wrist stability and function. The scapholunate ligament has three portions: volar, dorsal, and membranous. The dorsal portion is most resistant to tearing, followed by the volar and then the membranous.[19] The lunotriquetral interosseous ligament is credited with maintaining stability between the lunate and triquetrum. Unlike the scapholunate ligament, the volar aspect is more resistant to tearing.

The intrinsic transverse carpal ligament attaches the pisiform and hook of hamate medially to the scaphoid and trapezial tubercles laterally **(Fig. 9–13)**. It is continuous with, and often considered part of, the extrinsic flexor retinaculum. The transverse carpal ligament and the carpal bones form the **carpal tunnel**, which is a tightly confined space containing the median nerve and nine extrinsic tendons that pass from the forearm to the hand (see **Fig. 9–13B**). The tendons that pass through the carpal tunnel are encased in synovial sheaths (also known as the radial and ulnar bursae) to minimize tendon-on-ligament friction. The hook of the hamate and pisiform form the borders of the **ulnar tunnel**, or canal of Guyon, through which the ulnar nerve and artery pass.

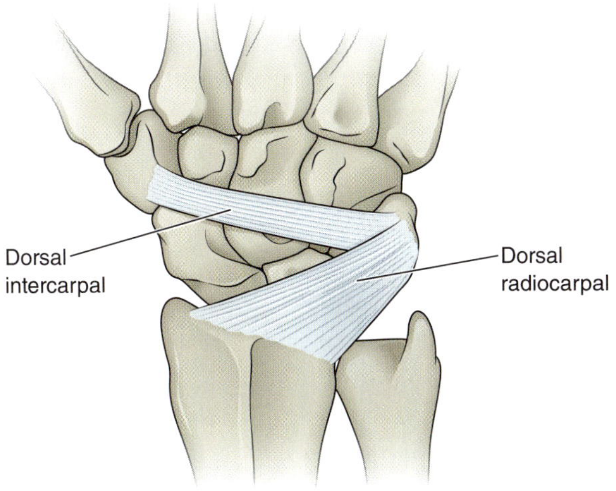

Figure 9–11 The dorsal radiocarpal and dorsal intercarpal ligaments form a horizontal V.

Expanded Concepts 9–1
Space of Poirier

There are no ligaments between the lunate and the capitate. The resulting gap between the lunate and capitate is known as the **space of Poirier** and is an area susceptible to injury. Perilunate instability can occur when radial/ulnar supporting structures are injured, such as the scapholunate and lunotriquetral ligaments. A full lunate dislocation requires injuries to the radial collateral and radioscaphocapitate ligaments and, on the ulnar side, the radiotriquetral and ulnotriquetral ligaments.[23]

Muscle Function

Dorsal Wrist Muscles—Extensors

The tendons from nine muscles cross the dorsal aspect of the wrist **(Fig. 9–14)**. Three of the nine muscles are primary wrist extensor muscles: the **extensor carpi radialis longus**, the **extensor carpi radialis brevis**, and the **extensor carpi ulnaris** (see **Fig. 9–14A**). The other six muscles are finger and thumb muscles that act secondarily on the wrist: the **extensor digitorum communis**, the **extensor indicis proprius**, the

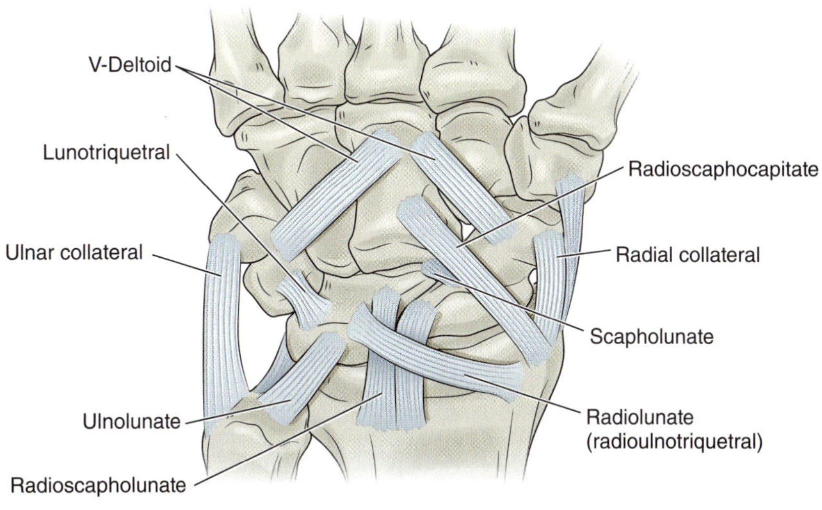

Figure 9–12 Volar ligaments of the wrist complex, including the radioscaphocapitate, the radiolunotriquetral (long and short radiolunate), the radioscapholunate, and the radial collateral ligament in addition to two intrinsic ligaments (scapholunate and lunotriquetral) that are particularly credited with maintaining scaphoid stability.

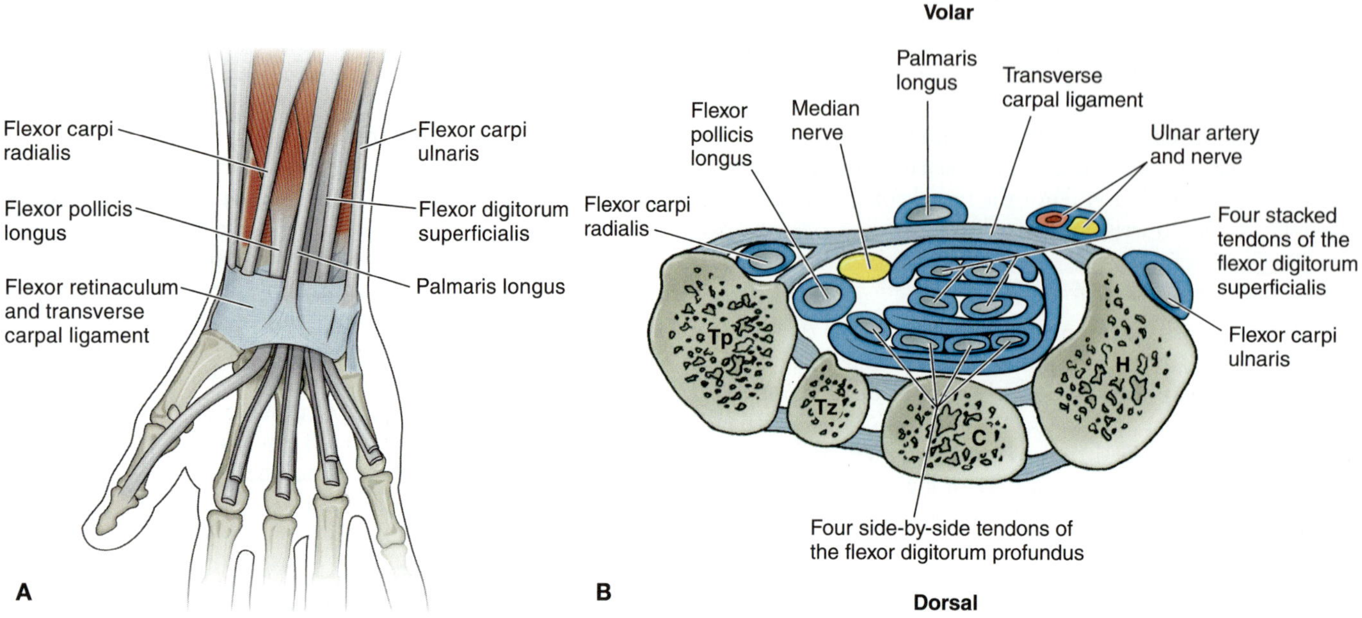

Figure 9–13 **A.** The tendons of the primary and secondary wrist flexors lie on the volar aspect of the wrist. All but the palmaris longus tendon and the flexor carpi ulnaris muscle pass beneath the flexor retinaculum. **B.** On cross section, the relationship of the tendons and nerves to the transverse carpal ligament is more evident. The flexor pollicis longus is encased in its own tendon sheath (also known as the **radial bursa**), whereas the four deep tendons of the flexor digitorum profundus and the four more superficial stacked tendons of the flexor digitorum superficialis are wrapped by folds in the **ulnar bursa**.

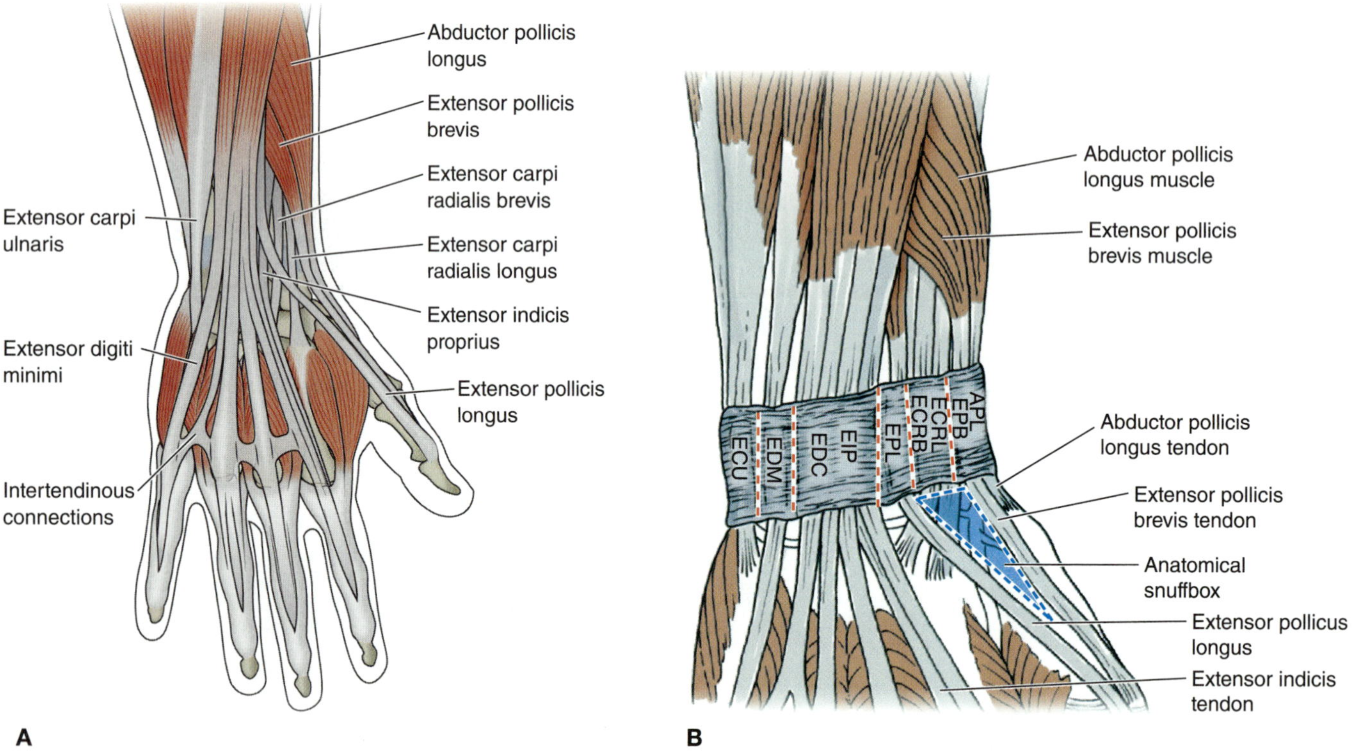

Figure 9–14 Dorsal aspect of the hand. **A.** The primary wrist extensors (extensor retinaculum removed) are the extensor carpi ulnaris and the extensor carpi radialis longus and brevis (ECRL and ECRB, respectively). Finger muscles that can assist with wrist extension include the extensor digitorum communis (EDC), the extensor indicis proprius (EIP), the extensor digiti minimi (EDM), the extensor pollicus longus and brevis (EPL and EPB, respectively), and the abductor pollicus longus (APL). The intertendinous connections serve to connect the long finger extensor tendons. **B.** The dorsally located extensor tendons pass beneath the extensor retinaculum, beneath which the tendons are compartmentalized. The anatomic snuff box is shown as a dotted triangle between the extensor pollicus brevis and abductor pollicus longus on the radial side of the triangle, and the extensor pollicus longus on the ulnar side of the triangle.

extensor digiti minimi, the **extensor pollicis longus**, the **extensor pollicis brevis**, and the **abductor pollicis longus**. The extensor digitorum communis and extensor indicis proprius muscles are (and more simply) known as the *extensor digitorum* and the *extensor indicis*, respectively. At the wrist, the tendons of all nine muscles pass under the **extensor retinaculum**, a fibrous band across the dorsal radius and ulna that is divided into six distinct fibro-osseous tunnels (see **Fig. 9–14B**). These tunnels, formed by septa beneath the retinaculum, maintain the relationship between the extensor tendons and the axis of wrist motion. The retinaculum also provides a dorsal pulley to maintain the position of the tendons when the wrist is extended to prevent bowstringing.[24] As the tendons pass deep to the extensor retinaculum, each tendon is encased within its own tendon sheath to reduce friction between the tendons and the retinaculum.

Muscles that extend the wrist make up a significant portion of the posterior forearm musculature[25] (see Fig. 9–14). The extensor carpi radialis brevis shares a proximal attachment on the lateral epicondyle with the extensor carpi ulnaris and extensor digitorum, resulting in a strong, conjoined tendon known as the **common extensor tendon**.[26] The extensor carpi radialis brevis is somewhat smaller than the extensor carpi radialis longus muscle, but has a more central location as it inserts distally into the third metacarpal. The sagittal plane moment arm for extension is greater for the extensor carpi radialis brevis than that of the extensor carpi radialis longus;[27] thus, the brevis is considered the primary extensor of the wrist.[28] In addition, the extensor carpi radialis brevis muscle appears to be necessary during forearm rotation. One study showed significant muscle activation during pronation with EMG values between 43% and 53% of the muscle's maximum voluntary isometric contraction. In contrast, the muscle's activation was lowest during supination.[29] Clinically, this muscle is often involved in lateral elbow tendinopathy, or **tennis elbow**.[28] Of the three muscles originating from the lateral epicondyle, the extensor carpi radialis brevis is the deepest and most susceptible to injury, especially as it becomes active during wrist extension. Understanding its activation may help in designing ergonomic and exercise interventions.

The extensor carpi radialis longus has a smaller moment arm for wrist extension than does the brevis.[27] However, its attachment on the second metacarpal provides the muscle with a longer moment arm for radial deviation compared to the centrally located extensor carpi radialis brevis.[27] The extensor carpi radialis longus and brevis have a significant role in forceful grip[30] because the wrist extensor muscles must be capable of providing sufficient force to maintain the wrist in a neutral or slightly extended position when gripping. Otherwise, the long finger flexors responsible for gripping may also flex the wrist, weakening grip due to active insufficiency. Therefore, the extensor carpi radialis muscles must neutralize the flexor moment at the wrist provided by the long finger flexors so that a strong grip can be achieved. Notably, when wrist position changes between extension, neutral, and flexion, the extensor carpi radialis force output varies considerably (36% between minimum and maximum values). For example, the extensor carpi radialis longus and brevis muscles lose ~60% of their maximum capacity when the wrist is in flexion.[31] This suggests the extensor carpi radialis muscles are critical for the interaction between wrist position and grip force.[30] This is an important point for designing exercise interventions to improve grip strength.

The extensor carpi ulnaris muscle crosses the wrist on the ulnar side of the dorsum (see Fig. 9–14). It acts synergistically with the extensor carpi radialis longus and brevis to achieve neutral wrist extension.[25] The extensor carpi ulnaris crosses the wrist close to the wrist flexion-extension axis. While the extensor carpi ulnaris is considered a wrist extensor and ulnar deviator, the moment arm for extension is much smaller than that of the more radially located wrist extensors.[32] In addition, its extension moment arm is dependent on forearm position.[27] For example, when the forearm is pronated, the tendon shifts more toward the ulnar aspect of the wrist, and there is a marked decrease in the extension moment arm that limits the muscle's ability to act as a wrist extensor. In this pronated position of the forearm, the extensor carpi ulnaris is more suited to act as an ulnar deviator. It also opposes the radial deviation moment created by the radially located wrist extensors.[32] When the forearm is supinated, the extensor carpi ulnaris exits its fibro-osseous tunnel at a 30° angle as it inserts onto the fifth metacarpal. This angulation of the tendon allows the extensor carpi ulnaris to function more as a wrist extensor. The extensor carpi ulnaris is tethered to its location by a subsheath and attachment to the extensor retinaculum.[33] Its subsheath is also a component of the triangular fibrocartilage complex.

The extensor indicis and extensor digiti minimi (see Fig. 9–14) attach distally to the extensor expansion of the second and fifth digit, respectively. The extensor indicis and extensor digiti minimi muscles are capable of extending both the wrist and the metacarpophalangeal (MCP) joints that they cross.[34] The extensor indicis can function alone, allowing the index finger to move independently, or it can work with the extensor digitorum to extend the index finger with the other fingers.[34] Likewise, the extensor digiti minimi provides independent action to the fifth digit, allowing it to extend the digit even if the other digits are flexed.

The extensor digitorum crosses the wrist deep to the extensor retinaculum. Once past the retinaculum, the four slips of the extensor digitorum are held together on the dorsum of the hand by intertendinous connections[34] (see Fig. 9–14A). Of the three finger extensors, wrist extension is credited more to the extensor digitorum muscle than the two independent finger extensors (the extensor indicis and extensor digiti minimi). The extensor digitorum is important for wrist extension because its central location allows it to function without radial or ulnar deviation. It also extends the carpometacarpal and MCP joints that it crosses before blending into the extensor mechanisms of each finger (see **Fig. 9–15**). Like other wrist extensors, the extensor digitorum force output decreases with changes in wrist position but to a lesser amount than the extensor carpi radialis.[31] Authors reported a 20% reduction in force output when the wrist was flexed. The extensor digitorum reaches its maximal force output with the MCP joints flexed ~25° and the wrist in a neutral position, but this position can vary and still produce near-optimal output. This is important because grip

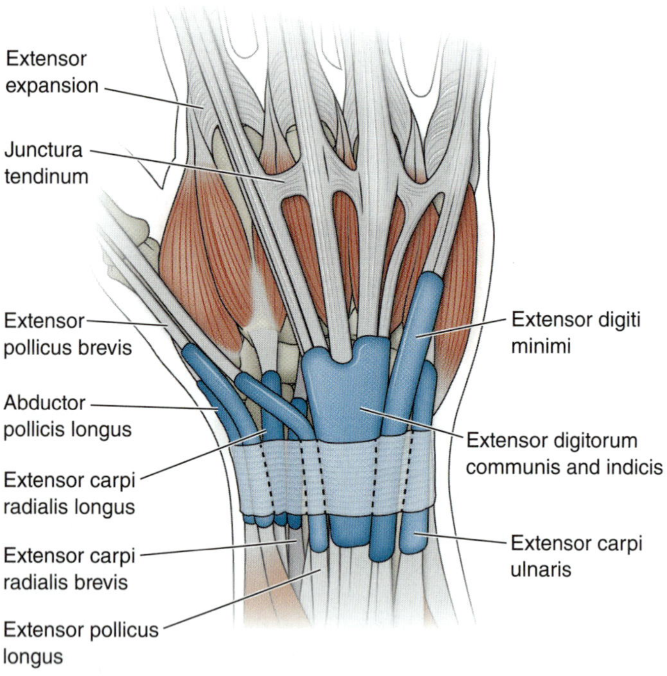

Figure 9–15 Dorsal view of the hand, illustrating the six compartments of the extensor retinaculum at the wrist, the synovial sheaths, and the finger extensors (extensor digitorum communis, extensor indicis proprius, and extensor digiti minimi muscles) that merge with the extensor expansion at the metacarpophalangeal joint. The junctura tendinae of the extensor digitorum communis muscle lies just proximal to the metacarpophalangeal joints.

tasks require various finger flexion angles based on the size of the object being gripped. Like the extensor carpi radialis muscles, the extensor digitorum is important to balance the finger flexor forces during grip. Together, these three muscles contribute to an optimal posture in which to place the wrist and finger muscles for the most advantageous position for force production.[31] Due to the proximal attachment of the extensor digitorum on the lateral epicondyle, it also has been implicated in development of lateral elbow tendinopathy.[35] A study showed that there is a reduction in extensor digitorum muscle activity at faster wrist movements and when wrist extension is combined with extremes of radial or ulnar deviation. Some have suggested that this may alter the balance in force production between the extensor digitorum and the digital flexor muscles, resulting in injury.[36]

Three extrinsic thumb muscles cross the dorsal aspect of the wrist. The abductor pollicis longus and extensor pollicis brevis cross the wrist in the first (most radial) fibro-osseous compartment of the extensor retinaculum (see Fig. 9–14B). These two tendons make up the radial border of the **anatomic snuffbox** (see 9–14B), an important anatomic landmark for identifying the scaphoid. The abductor pollicis longus attaches distally to the first metacarpal. Unlike other dorsal muscles, its position at the wrist causes this muscle to act as a secondary wrist *flexor*, although its moment arm for that action is smaller than that of other wrist flexors.[27] The abductor pollicus longus is a radial deviator of the wrist.[37] The extensor pollicis brevis extends, and can also radially deviate the wrist. There are several anatomic variations such as extra tendon slips, or an additional septum that may separate the abductor pollicis longus and the extensor pollicis brevis tendons into separate compartments as opposed to sharing a compartment.[38,39] Additional abductor pollicis longus tendon slips may be found that can influence the moment arm of the tendon[27] and may contribute to **De Quervain's tenovaginitis**, a thickening of the fibrous sheath around a tendon(s) that occurs on the radial side of the wrist near the radial styloid process.[39] Biomechanical studies show the additional septum resists the gliding of the abductor pollicis longus and extensor pollicis brevis in various wrist positions[40] and elevates tendon pressures on the side of the extensor pollicis brevis.[41]

The extensor pollicis longus muscle crosses the wrist closer to the midline of the wrist than the extensor pollicis brevis. The extensor pollicis longus makes a sharp trajectory around the **tubercle of Lister,** using the bony prominence as a pulley to change the direction of the tendon (Fig. 9–15). It enters the hand through the third fibro-osseous compartment and crosses over the extensor carpi radialis longus and brevis tendons, forming the ulnar side of the anatomic snuffbox opposite the abductor pollicis longus and extensor pollicis brevis. The extensor pollicis longus muscle has the most complicated movements and influences all the joints it crosses.[42] The extensor pollicis longus extends the wrist, first carpometacarpal joint, and the thumb MCP and interphalangeal joints.[34]

Volar Wrist Muscles—Flexors

Six muscles have tendons crossing the volar aspect of the wrist and, therefore, can flex the wrist (see Fig. 9–13A). Primary wrist flexors include the **palmaris longus,** the **flexor carpi radialis,** and the **flexor carpi ulnaris.** The secondary wrist flexors include the **flexor digitorum superficialis,** the **flexor digitorum profundus,** and the **flexor pollicis longus** muscles. The finger flexors and the flexor pollicis longus pass beneath the **flexor retinaculum** at the wrist through the carpal tunnel along with the median nerve (see Fig. 9–13B). The flexor retinaculum prevents bowstringing of the long flexor tendons, thereby maintaining an appropriate length-tension relationship. The flexor retinaculum is often considered to have a proximal portion and a distal portion, with the distal portion being the transverse carpal ligament**.** The average torque produced by the wrist flexors is more than twice that of the extensors.[43]

The flexor carpi radialis muscle is one of the superficial, anterior forearm muscles. Its distal attachment on the bases of the second and third metacarpals places it in line with the long axis of the hand. Based on where it crosses the wrist, it should be capable of both wrist flexion and radial deviation. It has a large wrist flexion moment arm, with a peak tendon force during flexion motions.[27,44] However, the flexor carpi radialis muscle does not appear to be effective as a radial deviator in an isolated contraction. Like the extensor carpi radialis brevis, its attachment to the second and third metacarpals results in a short moment arm for radial deviation. However, the flexor carpi radialis' poor radial deviation may also be attributed in part to contact between the scaphoid and radial styloid. The flexor carpi radialis can work synergistically with the extensor carpi radialis longus to add to radial deviation force, while also offsetting what may be undesired wrist extension moment. The greatest tendon force produced by the flexor carpi radialis is during wrist circumduction, an elliptical motion created with 30° wrist extension and flexion and 10° of ulnar and radial deviation.[44]

The flexor carpi ulnaris crosses the radiocarpal joint and attaches to the pisiform, a sesamoid bone that increases the moment arm of the flexor carpi ulnaris muscle for wrist flexion.[45] The importance of the increased moment arm from the pisiform can be seen following pisiform excision, in which case the flexor carpi ulnaris must generate nearly 30% more force to achieve the same wrist motion.[46] The flexor carpi ulnaris is the only muscle that attaches to a bone in the proximal carpal row; however, the pisiform is only loosely connected to the triquetrum below it.[47] After crossing the pisiform, the flexor carpi ulnaris attaches both to the hook of hamate (part of the distal carpal row) and to the fifth metacarpal.[34] Consequently, forces applied to the pisiform by the flexor carpi ulnaris muscle are translated not to the triquetrum on which the pisiform sits but to the hamate and fifth metacarpal via pisiform ligaments. The flexor carpi ulnaris tendon crosses the wrist at a greater distance from the wrist axis for radial/ulnar deviation than does the flexor carpi radialis muscle, creating a rather large ulnar deviation moment arm. Consequently, the flexor carpi ulnaris muscle is more effective in producing ulnar deviation than the flexor carpi radialis muscle is in producing radial deviation.[48] The flexor carpi ulnaris muscle is able to exert the greatest tension of all the wrist muscles, giving it particular functional relevance, especially with activities requiring high ulnar deviation forces.[48] The flexor carpi ulnaris is active during grip tasks and can be affected by wrist position. Roman-Liu and Bartuzi demonstrated a significant increase in muscle activation during grip tasks when the wrist was flexed compared to an extended or neutral position, suggesting that more activation is needed to maintain the same force output when the muscle is shortened.[49]

The palmaris longus muscle is the most superficial wrist flexor located at the approximate midline of the wrist; therefore, it does not produce radial or ulnar deviation. The presence of the palmaris longus muscle is variable among individuals, with between 1.5% and 63.9% prevalence.[50] Given its apparent redundancy with other muscles as a wrist flexor, the palmaris longus tendon (when present) may be "sacrificed" for surgical reconstruction of other structures.[11] Due to its insertion on the palmar fascia and relationship to the transverse carpal ligament, its presence has been implicated in carpal tunnel syndrome because contraction of the muscle is thought to increase carpal tunnel pressure.[51]

The flexor digitorum superficialis and flexor digitorum profundus muscles are predominantly finger flexors, and the flexor pollicis longus muscle is predominantly a thumb flexor. Their effect other than on the wrist will be described in the section on finger function. As multi-joint muscles, their capacity to effectively contribute to wrist flexion force depends on synergistic stabilization of the joints of the fingers these muscles cross. If these muscles attempt to shorten over both the wrist and the more distal joints, the muscles will become actively insufficient. The flexor digitorum superficialis and flexor digitorum profundus muscles show varied activity in wrist radial/ulnar deviation, as might be anticipated from the central location of the tendons. The flexor digitorum superficialis muscle seems to function more consistently as a wrist flexor than does the flexor digitorum profundus muscle.[52] This is logical because the flexor digitorum profundus muscle is a longer, deeper muscle, and crosses more joints, so it is more likely to become actively insufficient. The effect of the flexor pollicis longus muscle on the wrist has received relatively little attention. The position of this tendon at the wrist suggests the ability to contribute to wrist flexion and radial deviation if its more distal joints are stabilized.

Wrist Kinematics

Wrist ROM varies between individuals and reflects differences in carpal movement that arise from ligamentous laxity, shape of the articular surfaces, and the constraining effects of muscles.[53] There are also variations due to hand dominance, sex, and age.[54] Two recent studies examined wrist ROM, where maximum flexion angles ranged from 53° to 64° and maximum extension values ranged from 65° to 80°; the maximum radial deviation ROM was ~20° whereas ulnar deviation was ~30° to 32°.[55,56]

During flexion and extension, the radiocarpal and midcarpal joints each contribute approximately half of the full active wrist ROM. According to one study in which the typical flexion-extension arc was 111°, the average radiocarpal joint contribution was 63°and the midcarpal joint contribution was 47°.[57]

There is controversy over the location of the combined center of rotation for the wrist joint motion. Many authors suggest that it is the head of the capitate.[4] Neu et al studied capitate kinematics with wrist motion and concluded that the location of the axes of motion are not constant.[58] Badida et al showed that the center of rotation was on the proximal surface of the capitate during flexion and extension but shifted to the mid-capitate during radial and ulnar deviation.[59] Regardless, combined motion of the radiocarpal and midcarpal joints appear centered on the capitate in both flexion/extension and radial/ulnar deviation.

Expanded Concepts 9–2
The Dart-Thrower's Motion

One recent study showed that the orientation envelope of wrist motion is oblique and oriented toward ulnar deviation and flexion.[59] Another described the wrist commonly following a dart-thrower's motion (extension with radial deviation and flexion with ulnar deviation), with a third study describing the wrist as having an elliptical envelope of functional ROM made up ~60% of maximal circumduction.[56,60]

Flexion/Extension

There are a number of biomechanical theories available to describe wrist and intercarpal motion, but there is a lack of consensus on which theory most accurately represents typical motion.[4] Here, we will discuss two theories (the "row theory" and the "link theory") frequently described in rehabilitation literature to provide an overview of radiocarpal, midcarpal, and intercarpal ROM and their importance in wrist stability.

The "row theory," describes the distal and proximal carpal rows separately.[4] The distal carpal row (with its attached metacarpal bones) moves as an almost fixed unit in response to musculotendinous forces imposed by wrist muscle contractions, while strong ligamentous connections between the carpal bones of the distal row limit intercarpal motion.[61] In support of this theory, Norman et al showed that the motion of the bones of the distal carpal row on the proximal row does not differ from each other, except for the motion between the hamate and trapezium at 40° of flexion.[62]

There are no muscular forces applied directly to the bones of the proximal row. Therefore, the proximal carpals move on the radius, ulna, and radioulnar disc, guided and restrained by the connecting ligaments and joint capsule.[61] The intercarpal motions of the scapholunate and lunotriquetral joints in the proximal carpal row move more than those of the distal row. However, the type and amount of motion has been difficult to quantify.

Dynamic computed tomography (4D-CT) has improved the visualization of carpal kinematics.[55,62] While moving from extension to flexion, the amount of flexion between bones of the proximal row appears to differ, with the scaphoid flexing the most (more than 50°) followed by the triquetrum.[55,62] Moving in the opposite direction from extreme flexion to extreme extension, the scaphoid continues to undergo more angular displacement, or "out-of-plane" motion, as it rotates compared to the lunate. The dissimilar motions of the scaphoid and lunate opens, or creates separation, in the palmar surfaces of the two bones during extension, and coapts (close-packs) the two bones during flexion.[1]

The "link joint-theory"[4] was originally proposed by Gilford et al.[63] In this theory, the proximal carpal row serves as a mechanical link interposed between the radius and distal carpal row, often referred to as an **intercalated segment.**[64] In an intercalated segment, the middle segment (the proximal carpal row) tends to collapse between the segments on either side if not held together by a control rod or stop mechanism.[64] This stop mechanism is thought to be provided by the large scaphoid that is part of the proximal carpal row but projects into the distal carpal row (see Fig. 9-9), thus serving as a bridge between the radius and the distal carpal row.[4,64]

An injury to the scaphoid, such as a fracture or injury to the scapholunate interosseous ligament, could disrupt the "bridging effect" of the scaphoid, diminishing or removing the synergistic stabilization between the lunate and scaphoid.[65,66] When this occurs, the scaphoid behaves as an unconstrained middle segment, following its natural tendency to collapse into flexion on the volarly inclined surface of the distal radius (radioscaphoid articulation). The base of the flexed scaphoid slides dorsally on the radius and may sublux. Once released from stabilization of the contiguous scaphoid, the lunate and triquetrum together follow their natural tendency to extend (rotate dorsally) on the radiolunate articulation and triangular fibrocartilage disc. The resulting zigzag pattern of the scaphoid and lunate/triquetrum on the radiocarpal joint proximally and the distal carpal row is known as *intercalated segmental instability.*[67,68]

If the lunate assumes an atypical extended (dorsally tilted) posture when released from its scaphoid attachments, the presentation is referred to as **dorsal intercalated segmental instability** (DISI) **(Fig. 9–16A)**. The scaphoid's subluxation into flexion (volar tilt) may be dynamic, occurring only with compressive loading of the wrist by muscle forces, or the

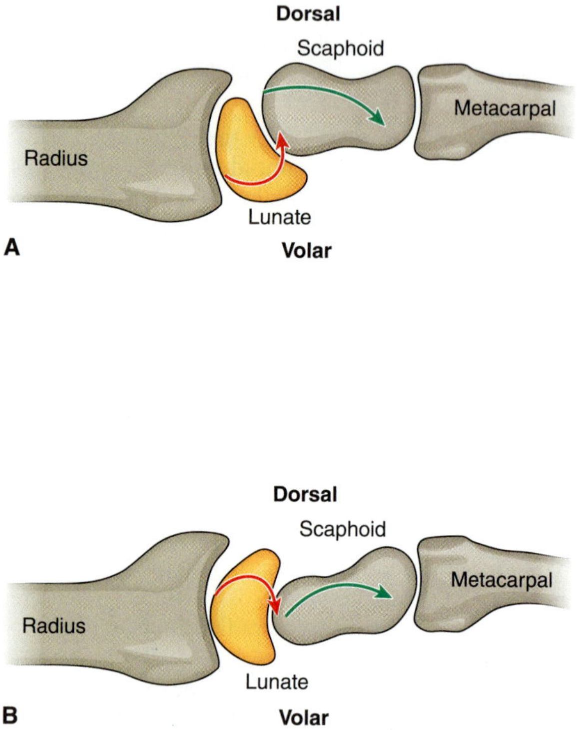

Figure 9–16 **A.** Dorsal intercalated segmental instability (DISI). The lunate, released by ligamentous laxity or a tear from the flexed scaphoid, extends (rotates dorsally) on the radius. **B.** Volar intercalated segmental instability (VISI). The lunate and scaphoid both flex (rotate volarly) on the radius when ligamentous laxity or tear separates the lunate from the triquetrum.

subluxation may become fixed or static.[69] With subluxation of the scaphoid, the pressure of the scaphoid on the lateral facet of the radius increases because the contact occurs over a smaller area.[70,71] Over time, DISI may contribute to degenerative changes at the radioscaphoid joint and ultimately, at the other intercarpal joints.[16] With sufficient intercarpal ligamentous laxity, the capitate, now relatively flexed on the extended lunate, may sublux dorsally off the extended lunate **(Fig. 9–17A)** or, more commonly, migrate into the gap between the flexed scaphoid and extended lunate (see **Fig. 9–17B** and **9–17C**). The progressive degenerative problem from an untreated dorsal intercalated segmental instability is known as **scapholunate advanced collapse (SLAC).**[71,72] The progressive stages have been identified on the basis of radiographs taken over time after injury.[61,72,73] Although it is arguable whether the load between the scaphoid and the lunate increases or decreases with dorsal intercalated segmental instability, there is agreement that the radiolunate articulation is less likely to show degenerative changes than is the radioscaphoid joint.[47,70,74] The lesser tendency toward degenerative changes in the radiolunate joint has been attributed to a more spherical configuration of the radiolunate facets that better distributes the applied loads across the articular surfaces.[71]

The other common form of carpal instability occurs when the ligamentous union of the lunate and triquetrum is disrupted through injury.[67,69] The lunate and triquetrum typically tend to move together toward extension, together offsetting the tendency of the scaphoid to flex. When the lunate is no longer

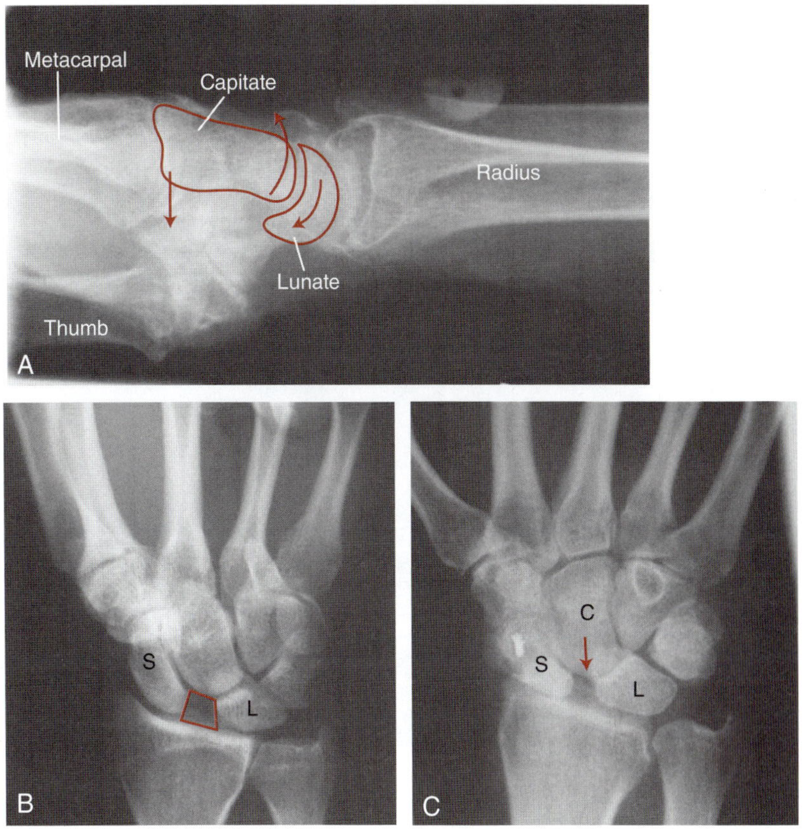

Figure 9–17 **A.** Dorsal intercalated segmental instability (DISI) results in dorsal tilt of the lunate (shown), as well as a less evident volar tilt of the scaphoid and capitate. **B.** With disruption of the scapholunate ligaments through trauma, the scaphoid and lunate migrate apart, leaving a gap (diastasis). **C.** Scapholunate advance collapse (SLAC) with migration of the capitate proximally and erosion of the radioscaphoid and capitate-lunate joints.

linked with the triquetrum, the lunate and scaphoid together fall into flexion, and the triquetrum and distal carpal row extend (see **Fig. 9–16B**). This ulnar perilunate instability is known as **volar intercalated segmental instability (VISI).**[75] This condition is not as common as dorsal intercalated segmental instability. Segmental instabilities and their sequelae illustrate the importance between proximal carpal row stabilization and wrist function, as well as the need to maintain the scaphoid as an intact bridge between the distal carpal row, the other bones of the proximal row, and the radius and disc.

Patient Application 9–2

Jon Chin is a 32-year-old glazier who plays in a men's softball league. When he was 27 years old, he sustained a fall on an outstretched hand FOOSH that resulted in pain and swelling on the dorsum of the wrist. A radiograph taken in a walk-in clinic a week later showed a separation between his scaphoid and lunate (see Fig. 9–16B) that is indicative of ligamentous damage, including a tear of the scapholunate interosseous ligament. It was recommended that he see a hand specialist. A follow-up radiograph with the hand surgeon showed dorsal intercalated segmental instability or DISI (see Fig. 9–16A). Jon made the decision not to pursue any kind of treatment beyond a period of immobilization. The problem appeared to resolve with time. However, he is now finding that pain in his wrist has increased to the point where he has decided once again to seek medical attention from the hand surgeon. The hand surgeon diagnosed SLAC. Repetitive loading of the wrist (grasping, lifting) caused wrist instability marked by proximal migration of the capitate into the space between the scaphoid and lunate, with degenerative changes in the radioscaphoid and capitate-lunate joints (see Fig. 9–17C). A partial wrist fusion (scaphocapitate arthrodesis) was recommended to improve stability (removing one source of pain) while allowing some remaining mobility to minimize loss of wrist function.

Radial/Ulnar Deviation

During radial/ulnar deviation, the distal carpal row moves as a fixed unit at the midcarpal joint. The proximal carpal row displays a unique "reciprocal" motion with radial and ulnar deviation **(Fig. 9–18)**.[1] In **radial deviation,** the proximal carpal row slides in an *ulnar* direction, as is expected arthrokinematically. The convex proximal carpal row is sliding on the concave radioulnar articulation in the direction opposite to osteokinematic motion. Less expectedly, there is simultaneous flexion of the proximal row carpals with radial deviation (see **Fig. 9–18A**). Focusing on the large scaphoid, Amarasooriya et al showed 19° of scaphoid flexion as the wrist moved from ulnar to radial deviation, and 17° of radial angulation in the frontal plane.[55] The opposite arthrokinematics take place during **ulnar deviation**; the convex proximal row slides *radially* on the concave radioulnar surfaces while the scaphoid and lunate extend and ulnarly deviate[76] (see **Fig. 9–18B**).

During wrist radial/ulnar deviation, there is also rotation around a longitudinal axis between bones of the proximal row.[1,76] That rotation is responsible for separating the scaphoid and lunate during ulnar deviation, and coaptating the scaphoid and lunate during radial deviation.[1] The magnitude of individual carpal motion during radial/ulnar deviation is influenced by individual ligament laxity.[53,77]

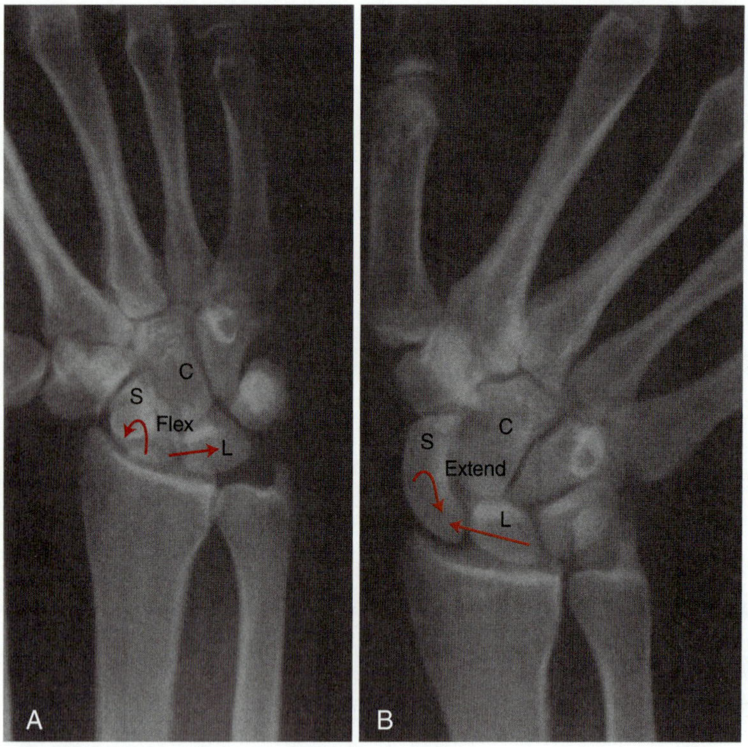

Figure 9–18 **A.** During radial deviation, the proximal row slides ulnarly on the radioulnar surfaces with the scaphoid also flexing. **B.** During ulnar deviation, the proximal row slides radially on the radioulnar surfaces while the scaphoid extends.

Radial and ulnar deviation ROM are greatest when the wrist is in neutral flexion/extension.[78] In full radial deviation, the radiocarpal and midcarpal joints are in closed-packed position, locking the carpal to each other with very little flexion/extension possible.[79,80] Wrist extension is also in the close-packed position. In wrist flexion, the intercarpal joints are loose-packed, but the splaying of the bones of the proximal row limit radial/ulnar deviation in that position.[81]

Wrist Kinetics

There is general agreement that when a longitudinal compressive load is applied to the typical wrist joint, the scaphoid and lunate receive 80% of the load, whereas the triangular fibrocartilage complex receives approximately 20%.[1] This changes when the forearm is in pronation. In pronation, the load across the ulnocarpal joint increases to 37% and is likely due to the relative shortening of the radius compared to the ulna that results in a negative ulnar variance.[1]

Gripping can add additional forces across the wrist joint. When gripping an object, an individual is subject to both compressive and shear forces resulting from externally applied forces and contraction of different muscles used to stabilize the wrist and digits. Forces at the wrist during grip can be up to 10 times higher than the forces applied at the fingertips.[19] At the intercarpal joints, 60% of the load is transmitted through the capitate, to the scaphoid, and lunate, but this distribution can vary substantially depending on the position of the wrist and the amount of ulnar variance.[19] One should consider these important kinetics when designing exercise programs for individuals with wrist injuries.

Structure and Function of the Hand Complex

The "hand" consists of the palm and five digits numbered 1–5, with the thumb being number 1. Digits 2-5 are commonly referred to as "fingers" with different assigned numbers because there are only 4 fingers; we will refer to "digits" in the chapter to avoid confusion between the numbering systems. Each digit has a carpometacarpal joint, an MCP joint, with digits 2–5 each having two interphalangeal joints—one proximal and one distal; the thumb has one interphalangeal joint **(Fig. 9–19)**. Digits 2–5 are similar to each other, but the structure and function of the thumb is substantially different and shall be considered separately.

Digits 2–5

Carpometacarpal Joints 2–5

Carpometacarpal joints are composed of articulations between the distal carpal row and the proximal bases of metacarpals 2–5 (see Fig. 9–19). The second metacarpal articulates primarily with the trapezoid and secondarily with the trapezium and capitate. The third metacarpal articulates primarily with the capitate, the fourth metacarpal articulates with the capitate and hamate, and the fifth metacarpal articulates with the hamate. Each of the metacarpals also articulates at its base with the adjacent metacarpal or metacarpals except for the second metacarpal because it does not articulate with the adjacent first metacarpal. Carpometacarpal joints 2–5 are plane, synovial joints that share a common synovial capsule. The carpometacarpal joints are held together by strong ligaments.[15]

PALMAR ARCHES

The metacarpals are flat posteriorly and concave anteriorly and laterally.[15] This shape, and the shape of the carpometacarpal joints, contribute (along with the thumb) to the **palmar arch system (Fig. 9–20)**. The arches allow the palm and the digits to conform to the shape of an object being held, maximize the amount of surface contact with the object, enhance stability, and increase sensory feedback.[82] The **longitudinal arch** runs longitudinally from carpals proximally to the distal digits. The **proximal transverse (carpal) arch**, as noted earlier in the chapter, is formed by the palmer concavity of the carpal bones (see Fig. 9–10). The transverse carpal ligament and the transversely oriented intercarpal ligaments help maintain the carpal arch, as may the several intrinsic hand muscles that attach to the transverse carpal ligament and bones of the distal carpal row.

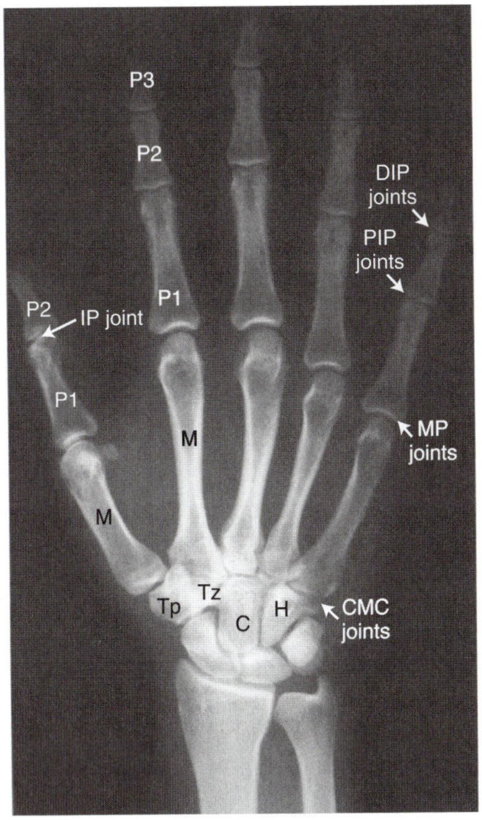

Figure 9–19 Bony anatomy of the thumb and fingers. DIP, distal interphalangeal joint; PIP, proximal interphalangeal joint; MP, metacarpophalangeal joint; CMC, carpometacarpal joint; M, metacarpal; P1, proximal phalanx; P2, middle phalanx; P3, distal phalanx; Tp, trapezium; Tz, trapezoid; C, capitate; H, hamate.

The last of the palmar arches, the **distal transverse arch,** is formed by the adjustable positions of the first, fourth, and fifth metacarpal heads, which is therefore more mobile than the typically fixed concavity of the proximal transverse arch. The deep transverse metacarpal ligament spans the distal portion of the metacarpal heads of the second through fourth metacarpals anteriorly. It tethers together the metacarpal heads, providing stability to the mobile distal palmar arch during grip activities.[83] Although the transverse metacarpal ligament contributes directly to carpometacarpal joint stability, it is structurally part of the MCP joint and will be discussed later in that context.

ROM

The carpometacarpal (CMC) joints of digits 2–5 have a small but variable ROM, with a slight but progressive increase from 2–5. The second and third carpometacarpal joints are essentially immobile and are referred to as the *fixed rays.* The restricted mobility provides a stable, central base upon which the thumb, fourth, and fifth rays move. The fourth and fifth carpometacarpal joints are capable of small amounts of flexion/extension and are consequently referred to as the *mobile rays.* Motion at the fourth and fifth carpometacarpal joints facilitates opposition between the fourth and fifth digits with the thumb while also allowing the fingers to conform to variously shaped and sized objects.

Metacarpophalangeal Joints 2–5

Metacarpophalangeal joints of digits 2–5 are comprised of the convex metacarpal head proximally and the concave base of the proximal phalanx distally (see Fig. 9–19). These MCP joints are condyloid synovial joints with two degrees

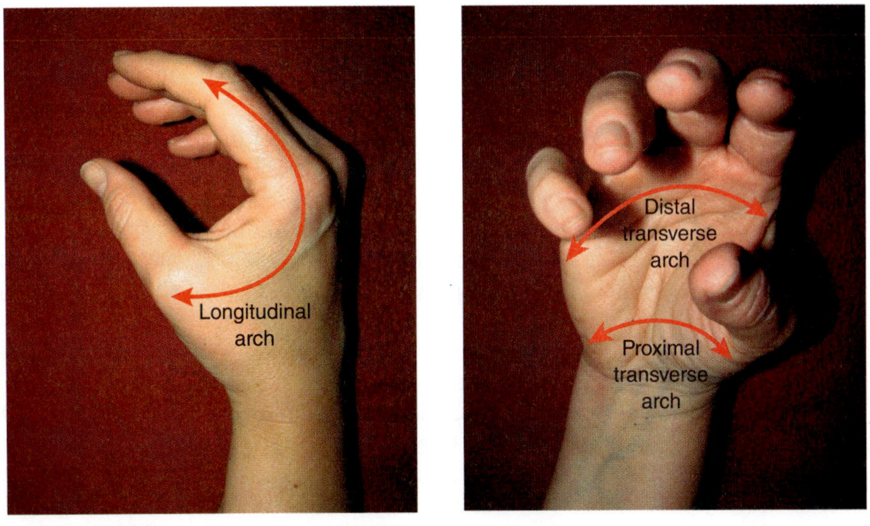

Figure 9–20 The palmar arch system assists with functional grasp. The proximal transverse arch is fixed, whereas the distal transverse arch and the longitudinal arch are mobile.

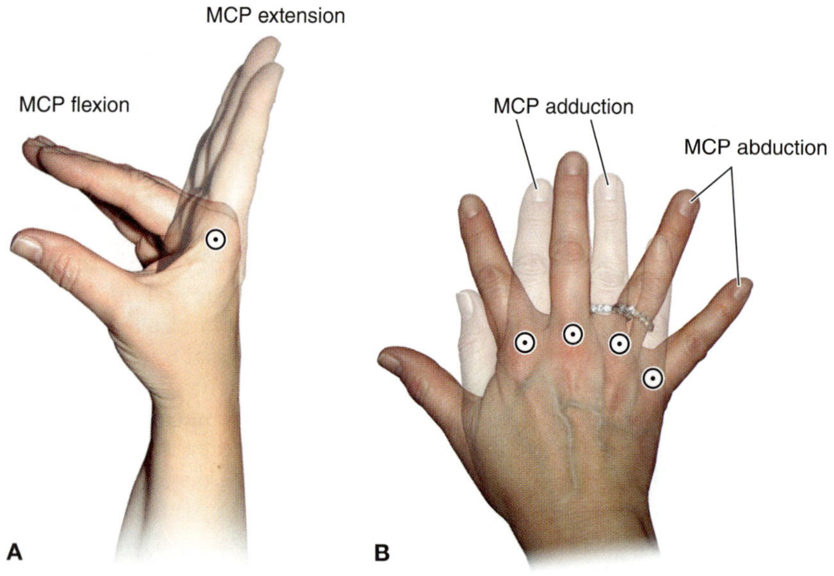

Figure 9–21 Two degrees of freedom at the metacarpophalangeal joints of digits 2–5. **A.** Flexion/extension around a coronal axis through the metacarpal head. **B.** Abduction/adduction around an A-P axis through the metacarpal heads.

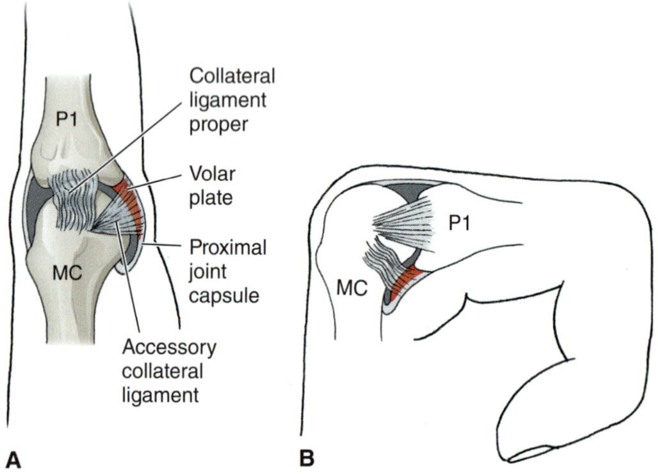

Figure 9–22 Metacarpophalangeal joint capsule, collateral ligaments and volar plate. **A.** The volar plate attaches firmly to the base of the proximal phalanx (P1), blending with the joint capsule to attach loosely to the neck of the metacarpal (MC) below. **B.** In metacarpophalangeal joint flexion, the loose and flexible attachments of the plate and capsule proximally allow the plate to slide down the metacarpal head without impeding motion.

of freedom: flexion/extension and abduction/adduction **(Fig. 9–21)**.[84] The large metacarpal head has 180° of articular surface in the sagittal plane, with the predominant portion lying volarly; the base of the proximal phalanx has only about 20° of articular surface **(Fig. 9–22)**. In the frontal plane, there is less articular surface than in the sagittal plane, and the articular surfaces are more congruent (see Fig. 9–18). Boccolari et al indicated that the head of the metacarpal is trapezoid shaped in the transverse plane, contributing to joint stability.[85]

Metacarpophalangeal joints 2–5 are each surrounded by a capsule that is generally considered to be lax in extension and taut in flexion, making flexion the close-packed position for the MCP joints. Additional noncontractile structures of each MCP joint include two **collateral ligaments** and a **volar plate**, as well as the deep transverse metacarpal ligament that connects the metacarpal heads; these structures all contribute to MCP joint stability. One cadaver study found that MCP joint stability can also be influenced by the extensor mechanism, the sagittal bands, and the extrinsic flexor tendons, each of which will be further discussed.[86]

COLLATERAL LIGAMENTS

The **radial and ulnar collateral ligaments** of the MCP joint are comprised of two parts: the **collateral ligament proper,** which is more dorsal and cordlike, and the **accessory collateral ligament,** which is more volar (see Fig. 9–22). According to a recent scoping review, the collateral ligaments demonstrate position-dependent tension, with the collateral ligament proper being under greater tension during flexion with the accessory collateral ligament typically taut in extension and more lax in flexion.[85] This process of reciprocal tightening between the portions of the collateral ligaments enables constant tension throughout the range of MCP joint motion, thereby providing excellent protection from varus-valgus forces.[85]

In spite of the incongruence of the MCP joint articulations, the accessory structures provide sufficient compensations that the metacarpophalangeal joints have the lowest overall incidence of osteoarthritis compared to other hand joints; unlike other joints in the hand, the osteoarthritic incidence is slightly higher in men than women.[87] This sex difference may be attributable to manual or heavy labor historically performed by men who are now older.[88] In an attempt to understand the lower incidence of osteoarthritis at this joint, authors of one cadaver study measured the fibrocartilage projections from the inner surface of the dorsally located extensor hood; the fibrocartilage was largest at the MCP joints compared to the interphalangeal joints and may contribute to increased surface area for the small base of the proximal phalanx as it articulates with the large metacarpal head.[89]

VOLAR PLATES

The volar plate (or **palmar plate**) is a fibrocartilage projection at MCP joints 2–5. Each plate attaches firmly to the base of the proximal phalanx, loosely to the neck of the metacarpal just below its volar articular surface, and blends with the joint capsule volarly (see Fig. 9–22).[86] The volar plate's function is to enhance joint congruence by adding to the articular surface of the proximal phalanx; it also helps limit MCP hyperextension. The fibrocartilage composition of the plate is consistent with its ability to resist tensile stresses during MCP hyperextension, and compressive forces on the metacarpal head that can occur from objects held in the palm.[90] The membranous attachment to the neck of the metacarpal is sufficiently lax that the plate can slide down the volar surface of the metacarpal head in flexion (see **Fig. 9–22B**) without restricting motion or pinching the long flexor tendons as they pass MCP joints. As we've seen with other accessory joint structures, the plates enhance MCP joint stability without limiting, in this case, flexion mobility. The deep transverse metacarpal ligament connects and blends with the volar MCP joint capsules and their associated volar plates of digits 2–5 **(Fig. 9–23)**.

There are two **sagittal bands** located at each of MCP joints 2–5. These bands lie dorsal to the deep transverse metacarpal ligament, with one on each side of the metacarpal head. The sagittal bands lie superficial to the MCP collateral ligament and do not attach to either the proximal phalanx or the metacarpal, thus are not ligaments. The paired sagittal bands form a cylindrical tube that surrounds the metacarpal head and MCP joints, with their fibers joining the capsule and plate volarly to the extensor digitorum tendon and its associated extensor expansion dorsally **(Fig. 9–24)**.[91] The sagittal bands help stabilize the extensor digitorum tendon over the metacarpal heads, keeping the tendons in their central location on the metacarpal head without falling to either side, especially in MCP flexion. The bands vary in size depending on their associated digit, and move independent of the collateral ligaments during MCP joint flexion and extension.[91]

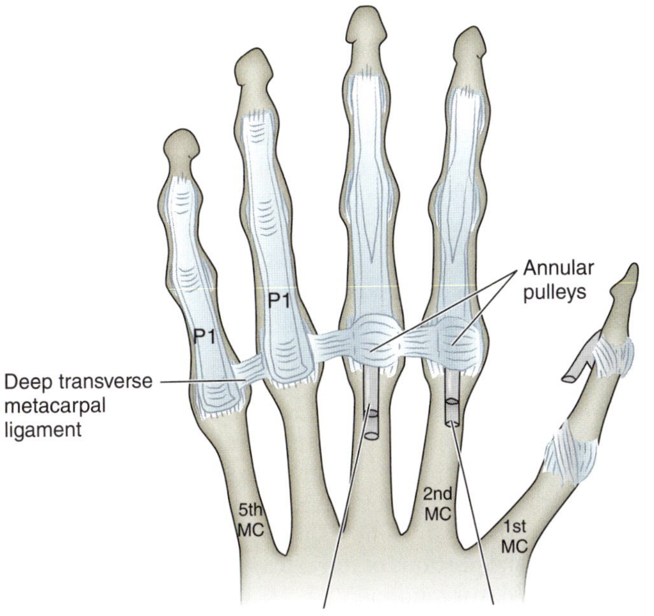

Figure 9–23 The deep transverse metacarpal ligament runs transversely across and joining metacarpal (MC) heads 2–5. The volar aspect of the transverse metacarpal ligament is grooved to hold the long finger flexor tendons (shown on fourth and fifth metacarpophalangeal joints where the more superficial annular pulleys and tendons are removed). P1, proximal phalanx.

ROM

The total available ROM for flexion and extension at MCP joints 2–5 varies with each digit. Flexion/extension increases incrementally from 2–5 **(Fig. 9–25)**, with the second MCP joint having approximately 90° to 100° of flexion.[92] Hyperextension is fairly consistent between digits but varies widely among individuals. The range of passive hyperextension has been used as a measure of generalized body flexibility.[93]

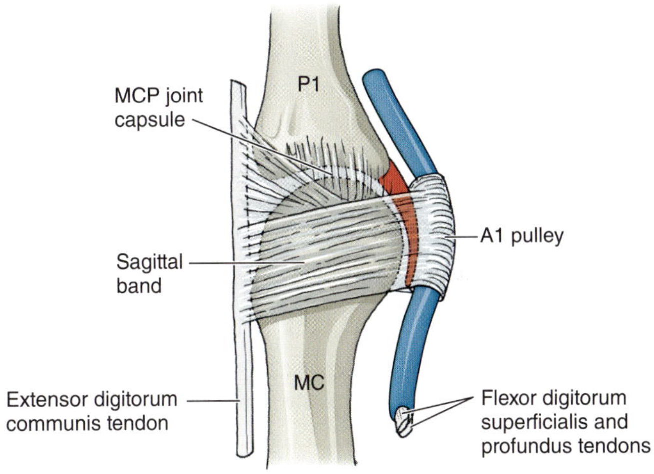

Figure 9–24 The paired sagittal bands lie on each side of metacarpal (MC) head, with attachments to the capsule and its plate volarly and to the extensor digitorum communis tendon and extensor expansion dorsally. The sagittal bands simultaneously help stabilize the volar plates via their capsular connections and the extensor digitorum communis tendons as each crosses the metacarpophalangeal joints. P1, proximal phalanx.

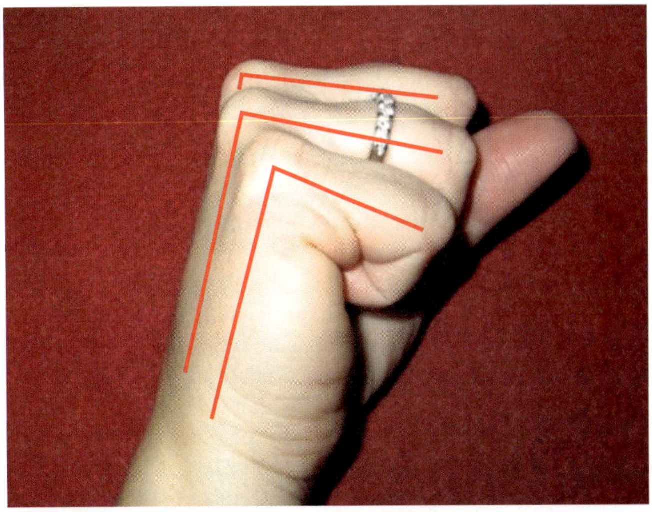

Figure 9–25 The available ROM at the metacarpophalangeal joints of the fingers increases incrementally from 2–5 (second metacarpophalangeal joint not visible), with the greatest metacarpophalangeal finger range at the fifth metacarpophalangeal joint.

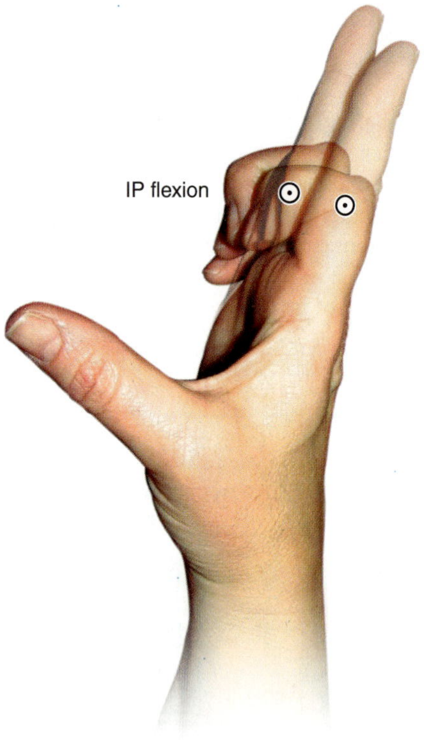

Figure 9–26 One degree of freedom (flexion/extension about a coronal axis) takes place at each of the proximal and distal interphalangeal (IP) joints.

Metacarpophalangeal joint abduction/adduction are named relative to movement toward or away from the third digit (also called the long or middle finger). During abduction, the proximal phalanges (P1s) of digits 2, 4, and 5 (index, ring, and small fingers) move away from the long digit; in adduction, they move toward the long digit. Abduction/adduction are greatest in MCP joint extension compared to flexion. This is due to both joint geometry and MCP joint collateral ligamentous tension. The MCP joints of digits 4 and 5 have more frontal plane mobility than do the middle and ring digits, which may also help in conforming the sides of the hand around different sized and shaped objects.

Interphalangeal Joints 2–5

The **proximal** and **distal interphalangeal joints** (**PIP** and **DIP joints**, respectively) of digits 2–5 are formed proximally by the head of a phalanx and distally by the base of an adjacent phalanx. The IP joints are synovial hinge joints with one degree of freedom (flexion/extension) **(Fig. 9–26)**. The convex head of the proximally located phalanx is bicondylar with an intercondylar groove, and is wider volarly than dorsally. The head of the proximally located phalanx is tilted volarly and has a large articular surface (160°–210°). The base of the more distal phalanx reverses the configuration of the adjacent phalangeal head, having two concave portions separated by a central ridge.[94] There is minimal dorsal articular surface at the PIP or DIP joints; therefore, the joints have minimal to no hyperextension.

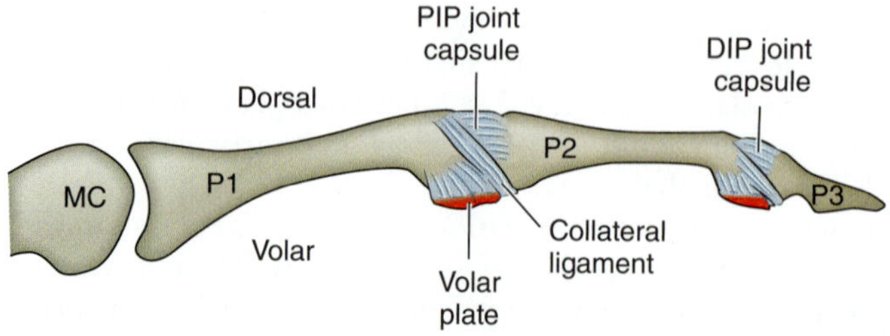

Figure 9–27 The proximal and distal interphalangeal joints (PIP and DIP joints, respectively), like the metacarpophalangeal joints, have volar plates that blend with the volar portion of the capsule. The orientation of the collateral ligaments at the proximal and distal joints, however, differs from that of the collateral ligaments at the metacarpophalangeal joints. MC, metacarpal, P1, proximal phalanx, P2, middle phalanx, P3, distal phalanx.

VOLAR PLATES AND COLLATERAL LIGAMENTS

The proximal and distal interphalangeal joints are similar in structure and soft tissue arrangement.[15] Each has a joint capsule, two collateral ligaments, and a volar plate **(Fig. 9–27)**. Due to these similarities between the PIP and DIP joints of digits 2–5, we will reference the interphalangeal (IP) joints collectively with application to the structural elements of all eight PIP and DIP joints. Like the MCP joint, the IP joint collateral ligaments attach to the more proximal phalanx and to its more distal adjacent phalanx. Each collateral ligament has both a proper and accessory component similar in fiber orientation to those of the MCP joint.[94] Unlike those of the MCP joint, the proper and accessory collateral ligaments are taut throughout the ROM, thus stabilizing the IP joints in all positions. Similar to what was described at the MCP joint, the accessory collateral at each IP joint also stabilizes the volar plates[15] (see Fig. 9–22).

The collateral ligaments are the primary stabilizers to varus/valgus forces at the IP joints. Dzwierzynski et al found the lateral collateral ligament of the second (index) digit to be the strongest, whereas the fifth IP joint had the weakest collateral ligaments.[95] The relative strengths of the lateral collateral ligaments meet functional expectations because the thumb is most likely to oppose the radial side of the index digit (creating a varus stress at the IP joint), and least likely to do so at the fifth digit. Injuries to the collateral ligaments of the IP joint are common, particularly in sports and in the workplace, with the radial collateral twice as likely to be injured as the ulnar collateral.[95] The volar plates of the interphalangeal joints mirror the structure and function described for the volar plates of the MCP joints (see Fig. 9–22). The volar plate increases the congruence (stability) of its respective IP joint without limiting the range of flexion. The more firmly attached distal portion of the plate provides the resistance for joint hyperextension.[94] The IP joints are further supported by the most distal portions of the extensor mechanism as well as by the long flexor tendons.[96]

RANGE OF MOTION

The total range of flexion/extension ROM available to the IP joints is not the same across digits 2–5. The ROM is greater at the PIP joints (e.g., ~100° to 110°) than at the DIP joints (e.g., ~80°). As we saw with both the CMC and MCP joints,

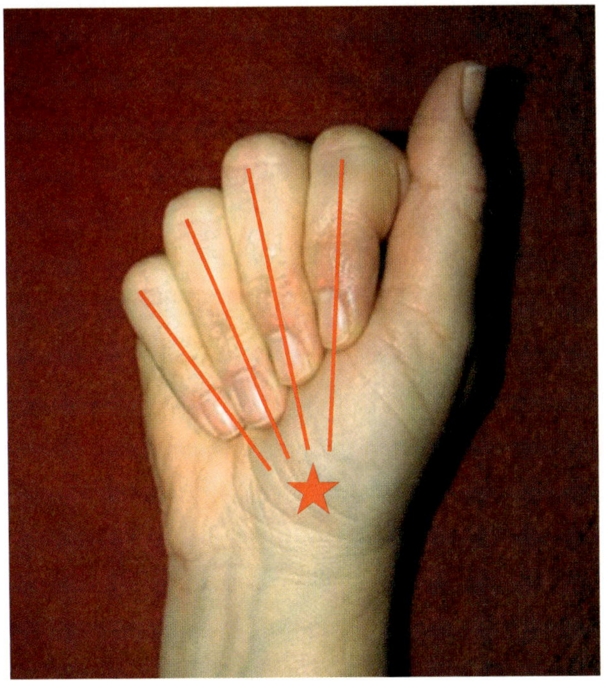

Figure 9–28 With flexion of digits into the palm, there is a convergence of the fingertips toward the scaphoid tubercle (star) and thumb. This obliquity is influenced by the increasing flexion mobility of the carpometacarpal, metacarpophalangeal, and proximal interphalangeal joints from the radial to the ulnar side of the hand.

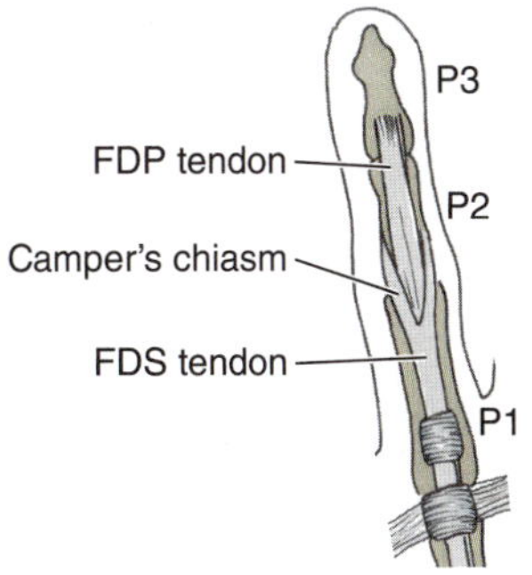

Figure 9–29 The flexor digitorum superficialis (FDS) tendon is superficial to the flex digitorum profundus (FDP) tendon as they cross the metacarpophalangeal joint. The FDS tendon splits at the proximal phalanx (P1) before attaching to the middle phalanx (P2). The deeper FDP tendon emerges through the split FDS tendon (Camper's chiasm) to become the more superficial tendon as it passes on to attach to the distal phalanx (P3).

flexion of the PIP and DIP joints increases incrementally from digit 2 through digit 5, with the PIP and DIP joints of the fifth digit achieving as much as 135° and 90° of flexion, respectively. The increase in DIP flexion is less obvious than that at the PIP joints.[97] The greater ROM available to the more ulnarly located digits, as well as their shorter metacarpals, favors angulation of the fingers toward the scaphoid (termed **flexion convergence**) and facilitates opposition of the fingers with the thumb **(Fig. 9–28)**. The greater ROM available to the fingers ulnarly also facilitates a tighter grip on that more mobile side of the hand. Many objects, such as a drinking glass, are constructed so that the shape is narrower where there is contact with the fourth and fifth digits, but wider at the less mobile second and third digits, thus optimizing contact with the gripped object.

Muscles of the Digits

Extrinsic muscles of the hand are those with proximal attachments on the humerus or forearm, whereas intrinsic muscles are those with all attachments distal to the radiocarpal joint; all, of course, cross the joints of the hand. Functionally, the extrinsic muscles are divided into flexors and extensors. We will discuss the extrinsic and intrinsic muscles of digits 2–5 and then the extrinsic and intrinsic muscles of the thumb separately. We will conclude with discussing the coordinated function of all the muscles together.

Extrinsic Flexors for Digits 2–5

There are two extrinsic muscles that contribute to flexion of the digits 2–5. These are the **flexor digitorum superficialis (FDS)** and the **flexor digitorum profundus (FDP)** muscles. The flexor digitorum superficialis muscle primarily flexes the PIP joint, but also creates flexion moments at the wrist and MCP joints. The flexor digitorum profundus creates flexion moments at these same joints as well as at the DIP joints. The flexor digitorum superficialis muscle can produce more torque at the MCP joint than can the flexor digitorum profundus muscle. Not only does the flexor digitorum superficialis muscle cross fewer joints (making it less likely to lose tension as it shortens over multiple joints), but the flexor digitorum superficialis tendon is also superficial to the flexor digitorum profundus tendon at the MCP joint, and consequently, has a greater moment arm for MCP joint flexion.[98]

Near the head of the proximal phalanx, the flexor digitorum superficialis tendon splits, and at this point the flexor digitorum profundus tendon emerges through the split (**tendinous chiasm,** or **Camper's chiasm**)[34] **(Fig. 9–29)**. The two slips of the flexor digitorum superficialis tendon insert onto the anterior surface of the middle phalanx, deep to the flexor digitorum profundus tendon. At the PIP joint, the flexor digitorum superficialis tendon lies deep to the flexor digitorum profundus tendon and, therefore, has a smaller moment arm at the PIP joint.[98] The switch in position between the flexor digitorum superficialis and flexor digitorum profundus tendons occurs just proximal to the PIP joint.

It is often thought that the flexor digitorum superficialis muscle is the stronger muscle during PIP joint flexion, but the change in its moment arm may influence its strength (torque production) at this joint. Nevertheless, the flexor digitorum superficialis tendon is important for balance at the PIP joint. For example, while estimates vary widely, the fifth digit is actually missing an FDS tendon in one or both hands up to 30% of the time. When the flexor digitorum superficialis tendon is absent, a forceful pinch using the flexor digitorum profundus muscle alone may create DIP joint flexion with accompanying PIP joint *hyper*extension because the middle phalanx is unstable, acting as an intercalated segment **(Fig. 9–30)**.[99]

A recent study examined flexor digitorum superficialis and profundus muscle forces during finger flexion against incrementally increasing resistance. The flexor digitorum

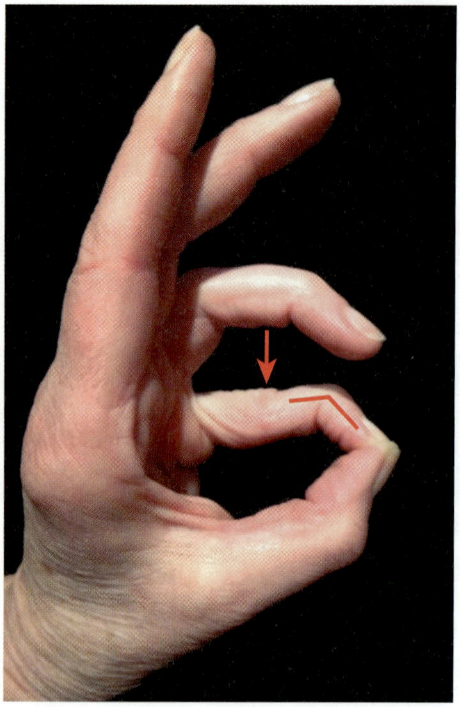

Figure 9–30 Forcefully pressing the pads of the thumb and little finger together activates the flexor digitorum profundus to flex both interphalangeal joints of the little finger against the flexed interphalangeal joint of the thumb. When the flexor digitorum superficialis is absent (as it often is in the little finger), a contraction of the profundus produces distal interphalangeal joint flexion with *proximal interphalangeal joint extension* (arrow). Without the stabilization of the proximal interphalangeal joint by the flexor digitorum superficialis muscle, the flexor digitorum profundus muscle cannot flex both joints.

superficialis consistently produced more force than the flexor digitorum profundus, but the profundus underwent a greater amount of excursion.[100]

As extrinsic muscles, the flexor digitorum superficialis and flexor digitorum profundus muscles are dependent on wrist position for maintaining an optimal length-tension relationship in each muscle.[101] During active finger flexion (as in grasp activities), there will be a counterbalancing wrist extensor force that prevents wrist flexion by the FDS and FDP. Without the synergy of the wrist extensor muscles, contraction of the FDS and FDP muscles will cause wrist flexion to occur, with a concomitant loss of flexor tension at the interphalangeal joints. In fact, it is almost impossible to fully flex the fingers actively if the wrist is also flexed.[102] Although the poor length-tension relationship in the flexor digitorum superficialis and flexor digitorum profundus muscles accounts for some of this phenomenon, the inability to completely flex the digits with wrist flexion is also attributable to the concomitant passive tension in the stretched finger extensors.

In general, muscles that cross the carpometacarpal joints can contribute to changes in the shape of the mobile longitudinal and distal transverse palmar arches (i.e., cupping, or conformation of the palm to an object) by acting on their distal attachments in the hand. Finger flexion tends to increase the curvature of the palmar arches while extension of the fingers tends to be accompanied by relative flattening of the palmar arches. Activity of the flexor carpi ulnaris and intrinsic hand muscles that cross or indirectly act on the midcarpal and carpometacarpal joints can also affect the shape of the arches.[103,104] The extrinsic flexors and extensors that attach distally to the bases of metacarpals 2 and 3 produce little or no motion because these carpometacarpal articulations are relatively fixed.

FLEXION GLIDING MECHANISMS

The flexor function of the flexor digitorum superficialis and the flexor digitorum profundus muscles depends on fibrous structures that stabilize the locations of the FDS/FDP tendons as they pass from the forearm, across the joints of the wrist and hand, to their distal attachments on the middle and distal phalanges.[105] These fibrous structures maintain stability of the tendons along their journey and may also serve as anatomic pulleys. The structures include the flexor retinacula of the wrist (including the transverse carpal ligament) and a series of fibro-osseous structures on the volar surface of each finger known as the **annular** and **cruciate pulleys** **(Fig. 9–31)**. The two most proximal annular pulleys lie closely together, with one (designated the A1 pulley) at the head of the metacarpal and a second larger one (A2 pulley) along the volar midshaft of the proximal phalanx (see **Fig. 9–31A**). The floor of the first (A1) pulley is formed by the previously referenced flexor groove in the transverse metacarpal ligament (see Fig. 9–23), whereas all the other annular pulleys attach directly to bone. The third annular pulley (A3) lies at the distal most part of the proximal phalanx, and the fourth (A4 pulley) lies centrally on middle phalanx. A variable fifth pulley (A5) may lie at the base of the distal phalanx. In addition to the annular pulleys, there are three cruciate (or cruciform) pulleys that also tether the extrinsic flexor tendons. One is located between the A2 and A3 pulleys and is designated as C1; the next cruciate pulley (C2) lies between the A3 and A4 pulleys; and the last cruciate pulley (C3) lies between the A4 and A5 pulleys. The A4, A5, and C3 structures contain only the flexor digitorum profundus tendon because the flexor digitorum superficialis tendon inserts on the middle phalanx, proximal to these structures.

Although the flexor retinaculum and fibro-osseous tunnels maintain the positions of the extrinsic flexor tendons close to the wrist and digital axes of rotation and prevent bowstringing that would result in loss of both excursion and work efficiency in the contracting muscles, these structures also create potential problems. As noted in discussion of the wrist, the extrinsic muscles crossing the wrist joints pass under either the flexor retinaculum (see Fig. 9–13B) or the extensor retinaculum (see Fig. 9–14B). Each tendon is encased in its own or a shared synovium-lined tendon sheath or bursa to minimize friction between the tendons and the fibrous structures that stabilize them. As the flexor digitorum superficialis and profundus pass through their respective annular and cruciate pulleys, the tendons in each finger share a continuous **synovial tendon sheath** containing synovial-like fluid to protect the tendons from friction, thus allowing the tendons to be anchored to the digits without interfering with their excursion.

Of the annular pulleys, the integrity of pulleys A2 and A4 is most critical to maintaining the flexor digitorum superficialis/flexor digitorum profundus muscle efficiency. Once the flexor digitorum profundus tendon passes through the last annular

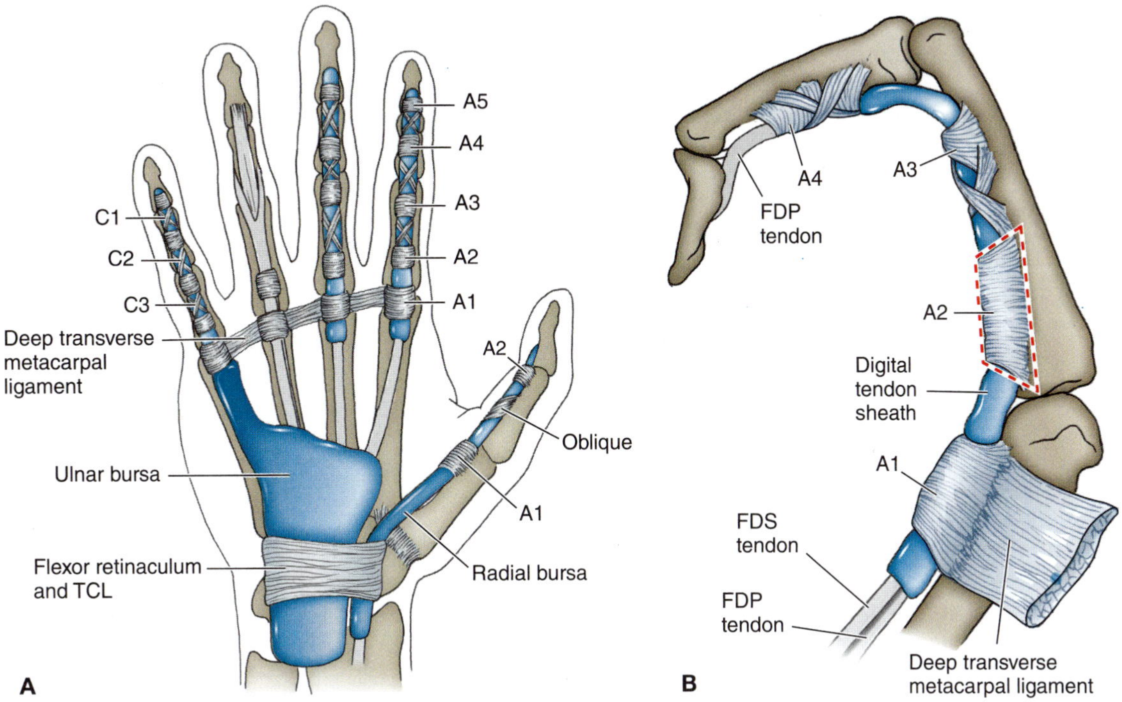

Figure 9–31 Flexor gliding mechanisms. **A.** The flexor mechanisms of the fingers and thumb include the fibro-osseous tunnels formed by the flexor retinaculum and transverse carpal ligament at the wrist, the annular pulleys (A1 to A5) shown on the index finger, and the cruciate pulleys (C1 to C3) shown on the little finger. The tendons are protected within the tunnels by the radial and ulnar bursae and the digital tendon sheaths. **B.** The annular pulleys are shorter on the roof of the tunnel than at its base (as shown at pulley A2) This shape avoids contact between contiguous pulleys during finger flexion, also more evenly distributing pressure on the tendon and sheath against the roof of the fibro-osseous tunnels.

pulley, the tendon sheath ends because lubrication of the tendon is no longer needed.

At the wrist, the tendon sheaths encase multiple tendons to all digits and, as noted earlier, are known as the ulnar and radial bursae (see Fig. 9–13B). All eight tendons of the flexor digitorum profundus and flexor digitorum superficialis muscles are contained within the ulnar bursa, with the bursa compartmentalized to prevent friction between tendons. The pattern of connections between bursae and tendon sheaths may vary among individuals; in the most common pattern, the tendon sheath for digit 5 is continuous with the ulnar bursa while the tendon sheaths for digits 2–4 are not. For digits 2–4, the ulnar bursa ends just distal to the proximal palmar crease, with the digital tendon sheaths beginning at the middle or distal palmar creases.[106]

Any interruption in the digital tendon sheaths or annular pulleys can result in substantial functional impairment of flexor digitorum superficialis and flexor digitorum profundus muscles or in structural deformity. **Trigger finger** is one example of such a pathology. Overuse of the finger flexors or comorbid conditions may lead to inflammation of the tendon sheath, impairing the ability of the flexor tendon to glide smoothly within the sheath, particularly at the annular pulleys (most commonly at the A1). The tendon itself may then become inflamed as well, thus narrowing the space within the annular pulley. This causes resistance to tendon gliding during active flexion of the affected finger, potentially leading to the finger getting "stuck" in flexion until a manual extension force is applied.

The vascular supply to the flexor tendon gliding mechanism is critical to tendon nutrition. Direct vascularization of each tendon occurs through vessels that reach the tendon via the **vincula tendinum.** The vincula are folds of synovial membrane (usually four in number) that carry blood vessels to the tendon and to the tendinous insertions of the flexor digitorum superficialis and profundus muscles of each finger.[15] The tendons also receive some of their nutrition directly from the synovial fluid within the sheath.

Expanded Concepts 9–3
Connection Between Bursae and Digital Tendon Sheaths

The connection between the ulnar bursa proximally and the digital tendon sheaths that may communicate with that bursa is clinically relevant. Infection within a tendon sheath can travel throughout its shared bursa and sheaths, producing painful tenosynovitis throughout. For example, if a tendon sheath for a digit is continuous with the ulnar (or radial) bursa, infection initiated at that digit can spread from the digit into the palm (or vice versa). The tendon sheaths for digits 2–5 terminate proximal to the insertion of the flexor digitorum profundus muscle, effectively ending at the distal aspect of the middle phalanx. Consequently, puncture wounds or injuries to the digital pads (distal phalanx), which are a fairly common site of trauma, are unlikely to introduce infection into the digital tendon sheaths and bursa.

Extrinsic Extensors for Digits 2–5

The extrinsic muscles that extend the digits are the extensor digitorum, the extensor indicis, and the extensor digiti minimi muscles. The extrinsic digital extensors are also wrist extensors, as previously described. The extensor indicis and extensor digiti minimi tendons attach distally to the extensor digitorum tendon at or just proximal to the extensor hood. Given their attachments to the extensor digitorum, the extensor indicis and extensor digiti minimi muscles add force and independent action to extension of the second and fifth digits, respectively.

The extensor digitorum tendons of one digit may be connected to the tendon(s) of adjacent digit(s) by junctura tendinae. The slips of connective tissue connect the extensor digitorum tendon for the second (index) digit to the third (middle) and fourth (ring) digits, with variable connections to the second (index) digit[24] (see Fig. 9–15). In general, the index digit has the most independent active extension, with extension of the fifth, fourth, and third digits in declining order of independence.[107]

Intrinsic Finger Muscles for Digits 2–5

DORSAL AND PALMAR INTEROSSEI MUSCLES

There are four **dorsal interossei** muscles (one to each digit) and three **palmar interossei** muscles. These intrinsic muscles attach proximally to the sides of contiguous metacarpals 1–4; distally some muscle fibers insert directly into the proximal phalanx of digits 2–4, while others join and become part of the extensor mechanism on the dorsal surface of the digit **(Fig. 9–32)**. The little finger (digit 5) does not have a dorsal interosseous muscle; instead, the abductor digiti minimi is the MCP abductor for the fifth digit. Although bearing a dissimilar name because it attaches to only one metacarpal, the abductor digiti minimi muscle otherwise has similar attachments and alignment to the dorsal interossei, with similar effects on the MCP and IP joints. While discussion will not include reference to the abductor digiti minimi, it should be assumed that descriptions of the dorsal interossei also apply to the abductor digiti minimi.

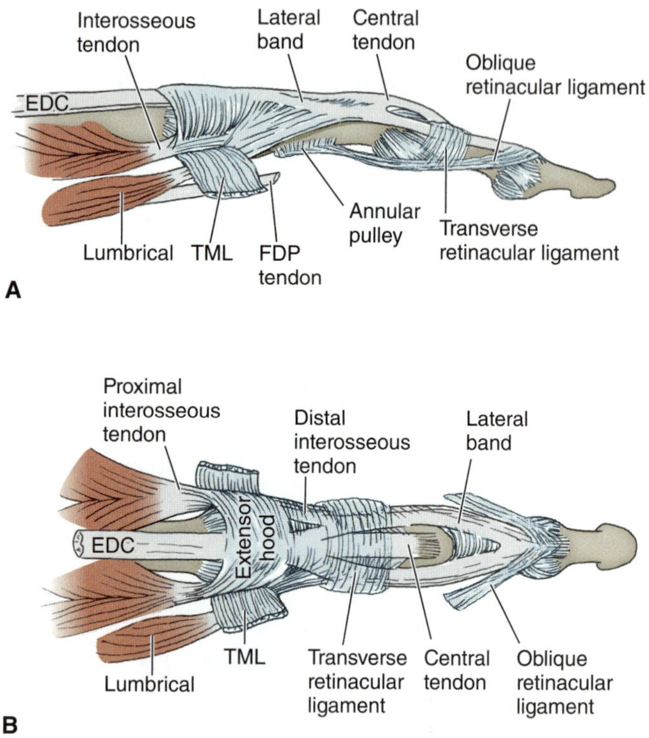

Figure 9–32 In both the lateral, **A**, and superior, **B**, views, one can see that the interossei muscles pass dorsal to the transverse metacarpal ligament (TML), typically with some fibers attaching directly to the base of the proximal phalanx while other fibers attach more distally to the central tendon and lateral bands of the extensor mechanism. The lumbrical muscles attach to the flexor digitorum profundus (FDP) tendon proximally and to the lateral bands of the extensor mechanism distally. The oblique retinacular ligament is attached to the A2 annular pulley proximally and to the lateral bands of the extensor mechanism distally. EDC, extensor digitorum communis.

The dorsal and palmar interossei muscle groups are often characterized by their ability to produce MCP joint abduction and adduction, respectively. However, all of the dorsal interossei and palmar interossei muscles pass *dorsal* to the transverse metacarpal ligament but *volar* to the axis for MCP joint flexion/extension. Therefore, the interossei can be characterized not only as abductors or adductors of their respective MCP joints but also as flexors of that joint. Changes in MCP joint position change the interossei muscle moment arms. Thus, their ability to produce abduction, adduction, or flexion changes based on the position of the MCP joint.

When the MCP joint is in extension, the tendons of the interossei muscles pass directly through (or very near to) the MCP axis for flexion/extension; consequently, there is a very small moment arm for MCP flexion with little or no flexion torque generated by an active contraction. While in MCP joint extension, the interossei muscles can also be effective MCP joint stabilizers (joint compressors) and are important in checking MCP joint hyperextension of the fingers by the intact extensors.[107,108] Further, when the MCP joints are in extension, the interossei (and abductor digiti minimi) muscles lie at a relatively large distance from the A-P axis for MCP joint abduction/adduction, making them very effective at those motions without the loss of tension that would occur if the muscles were to simultaneously produce MCP joint flexion.

As the MCP joint flexes, the tendons and action lines of the interossei muscles migrate volarly away from the MCP joint's coronal axis, increasing their moment arm for MCP flexion **(Fig. 9–33)**. In full MCP joint flexion, the action lines of the interossei muscles are nearly perpendicular to the proximal phalanx, with the palmar interossei possessing larger moment arms than the dorsal interossei.[109] Consequently, the ability of the interossei muscles to create an MCP flexion torque increases as the MCP joint moves toward full flexion. As the MCP joint approaches full flexion, the deep transverse metacarpal ligament limits any further volar migration of the interossei tendons; the collateral ligaments also become increasingly taut, thus limiting MCP abduction/adduction. The effect is that the MCP flexed position results in a large MCP joint flexion torque, now making the interossei muscles powerful MCP joint flexors capable of contributing to a coordinated and strong grip force.[101,109]

The portions of the dorsal and palmar interossei muscles that attach to the extensor mechanism of digits 2–5 (rather

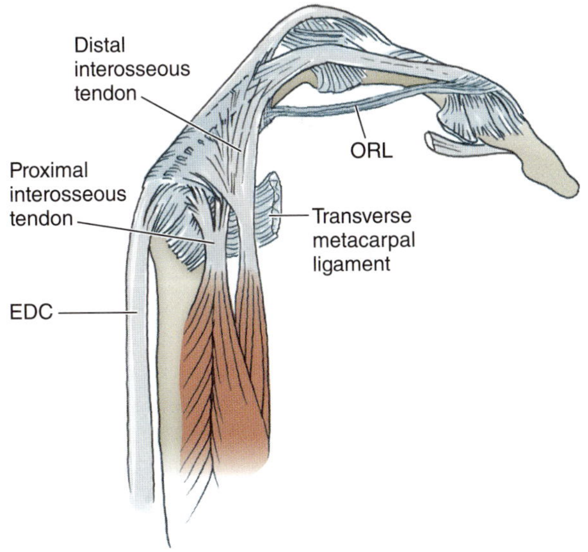

Figure 9–33 When the metacarpophalangeal joint is flexed, the interossei muscles migrate anteriorly away from the metacarpophalangeal joint axis for flexion/extension, resulting in a relatively large moment arm and a line of pull that is nearly perpendicular to the proximal phalanx. The anterior migration of the interossei muscles is limited by the deep transverse metacarpal ligament that prevents loss of tension and serves as an anatomic pulley for the interossei. EDC, extensor digitorum communis; ORL, oblique retinacular ligament.

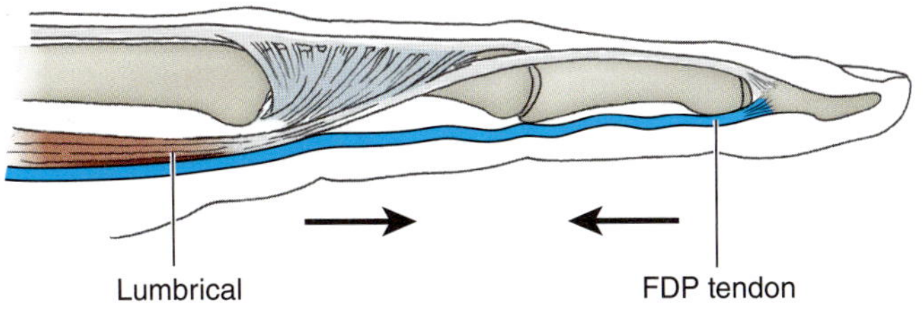

Figure 9–34 The lumbrical muscle attaches to the flexor digitorum profundus (FDP) tendon proximally and to the lateral band of the extensor expansion distally. A contraction of the lumbrical muscle will create tension in the lateral band, leading to proximal/distal interphalangeal joint extension, concomitantly pulling the tendon of the relaxed flexor digitorum profundus distally and releasing the passive flexor tension that could impede interphalangeal extension.

than directly to the bases of the proximal phalanx) are, for that reason, often referred to as the *distal interossei*. The distal interossei are instrumental in producing interphalangeal joint extension via their pull on the central tendon and lateral bands of the extensor mechanism (see Fig. 9–32). Interphalangeal joint extension torque produced by the distal interossei varies with changes in the MCP joint flexion angle. For example, when the MCP joint is extended, the action lines of the distal interossei attachments are capable of extending the interphalangeal joints through their active pull on the extensor mechanism. With the MCP joints in flexion, the volar migration of the interossei tendons is checked by the transverse metacarpal ligament (see Fig. 9–33). This ligament prevents the interossei tendons from becoming slack, providing a pulley effect on the now stretched interosseous tendons and enhancing the function of the distal interossei muscles as interphalangeal joint extensors.

In the position of combined MCP flexion and interphalangeal extension, both the proximal and distal attachments of the interossei muscles are effective active MCP joint flexors, while the distal components are also effective as interphalangeal (PIP and DIP) joint extensors. The consistent activity of both the dorsal and palmar interossei during combined MCP flexion and interphalangeal extension provides evidence of the optimal biomechanics for all elements of the interossei in this position.

LUMBRICAL MUSCLES

There are four intrinsic **lumbrical muscles**, one on each of digits 2–5. The lumbricals attach proximally to the flexor digitorum profundus before the profundus tendon crosses the MCP joint. The lumbricals attach distally to the radial side of the lateral bands of the extensor mechanism beyond the attachments of the distal interossei. Uniquely, the lumbricals are the only muscles that do not attach to a bone at either end.[110, 111] Like the interossei muscles, the lumbricals cross the MCP joint volar to its coronal axis and dorsal to the interphalangeal joints through their attachment to a lateral band.

The lumbrical muscles are more superficial than the interossei muscles (see Fig.9–32A), thus appearing to have a greater moment arm for MCP joint flexion. Functionally, however, the lumbrical muscles contribute little to the flexion torque at the MCP joint.[110] This relative weakness may be attributed to the small cross section of the lumbrical muscles compared to the somewhat larger interossei muscles, as well as to its proximal attachment to the mobile flexor digitorum profundus tendon. An active lumbrical contraction not only pulls on its lateral band to produce an extension torque at the IP joints but also shifts the mobile profundus tendon somewhat distally. This tendon shift releases some of the *flexor* tension in the profundus tendon at the IP joints while the lumbricals simultaneously *extend* the IP joints **(Fig. 9–34)**. If the profundus muscle belly does not maintain at least some active or passive tension in its tendon, the pull of the lumbrical may shift the profundus tendon so far distally that the lumbricals' MCP joint flexion and IP extension torques are impaired.

HYPOTHENAR MUSCLES

Muscles of the **hypothenar eminence** include the **abductor digiti minimi,** the **flexor digiti minimi,** and the **opponens digiti minimi.** As noted earlier, the abductor digiti minimi functions as a proximal interosseous muscle to flex and abduct the fifth MCP joint. The flexor digiti minimi arises from structures within the palm, crosses the fifth MCP joint, and attaches to the fifth proximal phalanx. According to Brand and Hollister,[101] the flexor digiti minimi—like the abductor digiti minimi—can abduct and flex the MCP joint of the fifth digit although the abductor digiti minimi has a greater moment arm for abduction. The opponens digiti minimi also arises from structures in the palm but attaches to the fifth metacarpal, crossing the fifth carpometacarpal joint but not its MCP joint. No other muscles cross or act on the finger carpometacarpal joints alone. The oblique line of pull of the opponens digiti minimi is optimally aligned to flex and rotate

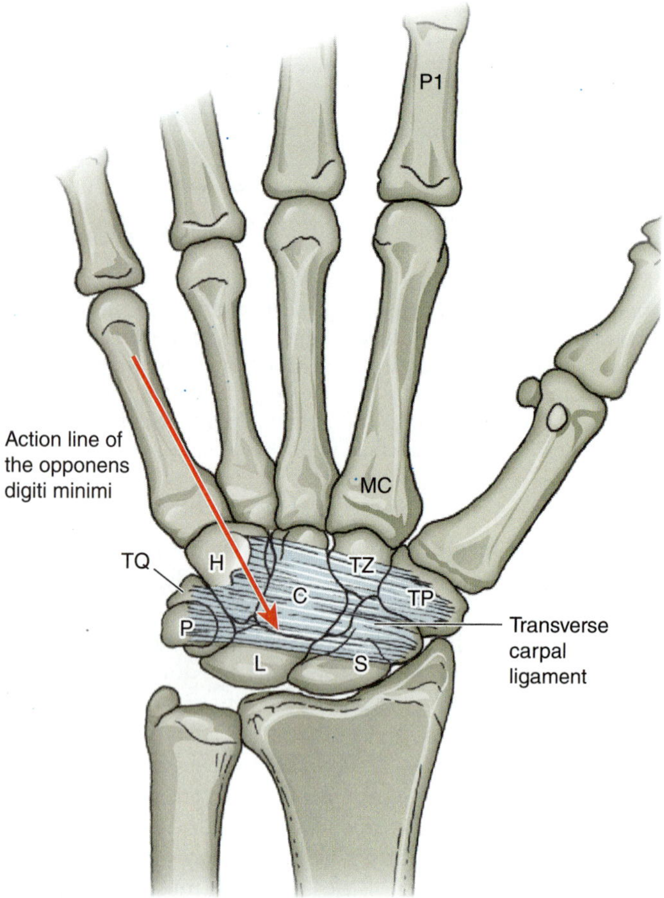

Figure 9–35 The opponens digiti minimi is the only muscle that acts exclusively on a carpometacarpal joint. As indicated by its action line, it is effective at flexion of the fifth metacarpal joint and rotation of the metacarpal joint around its long axis. The opponens digiti minimi muscle's attachment to the transverse carpal ligament may also contribute to supporting the proximal palmar arch.

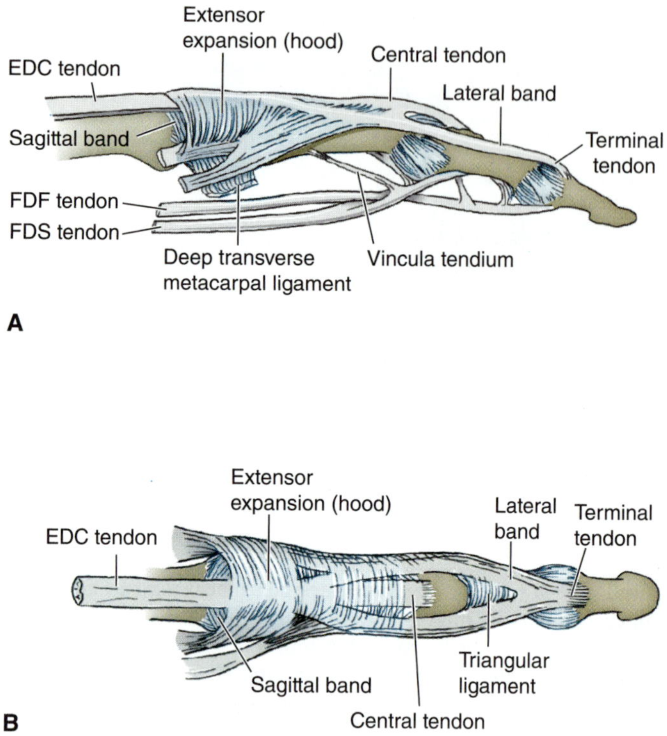

Figure 9–36 In the lateral, **A,** and superior, **B,** views, one can see the building blocks of the extensor mechanism. The elements include the extensor digitorum communis (EDC) tendon that merges with the extensor hood and sagittal bands and then continues distally to split into a central tendon inserting into the middle phalanx, and two lateral bands that merge into a terminal tendon that inserts into the distal phalanx. The two lateral bands are stabilized dorsally by the triangular ligament. The vincula tendium is composed of synovial folds that carry blood vessels to the long flexor tendons.

the fifth metacarpal about its long axis **(Fig. 9–35)**, with its primary function to oppose the fifth digit toward the thumb by rotating the metacarpal and turning the palm into a cup, with this action contributing *indirectly* to MCP flexion.[101]

The opponens digiti minimi and the flexor digiti minimi muscle activity pattern is more variable than that of the abductor digiti minimi; however, both tend to show activity in direct proportion to the amount of abduction and rotation of the *first* metacarpal required by a task. In fact, increased activity of the opponens pollicis muscle automatically results in increased activity of the opponens digiti minimi and flexor digiti minimi muscles.

Extensor Mechanism for Digits 2–5

ANATOMY

The extensor mechanism for digits 2–5 is comprised of the extensor digitorum tendon and active and passive interconnections at the MCP and interphalangeal joints. The foundation of each finger's extensor mechanism is the tendon of the extensor digitorum muscle along with its accompanying tendons of the extensor indicis and extensor digiti minimi muscles. As noted earlier, reference to the extensor digitorum tendon at the second and fifth digits will be assumed to include the extensor indicis and extensor digiti minimi, respectively. At the MCP joint, the extensor digitorum tendon flattens into a broad aponeurosis known as the **extensor expansion** and alternatively known as the **dorsal expansion** or **dorsal hood (Fig. 9–36)**. The extensor expansion is a triangle-shaped connective tissue structure fanning around the dorsum and sides of the metacarpal head and base of the proximal phalanx.[34] Here, the sagittal bands connect the dorsal surface of the extensor expansion to the volar plate (see Fig. 9–24), as well as to the deep transverse metacarpal ligament (see **Fig. 9–36A**).

Distal to the MCP joint, the extensor digitorum tendon splits into three bands: the central tendon that attaches to the base of the middle phalanx, and two lateral bands that cross the PIP joints before rejoining to form the terminal tendon that attaches to the base of the distal phalanx (see Fig. 9–36A and 9–36B). The connections of the distal interossei to these components of the extensor mechanism were previously discussed. At the PIP joint, the lateral bands are interconnected dorsally by a triangle-shaped band of superficial fibers known as the **triangular ligament**, or *triangular membrane*[15] (see **Fig. 9–36B**). When the PIP joint is flexed, the lateral bands might separate to either side of the joint, but the triangular ligament helps stabilize the lateral bands on the dorsal surface of the finger.

The final connective tissue structures that contribute to the extensor mechanism are the **oblique retinacular ligaments (ORLs)**. The oblique retinacular ligaments arise volarly from both sides of the proximal phalanx and it's A4 annual pulley volarly, continuing distally to attach to the lateral bands just distal to the PIP joint (see Fig. 9–32A and 9–32B).[112,113] The oblique retinacular ligaments lie volar to the PIP joint and dorsal to the DIP joint with its function described in the next section on biomechanics.

The structures of the extensor expansion are key components contributing to the delicate balance between finger flexors and extensors, thus affecting the quality of grasp and release and essential for maintaining force producing capability of the finger.[114, 115]

BIOMECHANICS

Extensor Mechanism Influence on Metacarpophalangeal Joint Function

The extensor digitorum, extensor indicis, and extensor digiti minimi are the only muscles capable of extending the MCP joints. These muscles extend the MCP joints via their connection to the extensor expansion. An active contraction of the muscle creates tension on the extensor expansion of the extensor mechanism, pulling the expansion proximally over the MCP joint, thus extending the proximal phalanx on the metacarpal head.

When the hand is completely relaxed (at rest), it typically assumes a position of at least slight flexion at all the finger joints. However, in the presence of an ulnar nerve injury, the hand will rest in MCP extension or hyperextension with flexion observed at the interphalangeal joints. This position of the fingers (MCP joint hyperextension with passive interphalangeal flexion) is known as **clawing** (**Fig. 9–37**). The interphalangeal flexion that accompanies MCP joint hyperextension in an ulnar nerve injury is produced by passive tension in the flexor digitorum superficialis and flexor digitorum profundus muscles that are stretched over the hyperextended MCP joint.

Clawing of the hand is typically seen when passive tension in the primary MCP flexors (the lumbricals and interossei) is absent due to the ulnar nerve injury—even if the flexor digitorum superficialis is intact in all fingers. The second (index) and third (middle) digits are extended, but not hyperextended, at the MCP joint (see Fig. 9–37) because the lumbrical and flexor digitorum profundus muscles of those two digits are intact (innervated by the radial rather than ulnar nerve); the passive tension in the intact lumbricals and profundus is sufficient to prevent MCP hyperextension. Clawing at rest demonstrates that the passive tension in the extensor digitorum provides more extension torque at the MCP joint than does passive flexion torque from the remaining flexors. The clawed position is also known as an **intrinsic minus position** because it is attributed to the absence of the finger intrinsic muscles (although the first and second lumbricals remain intact).

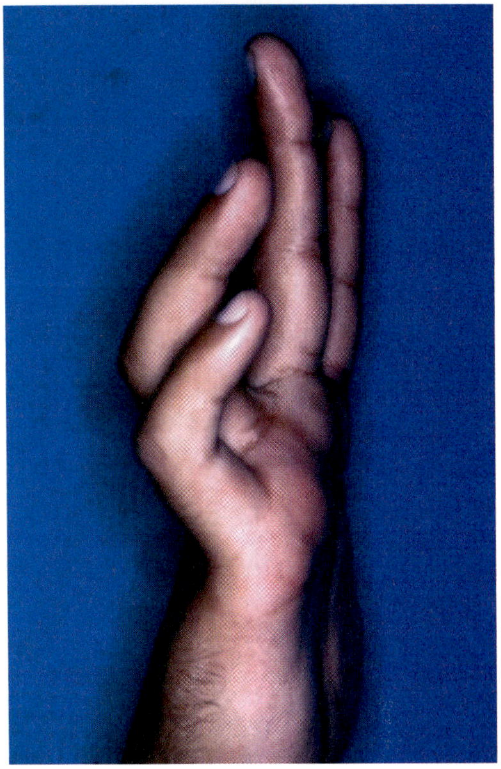

Figure 9–37 In the ulnar nerve–deficient hand (claw hand) at rest, the metacarpophalangeal joints of the ring and little finger are hyperextended because of relatively unopposed passive tension in the intact extensor digitorum communis muscle resulting from the loss of the interossei and lumbrical muscles; the interphalangeal joints of those fingers are flexed because of increased passive tension in the long flexors stretched over the extended metacarpophalangeal joints. The index and middle fingers are less affected because these fingers still have intact median nerve–innervated lumbricals.

Foundational Concepts 9–2
Intrinsic Muscles Summary

- The dorsal and palmar interossei produce MCP joint abduction and adduction torque, respectively; the abduction/adduction ROM is limited when the MCP joint is in flexion due to MCP joint structural limitations.
- Interossei that have attachments directly to the base of the proximal phalanx are known as *proximal* interossei, while those with attachments more distally on the extensor expansion are known as *distal* interossei.
- Proximal interossei are strong flexors of the MCP joint; distal interossei are strong extensors of the proximal and distal IP joints via their pull on the extensor expansion.
- The lumbrical muscles are strong extensors of the interphalangeal joints, regardless of MCP joint position.
- The lumbrical muscles are relatively weak MCP joint flexors, regardless of the MCP joint position.
- The ability of the lumbrical muscles to extend the interphalangeal joints appears to depend only on intact tension in the extensor mechanism and in the flexor digitorum profundus tendons.

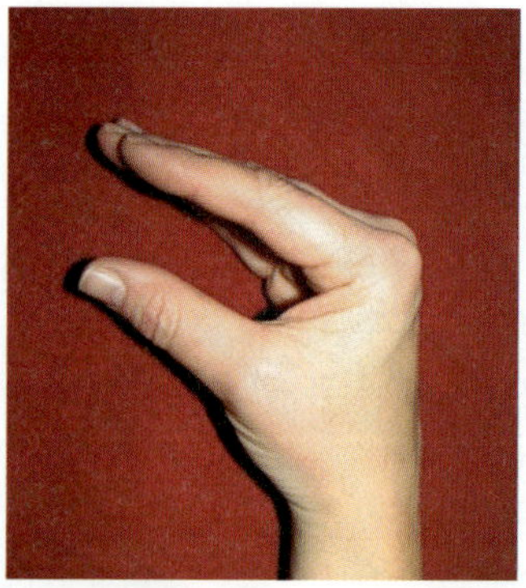

Figure 9–38 Activity of the lumbrical and interossei muscles without any *extrinsic* finger flexor or extensor activity produces the "intrinsic plus" position of the hand (metacarpophalangeal flexion and interphalangeal extension).

- When the lumbrical and interossei muscles are both active without any extrinsic finger flexor or extensor muscle activity, these intrinsic muscles produce MCP joint flexion and interphalangeal joint extension, the so-called **intrinsic plus** position of the hand (named because the intrinsics are intact) **(Fig. 9–38)**.
- When the extrinsic finger flexors and extensors are active without any concomitant activity of the intrinsic muscles, the hand assumes a claw position, or intrinsic minus position (see Fig. 9–37).

Extensor Mechanism and Interphalangeal Joint Extension

Extension of the proximal and distal interphalangeal (PIP and DIP) joints are interdependent. That is, PIP and DIP extension always occur together. This interdependence can be understood by examining structural relationships in the extensor mechanism.

The PIP joint is crossed dorsally by the central tendon and lateral bands of the extensor expansion and the DIP joint is crossed by the terminal tendon (see Fig. 9–36). The extensor digitorum, interossei, and lumbrical muscles all have attachments to one or more structures that make up the extensor expansion (see Fig. 9–32) and rely on each other to maintain function.

An extensor digitorum muscle contraction alone will produce MCP joint extension but not interphalangeal joint extension. An active contraction of a distal interosseous or lumbrical muscle alone *is* capable of extending the PIP and DIP joints but will produce simultaneous MCP joint flexion. Although it may appear that the intrinsic muscles are independently extending the interphalangeal joints, simultaneous passive tension in the extensor digitorum and extensor expansion (stretched over the flexed MCP joint) may be assisting the active intrinsic muscles by anchoring the proximal portion of the extensor mechanism. In addition to the need for some tension in the extensor digitorum to allow the intrinsics to produce IP joint extension, we've already seen that the lumbricals rely on some tension in the flexor digitorum profundus tendon to be effective in their IP joint extension function. Ranney and Wells confirmed this, finding that the lumbrical muscles did not begin to extend the interphalangeal joints until the tension within the lumbrical muscle equalled the tension in the flexor digitorum profundus tendon.[116] The distal interossei muscles, without the lumbricals, are less effective interphalangeal extensors. The interossei do not have the same ability to release the passive tension of the flexor digitorum profundus tendon; thus, the distal interossei have to extend the IP joints against the passive resistance of the profundus tendon.

The oblique retinacular ligaments also contribute to the interdependence of PIP and DIP joint extension. As a reminder, the two oblique retinacular ligaments on each finger pass just volar to the PIP joint axis and attach distally to the radial and ulnar sides of the lateral bands (see Fig. 9–32). When the PIP and DIP joints are both flexed, the oblique retinacular ligaments are slack at the PIP joint but still retain some tension from the passively stretched lateral bands (see Fig. 9–33). If extension is initiated at the PIP joint (whether actively or passively), the oblique retinacular ligaments will increase tension as the PIP joint extends; consequently, the ligaments will increase their pull on the taut lateral bands and the DIP joint will begin to extend as well. However, the length of each oblique retinacular ligament is such that the contribution of PIP joint extension to producing DIP extension via the oblique retinacular ligaments may be significant only during the first half of the DIP joint's return from flexion (90°–45° flexion) when the lateral bands and attached oblique retinacular ligaments are most stretched.[112,116]

Extensor Mechanism and Interphalangeal Joint Flexion

Just as PIP and DIP joint extension are typically coupled, flexion of the PIP and DIP joints is similarly linked by a complex combination of active and passive forces. When DIP joint flexion is initiated by a contraction of the flexor digitorum profundus muscle, there is a simultaneous flexor torque applied at the PIP joint that the tendon also crosses, so simultaneous DIP and PIP joint flexion is not surprising. However, the active force of the flexor digitorum profundus muscle on the distal phalanx might *not* be sufficient to produce simultaneous PIP flexion if extensor restraining forces at the PIP joint were not released at the same time.

When DIP flexion is initiated by the flexor digitorum profundus muscle, the terminal tendon and its lateral bands are stretched over the dorsal aspect of the DIP joint. The stretch in the lateral bands shifts the extensor expansion (from which the lateral bands arise) distally. This distal migration causes the central tendon to relax, thus releasing its extensor influence at the PIP joint and, thereby, facilitating PIP flexion. The simultaneous flexor torque and release of extensor torque still might not be adequate for the flexor digitorum profundus muscle to simultaneously flex the PIP joint if the lateral bands remained taut on the dorsal aspect of the PIP joint. The bands, however, are permitted to separate somewhat by the elasticity of the interconnecting triangular ligament (see Fig. 9–36) and by passive tension in the transverse retinacular ligament (see Fig. 9–32). Although the example used here was initiated by an active contraction of the flexor digitorum profundus muscle, the same set of mechanisms will tie passive DIP flexion (produced by an external flexor force) to passive PIP flexion.

The functional coupling of PIP/DIP joint action can be demonstrated by one other PIP/DIP joint relation.[57] When the PIP joint is fully flexed actively by the flexor digitorum superficialis muscle or passively by an external force, the DIP joint cannot be actively extended. When the PIP joint is flexed, the dorsally located central tendon is lengthened. The increasing tension in the central tendon pulls the extensor expansion (from which the central tendon arises) distally. This distal migration releases some of the tension in the lateral bands. The tension in the lateral bands is further released as the lateral bands separate slightly at the flexing PIP joint. Releasing tension in the lateral bands releases tension in the terminal tendon on the distal phalanx. At 90° of PIP joint flexion, loss of tension in the terminal tendon is sufficient to eliminate any extensor force at the DIP joint, including any potential contribution from the oblique retinacular ligaments because these ligaments have also been released by PIP flexion.[117] Although the DIP joint can be actively flexed by the flexor digitorum profundus muscle when the proximal phalanx is already fully flexed, the distal phalanx cannot be actively re-extended as long as the PIP joint remains fully flexed.

Foundational Concepts 9–3
Summary of Coupled Actions of the Proximal and Distal Interphalangeal Joints

- Active extension of the PIP joint will typically be accompanied by extension of the DIP joint.
- Active or passive flexion of the DIP joint will typically initiate flexion of the PIP joint.
- Full flexion of the PIP joint (actively or passively) will prevent the DIP joint from being actively extended.

The Thumb

Joints of the Thumb

CARPOMETACARPAL JOINT OF THE THUMB

The carpometacarpal (or trapeziometacarpal) joint of the thumb is the articulation between the trapezium and the base of the first metacarpal. Unlike the carpometacarpal joints of digits 2–5, the first carpometacarpal (CMC) joint is a saddle joint with two degrees of freedom allowing flexion/extension and abduction/adduction. The saddle-shaped portion of the trapezium is concave in the sagittal plane allowing abduction/adduction and convex in the frontal plane allowing flexion/extension. The base of the first metacarpal has a reciprocal shape to that of the trapezium **(Fig. 9–39)**. Flexion/extension of the first carpometacarpal joint occurs around a somewhat oblique A-P axis, with abduction/adduction occurring around a somewhat oblique coronal axis. This is a reversal of what is found at most other joints, with flexion/extension usually occurring around a coronal axis and abduction/adduction around an A-P axis. This reversal is due to the out-of-plane orientation of the trapezium such that flexion/extension of the proximal phalanx occurs nearly parallel to the palm, while abduction/adduction of the phalanx occurs nearly perpendicular to the palm. This orientation conveniently places the thumb in a position to contact the tips of digits 2–5 and perform pinch tasks. Extension has alternatively been referred to as *radial abduction*, whereas abduction has been referred to as *palmar abduction*. The joint also permits some axial, or internal, rotation that couples with flexion and abduction to complete a motion termed **opposition**.

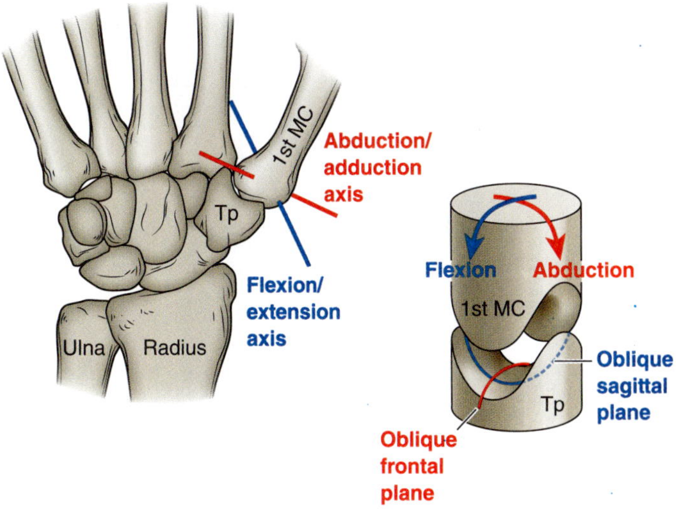

Figure 9–39 Flexion/extension of the saddle-shaped first carpometacarpal joint occurs in an oblique frontal plane as movement of the convex proximal metacarpal (MC) on the concavity of the trapezium (Tp). Flexion/extension occurs in an oblique sagittal plane as movement of the concave proximal metacarpal on the convexity of the trapezium. Atypically compared with other joint motions, flexion/extension takes place around an (oblique) A-P axis while abduction/adduction takes place around an (oblique) frontal axis.

During opposition, the tip of the thumb and digits can come into contact. This motion is accomplished through a combination of carpometacarpal joint abduction, flexion, adduction, and rotation of the first metacarpal. Metacarpal rotation locks the **metacarpal beak**, a small prominence at the base of the metacarpal, into the beak recess in the trapezium. The component movements resulting in opposition bring the thumb toward the other digits and provides a stable base for pinch tasks. Opposition is necessary in almost all forms of prehension (grasp and dexterity activities). Cooney et al measured the first carpometacarpal joint ROM as an average of 53° of flexion/extension, 42° of abduction/adduction, and 17° of rotation.[118]

The carpometacarpal joint capsule is relatively lax, allowing joint mobility while the reinforcing radial, ulnar, volar, and dorsal ligaments contribute to stability. The dorsal ligament complex (comprised of the dorsal radial ligament and posterior oblique ligaments) is the largest and thickest ligament of the carpometacarpal joint and serves as the primary stabilizer. During metacarpal rotation and opposition, when the metacarpal beak locks into the trapezium, the dorsal ligament complex is taut.[119] The anterior oblique ligament, often called the "beak ligament," is taut in the hitchhiker position.[119] There is also an intermetacarpal ligament that helps tether the bases of the first and second metacarpals and provide stability when the dorsal ligament complex and anterior oblique ligaments are injured.[119]

Expanded Concepts 9–4
First Carpometacarpal Osteoarthritis

Osteoarthritic changes are common at the first carpometacarpal joint and may be attributable to the large compressive and shear forces across the joint that occur with pinch. When the metacarpal beak is

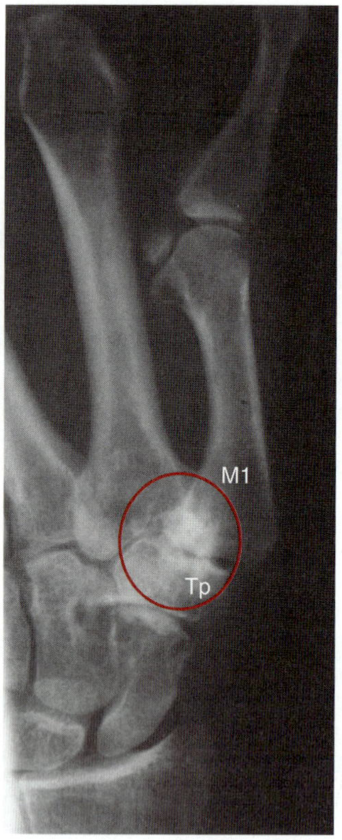

Figure 9–40 Degenerative changes at the first carpometacarpal joint between the trapezium (Tp) and first metacarpal (M1).

engaged with the trapezium beak recess, the joint contact area is small, resulting in only a small area to dissipate forces. Over time, this may lead to a breakdown in the metacarpal rotation that occurs with opposition[120] and may lead to radiodorsal subluxation of the base of the metacarpal. The first metacarpal can assume a posture of CMC flexion into the palm and consequent metacarpophalangeal joint hyperextension **(Fig. 9–40)**.

Patient Application 9–3

Megan Fiore is a 78-year-old woman referred to a hand surgeon by her primary care physician after she reported the progressive onset of thumb pain. Her symptoms of aching and tenderness were exacerbated by activities such as turning a key, opening a jar, and writing. Manual longitudinal compression of the first metacarpal joint into the trapezium produced pain and crepitation (positive Grind test), indicative of carpometacarpal osteoarthritis. Osteoarthritic changes and subluxation of the metacarpal were evident on radiograph (see Fig. 9–40). A custom thumb orthosis was fabricated and the patient was instructed in activity modifications along with general joint protection principles. These included avoiding forceful, repetitive, and sustained pinching, along with utilizing pens and kitchen utensils with larger grips or handles.

METACARPOPHALANGEAL AND INTERPHALANGEAL JOINTS OF THE THUMB

The MCP joint of the thumb is a condyloid joint, formed by the head of the first metacarpal and the base of its proximal phalanx. The joint is capable of flexion and extension around a coronal axis, and its main functional contribution is to provide additional flexion range to the thumb during opposition and to allow the thumb to grasp and contour to objects.

Despite the structural similarities between the MCP joints, the first MCP joint is far more restricted in motion than those of digits 2–5. On average, there is approximately 50° of flexion at the first MCP joint, just over half that of the MCP joints 2–5; there is little, if any, hyperextension. While the shape of the metacarpal head should allow abduction and adduction of the proximal phalanx, as is the case for digits 2–5, there are no muscle attachments capable of performing the action in the thumb.

Stability of the thumb MCP joint is provided by connective tissues around the joint including the joint capsule, collateral ligaments, and a volar plate.[121] The capsule is reinforced anteriorly by two **sesamoid bones**. Goldberg and Nathan proposed that the sesamoid bones develop over time as a result of friction force and pressure on the flexor tendons in which the sesamoid bones are embedded.[122] Once developed, the sesamoids may help in tendon function by maintaining tendon alignment, and reducing tendon friction and pressure.[123,124] Development of the sesamoids, however, is dependent on sex and ethnicity and appears to align with the period of puberty.[124] The sesamoids are held together by collagenous dense fibrous tissue that runs perpendicular to the long axis of the thumb **(Fig. 9–41)**, and laterally by additional tissues parallel to the thumb that blend with the radial and ulnar collateral ligaments.[125] The radial and ulnar collateral ligaments of the MCP joint can be injured (ulnar far more so than radial) and result in compromised joint stability.[126] The thumb's volar plate differs histologically from the plates of digits 2–5 in that it is composed of loose connective tissue rather than fibrocartilage, perhaps due to the presence of sesamoids that could provide additional joint stability, minimizing the need for a cartilaginous volar plate.[125]

The interphalangeal joint of the thumb is the articulation between the head of the proximal phalanx and the base of the distal phalanx. It is structurally and functionally similar to the interphalangeal joints of the fingers, so will not be described any further.

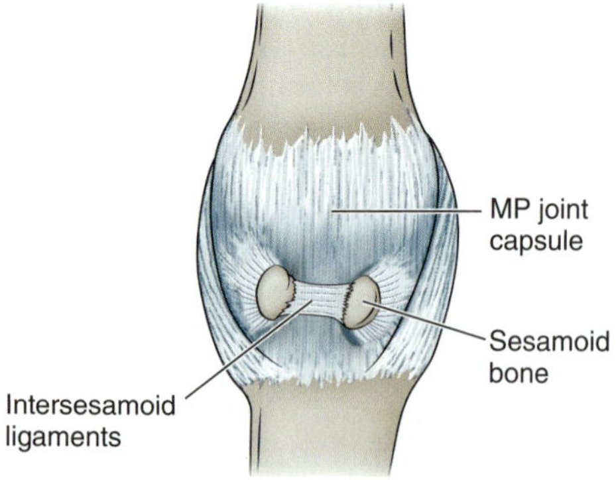

Figure 9–41 The metacarpophalangeal joint of the thumb has two sesamoid bones secured to the anterior aspect of the joint capsule by intersesamoid ligaments.

Thumb Muscles

During hand and thumb tasks, the muscles of the thumb must provide a continuous, effective pull in every direction to maintain stability. The first metacarpal and the proximal and distal phalanges form an articulated shaft that sits on the trapezium. Because the stability of the carpometacarpal joint comes from the muscles more than articular constraints, most muscles that attach to the thumb tend to be active during most thumb motions. There is also substantial individual variability in motor strategies among normal subjects.[127] Consequently, thumb muscle function is not really an issue of when a muscle is active but more so when the preponderance of muscle activity might be expected between differing tasks.

EXTRINSIC THUMB MUSCLES

There are four extrinsic thumb muscles: the **flexor pollicis longus** on the volar surface, and the **extensor pollicis brevis, extensor pollicis longus,** and **abductor pollicis longus** muscles on the dorsal surface (see Fig. 9–14A). At the wrist, the flexor pollicis longus tendon is enclosed within the radial bursa. This bursa is typically continuous with the digital tendon sheath (see Fig. 9–31A). After emerging from the carpal tunnel, the flexor pollicis longus passes ulnar to the trapezium tubercle on its way to insert in the distal phalanx. This muscle's function is independent of the extrinsic flexors for digits 2–5, and it is the only muscle capable of thumb interphalangeal joint flexion. The flexor pollicis longus tendon sits between the sesamoid bones at the head of the metacarpal and appears to derive some protection from those bones. Along with its tendon sheath, the flexor pollicis longus tendon runs through fibro-osseous tunnels formed by two annular pulleys and one oblique pulley (see Fig. 9–31A).

The remaining three of the thumb extrinsic muscles are located on the dorsoradial aspect of the hand (see Fig. 9–14A). In contrast to digits 2–5, there is a separate tendon to each of the CMC, MCP, and IP joints of the thumb. The abductor pollicis longus muscle attaches to the radial side of the first metacarpal base, the extensor pollicis brevis muscle inserts on the base of the proximal phalanx, and the extensor pollicis longus muscle inserts on the base of the distal phalanx. The abductor pollicis longus muscle abducts and extends the first carpometacarpal joint. The extensor pollicis brevis extends both the carpometacarpal and MCP joints.

The extensor pollicis longus muscle, at the level of the proximal phalanx of the thumb, is joined by expansions from the abductor pollicis brevis muscle, the first dorsal interossei muscle, and the adductor pollicis muscle. Muscles attaching to the extensor pollicis longus tendon, acting independently, can extend the interphalangeal joint to neutral but cannot complete the range of hyperextension of which the extensor pollicis longus is capable. The extensor pollicis longus muscle inserts on the base of the distal phalanx and can extend all of the joints it crosses, but it is the sole extensor of the interphalangeal joint. The extensor pollicis longus muscle can also contribute to adduction of the carpometacarpal joint of the thumb.[42]

Because the extrinsic thumb muscles span multiple joints, their force output is influenced by wrist position. Like other extrinsic digital flexors, the flexor pollicis longus muscle is less effective as a thumb interphalangeal joint flexor when the wrist is in flexion. The extensor pollicis longus muscle cannot complete thumb interphalangeal joint extension when the wrist, carpometacarpal, and MCP joints are simultaneously extended. Being radial deviators of the wrist, the abductor pollicis longus and extensor pollicis brevis muscles require the antagonistic action of a wrist ulnar deviator to prevent the muscles from creating a wrist radial deviation movement that would affect their ability to generate tension over the joints of the thumb.

INTRINSIC THUMB MUSCLES

There are four intrinsic muscles to the thumb that make up the **thenar eminence.** These muscles arise from the flexor retinaculum and the carpus to insert onto the thumb. The opponens pollicis is the only intrinsic thumb muscle to have its distal attachment on the first metacarpal. Its action line is nearly perpendicular to the long axis of the metacarpal and is applied to the lateral side of the bone. The opponens pollicis muscle, therefore, is very effective in positioning the metacarpal into an abducted, flexed, and rotated position. The **abductor pollicis brevis, flexor pollicis brevis,** and **adductor pollicis muscles** all insert on the thumb's proximal phalanx. The flexor pollicis brevis muscle has two heads of insertion. Its larger lateral head attaches distally with the abductor pollicis brevis muscle and also applies some abductor force. The flexor pollicis brevis muscle crosses the sesamoid bones at the MCP joint and, like other sesamoid bones, increases the flexor pollicus brevis' moment arm for MCP joint flexion. The medial head of the flexor pollicis brevis muscle attaches distally with the adductor pollicis muscle and assists in thumb adduction.

Although not generally considered a thenar muscle, the first dorsal interossei muscle may contribute to thumb function, along with its contributions to the index finger. The first dorsal interossei muscle is a bipennate muscle arising from both the first and second metacarpals and from the intercarpal ligament that joins these metacarpal bases. Brand and Hollister reported that the first dorsal interossei muscle provides a consistent distraction force on the first carpometacarpal joint that is atypical of most muscles **(Fig. 9–42)**; they proposed that a distraction force on the first carpometacarpal joint by the first interosseous muscle may offset the compressive and dorsoradially directed forces that the flexor/adductor muscles create across the carpometacarpal joint in lateral pinch and power grip. When flexor/adductor forces were created in laboratory specimens without tension in the first dorsal interossei muscle, the carpometacarpal joint subluxed.[101] More recent studies supported the earlier hypothesis, showing that the first dorsal interossei was able to reduce carpometacarpal joint subluxation in healthy subjects when examined under fluoroscopy,[128] and that concomitant activation of the opponens pollicis and the first dorsal interossei muscles was able to reduce carpometacarpal joint subluxation in a dose-dependent manner.[129]

The thenar muscles are active in most grasping activities, regardless of the precise position of the thumb. The opponens pollicis muscle works together most frequently with the abductor pollicis brevis and the flexor pollicis brevis muscles, although the intensity of the relation varies. When the thumb is *gently* brought into contact with any of the fingers, activity of the opponens pollicis muscle predominates in the thumb,

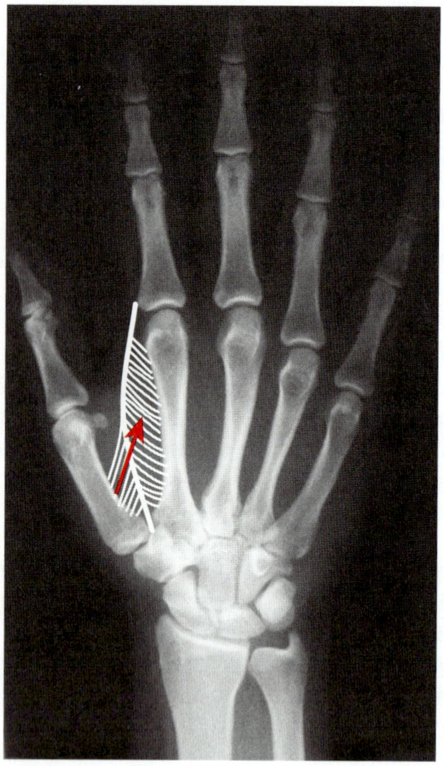

Figure 9–42 Brand and Hollister proposed that the attachment of the first dorsal interossei muscle to the first metacarpal can serve as a distractor of the first carpometacarpal joint, helping to offset the strong compressive forces that occur across the first carpometacarpal joint.[101]

with abductor pollicis brevis activity exceeding that of the flexor pollicis brevis muscle. When opposition to the index finger or middle finger is performed *firmly*, activity of the flexor pollicis brevis muscle exceeds that of the opponens pollicis muscle. As opposition moves from the index and middle fingers to the ring and little fingers, the proportion of opponens pollicus activity increases, equalling activity of the flexor pollicis brevis muscle with firm opposition to the little finger.[130] The change in balance of muscle activity with firm opposition and with increasingly ulnar opposition can be accounted for by the increased need for thumb abduction and metacarpal rotation. Increased pressure (firmness) in opposition additionally appears to bring in activity of the adductor pollicis muscle. The adductor pollicis muscle stabilizes the thumb against the opposed finger. In *firm* opposition to the index and middle fingers, adductor pollicis activity exceeds the very minimal activity of the abductor pollicis brevis muscle. With more ulnarly located opposition, the increased need for abduction of the thumb results in simultaneous activity of the thumb's intrinsic abductor and adductor.[130]

Activity of the extrinsic thumb musculature in grasp appears to be partially a function of helping to position the MCP and interphalangeal joints. The main function of the extrinsic thumb muscles is in release: returning the thumb to extension (out of the palm) from its position in the palm. Although release of an object is essentially an extrinsic function, some opponens pollicis and abductor brevis activity have been identified.[130] This muscular activity may assist in maintaining the thumb in abduction and in maintaining the first metacarpal rotation that facilitates the next move of the thumb back into opposition.

Prehension

Prehension, or grasp, involves taking hold of an object between any two surfaces in the hand. There are numerous ways that objects of varying sizes and shapes may be grasped, with strategies varying among individuals.[131] It is a highly coordinated skill requiring involvement of the musculoskeletal, visual, sensory, and neurological systems. The shoulder, elbow, radioulnar joint, and wrist are part of reach and grasp as they position the hand in space while the hand grasps and releases. Hand function further includes multiple important tasks, one being adapting the hand grip to the size, shape, and use of the object, and the second being the timing required so that finger movements are coordinated with forearm, humeral, and trunk movement toward the object.[132] Jeannerod[132] also described the need for anticipatory shaping of the hand, a visuomotor task that occurs during reach. Opening the hand during object approach and release is primarily an extensor function, calling in activity of the lumbrical, extensor digitorum, and thumb extrinsic muscles.

In another model of prehension, authors described the opposition space model,[133] where grasp requires opposing forces to come together.[134] According to Roy et al,[133] this model includes planning the opposition through to releasing the opposition at the completion of the task, and ties together the multiple subtasks associated with grasp such as transporting the hand, preshaping the hand, acquiring the object in a stable grasp, manipulating the object, and releasing the object.[133] When analyzing movement, both hand approach and placement are important considerations.

More specific to hand motion, Napier[135] described two basic patterns of hand movement, **power grip** and **precision grip**. In power grip, the object is held between the palm and flexed digits with a counter force provided by the thumb, and in precision grip, an object is held between the thumb and the flexor surface of a digit(s).[135] Slocum and Pratt, as cited by Mackenzie and Iberall, used the term **pinch** to describe the opposition of the pad of the thumb to the pads of the other digits.[134,136] Pad-to-pad opposition is now more commonly referred to as **pulp pinch,** or **pad-to-pad pinch,** while opposition between the thumb tip and the tip of another digit is referred to as **tip-to-tip pinch**, or **tip pinch,** for short.

Other classifications for prehension exist. A thorough discussion of each is beyond the scope of this chapter. Thus, an overview of frequently used power and precision grips will be provided. Knowledge of these positions allows one to have a general understanding of the different, coordinated positions of hand function.

During each type of prehension, synergy of the hand muscles results in almost constant activity of all intrinsic and extrinsic muscles.[101,137,138] Our task here, therefore, is more to identify when muscles are *not* working or when the balance of activity between muscles might shift. It should also be emphasized that the muscular activity documented by EMG studies is specific to the activity as performed in a given study. Even in studies using similar forms of prehension, variables such as size of the object, firmness of the hold on the object, timing, and instructions to the participant can cause substantial changes in reported muscle activity. However, studies do provide indications of general muscular activity patterns in which hand function can be understood.

Power Grip

Power grip has been described as having 5 sequential phases: (1) opening the hand, (2) positioning the fingers, (3) bringing the fingers to the object, (4) maintaining a static phase that actually constitutes the grip holding the object in place, and (5) release, which requires the opposite, yet coordinated action. The fingers in power grip usually function in concert to clamp onto and hold an object in the palm. The fingers assume a position of sustained flexion that varies in degree with the size, shape, and weight of the object. The palm is likely to contour to the object as the palmar arches and medial carpometacarpal joints flex to form around it. The thumb may be removed from the object, or positioned in a manner that it is available in the event the task requires a counter or stabilization force. When involved, the thumb is adducting (from an abducted position) to clamp the object to the palm. Four varieties of power grip studied by Long and associates exemplify the similarities and differences seen in power grip **(Fig. 9–43)**.[108] These are the cylindrical grip (A), the spherical grip (B), hook grip (C), and lateral prehension (described separately in the next section).

Cylindrical Grip

Cylindrical grip (see **Fig. 9–43A**) predominantly uses the extrinsic finger flexors to position the fingers around and maintain grasp on an object. Study results confirm the flexor digitorum profundus muscle is the workhorse for composite fist formation regardless of effort. However, contrary to prior studies, evidence suggests that there is more variability in flexor digitorum superficialis and interossei recruitment among individuals in the creation of a light fist although their recruitment is not predictable.[139] Another study showed differences in force output between digits, suggesting that some digits contribute more to grip than others. In addition, there is variability in the load distribution across the palm and digits between dominant and nondominant sides.[140]

Thumb position in cylindrical grip is the most variable of the digits. The thumb usually comes around the object, then flexes and adducts to close the vise. The flexor pollicis longus and thenar muscles are all active, but they will vary with the width of the web space, the amount of carpometacarpal joint rotation required, and the increased pressure or resistance needed. The thumb extensor muscles may be variably active as stabilizers.

Cylindrical grip is typically performed with the wrist in neutral flexion/extension and slight ulnar deviation. Wrist ulnar deviation puts the thumb in line with the long axis of the forearm to better align the object in the hand with the thumb.[141] It is also the position that optimizes force of the long finger flexors. The heavier an object is, the more likely it is that the wrist will ulnarly deviate. In addition, a strong contraction of the flexor carpi ulnaris muscle at the wrist will increase tension on the transverse carpal ligament, providing a more stable base for the active hypothenar muscles that originate from that ligament.

Spherical Grip

In **spherical grip** (see **Fig. 9–43B**), the extrinsic finger and thumb flexors and the thenar muscles follow similar patterns of activity and variability as those in cylindrical grip. The main distinction can be made by the greater spread of the fingers to encompass the object used in spherical grip.

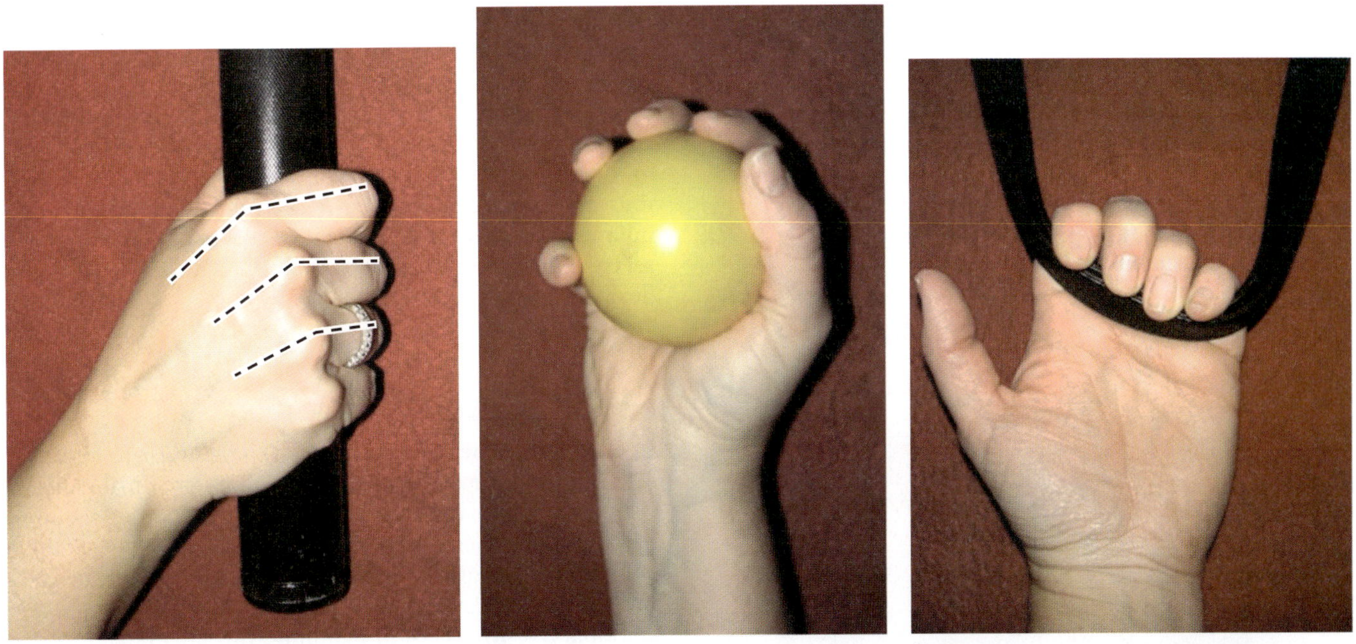

A B C

Figure 9–43 **A.** Cylindrical grip. The MCP joints may ulnar deviate using the interossei muscles to help orient the fingers toward the thumb. Ulnar deviation of the wrist may help this orientation. **B.** Spherical grip **C.** Hook grip.

This evokes more interosseous activity than is seen in other forms of power grip.[124] The MCP joints do not deviate in the same direction (e.g., ulnarly) but tend to abduct so that the phalanges are no longer parallel to each other as they commonly are in cylindrical grip. The MCP joint abductors must be joined by the adductors to stabilize the MCP joints that are in the loose-packed position near extension. Flexor activity predominates in the digits as it does in all forms of power grip; however the MCP and IP joint extensors also have a role providing a balancing force for the flexors and also are essential for smooth and controlled opening of the hand and release of the object.

Hook Grip

Hook grip (see **Fig. 9–43C**) is actually a specialized form of prehension. It is included in power grip because it has more characteristics of power grip than of precision grip. It is a function primarily of the fingers. It may include the palm but, by definition, never includes the thumb. This type of grip is used when a person carries a bag or briefcase at their side. The major muscular activity is provided by the flexor digitorum profundus and flexor digitorum superficialis muscles. The load may be sustained completely by one muscle or the other, or by both muscles in concert. This depends on the position of the load in relation to the phalanges. If the load is carried more distally (i.e., with the MCP joints in neutral) the flexor digitorum profundus muscle provides the required force to hold the object. If the load is carried more in the middle of the fingers (i.e., with the MCP joints in greater flexion), the flexor digitorum superficialis muscle may be sufficient. Some interosseous muscle activity has been demonstrated on an EMG, but its purpose is not fully understood. It may help prevent clawing in the MCP joints, although the activity is not evident in every finger.[124] In hook grip, the thumb is held in moderate to full extension by thumb extrinsic muscles.

Lateral Prehension

Lateral prehension is neither a power nor a precision grip. It is a unique grip in that contact occurs between the pulp of the thumb and a digit. When performed between the pad of the thumb and the radial side of the index digit, it is known as **key grip, key pinch,** or **lateral pinch (Fig. 9–44)**.

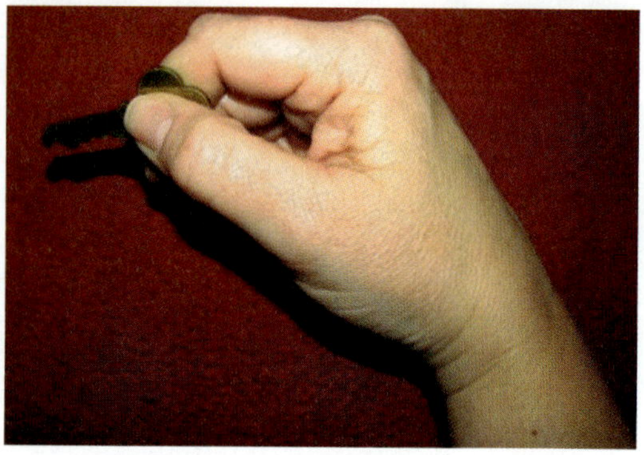

Figure 9–44 Lateral prehension, which is neither a power nor a precision grip.

In this position, the thumb is more adducted and less rotated. The activity level of the flexor pollicis brevis muscle increases and that of the opponens pollicis muscle decreases in comparison with other types of precision grip. Slight flexion of the distal phalanx of the thumb is required, thus recruiting the flexor pollicus longus. If the pad-to-side prehension is being used for something such as turning a key, the wrist will again assume neutral flexion/extension and drop into slight ulnar deviation to put the key in line with the forearm so that pronation or supination can be used to turn the key.

Lateral pinch can be performed by a person with paralysis of all hand muscles. If the hand muscles are paralyzed as they would be in a person with a spinal cord injury above the C7 level, active wrist extensors (assuming they are present) can create lateral pinch. Wrist extension provided by the intact and active extensor carpi ulnaris, extensor carpi radialis longus, and extensor carpi radialis brevis muscles results in MCP and interphalangeal joint flexion of the fingers and thumb because of passive tension in the extrinsic finger flexor tendons (flexor digitorum superficialis and profundus and flexor pollicis longus) that are stretched over the extending wrist. This wrist extension action also pulls the pad of the thumb to the radial side of the index digit, allowing lateral pinch. Lateral pinch is released by relaxing the wrist extensor muscles and allowing gravity to flex the wrist. As the wrist flexes, the extrinsic flexor tendons become slack and the extensor expansion is stretched, producing sufficient tension in the extensor digitorum and extensor expansion to partially extend both MCP and interphalangeal joints.

The phenomenon of using active wrist extension to passively close the fingers and passive wrist flexion to passively open the fingers is known as **tenodesis.** Individuals with low cervical cord injuries can use the same tenodesis action to achieve a cylindrical grip if the proper balance of tension exists in the extrinsic flexors. The flexors of the digits must be loose enough to permit the partially flexed fingers of the *open* hand to surround the object in wrist flexion, while still being tight enough to hold onto the object when the wrist is extended. Active control of at least one wrist extensor muscle is the minimal requirement for functional use of tenodesis in a person without any active control of finger or thumb musculature. Tenodesis can be seen in individuals without injury simply by actively extending the wrist in isolation, then relaxing the wrist extensors to allow the hand to fall back into flexion.

Precision Grip

Precision Handling

In power grip, the object is grasped so that the object can be moved through space by the wrist or more proximal joints.[143] The term **precision handling** was developed as a way to define grasp when the hand is moving an object, [143] such as during translation, manipulation, and rotation because previous classifications described grasp when the object was stationary.[134] In precision handling, the fingers and thumb grasp the object for the purpose of manipulating it between the fingers or within the hand. Although precision handling shares the first three steps of the sequence, it does not contain

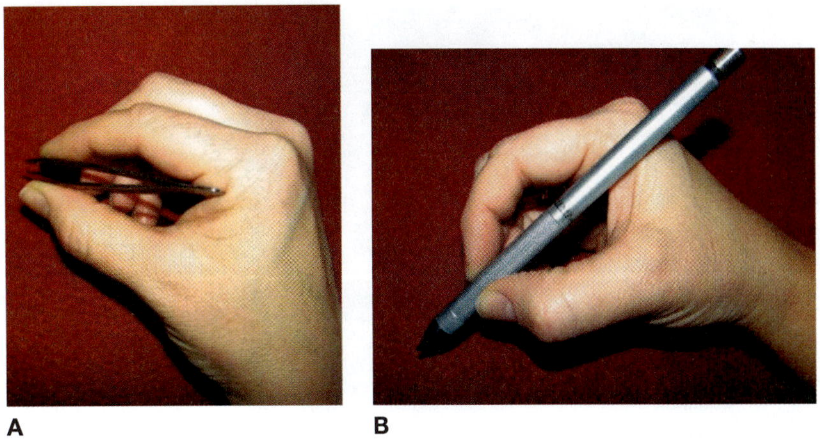

Figure 9–45 Two varieties of precision handling: **A.** Pulp pinch, which is also called *pad-to-pad prehension*. **B.** Tip pinch, which is also called *tip-to-tip prehension*.

a static phase. The positions and muscular requirements of precision handling are somewhat more variable than those of power grip, require much finer motor control, and are more dependent on intact sensation. Of all forms of precision handling, 80% are considered to fall into the category of pad to pad.[1] In dynamic manipulation, the palmar interossei and dorsal interossei muscles tend to work reciprocally, rather than in the synergistic co-contraction pattern observed during power grip.

Pulp Pinch

Pulp pinch involves opposition of the pad, or pulp, of the thumb to the pad, or pulp, of the finger **(Fig. 9–45)**. The pad of the distal phalanx of each digit has the greatest concentration of tactile corpuscles found in the body. The finger used in two-jaw chuck is usually the index; in three-jaw chuck, the middle finger is added. The MCP and PIP joints of the fingers are partially flexed, with the degree of flexion being dependent on the size of the object being held. The DIP joint may be fully extended or in slight flexion. When the DIP joint is extended, the flexor digitorum superficialis muscle can perform the MCP and PIP joint flexion alone without the assistance of the flexor digitorum profundus muscle. Extension of the DIP joint in this instance is caused by flexion of the middle phalanx (flexor digitorum superficialis muscle) against the upward force of the object or thumb on the distal phalanx in what is effectively a closed chain. When partial flexion of the DIP is required by the pad-to-pad task, the flexor digitorum profundus muscle must be active. Interosseous activity is often present to supplement MCP joint flexor force. With the increased force of pad-to-pad pinch, the interossei muscles may co-contract.[108]

In pulp pinch, the first carpometacarpal joint is held in abduction, flexion, and rotation (opposition). The first MCP and interphalangeal joints may be partially flexed or fully extended. The thenar muscle control is provided by the opponens pollicis, flexor pollicis brevis, and abductor pollicis brevis muscles. Adductor pollicis muscle activity (ulnar nerve innervated) increases with the increased pressure of the pinch. In ulnar nerve paralysis, loss of adductor pollicis function (as well as loss of function of the dorsal interossei and palmar interossei muscles) makes the thumb less stable and affects the precision of the activity.

Fine adjustments in the flexion angle of the DIP joint of the finger and the interphalangeal joint of the thumb control the points of contact on the pads of the digits. If the finger's DIP and thumb's interphalangeal joint are in extension, contact occurs on the more proximal portion of the pad of the finger. As flexion of the finger's DIP and thumb interphalangeal joints increase, the contact moves distally toward the fingertip. Flexion of the distal phalanx, when required, is provided by the flexor digitorum profundus muscle for the finger and by the flexor pollicis longus muscle for the thumb. DIP flexion in the finger is accompanied by a proportional flexion in the PIP joint.

As is found in power grip, the extensor musculature is used for opening the hand to grasp, for release, and for stabilization when necessary. In the thumb, the extensor pollicis longus muscle may be used to maintain the interphalangeal joint in extension when contact is light and on the proximal portion of the pad of the finger. Synergistic wrist activity must also occur to balance the forces created by the flexor digitorum superficialis and flexor digitorum profundus muscles.

Tip Pinch

Although the muscular activity found in tip pinch (see **Fig. 9–45B**) is nearly identical to that of pulp pinch, there are some key differences.[142] In tip pinch, the interphalangeal joints of the finger and thumb must have the range and available muscle force to create nearly full joint flexion. The MCP joint of the finger opposing the thumb must also be ulnarly deviated (with fingertip pointed radially) to present the tip of the finger to the thumb. In the index finger, ulnar deviation occurs because of MCP joint adduction. If opposition occurs with one of the other fingers, the ulnar deviation is produced by MCP abduction. If the flexion range for the distal phalanx in either the opposing finger or the thumb is not available, or if the active force for interphalangeal flexion and MCP joint ulnar deviation cannot be provided, tip pinch cannot be performed effectively. As the most precise form of grasp, it is also the most easily disrupted. Tip pinch has all the same muscular requirements as pulp pinch in both the digits and thumb. However, activity of the flexor digitorum profundus, flexor pollicis longus, and interossei muscles is a necessity in tip-to-tip prehension, whereas they are not a necessity in pulp pinch.

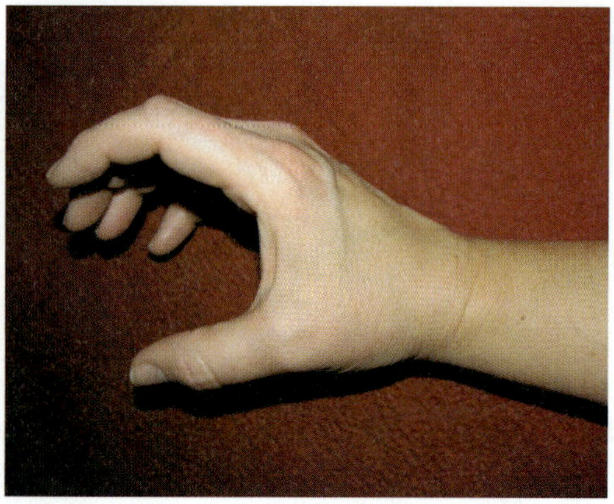

Figure 9–46 Functional position of the hand: wrist extension and ulnar deviation with moderate flexion of the metacarpophalangeal and minimal flexion of the interphalangeal joints of the finger and thumb.

Functional Position of the Wrist and Hand

The position from which optimal hand function is most likely to occur is known as the **functional position** of the wrist and hand. This position optimizes the power of the finger flexors so that hand closure can be accomplished with the least possible effort. It is also the position in which all wrist muscles are under equal tension. With similar considerations for the position of the joints of the digits, the functional position provides the best opportunity for a hand that is injured to interact with the environment. It is *not necessarily* the position in which a hand should be immobilized. Position for hand immobilization will be dependent upon the injury or disability. The functional position is as follows:

1. Wrist in slight extension (20°)
2. Wrist in slight ulnar deviation (10°)
3. Fingers moderately flexed at the MCP joints (45°)
4. Fingers moderately flexed at the PIP joints (30°)
5. Fingers slightly flexed at the DIP joints **(Fig. 9–46)**[4]

SUMMARY

- The wrist and hand are complex sets of joints and articulations with both mobile and stable components that provide the distal upper extremity with the ability to perform highly complex tasks.
- The balance of muscle forces across wrist and hand intrinsic and extrinsic muscles is required for fine and gross motor tasks.
- The wrist and hand require sensory feed-forward and feedback mechanisms to integrate with motor planning and motor control to carry out activities.

STUDY QUESTIONS

1. Name the bones of the wrist complex; describe the articulations that occur between these bones and the functional joints that are formed.
2. Describe the components and role of the triangular fibrocartilage complex (TFCC) in wrist function.
3. What is the total ROM typically available at the wrist complex? How are the motions distributed between the radiocarpal and midcarpal joints of the complex?
4. Describe the sequence of carpal motion occurring from full wrist flexion to full extension and radial to ulnar deviation, emphasizing the role of the scaphoid.
5. What effect does release of the scapholunate stabilizers or of the lunotriquetral stabilizers have on bony positions?
6. Identify the muscles that can extend the wrist; include the joints crossed, actions produced, and activity levels of each.
7. Describe the transverse carpal ligament, its attachments, and its role in wrist and hand function.
8. What is the function of the carpometacarpal joints of the fingers? How do the variations in ROM among the four carpometacarpal joints of the fingers contribute to function?
9. What role does the transverse metacarpal ligament play at the carpometacarpal joint? What role at the MCP joint?
10. Describe the locations and functions of the volar (palmar) fibrocartilage plates.
11. What MCP joint position is most prone to injury and why?
12. Compare the joint structure of the MCP joints with that of the interphalangeal joints of the fingers. Identify both similarities and differences.
13. Describe the mechanisms, joint motions, and muscles that are necessary for the fingers to gently close into the palm without friction or loss of the length-tension relationship.
14. How does the "pistol-grip" design of most tools (larger ulnarly) relate to the MCP joint ROM and muscular function of the four fingers?
15. When is the flexor digitorum superficialis muscle active as the primary finger flexor? When does it back up the flexor digitorum profundus muscle?
16. What muscles are active in gentle closure of the typical hand? What role, if any, do the intrinsic muscles play in this activity?
17. What wrist position is assumed when a person needs to optimize finger flexion strength? Which wrist position is least effective for grasp?
18. What are annular pulleys and cruciate ligaments in the digits? Where are they found, and what functions do they serve?
19. Identify the bursae of the hand. What are their functions and how are they most typically related to the digital tendon sheaths?
20. Describe the active and passive elements that make up the extensor mechanism. What are the specific functions of each?
21. What role do the extensor digitorum communis, extensor indicis proprius, and extensor digiti minimi muscles play in active extension of the PIP and DIP joints of the hand?
22. How do the proximal and distal attachments of the interossei muscles affect function at the MCP and interphalangeal joints?
23. Describe the attachments of the lumbrical muscles to the extensor mechanism. How do these muscles contribute to interphalangeal extension? What is their role at the MCP joint?
24. Why is active DIP joint flexion typically accompanied by PIP joint flexion at the same time?
25. Explain why the DIP joint cannot be actively extended if the PIP joint is fully flexed.

26. Why will an isolated contraction of the extensor digitorum communis muscle produce flexion of the PIP and DIP joints? What is this finger position called?
27. How are the extrinsic flexors and extensors stabilized at the MCP joints?
28. Why is finger extension weaker in the index and little fingers?
29. Why does MCP joint adduction weaken more quickly than abduction in a progressive ulnar nerve problem?
30. Which are stronger flexors of the MCP joint, the lumbrical or the interossei muscles?
31. Compare and contrast the MCP joint structure of the thumb with the MCP joint structure of the fingers.
32. What does the motion of thumb opposition require in terms of joint function and musculature?
33. What are the primary muscles of extension (release) in the wrist and hand?
34. In general, what is the difference between power grip and precision handling at the wrist, in the fingers, and in the thumb? What do these two forms of prehension have in common? Name two functional activities specific to each.
35. Cylindrical grip is generally referred to as an *extrinsic hand function*. Why is this true?
36. What requirement does spherical grip have that differentiates it from cylindrical grip?
37. Which form of prehension requires only intrinsic musculature?
38. Which forms of prehension do not require the thumb?
39. What roles do interossei muscles play in precision handling?
40. What requirements does tip-to-tip prehension have that are not necessary for pad-to-pad prehension?
41. What is the finest (most precise) form of prehension that can be accomplished by someone without intact hand musculature, assuming the availability of an active wrist extensor?
42. What is the functional position of the wrist and hand? Why is this the optimal resting position when there is no specific hand problem?
43. Why is an ulnar nerve injury called "claw hand"? What deficiency causes the clawing, and in which fingers does it occur?

REFERENCES

1. Zelouf SD, Wilson SM, Hussain H: Anatomy and kinesiology of the wrist, in Skirven TM (ed): Rehabilitation of the Hand and Upper Extremity (ed 7). Philadelphia, PA, Elsevier Inc., 2021
2. van der Post AS, Jens S, Daams JG, et al: The triangular fibrocartilage complex in the human wrist: a scoping review toward uniform and clinically relevant terminology. Clin Anat 35:626-48, 2022
3. Hagert E, Hagert CG: Understanding stability of the distal radioulnar joint through an understanding of its anatomy. Hand Clin 26:459-66, 2010
4. Eschweiler J, Li J, Quack V, et al: Anatomy, biomechanics, and loads of the wrist joint. Life 12, 2022
5. Taleisnik J: The ligaments of the wrist. J Hand Surg Am 1:110-18, 1976
6. McKinnis LM: Fundamentals of Musculoskeletal Imaging: Contemporary Perspectives in Rehabilitation (ed 5). Philadelphia, PA, FA Davis, 2020
7. Szabo RM, Weber SC: Comminuted intraarticular fractures of the distal radius. Clin Orthop Relat Res 230:39-48, 1988
8. Viegas SF, Patterson RM: Load mechanics of the wrist. Hand Clin 13:109-20, 1997
9. Chinen S, Okubo H, Onaka K, et al: Bone morphology in ulnar impaction syndrome: a radiographic evaluation. J Hand Surg Asian Pac Vol 27:491-8, 2022
10. Yoshioka H, Tanaka T, Ueno T, et al: Study of ulnar variance with high-resolution MRI: correlation with triangular fibrocartilage complex and cartilage of ulnar side of wrist. J Magn Reson Imaging 26:714-19, 2007
11. Kamal RN, Leversedge FJ: Ulnar shortening osteotomy for distal radius malunion. J Wrist Surg 3:181-6, 2014
12. Werner FW, Palmer AK, Fortino MD, et al: Force transmission through the distal ulna: effect of ulnar variance, lunate fossa angulation, and radial and palmar tilt of the distal radius. J Hand Surg 423-8, 1991
13. Asfuroğlu ZM, Güvenç K, Gümüşoğlu E, et al: Order of importance of anatomical risk factors in Kienböck's disease: an artificial neural network study. Hand Surg Rehabil 41:328-33, 2022
14. Pulos N, Bozentka DJ: Carpal ligament anatomy and biomechanics. Hand Clin 31:381-7, 2015
15. Erickson M, Smith FH, Waggy C, et al: Anatomy and kinesiology of the hand, in Skirven T (ed): Rehabilitation of the Hand and Upper Extremity (ed 7). Philadelphia, PA, Elsevier, 2021
16. Kijima Y, Viegas SF: Wrist anatomy and biomechanics. J Hand Surg 34:1555-63, 2009
17. Berger RA, Kauer JMG, Landsmeer JMF: Radioscapholunate ligament: a gross anatomic and histologic study of fetal and adult wrists. J Hand Surg Am 16:350-5, 1991
18. Leake RL, Mills MK, Allen H, et al: MRI of the wrist ligaments. Top in Magn Reson Imaging 29:209-20, 2020
19. Salva-Coll G, Lluch A, Esplugas M, et al: Scapholunate and lunotriquetral joint dynamic stabilizers and their role in wrist neuromuscular control and proprioception. J Hand Ther, 2023
20. Nowalk MD, Logan SE: Distinguishing biomechanical properties of intrinsic and extrinsic human wrist ligaments. J Biomech Eng 113:85-93, 1991
21. Vassa R, Garg A, Omar IM: Magnetic resonance imaging of the wrist and hand. Pol J Radiol 85:e461-88, 2020
22. Pulos N, Bozentka DJ: Carpal ligament anatomy and biomechanics. Hand Clin 31:381-7, 2015
23. Kapoor G, Heire P, Turmezei T, et al: Perilunate injuries: biomechanics, imaging, and classification. Clin Radiol 75:81-87, 2020
24. Lovy AJ, Elhassan BT: Surgical management of extensor tendon injuries, in Skirven TM (ed): Rehabilitation of the Hand and Upper Extremity (ed 7). Philadelphia, PA, Elsevier, 2021
25. Ramage JL, Varacallo M: Anatomy, shoulder and upper limb, wrist extensor muscles [Internet]. StatPearls, 2023 [cited 2024 Jun 27], Available from: https://www.ncbi.nlm.nih.gov/books/NBK534805/
26. Bunata RE, Brown DS, Capelo R: Anatomic factors related to the cause of tennis elbow. J Bone and Joint Surg 89:1955-63, 2007
27. Garland AK, Shah DS, Kedgley AE: Wrist tendon moment arms: quantification by imaging and experimental techniques. J Biomech 68:136-40, 2018
28. Walkowski AD, Goldman EM: Anatomy, shoulder and upper limb, forearm extensor carpi radialis brevis muscle [Internet]. StatPearls, 2023 [cited 2024 Jun 27], Available from: https://www.ncbi.nlm.nih.gov/books/NBK539719/
29. O'Sullivan LW, Gallwey TJ: Upper-limb surface electro-myography at maximum supination and pronation torques: the effect of elbow and forearm angle. J Electromyogr and Kinesiol 12:275-85, 2002
30. Caumes M, Goislard de Monsabert B, Hauraix H, et al: Complex couplings between joints, muscles and performance: the role of the wrist in grasping. Sci Rep 9, 2019
31. Goislard de Monsabert B, Hauraix H, Caumes M, et al: Modelling force-length-activation relationships of wrist and finger extensor muscles. Med Biol Eng Comput 58:2531-49, 2020
32. Fridén J, Lieber RL: Wrist extensor pathomechanics: implications for tendon and nerve transfer. J Hand Surg: European Volume, 2024
33. Dineen HA, Greenberg JA: Ulnar-sided wrist pain in the athlete. Clin Sports Med 39:373-400, 2020
34. Agur A, Dalley A: Moore's Clinically Oriented Anatomy (ed 9). Philadelphia, PA, Lippincott, Williams, and Wilkins, 2023
35. Fairbank SM, Corlett RJ: The role of the extensor digitorum communis muscle in lateral epicondylitis. J Hand Surg 27 B:405-9, 2002
36. Lee SY, Chieh HF, Lin CJ, et al: The potential risk factors relevant to lateral epicondylitis by wrist coupling posture. PLoS One 11, 2016
37. Shah DS, Middleton C, Gurdezi S, et al: The importance of abductor pollicis longus in wrist motions: a physiological wrist simulator study. J Biomech 77:218-22, 2018
38. Lee ZH, Stranix JT, Anzai L, et al: Surgical anatomy of the first extensor compartment: a systematic review and comparison of normal cadavers vs. De Quervain syndrome patients. J Plast, Reconstr and Aesthetic Surg 70:127-31, 2017
39. Bonczar M, Walocha J, Pasternak A, et al: Anatomical variations in the first dorsal compartment of the wrist: meta-analysis. Folia Morphol 82:766-76, 2023

40. Kutsumi K, Amadio PC, Zhao C, et al: Gliding resistance of the extensor pollicis brevis tendon and abductor pollicis longus tendon within the first dorsal compartment in fixed wrist positions. J Orthop Res 23:243-8, 2005
41. Sugiura S, Matsuura Y, Suzuki T, et al: Biomechanical assessment of the first dorsal compartment of the wrist: a fresh cadaver study with relevance to de Quervain's disease. Clin Anat 35:1058-63, 2022
42. Li ZM, Tang J, Chakan M, et al: Complex, multidimensional thumb movements generated by individual extrinsic muscles. J of Orthop Res 26:1289-95, 2008
43. Unyó C, Chaler J, Rojas-Martínez M, et al: A cross-sectional study comparing strength profile of dorsal and palmar flexor muscles of the wrist in epicondylitis and healthy men. Eur J Phys Rehabil Med 49:507-15, 2013
44. Werner FW, Short WH, Palmer AK, et al: Wrist tendon forces during various dynamic wrist motions. J Hand Surg 35:628-32, 2010
45. Carratalá Baixauli V, Pereira AD, Lucas García FJ, et al: Arthroscopic pisiform excision in pisotriquetral osteoarthritis technique using a direct pisotriquetral portal. Tech Hand Up Extrem Surg 25:264-68, 2021
46. O'Keefe KD, Werner FW, Boyette M, et al: Effect of pisiform excision or pisotriquetral arthrodesis as a treatment for pisotriquetral arthritis: a biomechanical study. J Hand Surg 38:1913-18, 2013
47. Pevny T, Rayan GM, Egle D: Ligamentous and tendinous support of the pisiform, anatomic and biomechanical study. J Hand Surg 20:299-304, 1995
48. Brand PW, Hollister A: Clinical Mechanics of the Hand (ed 3). St. Louis, MO, Mosby Year Book, 1999
49. Roman-Liu D, Bartuzi P: The influence of wrist posture on the time and frequency EMG signal measures of forearm muscles. Gait Posture 37:340-4, 2013
50. Javaid Q: Prevalence of agenesis of palmaris longus in male and female genders on clinical examination—a review. J Pak Med Assoc 72:733-7, 2022
51. Boltuch AD, Marcotte MA, Treat CM, et al: The palmaris longus and its association with carpal tunnel syndrome. J Wrist Surg 9:493-7, 2020
52. Backdahl M, Carlson S: Distribution of activity in muscles acting on the wrist (an electromyographic study). Acta Morphol Neerl Scand 4:136-44, 1961
53. Garcia-Elias M, Ribe M, Rodriguez J, et al: Influence of joint laxity on scaphoid kinematics. J Hand Surg 20:379-82, 1995
54. Moromizato K, Kimura R, Fukase H, et al: Whole-body patterns of the range of joint motion in young adults: masculine type and feminine type. J Physiol Anthropol 35, 2016
55. Amarasooriya M, Al-Dirini R, Bryant K, et al: Scaphoid kinematics in scapholunate instability: a dynamic CT study. Skeletal Radiol 52: 1557-66, 2023
56. Nadeem M, Loss JG, Li ZM, et al: Ulnar extension coupling in functional wrist kinematics during hand activities of daily living. J Hand Surg 47:187. e1-.e13, 2022
57. Arimitsu S, Sugamoto K, Hashimoto J, et al: Analysis of radiocarpal and midcarpal motion in stable and unstable rheumatoid wrists using 3-dimensional computed tomography. J Hand Surg 33:189-97, 2008
58. Neu CP, Crisco JJ, Wolfe SW: In vivo kinematic behavior of the radio-capitate joint during wrist flexion-extension and radio-ulnar deviation. J Biomech 34:1429-38, 2001
59. Badida R, Akhbari B, Vutescu E, et al: The role of scapholunate interosseous, dorsal intercarpal, and radiolunate ligaments in wrist biomechanics. J Biomech 125, 2021
60. Anderton W, Tew S, Ferguson S, et al: Movement preferences of the wrist and forearm during activities of daily living. J Hand Ther 36:580-92, 2023
61. Kuo CE, Wolfe SW: Scapholunate instability: current concepts in diagnosis and management. J Hand Surg 33:998-1013, 2008
62. Norman E, Mistry MR, Lalone E, et al: A kinematic analysis of wrist and carpal function using four-dimensional computed tomography technology: a dynamic perspective. J Hand Surg, 2023
63. Gilford V, Bolton R, Lambrinudi C: The mechanism of the wrist joint. Guy's Hosp Rep 92:52-9, 1943
64. Linscheid RL, Dobyns JH, Beabout JW, Bryan RS: Traumatic instability of the wrist: diagnosis, classification, and pathomechanics. J Bone Joint Surgical 54(8):1612-32, 1972
65. Gardner MJ, Crisco JJ, Wolfe SW: Carpal kinematics. Hand Clin 22: 413-20, 2006
66. Carlsen BT, Shin AY: Wrist instability. Scand J Surg 97:324-32, 2008
67. Taleisnik J: Current concepts review carpal instability. J Bone Joint Surgical 70A:1262-68, 1988
68. Linscheid RL: Kinematic considerations of the wrist. Clin Orthop Relat Res 202:27-39, 1986
69. Cooney W: The Wrist: Diagnosis and Operative Treatment (ed 2). St Louis, MO, Mosby Year Book, 2010
70. Patterson R, Viegas SF: Biomechanics of the wrist. J Hand Ther 8:97-105, 1995
71. Blevens AD, Light TR, Jablonsky WS, et al: Radiocarpal articular contact characteristics with scaphoid instability [Internet]. J Hand Surg Am 14:781-90, 1989 [cited 2024 Jun 27], Available from: https://pubmed.ncbi.nlm.nih.gov/2794392/
72. Watson HK, Ballet FL: The SLAC wrist: scapholunate advanced collapse pattern of degenerative arthritis. J Hand Surg 9:358-65, 1984
73. Stäbler A, Heuck A, Reiser M: Imaging of the hand: degeneration, impingement and overuse. Eur J Radiol 25:118-28, 1997
74. Short WH, Werner FW, Green JK, et al: Biomechanical evaluation of the ligamentous stabilizers of the scaphoid and lunate: Part II. J Hand Surg 30:24-34, 2005
75. Taleisnik J: The Wrist. New York, NY, Churchill Livingstone, 1985
76. Tang JB, Xu J, Xie RG: Scaphoid and lunate movement in different ranges of carpal radioulnar deviation. J Hand Surg Am 36:25-30, 2011
77. Mack ZE, Kamal RN, Best GM, et al: The intercalated segment: does the triquetrum move in synchrony with the lunate? J Hand Surg 47:762-71, 2022
78. Li ZM, Kuxhaus L, Fisk JA, et al: Coupling between wrist flexion-extension and radial-ulnar deviation. Clin Biomech 20:177-83, 2005
79. Youm Y, McMurtry RY, Flatt AE, et al: Kinematics of the wrist. I. An experimental study of radial-ulnar deviation and flexion-extension. J Bone and Joint Surg—Series A 60:423-31, 1978
80. Fisk G: Carpal instability and the fractured scaphoid. Ann R Cell Surg Engl 46:63-76, 1970
81. MacConaill MA: The mechanical anatomy of the carpus and its bearings on some surgical problems. J Anat 75:166-75, 1941
82. Sangole AP, Levin MF: Arches of the hand in reach to grasp. J Biomech 41:829-37, 2008
83. al-Qattan MM, Robertson G: An anatomical study of the deep transverse metacarpal ligament. [Internet]. J Anat 182, Pt 3:443-6, 1993 [cited 2024 Jun 22], Available from: http://www.pubmedcentral.nih.gov/articlerender.fcgi?artid=1259819&tool=pmcentrez&rendertype=abstract
84. Degeorges R, Parasie J, Mitton D, et al: Three-dimensional rotations of human three-joint fingers: an optoelectronic measurement. preliminary results. Surg and Radiol Anat 27:43-50, 2005
85. Boccolari P, Pantaleoni F, Tedeschi R, et al: The mechanics of the collateral ligaments in the metacarpophalangeal joints: a scoping review. Morphologie 108, 2024
86. Widgerow AD, Ladas CS: Anatomical attachments to the proximal phalangeal base—a case for stability. Scand J Plast Reconstr Surg Hand Surg. 35(1):85-90, 2001
87. Snyder EA, Alvarez C, Golightly YM, et al: Incidence and progression of hand osteoarthritis in a large community-based cohort: the johnston county osteoarthritis project. Osteoarthritis Cartilage 28:446-52, 2020
88. Davis JE, Schaefer LF, McAlindon TE, et al: Characteristics of accelerated hand osteoarthritis: data from the osteoarthritis initiative. J Rheumatol 46:422-28, 2019
89. Fisher DM, Elliott S, Cooke TDV, et al: Descriptive anatomy of fibrocartilaginous menisci in the finger joints of the hand. J Orthop Res 3:484-91, 1985
90. Benjamin M, Ralphs JR, Shibu M, et al: Capsular tissues of the proximal interphalangeal joint: normal composition and effects of Dupuytren's disease and rheumatoid arthritis. J Hand Surg (British and European Volume) 18:371-6, 1993
91. Young CM, Rayan GM: The sagittal band: anatomic and biomechanical study. J Hand Surg 25:1107-13, 2000
92. Norkin CC, White DJ: Normative range of motion values, in Measurement of Joint Motion: A Guide to Goniometry (ed 5). Philadelphia, PA, F.A Davis, 2016, pp 537-41
93. Armstrong R, Greig M: Classifying joint hypermobility: a comparison of three current classification systems. Int J Th Rehab. 25:340-5, 2018
94. Pang EQ, Yao J: Anatomy and biomechanics of the finger proximal interphalangeal joint. Hand Clin 34:121-6, 2018
95. Dzwierzynski WW, Pintar F, Matloub HS, et al: Biomechanics of the intact and surgically repaired proximal interphalangeal joint collateral ligaments. J Hand Surg 21:679-83, 1996
96. Kamnerdnakta S, Huetteman HE, Chung KC: Complications of proximal interphalangeal joint injuries: prevention and treatment. Hand Clin 34:267-88, 2018
97. Mallon WJ, Brown HR, Nunley JA: Digital ranges of motion: normal values in young adults. J Hand Surg 16:882-7, 1991
98. Yang TH, Lu SC, Lin WJ, et al: Assessing finger joint biomechanics by applying equal force to flexor tendons in vitro using a novel simultaneous approach. PLoS One 11, 2016

99. Hamman J, Ali A, Phillips C, et al: A biomechanical study of the flexor digitorum superficialis: effects of digital pulley excision and loss of the flexor digitorum profundus. J Hand Surg 22:328-35, 1997
100. Lv Y, Zheng Q, Chen X, et al: Analysis on synergistic cocontraction of extrinsic finger flexors and extensors during flexion movements: a finite element digital human hand model. PLoS One 17, 2022
101. Brand PW, Hollister AM: Clinical Mechanics of the Hand (ed 3). St. Louis, MO, Mosby, 1999
102. Gehrmann S V, Kaufmann RA, Li ZM: Wrist circumduction reduced by finger constraints. J Hand Surg 33:1287-92, 2008
103. Cailliet R: Hand Pain and Impairment. Philadelphia, PA, FA Davis, 1994
104. Kaplan EB: The participation of the metacarpophalangeal joint of the thumb in the act of opposition. Bull Hosp Jt Dis 27:39-45, 1966
105. Idler RS: Anatomy and biomechanics of the digital flexor tendons. Hand Clin 1:3-11, 1985
106. Kapandji I: The Physiology of the Joints (ed 6). Edinburgh, Scotland, Churchill Livingstone, 2009
107. Ranney D: The hand as a concept: digital differences and their importance. Clin Anat 8:281-7, 1995
108. Long C: Intrinsic-extrinsic muscle control of the fingers: electromyographic studies. J Bone and Joint Surg—Series A 50:973-84, 1968
109. Kozin SH, Porter S, Clark P, et al: The contribution of the intrinsic muscles to grip and pinch strength. J Hand Surg 24:64-72, 1999
110. Palti R, Vigler M: Anatomy and function of lumbrical muscles. Hand Clin 28:13-17, 2012
111. Siegel DB, Kuzma G, Eakins D: Anatomic investigation of the role of the lumbrical muscles in carpal tunnel syndrome [Internet]. J Hand Surg Am 20:860-3, 1995 [cited 2024 Aug 11], Available from: https://pubmed.ncbi.nlm.nih.gov/8522757/
112. El-Gammal TA, Steyers CM, Blair WF, et al: Anatomy of the oblique retinacular ligament of the index finger. J Hand Surg 18:717-21, 1993
113. Liss FE: The interosseous muscles: the foundation of hand function. Hand Clin 28:9-12, 2012
114. Wei Y, Zou Z, Qian Z, et al: Biomechanical analysis of the effect of the finger extensor mechanism on hand grasping performance. IEEE Trans on Neural Syst and Rehabil Eng 30:360-8, 2022
115. Synek A, Pahr DH: The effect of the extensor mechanism on maximum isometric fingertip forces: a numerical study on the index finger. J Biomech 49:3423-29, 2016
116. Ranney D, Wells R: Lumbrical muscle function as revealed by a new and physiological approach. Anat Rec 222:110-14, 1988
117. Landsmeer JM: The anatomy of the dorsal aponeurosis of the human finger and its functional significance. Anat Rec 104:31-44, 1949
118. Cooney WP, Lucca MJ, Chao EYS, et al: The kinesiology of the thumb trapeziometacarpal joint. J Bone and Joint Surg—Series A 63:1371-81, 1981
119. Nichols DS, Oberhofer HM, Chim H: Anatomy and biomechanics of the thumb carpometacarpal joint. Hand Clin 38:129-39, 2022
120. Komatsu I, Lubahn JD: Anatomy and biomechanics of the thumb carpometacarpal joint. Oper Tech Orthop 28:1-5, 2018
121. Schroeder NS, Goldfarb CA: Thumb ulnar collateral and radial collateral ligament injuries. Clin Sports Med 34:117-26, 2015
122. Goldberg I, Nathan H: Anatomy and pathology of the sesamoid bones—the hand compared to the foot. Int Orthop 11:141-7, 1987
123. Ergen E, Yılmaz Ö, Arı B, et al: Prevalence of metacarpophalangeal sesamoid bones of the hand in Turkish population. Jt Dis Relat Surg 32:391, 2021
124. Sahin R, Kazdal C: The relationship between ossification in metacarpophalangeal sesamoids of the thumb and the period of puberty: a radiographic study. Medeni Med J 37:300-5, 2022
125. Tan SHS, Pan F, Sirisena R, et al: Histology of the volar plate of the thumb metacarpophalangeal joint. Hand Surg Rehabil 42:141-6, 2023
126. Mitchell TW, Mitchell SA, Wu C: Radial collateral ligament injuries of the thumb metacarpophalangeal joint. Curr Rev Musculoskelet Med 15:581-9, 2022
127. Johanson ME, Skinner SR, Lamoreux LW: Phasic relationships of the intrinsic and extrinsic thumb musculature. Clin Orthop Relat Res 322:120-30, 1996
128. McGee C, O'Brien V, Van Nortwick S, et al: First dorsal interosseous muscle contraction results in radiographic reduction of healthy thumb carpometacarpal joint. J Hand Ther 28:375-81, 2015
129. Adams JE, O'Brien V, Magnusson E, et al: Radiographic analysis of simulated first dorsal interosseous and opponens pollicis loading upon thumb CMC joint subluxation: a cadaver study. Hand (NY) 13:40-44, 2018
130. MacConaill M, Basmajian J: Muscles and Movement: A Basis for Human Kinesiology. Baltimore, MD, Williams & Wilkins, 1969
131. Al-Sukaini A, Singh HP, Dias JJ: Extrinsic versus intrinsic hand muscle dominance in finger flexion. J Hand Surg: European Volume 41:392-9, 2016
132. Jeannerod M: The Neural and Behavioral Organization of Goal-Directed Movements. Oxford, England, Clarendon Press, 1988
133. Roy EA, Leavitt JL: Changes in sensory motor behavior in aging, in Advances in Psychology. Amsterdam; Lausanne: North-Holland/Elsevier, 1996
134. Mackenzie CL, Iberall T: The grasping hand. Amsterdam; New York: North-Holland, 1994
135. Napier JR: The prehensile movements of the human hand. J Bone Joint Surg 38:902-13, 1956
136. Slocum DB, Pratt DR: Disability evaluation for the hand. J Bone Joint Surg Am 491-95, 1946
137. Kamper DG, George Hornby T, Rymer WZ: Extrinsic flexor muscles generate concurrent flexion of all three finger joints. J Biomech 35: 1581-89, 2002
138. Milner TE, Dhaliwal SS: Activation of intrinsic and extrinsic finger muscles in relation to the fingertip force vector. Exp Brain Res 146:197-204, 2002
139. Fox PM, Oliver JD, Nguyen V, et al: Electromyographic analysis of grip. Orthopedics 42:E555-8, 2019
140. Cai A, Pingel I, Lorz D, et al: Force distribution of a cylindrical grip differs between dominant and nondominant hand in healthy subjects. Arch Orthop Trauma Surg 138:1323-31, 2018
141. Barr A, Bear-Lehman J: Biomechanics of the wrist and hand, in Nordin M, Frankel V (eds): Basic Biomechanics of the Musculoskeletal System (ed 4). Baltimore, MD, Lippincott Williams, and Wilkins, 2012
142. Long C, Conrad PW, Hall EA, et al: Intrinsic-extrinsic muscle control of the hand in power grip and precision handling: an electromyographic study. J Bone Joint Surg Am 52:853-67, 1970
143. Landsmeer JM: Power grip and precision handling. Ann Rheum Dis 21:164-70, 1962

SECTION 4

Lower Extremity Joint Complexes

CHAPTER 10 **The Hip Complex** 310

CHAPTER 11 **The Knee** 351

CHAPTER 12 **The Ankle and Foot Complex** 397

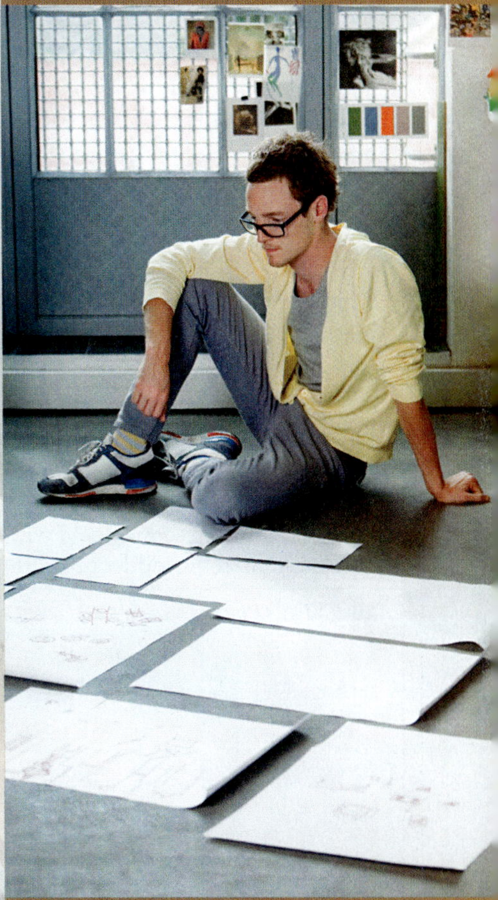

CHAPTER

10 The Hip Complex

Yongni Zhang PT, PhD | RobRoy L. Martin PT, PhD, CSCS

CHAPTER OUTLINE

INTRODUCTION 312

STRUCTURE AND FUNCTION OF THE HIP JOINT 312

- Structure 312
  - Proximal Articular Surface 312
  - Distal Articular Surface 314
  - Articular Congruence 319
  - Hip Joint Capsule and Ligaments 320
  - Structural Adaptations to Weight-Bearing 323
- Function 325
  - Motion of the Femur on the Acetabulum 325
  - Motion of the Pelvis on the Femur 326
  - Coordinated Motions of the Femur, Pelvis, and Lumbar Spine 329
  - Hip Joint Musculature 332

HIP JOINT FORCES AND MUSCLE FUNCTION IN STANCE 337

- Bilateral Stance 337
- Unilateral Stance 338
  - Compensatory Lateral Lean of the Trunk 340
  - Use of a Cane Ipsilaterally 341
  - Use of a Cane Contralaterally 342

HIP PAIN ACROSS THE LIFE SPAN 344

- Femoroacetabular Impingement Syndrome 344
- Acetabular Dysplasia 345
- Hip Osteoarthritis 345

SUMMARY 346

STUDY QUESTIONS 346

REFERENCES 346

ANATOMY OVERVIEW

MUSCLE ACTIONS OF THE HIP (FEMOROACETABULAR JOINT)

Muscle actions are considered with the hip beginning from anatomic position. Muscle actions can change if activated from a different position.

TABLE KEY: Primary muscle | Secondary muscles | Dependent on hip position

Sagittal Plane	Flexion	Extension
	Iliopsoas	Gluteus maximus
	Rectus femoris	Semitendinosus
	Tensor fascia latae	Semimembranosus
	Sartorius	Biceps femoris, long head
	Pectineus	Gluteus medius (posterior fibers)
	Adductor longus	Adductor magnus (posterior fibers)
	Adductor magnus	Piriformis
	Gracilis	
	Gluteus minimus (anterior fibers)	
Frontal Plane	**Abduction**	**Adduction**
	Gluteus medius	Adductor magnus
	Gluteus minimus	Pectineus
	Tensor fascia latae	Adductor longus
	Piriformis	Adductor brevis
	Sartorius	Gracilis
	Rectus femoris	Obturator externus
Transverse Plane	**Medial Rotation**	**Lateral Rotation**
	Tensor fascia latae	Gluteus maximus
	Gluteus minimus	Piriformis
	Gluteus medius (anterior fibers)	Quadratus femoris
	Pectineus	Obturator internus and externus
	Adductor longus and brevis	Gemellus superior and inferior
	Adductor magnus (posterior fibers)	Sartorius
	Semimembranosus	Gluteus medius (posterior fibers)
	Semitendinosus	Biceps femoris, long head

ANATOMY OVERVIEW

Muscle	Proximal Attachment	Distal Attachment
Iliopsoas	*Psoas major* and *minor*: Transverse processes and lateral aspect of T12–L5 vertebral bodies and discs *Iliacus:* Iliac crest, iliac fossa, sacral ala and anterior SI ligaments	Lesser trochanter
Rectus femoris	Anterior inferior iliac spine (AIIS)	Quadriceps tendon to patella and ultimately tibial tuberosity
Tensor fascia latae	Anterior superior iliac spine (ASIS)	Iliotibial (IT) band to lateral condyle of tibia
Sartorius	ASIS	Superior aspect of medial tibia
Pectineus	Superior ramus of pubis	Pectineal line (femur), just inferior to lesser trochanter
Adductor longus	Body of pubis, inferior to pubic crest	Middle third of linea aspera (femur)
Adductor brevis	Body and inferior ramus of pubis	Pectineal line and proximal part of linea aspera (femur)
Adductor magnus	Inferior ramus of pubis to ischial tuberosity	Gluteal tuberosity to adductor tubercle of femur via linea aspera (femur)
Gracilis	Body and inferior ramus of pubis	Superior aspect of medial tibia
Gluteus maximus	Posterior ilium, sacrum and coccyx	IT band to lateral condyle of tibia
Gluteus medius	Lateral surface of ilium between anterior and posterior gluteal lines	Greater trochanter (femur)
Gluteus minimus	Lateral surface of ilium between anterior and inferior gluteal lines	Greater trochanter (femur)
Semimembranosus	Ischial tuberosity	Posterior aspect of medial tibial condyle
Semitendinosus	Ischial tuberosity	Superior aspect of medial tibia
Biceps femoris, long head	Ischial tuberosity	Lateral aspect of fibular head
Piriformis	Anterior surface of sacrum	Greater trochanter (femur)
Obturator externus	Edge of obturator foramen	Trochanteric fossa (femur)
Obturator internus	Pelvic edge of obturator foramen	Greater trochanter to trochanteric fossa (femur)
Gemellus superior and inferior	*Superior:* Ischial spine *Inferior:* Ischial tuberosity	Greater trochanter to trochanteric fossa (femur)
Quadratus femoris	Ischial tuberosity	Inter-trochanteric crest (femur)

Introduction

The hip joint, also called the **coxofemoral** or **femoroacetabular joint**, is the articulation of the acetabulum of the pelvis and the head of the femur **(Fig. 10–1)**. These two segments form a synovial ball-and-socket joint with three degrees of freedom: flexion/extension in the sagittal plane, abduction/adduction in the frontal plane, and medial/lateral rotation in the transverse plane. Although the hip joint and the shoulder complex have some common features, each has undergone such extensive functional and structural adaptations to support their respective roles that comparisons between these joints are more for general interest than functional relevance. For example, the role of the shoulder complex is to provide a stable base on which a wide range of mobility for the hand can be superimposed. Shoulder complex structure gives precedence to this open-chain function. Instead, the primary function of the hip joint is to support the weight of the head, arms, and trunk (**HAT**) in static erect posture and dynamic postures such as ambulation, running, and stair climbing. The interaction between the hip and lumbosacral spine and the influence they have on each other's ability to function are important to understand. The hip joint, like the other joints of the lower extremity, is structured primarily to serve its weight-bearing function. Although we examine hip joint structure and function as if the joint were designed to move the foot through space in an open chain, hip joint structure is more influenced by the demands placed on the joint when the limb is bearing weight as well as shifting weight. As we shall see later in this chapter, weight-bearing function of the hip joint and its related weight-bearing responses are key to understanding the hip joint and the interactions that occur between the hip and the other joints of the lower extremity and spine.

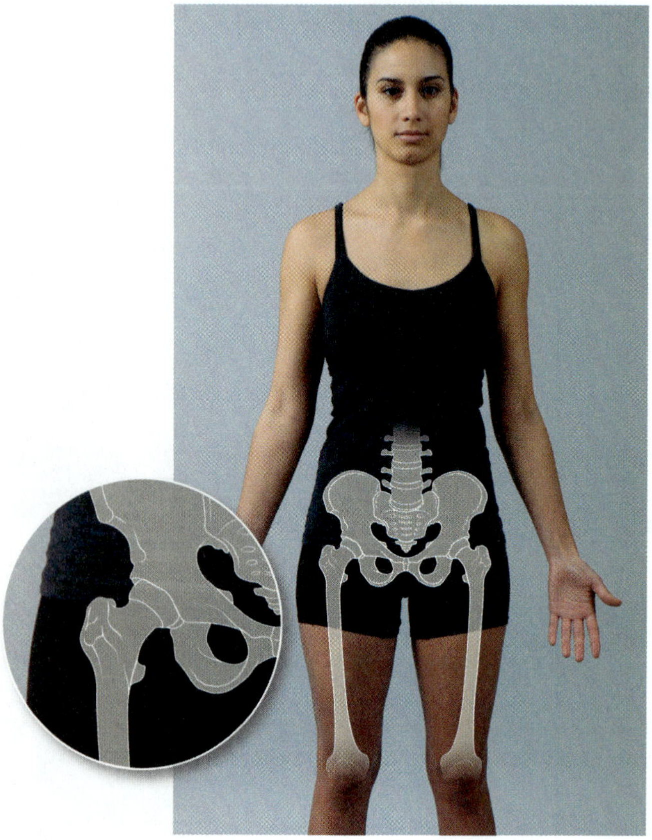

Figure 10–1 The hip joint is the connection between the leg and the trunk and is important during many functional activities.

Patient Application 10–1

Gabriella Martinez is a 32-year-old woman currently teaching kindergarten, a position she has held for the past 10 years. Gabriella has been bothered with recurrent left hip pain that has been intermittent throughout her young adult life. She recalls several instances of hip pain that interrupted her participation in gymnastics and dance as a teenager. Although Gabriella no longer participates in dance or gymnastics, she has remained physically active by running as well as taking Pilates and yoga classes until recently being limited by pain.

Over the past few months, she has experienced increasing problems, predominantly on her left side, that interfere with climbing the stairs in her two-story home, performing activities with her kindergarten class, and caring for her 3-year-old daughter. In addition to pain complaints, she also reports feeling as though her hip may "pop out of the socket" when she is doing twisting poses in yoga and has an occasional painful "click" in the hip. It has become too painful for her to run, and she has stopped participating in her exercise classes. She remembers being told by a physician when she was in her teens that she would probably have problems with her hips when she was older because her hips were "shallow."

Gabriella localizes her primary pain to her left groin, although the lateral hip area can also be painful. On clinical examination, Gabriella is observed to walk with reduced hip extension on the left. Pain occurs during mid to late stance phase and swing phase on the left. She also has a slight left lateral lean during left stance. During examination, you find that Gabriella has pain with the flexion-adduction-internal rotation (FADIR) test on the left.[1] In the supine position, there is an increase in medial rotation and decrease in lateral rotation at the left hip.

Structure and Function of the Hip Joint

Structure

Proximal Articular Surface

The cuplike concave socket of the hip joint is called the **acetabulum** and is located on the lateral aspect of the **innominate** or **os coxa** (pelvic bone) **(Fig. 10–2)**. Three bones form the pelvis: the ilium, the ischium, and the pubis. Each of the three bones contributes to the structure of the acetabulum **(Fig. 10–3A)**. The pubis forms one-fifth of the acetabulum, the ischium forms two-fifths, and the ilium forms the remainder (see Fig. 10–3A). Until full ossification of the pelvis occurs between 20 and 25 years of age, the separate segments of the acetabulum may remain visible on radiograph as in a typical two-year-old (see **Fig. 10–3B**).[2]

The **lunate surface** (the periphery of the acetabulum) is covered with hyaline cartilage. This horseshoe-shaped area of cartilage articulates with the head of the femur (see Fig. 10–3A) and allows for contact stress to be uniformly distributed.[3] The inferior aspect of the lunate surface (the base of the horseshoe) is interrupted by a deep notch called the **acetabular notch**, and is spanned by a fibrous band, the **transverse acetabular ligament**, which connects the two inferior ends of the lunate surface **(Fig. 10–4A)**. As the transverse acetabular ligament spans the acetabular notch, it creates a fibro-osseous tunnel that contains fibroelastic fat covered with synovial membrane

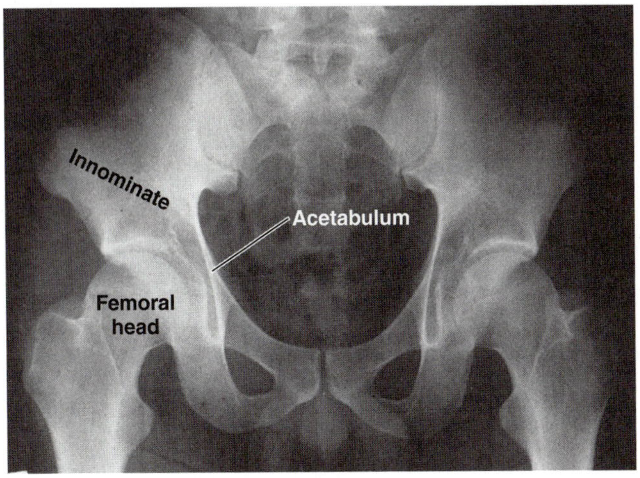

Figure 10–2 The hip joint is formed by the head of the femur and the acetabulum of the innominate bone (one half) of the pelvis.

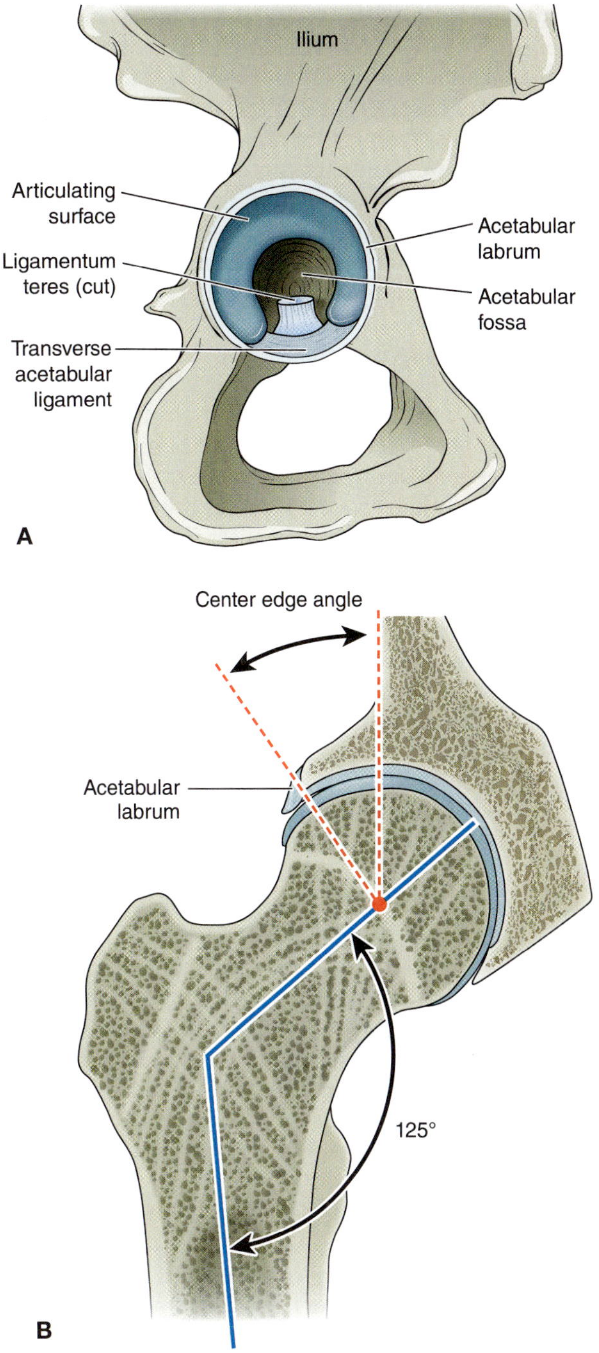

Figure 10–4 **A.** The transverse acetabular ligament connects the two inferior ends of the lunate surface, while the acetabular labrum deepens the acetabulum. **B.** The center edge angle of the acetabulum is formed between a vertical line through the center of the femoral head and a line connecting the center of the femoral head and the bony edge of the acetabulum.

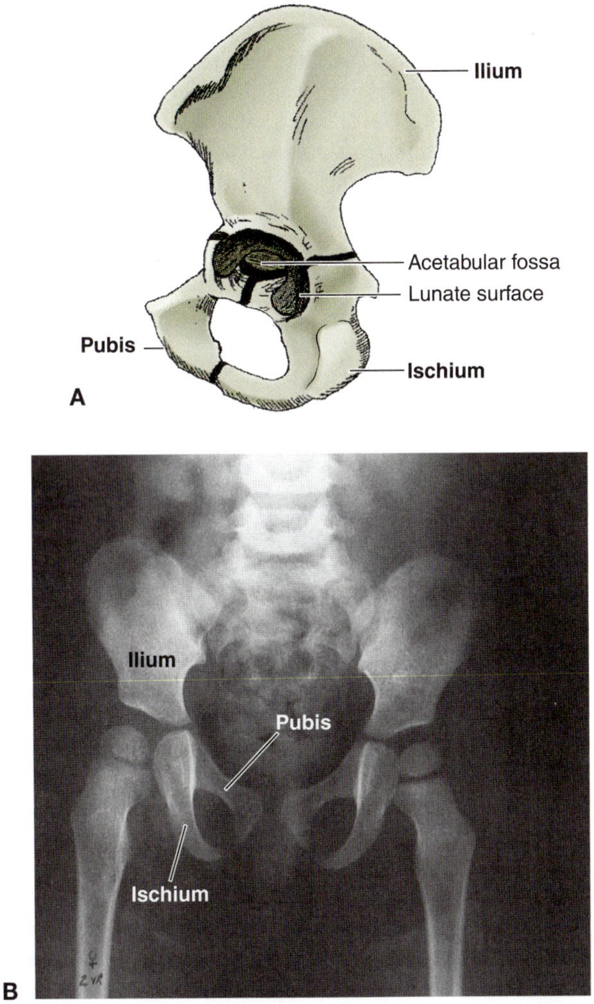

Figure 10–3 **A.** The acetabulum is formed by the union of the three bones of the pelvis, with only the upper horseshoe-shaped area (the lunate surface) being articular. **B.** In this radiograph of a typical 2-year-old child without impairments, the cartilaginous rather than bony union of the acetabulum is clearly evident as spaces between the three bones of the innominate.

through which blood vessels pass into the central and deepest portion of the acetabulum, called the **acetabular fossa**. Unlike the lunate surface, the acetabular fossa does not articulate with the femoral head.

ACETABULUM

Although appearing to be spherical, only the upper margin of the acetabulum has a true circular contour.[4] The opening of the acetabulum faces inferiorly by 50° and is rotated anteriorly (anteverted) 20°.[5-8] Women will generally have a few degrees greater acetabular inclination and anteversion compared with men.[4] The articular surface area of the acetabulum tends to be smaller in women than it is in men.[7] Typical functioning of the hip joint requires optimal femoral head coverage by the acetabulum. Femoral head coverage is largely determined by acetabular depth. Acetabular dysplasia, coxa profunda, acetabular protrusio, anteversion, and retroversion are terms used to describe acetabular abnormalities that can potentially lead to pathology, including excessive cartilage wear and osteoarthritis.[9]

Acetabular dysplasia is an abnormally shallow acetabulum that results in a *lack of* femoral head coverage.[10] It may contribute to instability of the hip joint or lead to disproportionate loading of the superior acetabular rim. **Coxa profunda** and **acetabular protrusio** are terms used to describe conditions in which the acetabulum *excessively* covers the femoral head. Acetabular over-coverage can lead to mechanical restrictions of range of motion (ROM) and impingement between the femoral head–neck junction and the acetabulum.[11] Acetabular depth can be measured as the **center edge angle** (see **Fig. 10–4B**).[12] The center edge angle is formed by a line connecting the lateral rim of the acetabulum and the center of the femoral head and a vertical line from the center of the femoral head. Center edge angles are classified as follows: definite dysplasia (less than 16°), possible dysplasia (16° to 25°), and typical (greater than 25°).[12] Lateral center edge angles greater than 45° may indicate excessive acetabular over-coverage.[13]

Abnormalities in acetabular depth, inclination, and version (abnormal positioning in the transverse plane) affect femoral head coverage. **Anteversion** of the acetabulum exists when the acetabulum is positioned anteriorly in the transverse plane an excessive amount; **retroversion** exists when the acetabulum is positioned posteriorly in the transverse plane. An acetabulum that is positioned with less inclination or more anteversion can lead to instability. Likewise, an acetabulum that is positioned with more inclination or retroversion can lead to over-coverage and impingement between the acetabulum femoral head–neck junction.[14]

ACETABULAR LABRUM

The acetabular labrum is a ring of wedge-shaped fibrocartilage attached to the outer periphery of the acetabulum (see labrum cross section in Fig. 10–4B). The labrum is attached to the periphery of the acetabulum by a zone of calcified cartilage.[15] The labrum of the hip is analogous to the meniscus of the knee and the labrum of the glenohumeral joint. The acetabular labrum deepens the socket and increases the concavity of the acetabulum through its triangular shape, grasping the head of the femur to maintain contact with the acetabulum. The labrum also acts as a seal to maintain negative intra-articular pressure *within* the hip joint, enhancing stability.[16] Nerve endings within the labrum may provide proprioceptive feedback to further enhance joint stability.[17] However, the nerve endings may also be a source of pain.[17] When the labrum is compromised, friction stresses increase—potentially leading to altered loads on the articular cartilage of the hip joint. Although the typical hip is intrinsically stable because of the deeply recessed acetabulum, an abnormally shallow acetabulum will increase stress on the surrounding capsule and labrum.

The transverse acetabular ligament (see Fig. 10-4A) is considered a continuation of the acetabular labrum. Histologically, it is predominantly ligamentous, but contains cartilaginous cells believed to withstand compressive loads.[18] However, experimental data do not support the transverse acetabular ligament as a load-bearing structure.[19] The ligament is believed to serve primarily as a tension band between the anteroinferior and posteroinferior aspects of the acetabulum (the "feet" of the horseshoe-shaped articular surface) that protects the blood vessels traveling beneath it to reach the head of the femur.[19]

Patient Application 10–2

Gabriella's left groin pain is provoked by FADIR test that involves passive hip flexion and medial rotation.[1] This clinical finding may be indicative of damage to the anterosuperior labrum and possibly a site of osteoarthritic changes.[20,21] Due to her age, history of hip pain, and clinical findings, her physician ordered a magnetic resonance arthrogram (MRA) to identify the pathoanatomic source of her pain. After reviewing her MRA, Gabriella's physician confirmed the presence of a superior anterior labral tear and early-stage osteoarthritis. Acetabular labral tears are increasingly recognized as a source of hip pain and a starting point for degenerative changes at the acetabular rim.[17,22] Damage to the labrum was evident in 96% of postmortem and cadaveric hip joints in persons 61 to 98 years of age, with 74% showing damage in the anterosuperior quadrant.[11] Isolated labral tears are uncommon and usually occur in conjunction with bony abnormalities of the acetabulum or femoral neck junction.[23] Although a labral tear is not always symptomatic, a torn labrum can potentially cause anterior groin pain, clicking, locking, catching, instability, giving way, or joint stiffness.[24]

Distal Articular Surface

The head of the femur is a rounded hyaline cartilage–covered surface.[25] The articular area of the femoral head forms approximately two-thirds of a sphere and is more circular than the acetabulum[4,26] **(Fig. 10–5)**. Femoral shape and dimensions

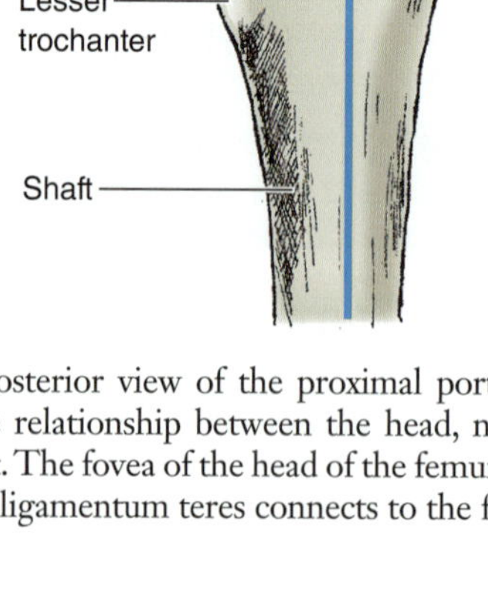

Figure 10–5 Posterior view of the proximal portion of the right femur shows the relationship between the head, neck, trochanters, and femoral shaft. The fovea of the head of the femur is non-articular, and is where the ligamentum teres connects to the femoral head.

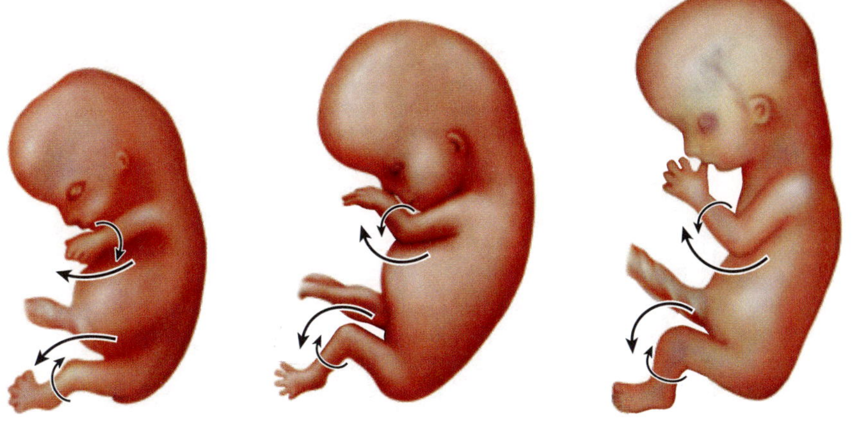

Figure 10-6 During fetal development from approximately the seventh through ninth weeks, the upper and lower extremities rotate in opposite directions.

can be variable even in bones of the same overall size.[26] The radius of curvature of the femoral head is smaller in women than in men relative to the dimensions of the pelvis.[26,27] Just inferior to the most medial point on the femoral head is a small, roughened pit called the **fovea** or **fovea capitis**. The fovea is not covered with articular cartilage and is the point at which the **ligamentum teres** (the ligament of the head of the femur) is attached.

The femoral head is attached to the femoral neck, which in turn is attached to the shaft of the femur between the greater and lesser trochanters (see Fig. 10-5). The femoral neck is, in general, only about 5 cm long and may vary slightly based on gender and ethnicity.[28,29] The femoral neck is angulated so that the femoral head faces medially, superiorly, and anteriorly with respect to the femoral shaft and distal femoral condyles.[30]

ANGULATION OF THE FEMUR

There are two angulations made by the head and neck of the femur in relation to the shaft. The **angle of inclination** occurs in the frontal plane between an axis through the femoral head and neck and the longitudinal axis of the femoral shaft. The **angle of torsion** occurs in the transverse plane between an axis through the femoral head and neck and an axis through the distal femoral condyles. The origin and variability of these angulations can be understood in the context of the embryonic development of the lower limb.

In the early stages of fetal development, both upper extremity and lower extremity limb buds project laterally from the body as if in full abduction. During the seventh and eighth weeks of gestational age and before full definition of the joints, adduction of the buds begins **(Fig. 10-6)**. At the end of the eighth week, the "fetal position" has been achieved, but the upper and lower limbs are no longer positioned similarly. Although the upper limb buds have undergone torsion somewhat *laterally* (so that the ventral surface of the limb bud faces anteriorly), the lower limb buds have undergone torsion *medially*, so that the ventral surface faces posteriorly.[28] The result for the lower limb is critical to understanding function. The knee flexes in the opposite direction from the elbow, and the extensor (dorsal) surface of the lower limb is located anteriorly rather than posteriorly. Although the head and neck of the femur retain the original position of the limb bud, the femoral shaft is inclined medially and undergoes medial torsion with regard to the head and neck. The magnitude of medial inclination and torsion of the distal femur (with regard to the head and neck) is dependent on embryonic growth and, presumably, fetal positioning during the remaining months of uterine life. The development of the angulations of the femur appears to continue after birth and through the early years of development. Both typical and abnormal angles of inclination and torsion of the femur are *properties of the femur alone*. However, abnormalities in the angulations of the femur can substantially alter hip joint stability, weight-bearing biomechanics of the hip joint, and muscle biomechanics. Likewise, such abnormalities in femoral angulation can influence compensatory changes in the remainder of the lower extremity and spine.

ANGLE OF INCLINATION OF THE FEMUR

The angle of inclination of the femur is approximately 125° (referencing the medial angle formed by the axes of the head–neck and the shaft) **(Fig. 10-7A)**.[21,31] This value can have a typical range from 110° to 144° in the unimpaired adult (see Fig. 10–7A).[26,27,32-34] As with the angle of inclination of the humerus, there are variations not only among individuals but also from side to side. In women, the angle of inclination is somewhat smaller than it is in men, owing to the greater width of the female pelvis.[28] With a typical angle of inclination, the greater trochanter lies at the level of the center of the femoral head.[35] The angle of inclination of the femur changes across the life span; it approximates 150° at birth (see Fig. 10–3B) and gradually declines to about 125° at skeletal maturity.[21,31] This angle can continue to decline again in the elderly.[33] A pathologically greater medial angulation between the neck and shaft is called **coxa valga** (see **Fig. 10-7B**) and a pathologically smaller angle is called **coxa vara**. **Figure 10-8** shows coxa valga (Fig. 10–8A) and coxa vara (Fig. 10-8B) radiographically.

Both coxa vara and coxa valga can lead to abnormal lower extremity biomechanics, altered muscle function, and gait abnormalities that contribute to pathologies such as labral pathology, hip and knee osteoarthritis, and slipped capital femoral epiphysis.[36-39]

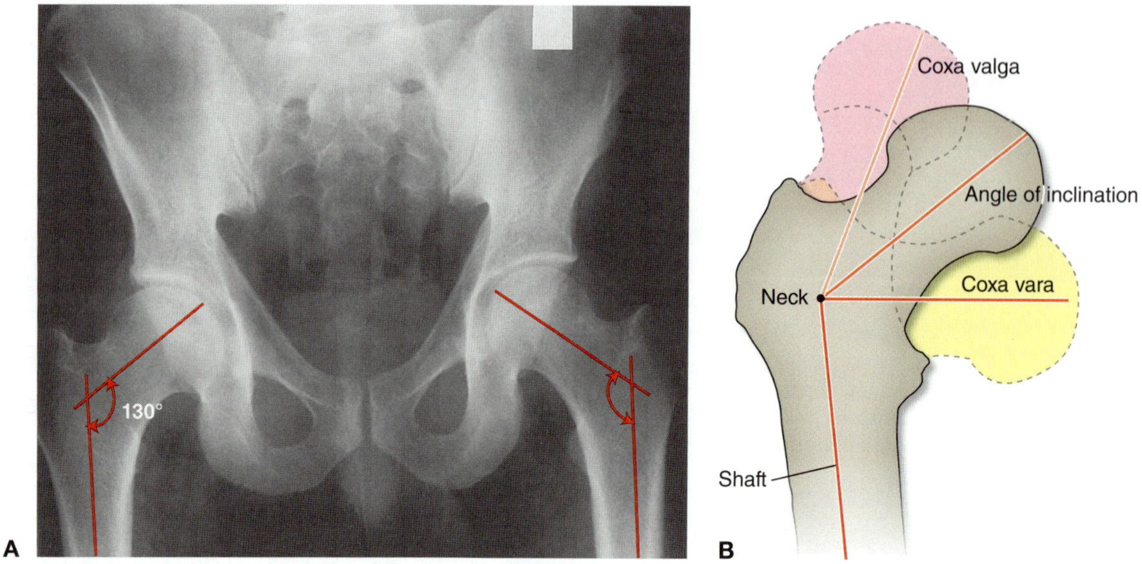

Figure 10–7 The axis of the femoral head and neck forms an angle with the axis of the femoral shaft called the *angle of inclination*. **A.** In this adult subject without impairments, the angle is slightly less than 130°, with a couple of degrees of variation from side to side. **B.** Greater medial angles are called coxa valga, whereas a smaller medial angle is called coxa vara.

In coxa valga (see Fig. 10–8A), the angle of inclination in the femur is greater than the typical adult angle of 125°. The increased angle brings the vertical weight-bearing line closer to the shaft of the femur, diminishing the shear, or bending, force across the femoral neck. The reduction in force across the femoral neck is reflected in a reduction in density of the lateral trabecular system.[40] However, the decreased distance between the femoral head and the greater trochanter also decreases the length of the moment arm of the hip abductor muscles. The decreased muscular moment arm results in an increased demand for muscular force generation to maintain sufficient abduction torque to counterbalance the gravitational adduction moment acting around the supporting hip joint during single-limb support. Either the additional muscular force requirement will increase the total joint reaction force within the hip joint, or the abductor muscles will be unable to meet the increased demand and will be functionally weakened. Although the strength of the abductors may be otherwise typical, the reduction in biomechanical effectiveness may produce the compensations typical of primary abductor muscle weakness. As the femoral head points more superiorly, coxa valga leads to a decreasing amount of coverage from the acetabulum superiorly. Consequently, coxa valga decreases the stability of the hip and predisposes the hip to dislocation.[8,41] This may further lead to femoroacetabular impingement and the progression of labral tearing, loss of joint stability, and eventual arthrosis.[42]

Coxa vara (see **Fig. 10–8B**) is considered to give the advantage of improved hip joint stability (if angle reduction is not too extreme). The apparent improvement in congruence occurs because the decreased angle between the neck and shaft of the femur will place the femoral head deeper into the acetabulum, decreasing the amount of articular surface usually exposed superiorly and increasing coverage from the acetabulum. A varus femur, if not caused by trauma, may also increase the length of the moment arm of the hip abductor muscles by increasing the distance between the femoral head and the greater trochanter.[43] The increased moment arm decreases the amount of force that must be generated by the abductor muscles in single-limb support which, in turn, reduces the joint reaction force. However, coxa vara has the disadvantage of increasing the bending moment along the femoral head and neck. This increase in bending force, evidenced by increased density of trabeculae laterally in the femur, is caused by the increase in tensile stresses.[40] The increased shear force along the femoral neck will also increase the predisposition toward a femoral neck fracture.[44]

Coxa vara in an adolescent who is not yet skeletally mature may increase the likelihood that the femoral head will slide on its cartilaginous growth plate, called the femoral capital epiphysis. In childhood, the epiphysis is fairly horizontal as seen in **Fig. 10–8C**.[8] Consequently, the superimposed weight merely compresses the head into its epiphyseal plate. In adolescence, growth of the bone results in a more oblique orientation of the epiphyseal plate.[45] The epiphyseal obliquity makes the plate more vulnerable to shear forces at a time when the plate is already weakened by the rapid growth that occurs during this period of life.[38] Weight-bearing forces may slide the femoral head inferiorly, resulting in a **slipped capital femoral epiphysis**. The surgical interventions to correct coxa vara deformities in children may come with inherent complications.[46,47] Despite correction of the deformity, a common complication and resultant failure of the procedure is an unstable femoral epiphysis. Optimal results require addressing the stability of the proximal femoral epiphysis and exemplifies the vulnerability of the growth plate of the femur in patients with a preexisting coxa vara deformity. As is true for a hip

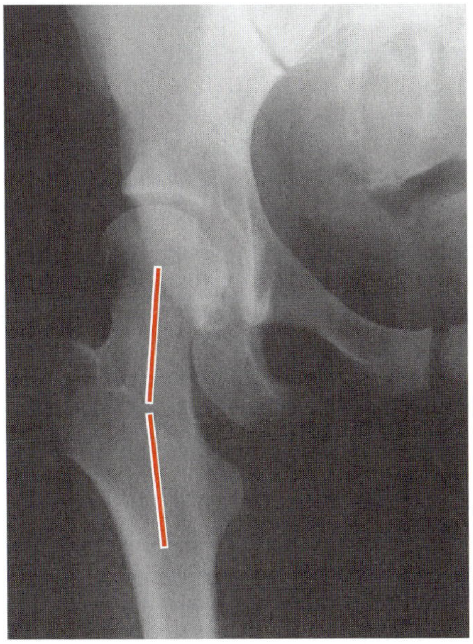

A Coxa valga

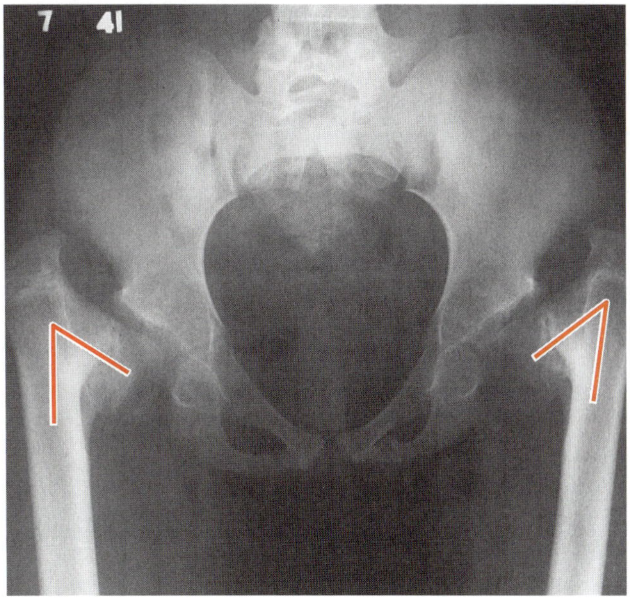

B Coxa vara

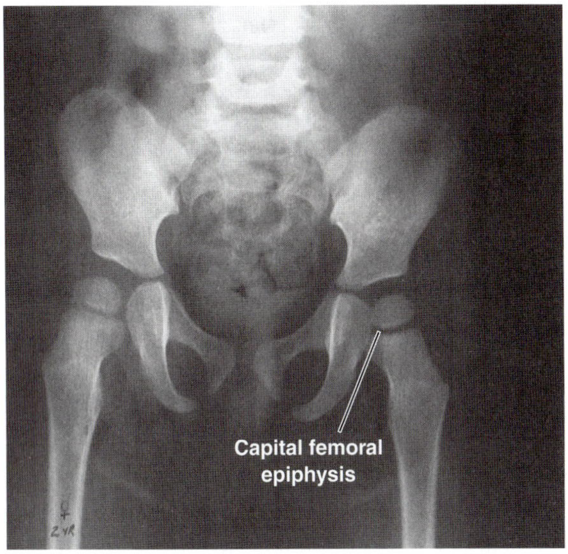

C

Figure 10–8 Abnormal angles of inclination found in two young adults with developmental hip dysplasia. **A.** A pathological increase in the angle of inclination is called coxa valga. **B.** A pathological decrease in the angle is called coxa vara. **C.** Cartilaginous femoral capital epiphyses shown radiographically in a typically developing 2-month-old.

fracture, the altered biomechanics and at-risk blood supply necessitate restoration of typical alignment before secondary degenerative changes can occur.

Foundational Concepts 10–1
Angle of Inclination of the Femur

- The normal angle of inclination of the femur in an adult is approximately 125°.
- A pathological increase in the angle of inclination is called coxa valga and often creates a "longer" limb, and may be associated with joint instability, particularly when the hip is in adduction. Individuals who present with coxa valga are often observed to adopt positions of hip abduction (to increase joint surface alignment and congruency) and are commonly accompanied by genu vara.
- A pathological decrease in the angle of inclination is called coxa vara and often creates a "shorter" limb length. Coxa vara is associated with greater hip stability, but the low angle of the femoral neck makes it susceptible to femoral neck fractures or a higher incidence of a slipped capital femoral epiphysis. Cases of coxa vara are often accompanied by a position of increased hip adduction (to increase joint surface alignment and congruency) and genu valgum.

Expanded Concepts 10–1
Slipped Capital Femoral Epiphysis

Slipped capital femoral epiphysis (SCFE) is the most common adolescent hip disorder occurring when the femoral head displaces posteriorly on the femoral neck at the level of the growth plate (physis). A decrease in femoral neck–shaft angle (coxa vara) and a high body mass index increase the shear force across the physis.[38,48] The risk can be reduced with weight loss to lower the body mass index.[49] Slipped capital femoral epiphysis can cause widening of the femoral head–neck junction and lead to internal impingement with the acetabulum.[50]

ANGLE OF TORSION OF THE FEMUR

The angle of torsion of the femur can best be viewed by looking down the length of the femur from top to bottom. An axis through the femoral head and neck in the transverse plane will lie at an angle to an axis through the femoral condyles, with the head and neck torsioned anteriorly (anteverted or laterally rotated) with regard to an angle through the femoral condyles **(Fig. 10–9)**. This angulation within the femur reflects the medial rotational migration of the lower limb bud that occurred during fetal development (see Fig. 10–6). The apparent contradiction between medial torsion of the embryonic limb bud and lateral torsion of the femoral head and neck simply reflects a shift in reference. In medial torsion of the limb bud, *the proximal end is fixed* and the distal end migrates medially in the transverse plane. When assessing femoral torsion in a child or adult, the working assumption is that the *distal end is fixed*, with an axis through the femoral condyles presumed to lie in the frontal plane (see **Fig. 10–9A**), and that the femoral head and neck are torsioned anteriorly with respect to the condyles. The angle of anterior torsion decreases with age. In the newborn, femoral neck anteversion averages 30° to 40°.[51] This angle decreases approximately 1.5° per year until skeletal maturity occurs and is usually symmetrical in the right and left sides.[40,51,52] In the adult, the typical angle of torsion is considered to be 10° to 20°: 15° for males and 18° for females.[51,53,54]

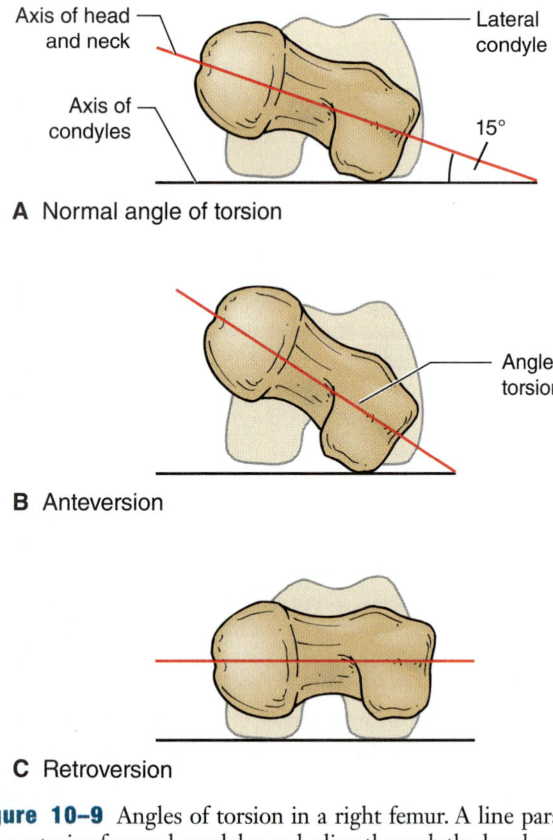

Figure 10–9 Angles of torsion in a right femur. A line parallel to the posterior femoral condyles and a line through the head and neck of the femur typically make an angle with each other that averages 10° to 20° in an adult without impairments. The femoral head and neck are in torsion anteriorly (laterally) with respect to the femoral condyles. **A.** An angle of torsion within typical limits. **B.** A pathological increase in the angle of torsion is called *anteversion.* **C.** A pathological decrease in the typical angle of torsion is called *retroversion.*

Femoral antetorsion (or **anteversion**) is considered to exist when the angle of anterior torsion is greater than 15° to 20° (see **Fig. 10–9B**). A reversal of anterior torsion, known as **femoral retrotorsion** (or **retroversion**), occurs when angles are less than 15° to 20° (see **Fig. 10–9C**). There may not be one angulation at which pathological femoral torsion may be diagnosed, given the substantial typical variability.[55] Variations in the degree of anteversion or retroversion may also be dependent on the method used to assess it, because computed tomography (CT) scan, magnetic resonance imaging (MRI), radiograph, ultrasound, and computer preplanning systems for robot-assisted orthopedic surgery have each been used to measure the angle of femoral torsion.[55-58] Clinical measures of anteversion have correlated with imaging measurements. It is important to note that the torsional angulation of the femur is a property *of the femur*; however, anteversion or retroversion affect how the femoral head sits in the acetabulum, so may affect hip joint function. For example, an anteverted femur exposes more articular surface anteriorly as it sits in the acetabulum; therefore, femoral anteversion tends to be associated with increased medial rotation ROM and concurrent decreased lateral rotation although the total excursion of hip rotation motion remains the same.[59]

Although some structural deviations such as femoral anteversion and coxa valga are commonly found together, each may occur independently of the other. Each structural deviation warrants careful consideration as to the effect on hip joint function as well as function of the joints both proximal and distal to the hip joint. As shall be evident when the knee and foot are discussed in subsequent chapters, femoral anteversion is often implicated in dysfunction at both the knee and foot. The other pathological angulations of the femur (retroversion, coxa vara, and coxa valga) similarly affect the hip joint and other joints proximally and distally.

Variations in the angle of torsion also affect hip biomechanics and function. Anteversion of the femoral head reduces hip joint stability because the femoral articular surface is more exposed anteriorly **(Fig. 10–10A)**. The line of pull for the hip abductors may fall more posterior to the joint, reducing the moment arm for abduction.[60] As is true for coxa valga, the resulting need for additional abductor muscle force may predispose the joint to arthrosis or may produce more energy-consuming gait deviations. The effect of femoral anteversion may also be seen at the knee joint. When the femoral head is anteverted, femoroacetabular congruency is diminished. To improve this congruency, pressure from the anterior capsuloligamentous structures and the anterior musculature may rotate the entire femur medially (see **Fig. 10–10B**). Although this medial rotation of the femur improves the congruence in the acetabulum, the knee joint axis through the femoral condyles is now turned

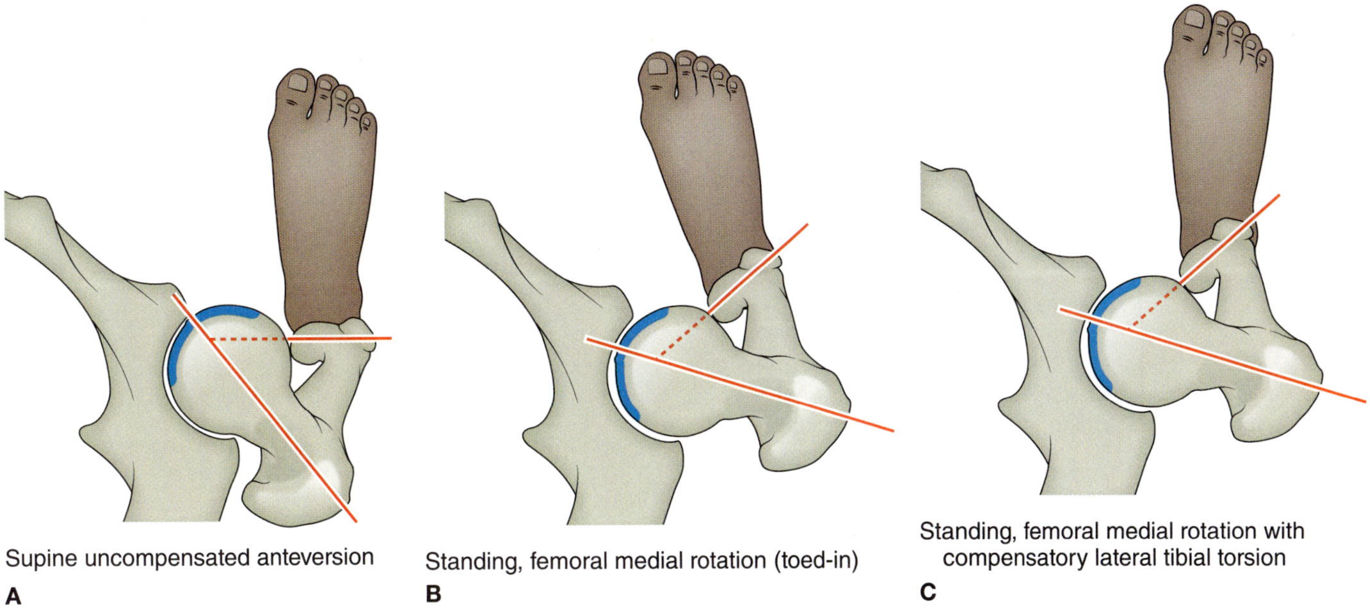

Figure 10–10 **A.** With the femoral condyles aligned in the frontal plane (in supine), the anteverted femoral head is exposed anteriorly. Lateral rotation will be limited, but medial rotation is relatively excessive. **B.** In standing, the anteverted femur tends to medially rotate within the acetabulum for improved joint congruency. The result is medial rotation of the femoral condyles in relation to the plane of progression. The torsional deformity of the femur, when assessed in standing, is referred to as *medial femoral torsion.* **C.** If there is an accompanying lateral tibial torsion, the expected toe-in may be minimized or reversed.

medially such that the patella is no longer facing anteriorly, but rather anteromedially. Medial rotation of the femoral condyles alters the plane of knee flexion/extension and results, at least initially, in a toe-in gait.[61] However, the toe-in position of the foot may appear to diminish over time because it is not uncommon to see a compensatory lateral tibial torsion develop (see **Fig. 10–10C**). Although the foot placement appears more "typical," the underlying hip problem generally remains (with some developmental reduction). The abnormal position of the knee joint axis is commonly labeled **medial femoral torsion.** Medial femoral torsion and femoral anteversion are the same abnormal condition of the femur. The label designates whether the exaggerated twist in the femur is altering the mechanics at the hip joint (femoral anteversion) or at the knee joint (medial femoral torsion) and simply represents which end of the segment is being referenced. Excessive femoral anteversion may be noted with increased knee abduction (i.e., varus), hip flexion and medial rotation, and increased anterior pelvic tilt during gait.[62] As shall be seen in the next two chapters, an anteverted femur will also affect the biomechanics of the patellofemoral joint at the knee and the subtalar joint in the foot.

Femoral retroversion is the opposite of anteversion (see Fig. 10-9C) and may create problems opposite those of femoral anteversion. Studies have shown patients with symptomatic labral tears have significantly *reduced* femoral anteversion compared with healthy controls.[63,64] This has led some to believe that femoral anteversion serves as a protective measure against impingement and subsequent labral pathology. However, recent research has shown larger labral tears are associated with greater femoral anteversion.[65,66] Thus, excessive femoral anteversion or retroversion compared with "typical" femoral torsion may be a factor in progressive hip joint disease.

Expanded Concepts 10–2
Femoral Rotation and Effect on Gait

Individuals with excessive femoral anteversion will often medially rotate the femur to center the femoral head in the acetabulum. By maintaining this medially rotated hip position, the medial rotators may become shortened, ultimately limiting the amount of lateral rotation available for passive ROM. Likewise, it is possible that this position leads to stretch weakness of the hip lateral rotators. Individuals who maintain a medially rotated position at the hip because of the presence of excessive anteversion can also present with a "toeing-in" type of gait; in a similar fashion, individuals with decreased femoral anteversion, or relative femoral retroversion, will often present with a "toeing-out" type of deviation as the femur laterally rotates to center the femoral head in the acetabulum. Toe-in with femoral anteversion and toe-out with femoral retroversion is most likely when there has not been compensatory tibial torsion.

Articular Congruence

The shape of the hip joint helps to decrease the peak contact stress.[3] The hip joint is considered to be a highly congruent joint. However, there is substantially more articular surface on the head of the femur than there is on the acetabulum (**Fig. 10–11**). In the neutral or standing position, the articular surface of the femoral head remains exposed anteriorly and somewhat superiorly (see **Fig. 10–11A**). The acetabulum does

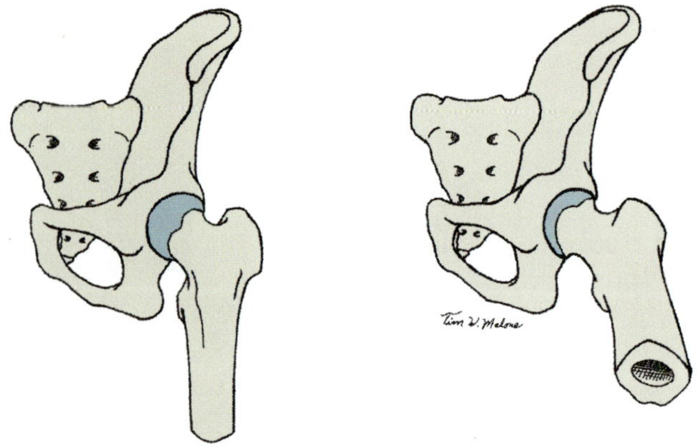

A Neutral hip joint, standing **B** Frog-leg position

Figure 10–11 **A.** In the neutral hip joint, articular cartilage from the head of the femur is exposed anteriorly and, to a lesser extent, superiorly. **B.** Maximum articular contact of the head of the femur with the acetabulum is obtained when the femur is flexed, abducted, and slightly rotated laterally.

not fully cover the head superiorly, and the anterior torsion of the femoral neck exposes a substantial amount of the femoral head's anterior articular surface. Combined abnormalities of femoral version and acetabular version, such as increased femoral anteversion and increased acetabular anteversion, can lead to overall joint instability and altered hip biomechanics.[67] In the typical non–weight-bearing hip joint, articular contact between the femur and the acetabulum can be increased by a combination of flexion, abduction, and slight lateral rotation (see **Fig. 10–11B**).[68] This position (also known as the *frog-leg position*) corresponds to that assumed by the hip joint in a quadruped position and is the true physiological position of the hip joint.[68]

Congruency of the hip joint is greater in weight-bearing and is less when in non–weight-bearing positions.[19] In weight-bearing, the elastic deformation of the acetabulum increases contact with the femoral head, with primary contact at the anterior, superior, and posterior articular surfaces of the acetabulum.[19] An additional contribution to articular congruence and coaptation (joining together) of joint surfaces may be made by the nonarticular and non–weight-bearing acetabular fossa. The acetabular fossa may be important in setting up a partial vacuum in the joint so that atmospheric pressure contributes to stability by helping maintain contact between the femoral head and the acetabulum. Atmospheric pressure in hip flexion activities has shown to have a greater role in stabilization of the hip joint than capsuloligamentous structures.[69] Intra-articular pressure keeps the femoral head and acetabulum together even after the joint capsule has been opened surgically. The pressure within the joint must be broken before the hip can be purposefully dislocated to access the femoral head.[68] The labrum enhances joint stability by both deepening the acetabulum and by acting as a seal to maintain negative intra-articular pressure.[16] When a labral tear is present, the labrum's ability to act as a buttress to prevent excessive movement and to act as a seal to maintain negative intra-articular pressure may be compromised, placing increased stress on the surrounding joint capsule.[68,70]

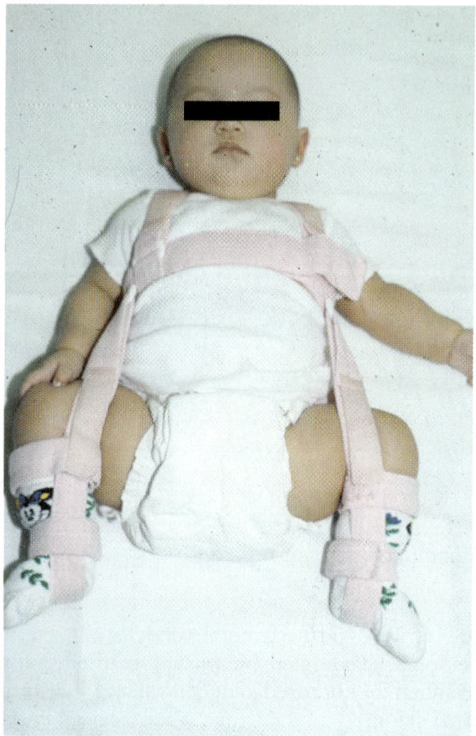

Figure 10–12 An infant can easily be maintained at the hip joint position of flexion, abduction, and lateral rotation (frog-leg position) by using a positioning device, creating maximal contact between the femoral head and acetabulum.

Patient Application 10–3

Gabriella's history may be consistent with her diagnosis of hip dysplasia. Current radiographs and MRI showed a valgus, anteverted femur, and a shallow acetabulum of her left hip. Gabriella's structural deviations of femoral anteversion, coxa valga, and a shallow acetabulum (decreased center edge angle) can result in increased articular exposure of the femoral head, less congruence, and reduced stability of the hip joint in the neutral weight-bearing position.

If Gabriella's hip dysplasia had been diagnosed in infancy, frog-leg positioning might have been maintained using a Frejka pillow or Pavlik harness **(Fig. 10–12)**.[71] These devices may decrease the deformities by increasing the contact between the femoral head and acetabulum. The position of combined flexion, abduction, and lateral rotation is commonly used for immobilization of the hip joint when the goal is to improve articular contact and joint congruence in developmental dysplasia of the hip joint.[71] Whether this was done or not, Gabriella's deformities of the femur and acetabulum persisted. Considering the reduction in center edge angle alone, the stress distribution within the joint is now concentrated in a smaller weight-bearing area throughout the gait cycle, compared with a typical center edge angle.[72] This increase in stress is likely to lead to degenerative changes over time. A reduced center edge angle in addition to age and the presence of a labral tear has been associated with joint degeneration.[65] It appears that Gabriella's history of hip dysplasia may predispose her to progressive intra-articular joint pathology and subsequent osteoarthritis of the hip.

Hip Joint Capsule and Ligaments

HIP JOINT CAPSULE

Unlike the relatively weak articular capsule of the shoulder, the hip joint capsule is a substantial contributor to joint stability.

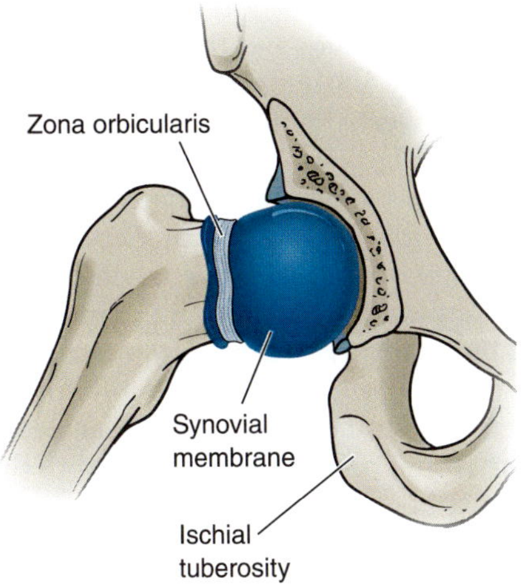

Figure 10–13 The zona orbicularis is composed of collar-like fibers that encircle the femoral neck and help to prevent distraction of the femoral head from the acetabulum.

The articular capsule of the hip joint is an irregular, dense fibrous structure with longitudinal and oblique fibers and three thickened regions that constitute the capsular ligaments.[73,74] The more extensive longitudinal fibers of the capsule are attached to the periosteum proximal to the acetabular rim and to the acetabular labrum.[74] The oblique fibers are aligned near the proximal attachment in a circumferential manner just distal to the femoral head, forming a collar-like structure around the femoral neck.[27,73,74] This area is known as the **zona orbicularis**. These collar-like fibers help to prevent distraction of the femoral head from the acetabulum **(Fig. 10–13)**.[75] The capsule is thickened anterosuperiorly, where there is little bony support and the predominant stresses occur. Posteroinferiorly, the capsule is relatively thin and redundant, with some areas of the capsule thin enough to be nearly translucent.[28,76] The capsule covers the femoral head and neck like a cylindrical sleeve and attaches to the base of the femoral neck. The femoral neck is intracapsular, whereas both the greater and lesser trochanters are extracapsular. The synovial membrane lines the inside of the capsule. Anteriorly, there are longitudinal retinacular fibers deep in the capsule that travel along the neck toward the femoral head.[28] The retinacular fibers carry blood vessels that are the major source of nutrition to the femoral head and neck. The retinacular blood vessels arise from a vascular ring located at the base of the neck formed by the medial and lateral circumflex arteries (branches of the deep femoral artery). The superior and inferior gluteal arteries supply more proximal and posterior portions of the joint capsule, whereas the medial and lateral circumflex arteries supply the more distal and anterior aspect of the joint capsule.[77] The femoral head is most commonly supplied through the medial femoral circumflex artery.[77]

As with the other joints already described, there are numerous bursae associated with the hip joint. Although as many as 20 bursae have been described, there are commonly recognized to be three primary or important bursae.[78,79] Because the bursae are more strongly associated with the hip joint muscles rather than its capsule, the bursae will be described with their corresponding musculature.

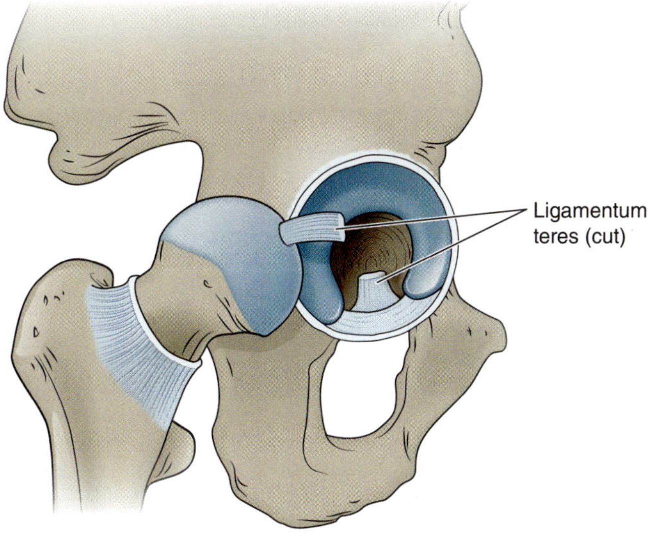

Figure 10–14 The ligamentum teres is an intra-articular but extrasynovial accessory joint structure that extends from the peripheral edge of the acetabular notch to the femoral fovea. It is also called *ligament of the head of the femur.*

HIP JOINT LIGAMENTS

The ligament of the head of the femur, or the ligamentum teres, is an *intra-articular* but *extrasynovial* accessory joint structure. The ligament is a triangular band that attaches to the peripheral edge of the acetabular notch. The ligament then passes under the transverse acetabular ligament (with which it blends) to attach at its other end to the fovea of the femur **(Fig. 10–14)**. The ligamentum teres is encased in a flattened sleeve of synovial membrane so that this connective tissue structure does not communicate with the synovial cavity of the joint. The material properties of the ligament of the head are similar to those of other ligaments.[80] Traditionally, it has been believed that the sole purpose of the ligamentum teres was to serve as a conduit for blood vessels to the femoral head and that it did not play a significant role in joint stabilization.[81] However, recent information suggests the ligamentum teres has a role in stabilizing the hip.[82-86] Specifically, the ligamentum teres has been shown to provide restraint of hip medial and lateral rotation when the hip is positioned in greater than 90° of flexion.[83-85] Individuals with acquired anterior hip instability and abnormally increased medial/lateral rotation of the hip joint may put excessive strain on the ligamentum teres that may compromise the integrity of the ligament. Once the ligament becomes compromised or lax, it may become pinched between the femoral head and acetabulum, which may result in painful clicking and catching within the joint. As a result, individuals with ligamentum teres deficiency may have apprehension going into a deep squat position. A lesion of the ligamentum teres was found to be the third most common finding in athletes undergoing arthroscopic surgery, with occurrence ranging from 8% to 51% of individuals.[87] It should be noted that ligamentum teres tears rarely occur in isolation and are frequently associated with labral tears, articular cartilage lesions, femoral acetabular impingement syndrome, and/or capsular laxity.[86-88]

Expanded Concepts 10–3
Blood Supply to the Femoral Head

The importance of the secondary blood supply carried by the ligamentum teres will vary across the life span, with a greater contribution to be made in childhood. While a child is still growing, the primary retinacular vessels (the medial and lateral circumflex arteries) cannot travel through the avascular cartilaginous epiphysis but must travel across the surface of the epiphysis, where the vessels are more vulnerable to disruption. Crock proposed that the femoral head was supplied predominantly by the blood vessels of the ligamentum teres until bony maturation and epiphyseal closure.[89] However, Tan and Wong found the ligament was absent in 10% of their examined specimens.[90] The vessels of the ligament of the head are commonly sclerosed in elderly persons.[91] Therefore, the secondary blood supply cannot be counted on to back up the primary retinacular supply when it is disrupted by such problems as femoral neck fracture.[90] The absence of a secondary blood supply to the head increases the risk of avascular necrosis of the femoral head if there is femoral neck trauma.

Expanded Concepts 10–4
Legg-Calvé-Perthes Disease

Legg-Calvé-Perthes disease is characterized by collapse of the femoral head, resulting in flattening of the head from loss of blood supply. This poorly understood childhood disorder is usually a self-limiting condition with a variable natural history. Impaired growth and abnormal development can result in deformity, joint incongruity, and the early onset of osteoarthritis over the long term if not properly treated.[92,93]

The hip joint capsule is typically considered to have three reinforcing capsular ligaments: two anteriorly and one posteriorly **(Fig. 10–15)**.[68,73,81] The two anterior ligaments are the iliofemoral ligament and the pubofemoral ligament (see **Fig. 10–15A**). The **iliofemoral ligament** is fan shaped and resembles an inverted letter *Y*; it is often referred to as the **Y ligament of Bigelow**. The apex of the ligament is attached to the anterior inferior iliac spine, and the two arms of the Y fan out to attach along the intertrochanteric line of the femur. The superior band of the iliofemoral ligament is the strongest and thickest of the hip joint ligaments.[68,73,94] The **pubofemoral ligament** is also anteriorly located, arising from the pubic portion of the acetabular rim inferior and medial to the iliopectineal eminence. The pubofemoral ligament forms a sling that supports the inferior aspect of the femoral neck and connects fibers of the iliofemoral and ischiofemoral ligaments.[73] The **ischiofemoral ligament** is the posterior capsular ligament (see **Fig. 10–15B**) and attaches to the posterior surface of the acetabular rim and the acetabular labrum. Some of its fibers spiral around the femoral neck and blend with the fibers of the circumferential fibers of the capsule. Other fibers are arranged horizontally and attach to the inner surface of the greater trochanter.

There is at the hip joint, as at other joints, some conflicting evidence as to the roles of the joint ligaments. There is consensus, however, that each of the hip joint motions will be restrained by at least one portion of one of the three major hip joint ligaments.[81] The forces transmitted by the ligaments (and capsule) are dependent on orientation of the femur in relation to the acetabulum.[73,76] The anterior capsuloligamentous structures tend to be stronger (stiffer and withstanding greater force at failure) than the posterior structures.[79] The primary stabilizing component of the anterior hip joint is the iliofemoral ligament. This ligament is capable of providing resistance to excessive lateral rotation.[73] In particular, the

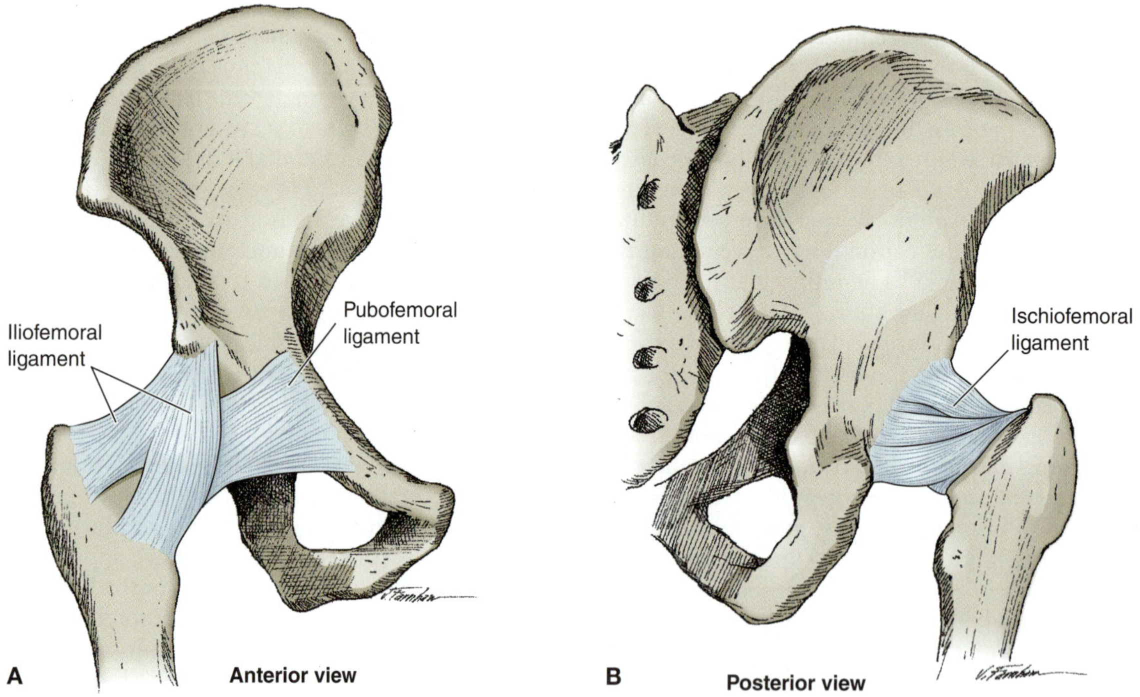

Figure 10–15 **A.** Anterior view of the right hip joint shows the two bands of the iliofemoral (Y) ligament and the more inferiorly located pubofemoral ligament. **B.** Posterior view of a right hip joint shows that the spiral fibers of the ischiofemoral ligament are tightened during full hip extension and, therefore, limit hyperextension.

more lateral portion of the iliofemoral ligament is the most significant restraint to lateral rotation when the hip is in neutral or flexed positions.[73,95] The pubofemoral ligament controls lateral rotation in an extended hip position and controls medial rotation in a flexed hip position.[73,96] The posteriorly located ischiofemoral ligament is the primary restraint to medial rotation of the hip regardless of hip position in flexion or extension.[95,97] The capsule and ligaments permit little or no joint distraction even under strong traction forces.

Under typical circumstances, the hip joint, its capsule, and ligaments routinely support two-thirds of the body weight (the weight of the HAT). In bilateral stance, the hip joint is typically in neutral position or slight extension. In this position, the capsule and ligaments are under some tension.[68] The typical line of gravity (LoG) in bilateral stance falls posterior to the hip joint axis, creating a gravitational extension moment. At end-range hip extension, additional passive tension is created in the capsuloligamentous complex that is sufficient to offset that extension moment. As the LoG falls farther posterior to the hip joint axis, the passive capsuloligamentous structures can provide greater contribution to the support of the superimposed body weight in symmetrical bilateral stance with minimal active assistance from the muscles crossing the hip.

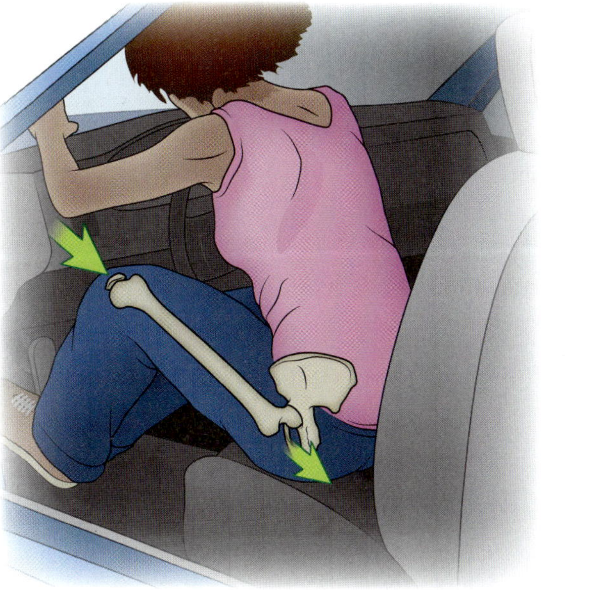

Figure 10–16 With the hip positioned in flexion, a large force applied along the shaft of the femur (as in a dashboard injury) may cause a posterior hip dislocation.

CAPSULOLIGAMENTOUS TENSION

Hip joint extension, with slight abduction and medial rotation, is the close-packed position for the hip joint.[28] With increased extension, the ligaments twist around the femoral head and neck, drawing the head into the acetabulum. In contrast to most other joints in the body, the close-packed and most stable position for the hip joint is *not* the position of optimal articular contact (congruence). As already noted, optimal articular contact occurs with combined flexion, abduction, and lateral rotation. Under circumstances in which the joint surfaces are neither maximally congruent nor close-packed, the hip joint is at greatest risk for traumatic dislocation. A position of particular vulnerability occurs when the hip joint is flexed and adducted (as it is when sitting with the thighs crossed). In this position, a strong axial force through the femoral shaft toward the hip joint (as when an unconstrained passenger's knee hits the dashboard in a car accident) may push the femoral head out of the acetabulum **(Fig. 10–16)**.[68] Macrotraumatic injuries associated with high impact are known to cause capsular laxity. Microtrauma associated with sports that involve repeated and forceful end-range movements may also be a cause of laxity.[98] Focal rotational anterior microinstability with repetitive forced external rotation that causes stretching of the anterior capsuloligamentous structures is a recognized condition. This type of instability may occur with sports such as golf, baseball, gymnastics, and figure skating.[99]

The capsuloligamentous tension at the hip joint is *least* when the hip is in midrange flexion, slight abduction, and midrotation. In this position, the typical intra-articular pressure is minimized, and the capacity of the synovial capsule to accommodate abnormal amounts of fluid is greatest.[69] This is the position assumed by the hip when there is pain arising from capsuloligamentous problems or from excessive intra-articular pressure caused by extra fluid (blood or synovial fluid) in the joint, which may be a result of such conditions as **synovitis** of the hip joint or bleeding into the joint from tearing of blood vessels with a femoral neck fracture. Minimizing intra-articular pressure not only decreases pain in the joint but also prevents compression of the intra-articular blood vessels that supply the femoral head.[69]

Structural Adaptations to Weight-Bearing

The internal architecture of the pelvis and femur reveals the remarkable interaction between mechanical stresses and structural adaptation created by the transmission of forces between the femur and the pelvis. The trabeculae (calcified plates of tissue within the cancellous bone) line up along lines of stress and form systems that typically adapt to stress requirements and changes in stresses. The trabeculae are quite evident on bony cross section, as seen in **Figure 10–17**, along with some of the other structural elements of the hip joint.

In Chapter 4, we followed the line of weight-bearing through the vertebrae of the spinal column to the sacral promontory and on through the sacroiliac joints. Most of the weight-bearing stresses in the pelvis pass from the sacroiliac joints to the acetabulae.[28] In standing or upright weight-bearing activities, at least half the weight of the HAT (the gravitational force) passes down through the pelvis to each femoral head. Because the compressive force of HAT passes medially to each of the femoral necks, a moment arm exists that creates a bending moment across each femoral neck in bilateral stance **(Fig. 10–18)**. This moment arm is the perpendicular distance between the superimposed body weight on the femoral head (a downwardly directed force) and the intertrochanteric area.[100] As a result of this bending moment, the femoral neck is subjected to a tensile force on the superior aspect of the femoral neck and a compressive force on the inferior aspect. Bone naturally responds better to compressive forces than tensile forces. Fractures occur in the area where the bone cannot sufficiently handle the applied load. If the bone cannot handle the bending moment across the femoral neck due to the presence of a large

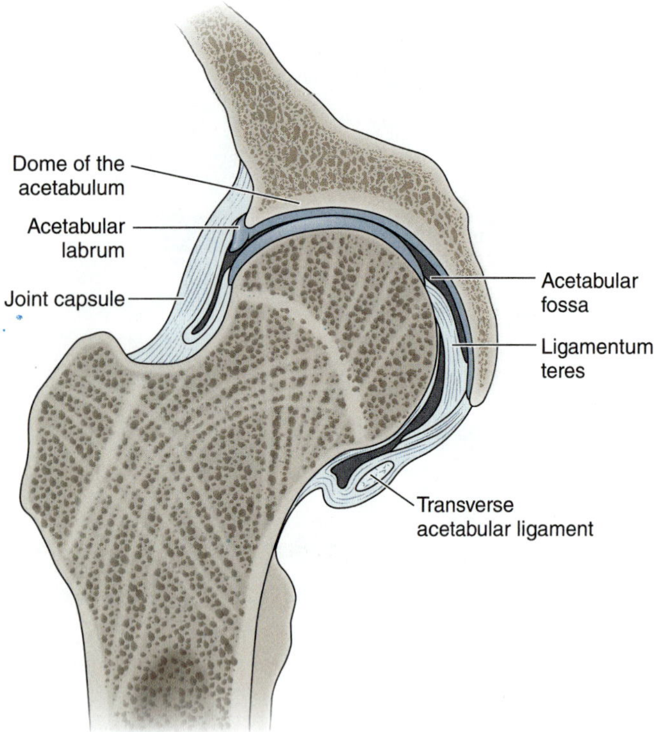

Figure 10–17 The trabeculae of the femur line up along lines of stress in the cancellous bone and can be seen on cross section.

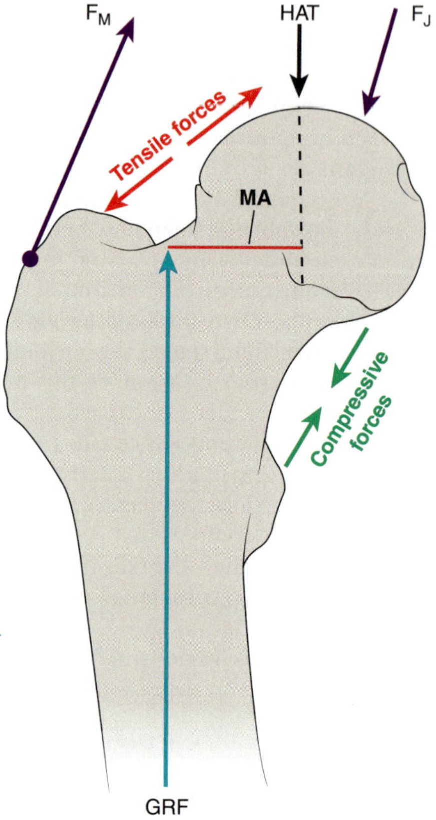

Figure 10–18 The weight-bearing line of the head, arms, and trunk (HAT) loads the head of the femur, whereas the ground reaction force (GRF) comes up the shaft of the femur, resulting in a force couple that creates a bending moment, with a moment arm (MA) that is dependent on the length and angle of the neck of the femur. The bending moment creates tensile stress on the superior aspect of the femoral neck and compressive stress on the inferior aspect.

tensile load across the superior portion of the femoral neck, then a fracture will occur. The body is able to minimize this tensile load by the incorporation of muscle activity across the hip (see Fig. 10–18), which can create large compressive forces across the femoral neck to offset the imposed tensile force due to the weight of the HAT. In addition, a complex set of forces within the femoral neck prevents the rotation of the neck on the shaft; among these forces are the structural resistance of two major and three minor **trabecular systems (Fig. 10–19)**.

The medial (or principal compressive) trabecular system arises from the medial cortex of the upper femoral shaft and radiates through the cancellous bone to the cortical bone of the superior aspect of the femoral head. The medial system of trabeculae is oriented along the vertical compressive forces passing through the hip joint.[68] The lateral (or principal tensile) trabecular system of the femur arises from the lateral cortex of the upper femoral shaft and, after crossing the medial system, terminates in the cortical bone on the inferior aspect of the head of the femur. The lateral trabecular system is oblique and may develop in response to parallel (shear) forces of the weight of HAT and the ground reaction force (GRF).[68] There are two accessory (or secondary) trabecular systems, of which one is considered compressive and the other is considered tensile.[68] Another secondary trabecular system is confined to the trochanteric area of the femur.[68,101] The loading environment in the femur during physical activity is mostly compressive in nature, with relatively small amounts of shear forces.[102]

The areas in which the trabecular systems cross each other at right angles are areas that offer the greatest resistance to stress and strain. There is an area in the femoral neck in which the trabeculae are relatively thin and do not cross each other. This **zone of weakness** (see Fig. 10–19) has less reinforcement and thus more potential for failure. The zone of weakness of the femoral neck is particularly susceptible to the bending forces across the area and can fracture either when forces are excessive or when compromised bony composition reduces the tissue's ability to resist typical forces.

Expanded Concepts 10–5
Femoral Neck Stresses

Although the zone of weakness in the cancellous bone has received a great deal of attention as a factor in hip fracture, Crabtree and colleagues used data from patients and cadavers with a hip fracture to conclude that the cortical bone, rather than trabecular (cancellous) bone, in the femoral neck supports at least 50% of the load placed on the proximal femur.[103] They suggested that compromise of cortical bone may be more of a factor in fracture than diminished cancellous bone. A more detailed description of the problems of hip fracture will be presented later in the chapter.

The primary weight-bearing surface of the acetabulum, or **dome** of the acetabulum, is located on the superior portion of the lunate surface (see Fig. 10–17).[100,104] In the normal hip, the dome

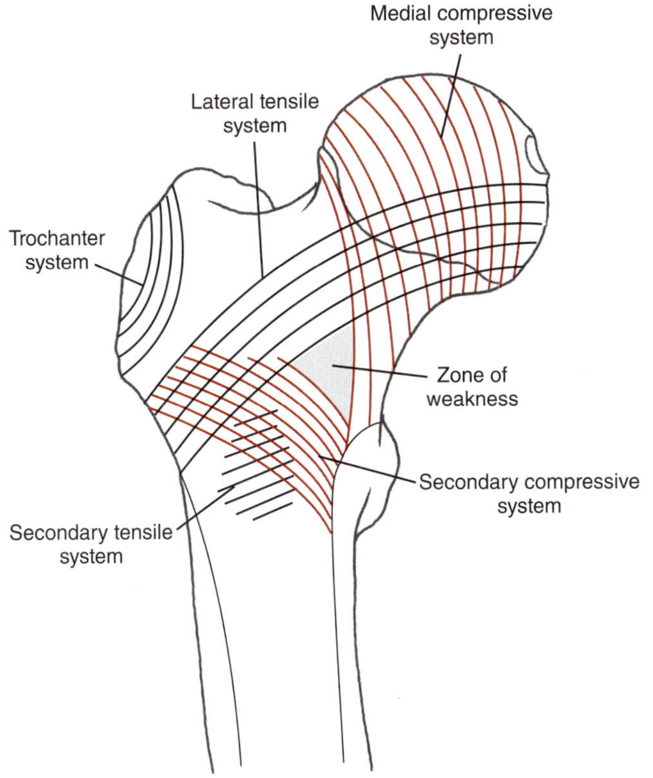

Figure 10–19 Two major (the medial compressive and lateral tensile) trabecular systems show the primary transmission of forces. Additional lines of stress are evident at the secondary compressive and tensile systems and at the trochanteric system. A distinct zone of weakness can be observed in which the trabeculae are thin and do not cross each other.

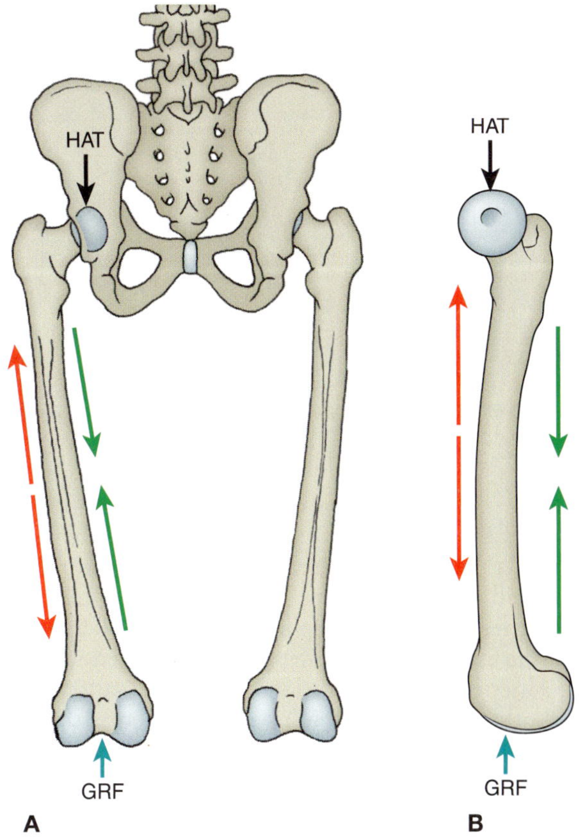

Figure 10–20 The weight-bearing line (HAT) from the center of rotation of the femoral head and the ground reaction force (GRF) cause a bending force on the shaft of the femur. **A.** In the frontal plane this results in compressive forces medially and tensile forces laterally. **B.** In the sagittal plane, the compressive forces are seen posteriorly and the tensile forces are anterior.

lies directly over the center of rotation of the femoral head.[104] Peak contact pressures during unilateral stance are located near the superior aspect of the dome.[27] Stress distribution can be altered with a lack of femoral head coverage by the acetabulum (decreased center edge angle) as well as excessive acetabular anteversion and femoral anteversion.[3,27,105] Contact area was found to be significantly smaller in women than in men with associated higher peak contact stress.[27] The dome shows the greatest prevalence of degenerative changes in the acetabulum, which corresponds to the area of greatest stress. The primary weight-bearing area of the femoral head is, correspondingly, its superior portion.[82,87] Degenerative changes of the femoral head include loss of the regular "ball" shape, with flattening of the superior portion. Degenerative changes of the femoral head are also consistently noted near the attachment of the ligamentum teres.[26]

Full loading of the hip joint is presumably necessary to achieve congruence and optimize load distribution between the larger femoral head and the acetabulum.[19] Incongruence of the acetabular dome in the moderately loaded hip (especially in young adults) could result in incomplete compression of the dome cartilage and, therefore, inadequate fluid exchange to maintain cartilage nutrition.[100] The superior femoral head receives compression from the dome in standing, from the posterior acetabulum in sitting, and the anterior acetabulum when the hip is in extension. More frequent and complete compression of the cartilage of the superior femoral head, according to this premise, leads to better nutrition within the cartilage. It must be remembered, however, that avascular articular cartilage is dependent on both *compression* and *release* to move nutrients through the tissue; too little compression and excessive compression (magnitude and frequency of loading) can each limit nutrient exchange that may lead to compromise of the cartilage structure.

The forces of HAT and the GRF that act on the articular surfaces of the hip joint and on the femoral head and neck also act on the femoral shaft. The shaft of the femur is not vertical but lies at an angle that varies considerably among individuals. However, the relatively vertical loading on the oblique femur results in bending stresses in the shaft.[68] The medial cortical bone in the shaft (diaphysis) therefore must resist compressive stresses, whereas the lateral cortical bone of the shaft must resist tensile stresses **(Fig. 10–20)**.

Function

Motion of the Femur on the Acetabulum

The motions of the hip joint are easiest to visualize as movement of the convex femoral head within the concavity of the acetabulum as the femur moves through its three degrees of freedom: flexion/extension, abduction/adduction, and medial/lateral rotation **(Fig. 10–21)**. The femoral head will slide within the acetabulum in a direction opposite to the motion of the

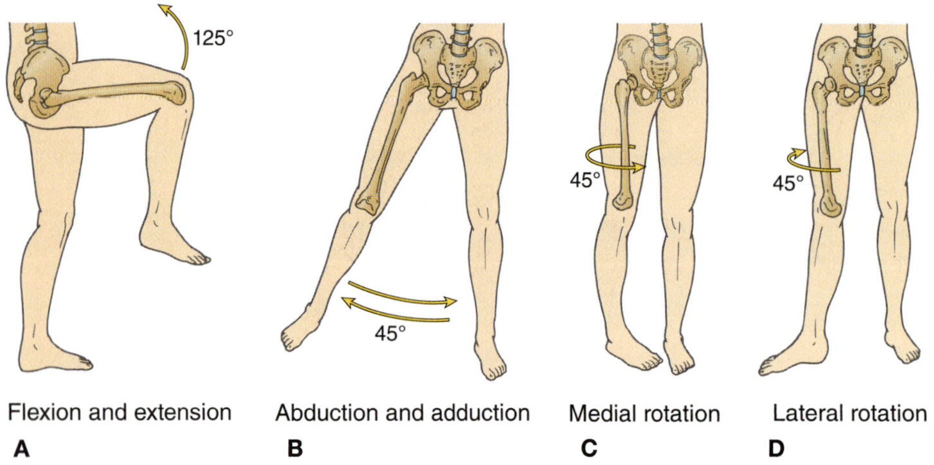

Figure 10–21 Hip joint kinematics depicted as the convex femur moving on the concave acetabulum. **A.** Flexion of the hip joint with extension occurring as the limb returns to vertical. **B.** Abduction (lower arrow) and adduction (upper arrow). **C.** Medial rotation. **D.** Lateral rotation.

distal end of the femur. Flexion and extension of the femur occur from a neutral position as an almost pure spin of the femoral head around a coronal axis through the head and neck of the femur. The head spins posteriorly in flexion and anteriorly in extension. However, flexion and extension from other positions (e.g., in abduction or medial rotation) must include both spinning and gliding of the articular surfaces, depending on the combination of motions. The motions of abduction/adduction and medial/lateral rotation must include both spinning and sliding of the femoral head within the acetabulum, but the intra-articular (arthokinematics) motion again occurs in a direction opposite to motion of the distal end of the femur (osteokinematics).

As is true at most joints, the ROM of the hip joint is influenced by structural elements, including whether the motion is performed actively or passively and whether passive tension in two-joint muscles is encountered or avoided. The following ranges of passive joint motion are typical of the hip joint.[106] Flexion of the hip is generally about 90° with the knee extended, and 120° when the knee is flexed so that passive tension in the two-joint **hamstrings** muscle group is released. Hip extension is considered to have a range of 10° to 30°. Hip extension ROM appears to diminish somewhat with age, whereas flexion remains relatively unchanged.[107] When hip extension is combined with knee flexion, passive tension in the two-joint **rectus femoris** muscle may limit the movement. The femur can be abducted 45° to 50° and adducted 20° to 30°. Abduction can be limited by the large group of adductor muscles or the two-joint **gracilis** muscle; adduction may be limited by the **tensor fascia latae (TFL)** muscle and the associated **IT band**. Medial and lateral rotation, with the hip joint in 90° of flexion, is typically 40° to 60°. Limited hip ROM can cause the lumbar spine to compensate with greater motion during activities that typically involve hip movement, leading to increased stress on the lumbar spine.[108] Thus, isolating hip movement from spine movement during exercises and assessments is essential to avoid compensatory patterns.

A normal gait on level ground requires at least the following hip joint ranges: 30° flexion, 10° extension, 5° of both abduction and adduction, and 5° of both medial and lateral rotation.[69,102] Walking on uneven terrain or stairs will increase the need for joint range beyond that required for level ground, as will activities such as sitting in a chair or sitting cross-legged.

Patient Application 10–4

Gabriella's passive ROM findings and asymmetries in her gait correspond to femoral anteversion on the left. In the supine position on the examination table (hip extended), she has more hip joint medial rotation than lateral rotation (although medial rotation with hip flexion is limited by pain). In her case, her shallow acetabulum increases the tendency for joint subluxation with lateral rotation of the extended hip. This would partially explain her complaints that her hip feels like it is "popping out of socket." When she walks, Gabriella's left foot is toed-in more than her right because her involved side is in greater hip medial rotation compared with her uninvolved side. This may be the body's way of maximizing congruence of the anteverted femur on the weight-bearing joint, or it may be to minimize the stretch on the proprioceptor-rich anterior capsule. The consequence for increased hip joint congruence is that the torsional deformity now appears as medial femoral torsion, resulting in a deviant positioning of the patella and femoral condyles.[109] Gabriella's foot would be more toed-in than she demonstrates, but it appears that Gabriella, like many persons with femoral anteversion (medial femoral torsion), also developed an excessive lateral tibial torsion. It is evident in Gabriella's case that altered biomechanical alignment of the hips relates directly to changes throughout the entire kinetic chain, specifically the knee, foot, and ankle.

Motion of the Pelvis on the Femur

Whenever the hip joint is weight-bearing, the femur is relatively fixed; motion, instead, is produced by movement of the pelvis on the femur. At all joints, the motion between articular surfaces is the same whether the distal or proximal lever moves. However, the proximal and distal levers move in opposite directions to produce the same articular motion. For example, elbow flexion can be a rotation of the distal forearm upward or, conversely, a rotation of the proximal humerus downward. In examinations of the upper extremity joint complexes thus far, motion of the distal lever tended to predominate functionally, and so this apparent reversal of motions was not a point of discussion. At the hip joint, this reversal of the moving lever is further complicated by the *horizontal* orientation and shape of the pelvis; thus, the "levers" of the hip joint lie essentially perpendicular to each other. In contrast to proximal segment motion at other joints, there is also a new set of terms to identify hip joint motion when the pelvis (rather than femur) is the moving segment. The terms for pelvic motions are used with weight-bearing hip joint motion because the motions of the pelvis are more apparent to the eye of the examiner and are, in fact, key to what occurs at the joints above and below the pelvis. It must be emphasized, however, that the motions of the pelvis presented in the next sections are *not new motions of the hip joint* but are simply how the same three degrees of freedom for the hip joint are accomplished by movement of the pelvis on the femur, rather than by movement of the femur on the pelvis.

ANTERIOR AND POSTERIOR PELVIC TILT

Anterior and **posterior pelvic tilts** are motions of the entire pelvic ring in the sagittal plane around a coronal axis **(Fig. 10–22)**. In the normally aligned pelvis, the **anterior superior iliac spines** (**ASISs**) of the pelvis lie on a horizontal line with the **posterior superior iliac spines** (**PSISs**) and on a vertical line with the symphysis pubis (see **Fig. 10–22A**).[110] Anterior and posterior tilting of the pelvis on the fixed femur produces hip flexion and extension, respectively. Hip flexion through anterior tilting of the pelvis moves the anterior superior iliac spines anteriorly and inferiorly; the inferior sacrum moves farther from the femur, rather than moving the femur away from the sacrum (see **Fig. 10–22B**). Hip joint extension via posterior tilting of the pelvis brings the symphysis pubis up and the sacrum of the pelvis closer to the femur, rather than moving the femur posteriorly on the pelvis (see **Fig. 10–22C**). Importantly, anterior and posterior tilting will result in flexion and extension of both hip joints simultaneously in bilateral stance, or can occur at the stance hip joint alone if the opposite limb is non–weight-bearing.

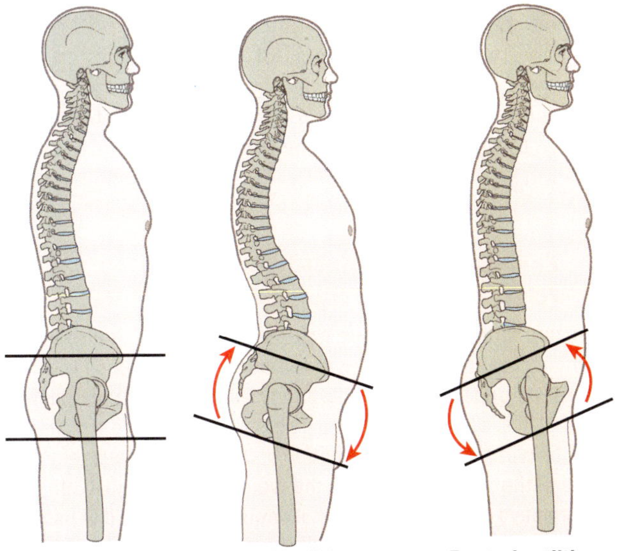

Figure 10–22 Flexion and extension of the hip occurring as tilting of the pelvis in the sagittal plane. **A.** The pelvis is shown in its typical position in erect stance. **B.** Anterior tilting of the pelvis moves the symphysis pubis inferiorly on the fixed femur. The hip joint flexes. **C.** In posterior tilting, the anterior superior iliac spines move superiorly on the fixed femur. The hip joint extends.

Foundational Concepts 10–2
Anterior Pelvic Tilt and Femoroacetabular Impingement Syndrome

Anterior pelvic tilt occurs when the pelvis tilts forward, causing an exaggerated curve in the lower back (see Fig. 10-22B). This misalignment can significantly affect the biomechanics of the hip. The anterior tilt of the pelvis affects the alignment and coverage of the femoral head by the acetabulum. As the degree of anterior pelvic tilt increase, the anterior aspect of the femoral head can be more covered.[111] This altered alignment can increase the risk of femoroacetabular impingement syndrome (FAIS) during hip flexion activities.[112] A key factor in addressing the effect of anterior pelvic tilt is evaluating the loss of hip extension. Tight hip flexors, a tight hip anterior capsule, or bone limitations can all contribute to the loss of hip extension. The anterior capsule of the hip joint can become tight due to prolonged sitting or poor posture, further restricting hip extension and contributing to the anterior tilt of the pelvis. Tightness in the hip flexors, particularly the iliopsoas, can pull the pelvis into an anterior tilt. Structural abnormalities or variations in bone anatomy can also limit hip extension. These factors should be assessed and addressed to improve hip extension and reduce the risk of FAIS.

LATERAL PELVIC TILT

Lateral pelvic tilt is a frontal plane motion of the entire pelvis around an anteroposterior axis **(Fig. 10–23)**. In the typically aligned pelvis in bilateral stance, a line through the anterior superior iliac spines is horizontal. In unilateral stance, however, the pelvis will often laterally tilt. Lateral pelvic tilt is named by what is happening to the side of the pelvis *opposite* to the weight-bearing hip in unilateral stance. The weight-bearing hip joint (e.g., the left hip joint) serves as the pivot point or axis for motion of the pelvis as the pelvis either elevates **(pelvic hike)** or drops **(pelvic drop)** in the frontal plane. If a person stands on the left limb and hikes the pelvis (i.e., the right iliac crest rises), the left hip joint is being abducted because the medial angle between the femur and a line through the anterior superior iliac spines increases (see **Fig. 10–23A**). If a person stands on the left leg and drops the pelvis (i.e., the right iliac crest drops), the left hip joint will adduct because the medial angle formed by the femur and a line through the anterior superior iliac spines will decrease (see **Fig. 10–23B**).

The weight-bearing hip joint *in unilateral stance* will always be the axis of rotation, and the opposite side of the pelvis will always be the reference side for naming the movement. In descriptions of the hip joint motions that occur in unilateral stance, the hip joint of the non–weight-bearing limb is in an open chain and has no *imposed* motions on it. However, the non–weight-bearing leg typically hangs straight down as the pelvis moves. If the non–weight-bearing limb continues to hang vertically, the non–weight-bearing hip will adduct and abduct with hike and drop of the pelvis, respectively, around the weight-bearing hip joint (see Fig. 10–23).

LATERAL SHIFT OF THE PELVIS

Lateral pelvic tilt can also occur in bilateral stance. If both feet are on the ground and the hip and knee of one limb are flexed, the opposite limb is largely the weight-bearing limb and the terminology is the same as for unilateral stance. However, if both limbs are weight-bearing, lateral tilt of the pelvis will

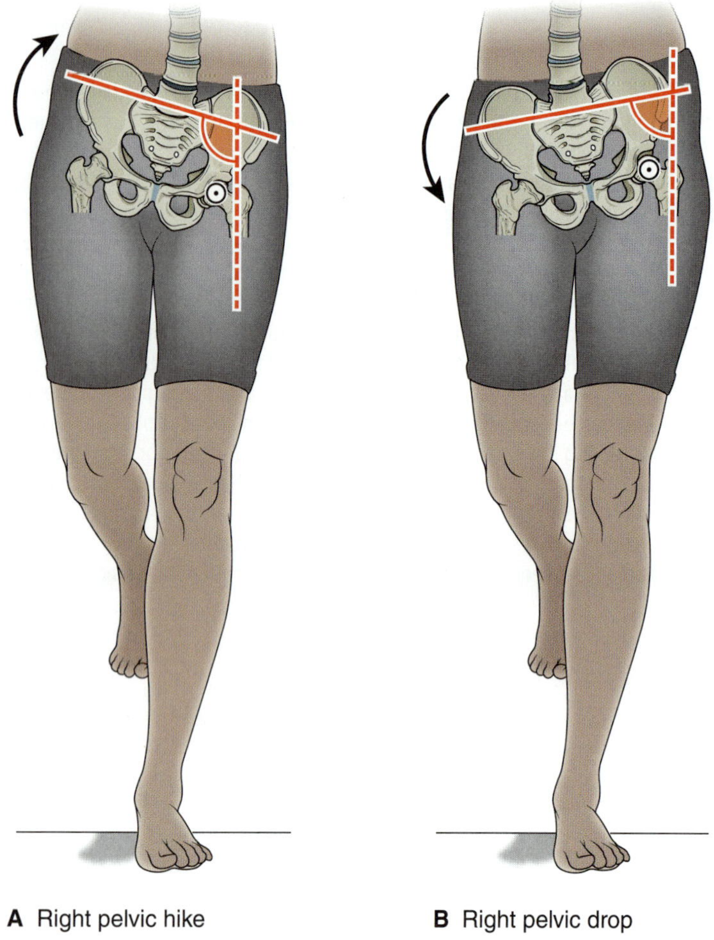

Figure 10–23 Lateral tilting of the pelvis around the left hip joint axis can occur either as hip hiking (elevation of the opposite side of the pelvis) or as pelvic drop (drop of the opposite side of the pelvis). **A.** Hiking of the pelvis around the left hip joint results in left hip abduction. **B.** Dropping of the pelvis around the left hip joint results in left hip joint adduction. Although it is visually tempting to name the direction of lateral tilt by the motion of the side of the pelvis *nearest* the hip, this is incorrect.

cause the pelvis to shift to one side or the other. With **pelvic shift**, the pelvis cannot hike; it can only drop. Because there is a closed chain between the two weight-bearing feet and the pelvis, both hip joints will move in the frontal plane in a predictable way as the pelvic tilt (or pelvic shift) occurs. If the pelvis is shifted to the right in bilateral stance, the left side of the pelvis will drop, the right hip joint will be adducted, and the left hip joint will be abducted **(Fig. 10–24)**. Right hip abductor and left hip adductor synergistic activity can shift the pelvis back to neutral.

FORWARD AND BACKWARD PELVIC ROTATION

Pelvic rotation is motion of the entire pelvic ring in the transverse plane around a vertical or longitudinal axis. Although rotation can occur around a vertical axis through the middle of the pelvis in a bilateral stance, it most commonly and more importantly occurs in single-limb support around the axis of the supporting or weight-bearing hip joint **(Fig. 10–25)**. **Forward** (anterior) **rotation** of the pelvis occurs in unilateral stance when the side of the pelvis *opposite* to the weight-bearing hip joint moves anteriorly (see **Fig. 10–25A**) from the neutral position (see **Fig. 10–25B**). Forward rotation of the pelvis produces medial rotation of the weight-bearing hip joint. **Backward** (posterior) **rotation** of the pelvis occurs when the side of the pelvis *opposite* the weight-bearing hip moves posteriorly (see **Fig. 10–25C**). Backward rotation of the pelvis produces lateral rotation of the weight-bearing hip joint.

Pelvic rotation can occur in bilateral stance as well as unilateral stance, as is true for lateral pelvic tilt. If both feet are bearing weight and the axis of motion occurs around a vertical axis through the *center* of the pelvis, the terms *forward rotation* and *backward rotation* must be used by referencing a side (e.g., forward rotation on the right and backward rotation on the left).

Foundational Concepts 10–3
Pelvic Rotation and Hip Joint Rotation

Similar to a lateral pelvic tilt (e.g., pelvic hike or pelvic drop), when referencing forward and backward rotation, the reference is the side of the pelvis opposite to the rotating (weight-bearing) hip joint (see Fig. 10–25). If it is known which leg a person is standing on in unilateral stance, forward or backward rotation of the pelvis always references the side of the pelvis opposite to the weight-bearing hip joint.

The relative rotation of the hip that occurs with forward or backward rotation of the pelvis in unilateral stance is often difficult for the novice to identify. The rotation of the hip joint that occurs during rotation of the pelvis can best be appreciated by performing the motion yourself. Standing on one leg and rotating the pelvis and trunk forward as much as possible will give a clear "feeling" of the relative medial rotation of the supporting limb. Similarly, rotating the pelvis backward as far as possible will give the feeling of the relative lateral rotation of the stance hip joint.

Expanded Concepts 10–6
Pelvic Rotation in Gait

In typical gait, the pelvis rotates forward around the weight-bearing hip in an alternating fashion to advance the lower extremity during each step (**Fig. 10–26**). Using the left limb as an example, the pelvis rotates forward around the left weight-bearing hip joint as the right non–weight-bearing limb advances (see **Fig. 10–26A**). By midstance on the left limb (see **Fig. 10–26B**), the pelvis has forwardly rotated to neutral. After the neutral position of the pelvis is reached, the *opposite* (right) side of the pelvis begins to advance to prepare the right limb for contact (see **Fig. 10–26C**). It may *appear* as if the right side of the pelvis is *backwardly* rotating (dotted line) but this is not the case. If forward rotation of one side of the pelvis was followed by actual backward rotation of the same side, the limbs could not alternatively advance to make forward progress during gait.

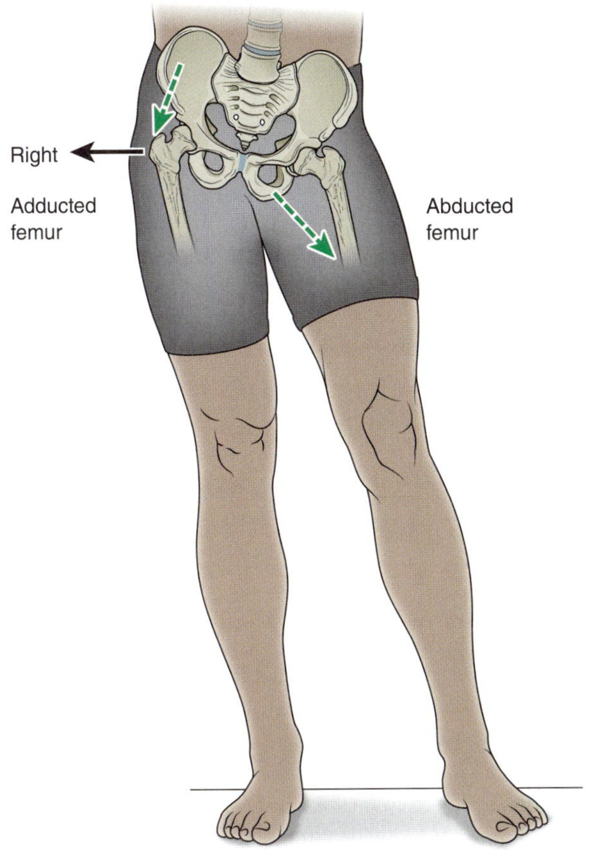

Figure 10–24 When the pelvis is shifted to the right in bilateral stance, the right hip joint will be adducted and the left hip joint will be abducted. To return to neutral position while continuing to bear weight on both feet, the right abductor muscles (on the side of hip adduction) and left adductor muscles (on the side of abduction) work synergistically to shorten and shift the weight back to center.

Coordinated Motions of the Femur, Pelvis, and Lumbar Spine

When the pelvis moves on a relatively fixed femur, there are two possible outcomes to consider. Either the head and trunk will follow the motion of the pelvis (moving the head through space) or the head will continue to remain relatively upright and vertical despite the pelvic motions. These are open- and "virtual" closed-chain responses, respectively. Each of these two situations produces very different reactions from the joints and segments proximal and distal to the hip joints and pelvis and must be examined separately.

PELVIFEMORAL MOTION

When the femur, pelvis, and spine move in a coordinated manner to produce a larger ROM than is available to one segment alone, the hip joint is participating in what will predominantly (but not exclusively) be an open-chain motion termed **pelvifemoral motion.** Pelvifemoral motion can be considered analogous to scapulohumeral motion because the combination of motions at several joints serves to increase the range available to the distal segment. In the case of scapulohumeral motion, the joints serve the hand. In the case of pelvifemoral motion, the joints may serve either end of the chain: the foot or head.

Foundational Concepts 10–4
Moving the Head and Arms Through Space

If the goal is to bend forward to bring the hands (and head) toward the floor, isolated flexion at the hip joints (anteriorly tilting the pelvis on the femurs) is generally insufficient to reach the ground. *If* the knees remain extended, the hips will typically flex no more than 90° (and often less, depending on extensibility of the hamstrings). The addition of flexion of the lumbar spine (and, perhaps, flexion of the thoracic spine) will add to the total ROM (**Fig. 10–27**). The combination of hip and trunk flexion is generally sufficient for the hands to reach the ground—as long as the hamstrings and lumbar extensors allow sufficient lengthening. This combination

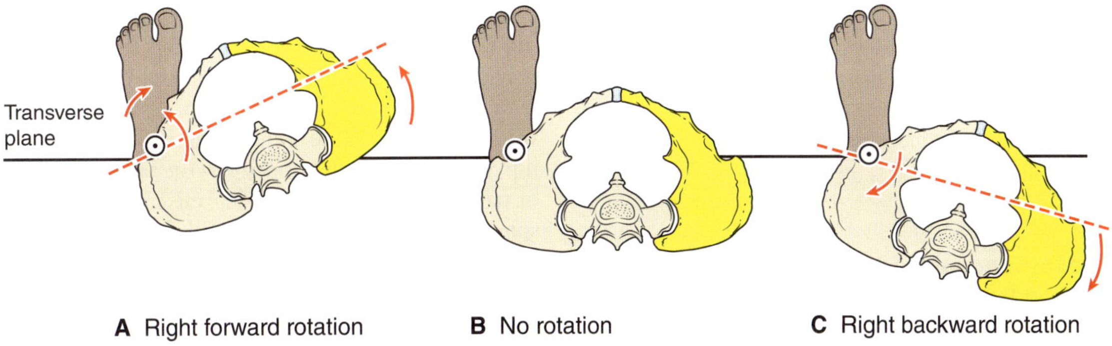

Figure 10–25 A superior view of rotation of the pelvis in the transverse plane. **A.** Forward rotation of the pelvis around the left hip joint results in medial rotation of the left hip joint. **B.** Neutral position of the pelvis and the left hip joint. **C.** Backward rotation of the pelvis around the left hip joint results in lateral rotation of the left hip joint.

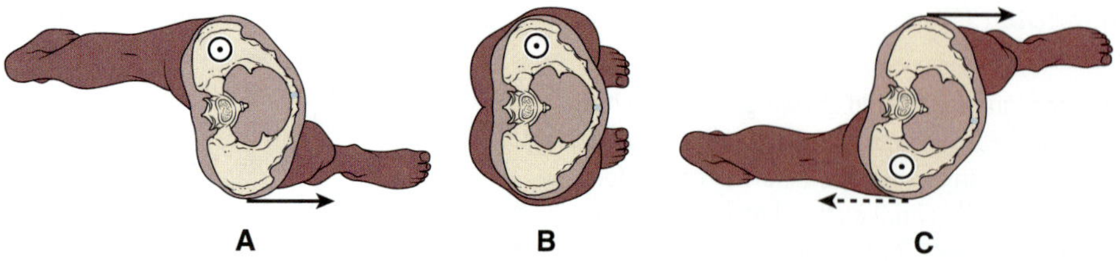

Figure 10–26 Representation of forward rotation of the pelvis during gait in a superior view. **A.** The pelvis is shown forwardly rotating around the weight-bearing left hip joint (the rotation is exaggerated to make the point more clearly). **B.** By midstance, the pelvis advances sufficiently around the left hip joint to return the pelvis to a neutral position. **C.** After midstance, the opposite side of the pelvis begins forward rotation to advance the right swing limb. However, observation of the right side of the pelvis alone will give the illusion of the pelvis forwardly and backwardly rotating sequentially.

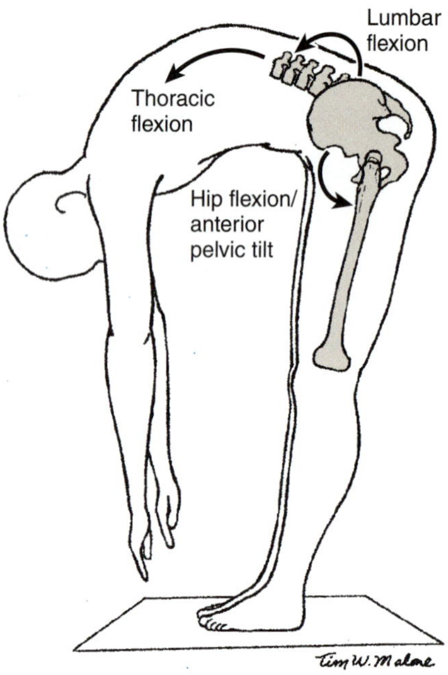

Figure 10–27 Pelvifemoral motion can increase the range of forward flexion of the head and arms by combining hip flexion, anterior pelvic tilt, and flexion of the lumbar spine (± the thoracic spine flexion). This combination permits the hands to maximize the reach toward the ground.

of hip and lumbar motion to achieve a greater ROM for the hands and head is an example of a largely open-chain response in the hips and trunk.

The open-chain response (the ability of each joint in the chain to move independently) is somewhat constrained (largely at the ankles) by the need to keep the line of gravity within the base of support.

Note: Please note that this is *not* an example of how to reach the floor to pick up an object!

Expanded Concepts 10–7

Moving the Foot Through Space

When a person is lying on the right side, the left foot may be moved upwards through an arc of motion approaching 90° (**Fig. 10–28**). This is clearly not all from the left hip joint, which can typically abduct only to 45°; motion of the foot through space also includes lateral tilting of the pelvis (hiking around the right hip joint) and lateral flexion of the lumbar spine to the left. The abducting limb is in an open chain; the lumbar spine (and potentially the thoracic spine) is constrained by the body weight and contact with the ground.

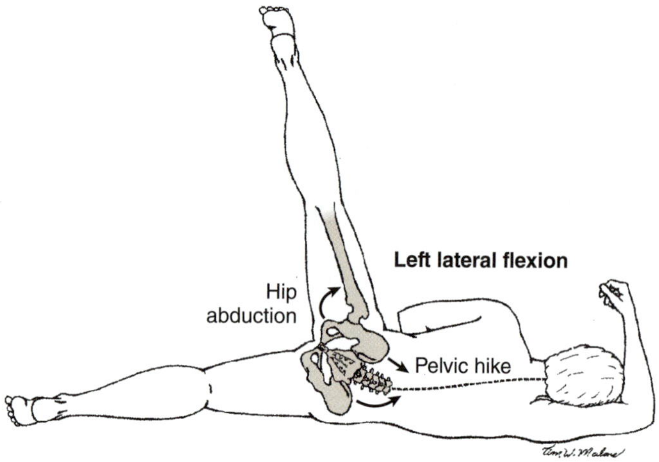

Figure 10–28 Pelvifemoral motion increases the range through which the foot can be moved in space by combining left hip abduction, lateral pelvic tilt (left hike), and lateral flexion of the lumbar spine to the left.

Pelvifemoral motion has also been referred to as **pelvifemoral "rhythm,"** which implies a continuous relationship between the two segments that somewhat contradicts the relative contributions that can vary widely among individuals and in different activities. Pelvic tilt contributes between 30% and 46% of the total range of a passive straight leg raise.[113] During active maximal hip flexion (knee flexed) in standing (e.g., marching in place), pelvic tilt contributed between 8% and 32% of the total motion, with an even greater variability among individuals (9% to 53%) when a 4.53-kg ankle weight was added.[114] The link between hip, pelvis, and lumbar motion is the basis of using provocation of pain with active straight-leg raising as a test for severity of spinal dysfunction in persons with low back pain.[115,116]

CLOSED-CHAIN HIP JOINT FUNCTION

The joints of the right and left lower limbs are part of a true closed chain when both lower limbs are weight-bearing and the chain is defined as all the segments between the right foot, up through the pelvis, and down through the left foot. A true closed chain is formed because both ends of the chain (both feet in this example) are "fixed" and movement at any one joint in the chain invariably involves movement at one or more other links in the chain. It is important not to confuse the idea of *weight-bearing* and *closed chain* as interchangeable terms. In *Foundational Concepts 10–4*, pelvic motion on the fixed femur results in moving the head and trunk through space. This is an open-chain movement despite the feet remaining securely to the floor in a weight-bearing position.

For the hips (and other lower limb joints) to be in a closed chain in standing, both ends of the chain (the head and feet) must be fixed. The feet are, in fact, fixed by weight-bearing. The head, however, is often (but not necessarily) functionally "fixed." Although the head is certainly free to move in space, it most often remains upright and vertically oriented during upright activities. The drive to keep the head upright is due, in part, to the influence of the tonic labyrinthine and optical righting reflexes that are typically evident almost immediately at birth and continue to operate throughout life.[117] The desire to keep the head upright and over the sacrum will effectively *fix the head in relative space;* that is, the head is functionally, rather than structurally, fixed. When the head (one end of the chain) is held upright and over the feet (the other end of the chain), all the segments in the axial skeleton and lower limbs function as part of a closed chain; movement at one joint will create movement in at least one other link in the chain. Consequently, in this functional closed-chain premise, hip flexion does not occur independently (which would move the head forward in space) but is accompanied by mandatory motion in one or more interposed segments to ensure that the head remains upright over the base of support and that the body remains stable. Table 10–1 presents the compensatory motions of the lumbar spine that accompany given motions of the pelvis and hip joint in a functional closed chain.

HIP-SPINE SYNDROME

The term **hip-spine syndrome** was introduced to acknowledge the frequent co-occurrence of symptoms in the hip and lumbar spine. Limitations in hip ROM can result in abnormal lumbopelvic mechanics.[118] Patients with abnormal femoral torsion may experience hip pain and exhibit an abnormal gait due to the rotational misalignment of the lower extremities. This abnormal femoral torsion affects the capsulolabral and musculotendinous structures of both the hip and lumbar spine, contributing to increased lumbopelvic pain. Additionally, a decreased range of hip flexion is likely to increase sacroiliac and lumbar spine stresses during hip flexion, while decreased hip extension ROM is likely to increase loading on the lumbar facet joints.[118]

Expanded Concepts 10–8
Closed-Chain Hip Joint Function

A common example of closed-chain (versus open-chain) function is seen when the hip flexor musculature is tight and the hip joint is maintained in flexion **(Fig. 10–29)**. A person standing with fixed hip flexion is shown in **Figure 10–29A** (an open-chain response) and **B** (a closed-chain response). A true open-chain response to isolated hip flexion would displace the head and trunk forward, with the line of gravity falling in front of the supporting feet if no other joints move concomitantly. More commonly, hip flexion in stance is not isolated to the hips but is accompanied by compensatory movements of the vertebral column (including extension or lordosis of the lumbar spine) that maintain the head in the upright position and keep the line of gravity within the base of support. In a functional closed chain, motion at the hip (one link in the chain) is accompanied by an essentially mandatory lumbar *extension*

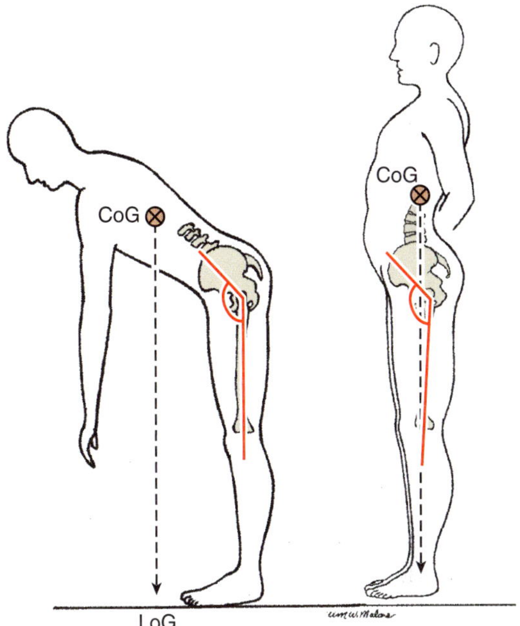

Figure 10–29 **A.** In an open-chain response to tight hip flexors that is isolated to the hip joints, the trunk will be inclined forward. The line of gravity (LoG), arising from the center of gravity (CoG) of HAT will fall outside the base of support if no other adjustments are made. **B.** In a functional closed-chain response to tight hip flexors, the head seeks to maintain a vertical position; the lumbar spine will extend (become lordotic) to return the head and CoG to a position over the sacrum and maintain the LoG within the base of support.

Table 10–1 Relationship of Pelvis, Hip Joint, and Lumbar Spine During Right Lower Extremity Weight-Bearing and Upright Posture

PELVIC MOTION	ACCOMPANYING HIP JOINT MOTION	COMPENSATORY LUMBAR SPINE MOTION
Anterior pelvic tilt	Hip flexion	Lumbar extension
Posterior pelvic tilt	Hip extension	Lumbar flexion
Lateral pelvic tilt (pelvic drop)	Right hip adduction	Right lateral flexion
Lateral pelvic tilt (pelvic hike)	Right hip abduction	Left lateral flexion
Forward rotation	Right hip medial rotation	Rotation to the left
Backward rotation	Right hip lateral rotation	Rotation to the right

to maintain the head over the sacrum (see Fig. 10–29B). In contrast, hip flexion in open-chain pelvifemoral motion may be accompanied by *lumbar flexion* because the goal is to achieve more range for the head in space (see Fig. 10–27).

Patient Application 10–5

Skeletal shortening of the limb with a developmental hip dysplasia is not unusual. As Gabriella stands with her weight evenly distributed between her feet, her pelvis will be laterally tilted (down on the left) as a result of a measured 1-in (2.54 cm) shortening of her left leg. To keep the line of gravity within the center of her base of support in bilateral stance, Gabriella's lumbar spine will be slightly laterally flexed to the right (away from the side of shortening). This is the opposite lumbar motion to what we saw in *Expanded Concepts 10–7* because Gabriella's goal is to keep her head upright, not to gain ROM. The lateral flexion of the spine with asymmetrical leg lengths puts a person at risk for low back pain, although this is not one of Gabriella's presenting complaints. Interestingly, the relative abduction of the left leg that occurs in stance with shortening of Gabriella's dysplastic left limb may reduce stress on the hip. The abducted position of the hip has the potential to increase congruence slightly, diminishing the peak pressure at the hip joint by distributing the forces over a larger contact area.

Hip Joint Musculature

There have been numerous studies of the muscles of the hip joint. Most confirm underlying principles of muscle physiology seen at the other joints we have examined so far. That is, hip joint muscles work best in the middle of their contractile range or on a slight stretch (at so-called optimal length-tension); two-joint muscles generate greatest force when not shortened or lengthened over both joints simultaneously. Tension generation is optimal with eccentric contractions, followed by isometric and then concentric contractions.

The muscles of the hip joint make their most important contributions to function during weight-bearing. In weight-bearing, the muscles are called on to move or support HAT (approximately two-thirds of body weight) rather than the weight of one lower limb (approximately one-sixth of body weight). Consequently, the hip joint muscles adapt their structure to support generation of large torques, as can be seen in their large areas of attachment, their length, and their large cross section. The alignment of the hip joint muscles and the large ROM available at the hip joint result in muscle functions that are strongly influenced by hip joint position. For example, the adductor muscles may assist with hip flexion in the neutral hip joint but will function as hip extensors when the hip joint is already flexed.[119] Delp and colleagues used computer modeling to determine that the medial rotators were capable of generating greater torque in positions of increased hip flexion, whereas the torque-generating capacity of the lateral rotators decreased in positions of increased hip flexion.[120] The investigators similarly determined that the piriformis muscle was a lateral rotator at 0° of hip flexion but a medial rotator at 90° of hip flexion. Such alterations in function are found in a few muscles at the shoulder (the clavicular portion of the pectoralis major, for example), but are fairly common in the hip joint. As a consequence, results of various studies may appear to be contradictory, but in fact, the different testing conditions can be used to explain the differing results. Some sex-related differences in study samples may also explain differential findings.[121]

It is best to examine muscle action at the hip joint in the context of specific functions such as single-limb support, posture, and gait. The next section will briefly review muscle function, but we will leave more detailed analyses for later in this and other chapters. Although the traditional action of each muscle on the distal femoral segment of the hip joint is described for the most part, it must be emphasized that any of the muscles are as likely (or more likely) to produce joint action by moving the proximal pelvic segment instead.

FLEXORS

The flexors of the hip joint function primarily as mobility muscles in open-chain function; that is, they function primarily to bring the swinging limb forward during ambulation or in various sports-specific movements. The flexors may function secondarily to resist strong hip extension forces that occur as the body passes in front of the weight-bearing foot. Nine muscles have action lines crossing the anterior aspect of the hip joint: **rectus femoris**, **iliacus**, **psoas major**, **tensor fascia latae**, **sartorius**, **pectineus**, **adductor longus**, **adductor magnus**, and **gracilis** **(Fig. 10–30)**. Of these, the primary muscles of hip flexion are the iliopsoas, rectus femoris, tensor fascia latae, and sartorius. The **iliopsoas** muscle is considered the most important of the primary hip flexors. It consists of two separate muscles, the iliacus muscle and the psoas major muscle, both of which attach to the femur by a common tendon. The two components of the iliopsoas muscle have many points of origin, including the iliac fossa as well as the discs, bodies, and transverse processes of the lumbar vertebrae. Given the attachments of the psoas major muscle to the anterior vertebrae and the iliacus muscle to the iliac fossa, activity of or passive tension in these muscles would anteriorly tilt the pelvis (iliacus muscle) and, apparently, pull the lumbar vertebrae anteriorly into flexion (psoas major muscle). In closed-chain function (head vertical), however, these muscles seem to create a paradoxical lumbar lordosis (lumbar extension) that results from the body's attempt to keep the head over the sacrum with anterior pelvic tilt and lower lumbar flexion. The role of the iliopsoas muscle in hip flexion may be particularly critical when active hip flexion from a sitting position is required. The hip may not be capable of actively flexing beyond 90° when the iliopsoas muscle is paralyzed, because the other hip flexor muscles are effectively actively insufficient in that position.[122] Both segments of the iliopsoas muscle, however, are likely active in various stages of hip flexion.[119] The moment arm of the iliopsoas muscle for medial or lateral rotation is very small and probably not functionally relevant.[119,120]

The rectus femoris muscle is the only portion of the quadriceps muscle that crosses both the hip and knee joints. It attaches proximally to the **anterior inferior iliac spine (AIIS)** and distally by way of a common tendon into the tibial tuberosity. The rectus femoris muscle flexes the hip joint and extends the knee joint. Because it is a two-joint hip flexor, the position of the knee during hip flexion will affect its ability to generate force at the hip. Simultaneous hip flexion and knee extension considerably shorten this muscle and increase the likelihood of active insufficiency. Consequently, the rectus femoris muscle makes its best contribution to hip flexion when the knee is maintained in flexion.

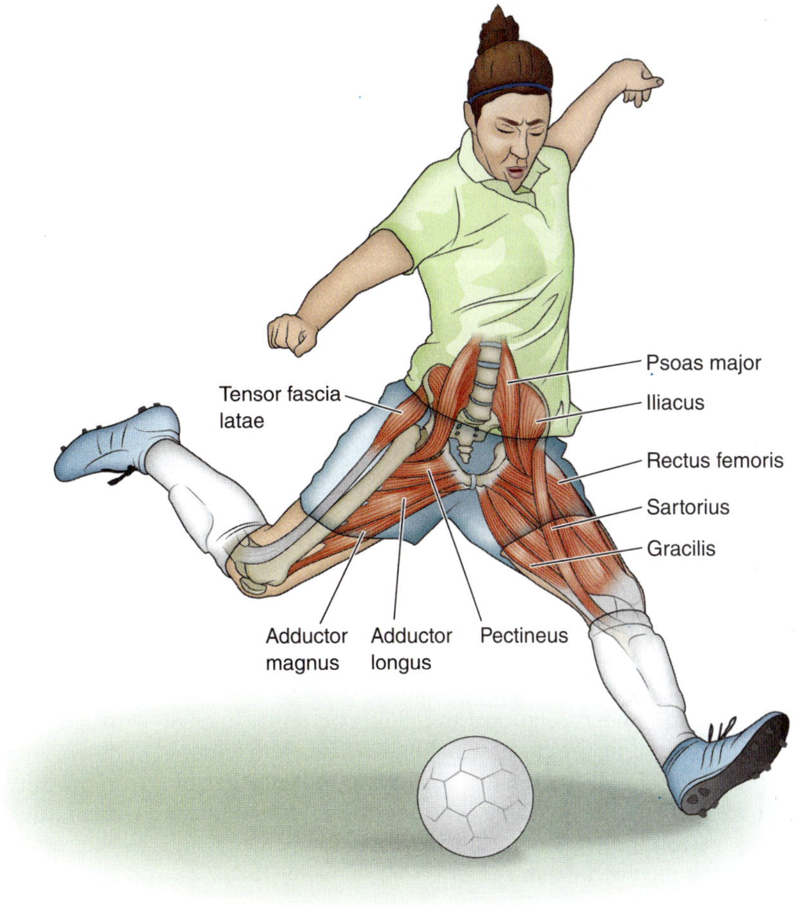

Figure 10–30 Nine muscles have action lines crossing the anterior aspect of the hip joint. The major muscles that contribute most of the flexion torque are the rectus femoris, iliopsoas (iliacus and psoas major), tensor fascia latae, and sartorius. In addition, the pectineus, adductor longus, adductor magnus, and gracilis have the capability of assisting with hip flexion.

The sartorius muscle is a strap-like muscle considered to be a flexor, abductor, and lateral rotator of the hip, as well as a flexor and medial rotator of the knee joint. The sartorius muscle, although a two-joint muscle, should be relatively unaffected by the position of the knee, given the relatively small proportional change in length with increased knee flexion.[123] Its function is probably most important when the knee and hip need to be flexed simultaneously (as in climbing stairs), but its small cross-sectional area argues against a critical role at the hip joint.[28]

The tensor fascia latae muscle has a proximal attachment that is more lateral than the sartorius muscle, on the anterolateral lip of the iliac crest. The muscle fibers attach distally into the **iliotibial (IT) band**, the thickened lateral portion of the **fascia lata** aponeurosis of the hip and thigh, about one-fourth of the way down the lateral aspect of the thigh. The IT band attaches proximally to the iliac crest lateral to the tensor fascia latae and **gluteus maximus** muscle.[124] The IT band continues distally on the lateral thigh to insert into the lateral condyle of the tibia. The tensor fascia latae muscle is considered to flex, abduct, and medially rotate the femur at the hip.[119] However, the tensor fascia latae's contribution to hip abduction may be dependent on simultaneous hip flexion.[125] The most important contribution of the tensor fascia latae muscle may be in maintaining tension in the IT band, in combination with the gluteus maximus. The IT band assists in relieving the lateral femur of some of the tensile stresses imposed on the shaft by weight-bearing forces[125,126] (see Fig. 10-20). Because bone more effectively resists compressive than tensile stresses, reduction of tensile stresses is important in maintaining integrity of the bone.

Although the importance of the tensor fascia latae muscle and IT band at the hip is controversial, evidence suggests they contribute to hip joint stability.[124] Excessive tension in the IT band may also contribute to reduced hip adduction ROM when the hip joint is extended. Gajdosik and colleagues performed the **Ober test**, presumed to test flexibility of the IT band, on men and women without impairments.[127] They found an average passive hip adduction of 9° for men and 4° for women when both the hip and knee were extended. When the knee was flexed during the maneuver, the hip did not get past neutral and remained in 4° of abduction for men and 6° of abduction for women, which implied that there was greater tension in the lateral hip joint structures (potentially with the IT band as a key factor) when the knee was flexed.[127] The Ober test presumably moves the IT band from its position anterior to the greater trochanter to a position posterior to the greater trochanter by extending the hip. Movement of the IT band anteriorly and posteriorly over the greater trochanter during functional activities has been implicated in **"snapping hip" syndrome** and in inflammation of the **trochanteric bursae**.[128]

The secondary hip flexors are the pectineus, adductor longus, adductor magnus, and the gracilis muscles. These muscles are described in the next section because they are predominantly adductors of the hip. Each, however, can contribute to hip joint flexion, but that contribution is dependent on hip joint position. These muscles are believed to contribute up to

40° to 50° of hip flexion.[68] The gracilis, a two-joint muscle, is active as a hip flexor when the knee is extended but not when the knee is flexed.[123]

ADDUCTORS

The hip adductor muscle group is generally considered to include the pectineus, **adductor brevis**, adductor longus, adductor magnus, and the gracilis muscles **(Fig. 10–31)**. These adductors are located anteromedially. The contribution of the adductor muscles to hip joint function has been debated for many years. One of the reasons for debate is a question concerning the degree to which the flexed, adducted, and medially rotated posture assumed by many individuals with cerebral palsy is attributable to adductor spasticity. Arnold and Delp (using kinematic data from children with cerebral palsy who showed excessive medial rotation of the hip, along with a "deformable femur" model) concluded that—in the typical hip in standing—the adductor brevis, adductor longus, pectineus, and posterior adductor magnus muscles had only small moment arms for medial rotation, whereas the gracilis and anterior adductor magnus muscles had small moment arms for lateral rotation.[53] With excessive femoral anteversion, the moment arms of the adductor brevis, pectineus, and the middle fibers of the adductor magnus muscles switched from medial rotational to lateral rotational lines of pull. After examining the changes in moment arms with femoral anteversion or combined hip medial rotation and knee flexion, the investigators concluded that the adductors were unlikely to have a strong influence on an excessively medially rotated hip position during the gait cycle.[53]

Basmajian and De Luca believed that the adductors function not as prime movers but by reflex response to gait activities.[119] As shall be seen in our discussion of muscle function in bilateral stance, the adductors may be synergists to the abductor muscles when both feet are on the ground, enhancing side-to-side stabilization of the pelvis. Although the role of the adductor muscles may be less clear than that of other hip muscle groups, the relative importance of the adductors should not be underestimated. The adductors as a group contribute 22.5% to the total muscle mass of the lower extremity, in comparison with only 18.4% for the flexors and 14.9% for the abductors.[129] The adductors are relevant in sports-related injuries because of the high frequency of adductor longus strains, particularly in sports such as hockey.[130]

EXTENSORS

The one-joint gluteus maximus muscle and the two-joint hamstrings muscle group are the primary hip joint extensors **(Fig. 10–32)**. These muscles may receive assistance from the posterior fibers of the **gluteus medius**, from the posterior fibers of the adductor magnus muscle, and from the piriformis muscle. The gluteus maximus is a large, quadrangular muscle that crosses the sacroiliac joint before its most superior fibers attach to the IT band (as do the fibers of the tensor fascia latae muscle) and its inferior fibers attach to the gluteal tuberosity. The gluteus maximus is the largest of the lower extremity muscles; this muscle alone constitutes 12.8% of the total muscle mass of the lower extremity.[129] The gluteus maximus is a strong hip extensor that appears to be active

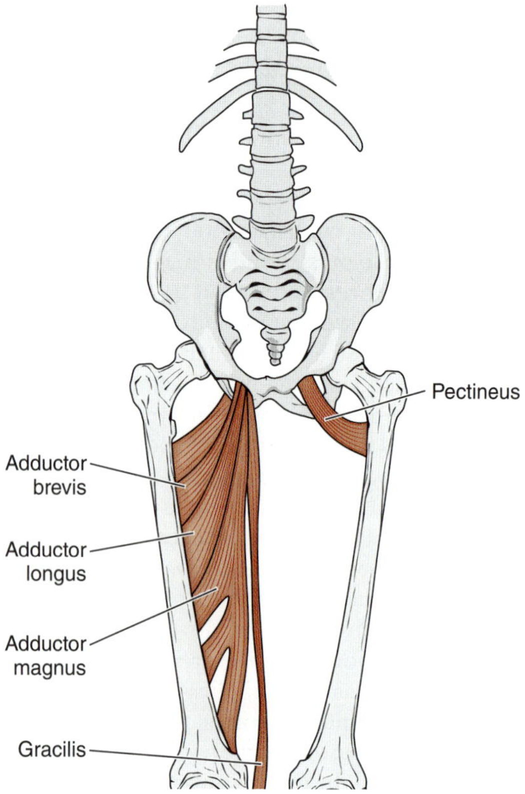

Figure 10–31 The hip adductor muscle group lies on the anteromedial aspect of the thigh and includes the pectineus, adductor brevis, adductor longus, adductor magnus, and the gracilis muscles.

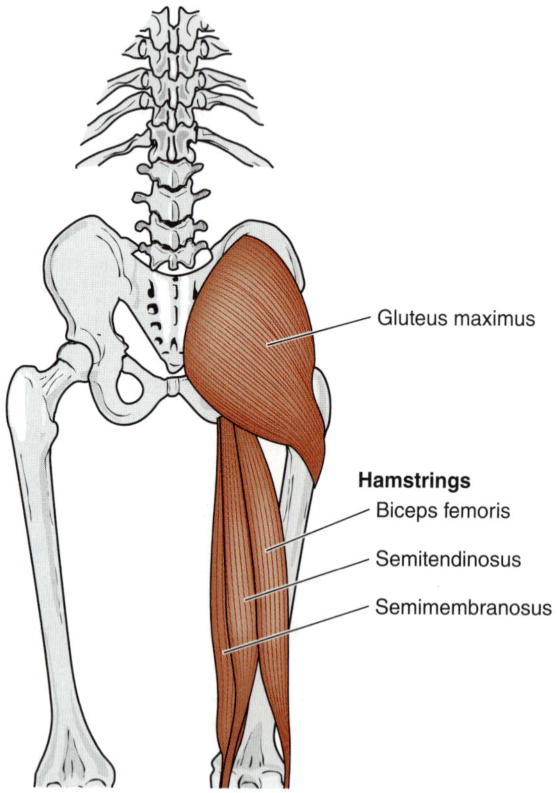

Figure 10–32 The primary hip extensors cross the joint posteriorly and include the one-joint gluteus maximus muscle and the two-joint hamstrings muscle group.

primarily against a resistance greater than the weight of the limb. Its moment arm for hip extension is considerably longer than that of either the hamstrings or the adductor magnus muscles and is maximal in the neutral hip joint position.[121] A favorable length-tension relationship, however, allows it to exert its peak extensor moment at 70° of hip flexion.[131] The fibers of the gluteus maximus have a substantial capacity to laterally rotate the femur, although the moment arms for lateral rotation diminish with increased hip flexion.[120]

The three two-joint extensors are the **long head of the biceps femoris**, the **semitendinosus**, and the **semimembranosus** muscles, known collectively as the **hamstrings**. All three hamstring muscles extend the hip with or without resistance, as well as serving as important knee flexors. The short head of the biceps femoris is excluded from this discussion of the hamstrings because it does not cross the hip joint. The hamstrings increase their moment arm for hip extension as the hip flexes to 35° and decrease it thereafter. This is somewhat in contrast to the moment arm of the gluteus maximus that is maximal at neutral position and decreases with any hip flexion thereafter.[121] Regardless of these changes in moment arm with joint position, the moment arm of the combined hamstrings for hip extension is smaller than that of the gluteus maximus at all points in the hip flexion/extension ROM. As two-joint muscles, the role of the hamstrings in hip extension is also strongly influenced by knee position. Chleboun and colleagues (using ultrasonography) determined that the moment arm for the long head of the biceps femoris was greater for hip extension than for knee flexion, with hip position affecting its excursion capability more than did knee position.[132] Although these investigators reported only on the long head of the biceps femoris, the anatomy of the medial hamstrings (semimembranosus and semitendinosus) makes it likely that these muscles have similar attributes. Importantly, if the hip is extended and the knee is flexed to 90° or more, the hamstrings may not be able to contribute much to hip extension force because of active insufficiency. Extension forces of the hip increase by 30% if the knee is extended.[131] The optimal length-tension relationship for the long head of the biceps is estimated to be at 90° of hip flexion and 90° of knee flexion, and it is likely that the medial hamstrings show similar behavior.[132] The medial hamstrings (semimembranosus and semitendinosus) have a small moment arm for medial rotation in the neutral hip but appear to switch to lateral rotators with the knee joint in flexion.[53] The biceps femoris (the lateral hamstring) may contribute to lateral rotation of the hip.[119]

ABDUCTORS

The abductors have been likened to the "rotator cuff of the hip," with the gluteus medius and **gluteus minimus** being analogous to the supraspinatus and subscapularis muscles, respectively **(Fig. 10–33)**.[133-135] The gluteus medius tendon attaches distally on the lateral and posterior superior portion of the greater trochanter, resulting in a moment arm similar in direction and force to the supraspinatus.[136] Active abduction of the hip is brought about predominantly by the gluteus medius and the gluteus minimus muscles. The superior fibers of the gluteus maximus and the sartorius muscles may assist when the hip is abducted against strong resistance. The tensor fascia latae muscle may be effective as an abductor only during simultaneous hip flexion. The gluteus medius has anterior, middle, and posterior parts that function asynchronously during movement at the hip.[137] Analogous to the deltoid muscle of the glenohumeral joint, the anterior fibers of the gluteus medius are active in hip flexion, whereas the posterior fibers assist with hip extension. In the neutral hip, the posterior portion of the gluteus medius will produce a lateral rotational moment, whereas the middle and anterior portions have small medial rotational moments. In hip flexion, all portions medially rotate the hip.[120] All portions of the gluteus medius are primary abductors of the hip joint, regardless of hip joint position.

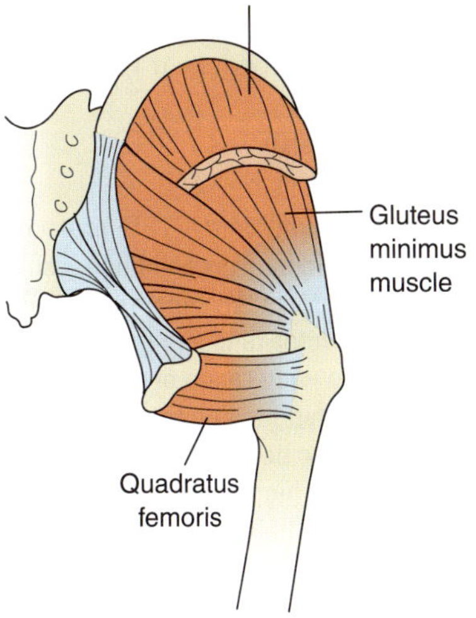

Figure 10–33 The muscles responsible for producing hip abduction lie on the lateral side of the joint. The prime abductors are the gluteus medius and the gluteus minimus muscles. The gluteus medius has been cut to show the gluteus minimus below it.

The gluteus minimus muscle lies deep to the gluteus medius, and it is best positioned to be an abductor and flexor of the hip joint but can exert several different moments including medial rotation or lateral rotation, depending on the position of the femur. There appears to be a consensus that the gluteus minimus has a tendinous insertion into the hip joint capsule as it passes to the greater trochanter. It is hypothesized that this attachment retracts the capsule during hip abduction to prevent entrapment, or tightens the capsule to add to the gluteus minimus's function of stabilizing the femoral head in the acetabulum.[138,139] Based on these observations, it follows that one of the primary functions of the gluteus minimus is to act as a femoral head stabilizer.[140]

The gluteus minimus and medius muscles function together either to abduct the femur (distal segment free as in non–weight-bearing) or, more important, to stabilize the pelvis (and superimposed HAT) in unilateral stance against the effects of gravity. As will be presented later, the gluteus medius and minimus muscles will offset the gravitation adduction torque on the pelvis (pelvis drop) around the weight-bearing hip in unilateral stance. The abductors are physiologically designed to work most effectively in a neutral or slightly adducted hip (slightly lengthened abductors).[141,142] Isometric abduction torque in the neutral hip position is 82% greater than abduction torque when the hip is in 25° of abduction (shortened abductors).[143] Because the gluteus medius is an important pelvic stabilizer, its weakness has been implicated in lower extremity overuse injuries such as bursitis and hip osteoarthritis, as well as disorders at the knee.[128,144,145]

Expanded Concepts 10–9
Greater Trochanteric Pain Syndrome

Greater trochanteric pain syndrome (GTPS) presents a challenge in orthopedic and sports medicine. This condition results from the interaction of various tissues under mechanical stress and includes greater trochanteric bursitis, abductor tendinopathy, and external snapping hip syndrome, leading to a wide range of clinical presentations.[146,147] Patients often report intermittent, debilitating pain across the lateral thigh and buttock, which can be exacerbated by daily activities such as sitting, stair climbing, or high-impact exercises. Historically, the primary source of lateral hip pain was thought to be inflammation of the peritrochanteric bursae.[148] Pfirrmann and colleagues used MRI, bursography, and conventional radiography to study the greater trochanter and its associated bursae in cadavers and asymptomatic volunteers.[79] They concluded that the greater trochanter consisted of four facets: the gluteus minimus attached to the anterior facet, with the **subgluteus minimus bursa** beneath the tendon; the gluteus medius attached to the posterosuperior and lateral facets, with the **subgluteus medius** bursa beneath the tendon at the lateral facet; and the large **trochanteric bursa** covered the posterior facet, which was free of tendinous attachments **(Fig. 10–34)**. Presumably, the trochanteric bursa serves to reduce friction between the posterior facet and the overlying gluteus maximus, as well as between the IT band and the trochanter.

However, recent imaging studies more frequently identify abductor muscle tears, tendinosis, and thickening of the IT band as the primary sources of pain rather than bursitis.[149] Although some patients with greater trochanteric pain syndrome exhibit bursitis, bursal inflammation is often a secondary complication resulting from repetitive friction between the greater trochanter and the IT band. This repetitive motion is thought to cause microtrauma at the attachment site of the gluteal tendons, mainly the gluteus medius and minimus, to the greater trochanter.[150,151] The injury and degeneration pattern of these muscles is similar to that observed in rotator cuff injuries, where abductor tears can vary from partial- to full-thickness tears due to altered cellular healing responses and diminished healing capability.

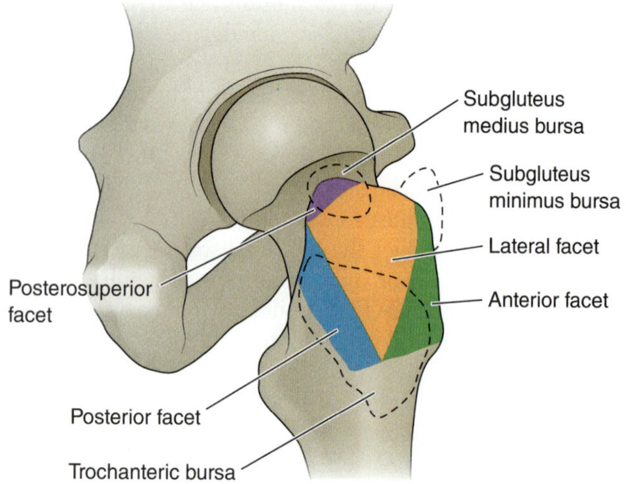

Figure 10–34 The greater trochanter has four facets: the anterior facet, the lateral facet, the posterior facet, and the posterosuperior facet. Also seen on cross section are three bursae, which can all become compressed due to muscle activity or a fall on the lateral hip.

Patient Application 10–6

In addition to her other problems, Gabriella reported lateral hip pain that was tender to palpation. Although other explanations for her pain exist, greater trochanter pain syndrome (GTPS) is a common complaint in middle-aged women (with a 4:1 ratio of women to men) and in those diagnosed with osteoarthritis.[43,78,152] The altered biomechanics associated with her leg length discrepancy may further predispose her to pathology of the lateral hip. Trochanteric bursitis and lesions of the abductor (gluteus medius and gluteus minimus) tendons commonly coexist and are analogous to rotator cuff tears and bursitis in the shoulder.[43,78,79,153] As we continue to explore the role of the hip abductors in standing and the possible effects of hip dysplasia on the hip abductors, it will become clear that Gabriella's hip abductors and associated bursae are likely at risk for overuse injury and perhaps the start of degenerative changes.

LATERAL ROTATORS

Six short muscles function primarily as lateral rotators of the hip joint. These muscles are the **obturator internus** and **externus**, the **gemellus superior** and **inferior**, the **quadratus femoris**, and the **piriformis muscles**. Other muscles that have fibers posterior to the axis of motion at the hip (the posterior fibers of the gluteus medius, minimus, and maximus) may produce lateral rotation combined with the primary action of the muscle (although it has already been noted that the lateral rotary function of these muscles decreases or reverses with increased hip flexion).[120] Of the primary lateral rotators, each inserts either on or in the vicinity of the greater trochanter **(Fig. 10–35)**. The piriformis and gluteus maximus are the only two muscles that cross the sacroiliac joint. The sciatic nerve, the largest nerve in the body, enters the gluteal region

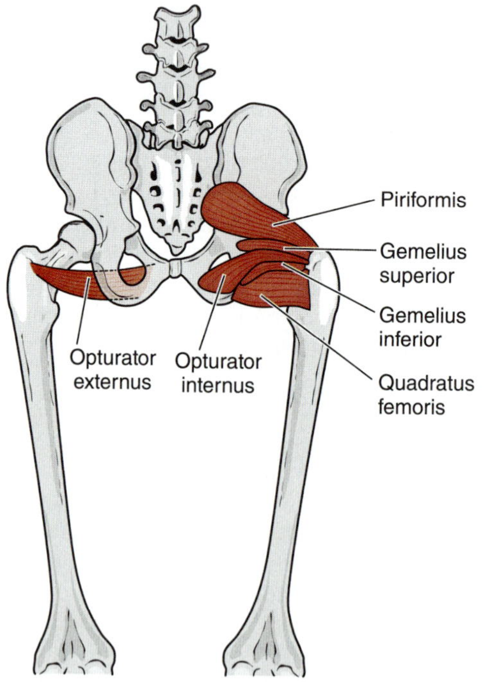

Figure 10–35 The lateral rotators pass posterior to the joint axis in a mediolateral direction. These short muscles include the obturator internus and externus, the gemellus superior and inferior, the quadratus femoris, and the piriformis muscles.

just inferior to the piriformis muscle as both structures pass through the greater sciatic notch. This close proximity of the piriformis to the sciatic nerve has the potential to contribute to radiating leg pain arising from impairments associated with the piriformis muscle. Sacroiliac joint dysfunction, hamstring tears, and intra-articular hip pathology may mimic sciatic nerve entrapment by presenting symptoms such as aching, burning sensations, or cramping in the buttock or posterior thigh.[154] To differentiate diagnoses, sitting pain with avoidance of seated activities is usually associated with sciatic nerve entrapment beneath the piriformis muscle.[155]

The lateral rotator muscles are positioned to perform their rotary function effectively, given the nearly perpendicular orientation to the shaft of the femur (see Fig. 10–35). However, exploration of function of these muscles has been restricted because of the relatively limited access to electromyography (EMG) surface or wire electrodes. Like their rotator cuff counterpart at the glenohumeral joint, these muscles would certainly appear to be effective joint compressors because their combined line of pull parallels the head and neck of the femur. The obturator internus, like the gluteal muscles, decreased its moment arm for lateral rotation with increased hip flexion.[98,120] The piriformis was estimated to have a large moment arm for lateral rotation with the hip joint at 0° but switched to a medial rotator with half the moment arm when the hip reached 90° of flexion. The obturator externus and quadratus femoris were the only lateral rotators that did not diminish their moment arm for lateral rotation with increased hip joint flexion.[120] Hypothetically, the lines of pull of the deep one-joint lateral rotators should make them ideal tonic (postural) stabilizers of the joint during most weight-bearing and non–weight-bearing activities. Although their ability to perform lateral rotation may decrease with hip flexion in some instances, the action lines of these muscles should remain largely compressive (parallel to the femoral neck) throughout the hip joint ROM.

MEDIAL ROTATORS

There are no muscles with a *primary* function of producing medial rotation of the hip joint. The more consistent medial rotators are the anterior portion of the gluteus medius, gluteus minimus, and the tensor fascia latae muscles. Although the role of the adductors in hip joint rotation is controversial, the majority of evidence appears to support the adductor muscles as medial rotators of the joint, with the possible exception of the gracilis muscle.[119,122] The ability of hip joint muscles to shift function with changing position of the hip joint is evident when medial rotation of the hip is examined. There is a trend toward increased medial rotation torques (or decreased lateral rotation torques) with increased hip flexion among many of the hip joint muscles, with three times more medial rotation torque in the flexed hip than in the extended hip.[53,120,122] Research has suggested that the medial rotation that may accompany a "crouched" gait seen in many individuals with cerebral palsy may be attributable more to hip flexion than to adductor spasticity.[120]

Expanded Concepts 10–10
"Rotator Cuff" of the Hip

The shoulder rotator cuff can be used to help understand the function of muscles around the hip. The lateral rotators of the shoulder (infraspinatus, teres minor, and supraspinatus) can be considered analogous to the lateral rotators of the hip, including the piriformis, obturator externus and internus, and superior and inferior gemelli, along with the posterior gluteus medius at the hip. The anterior fibers of the gluteus medius and gluteus minimus medially rotate the hip and can be analogized to the subscapularis of the shoulder. Abduction of the hip performed by the gluteus medius is analogous to supraspinatus function at the shoulder.[156]

Hip Joint Forces and Muscle Function in Stance

Bilateral Stance

In erect bilateral stance, both hips are in neutral or slight extension, and weight is evenly distributed between both legs. The line of gravity falls just posterior to the axis for flexion/extension of the hip joint. The posterior location of the line of gravity creates an external (gravitational) extension moment around the hip that tends to tilt the pelvis posteriorly on the femoral heads. The gravitational extension moment can be checked by passive tension in the hip joint capsuloligamentous structures if close to end range, although slight or intermittent activity in the iliopsoas muscles in relaxed standing is necessary to assist the passive structures.[119] The intermittent muscle activity may help relieve the capsuloligamentous structures from constant stress in long periods of quiet standing.

In the frontal plane during bilateral stance, the superincumbent body weight is transmitted through the sacroiliac joints and pelvis to the right and left femoral heads. Hypothetically, the weight of the HAT (two-thirds of body weight) should be distributed so that each femoral head receives approximately half of the superincumbent weight.[157] As shown in **Figure 10–36**, the joint axis of each hip lies at an equal distance from the line of gravity of HAT (W); that is, the gravitational moment arms for the right hip (MA_R) and the left hip (MA_L) are equal. Because the body weight on each femoral head is the same ($W_R = W_L$), the magnitude of the gravitational torques around each hip must be identical ($W_R \times MA_R = W_L \times MA_L$). The gravitational torques on the right and left hips, however, occur in opposite directions. The weight of the body acting around the right hip tends to drop the pelvis down on the left (right adduction moment), whereas the weight acting around the left hip tends to drop the pelvis down on the right (left adduction moment). These two opposing gravitational moments of equal magnitude balance each other, and the pelvis is maintained in equilibrium in the frontal plane without the assistance of active muscles. Assuming that muscular forces are not required to maintain either sagittal or frontal plane stability at the hip joint in bilateral stance, the compression across each hip joint in bilateral stance should simply be half the superimposed body weight (or one half of HAT to each hip).

Hip joint compression can be altered by different means. This includes leaning over one lower extremity during single-limb stance and the use of a cane in either hand. The magnitude of hip joint compression as it relates to bilateral stance, unilateral stance, compensatory leaning, ipsilateral cane use, and contralateral cane use is presented in Examples 10–1, 10–2, 10–3, 10–4, and 10–5, respectively. A summary of the calculations is presented after the examples in Table 10–2 for direct comparison.

The rationale presented in Example 10–1 for assuming that each hip receives one-third of body weight in bilateral stance

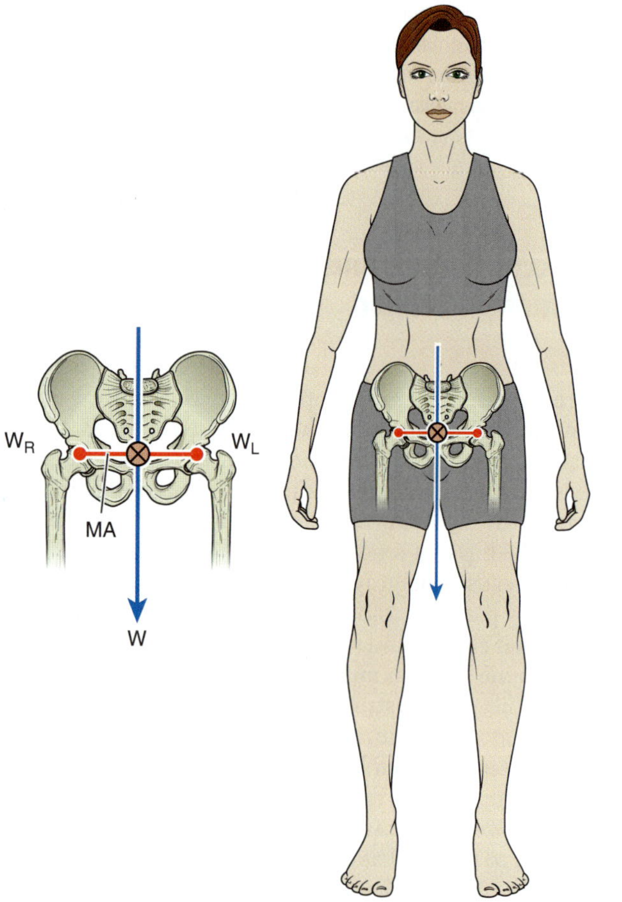

Figure 10–36 An anterior view of the pelvis in typical erect bilateral stance. The weight (W, the LoG of HAT) acting on the right hip joint (W_R) multiplied by the distance from the right hip joint axis to the body's center of gravity (MA_R) is equal to the weight acting at the left hip joint (W_L) multiplied by the distance from the left hip to the body's center of gravity (MA_L). Therefore, $W_R \times MA_R = W_L \times MA_L$. MA, moment arm.

is reasonable. However, Bergmann and colleagues showed in several subjects with instrumented pressure-sensitive hip prostheses that the joint compression across each hip in bilateral stance was 80% to 100% of body weight, rather than one-third (33%) of body weight, as commonly proposed.[158] When they added a symmetrically distributed load to the subject's trunk, the forces at both hip joints increased by the full weight of the load, rather than by half of the superimposed load as might be expected. Although the mechanics of someone standing who has a prosthetic hip may not fully represent typical hip joint forces, the findings of Bergmann and colleagues call into question the simplistic view of hip joint forces in bilateral stance. The slight activity in the iliopsoas muscle may account for more joint compression than previously thought. Alternatively, capsuloligamentous tension or activation of secondary stabilizing muscles may contribute to joint compression.

Example 10–1
Calculating Hip Joint Compression in Bilateral Stance

Using a hypothetical case of someone weighing 825 N (~185 lb), the weight of HAT (two-thirds body weight) will be 550 N (~124 lb). Of that 550 N, one-half will presumably be distributed through each hip. Because we are assuming no additional compressive force produced by hip muscle activity, the total hip joint compression at each hip in bilateral stance is estimated to be 275 N (~62 lb); that is, total hip joint compression through each hip in bilateral stance is one-third of body weight.

When bilateral stance is not symmetrical, frontal plane muscle activity will be necessary either to control the side-to-side motion or to return the hips to symmetrical stance. If the pelvis is shifted to the right (see Fig. 10–24), there is a relative adduction of the right hip and abduction of the left hip. To return to neutral position, an active contraction of the right hip abductors would be expected. However, a contraction of the left hip adductors would accomplish the same goal. Thus, in bilateral stance when both lower limbs bear at least some of the superimposed weight, the contralateral abductors and adductors may function as synergists to control the frontal plane motion of the pelvis. In unilateral stance, activity of the adductors either in the weight-bearing or non–weight-bearing hip *cannot* contribute to stability of the stance limb. Hip joint stability in unilateral stance is the sole domain of the hip joint abductors. In the absence of adequate hip abductor function, the adductors can contribute to stability—but only in bilateral stance.

Unilateral Stance

In **Figure 10–37**, the left leg has been lifted from the ground and the full superimposed body weight (HAT) is being supported by the right hip joint. Rather than sharing the compressive force of the superimposed body weight with the left limb, the right hip joint must now carry the full burden. In addition, the weight of the non–weight-bearing left limb that is hanging on the left side of the pelvis must be supported along with the weight of HAT. Of the one-third of the portion of body weight found in the lower extremities, the non–weight-bearing limb must account for one-half of that, or one-sixth of the full body weight.[159] The magnitude of body weight (W) compressing the right hip joint in right unilateral stance, therefore, is as follows:

$$\text{Right hip joint compression}_{\text{body weight}} = [2/3 \times W] + [1/6 \times W]$$

$$\text{Right hip joint compression}_{\text{body weight}} = 5/6 \times W$$

Our hypothetical subject from Example 10–1 weighs 825 N; thus, HAT accounts for 550 N. One lower extremity weighs one-sixth of body weight, or 137.5 N. Therefore, when this individual lifts one leg off the ground, the supporting hip joint will undergo 687.5 N (or five-sixths of body weight) of compression *from body weight alone*.[6]

Although we have accounted for the increase in hip joint compression from body weight as a person moves from double-limb support (bilateral stance) to single-limb support, the problem is more complex. Not only is the hip joint in unilateral stance being compressed by body weight (gravity), but body weight is also creating a torque around the stance limb hip joint that needs to be balanced.

Table 10–2 Summary of Calculations of Hip Joint Compression

Example:

BW = 825 N **HAT MA = 0.1 m** **Abductor MA = 0.05 m**	**UNILATERAL STANCE**	**LATERAL LEAN TOWARD STANCE LIMB**	**CANE IPSILATERAL**	**PROPOSED ANALYSIS OF A CANE CONTRALATERALLY**
		Lean decreases HAT MA	Pushing down with cane reduces BW	Pushing down with cane reduces BW Cane counter torque
BW compression = 5/6 × BW	687.50 N	687.50 N	563.75 N (BW x 15% through cane)	563.75 N (BW × 15% through cane)
HATLL $\text{torque}_{\text{Adduction}}$ = $\text{BW}_{\text{compression}}$ × HAT MA	68.75 Nm	17.2 Nm (HAT MA decreased to 0.025 m)	56.38 Nm	31.63 Nm (Latissimus dorsi pull offsets 24.75 Nm of adduction torque)
Force contraction $_{\text{Abductor}}$ = HATLL $\text{torque}_{\text{Adduction}}$ ÷ Abductor MA	1,375.00 N	343.75 N	1,127.60 N	632.6 N
Total joint compression = Force $\text{contraction}_{\text{Abductor}}$ + BW compression	2,062.50 N	1,031.25 N	1,691.35 N	1,193.35 N

BW: body weight; HAT: head, arms, and trunk; HATLL: head, arms, and trunk non–weight-bearing left lower limb; MA: moment arm.

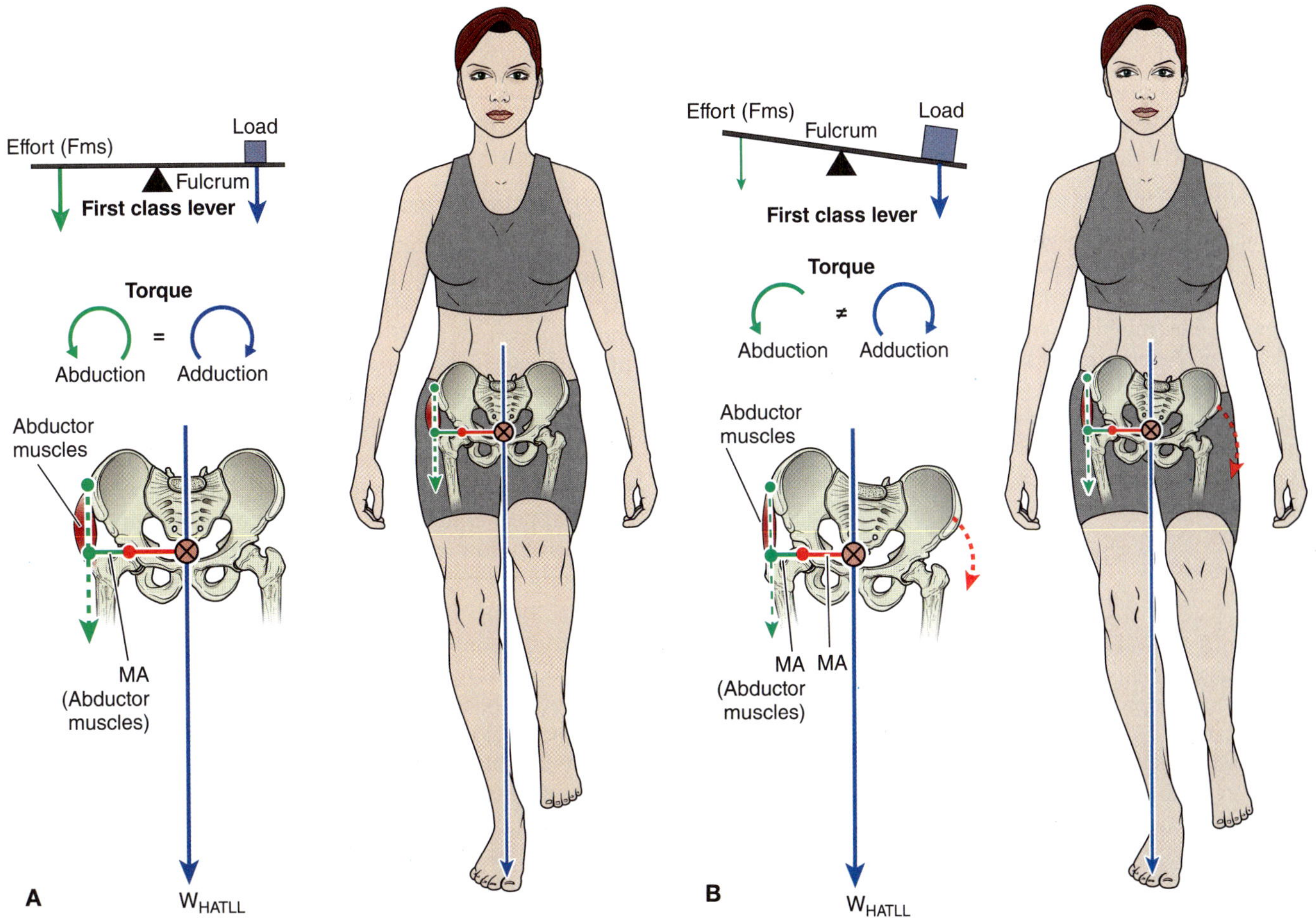

Figure 10–37 **A.** In right unilateral stance, the weight (W_{HATLL}) of HATLL (HAT plus left leg), as shown in the inset, acts 10 cm from the right hip joint (red dot). The hip abductors have a moment arm of approximately 5 cm and must be active to keep the pelvis level. **B.** If inadequate abduction torque is generated (e.g., from a weakened gluteus medius), the pelvis will drop on the contralateral side.

The combined force of gravity acting on HAT and the non–weight-bearing left lower limb (HAT + left leg, HATLL) will create an adduction torque around the weight-bearing hip joint; that is, gravity will attempt to drop the pelvis around the right weight-bearing hip joint axis. The abduction counter torque to maintain equilibrium will have to be supplied by the right hip abductor musculature. When muscles are active at a joint, they produce joint compression. Therefore, the total joint compression or joint reaction force is a combination of both body weight and abductor muscular compression. The total joint compression can be calculated for our hypothetical 825-N patient. The line of gravity of HATLL can be estimated to lie 10 cm (0.1 m, or ~4 in.) from the right hip joint axis. That is, the moment arm (MA) = 0.1 m (10 cm), although the actual distance will vary among individuals. The 10-cm estimate of the gravitational moment arm is for *symmetrical* stance. The actual moment arm is likely to be somewhat smaller, however, because the weight of the hanging left leg will pull the center of gravity of the superimposed weight slightly to the right, and a compensatory trunk lean will likely be needed to shift the line of gravity slightly right to get the line of gravity within the now smaller (i.e., single-foot) base of support.

Example 10–2
Calculating Hip Joint Compression in Unilateral Stance

For simplicity, the possible change in the moment arm of HATLL due to single limb support will be ignored, so our torque calculation here is simply an estimate of the actual gravitational torque. In our simplified hypothetical example, the magnitude of the gravitational adduction torque at the right hip will be as follows:

$$\text{HATLL torque}_{\text{adduction}}: 687.5\text{ N} \times 0.1\text{ m} = 68.75\text{ Nm}$$

To maintain the single-limb support position, there must be a counter torque (abduction moment) of equivalent magnitude. The counter torque must be produced by the force of the hip abductors (gluteus medius, minimus, and tensor fascia latae muscles) acting on the pelvis. Assuming that the abductor muscles act through a typical moment arm of 5 cm (0.05 m, or 2 in.) and knowing that the muscles must generate an abduction torque equivalent to the adduction torque of gravity (68.75 Nm), we can solve for the magnitude of muscle contraction (F_{ms}) needed to maintain equilibrium in our hypothetical example.[93]

$$\text{Torque}_{\text{abduction}}: 68.75\text{ Nm} = F_{ms} \times 0.05\text{ m}$$

$$F_{ms} = 68.75\text{ Nm} \div 0.05\text{ m} = 1{,}375\text{ N}$$

Assuming that all the abductor muscular force is transmitted through the acetabulum to the femoral head, the 1,375-N abductor muscular compressive force is now added to the 687.5 N of compression caused by body weight passing through the supporting hip. Thus, the total hip joint compression, or joint reaction force, at the stance hip joint in unilateral support can be estimated for our hypothetical patient as:

1,375 N abductor joint compression

+ 687.5 N body weight (HATLL) compression

2,062.5 N total joint compression

The hypothetical figures used in the examples oversimplify and underestimate the forces involved in hip joint stresses as already noted. However, this example illustrates nicely that the hip joint compressive force is heavily influenced by muscle activity, and that the joint compressive force increases substantially during unilateral stance compared with bilateral stance. Total hip joint compression, or joint reaction forces, are generally found to be two to three times body weight in unilateral stance.[131,157,160] Some investigators have found that peak forces are higher than typically calculated for unilateral stance and can achieve four times body weight depending on measurement technique and individual characteristics.[161,162] Individual differences in hip structure (i.e., angulation of the femur) may substantially alter forces and pressures across the hip joint.[72,102,163]

If total joint compression in unilateral stance is approximately three times body weight, a loss of 1 N (~4.5 lb) of body weight will reduce the joint reaction force by 3 N (13.5 lb). For painful hip joints, however, the reductions in compression generally required are greater than can be realistically achieved through weight loss. The solution must be in a reduction of abductor muscle force requirements. If less muscular counter torque is needed to offset the effects of gravity, there will be a decrease in the amount of *muscular compression* across the joint, although the body weight compression will remain unchanged. Several options are available when there is a need to decrease abductor muscle force requirements. Some compression reduction strategies occur automatically, but at a cost of extra energy expenditure and structural stress. Other strategies require intervention such as assistive devices but have the advantage of minimizing the energy cost and structural stress.

Compensatory Lateral Lean of the Trunk

We know that gravitational torque at the pelvis is the product of body weight (HAT and non–weight-bearing limb) and the distance that the line of gravity lies from the hip joint axis (its moment arm, MA). If there is a need to reduce the torque of gravity in unilateral stance and if body weight cannot be reduced, the moment arm of the gravitational force can be reduced by laterally leaning the trunk over the pelvis toward the side of pain or weakness when in unilateral stance on the painful limb. Although leaning toward the side of pain might appear counterintuitive, the compensatory lateral lean of the trunk toward the painful stance limb will shift the line of gravity *closer* to the hip joint, thereby reducing the gravitational moment arm. Because the weight of HATLL must pass through the weight-bearing hip joint regardless of trunk position, leaning toward the painful or weak supporting hip does not increase the joint compression caused by HATLL. However, it does reduce the torque of HATLL (gravity). If there is a smaller gravitational adduction torque at the stance hip joint, there will be an equivalent reduction in the need for an abductor counter torque. Although it is theoretically possible to laterally lean the trunk enough to bring the line of gravity through the weight-bearing hip (reducing the torque to zero) or to the opposite side of the supporting hip (reversing the direction of the gravitational torque), these are relatively extreme motions that require high energy expenditure and would result in excessive motions of the lumbar spine.

More energy efficient and less structurally stressful compensations can still yield dramatic reductions in the hip abductor force.

Example 10–3
Calculating Hip Joint Compression With Lateral Lean

Returning to our hypothetical patient weighing 825 N, let us assume that they can laterally lean to the right enough to bring the line of gravity within 2.5 cm (0.025 m) of the right hip joint axis **(Fig. 10–38)**. The gravitational adduction torque would now be as follows:

$$\text{HATLL torque}_{\text{adduction}} = [5/6\ (825\ \text{N})] \times 0.025\ \text{m}$$

$$\text{HATLL torque}_{\text{adduction}} = 17.2\ \text{Nm}$$

If only 17.2 Nm of adduction torque were produced by the superimposed weight, the abductor force needed would be as follows:

$$\text{Torque}_{\text{abduction}}\text{: } 17.2\ \text{Nm} = F_{ms} \times 0.05\ \text{m}$$

$$F_{ms}\text{: } 17.2\ \text{Nm} \div 0.05\ \text{m} = 343.75\ \text{N}$$

If only ~344 N (~77 lb) of abductor force were required, the total hip joint compression in unilateral stance using the compensatory lateral lean would now be as follows:

343.75 N abductor joint compression

+ 687.5 N body weight (HATLL) compression

1,031.25 N total joint compression

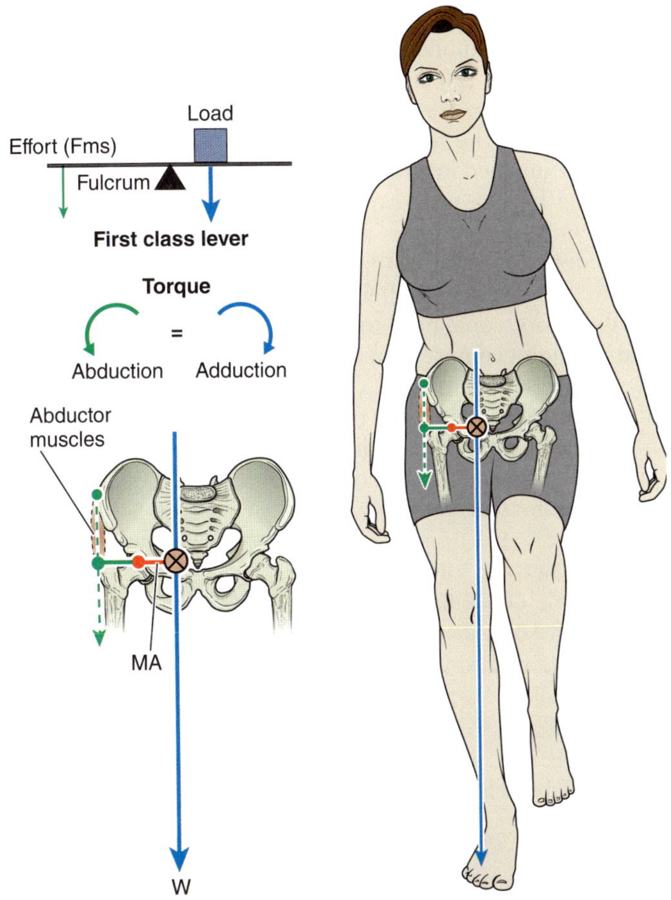

Figure 10–38 When the trunk is laterally flexed toward the right stance limb, the moment arm (MA) of HATLL is substantially reduced (e.g., 2.5 cm as compared to 10 cm with a neutral trunk), whereas that of the abductors' MA remains unchanged (e.g., 5 cm). The result is a substantially diminished torque from HATLL and, consequently, a substantially decreased need for hip abductor force to generate a counter torque.

The 1,031.25-N joint reaction force estimated in Example 10–3 is half the 2,062.5 N of hip joint compression previously calculated for our hypothetical patient in single-limb support (see Table 10–2 summary). This 50% reduction in joint compression may be enough to relieve some of the pain symptoms experienced by a person with arthritic changes in the hip joint or to provide some relief to a weak or painful set of abductors. The compensatory lean toward a painful stance limb is instinctive and commonly seen in people with hip joint disability.

Expanded Concepts 10–11
Pathological Gaits

When a lateral trunk lean toward the stance limb is seen during gait due to hip abductor muscle weakness, it is known as a **gluteus medius gait**. If the same compensation is due to hip joint pain, it is known as an **antalgic gait**. In some instances, the 344-N abductor force we calculated as necessary to stabilize the pelvis is still beyond the work capacity of very weak or completely paralyzed hip abductors. In such cases of extreme abductor muscle weakness, the pelvis will drop to the unsupported side even in the presence of a lateral trunk lean to the stance limb. If lateral lean and pelvic drop both occur during walking, the gait deviation is commonly referred to as a **Trendelenburg gait**. The lateral lean that accompanies the drop of the pelvis must be sufficient to keep the line of gravity within the supporting foot.

Whether a lateral trunk lean is due to muscular weakness or pain, a lateral lean of the trunk during walking still uses more energy than required for typical single-limb support and may result in stress changes within the lumbar spine if used over an extended time period. Use of a cane or some other assistive device offers a realistic alternative to the person with hip pain or weakness.

Use of a Cane Ipsilaterally

Pushing downward on a cane held in the hand on the side of pain or weakness should reduce the superimposed body weight by the amount of downward thrust; that is, some of the weight of HATLL would land on the cane, rather than on the weight-bearing hip joint. Inman and colleagues suggested that it is realistic to expect that someone can push down on a cane with approximately 15% of their body weight.[131] The proportion of body weight that passes through the cane will not pass through the hip joint and will not contribute to an adduction torque around the supporting hip joint.

Example 10–4
Calculating Hip Joint Compression With a Cane Ipsilaterally

If our 825-N patient can push down on the cane with 15% of their body weight, 123.75 N of body weight (825 N × 0.15) will pass through the cane. The magnitude of HATLL is thereby reduced to 563.75 N (687.5 N – 123.75 N). If the gravitational force of HATLL works through our estimated "typical" moment arm of 10 cm or 0.10 m (remember, the cane is intended to prevent the trunk lean), the torque of gravity is reduced to 56.38 Nm (563.75 N × 0.10 m). With a gravitational adduction torque of 56.38 Nm, the required force of the abductors acting through the usual 5-cm (0.05-m) moment arm is reduced to 1,127.6 N (56.38 Nm ÷ 0.05 m). The new hip joint reaction force using a cane *ipsilaterally* would then be as follows:

1,127.6 N abductor joint compression

+ 563.75 N body weight (HATLL-cane) compression

1,691.35 N total joint compression

Total hip joint compression of 1,691.35 N calculated in Example 10–4 when a cane is used ipsilaterally provides some relief over the total hip joint compression of 2,062.5 N ordinarily experienced in unilateral stance. The total hip joint compression when the cane is used ipsilaterally is still greater, however, than the total joint compression of 1,031.25 N found with a compensatory lateral trunk lean (see Table 10–2 summary). Although a cane used ipsilaterally provides some benefits in energy expenditure and structural stress reduction, it is not as effective in reducing hip joint compression as the undesirable lateral lean of the trunk. *Moving the cane to the opposite hand, however, produces substantially better results.*

Use of a Cane Contralaterally

When the cane is moved to the side opposite the painful or weak hip joint, the reduction in the magnitude of HATLL is the same as it is when the cane is used on the same side as the painful hip joint; that is, the superimposed body weight passing through the weight-bearing hip joint is reduced by approximately 15% of body weight. However, the cane is now substantially farther from the painful supporting hip joint than it would be if the cane is used on the same side; that is, in addition to relieving some of the superimposed body weight, the cane is now in a position to assist the abductor muscles in providing a counter torque to the torque of gravity.[164] A classic description of the benefit of using a cane in the hand opposite to the hip impairment presumes that the downward force on the cane acts through the full distance between the hand and the weight-bearing (impaired) hip joint.[164] We will first look at an example using the classic analysis and then determine how this analysis might be misleading.

According to the classic analysis of the value of a cane in the opposite hand in Example 10–5: Part 1, the hip joint reaction force would be due exclusively to body weight (563.75 N). This is, of course, an improvement over our calculated total hip compression with a lateral lean (1,031.25 N) and an even greater improvement over joint compression in typical unilateral stance (2,062.5 N) for a person weighing 825 N (see Table 10–2 summary).

Unfortunately, the classic treatment of biomechanics of cane use appears to overestimate substantially the effects of the cane. Krebs and colleagues (monitoring patients with an instrumented hip prosthesis) found reductions in peak pressure magnitudes of 28% to 40% during cane-assisted gait.[165] Although they reported pressures rather than forces, these values do not match the nearly 75% reduction in force that the classic calculation would indicate. Furthermore, Krebs and colleagues found a 45% reduction in gluteus medius electromyography (EMG), not an elimination of activity.[165] The discrepancy in the classic analysis and laboratory and modeling data can be resolved by examining *how* the force applied to the cane by a person provides a counter torque to gravity. Although this is conjectural, we propose that the force of the downward thrust on the cane arrives on the pelvis through an equivalent contraction of the latissimus dorsi muscle (123.75 N or 15% of body weight), which is necessary during cane use to maintain the shoulder in extension, and has an attachment to the pelvis on the posterior iliac crest, lateral to the erector spinae[28] **(Fig. 10–39)**.

Given the attachment site for the latissimus dorsi on the pelvis, the line of pull of the muscle can be approximated to have a point of application on the pelvis above the ipsilateral acetabulum (20 cm or 0.20 m from the right hip joint axis) as shown in Example 10-5: Part 2. If the adduction torque around the right weight-bearing hip continued but was of diminished magnitude because of the counter torque provided by the latissimus dorsi (123.75 × 0.20 m, or 24.75 Nm), contraction of the right hip abductors would still be needed to offset the remaining 31.63 Nm of adduction torque. Acting through their 0.05-M moment arm, the right hip abductors would need to contract with a force of 632.6 N. The total joint compression would be estimated as 1,193.35 N (see Table 10–2 summary). The hypothesized action of the latissimus dorsi on the side of the cane could account for the difference in compressive forces between classic calculations, with the cane used on the contralateral side and actual force measured in vivo.

Example 10–5
Part 1: Classic Calculation of Hip Joint Compression With a Cane Contralaterally

Our sample 825-N patient has a superimposed body weight (HATLL) of 687.5 N, of which 123.75 N (W × 0.15) passes through the cane. Consequently, 563.75 N of body weight will pass through the right stance hip joint and the gravitation adduction torque will be as follows:

$$\text{HATLL torque}_{\text{adduction}}\text{: } 563.75\ \text{N} \times 0.10\ \text{m} = 56.38\ \text{Nm}$$

The downward force on the cane of 123.75 N acts through an estimated moment arm of 50 cm (0.5 m) between the cane in the left hand and the right weight-bearing hip joint (see Fig. 10–37). The cane, therefore, would generate an opposing abduction torque as follows:

$$\text{Cane torque}_{\text{abduction}}\text{: } 123.75\ \text{N} \times 0.5 = 61.88\ \text{Nm}$$

The torque around the right stance hip produced by a cane in the left hand (61.88 Nm) exceeds the torque produced by the

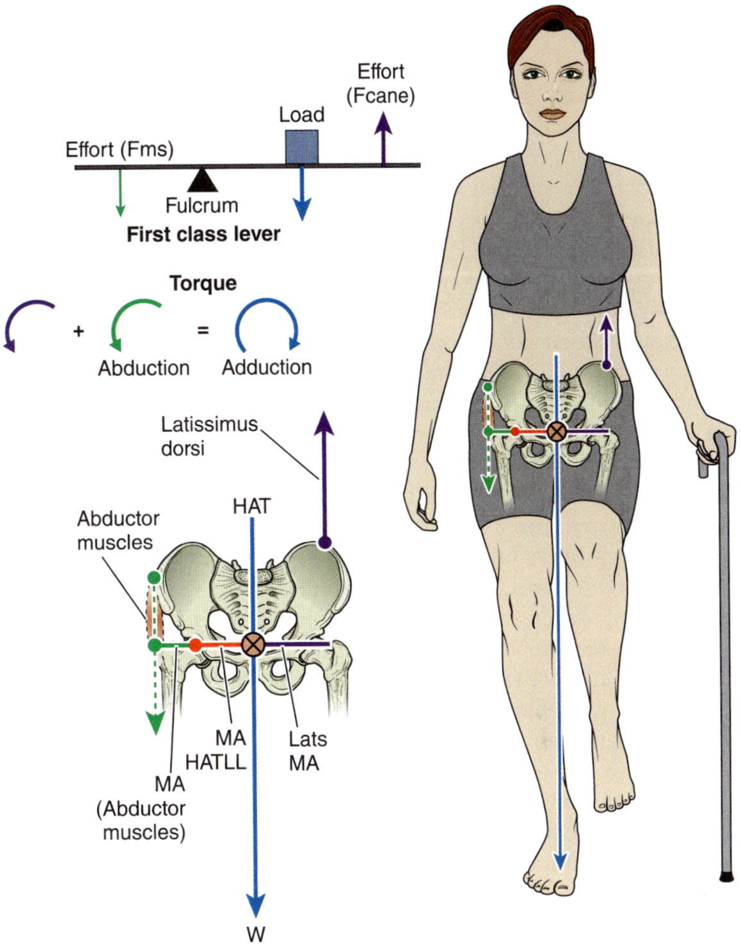

Figure 10–39 When a cane is placed in the hand opposite the painful supporting hip, the weight passing through the right hip joint is reduced, and activation of the left latissimus dorsi provides a counter torque to that of HATLL and diminishes the need for a contraction of the right hip abductors. The moment arm (MA) of the cane is erroneously estimated to be 50 cm, whereas the moment arm of the more relevant latissimus dorsi is estimated to be 20 cm.

remaining weight of HATLL (56.38 Nm). Because the gravitational torque (HATLL) may be underestimated, let us assume that the gravitational adduction torque and the counter torque provided by the cane offset each other. If the cane completely offset the adduction effect of gravity, there would be no need for hip abductor muscle force. The total hip joint compression in unilateral stance when a cane is used in the opposite hand would then be as follows:

0 N abductor joint compression

<u>+ 563.75 N body weight (HATLL-cane) compression</u>

563.75 N total joint compression

Example 10–5: Part B

Classic Calculation of Hip Joint Compression With a Cane Contralaterally Can Be Misleading

Assuming an estimated moment arm of 20 cm (0.2 m) for the latissimus dorsi muscle around the right weight-bearing hip joint, we would see an opposing abduction torque as follows:

$$\text{Latissimus dorsi torque}_{\text{abduction}}: 123.75 \text{ N} \times 0.2 = 24.75 \text{ Nm}$$

Subtracting this additional abduction torque from the HATLL $\text{torque}_{\text{adduction}}$ would leave us with 31.63 Nm of net torque for the hip abductor muscles to create. Consequently, the abductor muscle force would be 31.63 Nm ÷ 0.05 m = 632.6 N. Adding this compressive muscle force to the gravity compression force of HATLL would be as follows:

632.6 N abductor joint compression

<u>+ 563.75 N body weight (HATLL-cane) compression</u>

1,193.35 N total joint compression

This value aligns closer with experimental data (see text for further details).

Patient Application 10–7

Gabriella has osteoarthritic changes in her left hip that, if sufficient, can be a source of her pain. Furthermore, she has evidence of a labral tear, lateral hip pain, and a lean during left stance that may be at least partially attributable to degenerative changes in the gluteus medius/minimus tendons and trochanteric bursa inflammation. There is little doubt that Gabriella can benefit from reducing the demands on her left hip abductor muscles. Reduction in demand may minimize aggravation of any tears or inflammation as well as reduce hip joint compressive force that, with her hip dysplasia, are likely to be applied over a reduced area of articular contact. Using a cane in her right (i.e., contralateral) hand would be appropriate. Although a lateral lean actually reduces the demands on the hip abductors a bit more, the greater energy expenditure and structural stress on the spine must be considered.

Hip Pain Across the Life Span

Contributions to hip joint pain may arise from non-musculoskeletal, lumbosacral spine, intra-articular, and extra-articular sources.[166,167] Understanding of the complex interaction between the spine, pelvis, hip joint, and entire lower quarter is needed as lumbosacral, extra-articular, and intra-articular pathologies and impairments often coexist.[167,168] This interaction includes the labrum, articular cartilage, and the bony architecture of the acetabulum and femur, as well as the ligaments and muscles that support the hip region.

Extra-articular conditions may involve muscles, tendons, and/or nerves, while intra-articular conditions involve structures within the hip joint itself, including the labrum and articular cartilage. These hip conditions are often associated with age across the life span. Younger individuals involved in sports may be at risk for muscle-tendon injuries, particularly in muscles that cross two joints.[169] Examples of these two-joint muscles in the hip region include the hamstrings (biceps femoris long head, semitendinosus, and semimembranosus), rectus femoris, and gracilis. Middle-aged females are more likely to develop GTPS (greater trochanteric pain syndrome), while older adult females are at more risk for femoral neck fractures.[170,171] The most common intra-articular conditions include labral tears and hip arthritis.[172] Labral tears are frequently caused by abnormal bony architecture of the femur and acetabulum.[167,172] Examples of abnormal bony architecture include FAIS (femoroacetabular impingement syndrome) and acetabular dysplasia with a shallow acetabulum. Labral tears may become symptomatic in younger, more active individuals.[172] Over time, progressive overload of the labrum and articular cartilage may ultimately lead to hip osteoarthritis in older populations.[173-175] Because of the increasing interest in FAIS, acetabular dysplasia, and hip osteoarthritis, these topics will be expanded upon next.

Femoroacetabular Impingement Syndrome

FAIS is described as the dysfunctional abutment of the proximal femur and the acetabulum[176,177] **(Fig. 10–40)**. This impingement can cause a labral tear with overload of the chondrolabral and capsuloligamentous structures. Over time, this can progress to degenerative changes in the hip joint.[173,174,178,179] Individuals with FAIS commonly have motion- or position-related pain in the hip or groin, most notable in hip flexion and medial rotation. Individuals also may describe clicking, catching, locking, or giving way associated with the labral tear.[167,172] The two bony abnormalities described with FAIS syndrome are **cam- or pincer-type impingements**.[176-179] Radiographic measurements are essential in diagnosing these cam and pincer abnormalities.[167,172] Cam impingement originates from a bump or pistol-grip deformity of the femoral neck.[176-178] With this deformity, the femoral neck does not taper as it meets the femoral head laterally (see **Fig. 10–40A**). In a typical hip, the femoral head is round to allow for smooth and unrestricted movement. A cam impingement can cause excessive shear force on the acetabular rim as the bump on the femoral neck contacts the acetabular rim resulting in a labral tear.[176-178] In contrast to cam impingement, pincer impingement involves over-coverage of the acetabular rim (see **Fig. 10–40B**). This over-coverage is often caused by acetabular retroversion or a deeper acetabular fossa (coxa profunda), leading to the femoral head–neck junction directly pinching the acetabular labrum.[176-178] This contact between the femoral neck and acetabular rim in both cam and pincer deformities occurs most commonly in the position of hip flexion combined with medial rotation.[176,177] FAIS is analogous to primary subacromial impingement of the shoulder where a hooked acromion abnormally occupies more of the subacromial space to create a mechanical impingement.

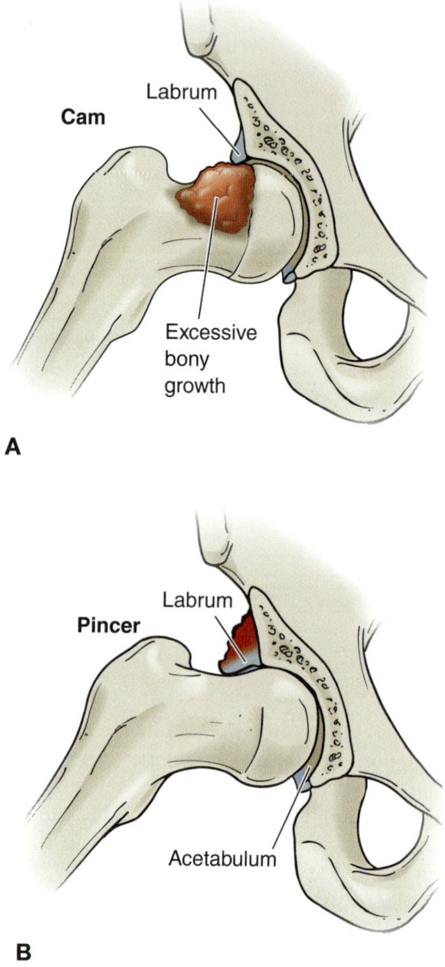

Figure 10–40 **A.** Cam impingement occurs as a result of an abnormal widening of the femoral neck that leads to the abutment of the anterior superior labrum and the articular cartilage of the acetabulum during flexion or abduction of the hip. **B.** Pincer impingement occurs as a result of an over-coverage of the acetabulum between the acetabular rim and the femoral head–neck junction with flexion or abduction.

Individuals with symptomatic FAIS present with limited motion and weakness, in addition to hip pain that limits typical function.[167,168] This presentation will be similar whether FAIS is a result of cam, pincer, or a mix of both types of deformity. Clinical practice guidelines and expert consensus statements support nonsurgical intervention as an initial intervention for those with FAIS, including physical therapist management.[167,168] This treatment should focus on neuromuscular re-education combined with stretching and strengthening exercises. While physical therapy will not be able to change the bony deformities, it may help individuals with FAIS move better to avoid the impingement. Individuals presenting with soft tissue–related ROM restrictions, strength deficits, and poor neuromuscular control are potentially good candidates for physical therapist management, particularly if they can avoid pain-provoking activities.[167,168]

There are surgical joint preservation options for those who fail conservative interventions. Hip arthroscopy with bone resection to reshape the cam and pincer, and either a labral repair or labral reconstruction to restore the suction seal, are surgical procedures that may prevent or slow down the articular cartilage degradation.[177] Significant improvements in hip pain and function during daily activities and sport have been reported following hip arthroscopy.[180,181] It has been noted that outcomes of hip arthroscopy can be negatively affected by the presence of more severe articular cartilage damage.[182]

Acetabular Dysplasia

A shallow acetabulum, a form of acetabular dysplasia, is a recognized cause of hip pain in young adults and particularly young females.[167,183] In those with acetabular dysplasia, the shallow acetabulum does not sufficiently cover the femoral head, leading to joint instability and pain during movement.[167] This instability and increased joint laxity can create a higher risk of subluxation during physical activities. Due to the inadequate coverage of the femoral head, there is an abnormal distribution of loads across the hip joint.[167] This increased pressure on the acetabular rim can lead to labral tears and progressive articular cartilage degradation.[175,184] Radiographic measurements can be used to identify those with acetabular dysplasia using the previously described center edge angle measurements (see Fig. 10–4).[12]

Treatment for acetabular dysplasia may include surgical or nonsurgical interventions. A consensus statement has outlined recommendations for a nonsurgical physical therapy program for individuals with acetabular dysplasia.[183] The program focuses on strengthening and neuromuscular control of the hip and lumbopelvic musculature with the objective of improving dynamic stability to offset the osseous instability.[183] Although physical therapy will not be able to change the bony deformities, it may improve the reliance on muscles for stability to offset the lack of bony stability. Physical therapy may play a more important role in those with mild deformities; however, even those with more severe acetabular dysplasia may undergo a trial of physical therapy.[183] Those who require surgery ultimately may have good outcomes with a periacetabular osteotomy (PAO) with concomitant hip arthroscopy. The PAO procedure reorients the acetabulum to improve femoral head coverage, while the hip arthroscopy repairs or reconstructs the labrum to restore the suction seal.[185-188]

Hip Osteoarthritis

Hip osteoarthritis (**OA**) is characterized by the degradation of articular cartilage resulting in pain and joint stiffness.[189] Radiographically, hip OA can be identified by joint space narrowing. OA is recognized as the most common cause of hip pain in those older than 50 years of age. In addition to age, previous injury to the hip joint, hip dysplasia, cam FAIS, reduced hip ROM, presence of osteophytes, lower socioeconomic status, higher bone mass, and higher BMI are risk factors for developing hip OA.[189] It was found that more than 90% of those with hip OA also had anatomic abnormalities.[190] Also, 25–50% of individuals with hip dysplasia develop OA by 50 years of age.[175] Those with hip OA clinically present with pain, decreased ROM, decreased strength, and reduced function. Specifically, this may include moderate anterior or lateral hip pain during weight-bearing activities, morning stiffness less than 1 hour in duration after wakening, hip medial rotation ROM less than 24° or medial rotation and hip flexion 15° less than the nonpainful side, and/or increased hip pain associated with passive hip medial rotation.[189]

A physical therapy clinical practice guideline provided evidence-based treatment recommendations of exercise, manual therapy, and patient education for those with a hip OA diagnosis.[189] Exercise is directed toward improving ROM, flexibility, strength, balance, and endurance as well as addressing function and gait limitations. Manual therapy aims to improve ROM deficits. Components of education include activity modification, weight reduction when overweight, and methods of unloading the arthritic joints. The overall goal of conservative therapy is to minimize joint reaction forces while improving function.[189] However, articular cartilage may continue to degrade with a progressive loss of function. Once an individual's quality of life becomes unsatisfactory and both nonsurgical and joint preservation options have been exhausted, surgery with total hip arthroplasty (**THA**) may be the final option. A THA involves replacing the articular cartilage on the femoral head and acetabulum with metal, plastic, and/or ceramic components. The outcomes of THA are good with significant pain relief, increase in hip joint mobility, and improvement in quality of life.[191,192]

Patient Application 10–8

Although we have probably covered the potential sources of Gabriella's problems fairly well at this point, it is worth reviewing the most likely underlying causes. Gabriella's persisting coxa valga and femoral anteversion are the likely sources of many, if not all, of her problems. With a valgus and anteverted femur, the articular contact within Gabriella's hip joint is substantially reduced, increasing the contact pressures and locating them atypically within the acetabulum and on the head of the femur. This is consistent with her complaints of instability and may also have contributed to her labral tear. Both her hip dysplasia and history of dance, gymnastics, and years of working at floor level with young children have exacerbated the likelihood of anterior impingement of the labrum, resulting in probable labral tear and chondral lesions. The mechanical disadvantage of her hip abductors is likely to contribute to overuse and degenerative lesions of the abductor mechanism, further affecting abductor function and resulting in a gluteus medius or antalgic gait. It appears that Gabriella's hip symptoms have been the result of an ongoing and progressive phenomenon that is leading to the early stages of joint degeneration. It likely began during repetitive movements and activities that required excessive and extremes of ROM. These repetitive movements, combined with altered hip mechanics due to her hip dysplasia, resulted in chronic and repeated trauma that damaged her anterior capsule and labrum. The degradation and plasticity of her capsule and labrum likely contributed to her feeling of instability of the hip. A labral tear can cause a leakage of joint fluid and disrupts the "seal" of the hip joint that creates intra-articular pressure that contributes to hip joint stabilization. Combined, all of these factors make an individual more susceptible to osteoarthritis. If Gabriella continues without intervention, it is likely that her pain will worsen and her joint may continue to deteriorate. This may lead to an eventual need for total joint arthroplasty. However, Gabriella is not without conservative treatment options for her current condition, including physical therapy. The emergence of hip arthroscopy combined with advancements in periacetabular osteotomy may allow postponement of the terminal procedure of a total hip arthroplasty.

SUMMARY

- The typical hip joint is well designed to withstand the large forces that act through and around it, assisted by the trabecular systems, labrum, cartilaginous coverings, muscles, and ligaments.
- Alterations in the direction or magnitude of forces acting around the hip create abnormal concentrations of stress that predispose the joint structures to injury and degenerative changes. The degenerative changes, in turn, can create additional alterations in function that not only affect the hip joint's ability to support the body weight in standing, in locomotor activities, and in other activities of daily living but may also result in adaptive changes at more proximal and distal joints.
- Consequently, the reader must understand both the dysfunction that might occur at the hip *and* the associated dysfunctions that may result in or from dysfunction elsewhere in the lower extremity and spine.

The remaining chapters of this text will focus not only on primary dysfunction at a joint complex but also on associated dysfunction related to proximal and distal joint problems.

STUDY QUESTIONS

1. Which side of the femoral neck and which side of the femoral shaft are subjected to compressive stresses during weight-bearing? How does the bone respond to these stresses?
2. What is the primary weight-bearing area of the femoral head? Of the acetabulum? Where are degenerative changes most commonly found in the femoral head and acetabulum?
3. Describe why using a cane on the side opposite hip joint pain or weakness is more effective than using the cane on the same side.
4. Demonstrate how variations in the angle of inclination affect the moment arm of the hip abductors by drawing the following: a typical angle of inclination at the hip, the angle in coxa vara, and the angle in coxa valga. Please include the action line and the moment arm of the hip abductors in the diagram.
5. Describe what would happen to the pelvis in left unilateral stance when the left hip abductors are paralyzed. How is equilibrium maintained in this situation?
6. Describe motion at the right and left hip joints and at the lumbar spine during hiking of the pelvis in right limb stance, assuming that the person is to remain upright.
7. Contrast the close-packed versus maximally congruent positions for the hip joint.
8. Calculate the minimum joint reaction force (total hip joint compression) at the right hip joint that would occur for a 200-lb person standing symmetrically on both legs versus one leg (assuming a gravitational moment arm of 4 in. and the abductor muscle moment arm of 2 in.).
9. Under what circumstances does the hip joint participate as part of an open chain? As part of a closed chain?
10. What bony abnormality or abnormalities of the femur or pelvis predispose the hip joint to the possibility of dislocation? Why?
11. Which structures at the hip joint, given their location, appear likely to limit the extremes of motion in flexion? In extension? In lateral rotation? In medial rotation? In abduction and adduction?
12. Which muscles of the hip joint are affected by knee joint position? Which position of the knee makes these muscles less effective at the hip joint?
13. If someone were in unilateral stance on the left limb, what hip joint motion would result from forward rotation of the pelvis?
14. If a person has a painful right hip, in which direction should they lean their trunk to reduce the forces on the right hip during right unilateral support? Explain the reasons for your answer.
15. What position does the hip joint tend to assume when there is joint pain? Why is this?
16. Identify several factors that might predispose someone to a femoral neck fracture.
17. How does the femoral head receive its blood supply? What problems might jeopardize that supply?
18. Relate femoral anteversion to medial femoral torsion.
19. Under what circumstances might the hip adductors work synergistically with the hip abductors?
20. Why is the acetabular notch nonarticular? In what ways does this serve hip joint function?
21. Explain the differences between cam and pincer impingement.
22. Describe how the presence of femoroacetabular impingement may lead to osteoarthritis of the hip.
23. What factors contribute to stability of the hip joint?
24. How are abnormalities at the femur and acetabulum related to femoroacetabular impingement, labral tears, and hip OA?

REFERENCES

1. Fernandes DA, Melo G, Contreras MEK, et al: Diagnostic accuracy of clinical tests and imaging exams for femoroacetabular impingement: an umbrella review of systematic reviews. Clin J Sport Med 32:635-47, 2022
2. Fabricant PD, Hirsch BP, Holmes I, et al: A radiographic study of the ossification of the posterior wall of the acetabulum: implications for the diagnosis of pediatric and adolescent hip disorders. J Bone Joint Surg Am 95:230-6, 2013
3. Daniel M, Iglic A, Kralj-Iglic V: The shape of acetabular cartilage optimizes hip contact stress distribution. J Anat 207:85-91, 2005
4. Gu D, Chen Y, Dai K, et al: The shape of the acetabular cartilage surface: a geometric morphometric study using three-dimensional scanning. Med Eng Phys 30:1024-31, 2008
5. Higgins SW, Spratley EM, Boe RA, et al: A novel approach for determining three-dimensional acetabular orientation: results from two hundred subjects. J Bone Joint Surg Am 96:1776-84, 2014

6. Köhnlein W, Ganz R, Impellizzeri FM, et al: Acetabular morphology: implications for joint-preserving surgery. Clin Orthop Relat Res 467: 682-91, 2009
7. Karachalios T, Karantanas AH, Malizos K: Hip osteoarthritis: what the radiologist wants to know. Eur J Radiol 63:36-48, 2007
8. Kim YJ, Bixby S, Mamisch TC, et al: Imaging structural abnormalities in the hip joint: instability and impingement as a cause of osteoarthritis. Semin Musculoskelet Radiol 12:334-45, 2008
9. Sautner J, Schueller-Weidekamm C: Radiological aspects of osteoarthritis. Wien Med Wochenschr 163:220-7, 2013
10. Savoye-Laurens T, Verdier N, Wettstein M, et al: Labral tears in hip dysplasia and femoroacetabular impingement: a systematic review. Orthop Traumatol Surg Res 109:103539, 2023
11. Lerch TD, Siegfried M, Schmaranzer F, et al: Location of intra- and extra-articular hip impingement is different in patients with pincer-type and mixed-type femoroacetabular impingement due to acetabular retroversion or protrusio acetabuli on 3D CT-based impingement simulation. Am J Sports Med 48:661-72, 2020
12. Wiberg G: A measuring method for distinguishing between a normal and a maldeveloped acetabulum. Acta Chir Scand 83, 1939
13. Chakraverty JK, Sullivan C, Gan C, et al: Cam and pincer femoroacetabular impingement: CT findings of features resembling femoroacetabular impingement in a young population without symptoms. AJR Am J Roentgenol 200:389-95, 2013
14. Grant AD, Sala DA, Schwarzkopf R: Femoro-acetabular impingement: the diagnosis—a review. J Child Orthop 6:1-12, 2012
15. Seldes RM, Tan V, Hunt J, et al: Anatomy, histologic features, and vascularity of the adult acetabular labrum. Clin Orthop Relat Res:232-40, 2001
16. Nepple JJ, Philippon MJ, Campbell KJ, et al: The hip fluid seal—Part II. The effect of an acetabular labral tear, repair, resection, and reconstruction on hip stability to distraction. Knee Surg Sports Traumatol Arthrosc 22:730-6, 2014
17. Alzaharani A, Bali K, Gudena R, et al: The innervation of the human acetabular labrum and hip joint: an anatomic study. BMC Musculoskelet Disord 15:41, 2014
18. Milz S, Valassis G, Büttner A, et al: Fibrocartilage in the transverse ligament of the human acetabulum. J Anat 198:223-8, 2001
19. Konrath GA, Hamel AJ, Olson SA, et al: The role of the acetabular labrum and the transverse acetabular ligament in load transmission in the hip. J Bone Joint Surg Am 80:1781-8, 1998
20. Arshad Z, Maughan HD, Sunil Kumar KH, et al: Over one third of patients with symptomatic femoroacetabular impingement display femoral or acetabular version abnormalities. Knee Surg Sports Traumatol Arthrosc 29:2825-36, 2021
21. Buller LT, Rosneck J, Monaco FM, et al: Relationship between proximal femoral and acetabular alignment in normal hip joints using 3-dimensional computed tomography. Am J Sports Med 40:367-75, 2012
22. Smith MV, Panchal HB, Ruberte Thiele RA, et al: Effect of acetabular labrum tears on hip stability and labral strain in a joint compression model. Am J Sports Med 39 Suppl:103s-10s, 2011
23. Kelly BT, Buly RL: Hip arthroscopy update. Hss j 1:40-8, 2005
24. Su T, Chen GX, Yang L: Diagnosis and treatment of labral tear. Chin Med J (Engl) 132:211-19, 2019
25. Lopes DS, Neptune RR, Gonçalves AA, et al: Shape analysis of the femoral head: a comparative study between spherical, (super)ellipsoidal, and (super) ovoidal shapes. J Biomech Eng 137:114504, 2015
26. Neilson M, White A, Malik U, et al: Changes in bone architecture in the femoral head and neck in osteoarthritis. Clin Anat 17:378-91, 2004
27. Genda E, Iwasaki N, Li G, et al: Normal hip joint contact pressure distribution in single-leg standing—effect of gender and anatomic parameters. J Biomech 34:895-905, 2001
28. Standring S: Gray's Anatomy: The Anatomical Basis of Clinical Practice (ed 42). New York, NY, Elsevier, 2020
29. Christensen AM, Leslie WD, Baim S: Ancestral differences in femoral neck axis length: possible implications for forensic anthropological analyses. Forensic Sci Int 236:193.e1-4, 2014
30. Rubin PJ, Leyvraz PF, Aubaniac JM, et al: The morphology of the proximal femur: a three-dimensional radiographic analysis. J Bone Joint Surg Br 74:28-32, 1992
31. Robertson DD, Britton CA, Latona CR, et al: Hip biomechanics: importance to functional imaging. Semin Musculoskelet Radiol 7:27-41, 2003
32. Lequesne M, Malghem J, Dion E: The normal hip joint space: variations in width, shape, and architecture on 223 pelvic radiographs. Ann Rheum Dis 63:1145-51, 2004
33. Noble PC, Box GG, Kamaric E, et al: The effect of aging on the shape of the proximal femur. Clin Orthop Relat Res:31-44, 1995
34. Noble PC, Kamaric E, Sugano N, et al: Three-dimensional shape of the dysplastic femur: implications for THR. Clin Orthop Relat Res:27-40, 2003
35. Iglic A, Antolic V, Srakar F: Biomechanical analysis of various operative hip joint rotation center shifts. Arch Orthop Trauma Surg 112:124-6, 1993
36. Redmond JM, Gupta A, Hammarstedt JE, et al: Labral injury: radiographic predictors at the time of hip arthroscopy. Arthroscopy 31:51-6, 2015
37. Coskun Benlidayi I, Guzel R, Basaran S, et al: Is coxa valga a predictor for the severity of knee osteoarthritis? A cross-sectional study. Surg Radiol Anat 37:369-76, 2015
38. Fishkin Z, Armstrong DG, Shah H, et al: Proximal femoral physis shear in slipped capital femoral epiphysis—a finite element study. J Pediatr Orthop 26:291-4, 2006
39. Kushare I, Wiltfong RE, Klingele KE: Acute, unstable slipped capital femoral epiphysis with associated congenital coxa vara. J Pediatr Orthop B 24:511-4, 2015
40. Kling TF, Jr, Hensinger RN: Angular and torsional deformities of the lower limbs in children. Clin Orthop Relat Res:136-47, 1983
41. Song KS, Choi IH, Sohn YJ, et al: Habitual dislocation of the hip in children: report of eight additional cases and literature review. J Pediatr Orthop 23:178-83, 2003
42. Wenger DE, Kendell KR, Miner MR, et al: Acetabular labral tears rarely occur in the absence of bony abnormalities. Clin Orthop Relat Res: 145-50, 2004
43. Bencardino JT, Palmer WE: Imaging of hip disorders in athletes. Radiol Clin North Am 40:267-87, vi-vii, 2002
44. Carpintero P, Leon F, Zafra M, et al: Stress fractures of the femoral neck and coxa vara. Arch Orthop Trauma Surg 123:273-7, 2003
45. Mirkopulos N, Weiner DS, Askew M: The evolving slope of the proximal femoral growth plate relationship to slipped capital femoral epiphysis. J Pediatr Orthop 8:268-73, 1988
46. Fassier F, Sardar Z, Aarabi M, et al: Results and complications of a surgical technique for correction of coxa vara in children with osteopenic bones. J Pediatr Orthop 28:799-805, 2008
47. Chotigavanichaya C, Leeprakobboon D, Eamsobhana P, et al: Results of surgical treatment of coxa vara in children: valgus osteotomy with angle blade plate fixation. J Med Assoc Thai 97 Suppl 9:S78-82, 2014
48. Gholve PA, Cameron DB, Millis MB: Slipped capital femoral epiphysis update. Curr Opin Pediatr 21:39-45, 2009
49. Nasreddine AY, Heyworth BE, Zurakowski D, et al: A reduction in body mass index lowers risk for bilateral slipped capital femoral epiphysis. Clin Orthop Relat Res 471:2137-44, 2013
50. Leunig M, Manner HM, Turchetto L, et al: Femoral and acetabular re-alignment in slipped capital femoral epiphysis. J Child Orthop 11: 131-7, 2017
51. Fabry G, MacEwen GD, Shands AR, Jr: Torsion of the femur: a follow-up study in normal and abnormal conditions. J Bone Joint Surg Am 55:1726-38, 1973
52. Svenningsen S, Apalset K, Terjesen T, et al: Regression of femoral anteversion: a prospective study of intoeing children. Acta Orthop Scand 60:170-3, 1989
53. Arnold AS, Delp SL: Rotational moment arms of the medial hamstrings and adductors vary with femoral geometry and limb position: implications for the treatment of internally rotated gait. J Biomech 34:437-47, 2001
54. Pitkow RB: External rotation contracture of the extended hip: a common phenomenon of infancy obscuring femoral neck anteversion and the most frequent cause of out-toeing gait in children. Clin Orthop Relat Res:139-45, 1975
55. Kuo TY, Skedros JG, Bloebaum RD: Measurement of femoral anteversion by biplane radiography and computed tomography imaging: comparison with an anatomic reference. Invest Radiol 38:221-9, 2003
56. Alghamdi A, Madan S, Shuweihdi F, et al: "The accuracy of the EOS imaging system to assess hip abnormalities in adolescents and adults": a systematic review and meta-analysis. Skeletal Radiol 53:29-42, 2024
57. Lee YS, Oh SH, Seon JK, et al: 3D femoral neck anteversion measurements based on the posterior femoral plane in ORTHODOC system. Med Biol Eng Comput 44:895-906, 2006
58. Blum S, Franken L, Hartmann A, et al: MRI-based static and functional assessment of complex hip deformities in comparison with CT: a validation study. Magma 33:829-38, 2020
59. Cibulka MT: Determination and significance of femoral neck anteversion. Phys Ther 84:550-8, 2004
60. Clark JM, Haynor DR: Anatomy of the abductor muscles of the hip as studied by computed tomography. J Bone Joint Surg Am 69:1021-31, 1987
61. Fabry G: Clinical practice: static, axial, and rotational deformities of the lower extremities in children. Eur J Pediatr 169:529-34, 2010
62. Bruderer-Hofstetter M, Fenner V, Payne E, et al: Gait deviations and compensations in pediatric patients with increased femoral torsion. J Orthop Res 33:155-62, 2015

63. Ito K, Minka MA, 2nd, Leunig M, et al: Femoroacetabular impingement and the cam-effect: a MRI-based quantitative anatomical study of the femoral head-neck offset. J Bone Joint Surg Br 83:171-6, 2001
64. Jackson TJ, Lindner D, El-Bitar YF, et al: Effect of femoral anteversion on clinical outcomes after hip arthroscopy. Arthroscopy 31:35-41, 2015
65. Heimann AF, Todorski IAS, Schmaranzer F, et al: What is the influence of femoral version on size, tear location, and tear pattern of the acetabular labrum in patients with FAI? Clin Orthop Relat Res 482:9, 2024
66. Ejnisman L, Philippon MJ, Lertwanich P, et al: Relationship between femoral anteversion and findings in hips with femoroacetabular impingement. Orthopedics 36:e293-300, 2013
67. Lerch TD, Antioco T, Meier MK, et al: Combined abnormalities of femoral version and acetabular version and McKibbin Index in FAI patients evaluated for hip preservation surgery. J Hip Preserv Surg 9:67-77, 2022
68. Kapandji IA: The Physiology of the Joints: Lower Limb. Philadelphia, PA, Elsevier Health Sciences, 1987
69. Wingstrand H, Wingstrand A, Krantz P: Intracapsular and atmospheric pressure in the dynamics and stability of the hip: a biomechanical study. Acta Orthop Scand 61:231-5, 1990
70. Bsat S, Frei H, Beaulé PE: The acetabular labrum: a review of its function. Bone Joint J 98-b:730-5, 2016
71. Gulati V, Eseonu K, Sayani J, et al: Developmental dysplasia of the hip in the newborn: a systematic review. World J Orthop 4:32-41, 2013
72. Mavcic B, Pompe B, Antolic V, et al: Mathematical estimation of stress distribution in normal and dysplastic human hips. J Orthop Res 20: 1025-30, 2002
73. Martin HD, Savage A, Braly BA, et al: The function of the hip capsular ligaments: a quantitative report. Arthroscopy 24:188-95, 2008
74. Wagner FV, Negrão JR, Campos J, et al: Capsular ligaments of the hip: anatomic, histologic, and positional study in cadaveric specimens with MR arthrography. Radiology 263:189-98, 2012
75. Ito H, Song Y, Lindsey DP, et al: The proximal hip joint capsule and the zona orbicularis contribute to hip joint stability in distraction. J Orthop Res 27:989-95, 2009
76. Stewart KJ, Edmonds-Wilson RH, Brand RA, et al: Spatial distribution of hip capsule structural and material properties. J Biomech 35:1491-8, 2002
77. Kalhor M, Beck M, Huff TW, et al: Capsular and pericapsular contributions to acetabular and femoral head perfusion. J Bone Joint Surg Am 91:409-18, 2009
78. Bird PA, Oakley SP, Shnier R, et al: Prospective evaluation of magnetic resonance imaging and physical examination findings in patients with greater trochanteric pain syndrome. Arthritis Rheum 44:2138-45, 2001
79. Pfirrmann CW, Chung CB, Theumann NH, et al: Greater trochanter of the hip: attachment of the abductor mechanism and a complex of three bursae—MR imaging and MR bursography in cadavers and MR imaging in asymptomatic volunteers. Radiology 221:469-77, 2001
80. Chen HH, Li AF, Li KC, et al: Adaptations of ligamentum teres in ischemic necrosis of human femoral head. Clin Orthop Relat Res:268-75, 1996
81. Fuss FK, Bacher A: New aspects of the morphology and function of the human hip joint ligaments. Am J Anat 192:1-13, 1991
82. Byrd JWT, Jones KS: Traumatic rupture of the ligamentum teres as a source of hip pain. Arthroscopy 20:385-91, 2004
83. Kivlan BR, Richard Clemente F, Martin RL, et al: Function of the ligamentum teres during multi-planar movement of the hip joint. Knee Surg Sports Traumatol Arthrosc 21:1664-8, 2013
84. Martin HD, Hatem MA, Kivlan BR, et al: Function of the ligamentum teres in limiting hip rotation: a cadaveric study. Arthroscopy 30:1085-91, 2014
85. Martin RL, Kivlan BR, Clemente FR: A cadaveric model for ligamentum teres function: a pilot study. Knee Surg Sports Traumatol Arthrosc 21:1689-93, 2013
86. O'Donnell JM, Devitt BM, Arora M: The role of the ligamentum teres in the adult hip: redundant or relevant? A review. J Hip Preserv Surg 5:15-22, 2018
87. Kaya M, Suziki T, Minowa T, et al: Ligamentum teres injury is associated with the articular damage pattern in patients with femoroacetabular impingement. Arthroscopy 30:1582-7, 2014
88. Perumal V, Woodley SJ, Nicholson HD, et al: Ligamentum teres lesions are associated with poorer patient outcomes in a large primary hip arthroscopy cohort of 1,935 patients. Arthrosc Sports Med Rehabil 4:e1363-72, 2022
89. Crock HV: An atlas of the arterial supply of the head and neck of the femur in man. Clin Orthop Relat Res:17-27, 1980
90. Tan CK, Wong WC: Absence of the ligament of head of femur in the human hip joint. Singapore Med J 31:360-3, 1990
91. Moore KL, Dalley AF, Agur AM: Clinically Oriented Anatomy. Philadelphia, PA, Lippincott Williams & Wilkins, 2013
92. Kocher MS, Tucker R: Pediatric athlete hip disorders. Clin sports med 25:241-53, viii, 2006
93. Pienkowski D, Resig J, Talwalkar V, et al: Novel three-dimensional MRI technique for study of cartilaginous hip surfaces in Legg-Calvé-Perthes disease. J Orthop Res 27:981-8, 2009
94. Hewitt JD, Glisson RR, Guilak F, et al: The mechanical properties of the human hip capsule ligaments. J Arthroplasty 17:82-9, 2002
95. Hidaka E, Aoki M, Izumi T, et al: Ligament strain on the iliofemoral, pubofemoral, and ischiofemoral ligaments in cadaver specimens: biomechanical measurement and anatomical observation. Clin Anat 27:1068-75, 2014
96. Martin HD, Khoury AN, Schröder R, et al: Contribution of the pubofemoral ligament to hip stability: a biomechanical study. Arthroscopy 33:305-13, 2017
97. Baba K, Chiba D, Mori Y, et al: Impacts of external rotators and the ischiofemoral ligament on preventing excessive internal hip rotation: a cadaveric study. J Orthop Surg Res 17:4, 2022
98. Domb BG, Philippon MJ, Giordano BD: Arthroscopic capsulotomy, capsular repair, and capsular plication of the hip: relation to atraumatic instability. Arthroscopy 29:162-73, 2013
99. Kivlan BR, Carroll L, Burfield A, et al: Length change of the iliofemoral ligament during tests for anterior microinstability of the hip joint: a cadaveric validity study. Int J Sports Phys Ther 14:613-22, 2019
100. Athanasiou KA, Agarwal A, Dzida FJ: Comparative study of the intrinsic mechanical properties of the human acetabular and femoral head cartilage. J Orthop Res 12:340-9, 1994
101. Greenspan A: Orthopedic Imaging: A Practical Approach. Philadelphia, PA, Lippincott Williams & Wilkins, 2011
102. Heller MO, Bergmann G, Deuretzbacher G, et al: Influence of femoral anteversion on proximal femoral loading: measurement and simulation in four patients. Clin Biomech (Bristol, Avon) 16:644-9, 2001
103. Crabtree N, Loveridge N, Parker M, et al: Intracapsular hip fracture and the region-specific loss of cortical bone: analysis by peripheral quantitative computed tomography. J Bone Miner Res 16:1318-28, 2001
104. Bombelli R, Santore RF, Poss R: Mechanics of the normal and osteoarthritic hip: a new perspective. Clin Orthop Relat Res:69-78, 1984
105. Sánchez Egea AJ, Valera M, Parraga Quiroga JM, et al: Impact of hip anatomical variations on the cartilage stress: a finite element analysis towards the biomechanical exploration of the factors that may explain primary hip arthritis in morphologically normal subjects. Clin Biomech (Bristol, Avon) 29:444-50, 2014
106. Norkin CC, White DJ: Measurement of Joint Motion: a Guide to Goniometry. Philadelphia, PA, FA Davis, 2009
107. Nonaka H, Mita K, Watakabe M, et al: Age-related changes in the interactive mobility of the hip and knee joints: a geometrical analysis. Gait Posture 15:236-43, 2002
108. Roach SM, San Juan JG, Suprak DN, et al: Passive hip range of motion is reduced in active subjects with chronic low back pain compared to controls. Int J Sports Phys Ther 10:13-20, 2015
109. Valmassy RL: Clinical Biomechanics of the Lower Extremities. Philadelphia, PA, Mosby Inc, 1995
110. Kendall F, McCreary E, Provance P: Muscles: Testing and Function. Baltimore, MD, Williams and Wilkins, 1993
111. Uemura K, Atkins PR, Peters CL, et al: The effect of pelvic tilt on three-dimensional coverage of the femoral head: a computational simulation study using patient-specific anatomy. Anat Rec (Hoboken) 304:258-65, 2021
112. Dandachli W, Ul Islam S, Richards R, et al: The influence of pelvic tilt on acetabular orientation and cover: a three-dimensional computerised tomography analysis. Hip Int 23:87-92, 2013
113. Bohannon R, Gajdosik R, LeVeau BF: Contribution of pelvic and lower limb motion to increases in the angle of passive straight leg raising. Phys Ther 65:474-6, 1985
114. Murray R, Bohannon R, Tiberio D, et al: Pelvifemoral rhythm during unilateral hip flexion in standing. Clin Biomech (Bristol, Avon) 17: 147-51, 2002
115. Mens JM, Vleeming A, Snijders CJ, et al: Validity of the active straight leg raise test for measuring disease severity in patients with posterior pelvic pain after pregnancy. Spine (Phila Pa 1976) 27:196-200, 2002
116. Scaia V, Baxter D, Cook C: The pain provocation-based straight leg raise test for diagnosis of lumbar disc herniation, lumbar radiculopathy, and/or sciatica: a systematic review of clinical utility. J Back Musculoskelet Rehabil 25:215-23, 2012
117. Gowitzke BA, Milner M: Scientific Bases of Human Movement. Philadelphia, PA, Williams & Wilkins, 1988
118. Khoury AN, Hatem M, Bowler J, et al: Hip-spine syndrome: rationale for ischiofemoral impingement, femoroacetabular impingement and

abnormal femoral torsion leading to low back pain. J Hip Preserv Surg 7:390-400, 2020
119. Basmajian JV, De Luca C: Muscles Alive: Their Functions Revealed by Electromyography. Baltimore, MD, Williams & Wilkins 1985
120. Delp SL, Hess WE, Hungerford DS, et al: Variation of rotation moment arms with hip flexion. J Biomech 32:493-501, 1999
121. Németh G, Ohlsén H: In vivo moment arm lengths for hip extensor muscles at different angles of hip flexion. J Biomech 18:129-40, 1985
122. Smith L, Weiss E, Lehmkuhl L: Muscle activity and strength. In Brunnstrom's Clinical Kinesiology. Philadelphia, PA, FA Davis, 1996
123. Wheatley MD, Jahnke WD: Electromyographic study of the superficial thigh and hip muscles in normal individuals. Arch Phys Med Rehabil 32:508-15, 1951
124. Birnbaum K, Siebert CH, Pandorf T, et al: Anatomical and biomechanical investigations of the iliotibial tract. Surg Radiol Anat 26:433-46, 2004
125. Kaplan EB: The iliotibial tract: clinical and morphological significance. J Bone Joint Surg Am 40-a:817-32, 1958
126. Radin EL: Biomechanics of the human hip. Clin Orthop Relat Res: 28-34, 1980
127. Gajdosik RL, Sandler MM, Marr HL: Influence of knee positions and gender on the Ober test for length of the iliotibial band. Clin Biomech (Bristol, Avon) 18:77-9, 2003
128. Walker P, Ellis E, Scofield J, et al: Snapping hip syndrome: a comprehensive update. Orthop Rev (Pavia) 13:25088, 2021
129. Ito J: Morphological analysis of the human lower extremity based on the relative muscle weight. Okajimas Folia Anat Jpn 73:247-51, 1996
130. Nicholas SJ, Tyler TF: Adductor muscle strains in sport. Sports Med 32:339-44, 2002
131. Inman VT, Ralston HJ, Todd F: Human Walking. Philadelphia, PA, Williams & Wilkins, 1981
132. Chleboun GS, France AR, Crill MT, et al: In vivo measurement of fascicle length and pennation angle of the human biceps femoris muscle. Cells Tissues Organs 169:401-9, 2001
133. Bunker TD, Esler CN, Leach WJ: Rotator-cuff tear of the hip. J Bone Joint Surg Br 79:618-20, 1997
134. Kagan A, 2nd: Rotator cuff tears of the hip. Clin Orthop Relat Res: 135-40, 1999
135. LaBan MM, Weir SK, Taylor RS: 'Bald trochanter' spontaneous rupture of the conjoined tendons of the gluteus medius and minimus presenting as a trochanteric bursitis. Am J Phys Med Rehabil 83:806-9, 2004
136. Robertson WJ, Gardner MJ, Barker JU, et al: Anatomy and dimensions of the gluteus medius tendon insertion. Arthroscopy 24:130-6, 2008
137. Soderberg GL, Dostal WF: Electromyographic study of three parts of the gluteus medius muscle during functional activities. Physical Therapy 58:691-6, 1978
138. Walters J, Solomons M, Davies J: Gluteus minimus: observations on its insertion. J Anat 198:239-42, 2001
139. Beck M, Sledge JB, Gautier E, et al: The anatomy and function of the gluteus minimus muscle. J Bone Joint Surg Br 82:358-63, 2000
140. Gottschalk F, Kourosh S, Leveau B: The functional anatomy of tensor fasciae latae and gluteus medius and minimus. J Anat 166:179-89, 1989
141. Jensen RH, Smidt GL, Johnston RC: A technique for obtaining measurements of force generated by hip muscles. Arch Phys Med Rehabil 52:207-15, 1971
142. Olson VL, Smidt GL, Johnston RC: The maximum torque generated by the eccentric, isometric, and concentric contractions of the hip abductor muscles. Phys Ther 52:149-58, 1972
143. Murray MP, Sepic SB: Maximum isometric torque of hip abductor and adductor muscles. Phys Ther 48:1327-35, 1968
144. Xie P, István B, Liang M: The relationship between patellofemoral pain syndrome and hip biomechanics: a systematic review with meta-analysis. Healthcare (Basel) 11, 2022
145. Amaro A, Amado F, Duarte JA, et al: Gluteus medius muscle atrophy is related to contralateral and ipsilateral hip joint osteoarthritis. Int J Sports Med 28:1035-9, 2007
146. Redmond JM, Chen AW, Domb BG: Greater trochanteric pain syndrome. J Am Acad Orthop Surg 24:231-40, 2016
147. Speers CJ, Bhogal GS: Greater trochanteric pain syndrome: a review of diagnosis and management in general practice. Br J Gen Pract 67: 479-80, 2017
148. Strauss EJ, Nho SJ, Kelly BT: Greater trochanteric pain syndrome. Sports Med Arthrosc Rev 18:113-9, 2010
149. Segal NA, Felson DT, Torner JC, et al: Greater trochanteric pain syndrome: epidemiology and associated factors. Arch Phys Med Rehabil 88:988-92, 2007
150. Lievense A, Bierma-Zeinstra S, Schouten B, et al: Prognosis of trochanteric pain in primary care. Br J Gen Pract 55:199-204, 2005
151. Silva F, Adams T, Feinstein J, et al: Trochanteric bursitis: refuting the myth of inflammation. J Clin Rheumatol 14:82-6, 2008
152. Williams BS, Cohen SP: Greater trochanteric pain syndrome: a review of anatomy, diagnosis and treatment. Anesthesia and Analgesia 108: 1662-70, 2009
153. Haliloglu N, Inceoglu D, Sahin G: Assessment of peritrochanteric high T2 signal depending on the age and gender of the patients. Eur J Radiol 75:64-6, 2010
154. Martin HD, Reddy M, Gómez-Hoyos J: Deep gluteal syndrome. J Hip Preserv Surg 2:99-107, 2015
155. Martin HD, Shears SA, Johnson JC, et al: The endoscopic treatment of sciatic nerve entrapment/deep gluteal syndrome. Arthroscopy 27:172-81, 2011
156. Fabrocini B MN: A comparison between the rotator cuffs of the shoulder and hip. Strength Con J 25, 2003
157. Nordin M, Frankel VH: Basic Biomechanics of the Musculoskeletal System. Philadelphia, PA, Lippincott Williams & Wilkins, 2001
158. Bergmann G, Graichen F, Rohlmann A, et al: Hip joint forces during load carrying. Clin Orthop and Related Res:190-201, 1997
159. LeVeau BF, Williams M: Williams & Lissner's Biomechanics of Human Motion. Philadelphia, PA, WB Saunders company, 1992
160. Davy DT, Kotzar GM, Brown RH, et al: Telemetric force measurements across the hip after total arthroplasty. J Bone Joint Surg Am 70:45-50, 1988
161. Anderson FC, Pandy MG: Static and dynamic optimization solutions for gait are practically equivalent. J Biomech 34:153-61, 2001
162. Fraysse F, Dumas R, Cheze L, et al: Comparison of global and joint-to-joint methods for estimating the hip joint load and the muscle forces during walking. J Biomech 42:2357-62, 2009
163. Lenaerts G, Bartels W, Gelaude F, et al: Subject-specific hip geometry and hip joint centre location affects calculated contact forces at the hip during gait. J Biomech 42:1246-51, 2009
164. Blount WP: Don't throw away the cane. J Bone Joint Surg Am 38-a:695-708, 1956
165. Krebs DE, Robbins CE, Lavine L, et al: Hip biomechanics during gait. J Orthop Sports Phys Ther 28:51-9, 1998
166. Gomez-Hoyos J, Martin RL, Martin HD: Current concepts review: evaluation and management of posterior hip pain. J Am Acad Orthop Surg 26:597-609, 2018
167. Enseki KR, Bloom NJ, Harris-Hayes M, et al: Hip pain and movement dysfunction associated with nonarthritic hip joint pain: a revision. J Orthop Sports Phys Ther 53:CPG1-70, 2023
168. Takla A, O'Donnell J, Voight M, et al: The 2019 International Society of Hip Preservation (ISHA) physiotherapy agreement on assessment and treatment of femoroacetabular impingement syndrome (FAIS): an international consensus statement. J Hip Preserv Surg 7:631-42, 2020
169. Mueller-Wohlfahrt HW, Haensel L, Mithoefer K, et al: Terminology and classification of muscle injuries in sport: the Munich consensus statement. Br J Sports Med 47:342-50, 2013
170. Disantis AE, Martin RL: Classification based treatment of greater trochanteric pain syndrome (GTPS) with integration of the movement system. Int J Sports Phys Ther 17:508-18, 2022
171. McDonough CM, Harris-Hayes M, Kristensen MT, et al: Physical therapy management of older adults with hip fracture. J Orthop Sports Phys Ther 51:CPG1-81, 2021
172. Griffin DR, Dickenson EJ, O'Donnell J, et al: The Warwick Agreement on femoroacetabular impingement syndrome (FAI syndrome): an international consensus statement. Br J Sports Med 50:1169-76, 2016
173. Agricola R, Heijboer MP, Bierma-Zeinstra SM, et al: Cam impingement causes osteoarthritis of the hip: a nationwide prospective cohort study (CHECK). Ann Rheum Dis 72:918-23, 2013
174. Thomas GE, Palmer AJ, Batra RN, et al: Subclinical deformities of the hip are significant predictors of radiographic osteoarthritis and joint replacement in women: a 20 year longitudinal cohort study. Osteoarthritis Cartilage 22:1504-10, 2014
175. Cooperman D: What is the evidence to support acetabular dysplasia as a cause of osteoarthritis? J Pediatr Orthop 33 Suppl 1:S2-7, 2013
176. Egger AC, Frangiamore S, Rosneck J: Femoroacetabular impingement: a review. Sports Med Arthrosc Rev 24:e53-8, 2016
177. Fortier LM, Popovsky D, Durci MM, et al: An updated review of femoroacetabular impingement syndrome. Orthop Rev (Pavia) 14:37513, 2022
178. Ganz R, Parvizi J, Beck M, et al: Femoroacetabular impingement: a cause for osteoarthritis of the hip. Clin Orthop Relat Res:112-20, 2003
179. Beck M, Kalhor M, Leunig M, et al: Hip morphology influences the pattern of damage to the acetabular cartilage: femoroacetabular

impingement as a cause of early osteoarthritis of the hip. J Bone Joint Surg Br 87:1012-8, 2005
180. Gohal C, Shamshoon S, Memon M, et al: Health-related quality of life after hip arthroscopy for femoroacetabular impingement: a systematic review and meta-analysis. Sports Health 11:209-17, 2019
181. Rahl MD, LaPorte C, Steinl GK, et al: Outcomes after arthroscopic hip labral reconstruction: a systematic review and meta-analysis. Am J Sports Med 48:1748-55, 2020
182. Spencer AD, Hagen MS: Predicting outcomes in hip arthroscopy for femoroacetabular impingement syndrome. Curr Rev Musculoskelet Med 17:59-67, 2024
183. Disantis AE, Martin RL, Enseki K, et al: Non-operative rehabilitation principles for use in individuals with acetabular dysplasia: a North American based Delphi study. Int J Sports Phys Ther 18:1331-45, 2023
184. Casartelli NC, Maffiuletti NA, Valenzuela PL, et al: Is hip morphology a risk factor for developing hip osteoarthritis? A systematic review with meta-analysis. Osteoarthritis Cartilage 29:1252-64, 2021
185. Jimenez AE, Lee MS, Owens JS, et al: Athletes undergoing concomitant hip arthroscopy and periacetabular osteotomy demonstrate greater than 80% return-to-sport rate at 2-year minimum follow-up. Arthroscopy 38:2649-58, 2022
186. Ellis T, Kohlrieser D, Rao B, et al: A comparison of 6-month outcomes between periacetabular osteotomy with concomitant hip arthroscopy to isolated hip arthroscopy for femoroacetabular impingement. Arch Orthop Trauma Surg 142:471-80, 2022
187. Lee MS, Fong S, Owens JS, et al: Outcomes after concomitant hip arthroscopy and periacetabular osteotomy: a systematic review. Orthop J Sports Med 11:23259671231160559, 2023
188. Maldonado DR, LaReau JM, Perets I, et al: Outcomes of hip arthroscopy with concomitant periacetabular osteotomy, minimum 5-year follow-up. Arthroscopy 35:826-34, 2019
189. Cibulka MT, Bloom NJ, Enseki KR, et al: Hip pain and mobility deficits—hip osteoarthritis: revision 2017. J Orthop Sports Phys Ther 47:A1-A37, 2017
190. Hunter DJ, Wilson DR: Role of alignment and biomechanics in osteoarthritis and implications for imaging. Radiol Clin North Am 47:553-66, 2009
191. Mei XY, Gong YJ, Safir O, et al: Long-term outcomes of total hip arthroplasty in patients younger than 55 years: a systematic review of the contemporary literature. Can J Surg 62:249-58, 2019
192. Callaghan JJ, Bracha P, Liu SS, et al: Survivorship of a Charnley total hip arthroplasty: a concise follow-up, at a minimum of thirty-five years, of previous reports. J Bone Joint Surg Am 91:2617-21, 2009

The Knee

Elanna K. Arhos, PT, DPT, PhD | Miriam F. Hazlett, PT, DPT, MBA | Laura C. Schmitt, PT, PhD, FAPTA

CHAPTER OUTLINE

INTRODUCTION 353

TIBIOFEMORAL JOINT STRUCTURE AND FUNCTION 353

- Structure 353
  - Femur 353
  - Tibia 354
  - Tibiofemoral Alignment and Weight-Bearing Forces 354
  - Menisci 356
  - Joint Capsule 358
  - Ligaments 361
  - Iliotibial Band 367
  - Bursae 368
- Function 368
  - Joint Kinematics 368
  - Muscles 374
  - Stabilizers of the Knee 380

PATELLOFEMORAL JOINT 380

- Tibiofemoral (Knee) Joint Motion and Patellar Contact 380
- Motions of the Patella 381
- Patellar Function 384
- Patellofemoral Joint Stress 384
- Quadriceps Strengthening Exercises and Patellofemoral Pain 386
- Patellar Motion and Medial/Lateral Patellar Restraints 387
- Lateral Bias of Patellar Motion 388

LIFE SPAN AND CLINICAL CONSIDERATIONS 390

- Tibiofemoral Joint Injury 390
- Patellofemoral Joint Injury 390

SUMMARY 391

STUDY QUESTIONS 391

REFERENCES 391

ANATOMY OVERVIEW

MUSCLE ACTIONS OF THE KNEE JOINT

TABLE KEY: Primary muscle | Secondary muscles

Sagittal Plane	Flexion	Extension
	Semimembranosus (primary) Semitendinosus (primary) Biceps femoris (long and short heads) (primary) Sartorius (secondary) Gracilis (secondary) Popliteus (secondary) Gastrocnemius (secondary)	Vastus lateralis (primary) Vastus medialis (primary) Vastus intermedius (primary) Rectus femoris (primary)
Transverse Plane	**Medial Rotation**	**Lateral Rotation**
	Popliteus (secondary) Semimembranosus (secondary) Semitendinosus (secondary) Sartorius (secondary) Gracilis (secondary)	Biceps femoris (secondary)

KNEE MUSCLE ATTACHMENT

Muscle	Proximal Attachment	Distal Attachment
Rectus femoris	Anterior inferior iliac spine (AIIS) and ilium superior to acetabulum	Quadriceps tendon to patella and ultimately tibial tuberosity
Vastus lateralis	Greater trochanter and lateral lip of linea aspera (femur)	Quadriceps tendon to patella and ultimately tibial tuberosity
Vastus medialis	Intertrochanteric line and medial lip of linea aspera (femur)	Quadriceps tendon to patella and ultimately tibial tuberosity
Vastus intermedius	Anterior and lateral surfaces of shaft of femur	Quadriceps tendon to patella and ultimately tibial tuberosity
Sartorius	Anterior superior iliac spine (ASIS) and superior part of notch inferior to it	Superior part of medial surface of tibia
Gracilis	Body and inferior ramus of pubis	Superior part of medial surface of tibia
Tensor faciae latae	ASIS; anterior part of iliac crest	Iliotibial (IT) band to lateral condyle of tibia
Semitendinosus	Ischial tuberosity	Medial surface of superior part of tibia
Semimembranosus	Ischial tuberosity	Posterior aspect of medial condyle of tibia; reflected attachment forms oblique popliteal ligament (to lateral femoral condyle)
Biceps femoris	Long head: Ischial tuberosity Short head: Linea aspera and lateral supracondylar line of femur	Lateral side of head of fibula
Gastrocnemius	Lateral head: Lateral aspect of lateral condyle of femur Medial head: Popliteal surface of femur; superior to medial condyle	Posterior surface of calcaneus via calcaneal tendon
Popliteus	Lateral surface of lateral condyle of femur and lateral meniscus	Posterior surface of tibia, superior to soleal line

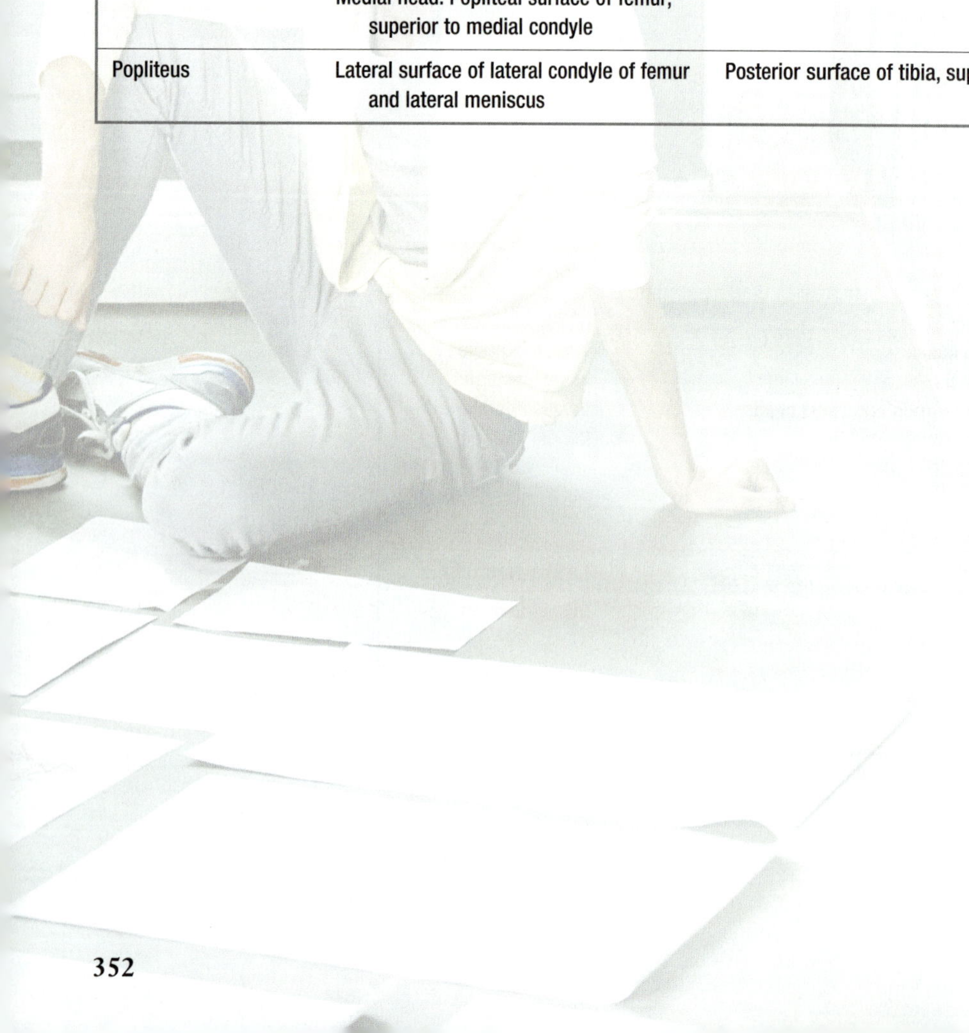

Introduction

The knee complex is one of the most often injured regions in the human body and the most frequently injured joint during sports activities.[1] The myriad ligamentous attachments, along with numerous muscles crossing the joint, provide insight into the joint's complexity. This anatomic complexity allows for elaborate interplay between the simultaneous mobility and stability roles required of the knee complex. The knee joint works in conjunction with the hip, ankle, and joints in the feet to support the body's weight during static erect posture. Dynamically, the knee complex is responsible for moving and supporting the body during a variety of both routine and difficult activities. The knee joint is a weight-bearing joint that works as part of closed and open chains, along with the hip and ankle, to transmit and absorb forces and to shorten and lengthen the lower extremity. The knee's complex structure and multiple functions reflect its major roles in stability and mobility that are needed to complete many human movements.

The knee complex is composed of two distinct articulations located within a single joint capsule: the tibiofemoral joint and the patellofemoral joint. The **tibiofemoral joint** is the articulation between the distal femur and the proximal tibia. Unlike the hip joint, the tibiofemoral articulation is incongruent, requiring the stability of the joint to come from soft tissue restraints rather than bony congruency. The **patellofemoral joint** is the articulation between the distal femur and the posterior patella. Although the patella enhances the effectiveness of the tibiofemoral mechanism, the characteristics, responses, and challenges of the patellofemoral joint are uniquely different from the tibiofemoral joint, warranting separate attention within this chapter. Also, despite its adjacent location, the superior tibiofibular joint is not considered to be a part of the knee complex because it is not contained within the knee joint capsule. Its function serves the ankle joint and will be discussed in Chapter 12.

Tibiofemoral Joint Structure and Function

The tibiofemoral, or knee, joint is a large synovial joint with three rotary degrees of freedom. The knee is classified as a double condyloid joint due to its two condyloid articulations between each condyle of the femur and the corresponding plateau of the tibia. Flexion and extension occur in the sagittal plane around a coronal axis through the epicondyles of the distal femur; medial/lateral rotation occurs in the transverse plane about a longitudinal axis and abduction and adduction occur in the frontal plane around an anteroposterior (A-P) axis.[2-4] The double condyloid knee joint is defined by its medial and lateral articular surfaces, also referred to as the **medial** and **lateral compartments** of the knee **(Fig. 11–1)**.

Structure

A full understanding of the tibiofemoral joint's common functions and dysfunctions requires careful examination of its articular surfaces, ligaments, and musculotendinous structures, along with an understanding of their relationship to each other.

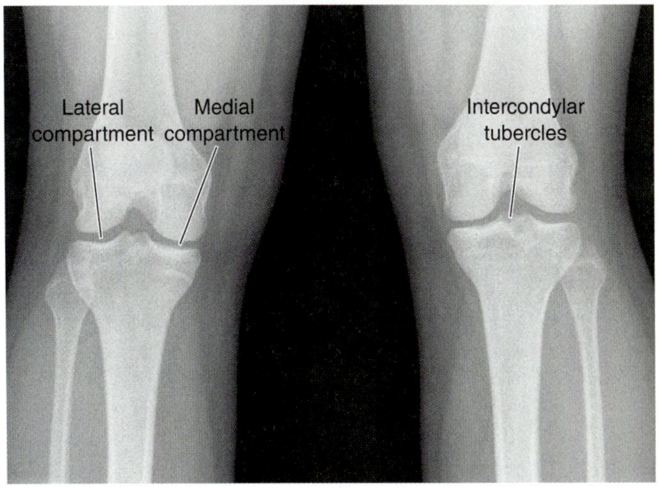

Figure 11–1 A weight-bearing knee radiograph showing the medial and lateral tibiofemoral (knee) compartments. The medial and lateral compartments are separated centrally by the intercondylar tubercles.

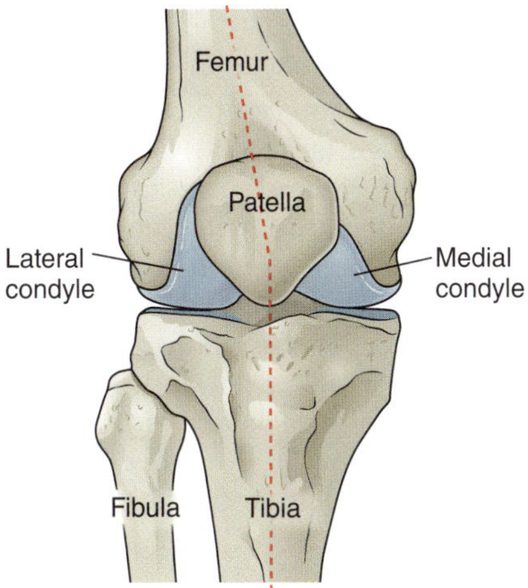

Figure 11–2 Because of the obliquity of the shaft of the femur, the medial condyle extends more distally to align horizontally with the lateral femoral condyle. The medial and lateral knee joint compartments can be appreciated, while only some of the concavity of the femoral condyles can be seen in this view.

Femur

The proximal articular surface of the knee joint is composed of the large medial and lateral condyles of the distal femur **(Fig. 11–2)**. If the shaft of the femur were observed in a true vertical position, it could be seen that the medial condyle extends farther distally than the lateral condyle.[5] However, because of the natural *oblique* angle of the shaft of the femur, the two femoral condyles sit horizontally on the tibial plateau, with both the medial and lateral condyles individually exhibiting a slight frontal plane convexity (see Fig. 11-2). In the sagittal plane, the condyles have a convex shape, with the radius of curvature posteriorly smaller and less spherically shaped than anteriorly[3,6] **(Fig. 11–3)**. There are also important size and positional differences between the medial and lateral femoral condyles **(Fig. 11–4)**. The lateral femoral articular

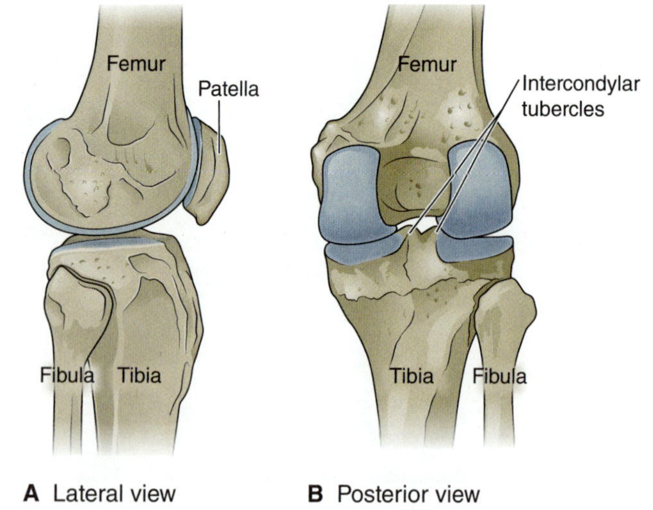

Figure 11–3 **A.** The lateral view of the tibiofemoral joint shows that the anteroposterior convexity of the condyles is not consistently spherical, having a smaller radius of curvature posteriorly. The tibial plateau is inclined posteriorly 7° to 10°. **B.** Viewed from the back, the large curvature of the femoral condyles can be easily distinguished, along with the interposed tibial tubercles on the tibial plateau.

surface is shorter from anterior to posterior than that of the medial femoral condyle (see **Fig. 11-4A**), as is also reflected on the corresponding articulating surfaces of the tibia[7] (see **Fig. 11-4B**). Although the lateral femoral condyle appears at first glance to be longer, when the patellofemoral surface is excluded, it is evident that the medial tibial surface of the femur extends farther anteriorly than the lateral condyle. The two femoral condyles are separated inferiorly by the **intercondylar notch** through most of their length but are joined anteriorly by an asymmetric, shallow groove called the **femoral sulcus, patellar groove**, or **patellar surface** (see Fig. 11–4A).

Tibia

The large convex femoral condyles sit on the relatively flat tibial condyles. The asymmetrical medial and lateral tibial condyles or plateaus compose the distal articular surface of the tibiofemoral joint (see Fig. 11–4B). Similar to the distal femur, the medial tibial articular surface is longer in the anteroposterior direction than the lateral; however, the lateral tibial articular cartilage is thicker than the articular cartilage of the medial tibial plateau.[6,8,9] The proximal tibia is larger than the tibial shaft, thus overhanging the tibial shaft posteriorly, with an associated posterior tilt of the tibial plateau 7° to 10° off horizontal (see Fig. 11–3A)—a factor that contributes to flexing the tibiofemoral (knee) joint as we shall see.[6,7] The medial and lateral tibial condyles are separated by a roughened area and two bony spines called the **intercondylar tubercles** (see Figs. 11–1 and 11–3B). These tubercles become lodged in the intercondylar notch of the femur when the knee is in an extended position. The predominantly flat tibial plateaus, with a slight convexity at the anterior and posterior margins, in combination with the convex femoral condyles, create a bony architecture that is very incongruent, thus necessitating accessory joint structures (menisci) to enhance joint congruency and stability.[3]

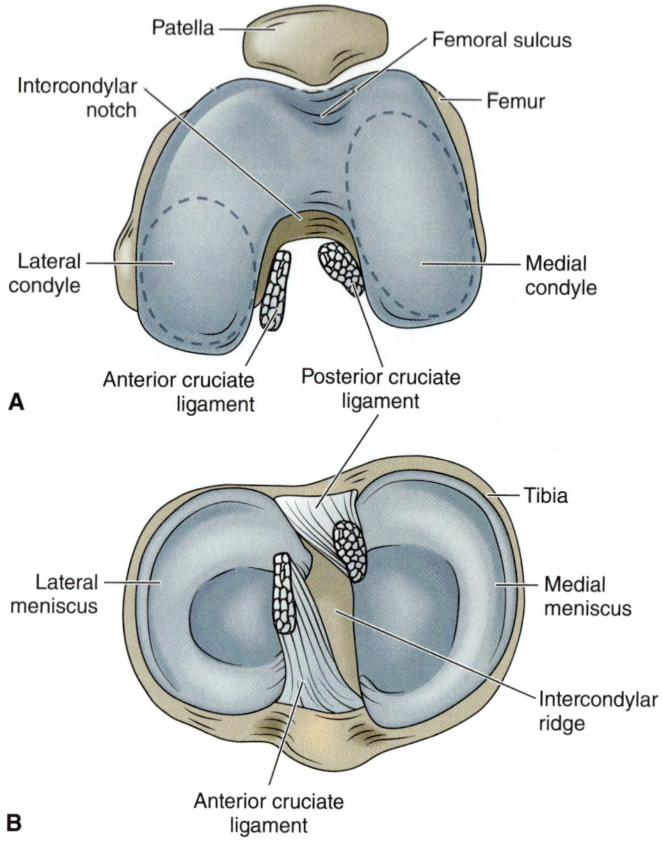

Figure 11–4 Knee complex articular surfaces. **A.** An inferior view of the femur shows the unequal lengths of the circumscribed medial and lateral articular surfaces, as well as the intercondylar notch of the femur that separates its articular surfaces. The articulating surfaces for the lateral and medial patellar facets are separated by the femoral sulcus. **B.** In this superior view of the tibial plateau, the larger medial plateau is separated from the smaller lateral surface by the intercondylar ridge.

Tibiofemoral Alignment and Weight-Bearing Forces

The **anatomic (longitudinal) axis** of the femur is oblique and directed inferiorly and medially from its proximal to distal end, while the longitudinal axis of the tibia is directed almost vertically **(Fig. 11–5)**. Consequently, the femoral and tibial anatomic axes typically form an angle medially at the knee joint of approximately 185°; that is, the femur is typically angled up to 5° off vertical, creating a slight physiological valgus angle at the knee (see **Fig. 11–5A**).[10] Genu valgum, or valgus malalignment, exists when the medial tibiofemoral angle is greater than 185°, resulting in a deviation of the knee joint toward the midline of the body commonly known as "knock-knees" (see **Fig. 11–5B**). Genu varum, or varus malalignment, exists when the medial tibiofemoral angle is 175° or less, resulting in deviation of the knee joint away from the midline of the body, commonly known as "bowlegs" (see **Fig. 11–5C**). Each condition alters the compressive stress on the medial and lateral compartments of the knee joint.

Frontal plane knee malalignment has important clinical implications due to its strong association with the incidence

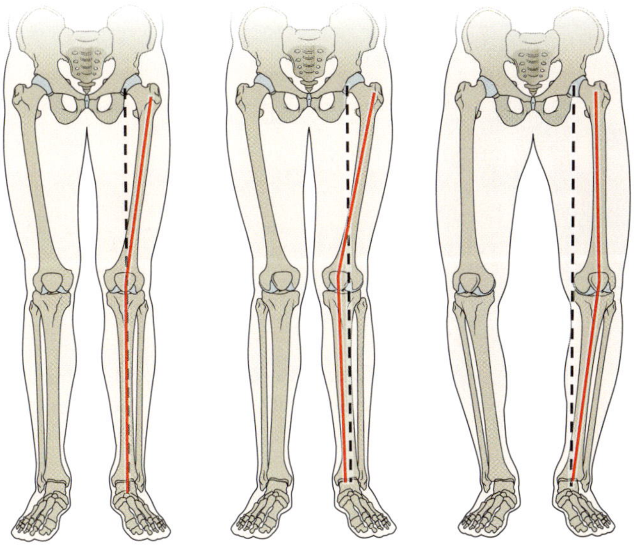

Figure 11–5 **A.** The anatomic axes of the femur and tibia result in a normal physiological valgus angulation of approximately 185° (red lines), with weight-bearing (compression) forces equally distributed on the medial and lateral aspects of the tibiofemoral joint as indicated by the dashed weight-bearing line at the knee joint. **B.** An increase in the typical tibiofemoral angle (red lines) results in genu valgum, or valgus malalignment of the knee joint. Weight-bearing forces are thereby increased on the lateral aspect of the tibiofemoral joint, as indicated by the location of the dashed weight-bearing line. **C.** A decrease in the typical tibiofemoral angle (red lines) results in genu varum, or varus malalignment of the knee joint. Here, weight-bearing forces are increased medially, as indicated by the location of the dashed weight-bearing line.

and progression of knee osteoarthritis.[11,12] The effect of knee alignment can be assessed by measuring the **mechanical axis**, or **weight-bearing line**, of the lower extremity. The weight-bearing line depicts the orientation of the **ground reaction force** (**GRF**) and is represented as a line drawn from the middle of the calcaneus to the head of the femur (see Fig. 11–5).[13]

In a neutrally aligned knee, the weight-bearing line will pass through the center of the knee joint, distributing load equally between the medial and lateral compartments (see Fig. 11–5A). In the presence of genu valgum, the weight-bearing line is shifted onto the lateral knee compartment (see Fig. 11–5B, dashed line), increasing the compression forces on the lateral knee articular cartilage compared with a neutrally aligned knee. In the case of genu varum, the weight-bearing line is shifted medially (see Fig. 11–5C, dashed line), increasing the compression force on the medial knee articular cartilage. The presence of genu valgum or genu varum creates a constant overload of joint compression on the lateral or medial articular cartilage, respectively, which may result in damage to the articular cartilage, progressive joint space narrowing, and potential progression to knee osteoarthritis.[14-18]

The weight-bearing forces applied to the knee joint differ in bilateral and unilateral stance **(Fig. 11–6)**. In bilateral stance, the weight-bearing (GRF) forces on the knee joint are equally distributed between the medial and lateral compartments in an individual with a neutral mechanical axis (see **Fig. 11–6A**).[19] However, in unilateral stance or when dynamic forces are applied to the joint, compartmental loading changes. In the case of unilateral stance (e.g., the opposite limb is in the swing phase of gait), the weight-bearing line (GRF) shifts toward the medial compartment to account for the now-smaller base of support (see **Fig 11–6B**). This shift increases the compressive forces on the medial compartment while reducing compression across the lateral compartment.[20] Although the medial compartment typically experiences greater joint compression than the lateral compartment during activities of daily living, the larger articular surface of the medial compartment helps minimize increases in joint stress by distributing the force over a broader surface.

Advances in technology allow both direct and indirect measurements of the mechanical loading across the knee's medial and lateral compartments. In vivo knee loading characteristics have been measured by instrumenting the prostheses used for total knee arthroplasty to directly measure load. Such direct measurements indicate that most activities of daily living place a greater load on the medial compartment compared with the lateral compartment, which may correspond to the higher rate of medial compartment osteoarthritis when compared with the lateral compartment.[21,22] Less invasive indirect measures can be used to estimate the compressive loads within the knee joint. Specifically, external forces through the leg can be measured from a force plate embedded in a walkway, allowing researchers to measure the GRFs during typical daily and sports activities (e.g., walking, running, jumping). These external forces can be used as surrogates for internal forces incurred by the knee joint and may be used to calculate torques (moments of force) around the joint. For example, if the GRF lies medial to the knee joint center (see Fig. 11–6B), an external adduction moment is created around the knee joint that imposes a varus stress. Thus, the magnitude of the knee adduction moment is often used as a surrogate measure for medial compartment loading during gait and other activities of daily living.[23] This is important because higher knee adduction moments are associated with the presence and severity of medial knee osteoarthritis.[24]

Expanded Concepts 11–1

Effects and Corrections of Malalignment

In the presence of frontal plane malalignment and unicompartmental osteoarthritis, orthopedic surgeons may perform a realignment procedure at the knee, called a *high tibial osteotomy*.[25] This procedure is intended to decrease the compressive force on the damaged, painful tibiofemoral compartment by realigning the limb and moving the weight-bearing line toward the opposite, unaffected tibiofemoral compartment.[26] High tibial osteotomies are also sometimes used in combination with meniscus and articular cartilage procedures when offloading of the structures being surgically repaired is needed.[25] In the case of either significant genu varum or genu valgum, the surgery creates a surgical fracture in the tibia (or sometimes in the femur) to realign the limb to a more neutral position. Other less invasive methods of attempting to diminish compartmental loads in the presence of malalignment include lateral/medial heel wedges or a knee brace ("unloader braces") to mechanically shift weight-bearing to the uninvolved compartment.

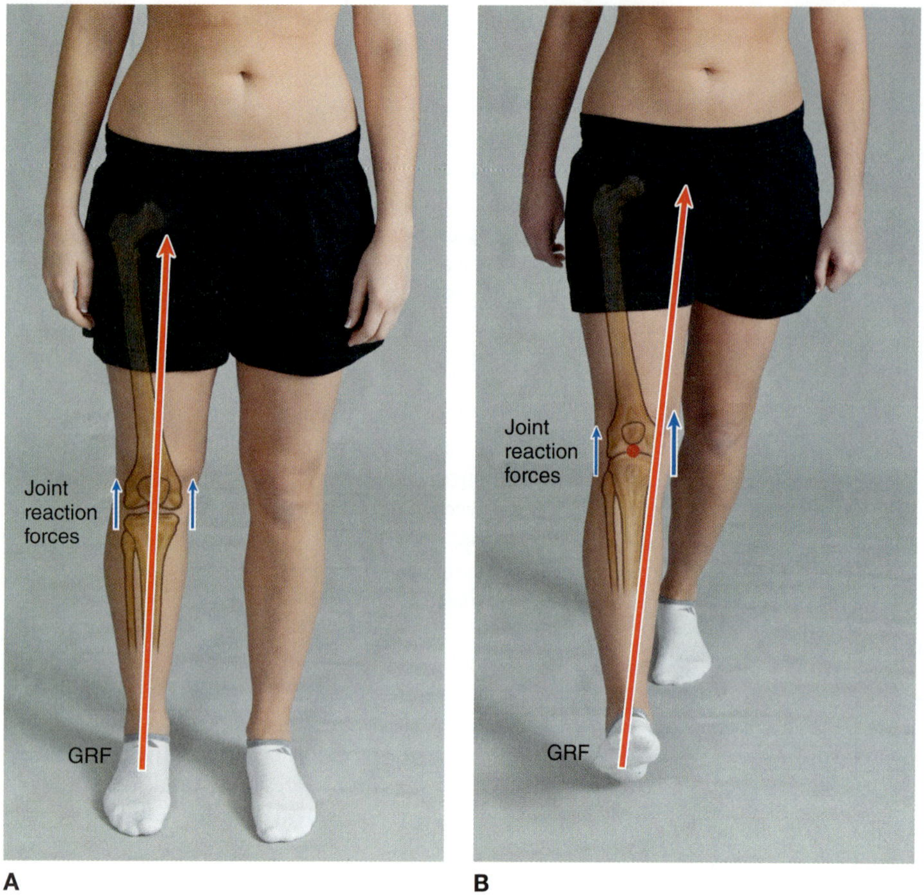

Figure 11–6 **A.** During bilateral stance in the neutrally aligned limb, the ground reaction force (GRF) vector (representing forces applied from the ground to the foot) passes through the center of the knee joint, resulting in joint reaction forces that are distributed somewhat equally between the medial and lateral compartments of the knee joint. **B.** During dynamic activities requiring unilateral stance, such as the early and middle phases of the gait cycle when weight shifts from both limbs to a single limb, the line of force shifts medially. This medial shift increases the joint reaction force through the medial compartment, as indicated by the larger blue arrow compared to the joint reaction force laterally.

Menisci

The relative tibiofemoral incongruence is improved by the presence of **medial** and **lateral menisci** **(Fig. 11–7)**. The menisci transform the fairly flat tibial articular surfaces into concavities for the femoral condyles. In addition to enhancing joint congruence and contact area, these accessory joint structures play important roles in transmitting and distributing weight-bearing loads, reducing friction between the tibia and the femur, providing shock absorption, enhancing joint stability, and aiding in joint proprioception.[27,28] The menisci are fibrocartilaginous discs with a semicircular shape. The medial meniscus is C-shaped, whereas the lateral meniscus forms four-fifths of a circle.[29] Lying *within* the tibiofemoral joint capsule, the menisci cover one-half to two-thirds of the articular surface of the tibial plateaus.[30] Both menisci are open toward the intercondylar tubercles (see Fig. 11-3B) and are thick peripherally and thin centrally (see Fig. 11-7). The lateral meniscus covers a greater percentage of the smaller lateral tibial articular surface than the medial meniscus does for the medial tibial articular surface.[31] As a result of its larger exposed tibial articular surface, the uncovered articular cartilage of the medial tibial plateau carries a greater load during routine daily activities than that of the lateral tibial plateau, making the medial cartilage more susceptible to injury.[32]

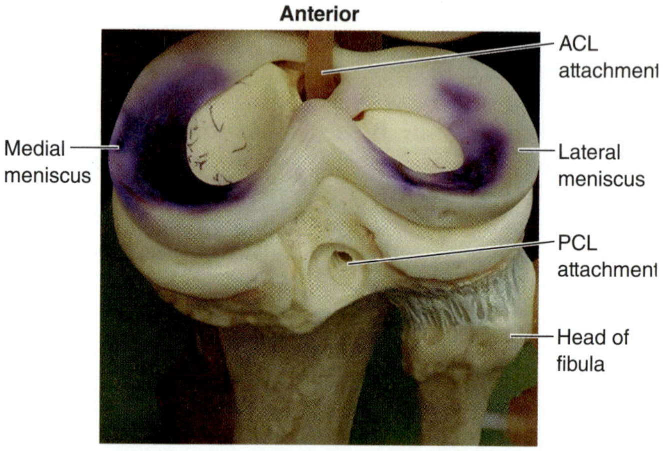

Figure 11–7 A posterosuperior view of the tibia with the menisci, with their wedge shape evident. The purple coloration emphasizes how the menisci deepen and contour the tibial articulating surface to accommodate the femoral condyles, thus distributing and transmitting weight-bearing loads, guiding arthrokinematics, and enhancing joint stability.

MENISCAL ATTACHMENTS

Menisci can translate across the tibial plateau but motion is limited by multiple attachments to surrounding structures. The medial meniscus has more ligamentous and capsular restraints than the lateral meniscus, resulting in more restricted translational movements.[33] The relative lack of mobility of the medial meniscus may contribute to its greater incidence of injury.[31,34]

The anterior and posterior ends of the menisci are called the **anterior** and **posterior horns,** each of which are firmly attached to the tibia[33,35] **(Fig. 11–8)**. Anteriorly, the menisci are connected to each other by the **transverse intermeniscal**

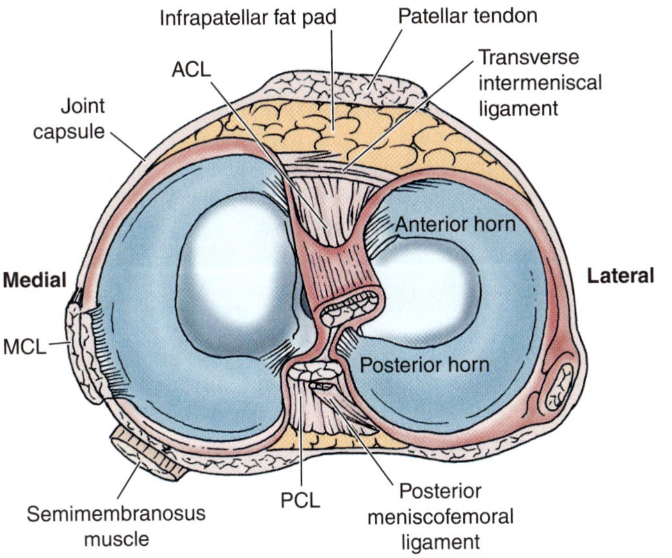

Figure 11–8 Structure and attachments of the menisci. A superior view of the menisci illustrates differences in size and configuration between the medial and lateral menisci. The medial meniscus is C-shaped, whereas the lateral meniscus is shaped like a nearly complete ring or circle. The anterior and posterior horns of the lateral meniscus are shown with the horns of the medial meniscus also attaching to the same locations. The medial meniscus also attaches to the medial collateral ligament (MCL) and the semimembranosus muscle. The location of the anterior cruciate ligament (ACL) and posterior cruciate ligament (PCL) on the tibial plateau is also shown; the synovial membrane of the joint capsule is shown in pink. All the structures in this view are within the circumferential fibrous layer of the capsule with the exception of the MCL and semimembranosus.

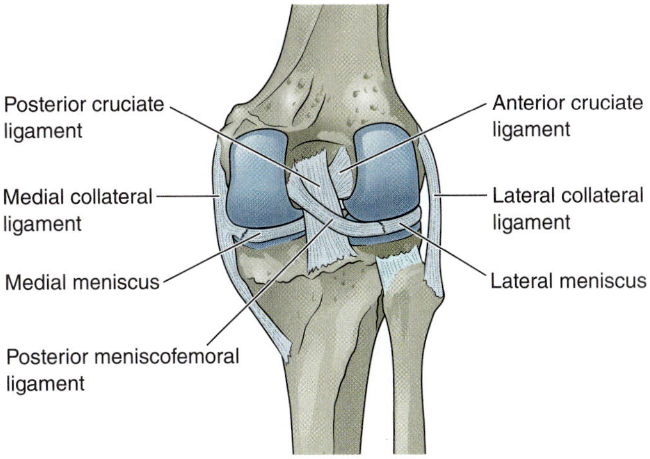

Figure 11–9 Posterior view (joint capsule removed for visualization) of the menisci showing the attachment of the medial meniscus with the MCL. Note the lack of meniscal attachment to the lateral collateral ligament. On the lateral side, the posterior meniscofemoral ligament is visualized.

ligament.[30,31] Both menisci are also attached directly or indirectly to the patella via the **patellomeniscal ligaments**, which are anterior capsular thickenings.[36] At the periphery, both menisci are connected to the tibial condyle by the **coronary ligaments**, which are composed of fibers from the knee joint capsule. The medial meniscus is firmly attached to the medial joint capsule through a capsular thickening extending from the femur to the tibia, referred to as the deep portion of the **medial collateral ligament (MCL)**. This connection to the MCL contributes to the restricted motion of the medial meniscus.[33] The anterior and posterior horns of the medial meniscus are attached on the tibia just anterior to the **anterior cruciate ligament (ACL)** and **posterior cruciate ligament (PCL),** respectively (see Fig. 11-8). Through capsular connections, the **semimembranosus muscle** connects to the medial meniscus.[37]

The anterior horn of the lateral meniscus and the anterior cruciate ligament share a common tibial insertion site.[38] Posteriorly, the lateral meniscus attaches to the PCL and the medial femoral condyle via the **meniscofemoral ligament**[39,40] **(Fig. 11–9)**. In much the same way that the semimembranosus tendon is attached to the medial meniscus, the tendon of the **popliteus muscle** attaches to the lateral meniscus.[30,40] The attachment to the popliteus tendon helps restrain or control the motion of the lateral meniscus.[41]

ROLE OF THE MENISCI

The morphology, structure, and composition of the menisci lead to their role and function within the knee joint. The primary functions of the menisci are to improve joint congruency and stability, disperse and transmit load, and aid joint nutrition and proprioception. The concave-shaped superior surface of each meniscus deepens and contours the flat tibial articulating surface to accommodate the convex femoral condyles (see Fig. 11–7), improving joint congruency. The strong attachments of the menisci prevent extrusion during axial compression of the tibiofemoral joint, allowing for greater contact area between the menisci and the femur. If the femoral condyles sat directly on the relatively flat tibial plateau, a small contact area would exist between the bony surfaces. With the addition of the menisci, the contact area at the tibiofemoral joint is increased and thus joint stress (force per unit area) is reduced[29,42] **(Fig. 11–10)**. The menisci assume 50% to 70% of the loads

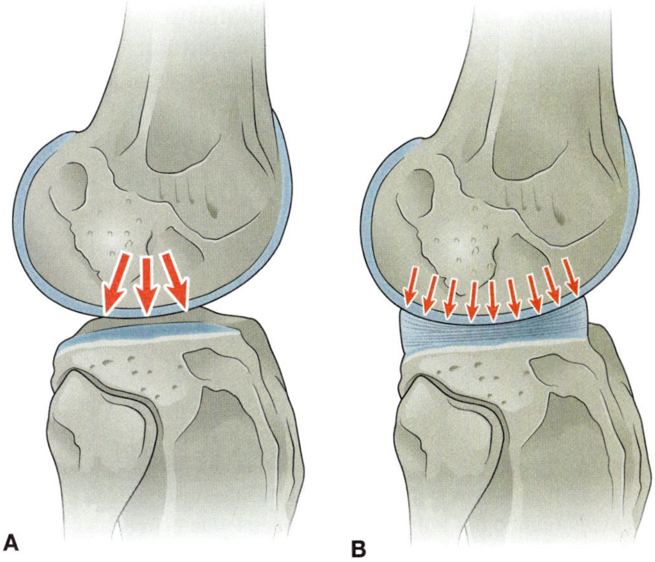

Figure 11–10 Stress distribution by the menisci. **A.** If the femoral condyles sit directly on the flat tibial plateau, the stress (force per unit area) would be high because of the limited contact area. **B.** With the addition of the wedge-shaped menisci, the contact area is increased, and the stress between the bony surfaces is reduced.

imposed through the knee; these forces can be considerable given that compressive forces in the knee may reach one to four times body weight during gait and stair climbing, three to four times body weight during running, and seven to eight times body weight during jumping and landing.[29,43-47]

After the removal of part or all of a meniscus (meniscectomy), the contact area in the tibiofemoral joint is reduced, resulting in increased joint stress that may lead to damage of the articular cartilage (and other degenerative changes) within the tibiofemoral joint. Removal of the menisci nearly doubles the articular cartilage stress on the femur and multiplies the stress by six or seven times on the tibial plateau.[48] Historically, partial meniscectomy has been a primary treatment option for meniscus injuries; however, the increased risk of articular cartilage damage and degeneration over time has increased the emphasis on meniscus preservation. For this reason, total meniscectomies are rarely performed after a meniscal tear; instead, care is taken to preserve as much of the meniscus as possible, either through debridement (removal of only damaged tissue) or meniscal repair procedures.[49] Transplantation of a meniscal allograft from an organ donor may be considered, especially in young and active individuals, when previous meniscal procedures have failed to eliminate pain or restore meniscus function. Currently, there is no uniform management strategy for meniscal injury, and an individualized approach is required with consideration of the meniscus injury (location, severity), concomitant injuries, patient characteristics, and patient goals.

Patient Application 11–1

Tina is a 43-year-old woman who presents with right knee pain during increased activity. Pain is 2/10 at best and 8/10 at worst. Aggravating factors include playing tennis and stair negotiation (ascending and descending). The medial aspect of her tibiofemoral joint line is tender to palpation, and she subjectively describes pain deep inside her knee. She is currently unable to jog, play tennis, or walk for more than 1 mile without discomfort. Tina's past medical history includes tearing her right medial meniscus when she was 24 years old, which was surgically treated with a partial medial meniscectomy. Clinical testing of her right knee revealed (1) full and pain-free passive range of motion (ROM), (2) 80% quadriceps strength compared to her left side, and (3) increased, but nonpainful, laxity with both varus and valgus stress testing of the knee.[50] Diagnostic images were obtained of Tina's lower extremities. Weight-bearing radiographs of the right limb revealed genu varum with moderate joint space narrowing in the right medial tibiofemoral compartment.

Tina's prior history of medial meniscus injury (with partial medial meniscectomy) increases her risk for right knee joint degeneration and osteoarthritis.[51-54] The partial removal of Tina's medial meniscus diminishes the contact area within the medial tibiofemoral compartment. The same force is now being focused through a smaller contact area, creating significantly higher joint stress and raising the potential for degenerative articular cartilage changes within the joint. Genu varum, according to measurements taken from her right limb radiographs, may alter the distribution of compartmental joint forces and increase the magnitude of compression force through the medial compartment during activities of daily living, resulting in subsequent articular cartilage degradation and the joint space narrowing evident on her radiograph.

The increased stress in her medial compartment, from the partial medial meniscectomy and genu varum, have likely damaged and irritated periarticular tissues, contributing to her medial knee pain. The chronic medial knee pain that she experiences may result in disuse atrophy, where, in this case, reduced use of the knee due to pain leads to quadriceps muscle weakness. Tina's knee pain and quadriceps weakness are consistent with her difficulties in performing dynamic, quadriceps-intensive functional activities.

MENISCAL NUTRITION AND INNERVATION

The location of a meniscal lesion, along with the age and health of the patient, influences the treatment options available after injury due to the capacity of the meniscus to heal. During the first year of life, blood vessels are contained throughout the meniscal bodies. Once weight-bearing is initiated, vascularity begins to diminish until only the outer 25% to 33% is vascularized by capillaries from the joint capsule and the synovial membrane.[55] After 50 years of age, only the periphery of the meniscal body is vascularized.[55] Therefore, the peripheral portion obtains its nutrition through blood vessels, but the central portion must rely on the diffusion of synovial fluid.[27,34] The process of fluid diffusion to support nutrition requires intermittent loading of the meniscus by either weight-bearing or muscular contractions.[55] Consequently, during prolonged non–weight-bearing conditions or periods of immobilization, the meniscus may not receive adequate nutrition. In addition, the avascular nature of the central portion of the meniscus reduces the potential for healing after an injury.[56] In adults, only the peripheral vascularized region of the meniscus is capable of inflammation, repair, and remodeling after a tearing injury. Historically, meniscal repair procedures were indicated only in younger patients with a lesion isolated to the peripheral margins of the meniscus. However, given the critical role of the meniscus in maintaining joint homeostasis, current indications for meniscal repair (vs. debridement) are broadening to include older, active patients and the repair of tears in avascular zones.[57]

The horns of the menisci and the peripheral vascularized portion of the meniscal bodies are well innervated with free nerve endings (nociceptors) and three different mechanoreceptors (Ruffini corpuscles, Pacinian corpuscles, and Golgi tendon organs), whereas the central portions are aneural.[27,55] The presence of nociceptors in the meniscus may explain some of the pain felt by patients after a meniscal tear if the lesion is located peripherally.[58] The potential for proprioceptive deficits exists after injury to the periphery of a meniscus as a result of injury to the mechanoreceptors within the meniscus.

Joint Capsule

Despite the additional support provided by the menisci, the incongruent knee joint is heavily dependent on the surrounding structures for joint stability. The balance between stability and mobility varies as the knee moves through its ROM. Bony congruence and overall ligament tautness are maximal in full extension, representing the close-packed position of the joint. In midrange knee flexion, the passive periarticular structures tend to be more lax, and the relative bony incongruence of the joint permits greater anterior and posterior translations, as well as rotation between the tibia and femur.[59]

Clinical Application 11–1

Objective assessment for ligamentous laxity is often performed in the open-packed position (approximately 25° of knee flexion) due to bony incongruence and increased laxity of passive structures that allows for greater translation between the femur and tibia. For example, testing the integrity of the ACL via the Lachman test, the MCL via valgus stress test, and the lateral collateral ligament (LCL) via varus stress test are all performed at approximately 20° to 30° of knee flexion.

A single, large joint capsule encloses both the tibiofemoral and patellofemoral joints. It is grossly composed of a superficial fibrous layer and a thinner, deep synovial membrane. In general, the outer fibrous portion of the capsule is firmly attached to the inferior aspect of the femur and the superior portion of the tibia.[60] Posteriorly, the capsule is attached proximally to the posterior margins of the femoral condyles and intercondylar notch, and distally to the posterior tibial condyle.[61] The anterior borders of the joint capsule consist of the tendon of the quadriceps muscles, the patella, and the **patellar tendon** (sometimes called the *infrapatellar tendon* or *infrapatellar ligament*). The anteromedial and anterolateral portions of the capsule that attach to the patella are often separately identified as the **medial** and **lateral patellar retinaculae**, or together as the **extensor retinaculum.**[62] The joint capsule is reinforced medially, laterally, and posteriorly by capsular ligaments, which will be discussed in detail later.

The knee joint capsule and its associated ligaments are critical in restricting excessive joint motions to maintain joint integrity and typical function. Although muscles clearly play a dominant role in stabilization (as we shall examine more closely later in the chapter), it is difficult to stabilize the knee with only active muscular forces in the presence of a disruption of the knee's capsule and ligaments. Beyond knee joint stability, the joint capsule plays important sensory and proprioceptive roles. The joint capsule is strongly innervated by both nociceptors as well as Pacinian and Ruffini corpuscles.[60] These mechanoreceptors may contribute to muscular stabilization of the knee joint by initiating reflex-mediated muscular responses. In addition, the joint capsule provides a tight seal to keep the lubricating synovial fluid within the joint space.[60]

SYNOVIAL LAYER OF THE JOINT CAPSULE

The synovial membrane lines much of the knee joint capsule.[63,64] The roles of the synovial tissue are to secrete and absorb synovial fluid into the joint for lubrication and to provide nutrition to avascular structures, such as portions of the menisci.[65] The synovial lining of the knee joint capsule is quite complex and is among the most extensive and involved in the body **(Fig. 11–11)**. Posteriorly, the synovium detaches from the inner wall of the fibrous joint capsule and folds anteriorly between the femoral condyles, where it adheres to the anterior aspect and sides of the ACL and PCL[64,66,67] (see Fig. 11-8). As a result of this invagination of the synovial member, both the ACL and the PCL are contained *within* the fibrous capsule (intracapsular), but remain *outside* of the synovial sheath (extrasynovial).[64,66,67] On the posterolateral side, the synovial lining slips between the popliteus muscle and lateral femoral condyle, whereas on the posteromedial side, it may fold between the semimembranosus tendon, the medial head of the **gastrocnemius** muscle, and the medial femoral condyle. The intricate folds of the synovium exclude several fat pads that lie *within* the fibrous capsule, rendering them intracapsular but extrasynovial, similar to the cruciate ligaments.[68] The anterior and posterior suprapatellar fat pads lie posterior to the **quadriceps tendon** and anterior to the distal femoral epiphysis, respectively. The **infrapatellar (Hoffa's) fat pad** lies deep to the patellar tendon (see Fig. 11–8).

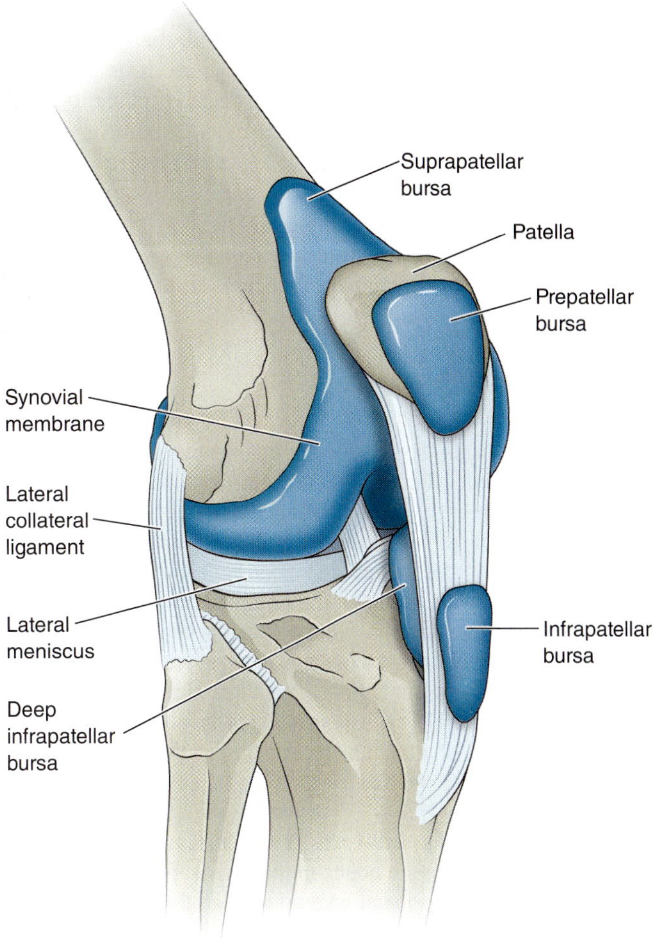

Figure 11–11 An anterolateral view of the knee complex (with the fibrous outer layer of the capsule removed) shows the complex course of the synovial layer of the knee joint capsule (blue), including the related bursae. The menisci, collateral ligaments, cruciate ligaments, and patellar tendon (white) are contained within the fibrous capsule (intracapsular) but are outside the synovial layer (extrasynovial).

Formation of the knee joint's synovial membrane occurs early in embryonic development, when it separates the medial and lateral articular surfaces into separate joint cavities.[69,70] By the 12th week of gestation, the synovial septae are somewhat resorbed, resulting in a single joint cavity but with retention of the posterior invagination of the synovium between the femoral condyles.[64] The failure of the synovial membrane to become fully resorbed can result in persistent folds in specific regions of the membrane. These folds are called **synovial plicae.**[70] Synovial plicae, when they exist, are generally composed of loose, pliant, and elastic fibrous connective tissue that easily passes back and forth over the femoral condyles as the knee flexes and extends.[71] On occasion, a plica may become irritated and inflamed leading to pain, effusion, and changes in joint function called **plica syndrome.**[71] There are four potential locations relative to the patella where plicae may be located: inferior (infrapatellar plica), superior (suprapatellar plica), medial (medial patellar plica), and lateral (lateral patellar plica).[69,70] The size, shape, and presence of these plicae vary among individuals, with infrapatellar plica most commonly present, lateral patellar plica least commonly present,[69] and medial patellar plica becoming the most common source of irritation.

Expanded Concepts 11–2
Synovial Plicae

The infrapatellar plica, also called the **ligamentum mucosum,** originates in the intercondylar area of the femur and courses parallel to the anterior border of the anterior cruciate ligament, passes through the infrapatellar fat pad (of Hoffa), and attaches distally to the inferior pole of the patella.[70] It is the most common plica present in the knee (found in 50% to 65% of knees).[70,71] The suprapatellar plica is generally located superior to the patella, forming from the undersurface of the quadriceps tendon, and often extending to the suprapatellar synovial pouch at the anterior aspect of the distal femoral shaft.[70] Despite its location above the patella, the suprapatellar plica rarely gets impinged between the patella and the femur.[71] In contrast, the medial patellar plica is more often implicated as a source of pain, although it is present less frequently (in only 25% to 30% of knees) than either the supra- or infrapatellar plica.[70,71] The medial patellar plica arises from the synovium lining the medial wall of the pouch of the extensor retinaculum and courses parallel to the medial edge of the patella to attach to the synovium of the infrapatellar fat pad and sometimes the infrapatellar plica.[70,71] Discomfort from the medial plica often occurs during knee movements that change the plical dimension and orientation stemming from their attachments to synovial lined structures.[70] For example, a typically thin and elastic medial plica can become impinged, beginning around 30° to 50° of knee flexion between the medial aspect of the patella and the medial femoral condyle, eventually leading to inflammation and thickening of the plica tissue.[70] The pain that occurs from the irritated synovial membrane can be attributed to its rich supply of Pacinian corpuscles and free nerve endings.[63]

FIBROUS LAYER OF THE JOINT CAPSULE

The fibrous joint capsule lies superficial to the synovial lining of the knee joint and provides passive support for the joint. The fibrous joint capsule itself is composed of two or three layers, depending on location. Several capsular thickenings (or capsular ligaments), as well as both intracapsular and extracapsular ligaments, provide additional structural support to the knee joint.

The anterior portion of the knee joint capsule is referred to as the *extensor retinaculum.* Superficially, the extensor retinaculum consists of a fascial layer that covers the quadriceps muscles distally, extending inferiorly to the quadriceps tendon. Deep to the extensor retinaculum, the anterior capsule also includes the medial and lateral retinacula **(Fig. 11–12)**, a series of transverse and longitudinal fibrous bands connecting the patella to the surrounding medial and lateral knee structures.[62] The thickest band within the medial retinaculum is the **medial patellofemoral ligament.**[72] Its fibers, oriented in a transverse manner, course anteriorly from the adductor tubercle of the femur to blend with the distal fibers of the vastus medialis and eventually insert onto the medial border of the patella.[72,73] The medial patellofemoral ligament is a clinically important stabilizer to maintain the patella in the femoral sulcus, and can rupture during lateral patellar subluxation or dislocation.[74] The lateral retinaculum is also deep to the extensor retinaculum and consists of less discrete fibrous bands compared with those of the medial retinaculum.[62] The transversely oriented fibers within the lateral retinaculum, called the **lateral patellofemoral ligament**, travel from the **iliotibial (IT) band** to the lateral border of the patella[75] (see Fig. 11-12). The remainder of the anterior retinacular bands include the obliquely oriented **medial patellomeniscal ligament**, the **lateral patellomeniscal ligament,** and the longitudinally positioned **medial** and **lateral patellotibial ligaments.**[62,75]

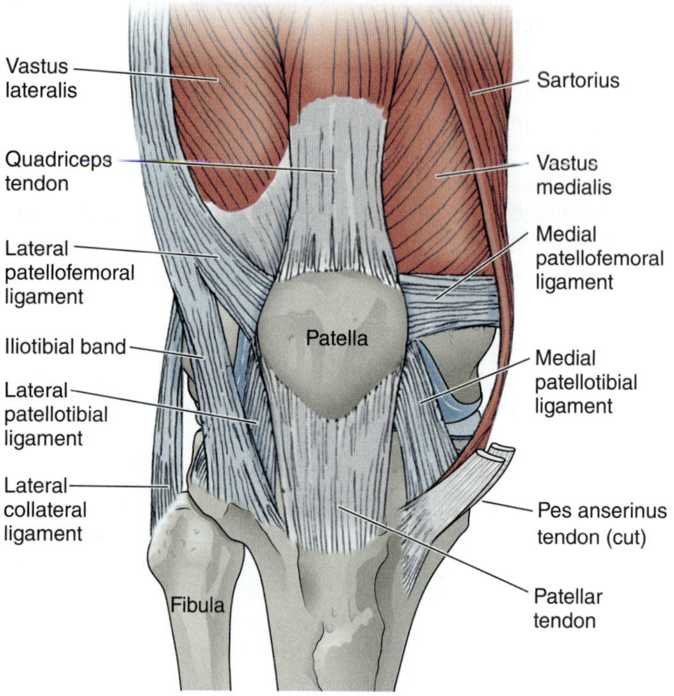

Figure 11–12 The extensor retinaculum is reinforced medially by the transversely oriented medial patellofemoral ligament and the longitudinally oriented medial patellotibial ligament. Laterally, the lateral patellofemoral ligament and lateral patellotibial ligament help resist an excessive medial slide of the patella.

Medially, the joint capsule also has deep and superficial portions arising from the medial collateral ligament. The superficial layer of the medial joint capsule blends with the fascial layers that cover the vastus medialis muscle anteriorly and the sartorius muscle posteriorly.[76] Laterally, the joint capsule is reinforced superficially by the IT band and its thick **fascia lata.**[77] Posteriorly, the capsule is reinforced by the oblique popliteal ligament and by the more laterally located **popliteofibular ligament** (previously called the *arcuate ligament*) **(Fig. 11–13)**; the **posterior oblique ligament** adds reinforcement posteromedially.[78-80] A more detailed discussion of knee ligaments and their function is below.

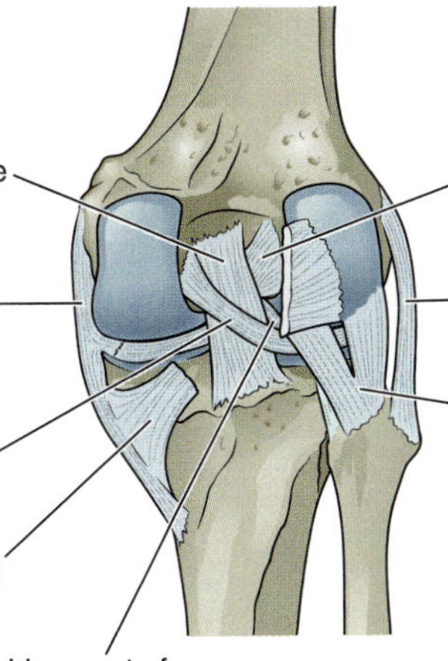

Figure 11–13 A posterior view of the knee shows reinforcement from the oblique popliteal ligament and popliteofibular ligament.

Ligaments

The roles of the various knee ligaments have received extensive attention in the literature, which reflects their importance for knee joint stability and the frequency with which function is disrupted following ligament injury. Given the lack of bony restraint to virtually any of the knee motions, the knee joint ligaments are variously credited with resisting or controlling excessive knee extension and motions of the tibia with respect to the femur, including adduction/abduction, anterior/posterior displacement, and medial/lateral rotation. When the position of the tibia is fixed (such as during weight-bearing), ligaments resist or control movement of the femur on the tibia (see Foundational Concepts 11–1). For every knee rotary or translatory motion, ligaments function as primary or secondary stabilizers, which will be discussed in more detail later.

Foundational Concepts 11–1 Weight-Bearing/Non–Weight-Bearing Versus Closed/Open-Chain

Weight-bearing activities (often called *closed-chain* activities) involve motion of the femur moving on a relatively fixed tibia. In contrast, non–weight-bearing activities (often termed *open-chain* activities) involve a moving tibia on a relatively fixed femur. As noted in earlier chapters, weight-bearing activities result in closed-chain effects on two or more joints only when the upright (vertically oriented) position of the head is maintained or from weight-shifting in bilateral stance. Consequently, we will refer to activities as weight-bearing or non–weight-bearing, rather than as "closed-chain" or "open-chain." The difference between weight-bearing and non–weight-bearing motions is important because the displacements and rotations of the tibia and the femur are expressed differently for each condition. For example, anterior displacement of the tibia on the femur during non–weight-bearing is equivalent to posterior displacement of the femur on the tibia during weight-bearing.

Our knowledge of the stresses (force per unit area) and strains (change in shape by an applied stress) on ligamentous tissues has been significantly advanced using cadaveric experiments. Two primary approaches have been used to reveal the relative roles of the knee ligaments. The first approach is to measure the amount of knee displacement in response to an applied load. Following the sectioning (cutting) of a particular ligament, joint displacement is measured again with the same applied load. The relative change in displacement (strain) provides evidence for the ligament's role in restricting motion against the magnitude and direction of the applied force. An alternative approach measures the force (stress) necessary to achieve a predetermined joint displacement. After a ligament is cut, the process is repeated. The change in the force required to displace the joint provides evidence of that ligament's role in resisting a given amount of joint displacement. A ligament's role in resisting motion will depend on the position of the knee joint, how the stresses are applied, and what active or passive structures are concomitantly intact.

MEDIAL COLLATERAL LIGAMENT

The medial collateral ligament (MCL), a flat band of connective tissue, can be divided into a superficial portion and a deep portion that are separated by a bursa. The superficial portion of the MCL arises proximally from the medial femoral epicondyle, anterior to the origin of the posterior oblique ligament and just distal to the femoral insertion of the medial patellofemoral ligament.[61,81] The MCL travels distally to insert into the medial aspect of the proximal tibia, distal to the **pes anserinus (Fig. 11–14)**.[61,81] The deep portion of the MCL is continuous with the joint capsule, originating from the inferior aspect of the medial femoral epicondyle and inserting on the proximal aspect of the medial tibial plateau.[61] Throughout its

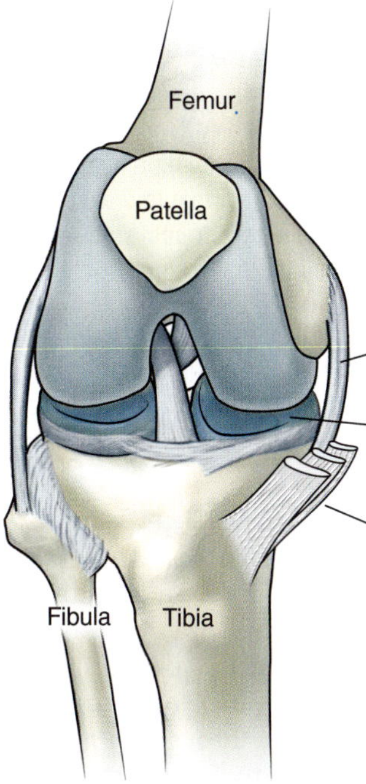

Figure 11–14 The superficial portion of the medial collateral ligament runs from the medial femoral condyle to the anteromedial tibial condyle, attaching posterior to the conjoined tendons of the pes anserinus.

course of travel, the deep portion of the MCL is rigidly affixed to the medial border of the medial meniscus (see Fig. 11–8).[61]

The MCL, specifically the superficial portion, is the primary restraint to excessive valgus and lateral tibial rotation stresses at the knee throughout most angles of knee flexion, whereas the deep portion serves as a secondary stabilizer to these stresses.[82] The superficial and deep portions of the MCL are also important in restraining medial tibial rotation.[82] The knee joint is better able to resist a valgus stress at full extension (i.e., closed-packed position) than in a flexed knee position. As joint flexion is increased, the MCL becomes more lax and bony congruence decreases, resulting in greater possible medial joint space opening (medial gapping) when a valgus force is applied.[83] Regardless of knee joint position, the MCL is the primary restraint to valgus forces.[82] Grood and colleagues explained that the MCL accounted for 57% of the restraining force against valgus gapping near full extension, but accounted for 78% of the restraining force at 25° of knee flexion.[84] This difference is likely due to the greater bony congruence and inclusion of other soft tissue structures (e.g., posteromedial capsule, ACL) at full extension that effectively assist with resisting a valgus stress in that position. The MCL also plays a secondary role in resisting anterior translation between the tibia and femur in the absence of the primary restraints.[85] An excessive valgus force at the knee, with or without tibial rotation, is the most common mechanism by which the MCL is torn.

Expanded Concepts 11–3
The Effect of MCL Tears on the ACL

Because of its secondary role as a restraint to anterior tibial translation, both partial and complete MCL tears will significantly increase the load on the ACL.[86] Conversely, injury to the anterior cruciate ligament can increase load on the MCL. Given this, and commonalities in the mechanisms of injury between the MCL and ACL, it is not uncommon to see injuries sustained to *both* ligaments simultaneously. When ACL tears or newly reconstructed ACL grafts coexist with an MCL injury, rehabilitation exercises with the tibia positioned neutrally (i.e., without rotation) are recommended to avoid excessive strain on the MCL until sufficient healing occurs. Surgical stabilization of an isolated MCL injury is rarely necessary and frequently not performed even with concomitant multi-ligament knee injuries because of the MCL's repair capacity.[87] The MCL has a rich blood supply providing it with the capability to heal when ruptured or damaged. Nevertheless, the remodeling process for the MCL can take up to a year.[87,88]

LATERAL COLLATERAL LIGAMENT

The **lateral collateral ligament (LCL)** attaches proximally at the lateral femoral epicondyle and distally to the fibular head **(Fig. 11–15)**, where it joins with the tendon of the **biceps femoris muscle** to form the conjoined tendon.[89,90] Unlike the MCL, the LCL is not a thickening of the capsule but is a separate cordlike structure throughout much of its length, and is therefore considered to be an extracapsular ligament. The LCL also lacks the meniscal attachments the MCL has. The LCL is the primary restraint to excessive varus stress at all degrees of knee flexion.[83,84,89] Grood and colleagues reported that the LCL accounted for 55% of the restraining force against varus stress at 5° of knee flexion, which increases to 69% of the restraining force with the knee flexed to 25°.[84] Although the LCL's primary role is to resist varus stresses, its orientation enables the LCL to also resist lateral rotation of the tibia in knee flexion along with other posterolateral knee structures (i.e., popliteofibular ligament, popliteus tendon).[91-93] As with other knee ligaments, the LCL assumes additional stabilization roles in the presence of injury to other knee ligaments. For example, the LCL acts as a weak secondary restraint to anterior tibial translation and medial rotation in an ACL-deficient knee.[94] An excessive varus force at the knee, with or without tibial rotation, is the common mechanism of injury to the LCL.

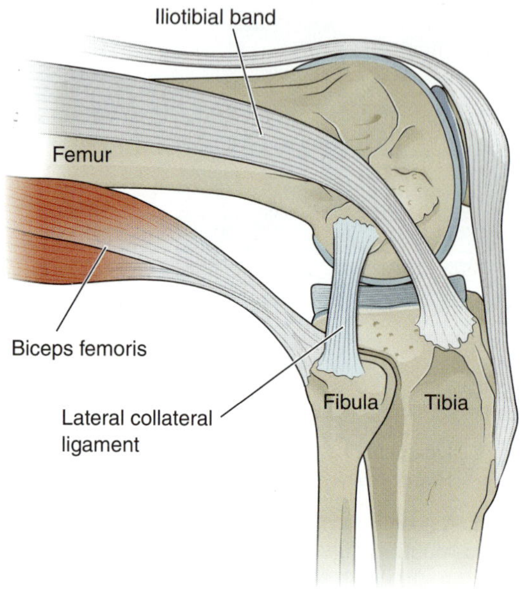

Figure 11–15 The LCL attaches proximally to the lateral femoral epicondyle and distally joins the tendon of the biceps femoris muscle to attach to the fibular head. The distal attachment of the IT band is to the anterolateral tibia.

ANTERIOR CRUCIATE LIGAMENT

The high injury rate to the ACL among athletes and other active individuals has resulted in a substantial amount of research related to the ligament's structure and function. The ACL originates at the posteromedial aspect of the lateral femoral condyle (see Fig. 11–13) and extends inferiorly, medially, and anteriorly to attach distally to the tibia on the lateral and anterior aspect of the medial intercondylar tibial spine[95] **(Fig. 11–16)**.

In addition, the ACL twists outwardly (laterally) before attaching distally.[66] The ACL consists of two separate bundles that wrap around each other as the knee flexes.[95,96] The **anteromedial bundle (AMB)** and **posterolateral bundle (PLB)** of the ACL are named for their tibial insertions.[97] The primary blood supply to both bundles of the ACL comes from the middle genicular artery.[97]

Given the position of the ACL within the knee joint, the ACL has a role in contributing to joint stability across all motions. The ACL functions as the primary restraint against anterior translation (anterior shear) of the tibia on the femur.[97] The AMB and PLB contribute differently to restraining anterior tibial translation depending on the knee flexion angle

(Fig. 11–17). The two bundles shift tension from one to the other to allow some portion of the ACL to remain relatively taut throughout the knee's ROM. For example, with the knee near full extension, the PLB is taut such that more anterior tibial translation force is resisted by the PLB than the AMB. As the knee flexes beyond 15°, however, the PLB loosens and the AMB becomes more taut, resulting in greater restraining forces by the AMB.[98,99]

Load-sharing by the AMB and PLB allows the ACL to resist anterior translation of the tibia on the femur through a larger range of knee motion than either bundle could do on its own. In the intact joint, forces producing an anterior translation of the tibia on the femur will result in maximal tibial anterior excursion at about 30° of flexion when neither of the ACL bundles is maximally tensed.[100] In contrast, the least amount of anterior translation of the tibia can occur in full extension when, in addition to the PBL of the ACL, many passive structures of the knee are taut.[99] Because the PLB is taut in full extension, the ACL is also responsible for resisting hyperextension of the knee.[101]

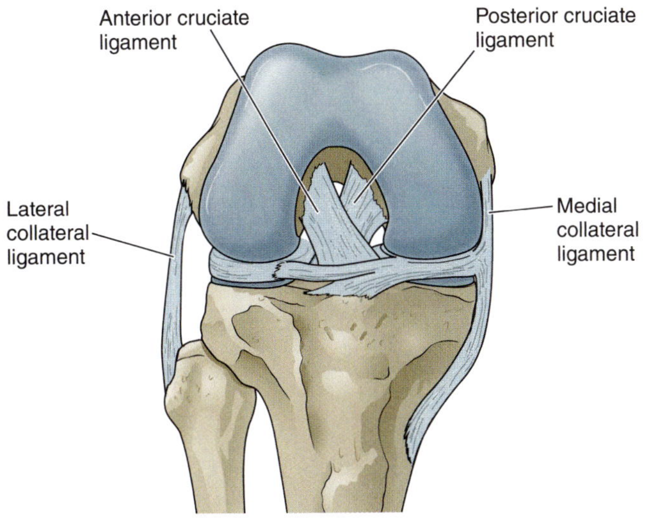

Figure 11–16 An anterior view of a flexed knee joint shows the course of the ACL from the posterior lateral femoral condyle to the anterior portion of the tibial plateau.

Clinical Application 11–2

Physical examination of ligament integrity often involves using "special tests" to identify passive laxity or abnormal movement when specific stresses are applied to a joint. The test position and stress applied are designed to isolate specific ligament structures. The Lachman test is a gold-standard clinical examination technique to evaluate ACL integrity and is performed with the patient in supine, the knee supported in 20° to 30° of flexion (open-packed position of the knee); the examiner pulls the proximal tibia anteriorly while stabilizing the distal femur—producing an anterior translational of the tibia. The Lachman test is considered positive if there is a lack of a firm endpoint and/or excessive anterior translation of the proximal tibia compared to the contralateral side. The anterior drawer test (performed similarly to the Lachman test but with the knee flexed to 90°) is also designed to evaluate ACL integrity; however, the Lachman test is considered the gold standard because it may better isolate the ACL, whereas the flexed position of the anterior drawer test may be a position where other structures also limit anterior tibial translation.

In addition to its primary restraint against anterior tibial translation on the femur, the ACL provides rotary stability of the knee during medial/lateral rotation, varus/valgus forces, and combinations thereof.[72,96,99,101,102] The PLB provides more rotational stability than the AMB, especially when the knee joint is extended which makes the PLB more taut.[95,96,99] The

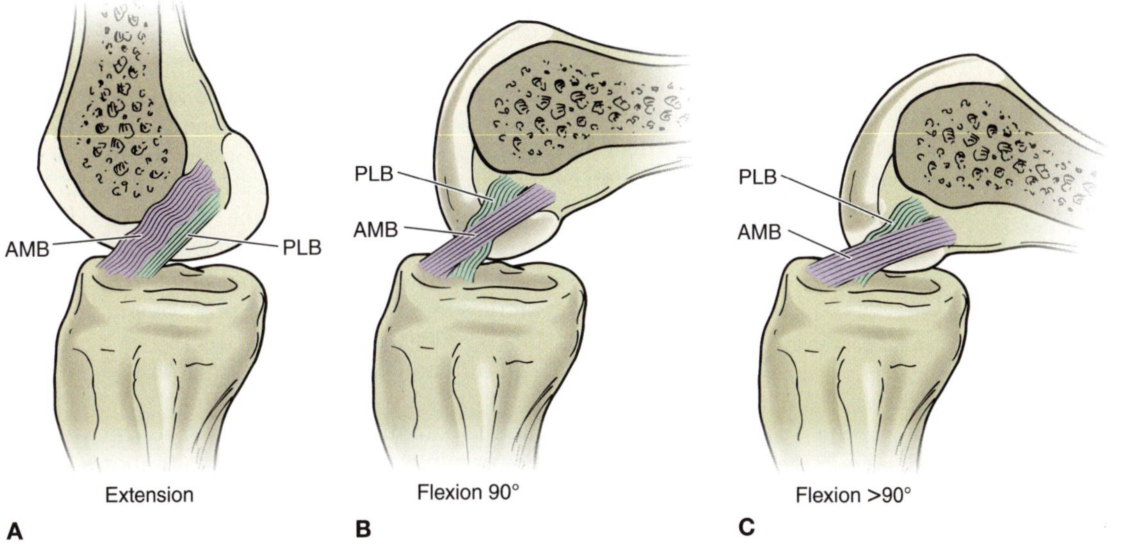

Figure 11–17 Anterior cruciate ligament tension shifts. **A.** The anteromedial bundle (AMB) of the ACL is slack in full knee extension while the posterolateral bundle (PLB) is taut. **B.** At 90° of knee flexion, the AMB tightens as the PLB loses tension. **C.** In knee flexion greater than 90°, the AMB is maximally taut while the PLB is relaxed. Some portion of the ACL remains fairly taut throughout the ROM.

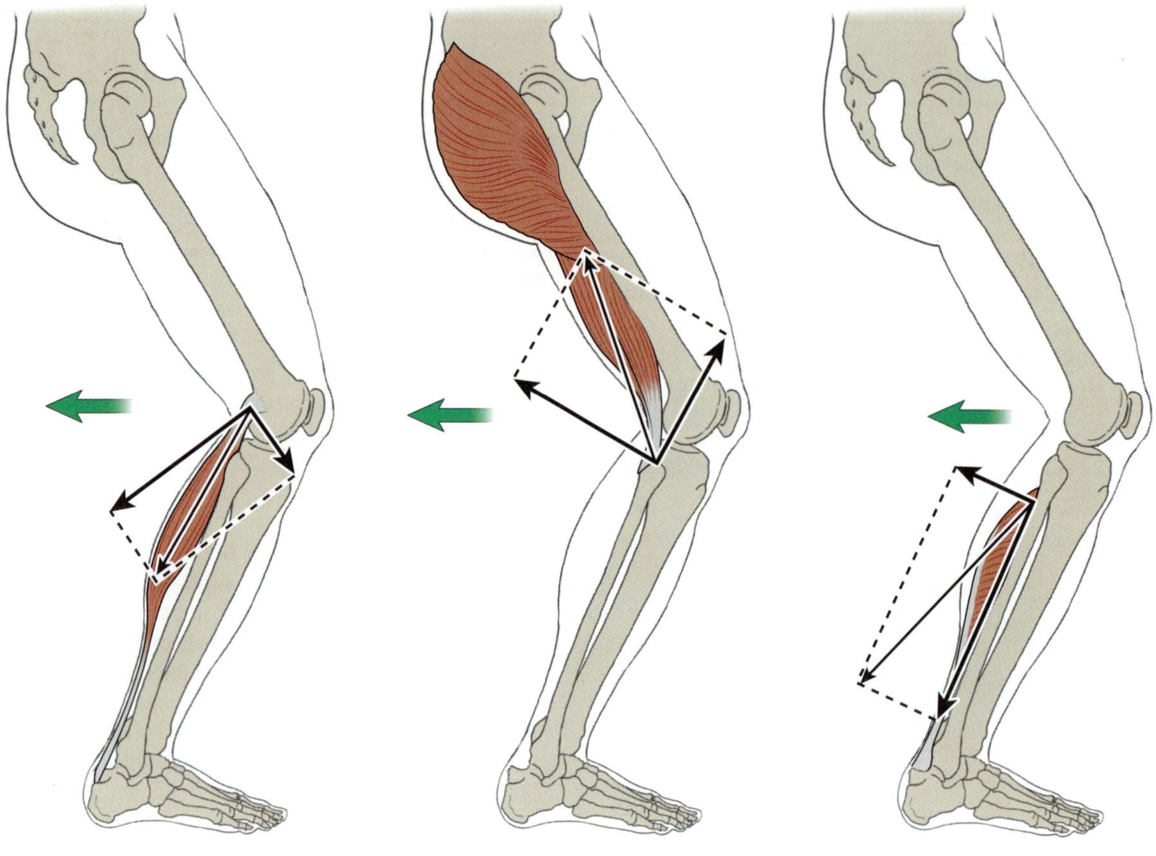

Figure 11–18 Muscles that surround the knee are capable of producing anterior/posterior shear forces (forces parallel to the tibial plateau) at the knee joint. **A.** The gastrocnemius produces a posterior *femoral* shear force (or anterior tibial shear) because of its proximal tendon wrapping around the posterior tibia. **B.** Similarly, a contraction of the hamstrings can produce a posterior tibial shear force. **C.** A contraction of the soleus muscle will produce posterior tibial shear at the knee.

ACL provides secondary stabilization to the MCL in resisting valgus loads. The strain in the ACL during a valgus load has been reported to increase 55% in the presence of a partial MCL tear, and 185% with a full MCL tear.[86] The ACL can also play a secondary role in limiting medial rotation of the tibia. Medial tibial rotation on the femur can increase the strain on the AMB of the ACL, with the peak strain occurring between 10° and 15° of knee flexion.[103-105] This is likely due to the orientation of the ACL winding its way medially around the PCL, becoming taut with medial rotation.

Expanded Concepts 11–4

Loading the ACL Through Combined Motions

Through cadaveric testing, Quatman and colleagues[106] demonstrated that combined translational and rotational movements can generate greater ACL strain than either movement individually. Importantly, the cadaveric testing was performed at 25° knee flexion to simulate landing from a jump, a common mechanism for ACL injury.[106] The authors determined that a combination of a valgus force with anterior translation and medial rotation of the tibia increases the strain on the ACL over three times as much as with either motion alone. Further, these three combined motions resulted in substantially greater strain in the ACL than in the MCL. This finding may explain the higher rate of reported isolated ACL injuries compared with concomitant ACL and MCL injuries.[107]

Although the ACL primarily resists anterior tibial translation, injuries to this ligament are not thought to occur during isolated instances of excessive anterior tibial translation. Rather, injury to the ACL occurs most commonly when the knee is slightly flexed and in a valgus position combined with anterior tibial translation, medial tibial rotation, or lateral tibial rotation during weight-bearing activities (see Expanded Concepts 11–4).[108] In flexion and medial tibial rotation, the ACL is tensed as it winds around the PCL, while in flexion and lateral tibial rotation the ACL is tensed as it is stretched over the lateral femoral condyle.[109]

The muscles surrounding the knee joint can alter (either increasing or decreasing) physiologic strain in the ACL (**Fig. 11–18**). Because the ACL's primary role is to resist an anterior translation of the tibia on the femur, any muscle action that produces a shear force at the tibiofemoral joint has the potential to influence physiologic strain on the ACL. For example, a muscle action that imposes an anterior shear force on the tibia (or posterior shear force on the femur) has potential to increase physiologic strain on the ACL, while a muscle action that induces a posterior tibial shear force has potential to reduce physiologic strain on the ACL. Specifically, with the tibiofemoral joint near full extension, an isolated **quadriceps muscle** contraction may generate an anterior shear force on the tibia as shown in the weight boot and leg press examples in Chapter 1, thereby increasing physiologic strain in the ACL.[103,110-113] Fleming and colleagues reported that the gastrocnemius muscle similarly has the potential to translate the tibia anteriorly because the proximal tendon of the gastrocnemius wraps around the posterior tibia, effectively *pushing the tibia forward* when the muscle becomes tense through active contraction or passive stretch[114] (see **Fig. 11-18A**). This anterior "push" by the gastrocnemius increases the strain on the ACL, although the gastrocnemius does not attach to the tibia. The hamstring muscles are capable of inducing a posterior shear force on the tibia throughout the range of knee flexion, becoming more effective in this role at greater knee flexion angles,[115-118] and assisting the ACL in restraining anterior tibial translation (see **Fig. 11-18B**). With the foot on the ground, the soleus muscle may also contribute to posterior translation of the tibia and assist the ACL in restraining anterior tibial translation[119] (see Fig. **11-18C**). During noninjurious performance of activities of daily living and dynamic tasks, the interplay of muscle action and tibial translation remains within physiologic levels of ACL strain. ACL injury occurs when joint loading exceeds the tensile capabilities of the ligament, most often through combined loading of the knee in valgus and rotation.

Given the potential of individual muscles to either increase or decrease loads on the ACL, it is not surprising that co-contraction of multiple muscles across the knee can also influence the strain on the ACL. For example, co-contraction of the *hamstrings* and quadriceps muscles allows the active hamstrings to counter the anterior translational force imposed by the active quadriceps, reducing strain on the ACL at knee flexion angles of 60° and greater.[113] In contrast, simultaneous activation of the *gastrocnemius* and the quadriceps muscles (both producing anterior tibial shear) results in *greater* strain on the ACL than either muscle would produce alone, unless hamstring co-contraction also occurs to mitigate the anterior translation imposed by the quadriceps and gastrocnemius.[114] Although muscular co-contraction of the quadriceps and hamstrings will limit the strain imposed on the ligaments of the knee, it is not fully understood how greater co-contraction may change the *compressive* loads experienced at the joint, thus affecting the injury potential in other joint structures sensitive to compressive loading (e.g., articular cartilage).[115,120-122]

Patient Application 11–2

James is a 20-year-old man who injured his left knee when he attempted to make a cut while playing soccer. Following physical examination and magnetic resonance imaging (MRI) testing, the patient was diagnosed with a complete ACL rupture and partial MCL rupture. In the weeks following his injury, James reported frequent episodes of his knee giving way, including buckling, shifting, or slipping of the knee during weight-bearing activities. James underwent ACL reconstruction using a bone-patellar tendon-bone autograft. No surgical procedures were performed on the partially torn MCL due to its rich blood supply and repair capacity. Three days after surgery, James started postoperative rehabilitation with the goal of returning to soccer. Primary postoperative impairments included knee joint effusion, decreased knee flexion and extension ROM, and decreased quadriceps activation and strength. Given these impairments, clinicians must consider various factors when choosing therapeutic exercises that both protect the healing ACL graft and facilitate restoration of quadriceps activation and strength.

The ultimate stress of the typical *in vivo* ACL is approximately 2,000 N, with an ultimate strain of approximately 15% (maximum stress and maximum strain before failure, respectively); however, during the first 2 to 4 weeks after reconstruction, the ACL graft and its fixation is at its weakest and may be injured by lesser forces.[123-125] Therapeutic exercises within a rehabilitation program after ACL reconstruction must not produce forces that exceed the tensile properties of the new graft to avoid graft stretching or rupture. Various activities are routinely prescribed to improve muscle strength and joint function after ACL reconstruction. It should be noted, however, that it is currently unclear as to how much strain can be detrimental to a healing graft. ACL strain is typically greatest between 10° and 30° of knee flexion for both weight-bearing and non–weight-bearing exercises, and 0% strain in positions of greater than 60° of knee flexion.[125]

Restoration of quadriceps activation and strength is critical for optimal joint function after ACL reconstruction. Current clinical practice guidelines recommend weight-bearing and non–weight-bearing quadriceps-strengthening exercises after ACL reconstruction.[126] Historically, the appropriateness of non–weight-bearing quadriceps exercise after ACL injury or reconstruction has been discussed in the literature given that isolated activation of the quadriceps can generate an anterior tibial shear force. Currently, there is broad consensus that non–weight-bearing exercises are safe and essential in effectively restoring quadriceps muscle function. Several studies have reported similar peak ACL strain values between non–weight-bearing knee extension and squatting.[125,127-129] During walking, ACL strain may reach up to 13% during midstance and late swing phases.[130,131] In comparison, peak ACL strain was measured at 4.4% during non–weight-bearing isometric knee extension at 15° knee flexion against a 30 N·m extension torque and 3.8% during non–weight-bearing knee extension from 0° to 90°.[128] This work informs recommendations that non–weight-bearing exercises can be safely implemented in postoperative rehabilitation if patients are independently walking or participating in weight-bearing exercise.[132,133]

For James, incorporating non–weight-bearing and weight-bearing knee extension exercise throughout the rehabilitation plan of care is needed to restore quadriceps activation and strength. In early phases of rehabilitation, consideration of low-load non–weight-bearing knee extension exercise is likely appropriate (e.g., multiangle isometrics). The patellar tendon bone-tendon-bone autograft is another consideration in quadriceps strengthening exercise prescription over the plan of care. Modification to exercise may be warranted based on graft-site pain and patellofemoral joint stress (discussed later in the chapter).

Expanded Concepts 11–5
Coping With ACL Deficiency

Certain individuals are capable of compensating successfully with a dynamic knee stabilization strategy in the presence of a complete ACL rupture.[134-137] Quadriceps strength training and neuromuscular re-education may help facilitate proper dynamic control and typical knee motion after ACL injury.[138-140] A percentage of athletes who cope well can even return to high-demand sports that require cutting and pivoting without reconstructing the ligamentous restraint to anterior tibial translation.[135,141,142] However, not all patients return to preinjury activity levels after sustaining an ACL rupture regardless of operative and rehabilitative interventions.[143] Evidence indicates that patients who choose a nonoperative approach are at no greater risk for developing knee osteoarthritis compared with those who undergo ACL reconstructions.[144,145]

Expanded Concepts 11–6
Anterolateral Ligament

Injury to the ACL and extra-articular structures on the anterolateral aspect of the knee contributes to rotatory knee instability. Anterolateral rotatory laxity of the knee following ACL injuries is often observed through a pivot shift test, a clinical test to appreciate the anterior subluxation and spontaneous reduction of the lateral tibial plateau during passive knee flexion and extension.[146] Anterolateral structures, in particular the **anterolateral ligament (ALL)**, has recently received a considerable increase in attention and research. Its presence, anatomy, biomechanical role, and need for surgical reconstruction have become topics of controversy and debate. The ALL is described as a broad fibrous band of the anterolateral joint capsule between the posterolateral epicondyle of the femur (posterior and proximal to the attachment of the lateral collateral ligament) and the anterior tibia (midway between the tibial attachment of the IT band and the fibular head).[147-151] A recent systematic review of ALL anatomic studies reported identification of the ALL in over 82% of cadaveric and MRI studies.[150] The potential role of the ALL and the anterolateral complex in providing anterior and rotational stability to the knee[152-155] has prompted consideration of extra-articular procedures, like a lateral external tenodesis procedure or ALL reconstruction procedure, concomitant with ACL reconstructions. Thus, some have suggested a reconstruction of the ALL concurrently with an ACL reconstruction to fully restore knee joint arthrokinematics.[148,156-159] Current indications for anterolateral augmentation procedures with anterior cruciate reconstruction and the effects on joint arthrokinematics, recurrent ACL injury and joint preservation, as well as patient outcomes are the focus of ongoing research.[148]

POSTERIOR CRUCIATE LIGAMENT

The PCL originates at the lateral aspect of the medial femoral condyle and travels inferiorly and somewhat posteriorly to attach distally to the posterior tibial surface, between the posterior horns of the two menisci (see Fig. 11–13).[160] The PCL blends with the posterior capsule and periosteum as it crosses to its tibial attachment.[161] Like the ACL, the PCL is *intracapsular* but *extrasynovial*.[160] The PCL is a shorter and less oblique structure than the ACL, with a cross-sectional area 120% to 150% greater than that of the ACL.[162] The large size and shape of the PCL along with its extensive femoral attachment help it to resist greater loads than the ACL before failing.[163] The vascular supply is provided by the middle genicular artery, like that of the ACL.[164] Also like the ACL, the PCL is typically divided into two bundles that are named for their tibial origins: the **posteromedial bundle (PMB)** and the **anterolateral bundle (ALB).**[165] These bundles function together to provide primary restraint to posterior tibial translation at all knee angles. When the knee is near full extension, the larger and stronger anterolateral bundle is lax, whereas the posteromedial bundle becomes taut, providing the main restraint to posterior tibial translation. At 80° to 90° of flexion, the posteromedial bundle is relaxed and the anterolateral bundle is maximally taut, providing primary restraint to posterior tibial translation.[166] Although these shifts in tension occur, biomechanical studies indicate that both bundles contribute to resisting posterior tibial translation across the range of knee flexion.[167-169] For example, the anterolateral bundle provides the main resistance to posterior translation between 70° and 105°; however, the more vertical orientation of the anterolateral bundle decreases its ability to resist posterior tibial displacement in full knee flexion.[160] Concurrently, as knee flexion increases, the femoral attachment of the posteromedial bundle translates anteriorly on the tibia, giving the posteromedial bundle a more horizontal orientation.[160,163] This translation creates greater tension and the necessary orientation for the posteromedial bundle to increase its ability to resist posterior displacement of the tibia in deep knee flexion angles.[160]

The PCL restrains approximately 90% of the posterior translatory force directed along the tibia across the majority of the knee flexion ROM.[160,170,171] In the fully extended knee, only minimal posterior displacements of the tibia can occur due to the multitude of ligaments that reinforce the posterior capsule (discussed next) that aid the PCL in resisting posterior tibial translation.[164,172] The PCL as a whole is more adept at restraining posterior tibial motion with the knee flexed, unlike the ACL, which resists force better at full extension.[101,164] Maximal posterior displacement of the tibia typically occurs at 75° to 90° of flexion; as the knee continues to flex, the secondary restraints against posterior translation become ineffective, enhancing the role of the PCL in resisting posterior translation at full knee flexion.[164] Like the ACL, the PCL has a role in restraining varus and valgus stresses at the knee and appears to play a role in both restraining and guiding rotation of the tibia.[172-174] When a posterior translatory force is applied to the tibia, the orientation of the PCL may create a concomitant *lateral rotary force* on the tibia as tension on the PCL increases. In the presence of PCL deficiency, *lateral tibial translation* is observed that may alter the contact locations of the knee joint, serving as a mechanism that may lead to articular cartilage degeneration similar to that postulated with an ACL injury.[173]

In the absence of the PCL, muscles must be recruited to actively stabilize against excessive posterior tibial translation. The popliteus muscle shares the PCL's role in resisting posteriorly directed forces on the tibia, and can thus contribute to knee stability following PCL rupture.[162] In contrast, hamstring contraction can destabilize a flexed knee joint in the absence of the PCL because the hamstrings produce rather than restrain a posterior shear force on the tibia (see Fig. 11–18B).[171] In contrast, a quadriceps contraction produces an anterior shear, thus reducing the strain in the PCL at knee flexion angles between 20° and 60°.[110,171]

LIGAMENTS OF THE POSTERIOR CAPSULE

Several structures reinforce the "corners" of the posterior knee joint capsule **(Fig. 11–19)**. The posteromedial corner of the capsule is reinforced by the semimembranosus muscle, given its tendinous expansion that contributes to the oblique popliteal ligament, and by the stronger and more superficial posterior oblique ligament (POL).[78,175] The oblique popliteal ligament is a large, broad, and flat posterior knee structure that extends laterally across the posterior aspect of the knee joint.[78] It attaches distally to the posterior margin of the posteromedial tibia, the posteromedial joint capsule, and the lateral expansion of the semimembranosus tendon; it attaches proximally to the posterolateral joint capsule and plantaris muscle.[78] The

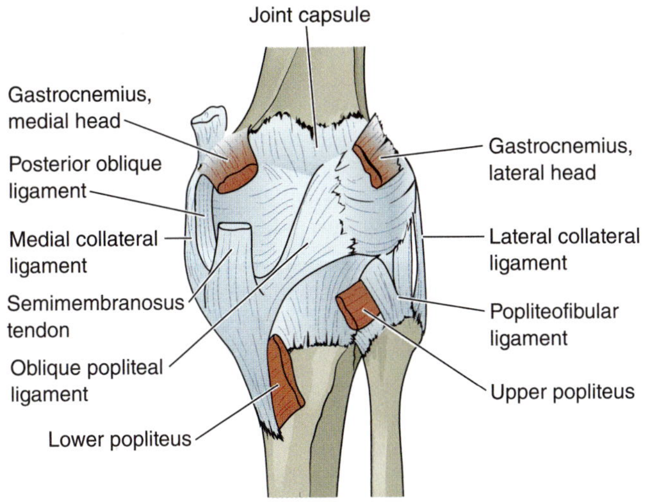

Figure 11-19 A view of the posterior capsule of the knee joint shows the reinforcing oblique popliteal ligament. Also seen are the collateral ligaments (MCL and LCL), the popliteofibular ligament, the posterior oblique ligament, and some of the reinforcing posterior musculature (cut), including semimembranosus, medial and lateral heads of the gastrocnemius, and the upper (femoral) and lower (tibial) attachments of the popliteus muscle.

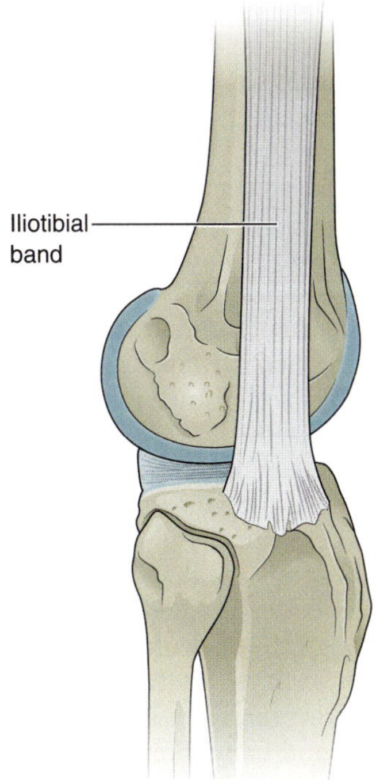

Figure 11-20 The IT band provides lateral support to the knee joint.

POL attaches proximally posterior to the adductor tubercle of the femur and anterior to the gastrocnemius tubercle on the femur.[72] Distally, the POL attaches to the posterior capsule and medial meniscus, helping to reinforce the deep portion of the MCL.[72] The posteromedial complex, specifically the POL, is taut in full extension and assists in checking posterior tibial translation and valgus forces.[176] The POL and posteromedial capsule become important stabilizers against posterior tibial translation and valgus loads, respectively, when there is injury to the ACL and PCL.[177]

The posterolateral corner of the capsule is primarily stabilized by the LCL, the popliteus tendon, and the popliteofibular ligament (see Fig. 11-19).[178,179] The popliteus tendon attaches to the lateral aspect of the femur just anterior to the LCL, courses underneath the LCL, and runs obliquely to the posteromedial tibia.[178,179] The popliteofibular ligament, previously identified as the arcuate ligament, attaches to the musculotendinous junction of the popliteus muscle and the posteromedial aspect of the fibular head.[178,179] Secondary structures that statically and dynamically support the posterolateral corner include the IT band, biceps femoris tendon, lateral gastrocnemius tendon, the fabellofibular ligament, and lateral joint capsule.[179-181] The fabellofibular ligament is a distal thickening of the capsular arm of the short head of the biceps femoris; it runs from the fabella (sesamoid bone or cartilaginous analog within the proximal lateral gastrocnemius tendon) to the lateral aspect of the fibular styloid process. Together, these structures protect the posterolateral corner of the knee by restraining tibial lateral rotation and providing varus stabilization, although an intact LCL provides the primary restraint to these forces.[178] The posterolateral corner and PCL work synergistically, as the posterolateral complex provides secondary stabilization to posterior tibial translation while the PCL provides secondary stabilization to tibial lateral rotation. Thus, after injury to the PCL, the posterolateral complex becomes an important stabilizer against posterior tibial translation, whereas an injury to both can result in significant posterior tibial instability.[178]

Expanded Concepts 11-7
Meniscofemoral Ligaments

The two meniscofemoral ligaments attach to the posterior horn of the lateral meniscus and to the lateral aspect of the medial femoral condyle, with one passing anterior to the PCL **(ligament of Humphry)** and the other posterior to the PCL (**ligament of Wrisberg**) (see Fig. 11-9).[29,39,160] Because of their attachment to the lateral meniscus at one end rather than to bone, they are not true ligaments. In addition, their presence within the knee is variable. In a review of the literature, Amis and colleagues reported that at least one of the meniscofemoral ligaments is present in 93% of knees, with only 50% of knees having both of the meniscofemoral ligaments.[163] The prevalence of having the posterior meniscofemoral ligament appears to be greater than the occurrence of the anterior meniscofemoral ligament.[163] Because the meniscofemoral ligaments assist the PCL in restraining posterior translation of the tibia on the femur, they are sometimes considered to be part of the PCL complex.[163] Nagasaki and colleagues have reported that, when present, the cross-sectional area of the mensicofemoral ligaments is 17.2% of the PCL.[182]

Iliotibial Band

The IT (iliotibial) band or tract is an extension of fascia covering the tensor fascia latae (TFL) and gluteus maximus muscles; it attaches proximally to the anterior superior iliac spine and external lip of the iliac crest.[179,180] The IT band continues distally with a primary attachment on the anterolateral tibia at Gerdy's tubercle **(Fig. 11-20)**, with additional attachments to the distal femur, lateral border of the patella, short head of the biceps femoris, and lateral head of the gastrocnemius—thus reinforcing the anterolateral aspect of the knee joint.[89] The IT band can be viewed as including (1) a tendinous portion between its proximal origin and its attachment to the lateral femoral epicondyle, and (2) a ligamentous portion between the lateral femoral epicondyle and Gerdy's tubercle on the tibia.

Despite the muscular attachments to the proximal end of the IT band, it functions as a passive structure at the knee joint. For example, a contraction of the TFL or the gluteus maximus muscles, to which the IT band attaches, produces only minimal longitudinal excursion of the band distally. Despite limited longitudinal movements, the IT band is often thought to shift anterior to the knee joint axis as the knee is extended and posterior as the knee is flexed.[183,184] However, cadaveric studies have challenged the concept that the IT band moves or "rolls" over the lateral femoral epicondyle with knee flexion/extension, given the observed fibrous connections to the femoral epicondyle that should check anterior/posterior shift of the band.[185] These studies also failed to identify a bursa between the IT band and the epicondyle of the femur that might become irritated, as is often suggested as a source of pain. However, there is adipose tissue present between the IT band and bony interface.[185-187] As the knee moves from full extension to 30° of flexion, compression of this highly vascularized and richly innervated adipose tissue increases between the iliotibial band and the lateral epicondyle. The adipose tissue is less compressed in full extension, which may account for the complaints of pain at the distal insertion of the IT band around 30° of flexion and not at full extension in patients with IT band symptoms.[185,188]

Additional fibrous connections from the IT band to the biceps femoris, lateral gastrocnemius, and **vastus lateralis** muscles form a sling behind the lateral femoral condyle, which assists the ACL in restraining posterior femoral (or anterior tibial) translation with the knee near full extension.[90,189] With the knee flexed, the combination of the IT band, the LCL, and the popliteal tendon can provide even greater assistance in resisting anterior displacement of the tibia on the femur as well as increased stability to the lateral side of the joint.[186] Despite its lateral location, the IT band alone provides only minimal resistance to varus loads and lateral joint space opening.[84,183] The IT band also attaches to the patella via the lateral patellofemoral ligament of the lateral retinaculum. This portion of the IT band becomes tighter as the knee moves into a flexed position.[185] As we shall see later in this chapter, the attachment of the IT band to the lateral border of the patella may have important implications for patellofemoral function.

Bursae

The extensive array of ligaments and muscles crossing the tibiofemoral joint, in combination with the large excursions of bony segments, creates the potential for substantial frictional forces among muscular, ligamentous, and bony structures. Numerous bursae, or fluid-filled sacs, however, prevent or limit such damaging forces (see Fig. 11–11). Three of the knee joint's bursae, the **suprapatellar bursa,** the **subpopliteal bursa,** and the **gastrocnemius bursa,** are not separate entities but rather are extensions of the capsule's synovium or communicate with the synovial lining of the joint capsule through small openings. The anteriorly located suprapatellar bursa lies between the quadriceps tendon and the anterior femur, superior to the patella. The posteriorly located subpopliteal bursa lies between the tendon of the popliteus muscle and the lateral femoral condyle. The gastrocnemius bursa lies between the tendon of the medial head of the gastrocnemius muscle and the medial femoral condyle. The gastrocnemius bursa continues beneath the tendon of the semimembranosus muscle to protect it from the medial femoral condyle.

The bursae that are part of or communicate with the synovial lining of the joint capsule allow the lubricating synovial fluid to move from recess to recess during flexion and extension of the knee. In extension, the posterior capsule and ligaments are taut, and the gastrocnemius and subpopliteal bursae are compressed. This shifts the synovial fluid anteriorly.[190,191] In flexion, the suprapatellar bursa is compressed, forcing the fluid posteriorly. When the knee joint is in the semiflexed position (e.g., open-packed position), the synovial fluid is under the least amount of pressure.

Clinical Application 11–3
Joint Effusion and the Open-Packed Position

When there is excess fluid within the joint cavity as a result of injury or disease (**joint effusion**), the semiflexed (open-packed) knee position helps to relieve tension in the capsule and, therefore, can minimize discomfort. For example, patients will often prefer to rest supine or semireclined with a pillow beneath their knee (promoting knee flexion of approximately 20° to 30°) after total knee arthroplasty, reporting it as their position of comfort.

Besides the bursae that communicate with the synovial capsule, there are several other bursae associated with the knee joint (see Fig. 11–11). **The prepatellar bursa,** located between the skin and the anterior surface of the patella, allows free movement of the skin over the patella during flexion and extension. The **infrapatellar bursa** lies inferior to the patella, between the patellar tendon and the overlying skin. Both the infrapatellar bursa and the prepatellar bursa may become inflamed as a result of direct trauma to the front of the knee or through activities such as prolonged kneeling. The **deep infrapatellar bursa,** located between the patellar tendon and the tibial tuberosity, helps to reduce friction between the patellar tendon and the tibial tuberosity.[192] This bursa is separated from the synovial cavity of the joint by the infrapatellar (Hoffa's) fat pad (see Fig. 11-8).[191,192] If the infrapatellar fat pad is removed, patellofemoral contact area decreases, thus increasing patellofemoral joint stress and the potential for degenerative changes.[193] There are also several small bursae that are associated with the ligaments of the knee joint. A bursa is often present between the LCL and the biceps femoris tendon.[194] On the medial side of the joint, small bursae can be found both superficial and deep to the superficial portion of the MCL to protect it from the deep portion of the MCL and the tendons of the **semitendinosus** and **gracilis** muscles, respectively.[37]

Function

Joint Kinematics

The primary rotary (osteokinematic) motion of the tibiofemoral joint is flexion/extension, although small amounts of both

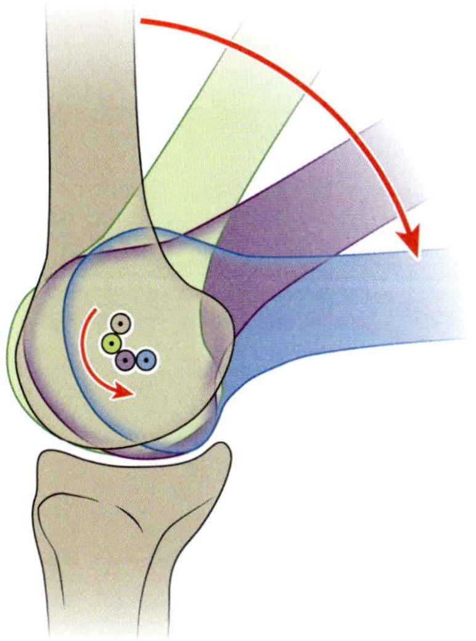

Figure 11–21 A lateral view of the knee demonstrating the changing knee center of rotation along a medial/lateral axis during knee flexion and extension.

medial/lateral rotation and varus/valgus motions also take place. Each of the knee joint motions occurs about changing, but definable, axes. The complex bony architecture results in both rotation and translation between the femoral condyles and the tibial plateau, producing a constantly changing center of rotation at the knee joint **(Fig. 11–21)**. Current advances in motion analysis tracking systems, musculoskeletal modeling techniques, and imaging modalities have permitted accurate representation of three-dimensional descriptions of motion, including all six degrees of freedom (three rotational, three translational) at the tibiofemoral joint. Understanding the three primary axes of motion will provide the necessary framework to comprehend typical knee kinematics and to diagnose and treat abnormal movement patterns. In addition to rotary motions at the knee, translation between the tibia and femur in an anteroposterior direction is common within the tibiofemoral compartments. Medial and lateral translations may also occur in response to varus and valgus forces, although to a substantially lesser extent. The small amounts of anteroposterior displacements that occur in the typical knee are the result of joint incongruence and variations in ligamentous tension. Importantly, these small anteroposterior translations are necessary for typical joint motions to occur. Excessive translational motions, however, should be considered abnormal and generally indicate some degree of ligamentous incompetence. We will focus on typical knee joint motions, including both osteokinematics and arthrokinematics.

FLEXION/EXTENSION

The axis for tibiofemoral flexion and extension can be simplified as a horizontal line passing through the femoral epicondyles.[2,195] Although this transepicondylar axis represents an accurate estimate of the axis for flexion and extension, it should be appreciated that this axis is not truly fixed but, as just noted, shifts throughout the ROM (see Fig. 11–21). The shift in rotational axes of the knee can be largely attributed to the changing radius of curvature of the distal end of the femur.

Sliding motions must occur between the large articular surfaces of the femur and the relatively small tibial condyles as one joint surface is rolling over the other to maintain adequate joint contact. If, in weight-bearing, the convex femoral condyles were permitted to roll posteriorly on a fixed, concave tibial plateau, the femur would "run out of" tibia to roll on, and limit flexion. For the femoral condyles to continue to roll posteriorly as flexion increases, the femoral condyles must simultaneously slide anteriorly on the tibial plateau **(Fig. 11–22A)**. The initiation of knee flexion (0° to 25°), therefore, occurs primarily as posterior rolling of the femoral condyles on the tibia that moves the contact of the femoral condyles posteriorly on the tibial plateau. As flexion continues, the rolling of the femoral condyles is accompanied by a simultaneous anterior slide that together create a nearly pure spin of the femur on the posterior tibia with little linear displacement of the contact point on the tibial plateau after 25° of flexion. Extension of the knee from a flexed position is essentially a reversal of this motion **(Fig. 11–22B)**. Knee joint extension occurs initially as an anterior rolling of the femoral condyles on the tibial plateau, displacing the femoral condyles back to a neutral position on the tibial plateau. After the initial forward rolling, the femoral condyles slide posteriorly just enough to continue extension of the femur, with the combined roll and slide occurring as an almost pure spin of the femoral condyles on the tibial plateau. Although the interdependent osteokinematic and arthrokinematic motions were described with the tibia fixed in weight-bearing, the tibia, of course, is also capable of moving on a fixed femur (e.g., during a seated knee extension or during the swing phase of gait) **(Fig. 11–23)**. In this case, the movements would be described somewhat differently but represent the same relative movements. When the tibia is flexing on a fixed femur, the tibia both rolls and slides posteriorly on the relatively fixed femoral condyles (see **Fig. 11–23A**). Extension of the tibia on a fixed femur incorporates an anterior roll and slide of the tibial plateau on the fixed femur (see **Fig. 11–23B**). It is important to recognize that an anterior slide of the tibia on the femur represents the same movement as a posterior slide of the femur on the tibia. In the first case, we are simply describing the movement of the tibia on a fixed femur (i.e., non–weight-bearing), whereas the second case describes the movement of the femur on a fixed tibia (i.e., weight-bearing).

Expanded Concepts 11-8
Tibiofemoral Contact Points

Advancements in diagnostic imaging techniques and biomedical modeling techniques have improved the ability to accurately predict the contact points of cartilage in the knee. Li and colleagues used advanced imaging techniques to model surface contact locations between the articular cartilage of the femur and tibia.[196] Three-dimensional motions were assessed to measure the contact points of the cartilage within the medial and lateral compartments of the knee joint. This investigation concluded that the contact points of the lateral tibial cartilage translated posteriorly with increased flexion, whereas the contact points of the medial tibial cartilage did not translate significantly during knee flexion. These results indicate that a greater amount of rolling motion occurs between the lateral femoral condyle and the lateral tibial plateau compared with that of the medial compartment, whereas more sliding motion occurs between the medial femoral condyle and the medial tibial plateau.[196]

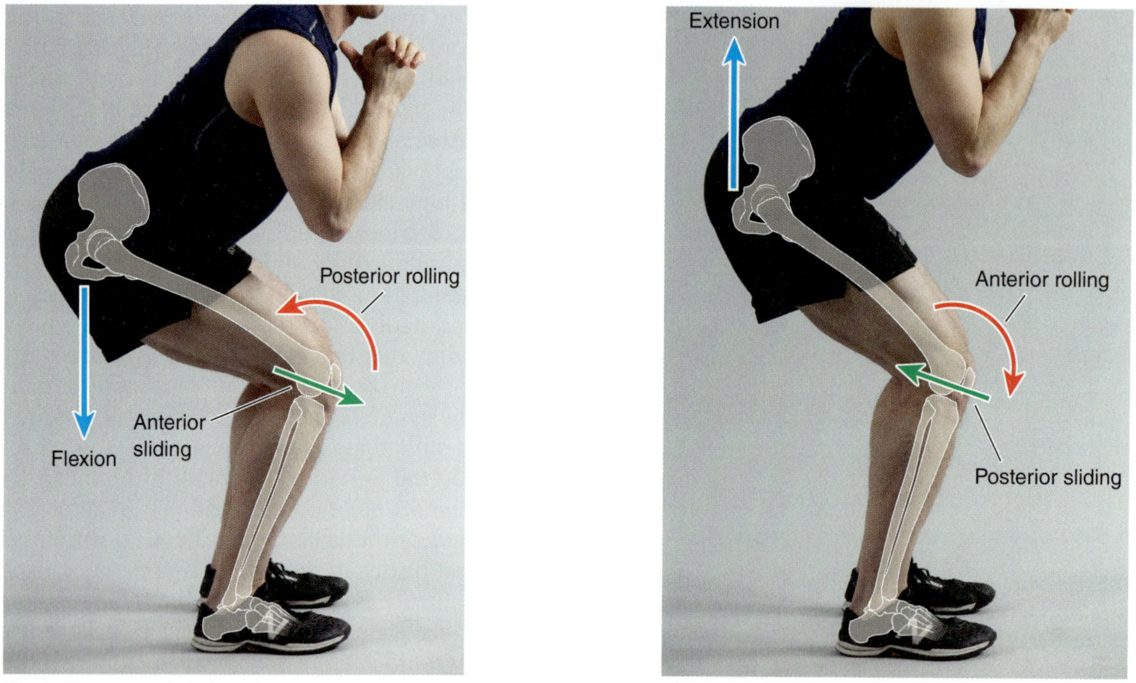

A B

Figure 11–22 **A.** A schematic representation of rolling and sliding of the femoral condyles on a fixed tibia during knee flexion in a weight-bearing position. The femoral condyles roll posteriorly while simultaneously sliding anteriorly. **B.** Motion of the femoral condyles during extension. The femoral condyles roll anteriorly while simultaneously sliding posteriorly.

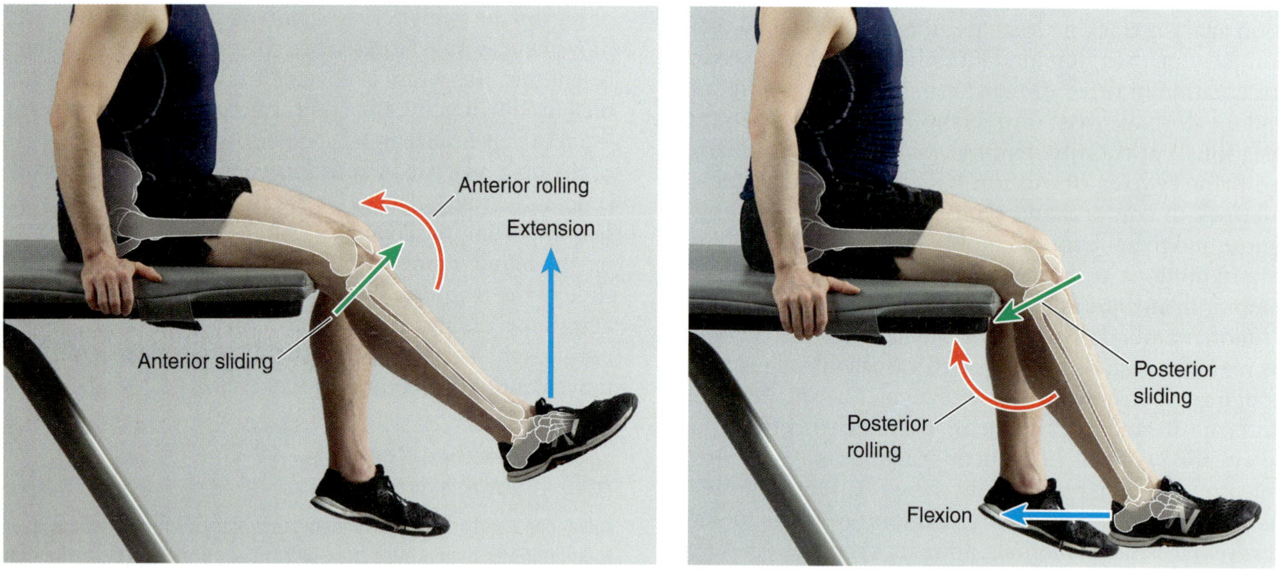

A B

Figure 11–23 **A.** A schematic representation of rolling and sliding of the tibial plateau during knee extension in a non–weight-bearing position. The tibial plateau roll anteriorly while simultaneously sliding anteriorly. **B.** Motion of the tibial plateaus during flexion. The tibial plateau roll posteriorly while simultaneously gliding posteriorly.

Role of the Cruciate Ligaments and Menisci in Flexion/Extension

The arthrokinematics associated with knee joint flexion and extension are somewhat dictated by the presence of the cruciate ligaments **(Fig. 11–24)**. If the cruciate ligaments are assumed to be rigid segments with a constant length, posterior rolling of the femur during weight-bearing knee flexion would cause the "rigid" ACL to tighten.[197] Continued rolling of the femur would result in the taut ACL simultaneously creating an anterior translational force on the femoral condyles (see **Fig. 11–24A**). The PCL would function in a similar manner during weight-bearing knee extension. The femoral

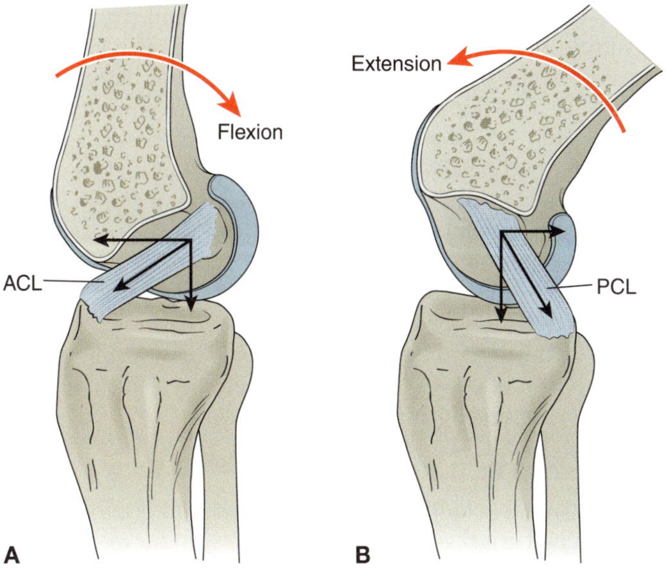

Figure 11–24 Cross-sectional, sagittal view of the knee. **A.** In flexion of the femur, posterior rolling of the femoral condyles creates tension in the "rigid" ACL that results in an anterior translational force imposed by the ACL on the femur. **B.** In extension of the femur, anterior rolling of the femoral condyles creates tension in the "rigid" PCL, which results in a posterior translational force imposed by the PCL on the femur. The ACL and PCL, of course, are not rigid. However, with increased tension in each of these ligaments, the force vectors will be similar.

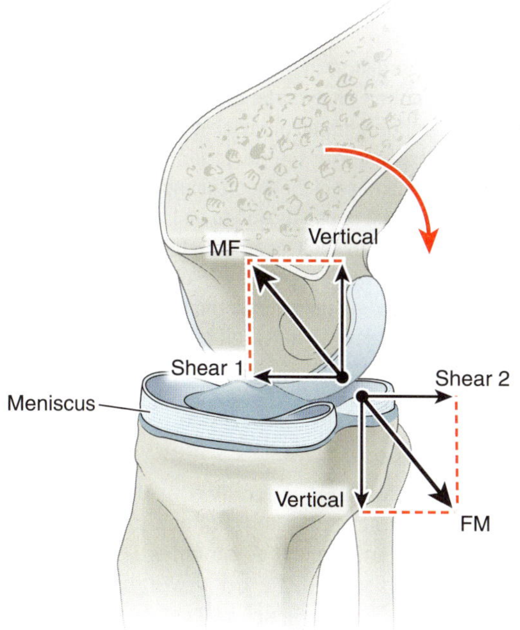

Figure 11–25 The oblique contact of the femur with the wedge-shaped meniscus results in the reaction forces of meniscus-on-femur (MF) and femur-on-meniscus (FM). Each reaction force can be resolved into vertical and shear components. Shear 1 assists the femur in its forward slide during flexion, and shear 2 assists in the posterior migration of the menisci that occurs with knee flexion.

condyles roll anteriorly on the tibial plateau until the "rigid" PCL checks further anterior progression of the femur, creating a posterior translational force on the femoral condyles (see **Fig. 11–24B**).

The anterior slide of the femur during weight-bearing flexion may be further facilitated by the shape of the menisci. As the femoral condyles roll posteriorly on the tibial plateau in weight-bearing, they must roll "uphill" on the "wedge" created by the menisci that are thicker peripherally. The oblique contact force of the thicker portion of the menisci on the femur creates an anterior shear component that helps guide the femur anteriorly during flexion, whereas the reaction force of the femur on the menisci contains a posterior shear component that deforms the menisci posteriorly on the tibial plateau **(Fig. 11–25)**.[198] Posterior deformation of the menisci occurs because the rigid attachments at the meniscal horns limit the ability of the menisci to move in their entirety.[198] Posterior deformation also allows the menisci to remain beneath the rounded femoral condyles during the rolling phase at the initiation of weight-bearing knee flexion as the condyles move on the relatively flat tibial plateau. As the knee joint begins to return to extension from full flexion, the posterior margins of the menisci return to their neutral position. As extension continues, the anterior margins of the menisci are deformed anteriorly by the femoral condyles.

The motion (or distortion) of the menisci is an important component of tibiofemoral flexion and extension. Given the need of the menisci to reduce friction and absorb the forces of the femoral condyles that are imposed on the relatively small tibial plateau, the menisci must remain beneath the femoral condyles to continue these functions. The posterior deformation of the menisci during flexion is assisted by muscular mechanisms to ensure that appropriate meniscal motion occurs. During knee flexion, for example, the semimembranosus muscle exerts a posterior pull on the medial meniscus to which it is attached **(Fig. 11–26)**, whereas the popliteus muscle assists with posterior deformation of the lateral meniscus.[37,41]

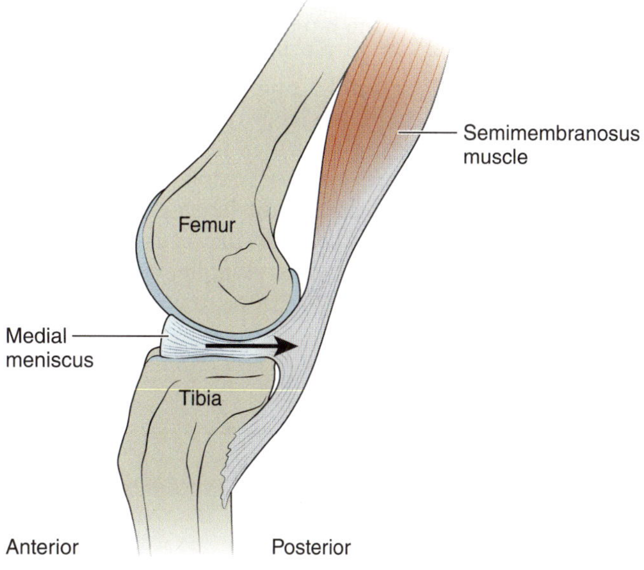

Figure 11–26 A schematic representation of the semimembranosus muscle and its attachment to the medial meniscus is shown. The arrow represents the direction of pull of the semimembranosus muscle on the medial meniscus during flexion.

Expanded Concepts 11-9
Meniscal Motion

Failure of the menisci to distort in the proper direction can result in impairments in joint motion or damage to the menisci. If the femur literally rolls up the wedge-shaped menisci in flexion (without either the anterior slide of the femur or the *posterior distortion* of the menisci), the increasing thickness of the menisci and the threat of rolling off the posterior margin will cause flexion to be limited. Alternatively, the atypical stress on the meniscus (especially the less mobile medial meniscus) may cause the meniscus to tear. Failure of the menisci to *distort anteriorly* during extension causes the thick anterior margins of the menisci to become wedged between the femur and tibia in the final stages of extension, thus limiting extension.

Flexion/Extension ROM

Passive range of knee flexion is generally considered to be 130° to 140°.[199] During an activity such as deep knee squatting, however, knee flexion may reach as much as 160° as the hip and knee are both flexed and the body weight is superimposed on the joint.[200] Normal gait on level ground requires approximately 60° to 70° of knee flexion, whereas ascending stairs requires about 80°, and sitting down into and arising from a chair requires 90° of flexion or more.[199] Over 90% of people demonstrate knee joint extension beyond 0° (knee joint hyperextension), and up to 5° to 10° of knee hyperextension is common.[201] A position of excessive knee hyperextension is termed **genu recurvatum**.[202]

Many of the muscles acting at the knee are two-joint (biarticulate) muscles crossing not only the knee but also the hip or ankle. Therefore, the hip or ankle joint position can influence the knee joint's ROM. For example, knee flexion can be limited to 120° or less if the hip joint is simultaneously extended, due to passive insufficiency of the **rectus femoris** **(Fig. 11-27A).** When the hip joint is in neutral position, the rectus femoris allows increased knee flexion (see **Fig. 11-27B**). When the lower extremity is in weight-bearing, ROM limitations at other joints, such as the ankle, may cause restrictions in knee flexion or extension. As an example, rigid ski boots generally hold the ankle in dorsiflexion, preventing full knee extension when the foot is flat on the ground **(Fig. 11-28A)**, resulting in a flexed knee gait pattern. A similar pattern is created in the presence of a fixed dorsiflexion deformity in the ankle. The opposite situation occurs with a limitation to dorsiflexion. A lack of ankle dorsiflexion (e.g., caused by tight plantarflexors) may limit the amount of knee flexion that can be performed before lifting the heel off the ground. For example, tight plantarflexors at the ankle can lead to the inability to bring the tibia forward in weight-bearing and result in knee hyperextension or genu recurvatum in standing **(Fig. 11-28B)**. The relationship between ankle and knee position when the foot is on the ground can be exploited by intentionally altering ankle joint motion (e.g., through a heel lift or an ankle–foot orthosis) to prevent or control knee ROM.

MEDIAL/LATERAL ROTATION

Medial/lateral **(axial)** rotation of the knee joint occurs about a longitudinal axis that runs through or close to the *medial* tibial intercondylar tubercle.[3] Consequently, the medial condyle acts as the pivot point, whereas the lateral condyles move through a greater arc of motion, regardless of the direction of rotation **(Fig. 11-29)**. For example, as the tibia *laterally rotates* on the femur, the medial tibial condyle moves only slightly on the relatively fixed medial femoral condyle, although the lateral tibial condyle moves a larger distance posteriorly on the relatively fixed lateral femoral condyle. During tibial *medial rotation*, the medial tibial condyle again rotates only slightly, whereas the lateral condyle moves anteriorly through a larger arc of motion. During both medial and lateral rotation, the knee joint's menisci will distort in the direction of movement of the corresponding femoral condyle and, therefore, will maintain their relationship to the femoral condyles just as they did in flexion and extension. For example, as the tibia medially rotates on the femur (or femur laterally rotates on the tibia in weight-bearing), the medial meniscus will distort anteriorly on the tibial condyle to remain beneath the relatively anteriorly moving medial femoral condyle, and the lateral meniscus will distort posteriorly to remain beneath the posteriorly moving lateral femoral condyle. In this way, the menisci continue to reduce friction and distribute forces without restricting motion of the femur.

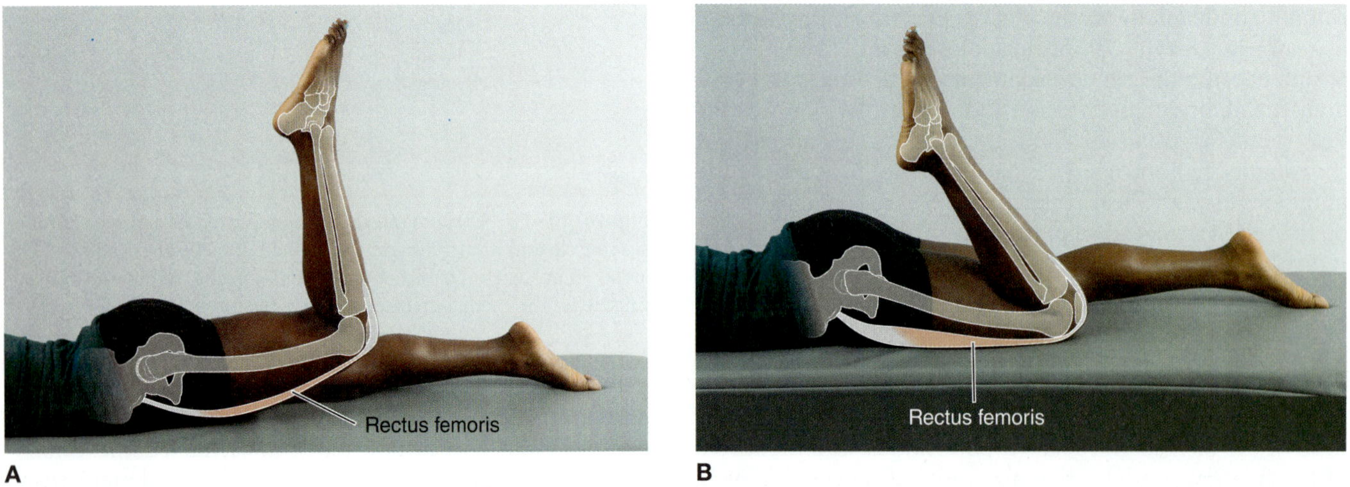

Figure 11-27 **A.** With the hip in an extended position, passive insufficiency in the rectus femoris limits flexion at the knee joint. **B.** With the hip in a neutral position, the rectus femoris is able to lengthen sufficiently to allow knee flexion range of motion.

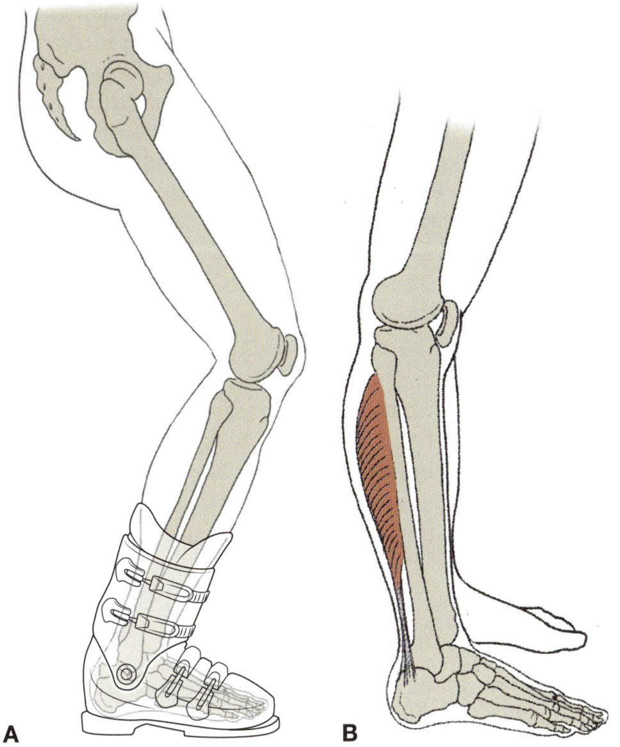

Figure 11–28 **A.** With the ankle fixed in dorsiflexion by the rigid ski boot, the knee cannot be fully extended without the forefoot being lifted from the ground. **B.** With a fixed plantarflexion deformity of the ankle, the knee is forced into hyperextension when the foot is flat on the ground.

Axial rotation is permitted by ligamentous laxity and the knee's unique bony anatomy, and its magnitude depends on the flexion/extension position of the knee. When the knee is in full extension, the ligaments are taut, the tibial tubercles are lodged in the intercondylar notch, and the menisci are tightly interposed between the articulating surfaces; consequently, very little axial rotation is possible. As the knee flexes toward 90°, capsular and ligamentous laxity increases, the tibial tubercles are no longer within the intercondylar notch, and the condyles of the tibia and femur are free to move on each other. Therefore, the greatest amount of axial rotation is available at 90° of knee flexion. At 90°, the total axial rotation available is approximately 35°, with the range for lateral rotation being slightly greater (0° to 20°) than the range for medial rotation (0° to 15°).[203] The magnitude of axial rotation again decreases as the knee approaches full flexion.

VALGUS (ABDUCTION)/VARUS (ADDUCTION)

Frontal plane motion at the knee (varus/valgus or adduction/abduction of the tibia, respectively), although minimal, does exist and contributes to typical functioning of the tibiofemoral joint. Frontal plane ROM is typically only 8° at full extension, and 13° at 20° of knee flexion.[59,204] Excessive frontal plane motion can indicate ligamentous insufficiency. Muscles that cross the knee joint have the capacity to both generate and control substantial valgus and varus torques.[205-207] When there is ligamentous laxity, the excessive frontal plane motion could increase peak stresses across the medial or lateral compartment (e.g., the lateral compartment would experience greater stress during valgus motion). Consequently, there could be an increase in activity of the muscles around the knee joint to control this excessive motion; however, greater muscle activity creates greater joint compression and thus may also precipitate greater peak stresses across the joint.[20,207]

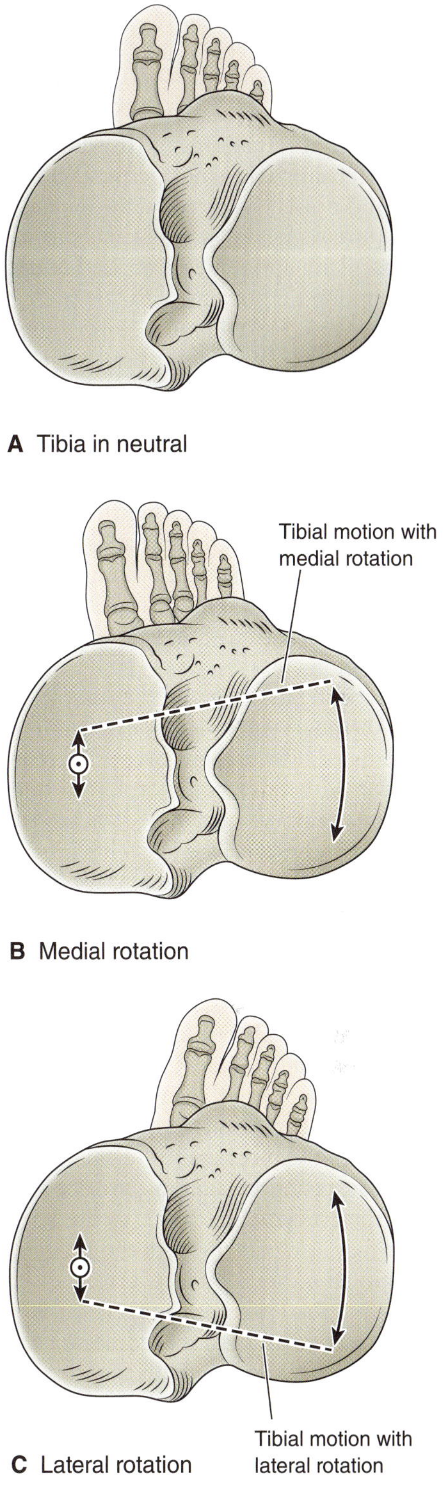

Figure 11–29 During axial rotation of the tibia, there is more motion of the lateral tibial condyle than of the medial tibial condyle in both directions; that is, the longitudinal axis for medial/lateral rotation appears to be located on the medial tibial plateau. **A.** Neutral knee joint rotation. **B.** Medial rotation of the knee joint. **C.** Lateral rotation of the knee joint.

COUPLED MOTIONS

Typical knee joint motions are not as straightforward as we have described. Biplanar intra-articular motions can occur because of the oblique orientation of the axes of motion with respect to the longitudinal axes of the femur and tibia. The true flexion/extension axis is not perpendicular to the shafts of the femur and tibia.[208] Therefore, flexion and extension do not occur as pure sagittal plane motions but include frontal and transverse plane components termed **coupled motions** (similar to coupling that occurs with lateral flexion and axial rotation in the vertebral column). As previously noted, the medial femoral condyle lies slightly distal to the lateral femoral condyle, which results in a physiological valgus angle in the extended knee that is similar to the physiological valgus angle that exists at the elbow. With knee flexion around the obliquely oriented axis, the tibia moves from a position oriented slightly lateral to the femur, to a position slightly medial to the femur in full flexion; that is, the foot approaches the midline of the body with knee flexion just as the hand may approach the midline of the body with elbow flexion. Therefore, extension is coupled with a valgus motion, whereas flexion is coupled with a varus motion.

There is an obligatory lateral rotation of the tibia that accompanies the final stages of knee extension that is not voluntary or produced by muscular forces. This coupled motion (lateral rotation with extension) is referred to as **automatic** or **terminal rotation**. We have already noted that the medial articular surface of the knee is longer (has more articular surface) than does the lateral articular surface (see Fig. 11-29A). Consequently, during the last 30° of non–weight-bearing knee extension (30° to 0°), the shorter lateral femoral condyle/tibial plateau articulation completes its rolling–sliding motion before the longer medial articular surfaces.[209] As extension continues, the longer medial plateau continues to roll and slide anteriorly after the lateral side of the plateau has halted. This continued anterior motion of the medial tibial plateau on the medial femoral condyle results in lateral rotation of the tibia on the femur, with the motion most evident in the final 5° of extension.[208] Increasing tension in the knee joint ligaments, in particular the cruciate ligaments, as the knee approaches full extension may also contribute to the obligatory rotational motion, bringing the knee joint into its close-packed or locked position with the tibial tubercles lodged in the intercondylar notch, the menisci tightly interposed between the tibial and femoral condyles, and the ligaments taut.[164,210]

The motions of the knee joint, exclusive of automatic rotation, are produced primarily by the muscles that cross the joint. We will complete our examination of the tibiofemoral joint by first examining the individual contribution of the muscles, emphasizing their role in producing and controlling knee joint motion. We will then reexamine the muscles in combination with the passive joint structures of the knee as stabilizers of this very complicated joint.

Foundational Concepts 11–2

Locking or Screw Home Mechanism

The automatic or terminal rotation is also known as the **locking** or **screw home mechanism** of the knee. To initiate knee flexion from full extension, the knee must first be "unlocked"; that is, the laterally rotated tibia cannot simply flex but must medially rotate simultaneously as flexion is initiated. Flexion motion will automatically result in medial rotation of the tibia because the longer medial side will move before the shorter lateral compartment. Automatic rotation or locking of the knee is thought to occur during both weight-bearing and non–weight-bearing knee joint function. In weight-bearing, this would require the freely moving femur to medially rotate on the relatively fixed tibia during the last 30° of extension. Unlocking would require lateral rotation of the femur on the tibia before flexion can proceed.

Muscles

The muscles that cross the knee are typically thought of as either flexors or extensors, because flexion and extension are the primary motions occurring at the tibiofemoral joint. Each of the muscles that flex and extend the knee also has a line of pull that can generate both frontal and transverse plane motions, although the moment arms for these latter motions are generally small. Therefore, each of the muscles, although grouped as flexors and extensors, will also be discussed regarding its role in controlling frontal and transverse plane motions.

KNEE FLEXOR GROUP

There are seven muscles that cross the knee joint posteriorly and can flex the knee. These are the semimembranosus, semitendinosus, biceps femoris (long and short heads), sartorius, gracilis, popliteus, and gastrocnemius muscles. The **plantaris muscle** may be considered an eighth knee flexor, but it is commonly absent. Except for the short head of the biceps femoris and the popliteus, all of the knee flexors are two-joint muscles. As biarticulate muscles, the ability to produce effective force at the knee is influenced by the relative position of the other joint that the muscle crosses. Five of the flexors (the semimembranosus, semitendinosus, sartorius, gracilis, and popliteus muscles) have the potential to medially rotate the tibia on a fixed femur, whereas the biceps femoris has a line of pull capable of laterally rotating the tibia.[211] The lateral muscles (biceps femoris, popliteus, and the lateral head of the gastrocnemius) are capable of producing valgus moments at the knee, whereas those on the medial side of the joint (semimembranosus, semitendinosus, sartorius, gracilis, and the medial head of the gastrocnemius) can generate varus moments.[206]

The three muscles of the hamstrings each attach proximally to the ischial tuberosity of the pelvis, except the short head of the biceps, which originates on the posterior femur. The semitendinosus muscle attaches distally to the anteromedial aspect of the tibia by way of a common tendon with the sartorius and the gracilis muscles. The common tendon is called the *pes anserinus* because of its shape (*pes anserinus* means "goose's foot") (see Fig. 11–14). The semimembranosus muscle inserts posteromedially on the tibia (and, as noted earlier, has fibers that attach to the medial meniscus that can facilitate posterior distortion of the medial meniscus during knee flexion).[37] Both heads of the biceps femoris muscle attach distally to the head of the fibula, with a slip to the lateral tibia. The short head of the biceps femoris muscle does not cross the hip joint and, therefore, acts only at the knee joint. The rest of the hamstring muscles cross both the hip (as extensors) and the knee (as flexors); therefore, their force-producing capability at the knee is affected by the angle of the hip joint. Greater hamstring force can be produced with the hip flexed because the hamstrings are lengthened across the hip, placing them at or near optimal length-tension.[178] When the two-joint hamstrings are required to contract with the hip extended and the knee flexed to 90° or more, the hamstrings are required to shorten across both the hip and the knee simultaneously. The hamstrings produce less force as knee flexion approaches the hamstring's maximal shortened (active insufficient) position, and the hamstrings must also overcome the increasing tension in the passively insufficient rectus femoris muscle.[212] In non–weight-bearing activities, the hamstrings generate a posterior shear force on the tibia that increases as knee flexion increases, peaking between 75° and 90° of knee flexion.[213] This posterior shear force can reduce strain on the ACL, although it increases the strain on the PCL.[171]

The two heads of the gastrocnemius muscle originate from the posterior aspects of the medial and lateral condyles of the femur and jointly attach distally to the calcaneal (or Achilles) tendon. Except for the small and often absent plantaris muscle, the gastrocnemius muscle is the only muscle that crosses both the knee and ankle joints. Much like the hamstrings' interaction with the hip joint, the gastrocnemius muscle's ability to produce knee flexor torque is dependent on the position of the ankle joint. The gastrocnemius muscle makes a relatively small contribution to knee flexion torque, especially when compared with the large ankle plantarflexor torque it can produce. The gastrocnemius generates the greatest knee flexion torque when the knee is in full extension.[214] As the knee is flexed, the ability of the gastrocnemius muscle to produce a knee flexion torque significantly decreases.[214]

The sartorius muscle arises anteriorly from the anterior superior iliac spine (ASIS) and crosses the femur to insert into the anteromedial surface of the tibial shaft (most often as part of the common pes anserinus tendon) (see Fig. 11–14). Variations in the distal attachment of the sartorius muscle are not uncommon and may be functionally relevant. When attached just anterior to its typical location, the sartorius muscle's line of action may fall anterior to the knee joint axis, serving as a mild knee joint extensor rather than as a knee flexor. Typically, however, the sartorius muscle functions as a flexor and medial rotator of the tibia. Despite its potential actions at the knee, activity within the sartorius muscle is more common during hip motion than with active knee motion. During gait, the sartorius muscle is typically active only during the swing phase. The gracilis muscle arises from the symphysis pubis and attaches distally to the common pes anserinus tendon (see Fig. 11–14). The gracilis muscle functions primarily as a hip joint flexor and adductor but also has the capability to produce weak flexion at the knee joint and produce slight medial rotation of the tibia. The three muscles of the pes anserinus appear to function effectively as a group to resist valgus forces and provide stability to the anteromedial aspect of the knee joint.

The popliteus muscle is a relatively small, single-joint muscle that attaches to the posterolateral aspect of the lateral femoral condyle and courses inferiorly and medially to attach to the posteromedial surface of the proximal tibia. The primary function of the popliteus muscle is to medially rotate the tibia on the femur.[211] The role of medially rotating the knee to unlock it during early knee flexion has been attributed to the popliteus muscle (see Foundational Concepts 11–2). However, it should be noted that unlocking is part of automatic rotation and is due in part to the obliquity of the joint axis and the anatomy of the articular surfaces. The popliteus muscle is also attached to the lateral meniscus and plays a role in deforming the lateral meniscus posteriorly during active knee flexion.[30] Together, the activity of both the semimembranosus and the popliteus muscles contribute to the posterior movement and deformation of their respective menisci on the tibial plateau while also generating a flexion torque at the knee. However, the menisci will move posteriorly on the tibial condyle even during passive flexion. Active assistance of the semimembranosus and popliteus muscles ensures that tibiofemoral congruence is maximized throughout the range of knee flexion assisting to keep both menisci beneath the femoral condyles. This actively assisted motion of the menisci reduces the potential for meniscal entrapment, which could limit knee flexion and increase the risk of meniscal injury.

The soleus and gluteus maximus muscles do not cross the knee joint; however, both can influence function at the knee during weight-bearing activities. The soleus muscle originates on the posterior aspect of the proximal tibia and fibula and attaches distally to the calcaneal (Achilles) tendon. With the foot fixed on the ground during weight-bearing activity, a soleus muscle contraction can assist with knee extension by pulling the tibia posteriorly (plantarflexing the ankle) **(Fig. 11–30)**. Additionally, as we've seen many times, the rotary (perpendicular) force of the soleus also creates a posterior

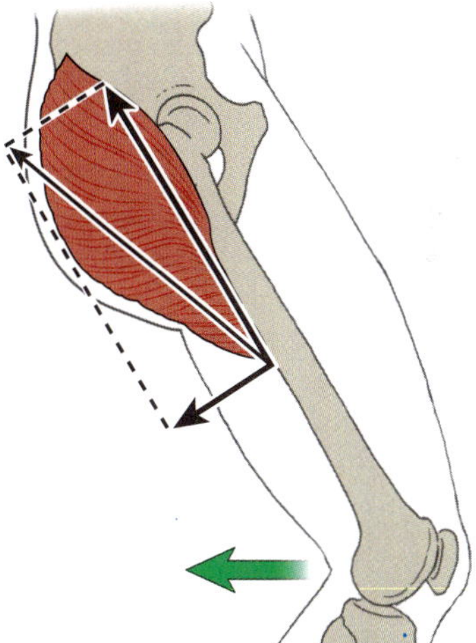

Figure 11–30 The actions of the gluteus maximus and soleus muscles can influence knee motion in weight-bearing. Although they do not cross the knee joint, these muscles can assist with knee extension with the foot on the ground.

shear on the weight-bearing leg, and can assist the hamstrings in restraining excessive anterior displacement of the tibia.[119] The gluteus maximus muscle, like the soleus muscle, can assist with knee extension during weight-bearing activities. It is well known that the large muscle mass of the gluteus maximus functions well as a hip extensor. With the foot flat on the ground and the knee bent, a contraction of the gluteus maximus extends the femur at the hip. Extension of the femur by the gluteus maximum in weight-bearing also produces knee extension and ankle plantarflexion by "continued action"—a closed-chain response. The rotary component of the gluteus maximus, however, also imposes a posterior shear of the femur on the tibia (or a relative anterior shear of the tibia on the femur), which would increase tension in the ACL without an offsetting co-contraction of other muscles.

KNEE EXTENSOR GROUP

The four extensors of the knee (rectus femoris, **vastus lateralis, vastus medialis,** and **vastus intermedius**) are known collectively as the quadriceps femoris muscle. The only portion of the quadriceps that crosses two joints is the rectus femoris muscle, which crosses the hip and knee from its proximal origin on the anterior inferior iliac spine. The vastus intermedius, vastus lateralis, and vastus medialis muscles originate on the femur and merge with the rectus femoris muscle into the common quadriceps tendon. The quadriceps tendon inserts into the *proximal aspect of the patella*; once the fibers reach the *distal patella*, they become the patellar tendon (or **patellar ligament**). The patellar tendon runs from the apex of the patella to the proximal portion of the tibial tuberosity. The vastus medialis and vastus lateralis also insert directly into the medial and lateral aspects of the patella by way of the retinacular fibers of the joint capsule (see Fig. 11–12).

Together, the four muscles of the quadriceps femoris function to extend the knee. Each muscle is oriented differently from the others, resulting in different lines of pull relative to the femoral shaft **(Fig. 11–31)**. Biomechanical testing has shown that the resultant pull of the vastus lateralis muscle on the long axis of the femur is 35° laterally, whereas the resultant pull of the vastus medialis muscle is 40° medially (see **Fig. 11–31A**).[215] The pull of the vastus intermedius muscle is parallel to the shaft of the femur, making it the purest knee extensor of the group.[216] Because of the pennate nature of the quadriceps muscles, not all fibers within each muscle are oriented in the same direction. For example, the upper fibers of the vastus medialis are angled 15° to 18° medially to the femoral shaft, whereas the distal fibers are angled as much as 50° to 55° medially.[216,217] Because of the drastically different orientation of the upper and lower fibers of the vastus medialis muscle, the upper fibers are sometimes referred to as the **vastus medialis longus (VML)**, and the lower fibers are referred to as the **vastus medialis oblique (VMO).** Despite the different orientation of the fibers of the vastus medialis oblique and the vastus medialis longus, these muscle fibers are simply portions of the same muscle innervated commonly by the femoral nerve, making selective, or isolated, activation of these fibers impossible.[217-219] Lieb and Perry found the resultant pull of the combined four portions of the quadriceps femoris muscle to be 7° to 10° in the lateral direction, and 3° to 5° anteriorly in relation to the long axis of the femur.[216] Powers and colleagues noted the posterior attachment site of the vastus lateralis and vastus medialis muscles which, together, have a posterior resultant that averages 55° in the extended knee and compresses the patellofemoral joint (see **Fig. 11–31B**).[215] The compressive force from these muscles on the patella is present throughout the ROM, but is minimized at full extension and increases as knee flexion continues.

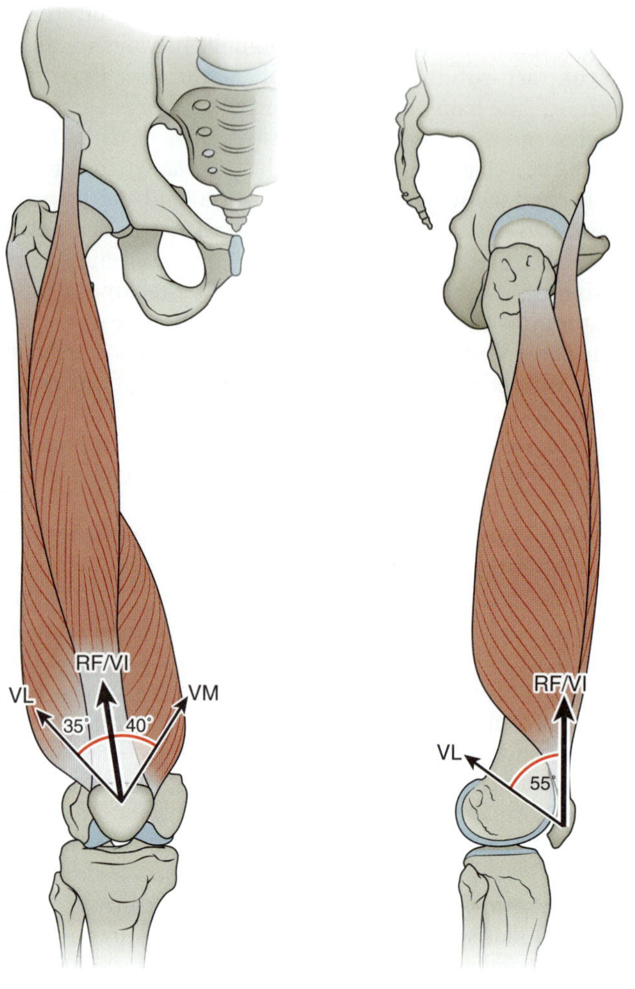

Figure 11–31 **A.** The orientation of the four components of the quadriceps muscle are shown, including the vastus lateralis (VL), vastus intermedius (VI), rectus femoris (RF), and vastus medialis (VM).[215] **B.** The posteriorly directed vectors of the VL and VM (VL shown) were found to result in net compression of the patella against the tibia, even in full extension.

Patellar Influence on Quadriceps Muscle Function

Function of the quadriceps muscle is strongly influenced by the patella (which, in turn, is strongly influenced by the quadriceps, as will be discussed later). From the perspective of mechanical advantage, the patella lengthens the moment arm of the quadriceps by increasing the distance of the quadriceps tendon and patellar tendon from the axis of the knee joint. The patella functions as an anatomic pulley, deflecting the action line of the quadriceps femoris muscle away from the

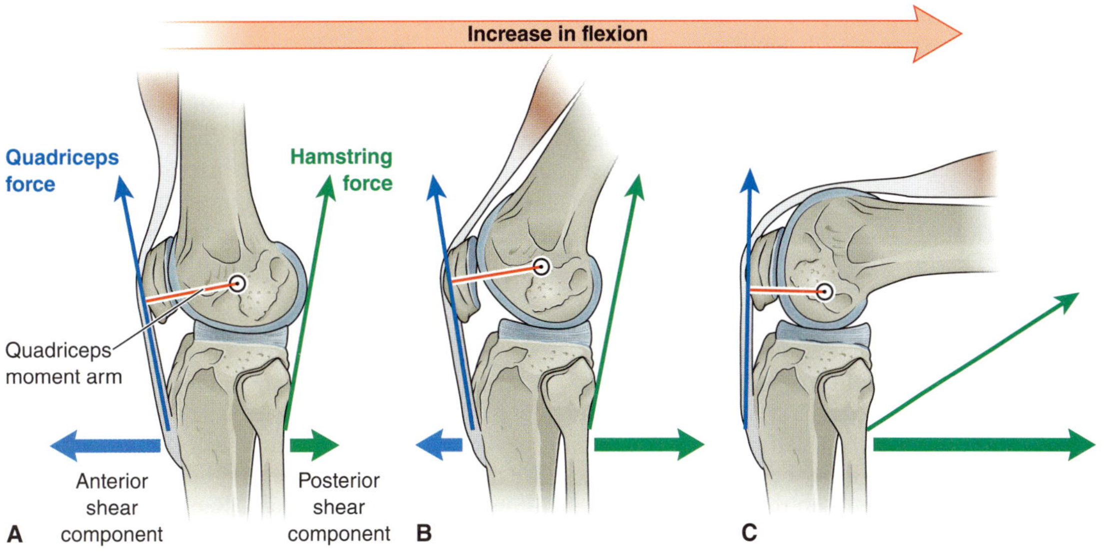

Figure 11–32 The patella acts as a pulley for quadriceps muscle force production. Changes in the knee joint center of rotation and position of the patella within the femoral trochlea influences the magnitude of the moment arm of the quadriceps muscle. **A.** Smallest moment arm with full knee extension. **B.** Increased moment arm with further flexion. **C.** Large moment arm at 90° of flexion due to pulley effect of femoral condyles and posterior shift of the joint axis.

knee joint axis and increasing the angle of pull on the tibia to enhance the ability of the quadriceps to generate extension torque **(Fig. 11–32)**. The patella does not, however, function as a simple pulley. In a simple pulley, the tension is equal on either side of the pulley; in contrast, the tension in the patellar tendon on the inferior aspect of the patella is rarely equal to the tension in the quadriceps tendon at the superior aspect of the patella.[220]

The knee joint geometry and the patella together dictate the quadriceps' angle of pull on the tibia as the knee flexes and extends. The patella plays a primary role in increasing the quadriceps' angle of pull when the knee is in extended positions (see **Fig. 11-32A** and **11-32B**). In full knee flexion, the patella's function as a pulley is significantly reduced because the patella is fixed firmly inside the intercondylar notch of the femur (see **Fig. 11-32C**). Despite this, the quadriceps maintains the ability to produce considerable torque in full knee flexion because of a large moment arm created by the rounded contour of the femoral condyles. The condyles deflect the muscle's line of action and, with the posteriorly shifted axis of rotation, a relatively large moment arm is present with little contribution from the patella. As the knee extends from full flexion, the moment arm of the quadriceps muscle lengthens as the patella leaves the intercondylar notch and begins to travel up and over the rounded femoral condyles. At about 50° of knee flexion, the femoral condyles have pushed the patella to its farthest distance from the knee's axis of rotation. With continued extension, the moment arm will once again diminish[221] (see Fig. 11-32). The influence of the changing moment arm on quadriceps torque production is readily apparent when knee extension strength is measured throughout the ROM. Peak torques are often observed at approximately 45° to 60° of knee flexion, a region in which both the moment arm and the length-tension relationship of the muscle are maximized.[222]

Although the patella's effect on the quadriceps' moment arm is diminished in the final stages of knee extension, the small improvement in joint torque provided by the patella may be most important here. The quadriceps is in a shortened position near end range extension, which reduces its ability to generate active tension. The decreased ability of the quadriceps to produce active force makes the relative size of the moment arm critical to torque production in the last 15° of knee extension.

Expanded Concepts 11–10
Quadriceps Lag

The quadriceps may not be able to produce adequate torque to complete the last 15° of non–weight-bearing knee extension if there is substantial quadriceps weakness or if the patella has been removed because of trauma (a procedure known as a *patellectomy*). The inability of a patient to fully extend the knee actively is referred to clinically as *quadriceps lag, quad lag,* or *extension lag.* For example, the patient may have difficulty maintaining full knee extension while performing a straight-leg raise **(Fig. 11–33)**. With the knee joint in greater flexion, removal of the patella or the presence of quadriceps weakness will have less effect on the ability of the quadriceps to generate extension torque because (1) the femoral condyles also serve as a pulley to increase the quadriceps' moment arm and (2) the relatively lengthened muscle can produce greater force. The patient likely will not have a "quad lag" during weight-bearing activities because, with the foot on the ground, the soleus and gluteus maximus muscles can assist the quadriceps with knee extension.

The patella's role in increasing the quadriceps' angle of pull on the tibia enhances torque production but can also lead to negative side effects. The rotary (Fy) component of the quadriceps muscle group not only produces an extension torque but also creates an anterior shear of the tibia on the femur at various knee flexion angles, depending on the task **(Fig. 11–34A)**.[125] The anterior translational (shear) force imposed by the quadriceps requires a posterior shear to limit translation, which can be produced actively by muscles (e.g., the hamstrings) or passively by capsuloligamentous forces. The ACL represents the most prominent passive restraint to the imposed anterior tibial translation of the quadriceps. Increases and decreases in the angle of pull of the quadriceps are accompanied by concomitant increases and decreases in stress in the ACL.[125] The strain on both bundles of the ACL ordinarily increases as the knee joint approaches full extension. In the absence of passive stabilizers such as the ACL, a quadriceps contraction near full extension has the potential to generate a perceptible anterior translation of the tibia on the femur, which the patient may describe as the knee "giving way" or "buckling."[112] The strain on the ACL evoked by a quadriceps contraction is substantially diminished as the knee is flexed beyond 60° because the shear component (Fy) of the quadriceps diminishes substantially from its maximum value (see **Fig. 11–34B**).

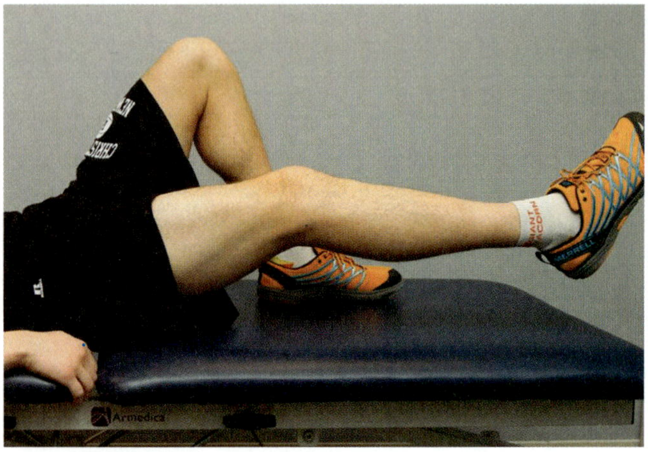

Figure 11–33 Severe quadriceps weakness can result in a quadriceps lag ("quad lag") during a straight-leg–raise exercise. Near full extension, the patella is only capable of increasing the moment arm slightly, and the decreased length-tension relationship of the already weakened quadriceps renders the quadriceps incapable of generating sufficient torque to complete the extension ROM.

During weight-bearing activities, the quadriceps' activity is influenced by several other factors. Muscles such as the soleus and gluteus maximus can assist with knee joint extension. During erect standing postures, activity of the quadriceps is minimal because the line of gravity passes just anterior to the knee axis for flexion/extension, creating an extension torque that maintains the joint in extension. The posterior joint capsule, ligaments, and posterior muscles offset the small external extension torque, preventing further knee joint extension. In weight-bearing with the knee flexed, as during a squat or when someone cannot fully extend the knee (e.g., flexion contracture), the line of gravity will pass posterior to the knee joint axis and create a flexion torque at the knee that necessitates activity of the quadriceps to maintain the knee joint in equilibrium. Because the quadriceps femoris muscle is responsible for supporting the body weight and resisting the force of gravity, it is often over 50% stronger than the hamstring muscles.[222] Although the hamstrings perform a similar function in supporting the body weight when there is a gravitational flexion moment at the hip, the hamstrings are assisted in this function by the large gluteus maximus. In contrast, the quadriceps is the primary muscle for supporting the knee joint against large external torques imposed by gravity.

The quadriceps muscle functions differently because of different biomechanical demands of various activity and exercise conditions. During seated (non–weight-bearing) knee extension, the moment arm of the resistance (e.g., weight of the leg plus external resistance) is minimal when the knee is flexed to 90° but increases as knee extension progresses **(Fig. 11–35)**. Therefore, greater quadriceps force is required to extend the knee as the knee approaches full extension. The opposite occurs during weight-bearing activities. In a standing squat, the moment arm of the resistance (e.g., the effect of gravity on the body's center of mass) is minimal when the knee is extended and increases as knee flexion increases. Therefore, during weight-bearing activities such as a squat, the quadriceps muscle must produce greater force in positions of greater knee flexion **(Fig. 11–36)**.[223]

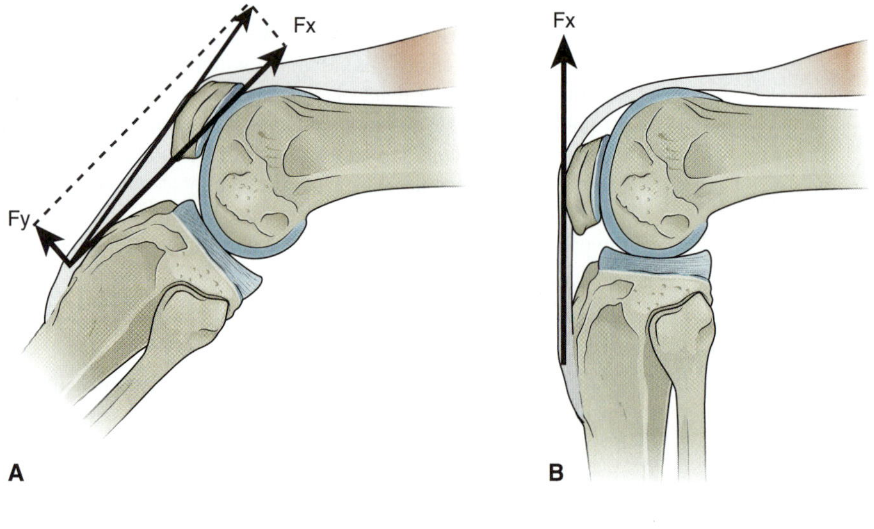

Figure 11–34 A. With the knee close to full extension, a forceful isolated quadriceps contraction can induce an anterior tibial translation (shear) because its rotary component (Fy) lies parallel to the tibial plateau. **B.** Once the knee is flexed to greater than 60°, little to no anterior translation occurs as the Fy component diminishes.

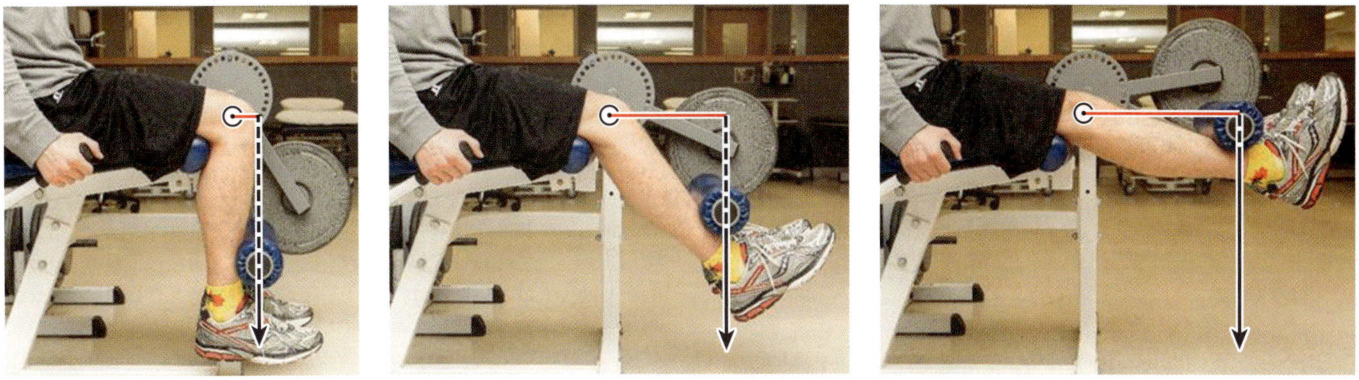

Figure 11–35 During open-chain exercises, the quadriceps muscle must generate more force (more torque) as the knee approaches full extension to overcome the increasing moment arm (and torque) of the external resistance.

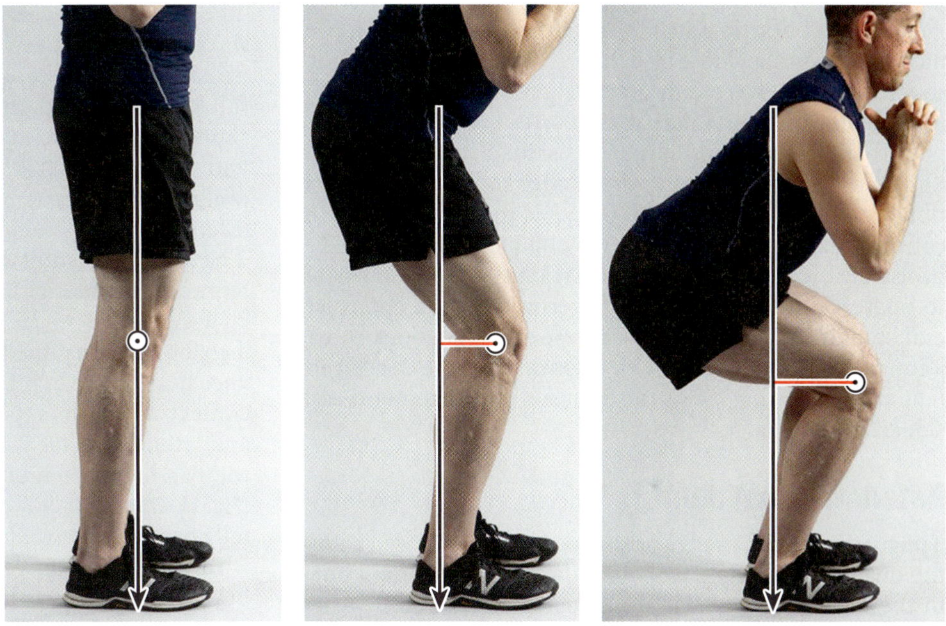

Figure 11–36 In a weight-bearing exercise, the quadriceps must generate more torque (and more force) as knee flexion increases to control the increasing moment arm (and torque) of the superimposed body weight at the knee joint.

Expanded Concepts 11–11

Quadriceps Strengthening: Weight-Bearing Versus Non–Weight-Bearing

Weight-bearing (closed-chain) exercises are often prescribed after anterior cruciate ligament, posterior cruciate ligament, or patellofemoral injury on the premise that these exercises are less stressful to the joints, more like functional movements, and safer than non–weight-bearing (open-chain) exercises. Wilk and colleagues computationally estimated anteroposterior shear force, compression force, and extensor torque at the knee during closed-chain and open-chain exercises that are commonly used for quadriceps muscle strengthening.[224] Closed-chain quadriceps exercises of a squat and leg press resulted in a *posterior* tibial shear force at the knee throughout the entire ROM, peaking at between 83° and 105° of knee flexion.[224,225] The posterior shear would presumably increase the stress on the PCL. In contrast, there was an *anterior* shear force in an open-chain knee extension exercise when the quadriceps actively extended the knee from 40° to 10°, with the maximal anterior shear force occurring between 20° and 10° of knee flexion. The anterior shear forces would presumably increase the stress on the ACL. Stresses on the posterior and ACL during certain types of open-chain and closed-chain exercises may be detrimental to the healing process if these ligaments are damaged or recently surgically reconstructed.[224,225]

Beynnon and colleagues measured ACL strain values in vivo to compare across commonly performed therapeutic exercises.[226,227] Similar ACL strain values were found regardless of whether the exercises were performed during weight-bearing or non–weight-bearing activities.[226,227] For example, weight-bearing one-legged sit-to-stands, lunges, step-ups, and step-downs produced ACL strain values similar to active non–weight-bearing knee extension exercises. ACL strains were higher when the quadriceps contracted between 50° to 0° of knee flexion regardless of whether the exercise was performed closed- or open-chain.[226,227]

The findings of these computationally derived forces and experimentally measured strains in the cruciate ligaments cast doubt on the rationale of basing rehabilitation exercises on the premise that either open-chain or closed-chain protocols are inherently better, safer, or more effective. Instead, a rehabilitation program incorporating both types of exercises and the functional requirements of the patient will likely maximize quadriceps strength gains.

Stabilizers of the Knee

Throughout the chapter, we have identified the role of both passive (capsuloligamentous) and active (muscular) forces in contributing to stability of the knee joint. The contributions of both capsuloligamentous and muscular structures to maintaining appropriate joint stability are dependent on the position of the knee joint as well as the surrounding joints, the magnitude and direction of the applied force, and the availability of secondary restraints. There can also be considerable variation among individuals (as well as between knees in the same individual) that contributes to the diversity of findings observed by both clinicians and researchers. Although admittedly an oversimplification, Table 11–1 summarizes the potential contribution of the different structures that limit anteroposterior translation, knee joint hyperextension, varus/valgus rotation, and medial/lateral rotation of the knee joint.

Table 11–1 describes stability in terms of single plane movements. As shown in Table 11–2, more complicated multiplanar stresses or motions typically occur, requiring multiplanar stabilization. For example, injury to the posterolateral corner (e.g., posterolateral joint capsule, popliteus muscle, popliteofibular ligament) can yield posterior instability and excessive lateral tibial rotation. This is termed **posterolateral instability.** In contrast, damage to the posterior oblique ligament, medial hamstrings, MCL, and posteromedial joint capsule contributes to **posteromedial instability**. Anteromedial and anterolateral stability is provided by the respective portions of the joint capsule, which fuses with extensions of the quadriceps femoris muscle that forms the extensor retinaculum on each side of the patella.

Patellofemoral Joint

The patella is a flat, triangularly shaped bone embedded within the quadriceps tendon, making it the largest sesamoid bone in the body **(Fig. 11–37A)**.[228] The patella sits as an inverted triangle, with its apex directed inferiorly, and attached inferiorly to the tibial tuberosity by the patellar tendon. As noted earlier in this chapter, there are also patellar connections to the medial and lateral extensor retinacular and via patellofemoral ligaments. The anterior surface of the patella is convex in both anterior-posterior and medial/lateral planes. The posterior surface, which articulates with the femur, is divided by a prominent central vertical ridge forming medial and lateral facets, with the lateral facet being slightly wider. Both the medial and lateral facets are flat to slightly convex side to side and superior to inferior to accommodate the concave trochlear groove (the patellofemoral articular facets of the femoral sulcus). Most patellae also have a less prominent second vertical ridge on the posterior surface toward the medial border that separates the medial facet from an extreme medial edge, known as the **odd facet** of the patella.[228] A majority of the posterior articulating surface of the patella is covered in a thick layer of articular cartilage, up to 7 mm thick,[229] to dissipate the large forces that develop between the articulating patella and femur (discussed next).

The posterior surface of the patella articulates with the **femoral trochlea** (see **Fig. 11–37B**). The trochlea is the portion of the femoral sulcus (the U-shaped groove) where the articular facets for the patella sit; the two terms (femoral sulcus and femoral trochlea) are often used interchangeably. The trochlea is composed of two facets separated by a central groove. The trochlear groove roughly corresponds with the central vertical ridge on the posterior patella and guides patellar motion during knee flexion and extension. The medial and lateral facets of the trochlea articulate with the medial and lateral facets of the patella, respectively. Importantly, the lateral trochlear facet is larger, slightly more convex, and has a steeper inclination angle compared to the medial facet (see Fig. 11-37B).[228] The steeper lateral trochlear facet is crucial for guiding the patella during knee joint motion and providing a bony buttress to prevent excessive lateral translation of the patella.

Tibiofemoral (Knee) Joint Motion and Patellar Contact

The contact between the patella and the femur changes throughout the knee's ROM, with minimal contact near full extension and increasing contact as the knee flexes. Near full knee extension, the patella sits high in the trochlea and slightly laterally, with only the inferior pole making contact with the femur.[228,230,231] As the knee flexes, the patellofemoral contact surface moves superiorly along the patella and inferior-posterior along the femoral condyles **(Fig. 11–38A)**. The first consistent contact between the patella and the femur occurs along the inferior margin of the lateral patellar facet at 15° to 20° of knee flexion, with contact evenly distributed across medial and lateral patellar facets by 30° of knee flexion (see Fig. 11-38B). As knee flexion progresses, the contact area shifts superiorly on the patella along the medial and lateral patellar facets, with maximum contact between the patella and femur between 60° to 90° of knee flexion **(Fig. 11–39)**.[231] By 90° of knee flexion, all portions of the patella have experienced some (although inconsistent) contact, with the exception of the odd facet. As flexion continues beyond 90°, the smaller odd facet makes contact with the medial femoral condyle for the first time.[231] At full knee flexion, the patella bridges the span of the intercondylar notch with patellar contact on the far medial and lateral edges of the superior patella through the odd and lateral facets, respectively.[228]

Expanded Concepts 11–12
Patellar Alignment

In the fully extended knee, the vertical position of the patella within the trochlea is related to the length of the patellar tendon. In typically aligned patellofemoral joints, the ratio of the length of the patellar tendon to the length of the patella, called the **Insall-Salvati index,** typically approximates 1:1.[232] A markedly short patellar tendon produces an abnormally low position of the patella on the trochlea known as **patella baja** and in contrast, a high-riding patella is termed **patella alta.**[228] With patella alta, the more superior position of the patella places the patella proximal to the lateral femoral facet, rendering the patella less constrained and easier to sublux compared to typical vertical position of the patella. In patients with patella alta, the tibiofemoral joint must be more flexed before the patella sufficiently translates inferiorly to engage with the trochlear groove, leaving a larger knee ROM within which the patella is less constrained.

Table 11–1 Summary of Knee Joint Stabilizers*

STABILIZERS	STRUCTURES Bolded structures indicate a primary restraint.	FUNCTION Function depends on whether action is open-chain (non–weight-bearing) or closed-chain (weight-bearing).
A-P/hyperextension stabilizers	**ACL** MCL LCL IT band Hamstring muscles Soleus muscle (in weight-bearing) Gluteus maximus muscle (in weight-bearing)	Limit anterior tibial (or posterior femoral) translation
	PCL Meniscofemoral ligaments Quadriceps muscle Popliteus muscle Medial and lateral heads of gastrocnemius	Limit posterior tibial (or anterior femoral) translation
Varus/valgus stabilizers	**MCL** ACL PCL POL Pes anserinus: Sartorius muscle Gracilis muscle Semitendinosus muscle Semimembranosus muscle Medial head of gastrocnemius muscle	Limit valgus of tibia
	LCL IT band ACL PCL Poplitealfibular ligament Biceps femoris muscle Lateral head of gastrocnemius muscle	Limit varus of tibia
Medial/lateral rotational stabilizers	ACL PCL Posterior medial capsule Meniscofemoral ligament Biceps femoris MCL LCL	Limit medial rotation of tibia
	Posterolateral capsule Popliteus muscle Pes anserinus: Sartorius muscle Gracilis muscle Semitendinosus muscle Semimembranosus muscle MCL LCL PCL	Limit lateral rotation of tibia

*The contribution of muscles and capsuloligamentous structures depends on the position of the knee and contiguous joints, the magnitude and direction of the applied force, and the availability of secondary restraints. Findings vary among investigators, given the testing conditions.
ACL, anterior cruciate ligament; A-P, anteroposterior; IT, iliotibial; LCL, lateral collateral ligament; MCL, medial collateral ligament; PCL, posterior cruciate ligament;.

Motions of the Patella

As the contact between the patella and the femur changes with knee joint motion, the patella simultaneously translates (slides) and rotates on the femur. These movements are influenced by and reflect the patella's relationship to both the femur and the tibia.

During knee flexion and extension, there is superior/inferior and medial/lateral motion of the patella. When the femur

Table 11–2 Components to Multiplanar Stability

	MEDIAL	LATERAL
Anterior	**Anteromedial Stability***	**Anterolateral Stability†**
	MCL POL Posteromedial capsule ACL	ACL LCL Posterolateral capsule Poplitealfibular ligament Popliteus IT band
Posterior	**Posteromedial Stability**	**Posterolateral Stability**
	PCL POL MCL Semimembranosus Posteromedial capsule ACL	PCL Poplitealfibular ligament Popliteus LCL Biceps femoris Posterolateral capsule

* Indicates that the following active and passive stabilizers can resist one or more of the following: anterior translation, valgus, or external rotation of the tibia.

† Indicates that the following active and passive stabilizers can resist one or more of the following: anterior translation, varus, or internal rotation of the tibia.

ACL, anterior cruciate ligament; IT, iliotibial; LCL, lateral collateral ligament; MCL, medial collateral ligament; PCL, posterior cruciate ligament; POL, posterior oblique ligament.

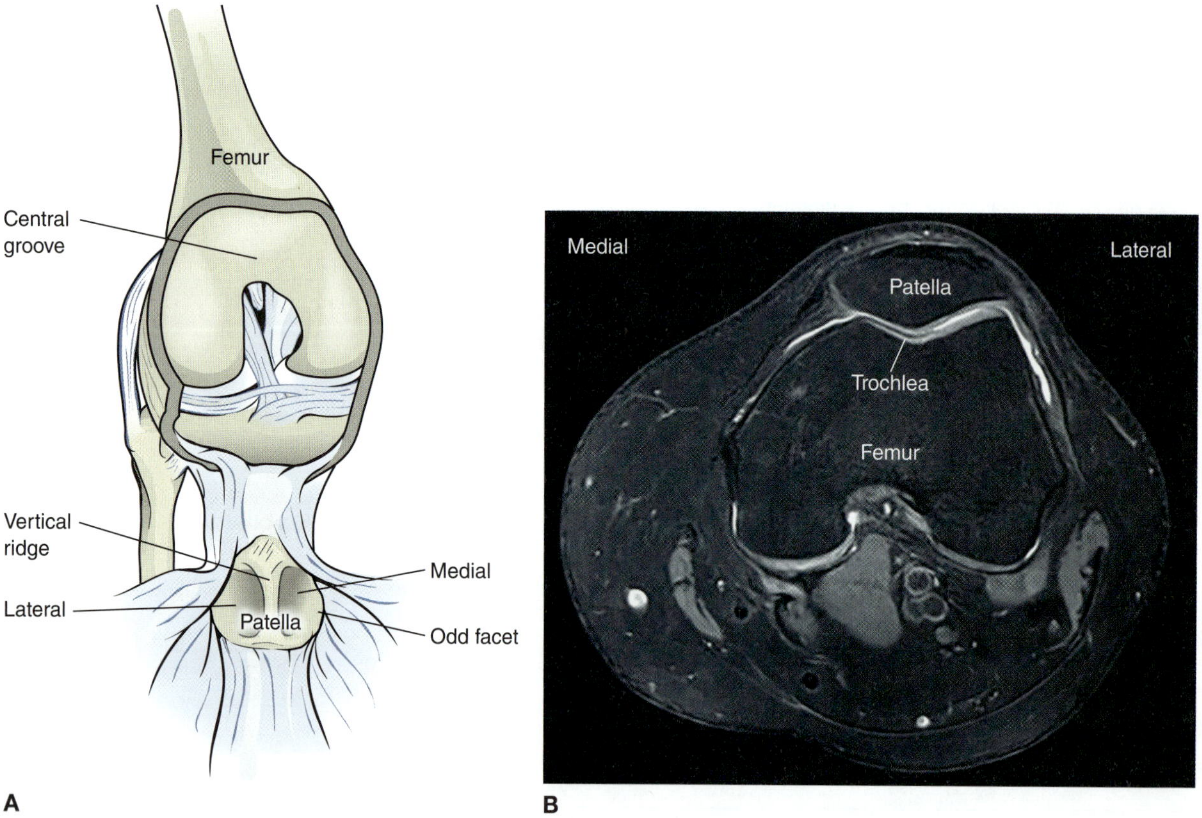

Figure 11–37 The patella. **A.** With the patella and retinacular fibers pulled away from the femur, the articulating surfaces on the posterior aspect of the patella and on the femoral sulcus can be seen. **B.** Cross section of the knee on an MRI shows the concave sulcus and the convex femoral condyles that articulate with the convex posterior aspect of the patella.

is fixed and the knee is flexing (i.e., non–weight-bearing), the patella is pulled inferiorly and medially into the trochlear groove of the femur via its attachment to the tibial tuberosity via the patellar tendon. The sagittal plane motion of the patella, as the patella slides (or "tracks") inferiorly in the trochlear groove during knee flexion, is termed **patellar flexion**. The medial patellar slide (or translation) that occurs in early knee flexion as the patella moving toward the medial femoral

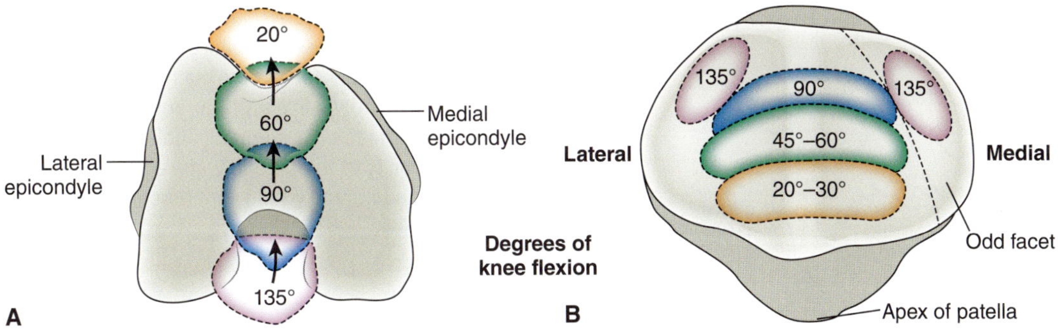

Figure 11–38 Patellofemoral articular contact. **A.** An inferior view of the femur shows how the position of the patella on the femur proceeds from early knee flexion to full knee flexion. **B.** Posterior view of the patella showing shifting contact with the femur. From 20° to 90° of knee joint flexion, the contact area on the patella moves superiorly and then laterally. By full flexion (135°), only the lateral and odd facets are contacting the femur.

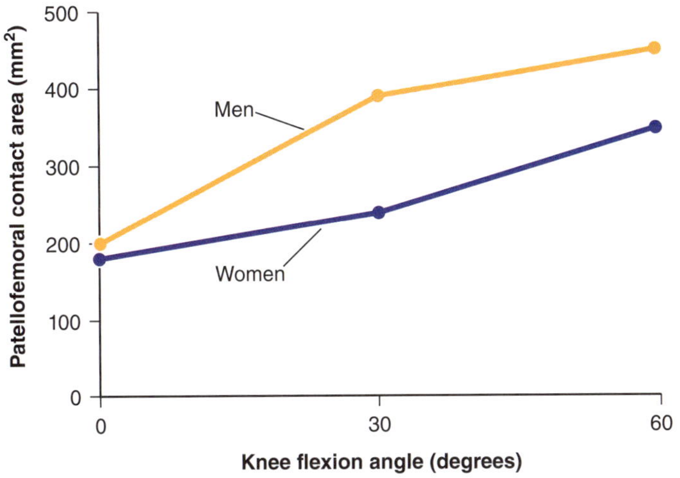

Figure 11–39 Contact between the articulating surfaces of the patella and femur is at a minimum in full knee extension. Patellofemoral contact area increases as the knee progresses from knee extension into knee flexion. *(Data from Besier TF, Draper CE, Gold GE, et al: Patellefemoral joint contact area increases with knee flexion and weightbearing. J Orthop Res 23:345, 2005.)*

condyle *in the frontal plane* is called a **medial patellar shift**[233] **(Fig. 11–40)**. With increasing knee flexion, there is increasing lateral patellar translation,[234,235] or **lateral patellar shift,** defined as the patella moving toward the lateral femoral condyle in the frontal plane. Of note, a lateral patellar shift is commonly used during the patella apprehension test to evaluate the integrity of medial patellar tissues in restraining the patella within the trochlea.[236] During knee extension, the patella slides superiorly on the femoral condyles, referred to as **patellar extension,** via the pull of the quadriceps tendon back to its original position on the femur. In weight-bearing knee flexion and extension (i.e., fixed tibia), it is the femoral surface that slides behind the patella as the patella is tethered to the tibia within the quadriceps tendon.[237]

In addition to patellar translations, the patella also tilts around a longitudinal axis (proximal to distal through the patella). Tilting about the longitudinal axis is termed **lateral/medial patellar tilt** and is named for the direction toward which the anterior surface of the patella is tipping **(Fig. 11–41)**.

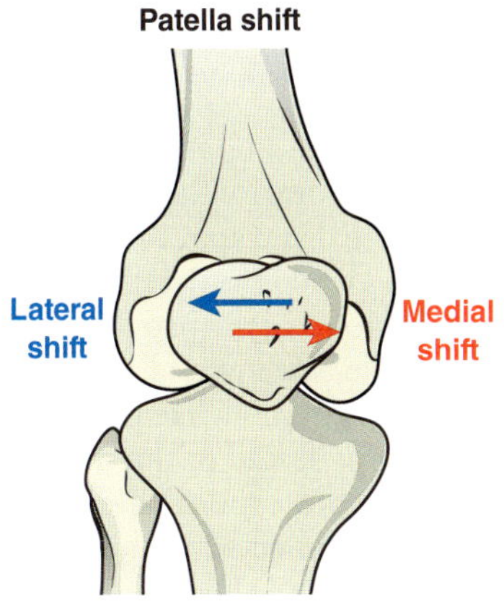

Figure 11–40 Medial and lateral shifts are named according to the direction in which the patella moves toward the medial or lateral femoral condyle.

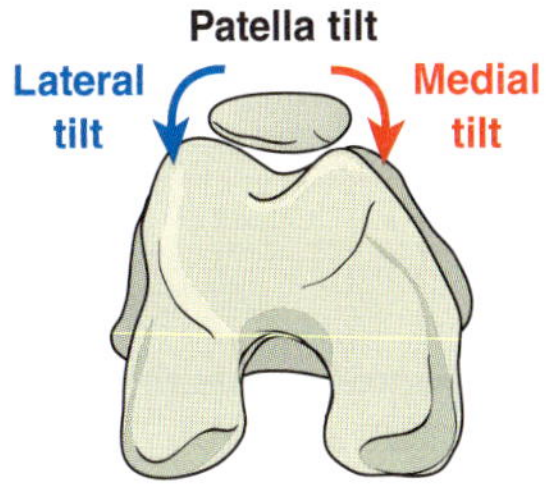

Figure 11–41 A superior view of the patellofemoral articulation. Medial and lateral tilt is named for the direction toward which the anterior surface of the patella is tipping, with the medial surface approximating the medial femoral condyle during medial tilt and vice versa during lateral tilt.

Lateral patella tilt occurs when the lateral edge of the patella tips toward the surface of the lateral femoral condyle, and medial patella tilt occurs when the medial edge of the patella tips toward the medial femoral condyle.[233] The direction and amount of patellar tilt is influenced by surrounding knee structures, such as the asymmetrical femoral condyles, the degree of medial or lateral tibial rotation, and tightness in soft tissues such as the knee's lateral extensor retinaculum.[238-240]

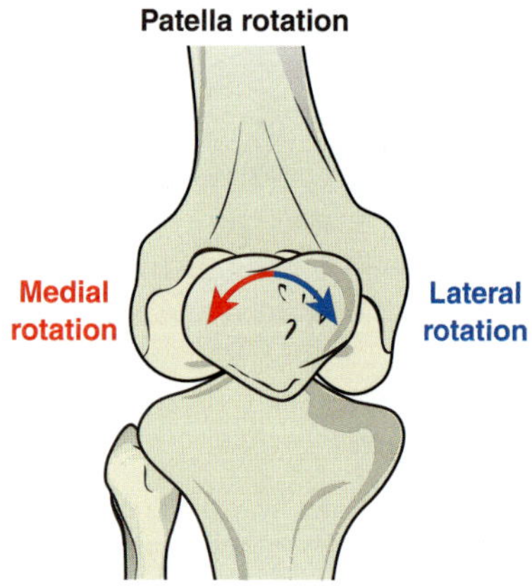

Figure 11–42 Medial rotation of the patella is shown in red. The inferior pole of the patella follows the tibial tuberosity during medial rotation of the tibia. Lateral rotation of the patella is shown in blue. The inferior pole of the patella follows the tibial tuberosity during lateral rotation of the tibia.

Rotation of the patella about an anteroposterior axis (termed **medial/lateral rotation** of the patella) is referenced by the movement of the distal apex of the patella **(Fig. 11–42)**. Medial rotation occurs when the patella spins around it's A-P axis with the apex (bottom) of the patella pointing toward the medial femoral condyle, with lateral patellar rotation being the opposite.[233] Patellar rotation, like patellar tilt, is necessary for the patella to remain seated in the trochlea as the femur undergoes axial rotation on the tibia. Because the inferior aspect of the patella is connected to the tibia via the patellar tendon, the inferior apex of the patella continually points toward the tibial tuberosity while moving with the femur.[241] Therefore, when the knee is in some flexion and there is medial rotation of the tibia on the fixed femur, the apex of the patella will point medially as the patella medially rotates. Similarly, as the tibia rotates laterally, the patella will rotate laterally to keep the apex aligned with the tibial tuberosity. During knee flexion, the patella medially rotates as the tibia medially rotates to "unlock" the knee. The patella then laterally rotates approximately 5° as the knee flexes from 20° to 90° because of the asymmetrical configuration of the femoral condyles.[239]

Clinical Application 11–4

The patella, although firmly attached to soft tissue stabilizers (e.g., the extensor retinaculum), undergoes translational motions that are dependent on the degree of tibiofemoral ROM. The patella translates superiorly and inferiorly with knee extension and flexion, respectively. Understanding these motions is important because they can influence knee joint function. During active knee extension, for example, if superior gliding of the patella is restricted, quadriceps function can be compromised, and knee extension may be limited. During tibiofemoral flexion, the patella slides inferiorly. A restricted inferior slide could therefore limit knee flexion. Simultaneous medial/lateral shifting of the patella accompanies superior-inferior patellar gliding.[239] In full knee extension, the patella sits high in the femur's trochlea and slightly laterally. As knee flexion is initiated, the patella is pushed medially by the large lateral femoral condyle. As knee flexion proceeds past 30°, the patella may shift slightly laterally or remain fairly stable as the patella is firmly engaged within the trochlea. Consequently, the patella shifts first medially and then laterally as the knee moves from full extension into flexion. Failure of the patella to slide, tilt, rotate, or shift appropriately can lead to maltracking of the patella, restrictions in knee joint ROM, or pain from compression of the patellofemoral articular surfaces. As such, clinical evaluation of both passive and active mobility of the patella with respect to the femur is necessary to better understand whole joint function.

Patient Application 11–3

Steven is a 68-year-old male patient with a 10-year history of progressing right knee pain. Radiographic imaging completed 3 years prior revealed osteoarthritis in the patellofemoral and medial tibiofemoral compartments. Steven reports difficulty flexing his knee during activities of daily living, such as tying his shoe or squatting to retrieve objects from the floor. During the initial evaluation, physical examination included assessment of tibiofemoral ROM and patellofemoral joint mobility.

Steven is likely to demonstrate an impairment in right knee flexion ROM. A deficit in passive ROM similar in magnitude to the deficit in active ROM would indicate that muscle activation and strength are probably not contributing to the lack of ROM. Instead, restrictions in joint mobility may be present at the tibiofemoral or patellofemoral joint—or both. An impairment in inferior patellar slide with accompanying impairments in either medial or lateral patellar gliding could be contributing to Steven's impairment in knee flexion ROM and activity limitations (difficulty completing activities of daily living that require knee flexion). If this were the case, then targeted patellar mobilizations aimed at restoring joint mobility may result in improved tibiofemoral and patellofemoral flexion ROM and improved patient function. The key takeaway is to be sure to assess both tibiofemoral and patellofemoral joint ROM for patients who have restrictions in knee flexion or extension. As Steven restores ROM, ongoing assessment should ensure that he is able to stabilize and use the new range, i.e., that he has sufficient strength so that active ROM continues to match the new gains in passive ROM.

Patellar Function

The patella's primary function is as an anatomic pulley for the quadriceps muscle, as previously discussed (see Fig. 11–32).[228] Additionally, interposing the patella between the quadriceps tendon and the femur prevents excessive friction between the tendon and bone. However, the joint's complex articulating surfaces can lead to many potential problems during typical joint function. The patellofemoral joint is exposed to significant forces during common activities of daily living, which can lead to pain and disability. When in relatively extended knee positions, the stability and constraint of the patellofemoral joint are primarily maintained by static and dynamic soft tissues rather than bony structures, which increases the joint's susceptibility to injury. Understanding the structures and forces that influence patellofemoral function provides valuable insight into the common clinical issues associated with this joint.

Patellofemoral Joint Stress

The patellofemoral joint experiences very high stresses during typical activities of daily living, making it a common location for pain, degenerative articular cartilage changes, and osteoarthritis to occur.[242-244] Joint stress (force per unit area) can be influenced by altering either patellofemoral joint reaction force magnitudes or joint surface contact areas. The patellofemoral joint reaction force is the resultant contact force acting on the joint and is influenced by both the magnitude of the quadriceps force and the knee angle. As the quadriceps contracts, the patella is pulled superiorly by the quadriceps tendon, with the pull resisted inferiorly by the patellar tendon. The combination of these pulls produces a posterior compression force of the patella on the femur that varies with the amount of knee flexion.[228] At full extension, the quadriceps posterior compressive force on the patella is minimized, with any compressive force due exclusively to the attachments of the vastus medialis and vastus lateralis muscles on the posterior femur[215] **(Fig. 11-43A)**. Despite the small contact area between the patella and the femur in full extension, this minimal posterior compressive force allows for low patellofemoral joint stress with the knee at full extension. These low joint stress levels provide rationale for the use of straight-leg–raising exercises as a way of improving quadriceps muscle strength without creating or exacerbating patellofemoral compression and pain.

Assuming the angle between the quadriceps tendon and the patellar tendon is 180° in full extension, the angle of pull between the two tendons decreases as knee flexion increases. The decreased angle of pull increases the joint reaction force that, in turn, produces greater patellofemoral joint compressive forces[228] (see **Fig. 11-43B**). This increased compression occurs whether or not the quadriceps muscle is active during knee flexion. If the quadriceps muscle is inactive, the passive tension of the stretched tissues alone will increase within the quadriceps and patellar tendons as knee joint flexion increases, thus increasing the posterior patellofemoral compressive force. If the quadriceps muscle is active, then both the active tension and passive elastic tension will contribute to increasing the posterior compressive force between the patella and femur. The joint reaction force between the patella and femur, therefore, is influenced by the magnitude of active tension of the quadriceps, passive elastic tension within the quadriceps and patellar tendons, and the angle of knee flexion.

Patellofemoral joint reaction forces can become very high during routine daily activities. During the stance phase of walking, when peak knee flexion is only approximately 20°, the patellofemoral joint reaction force is approximately 25% to 50% of body weight.[175] With greater knee flexion and greater quadriceps activity, as during running, patellofemoral joint reaction forces have been estimated to reach over 10 times body weight.[245] Deep knee flexion exercises that require large magnitudes of quadriceps activity can also substantially increase these compressive forces.[245] The large compressive forces created by activation of the quadriceps are distributed

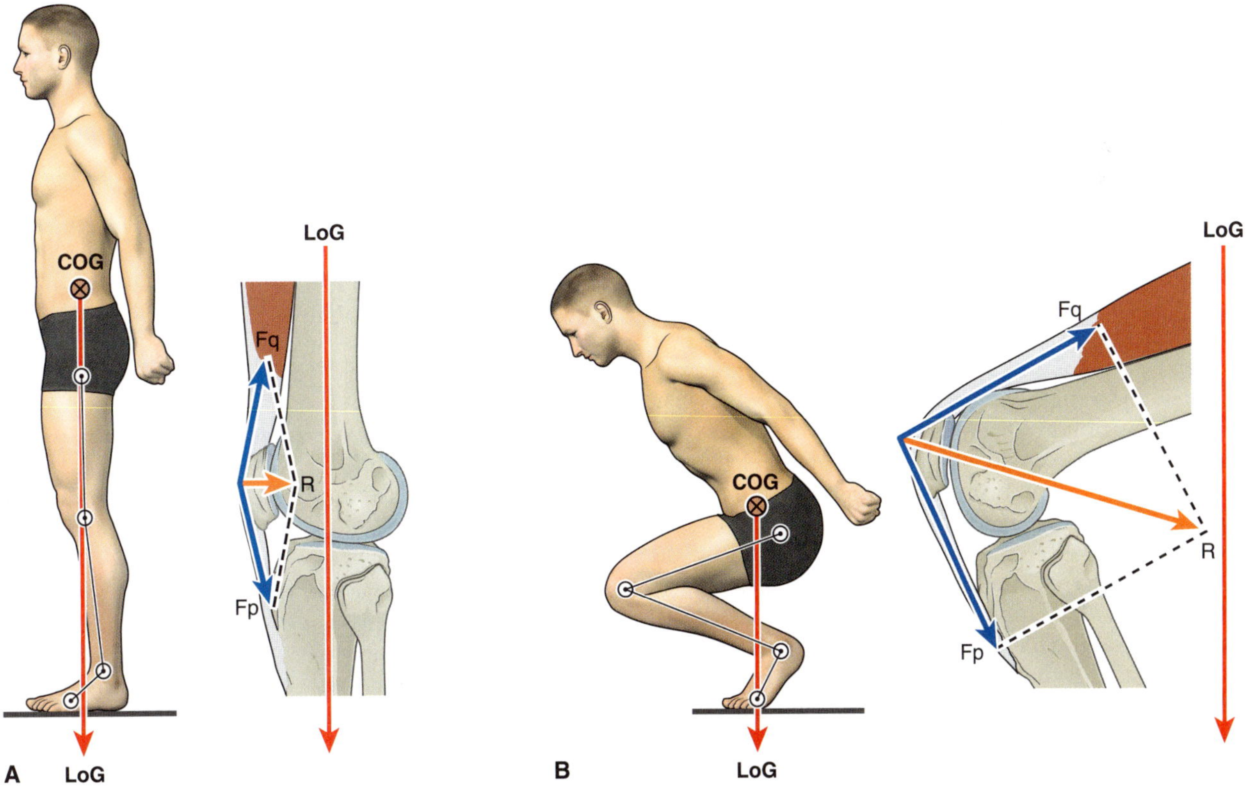

Figure 11-43 Knee flexion angle influences the magnitude of patellofemoral joint reaction forces. **A.** In full weight-bearing knee extension, the compressive force (R) between the pull of the quadriceps tendon (Fq) and the patellar tendon (Fp) is minimal. The quadriceps activity is minimal because the line of gravity (LoG) falls through or anterior to the knee joint axis. **B.** In full flexion, the compression force (R) is substantially increased as the angle of pull between Fq and Fp decreases. The LoG falls substantially posterior to the knee joint axis, increasing demand on the quadriceps when controlling flexion and attempting to re-extend the knee. COG = center of gravity.

over relatively small patellofemoral contact areas and can lead to large joint reaction forces. Several mechanisms help minimize or dissipate the patellofemoral joint stress on the patella. In full extension, minimal compressive forces are present on the patella; therefore, no compensatory mechanisms are necessary. As knee flexion increases, the area of patellar contact also gradually increases, thus dispersing the increased compressive force.[215,228] This simultaneous increase in contact area and compressive force helps to minimize patellofemoral joint stress until approximately 90° of flexion. Additionally, from 30° to 70° of flexion, the large contact force is higher in a knee flexion range where patellofemoral contact is on the thick cartilage of the medial facet near the central ridge. This articular cartilage is among the thickest hyaline cartilage in the human body, enabling it to withstand the substantial compressive forces transmitted across the medial facet of the patella. Within this same ROM, the patella has its greatest effect as a pulley because the moment arm of the quadriceps is maximized. The larger moment arm requires less quadriceps muscle force to produce the same torque, thereby somewhat mitigating an otherwise even larger patellofemoral joint compression force. As flexion proceeds, however, the moment arm diminishes, necessitating an increase in force production by the quadriceps to generate sufficient torque. As knee flexion continues beyond 90°, patellofemoral stress will increase across a now diminishing area of patellar contact. However, some of this increasing compressive force on the patella is taken on by the contact of the patellar tendon with femoral condyles.[246]

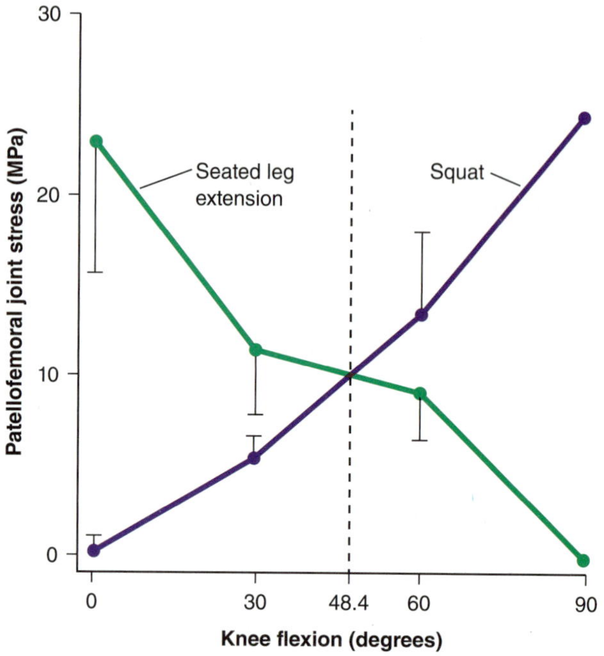

Figure 11–44 Patellofemoral joint stresses in non–weight-bearing seated leg extension with ankle weights and weight-bearing squat activities. At full knee extension (0°) and early flexion, patellofemoral joint stress is greater during non–weight-bearing leg extension (green) than weight-bearing exercises (purple). However, at approximately 50° of knee flexion, higher patellofemoral joint stresses are incurred by weight-bearing squat exercise. *(Data from Powers CM, Ho KY, Chen YJ, et al: Patellofemoral joint stress during weightbearing and non-weightbearing quadriceps exercises. J Orthop Sports Phys Ther 44: 320, 2014.)*

Quadriceps Strengthening Exercises and Patellofemoral Pain

Both weight-bearing and non–weight-bearing strengthening exercises for the quadriceps result in differential patterns of patellofemoral joint loading,[223,237] which should be considered when planning interventions to improve pain and function.[247] Different exercise modes affect the patellofemoral joint based on the knee's position within the ROM **(Fig. 11–44)**. This highlights the importance of tailoring exercises to focus on strengthening within pain-free knee ROMs. Non–weight-bearing extension exercises, such as the seated knee extension with an ankle weight, require increased quadriceps torque as extension progresses (quadriceps force must increase with decreasing knee flexion angle—see Fig. 11–35). However, the greater compressive force generated by the increased quadriceps contraction can be detrimental for an individual with patellofemoral pain, especially if the irritated tissue is located on the inferior aspect of the patella that is in greatest contact with the femur near extension. In contrast, a closed-chain exercise typically requires greater quadriceps activity with greater knee flexion (e.g., at the bottom of a squat—see Fig. 11–36). During closed-chain exercises, greater knee flexion results in increased compressive force across the patellofemoral joint, both because of increased active force demands on the quadriceps muscle and because of the increased patellofemoral compression that occurs in positions of greater knee flexion (from the greater passive tension of the now lengthened quadriceps). Substantial patellofemoral compression may aggravate patellofemoral pain. Closed-chain exercises may lead to higher joint stress in higher degrees of knee flexion whereas open-chain exercises may increase joint stress closer to full extension (see Fig. 11-44). Balancing these variables, with respect to each patient's unique symptoms and functional needs, can enhance effectiveness of interventions and optimize functional outcomes for patients experiencing patellofemoral pain.

Clinical Application 11–5
Quadriceps Strengthening: Weight-Bearing Versus Non–Weight-Bearing Exercises

The use of weight-bearing (closed-chain) exercises has occasionally been promoted as safer and more "functional" than non–weight-bearing (open-chain) exercises.[248] There are, however, numerous activities performed throughout the day in a non–weight-bearing position. Although other muscles are forced to work concomitantly during weight-bearing situations to control other joints, this is not always the best strategy for strengthening. The use of open-chain exercise isolates the target muscle, which may make strengthening more effective.[249,250] Rehabilitation programs using both open-chain and closed-chain quadriceps strengthening exercises have resulted in substantial decreases in pain levels in patients with patellofemoral pain, and the use of both strategies is recommended to provide both quadriceps-specific strengthening and functionally specific training.[251,252]

Patellar Motion and Medial/Lateral Patellar Restraints

In a well-functioning patellofemoral joint, the medial/lateral forces acting on the patella balance each other, allowing for pain-free motion of the patella with the femur. When there is a medial/lateral imbalance, optimal patellar tracking does not occur. Consequently, the patient may experience unconstrained medial/lateral patellar motion (with possible subluxation or dislocation) and/or altered patellar contact with the femur that may increase patellofemoral joint stress, potentially leading to patellofemoral pain and articular cartilage damage.

A slight lateral pull of the patella is often evident because the action lines of the quadriceps and the patellar tendon do not coincide due to the physiological valgus that typically exists between the tibia and femur **(Fig. 11–45)**. Soft tissue stabilizers must therefore assume more responsibility for medial/lateral stability in extension due to the resultant lateral pull of the patella where bony stability is reduced. Once knee flexion is initiated and the patella begins to slide down into the femoral sulcus (at about 20° of flexion), medial/lateral restraint is substantially increased by the presence of bony stability.

Both longitudinal and transverse soft structures influence medial/lateral patellar tracking into and along the femoral trochlea. The longitudinal soft tissue stabilizers of the patella, of course, include the quadriceps tendon superiorly and the patellar tendon inferiorly. The patellotibial ligaments that are part of the extensor retinaculum and reinforce the joint capsule are also considered longitudinal stabilizers[77] **(Fig. 11–46)**. The longitudinal stabilizers provide passive increases in patellofemoral compression that, in turn, helps to constrain the patella in the medial/lateral direction. However, in the extended knee, where patellofemoral compression is minimal, restraint of excessive medial/lateral patellar motion relies more on transverse soft tissue stabilizers. When knee extension is excessive, as in genu recurvatum, the pull of the quadriceps muscle and patellar tendon may actually distract the patella away from the femoral sulcus, further increasing the potential for excessive frontal plane patellar motion. The transverse soft tissue stabilizers of the patellofemoral joint are primarily composed of the superficial portion of the extensor retinaculum. The retinaculum provides active stabilization to the patella through direct connections of the vastus medialis and vastus lateralis muscles (see Fig. 11-46). The thickest portion of the medial retinaculum is the medial patellofemoral ligament, which provides approximately 60% of the passive restraining force against lateral translation of the patella.[73] Excessive medial translation is limited by the lateral patellofemoral ligament, which attaches the patella to the IT band laterally[77] (see Fig. 11-46).

In addition to soft tissue restraints, the femoral articular joint surfaces also stabilize the patella. As discussed above, the lateral trochlear facet is larger and has a steeper inclination angle compared to the medial facet[228] (see Fig. 11-37B). The steeper lateral trochlear facet effectively guides patellar motion and provides a bony buttress to prevent excessive lateral translation of the patella. However, the bony morphology of the trochlea and patella can vary greatly between people, varying the effectiveness of this osseous restraint. A flattened or domed shape of the femoral trochlea, called *trochlear dysplasia*, can lead to patellar subluxation or complete dislocation from relatively small lateral forces imposed on the patella.[228,253] Additionally, variations in patellar shape exist and correlate with trochlear morphology.[254] Bony morphology underlying

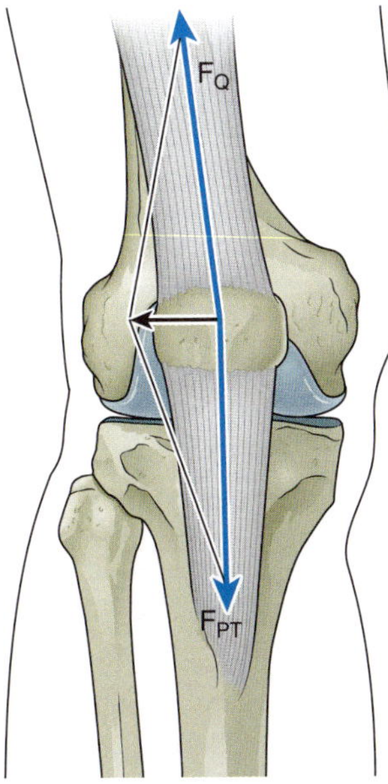

Figure 11–45 Because of the obliquity (physiological valgus angle) between the long axis of the femur and the tibia, the pull of the quadriceps (F_Q) and the pull of the patellar tendon (F_{PT}) lie at a slight angle to each other, producing a slight lateral force on the patella.

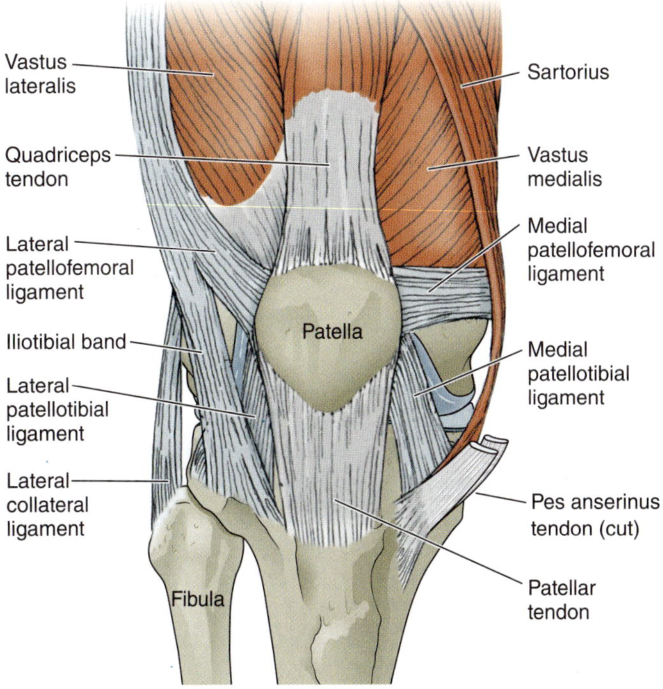

Figure 11–46 The longitudinal and medial/lateral stabilizers of the patellofemoral joint.

recurrent patellar subluxations or dislocations may require surgical intervention (such as soft tissue reconstruction, trochleoplasty, tibial tubercle transfer, or tibial/femoral/patellar osteotomy) to restore the underlying bony anatomy or modify angles of pull.[255]

Patellar hypermobility may result in patellar subluxations or dislocations, whereas hypomobility may yield pain due to greater patellofemoral stresses. The amount of passive patellar mobility is maximized when the knee is fully extended and the quadriceps are relaxed. A frontal plane imbalance in the passive tension (e.g., lax medial patellofemoral ligament) or a change in the line of pull of the dynamic structures can influence and change the orientation of the patella, often most notable when the knee joint is in extension and the patella sits on the relatively shallow superior femoral sulcus. Abnormal forces, however, may influence the excursion of the patella even in its more secure location within the intercondylar groove with the knee in flexion.

Clinical Application 11–6
Quadriceps Strength and Patellofemoral Pathology

Tension in the active or stretched quadriceps muscle creates compression between the patella and the femur, which increases patellofemoral restraint. The net force on the patella is determined by the resultant pull of the four muscles that constitute the quadriceps femoris and by the pull of the patellar tendon. Each of the segments of the quadriceps contributes to frontal plane mobility and stability due to their varying orientations along the femur (see Fig. 11–31A).[215,216] Because the vastus medialis and vastus lateralis muscles not only pull on the quadriceps tendon but also exert a pull on the patella through their retinacular connections, complementary function is critical. Weakness of the quadriceps muscle may substantially increase the resultant medial/lateral forces on the patella.[219]

It was previously assumed that a weak vastus medialis oblique contributed to diminished medial slide of the patella during activities. This assumption resulted in attempts to devise exercise regimens to selectively strengthen the vastus medialis oblique, commonly referred to as the VMO. However, both portions of the vastus medialis muscle (VM and VMO), like the other components of the quadriceps, are innervated by the femoral nerve, and preferential activation of one portion of a muscle or one portion of the quadriceps is not possible.[256] Further, atrophy of the entire quadriceps muscle, not just the vastus medialis, is present in patients with patellofemoral pain.[219] As such, exercise therapies targeting strength of the whole quadriceps muscle is recommended to address quadriceps weakness in patients with patellofemoral pathology.

Patient Application 11–4

Layla is a 16-year-old adolescent with a history of recurrent right patellar subluxations and instability. She plays volleyball competitively; however, due to increasing frequency of patellar subluxations, she elected not to join her travel team for this upcoming season. Most recently, she had to be seen in the emergency department for a right patellar dislocation that did not reduce on its own. She underwent medial patellofemoral ligament (MPFL) reconstruction surgery and now presents to physical therapy 1 week after.

Primary goals of early rehabilitation after MPFL reconstruction include restoring full active and passive extension ROM, gradually progressing flexion ROM (to greater than 90°), and restoring quadriceps activation. The emphasis on regaining quadriceps neuromuscular control is critically important. Exercises common in the early phases of rehabilitation include quadriceps setting (isometric quadriceps contraction in knee extension) and may need to include an assisted superior patellar slide toward the end of knee joint extension to improve simultaneous patellar mobility and restore extension ROM. Straight-leg raises may also be utilized in the early phases of rehabilitation once the patient demonstrates sufficient quadriceps strength and stability such that there is not a quadriceps lag (extension lag) present. As mentioned earlier, the open-packed position (with the knee slightly flexed) will likely maximize patient comfort after surgery. However, education to avoid prolonged periods of rest with the knee propped in the open-packed position is important. Regaining full knee extension is critical; therefore, resting with the knee in an extended position (minimizing time spent resting with the knee in slight flexion) will help to achieve and maintain full knee extension ROM. In some cases, prolonged extension stretches such as a prone hang (where the patient lays prone with their knee and lower leg extended off the bed allowing gravity to gradually increase knee extension) may be indicated. Additionally, exercises such as heel slides or standing hamstring curls can be useful for restoring active and passive knee flexion ROM as well as assist with early hamstring strengthening.

Lateral Bias of Patellar Motion

The orientation of the quadriceps' resultant pull with respect to the pull of the patellar tendon provides information about the net force on the patella in the frontal plane. The net effect of the pull of the quadriceps and the patellar tendon can be assessed clinically using a measurement called the **Q angle** (quadriceps angle). The Q angle is the angle formed between a line connecting the anterior superior iliac spine to the midpoint of the patella (representing the direction of pull of the quadriceps) and a line connecting the tibial tuberosity and the midpoint of the patella **(Fig. 11–47)**. A Q angle of 10° to 15° measured with the knee either in full extension or slight flexion is considered typical.[257] The Q angle is usually measured with the knee at or near full extension because lateral forces on the patella are typically more problematic in this position. With the knee flexed, the posterior compressive force is greater, and the patella is set more firmly engaged with the trochlea. Additionally, the Q angle will diminish with knee flexion as the tibia rotates medially in relation to the femur. Alterations in lower extremity alignment that *increase* the Q angle may increase the lateral force on the patella. An increase in this lateral force may increase the compression between the lateral patellar facet and the lateral facet of the trochlea. In the presence of a large enough lateral force, the patella may sublux or dislocate when the quadriceps muscle is activated with an extended knee.

It is generally thought that women have a slightly greater Q angle than do men because of the presence of a wider pelvis, increased femoral anteversion, and a relatively greater knee valgus angle.[257-259] Although an excessively large Q angle of 20° or more can be an indicator of structural malalignment,

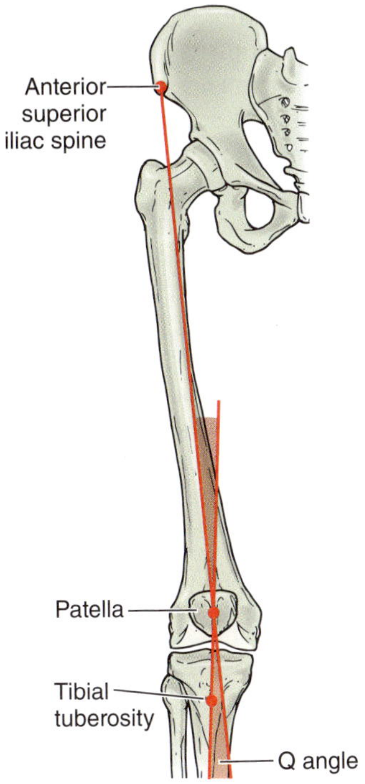

Figure 11–47 The Q angle is the angle between a line connecting the anterior superior iliac spine to the midpoint of the patella and the extension of a line connecting the tibial tubercle and the midpoint of the patella.

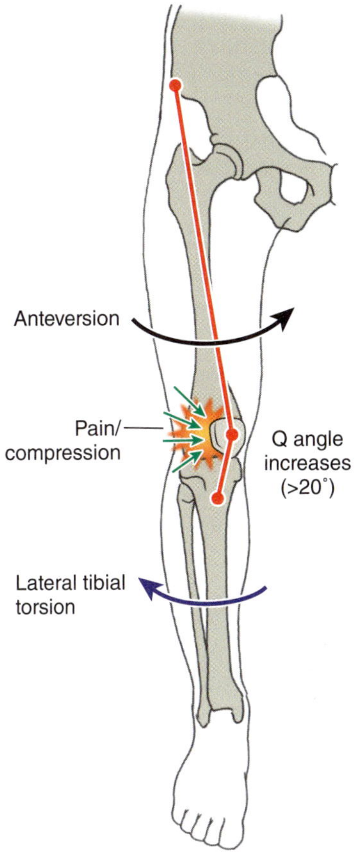

Figure 11–48 A simultaneous increase in medial femoral torsion (femoral anteversion) and lateral tibial torsion will result in a larger Q angle and an increased lateral force on the patella. This pairing can lead to articular deterioration and pain.

a typical Q angle will not necessarily ensure the absence of problems. Large Q angles are thought to create excessive lateral forces on the patella that may predispose the patella to pathological changes. One problem with using the Q angle as a static measure of the lateral pull on the patella is that the line between the anterior superior iliac spine and the mid patella is only an *estimate* of the line of pull of the quadriceps and does not necessarily reflect the actual line of pull during movement. Resting patellar position on the femur will also affect the Q angle. For example, a patella subjected to unbalanced forces that sits in an excessively lateral position in the femoral sulcus will yield a smaller Q angle because the atypically positioned patella lies more in line with the anterior superior iliac spine and tibial tuberosity. It is important to keep in mind that the etiology of patellofemoral dysfunction is multifactorial, and the Q angle provides only one measure of the many static and dynamic factors that influence patellofemoral joint function.

In addition to the pull of the quadriceps, there are several other factors that contribute increased lateral forces on the patella. The presence of a tight IT band could limit the typical patellar medial translation during flexion, contributing to increased stress under the lateral facet of the patella.[75] With knee flexion, the IT band exerts a lateral pull on the patella. An IT band under increased tension from a tensor fascia lata or gluteus maximus contraction can cause lateral shifting and tilting of the patella in mid ranges of knee flexion.[75] The increased lateral tilt could focus the patellofemoral load on the lateral facet, increasing joint stress. Genu *valgum* can further increase the obliquity of the femur and, concomitantly, the lateral pull of the quadriceps. In contrast, individuals with genu *varum* exhibit less obliquity of the femur and therefore should have a diminished lateral pull of the quadriceps. The transverse plane deviation of medial femoral torsion (or femoral anteversion) generally results in the femoral condyles being turned in (medially rotated) in weight-bearing. The medially oriented distal femur's trochlea carries the patella medially as well, thus increasing the Q angle. Likewise, lateral tibial torsion increases the Q angle due to the increased obliquity of the patellar tendon as the tibial tuberosity turns laterally. When medial femoral torsion and lateral tibial torsion coexist, the Q angle will increase substantially, resulting in a considerable lateral force on the patella **(Fig. 11–48)**. As we will see in Chapter 12, the presence of excessive or prolonged pronation in the foot can contribute to excessive or prolonged medial rotation of the lower extremity that moves the patella medially, increasing the Q angle and promoting a greater lateral force on the patella in a manner similar to that of medial femoral torsion. In addition to static contributors, the influence of lower extremity kinematics during dynamic movement in some patients may affect patellofemoral joint mechanics. Excessive motions of the femur and/or tibia in the frontal and transverse planes during dynamic movement may contribute to increased patellofemoral stress or lateral pull of the patella.[260,261] Movement deviations resulting from muscle weakness and/or poor neuromuscular control are responsive to intervention, with interventions appropriately aimed at either proximal contributors (trunk, pelvis, hip) or distal contributors (ankle, foot) as warranted.[261] Thorough evaluation of static and dynamic proximal and distal contributors to patellofemoral joint dysfunction is necessary to guide treatment decision making in patients with patellofemoral disorders.

Life Span and Clinical Considerations

The joints of the knee complex, like other joints in the body, are subject to developmental defects, injury, and disease processes. Several factors, however, make the knee joint unique in its susceptibility to various pathologies. The knee, unlike the shoulder, elbow, and wrist, must support the body weight while *also* providing considerable mobility. Further, the knee's anatomic complexity is necessary to dissipate the enormous forces applied through the joint, as two of the longest levers in the body meet at the knee complex.

Tibiofemoral Joint Injury

The tremendous forces applied through the knee have the potential to contribute to numerous injuries and degenerative damage. In addition, participation in physical fitness and sports activities that involve jumping, pivoting, cutting, or repetitive cyclic loading among all age groups and both sexes can increase the risk of injury to the menisci, ligaments, bones, bursae, and musculotendinous structures.

Meniscal injuries are common and usually occur as a result of sudden rotation of the femur on the fixed tibia when the knee is in flexion. Medial meniscus injuries are more prevalent than lateral meniscus injuries, in part because the pivot point during axial rotation in the flexed knee occurs through the medial meniscus, and also because the more rigidly attached medial meniscus makes it more susceptible to failure with large or unexpected loads. Ligamentous injuries may occur as a result of a force that causes the joint to exceed its typical ROM. Although excessive forces may cause ligamentous tears, lower-energy forces may similarly cause plasticity or failure in ligaments weakened by aging, disease, immobilization, steroids, or vascular insufficiency. Cyclic loading (whether short-term and intense or over a prolonged period) may also affect a ligament's viscoelasticity and stiffness. A weakened ligament may take 10 months or more to return to typical stiffness after injury or repair, with the new or damaged tissue requiring protection to minimize excessive stress through the healing tissue. Absence of tissue stress, however, is also detrimental, because the new tissue will not adapt and become stronger under prolonged unloaded conditions. Rehabilitation of a repaired or reconstructed ligament, therefore, is a balance in avoiding either too much or too little applied stress.

Knee osteoarthritis is often seen in older adults and is particularly common in women. This progressive erosion of articular cartilage may be initiated and progressed by things such as a previous traumatic joint injury, obesity, malalignment, instability, or quadriceps muscle weakness. Tibial plateau fractures can occur when large axial loads are applied through the joint such as landing on one or both legs from a height. Knee joint instability, as frequently seen in the knee after ACL injury, can lead to progressive changes in the articular cartilage, menisci, and other ligaments attempting to restrain the increased joint mobility. The presence of ligamentous instability induces abnormal forces through the joint as well as excessive shearing across articular surfaces. The excessive laxity present after ligamentous injuries must be controlled to avoid episodes of giving way. Because the knee has poor bony congruency, there is an increased demand on muscles for greater dynamic control of all fine and gross movements of the knee joint in the absence of one or more ligaments. The necessary increase in muscular co-contraction, however, may generate greater compressive forces through the joint, contributing to articular cartilage degeneration. An improved method of providing dynamic stability to a lax joint, therefore, is to generate isolated muscle contractions as needed, rather than a massive co-contraction to stiffen the joint.

The numerous bursae and tendons at the knee are also subject to injury. The cause of injuries to these structures may be either a direct blow or prolonged compressive or tensile stresses. Inflammation of bursa, or **bursitis**, is common after either blunt trauma or repetitive low-level compressions that can irritate the tissue. The prepatellar bursa, the superficial infrapatellar bursa, and the bursa beneath the pes anserinus are common locations for inflammation and injury. Acute inflammation of a tendon, or **tendinitis**, results from repetitive low-level stresses to the tendon tissues. It is frequently caused by overuse of the affected muscle and can occur in response to a previous ligamentous injury. **Tendinosis** is a chronic degeneration of a tendon, without the presence of inflammation, and may result from unhealed tendonitis. Another potential source of pain and dysfunction in the knee joint is the irritation of a patellar plica. Classic symptoms include pain with prolonged sitting, stair climbing, and during resisted knee extension exercises. In flexion, the medial patellar plica is drawn over the medial femoral condyle and can become compressed beneath the patella, causing inflammation.

Patellofemoral Joint Injury

Abnormal pathomechanics of the patellofemoral joint can predispose the knee to patellofemoral dysfunctions such as excessive stress on the lateral facets of the patella, lateral subluxation, or lateral dislocation. Both excessive patellar motion and increased patellofemoral compression are commonly associated with knee pain, poor tolerance of sustained passive knee flexion (as in sitting for long periods), "giving way" of the knee, and exacerbation of symptoms by repeated use of the quadriceps on a flexed knee. Avoidance of pain may lead to diminished use of the quadriceps that may then result in muscle atrophy and further deterioration of patellar control. As muscle function declines, patellofemoral dysfunction may progress, necessitating a series of controlled situations to generate hypertrophy of the quadriceps through knee ranges with minimized pain.

Increased lateral patellar compression can be caused by a tight IT band, large Q angle (e.g., as in genu valgum or femoral anteversion with lateral tibial torsion), or patellar hypomobility. Patellar hypermobility may be due to lax medial structures or alterations in underlying bony morphology, both of which increase the risk of lateral patellar subluxation or dislocation. Lateral patellar subluxation or dislocation often results in a torn or stretched medial extensor retinaculum. The return of the laterally dislocated patella into the trochlea may also affect the medial surface of the patella (occasionally causing an osteochondral fracture) if the patella snaps back with excessive force. There are a host of other pathologies, due to irritation or inflammation of peripatellar structures, that can affect the patellofemoral joint.

Cartilaginous changes seen on the lateral patellar facet were once considered to be diagnostic of patellofemoral dysfunction, and the term *chondromalacia patella* (softening of the cartilage) was assigned. With the knowledge that similar cartilaginous changes can be found in asymptomatic knees and that the medial patellar facet can show greater change without symptoms or progressive cartilage deterioration, the term "chondromalacia patella" has fallen from favor; more general diagnoses have been used, including **patellofemoral arthralgia** or **patellofemoral pain syndrome**. The more general terminology suggests that the damage extends beyond the articular cartilage. Cartilage is aneural and therefore cannot be the cause of pain.[262] Instead, patients with patellofemoral pain can experience discomfort from damage to subchondral bone, the synovial membrane, or ligamentous or musculotendinous structures. Advances in diagnostic imaging techniques allow for imaging of patellar tracking during dynamic tasks. The effects that femoral and tibial rotation have on patella position have warranted interventions that control the hip, pelvis, and ankle motion when treating patients with patellofemoral joint injury and pain. A comprehensive multijoint evaluation is therefore necessary to identify the pathomechanics underlying the myriad knee problems that might develop.

SUMMARY

- A thorough knowledge of typical structure and function of the knee joint can be used to predict or understand the immediate effect of a specific injury and the secondary effects on intact structures.
- The variety of forces transmitted through the knee complex arises from gravity (weight-bearing forces), muscles, ligaments, and other passive soft tissue structures. Any alteration of the knee's anatomy can substantially influence these forces and have a dramatic effect on the function of the knee joint.
- Damage to the tibiofemoral joint or the patellofemoral joint can result from either a large rapid load or the accumulation of smaller repetitive loads.
- An understanding of both the primary and secondary effects of injury is important to gain a full appreciation for the pathogenesis of knee disorders.

STUDY QUESTIONS

1. Describe the congruency of the tibiofemoral joint. What bony and soft tissue factors enhance or reduce its stability?
2. How does genu valgum alter the mechanical axis of the lower extremity? What effect can this have on the compressive loading of the articular cartilage in each tibiofemoral compartment?
3. Describe the menisci of the knee, including their function, shape, and attachments.
4. Which ligaments of the knee are considered capsular ligaments? Which ligaments of the knee are extracapsular?
5. What are the patella plicae, and what implications do they have in knee joint dysfunction?
6. Which knee joint ligaments contribute to anteroposterior stability of the knee joint?
7. Which ligaments contribute to medial/lateral stability of the knee joint?
8. Identify and describe which muscles are capable of altering strain on the ACL.
9. Identify the major bursae of the knee joint. Which of these are continuous with the synovial capsule of the knee?
10. Describe the arthokinematic movement of the femur and the tibia as the knee moves from full extension into flexion in both the weight-bearing and non–weight-bearing position.
11. Describe the movement and change in the shape of the menisci during knee motion. How do the attachments of each meniscus contribute to meniscal movement?
12. Describe the automatic axial rotation (locking) mechanism of the knee, including the structures responsible for its occurrence.
13. At which point in the knee's ROM is axial rotation greatest? Which muscles produce active medial rotation? Lateral rotation?
14. Which muscles that cross the knee joint are biarticulate? How does the position of the hip joint and ankle joint alter each of these muscle's function at the knee?
15. What function(s) does the patella serve at the knee joint?
16. How does the patella move in relation to the femur in typical motions? How is knee function affected if the patella is hypomobile? Hypermobile?
17. Describe the contact of the patella with the femur at rest in full extension. How does the contact location and resultant joint contact stress change as flexion progresses?
18. Is the patella equally effective as an anatomic pulley at all points in the knee ROM? At which point(s) is it most effective? Least effective?
19. What is the Q angle of the knee joint? How does it and other muscular and ligamentous features of the knee affect the medial/lateral motion of the patella? What musculoskeletal deviations have the potential to increase the Q angle?
20. Why are ascending stairs commonly cited as producing knee pain? Relate this to patellofemoral joint compression.

REFERENCES

1. Majewski M, Susanne H, Klaus S: Epidemiology of athletic knee injuries: a 10-year study. Knee 13:184-8, 2006
2. Churchill DL, Incavo SJ, Johnson CC, et al: The transepicondylar axis approximates the optimal flexion axis of the knee. Clin Orthop Relat Res:111-8, 1998
3. Iwaki H, Pinskerova V, Freeman MA: Tibiofemoral movement 1: the shapes and relative movements of the femur and tibia in the unloaded cadaver knee. J Bone Joint Surg Br 82:1189-95, 2000
4. Dhaher YY, Francis MJ: Determination of the abduction-adduction axis of rotation at the human knee: helical axis representation. J Orthop Res 24:2187-200, 2006
5. Smith PN, Refshauge KM, Scarvell JM: Development of the concepts of knee kinematics. Arch Phys Med Rehabil 84:1895-902, 2003
6. Martelli S, Pinskerova V: The shapes of the tibial and femoral articular surfaces in relation to tibiofemoral movement. J Bone Joint Surg Br 84:607-13, 2002

7. Siu D, Rudan J, Wevers HW, et al: Femoral articular shape and geometry: a three-dimensional computerized analysis of the knee. J Arthroplasty 11:166-73, 1996
8. Cicuttini FM, Wluka AE, Wang Y, et al: Compartment differences in knee cartilage volume in healthy adults. J Rheumatol 29:554-6, 2002
9. Bowers ME, Trinh N, Tung GA, et al: Quantitative MR imaging using "LiveWire" to measure tibiofemoral articular cartilage thickness. Osteoarthritis Cartilage 16:1167-73, 2008
10. Harvey WF, Niu J, Zhang Y, et al: Knee alignment differences between Chinese and Caucasian subjects without osteoarthritis. Ann Rheum Dis 67:1524-8, 2008
11. Heijink A, Gomoll AH, Madry H, et al: Biomechanical considerations in the pathogenesis of osteoarthritis of the knee. Knee Surg Sports Traumatol Arthrosc 20:423-35, 2012
12. Sharma L, Song J, Dunlop D, et al: Varus and valgus alignment and incident and progressive knee osteoarthritis. Ann Rheum Dis 69:1940-5, 2010
13. Babazadeh S, Dowsey MM, Bingham RJ, et al: The long leg radiograph is a reliable method of assessing alignment when compared to computer-assisted navigation and computer tomography. Knee 20:242-9, 2013
14. Teichtahl AJ, Davies-Tuck ML, Wluka AE, et al: Change in knee angle influences the rate of medial tibial cartilage volume loss in knee osteoarthritis. Osteoarthritis Cartilage 17:8-11, 2009
15. Brouwer GM, van Tol AW, Bergink AP, et al: Association between valgus and varus alignment and the development and progression of radiographic osteoarthritis of the knee. Arthritis Rheum 56:1204-11, 2007
16. Lewek MD, Rudolph KS, Snyder-Mackler L: Control of frontal plane knee laxity during gait in patients with medial compartment knee osteoarthritis. Osteoarthritis Cartilage 12:745-51, 2004
17. Felson DT, Niu J, Gross KD, et al: Valgus malalignment is a risk factor for lateral knee osteoarthritis incidence and progression: findings from the Multicenter Osteoarthritis Study and the Osteoarthritis Initiative. Arthritis Rheum 65:355-62, 2013
18. Sharma L, Song J, Felson DT, et al: The role of knee alignment in disease progression and functional decline in knee osteoarthritis. JAMA 286:188-95, 2001
19. Johnson F, Leitl S, Waugh W: The distribution of load across the knee: a comparison of static and dynamic measurements. J Bone Joint Surg Br 62:346-9, 1980
20. Andriacchi TP: Dynamics of knee malalignment. Orthop Clin North Am 25:395-403, 1994
21. Mundermann A, Dyrby CO, D'Lima DD, et al: In vivo knee loading characteristics during activities of daily living as measured by an instrumented total knee replacement. J Orthop Res 26:1167-72, 2008
22. Yamabe E, Ueno T, Miyagi R, et al: Study of surgical indication for knee arthroplasty by cartilage analysis in three compartments using data from Osteoarthritis Initiative (OAI). BMC Musculoskelet Disord 14:194, 2013
23. Foroughi N, Smith R, Vanwanseele B: The association of external knee adduction moment with biomechanical variables in osteoarthritis: a systematic review. Knee 16:303-9, 2009
24. Mundermann A, Dyrby CO, Andriacchi TP: Secondary gait changes in patients with medial compartment knee osteoarthritis: increased load at the ankle, knee, and hip during walking. Arthritis Rheum 52:2835-44, 2005
25. Bonasia DE, Governale G, Spolaore S, et al: High tibial osteotomy. Curr Rev Musculoskelet Med 7:292-301, 2014
26. Amis AA: Biomechanics of high tibial osteotomy. Knee Surg Sports Traumatol Arthrosc 21:197-205, 2013
27. Fox AJ, Wanivenhaus F, Burge AJ, et al: The human meniscus: a review of anatomy, function, injury, and advances in treatment. Clin Anat 28:269-87, 2015
28. Markes AR, Hodax JD, Ma CB: Meniscus form and function. Clin Sports Med 39:1-12, 2020
29. Messner K, Gao J: The menisci of the knee joint: anatomical and functional characteristics, and a rationale for clinical treatment. J Anat 193 (Pt 2):161-78, 1998
30. Rath E, Richmond JC: The menisci: basic science and advances in treatment. Br J Sports Med 34:252-7, 2000
31. Greis PE, Bardana DD, Holmstrom MC, et al: Meniscal injury: I. Basic science and evaluation. J Am Acad Orthop Surg 10:168-76, 2002
32. Gilbert S, Chen T, Hutchinson ID, et al: Dynamic contact mechanics on the tibial plateau of the human knee during activities of daily living. J Biomech 47:2006-12, 2014
33. Masouros SD, McDermott ID, Amis AA, et al: Biomechanics of the meniscus-meniscal ligament construct of the knee. Knee Surg Sports Traumatol Arthrosc 16:1121-32, 2008
34. McCarty EC, Marx RG, DeHaven KE: Meniscus repair: considerations in treatment and update of clinical results. Clin Orthop Relat Res:122-34, 2002
35. Wang YJ, Yu JK, Luo H, et al: An anatomical and histological study of human meniscal horn bony insertions and peri-meniscal attachments as a basis for meniscal transplantation. Chin Med J (Engl) 122:536-40, 2009
36. Dirim B, Haghighi P, Trudell D, et al: Medial patellofemoral ligament: cadaveric investigation of anatomy with MRI, MR arthrography, and histologic correlation. AJR Am J Roentgenol 191:490-8, 2008
37. De Maeseneer M, Shahabpour M, Lenchik L, et al: Distal insertions of the semimembranosus tendon: MR imaging with anatomic correlation. Skeletal Radiol 43:781-91, 2014
38. Fujishiro H, Tsukada S, Nakamura T, et al: Attachment area of fibres from the horns of lateral meniscus: anatomic study with special reference to the positional relationship of anterior cruciate ligament. Knee Surg Sports Traumatol Arthrosc 25:368-73, 2017
39. Gupte CM, Bull AM, Thomas RD, et al: A review of the function and biomechanics of the meniscofemoral ligaments. Arthroscopy 19:161-71, 2003
40. Osti M, Tschann P, Kunzel KH, et al: Posterolateral corner of the knee: microsurgical analysis of anatomy and morphometry. Orthopedics 36:e1114-20, 2013
41. Simonian PT, Sussmann PS, Wickiewicz TL, et al: Popliteomeniscal fasciculi and the unstable lateral meniscus: clinical correlation and magnetic resonance diagnosis. Arthroscopy 13:590-6, 1997
42. Makris EA, Hadidi P, Athanasiou KA: The knee meniscus: structure-function, pathophysiology, current repair techniques, and prospects for regeneration. Biomaterials 32:7411-31, 2011
43. Riener R, Rabuffetti M, Frigo C: Stair ascent and descent at different inclinations. Gait Posture 15:32-44, 2002
44. Robon MJ, Perell KL, Fang M, et al: The relationship between ankle plantar flexor muscle moments and knee compressive forces in subjects with and without pain. Clin Biomech (Bristol) 15:522-7, 2000
45. D'Lima DD, Steklov N, Patil S, et al: The Mark Coventry Award: in vivo knee forces during recreation and exercise after knee arthroplasty. Clin Orthop Relat Res 466:2605-11, 2008
46. Kuitunen S, Komi PV, Kyrolainen H: Knee and ankle joint stiffness in sprint running. Med Sci Sports Exerc 34:166-73, 2002
47. Cleather DJ, Goodwin JE, Bull AM: Hip and knee joint loading during vertical jumping and push jerking. Clin Biomech (Bristol) 28:98-103, 2013
48. Radin EL, de Lamotte F, Maquet P: Role of the menisci in the distribution of stress in the knee. Clin Orthop Relat Res:290-4, 1984
49. Weiss WM, Johnson D: Update on meniscus debridement and resection. J Knee Surg 27:413-22, 2014
50. Thorlund JB, Creaby MW, Wrigley TV, et al: Knee joint laxity and passive stiffness in meniscectomized patients compared with healthy controls. Knee 21:886-90, 2014
51. Hunter DJ, Niu J, Felson DT, et al: Knee alignment does not predict incident osteoarthritis: the Framingham osteoarthritis study. Arthritis Rheum 56:1212-8, 2007
52. Sharma L, Dunlop DD, Cahue S, et al: Quadriceps strength and osteoarthritis progression in malaligned and lax knees. Ann Intern Med 138:613-9, 2003
53. Lamplot JD, Tompkins WP, Friedman MV, et al: Radiographic and clinical evidence for osteoarthritis at medium-term follow-up after arthroscopic partial medial meniscectomy. Cartilage 13:588S-94S, 2021
54. Rangger C, Klestil T, Gloetzer W, et al: Osteoarthritis after arthroscopic partial meniscectomy. Am J Sports Med 23:240-4, 1995
55. Gray JC: Neural and vascular anatomy of the menisci of the human knee. J Orthop Sports Phys Ther 29:23-30, 1999
56. Hauger O, Frank LR, Boutin RD, et al: Characterization of the "red zone" of knee meniscus: MR imaging and histologic correlation. Radiology 217:193-200, 2000
57. Karia M, Ghaly Y, Al-Hadithy N, et al: Current concepts in the techniques, indications and outcomes of meniscal repairs. Eur J Orthop Surg Traumatol 29:509-20, 2019
58. Mine T, Kimura M, Sakka A, et al: Innervation of nociceptors in the menisci of the knee joint: an immunohistochemical study. Arch Orthop Trauma Surg 120:201-4, 2000
59. Markolf KL, Graff-Radford A, Amstutz HC: In vivo knee stability: a quantitative assessment using an instrumented clinical testing apparatus. J Bone Joint Surg Am 60:664-74, 1978
60. Ralphs JR, Benjamin M: The joint capsule: structure, composition, ageing and disease. J Anat 184 (Pt 3):503-9, 1994
61. LaPrade RF, Engebretsen AH, Ly TV, et al: The anatomy of the medial part of the knee. J Bone Joint Surg Am 89:2000-10, 2007
62. Thawait SK, Soldatos T, Thawait GK, et al: High resolution magnetic resonance imaging of the patellar retinaculum: normal anatomy, common injury patterns, and pathologies. Skeletal Radiol 41:137-48, 2012
63. Berumen-Nafarrate E, Leal-Berumen I, Luevano E, et al: Synovial tissue and synovial fluid. J Knee Surg 15:46-8, 2002

64. Lee SH, Petersilge CA, Trudell DJ, et al: Extrasynovial spaces of the cruciate ligaments: anatomy, MR imaging, and diagnostic implications. AJR Am J Roentgenol 166:1433-7, 1996
65. Smith MD: The normal synovium. Open Rheumatol J 5:100-6, 2011
66. Dodds JA, Arnoczky SP: Anatomy of the anterior cruciate ligament: a blueprint for repair and reconstruction. Arthroscopy 10:132-9, 1994
67. Petersen W, Tillmann B: Structure and vascularization of the cruciate ligaments of the human knee joint. Anat Embryol (Berl) 200:325-34, 1999
68. Diepold J, Ruhdorfer A, Dannhauer T, et al: Sex-differences of the healthy infra-patellar (Hoffa) fat pad in relation to intermuscular and subcutaneous fat content—data from the Osteoarthritis Initiative. Ann Anat 200: 30-6, 2015
69. Garcia-Valtuille R, Abascal F, Cerezal L, et al: Anatomy and MR imaging appearances of synovial plicae of the knee. Radiographics 22:775-84, 2002
70. Schindler OS: "The Sneaky Plica" revisited: morphology, pathophysiology and treatment of synovial plicae of the knee. Knee Surg Sports Traumatol Arthrosc 22:247-62, 2014
71. Dupont JY: Synovial plicae of the knee: controversies and review. Clin Sports Med 16:87-122, 1997
72. LaPrade MD, Kennedy MI, Wijdicks CA, et al: Anatomy and biomechanics of the medial side of the knee and their surgical implications. Sports Med Arthrosc Rev 23:63-70, 2015
73. Nomura E, Horiuchi Y, Inoue M: Correlation of MR imaging findings and open exploration of medial patellofemoral ligament injuries in acute patellar dislocations. Knee 9:139-43, 2002
74. Tom A, Fulkerson JP: Restoration of native medial patellofemoral ligament support after patella dislocation. Sports Med Arthrosc Rev 15:68-71, 2007
75. Merican AM, Amis AA: Anatomy of the lateral retinaculum of the knee. J Bone Joint Surg Br 90:527-34, 2008
76. De Maeseneer M, Van Roy F, Lenchik L, et al: Three layers of the medial capsular and supporting structures of the knee: MR imaging-anatomic correlation. Radiographics 20 Spec No:S83-9, 2000
77. Fulkerson JP, Gossling HR: Anatomy of the knee joint lateral retinaculum. Clin Orthop Relat Res:183-8, 1980
78. LaPrade RF, Morgan PM, Wentorf FA, et al: The anatomy of the posterior aspect of the knee: an anatomic study. J Bone Joint Surg Am 89:758-64, 2007
79. D'Ambrosi R, Corona K, Guerra G, et al: Posterior oblique ligament of the knee: state of the art. EFORT Open Rev 6:364-71, 2021
80. Chahla J, Moatshe G, Dean CS, et al: Posterolateral corner of the knee: current concepts. Arch Bone Jt Surg 4:97-103, 2016
81. Wijdicks CA, Griffith CJ, LaPrade RF, et al: Radiographic identification of the primary medial knee structures. J Bone Joint Surg Am 91:521-9, 2009
82. Griffith CJ, LaPrade RF, Johansen S, et al: Medial knee injury: Part 1, static function of the individual components of the main medial knee structures. Am J Sports Med 37:1762-70, 2009
83. Harfe DT, Chuinard CR, Espinoza LM, et al: Elongation patterns of the collateral ligaments of the human knee. Clin Biomech (Bristol) 13:163-75, 1998
84. Grood ES, Noyes FR, Butler DL, et al: Ligamentous and capsular restraints preventing straight medial and lateral laxity in intact human cadaver knees. J Bone Joint Surg Am 63:1257-69, 1981
85. Kanamori A, Sakane M, Zeminski J, et al: In-situ force in the medial and lateral structures of intact and ACL-deficient knees. J Orthop Sci 5:567-71, 2000
86. Battaglia MJ, 2nd, Lenhoff MW, Ehteshami JR, et al: Medial collateral ligament injuries and subsequent load on the anterior cruciate ligament: a biomechanical evaluation in a cadaveric model. Am J Sports Med 37:305-11, 2009
87. Miyamoto RG, Bosco JA, Sherman OH: Treatment of medial collateral ligament injuries. J Am Acad Orthop Surg 17:152-61, 2009
88. Frank CB, Hart DA, Shrive NG: Molecular biology and biomechanics of normal and healing ligaments—a review. Osteoarthritis Cartilage 7:130-40, 1999
89. James EW, LaPrade CM, LaPrade RF: Anatomy and biomechanics of the lateral side of the knee and surgical implications. Sports Med Arthrosc Rev 23:2-9, 2015
90. Recondo JA, Salvador E, Villanua JA, et al: Lateral stabilizing structures of the knee: functional anatomy and injuries assessed with MR imaging. Radiographics 20 Spec No:S91-S102, 2000
91. Coobs BR, LaPrade RF, Griffith CJ, et al: Biomechanical analysis of an isolated fibular (lateral) collateral ligament reconstruction using an autogenous semitendinosus graft. Am J Sports Med 35:1521-7, 2007
92. LaPrade RF, Tso A, Wentorf FA: Force measurements on the fibular collateral ligament, popliteofibular ligament, and popliteus tendon to applied loads. Am J Sports Med 32:1695-701, 2004
93. Lim HC, Bae JH, Bae TS, et al: Relative role changing of lateral collateral ligament on the posterolateral rotatory instability according to the knee flexion angles: a biomechanical comparative study of role of lateral collateral ligament and popliteofibular ligament. Arch Orthop Trauma Surg 132:1631-6, 2012
94. Wroble RR, Grood ES, Cummings JS, et al: The role of the lateral extraarticular restraints in the anterior cruciate ligament-deficient knee. Am J Sports Med 21:257-62; discussion 263, 1993
95. Kopf S, Musahl V, Tashman S, et al: A systematic review of the femoral origin and tibial insertion morphology of the ACL. Knee Surg Sports Traumatol Arthrosc 17:213-9, 2009
96. Siegel L, Vandenakker-Albanese C, Siegel D: Anterior cruciate ligament injuries: anatomy, physiology, biomechanics, and management. Clin J Sport Med 22:349-55, 2012
97. Giuliani JR, Kilcoyne KG, Rue JP: Anterior cruciate ligament anatomy: a review of the anteromedial and posterolateral bundles. J Knee Surg 22:148-54, 2009
98. Bach JM, Hull ML, Patterson HA: Direct measurement of strain in the posterolateral bundle of the anterior cruciate ligament. J Biomech 30:281-3, 1997
99. Gabriel MT, Wong EK, Woo SL, et al: Distribution of in situ forces in the anterior cruciate ligament in response to rotatory loads. J Orthop Res 22:85-9, 2004
100. Torzilli PA, Greenberg RL, Insall J: An in vivo biomechanical evaluation of anterior-posterior motion of the knee: roentgenographic measurement technique, stress machine, and stable population. J Bone Joint Surg Am 63:960-8, 1981
101. Wascher DC, Markolf KL, Shapiro MS, et al: Direct in vitro measurement of forces in the cruciate ligaments. Part I: the effect of multiplane loading in the intact knee. J Bone Joint Surg Am 75:377-86, 1993
102. Li G, Papannagari R, DeFrate LE, et al: The effects of ACL deficiency on mediolateral translation and varus-valgus rotation. Acta Orthop 78:355-60, 2007
103. Arms SW, Pope MH, Johnson RJ, et al: The biomechanics of anterior cruciate ligament rehabilitation and reconstruction. Am J Sports Med 12:8-18, 1984
104. Markolf KL, Burchfield DM, Shapiro MM, et al: Combined knee loading states that generate high anterior cruciate ligament forces. J Orthop Res 13:930-5, 1995
105. Markolf KL, Gorek JF, Kabo JM, et al: Direct measurement of resultant forces in the anterior cruciate ligament. An in vitro study performed with a new experimental technique. J Bone Joint Surg Am 72:557-67, 1990
106. Quatman CE, Kiapour AM, Demetropoulos CK, et al: Preferential loading of the ACL compared with the MCL during landing: a novel in sim approach yields the multiplanar mechanism of dynamic valgus during ACL injuries. Am J Sports Med 42:177-86, 2014
107. Kaeding CC, Pedroza AD, Parker RD, et al: Intra-articular findings in the reconstructed multiligament-injured knee. Arthroscopy 21:424-30, 2005
108. Quatman CE, Kiapour A, Myer GD, et al: Cartilage pressure distributions provide a footprint to define female anterior cruciate ligament injury mechanisms. Am J Sports Med 39:1706-13, 2011
109. Feagin JA, Jr., Lambert KL: Mechanism of injury and pathology of anterior cruciate ligament injuries. Orthop Clin North Am 16:41-5, 1985
110. Durselen L, Claes L, Kiefer H: The influence of muscle forces and external loads on cruciate ligament strain. Am J Sports Med 23:129-36, 1995
111. Withrow TJ, Huston LJ, Wojtys EM, et al: The relationship between quadriceps muscle force, knee flexion, and anterior cruciate ligament strain in an in vitro simulated jump landing. Am J Sports Med 34:269-74, 2006
112. Hirokawa S, Solomonow M, Lu Y, et al: Anterior-posterior and rotational displacement of the tibia elicited by quadriceps contraction. Am J Sports Med 20:299-306, 1992
113. Fujiya H, Kousa P, Fleming BC, et al: Effect of muscle loads and torque applied to the tibia on the strain behavior of the anterior cruciate ligament: an in vitro investigation. Clin Biomech (Bristol) 26:1005-11, 2011
114. Fleming BC, Renstrom PA, Ohlen G, et al: The gastrocnemius muscle is an antagonist of the anterior cruciate ligament. J Orthop Res 19:1178-84, 2001
115. MacWilliams BA, Wilson DR, DesJardins JD, et al: Hamstrings cocontraction reduces internal rotation, anterior translation, and anterior cruciate ligament load in weight-bearing flexion. J Orthop Res 17:817-22, 1999
116. O'Connor JJ: Can muscle co-contraction protect knee ligaments after injury or repair? J Bone Joint Surg Br 75:41-8, 1993
117. Withrow TJ, Huston LJ, Wojtys EM, et al: Effect of varying hamstring tension on anterior cruciate ligament strain during in vitro impulsive knee flexion and compression loading. J Bone Joint Surg Am 90:815-23, 2008
118. Pandy MG, Shelburne KB: Dependence of cruciate-ligament loading on muscle forces and external load. J Biomech 30:1015-24, 1997

119. Elias JJ, Faust AF, Chu YH, et al: The soleus muscle acts as an agonist for the anterior cruciate ligament: an in vitro experimental study. Am J Sports Med 31:241-6, 2003
120. Tsai LC, McLean S, Colletti PM, et al: Greater muscle co-contraction results in increased tibiofemoral compressive forces in females who have undergone anterior cruciate ligament reconstruction. J Orthop Res 30:2007-14, 2012
121. Alfayyadh A, Williams JR, Neal K, et al: Unbalanced medial-to-lateral knee muscle co-contractions are associated with medial tibiofemoral underloading during gait three months after anterior cruciate ligament reconstruction. J Biomech 163:111925, 2024
122. Khandha A, Manal K, Capin J, et al: High muscle co-contraction does not result in high joint forces during gait in anterior cruciate ligament deficient knees. J Orthop Res 37:104-112, 2019
123. Woo SL, Hollis JM, Adams DJ, et al: Tensile properties of the human femur-anterior cruciate ligament-tibia complex: the effects of specimen age and orientation. Am J Sports Med 19:217-25, 1991
124. Butler DL, Kay MD, Stouffer DC: Comparison of material properties in fascicle-bone units from human patellar tendon and knee ligaments. J Biomech 19:425-32, 1986
125. Escamilla RF, Macleod TD, Wilk KE, et al: Anterior cruciate ligament strain and tensile forces for weight-bearing and non-weight-bearing exercises: a guide to exercise selection. J Orthop Sports Phys Ther 42:208-20, 2012
126. Logerstedt DS, Scalzitti D, Risberg MA, et al: Knee stability and movement coordination impairments: knee ligament sprain revision 2017. J Orthop Sports Phys Ther 47:A1-A47, 2017
127. Beynnon B, Howe JG, Pope MH, et al: The measurement of anterior cruciate ligament strain in vivo. Int Orthop 16:1-12, 1992
128. Beynnon BD, Fleming BC, Johnson RJ, et al: Anterior cruciate ligament strain behavior during rehabilitation exercises in vivo. Am J Sports Med 23:24-34, 1995
129. Fleming BC, Oksendahl H, Beynnon BD: Open- or closed-kinetic chain exercises after anterior cruciate ligament reconstruction? Exerc Sport Sci Rev 33:134-40, 2005
130. Englander ZA, Garrett WE, Spritzer CE, et al: In vivo attachment site to attachment site length and strain of the ACL and its bundles during the full gait cycle measured by MRI and high-speed biplanar radiography. J Biomech 98:109443, 2020
131. Taylor KA, Cutcliffe HC, Queen RM, et al: In vivo measurement of ACL length and relative strain during walking. J Biomech 46:478-83, 2013
132. Brinlee AW, Dickenson SB, Hunter-Giordano A, et al: ACL reconstruction rehabilitation: clinical data, biologic healing, and criterion-based milestones to inform a return-to-sport guideline. Sports Health 14:770-9, 2022
133. Noehren B, Snyder-Mackler L: Who's afraid of the big bad wolf? Open-chain exercises after anterior cruciate ligament reconstruction. J Orthop Sports Phys Ther 50:473-5, 2020
134. Eastlack ME, Axe MJ, Snyder-Mackler L: Laxity, instability, and functional outcome after ACL injury: copers versus noncopers. Med Sci Sports Exerc 31:210-5, 1999
135. Moksnes H, Snyder-Mackler L, Risberg MA: Individuals with an anterior cruciate ligament-deficient knee classified as noncopers may be candidates for nonsurgical rehabilitation. J Orthop Sports Phys Ther 38:586-95, 2008
136. Noyes FR, Matthews DS, Mooar PA, et al: The symptomatic anterior cruciate-deficient knee. Part II: the results of rehabilitation, activity modification, and counseling on functional disability. J Bone Joint Surg Am 65:163-74, 1983
137. Rudolph KS, Eastlack ME, Axe MJ, et al: 1998 Basmajian Student Award Paper: movement patterns after anterior cruciate ligament injury: a comparison of patients who compensate well for the injury and those who require operative stabilization. J Electromyogr Kinesiol 8:349-62, 1998
138. Chmielewski TL, Hurd WJ, Rudolph KS, et al: Perturbation training improves knee kinematics and reduces muscle co-contraction after complete unilateral anterior cruciate ligament rupture. Phys Ther 85:740-9; discussion 750-4, 2005
139. Hartigan E, Axe MJ, Snyder-Mackler L: Perturbation training prior to ACL reconstruction improves gait asymmetries in non-copers. J Orthop Res 27:724-9, 2009
140. Risberg MA, Holm I, Myklebust G, et al: Neuromuscular training versus strength training during first 6 months after anterior cruciate ligament reconstruction: a randomized clinical trial. Phys Ther 87: 737-50, 2007
141. Fitzgerald GK, Axe MJ, Snyder-Mackler L: The efficacy of perturbation training in nonoperative anterior cruciate ligament rehabilitation programs for physically active individuals. Phys Ther 80:128-40, 2000
142. Grindem H, Eitzen I, Moksnes H, et al: A pair-matched comparison of return to pivoting sports at 1 year in anterior cruciate ligament-injured patients after a nonoperative versus an operative treatment course. Am J Sports Med 40:2509-16, 2012
143. Ardern CL, Taylor NF, Feller JA, et al: Fifty-five per cent return to competitive sport following anterior cruciate ligament reconstruction surgery: an updated systematic review and meta-analysis including aspects of physical functioning and contextual factors. Br J Sports Med 48:1543-52, 2014
144. Frobell RB, Roos HP, Roos EM, et al: Treatment for acute anterior cruciate ligament tear: five year outcome of randomised trial. BMJ 346:f232, 2013
145. Smith TO, Postle K, Penny F, et al: Is reconstruction the best management strategy for anterior cruciate ligament rupture? A systematic review and meta-analysis comparing anterior cruciate ligament reconstruction versus non-operative treatment. Knee 21:462-70, 2014
146. Galway HR, MacIntosh DL: The lateral pivot shift: a symptom and sign of anterior cruciate ligament insufficiency. Clin Orthop Relat Res:45-50, 1980
147. Kennedy MI, Claes S, Fuso FA, et al: The anterolateral ligament: an anatomic, radiographic, and biomechanical analysis. Am J Sports Med 43:1606-15, 2015
148. Meena A, Attri M, Farinelli L, et al: Anterolateral corner of knee: current concepts. J Exp Orthop 12:e70172, 2025
149. Ariel de Lima D, Helito CP, Daggett M, et al: Anterolateral ligament of the knee: a step-by-step dissection. BMC Musculoskelet Disord 20:142, 2019
150. Ariel de Lima D, Helito CP, Lacerda de Lima L, et al: Anatomy of the anterolateral ligament of the knee: a systematic review. Arthroscopy 35:670-81, 2019
151. Park JG, Han SB, Rhim HC, et al: Anatomy of the anterolateral ligament of the knee joint. World J Clin Cases 10:7215-23, 2022
152. Monaco E, Ferretti A, Labianca L, et al: Navigated knee kinematics after cutting of the ACL and its secondary restraint. Knee Surg Sports Traumatol Arthrosc 20:870-7, 2012
153. Parsons EM, Gee AO, Spiekerman C, et al: The biomechanical function of the anterolateral ligament of the knee. Am J Sports Med 43:669-74, 2015
154. Rasmussen MT, Nitri M, Williams BT, et al: An in vitro robotic assessment of the anterolateral ligament, Part 1: secondary role of the anterolateral ligament in the setting of an anterior cruciate ligament injury. Am J Sports Med 44:585-92, 2016
155. Pomajzl R, Maerz T, Shams C, et al: A review of the anterolateral ligament of the knee: current knowledge regarding its incidence, anatomy, biomechanics, and surgical dissection. Arthroscopy 31:583-91, 2015
156. Smith JO, Yasen SK, Lord B, et al: Combined anterolateral ligament and anatomic anterior cruciate ligament reconstruction of the knee. Knee Surg Sports Traumatol Arthrosc 23:3151-6, 2015
157. Tavlo M, Eljaja S, Jensen JT, et al: The role of the anterolateral ligament in ACL insufficient and reconstructed knees on rotatory stability: a biomechanical study on human cadavers. Scand J Med Sci Sports 26:960-6, 2016
158. Sonnery-Cottet B, Thaunat M, Freychet B, et al: Outcome of a combined anterior cruciate ligament and anterolateral ligament reconstruction technique with a minimum 2-year follow-up. Am J Sports Med 43:1598-605, 2015
159. Weber AE, Zuke W, Mayer EN, et al: Lateral augmentation procedures in anterior cruciate ligament reconstruction: anatomic, biomechanical, imaging, and clinical evidence. Am J Sports Med 47:740-52, 2019
160. Voos JE, Mauro CS, Wente T, et al: Posterior cruciate ligament: anatomy, biomechanics, and outcomes. Am J Sports Med 40:222-31, 2012
161. Saddler SC, Noyes FR, Grood ES, et al: Posterior cruciate ligament anatomy and length-tension behavior of PCL surface fibers. Am J Knee Surg 9:194-9, 1996
162. Harner CD, Hoher J, Vogrin TM, et al: The effects of a popliteus muscle load on in situ forces in the posterior cruciate ligament and on knee kinematics: a human cadaveric study. Am J Sports Med 26:669-73, 1998
163. Amis AA, Gupte CM, Bull AM, et al: Anatomy of the posterior cruciate ligament and the meniscofemoral ligaments. Knee Surg Sports Traumatol Arthrosc 14:257-63, 2006
164. Fanelli GC, Beck JD, Edson CJ: Current concepts review: the posterior cruciate ligament. J Knee Surg 23:61-72, 2010
165. Matava MJ, Ellis E, Gruber B: Surgical treatment of posterior cruciate ligament tears: an evolving technique. J Am Acad Orthop Surg 17:435-46, 2009
166. Kurosawa H, Yamakoshi K, Yasuda K, et al: Simultaneous measurement of changes in length of the cruciate ligaments during knee motion. Clin Orthop Relat Res:233-40, 1991
167. Ahmad CS, Cohen ZA, Levine WN, et al: Codominance of the individual posterior cruciate ligament bundles: an analysis of bundle lengths and orientation. Am J Sports Med 31:221-5, 2003
168. Kennedy NI, LaPrade RF, Goldsmith MT, et al: Posterior cruciate ligament graft fixation angles, Part 1: biomechanical evaluation for anatomic single-bundle reconstruction. Am J Sports Med 42:2338-45, 2014

169. Harner CD, Xerogeanes JW, Livesay GA, et al: The human posterior cruciate ligament complex: an interdisciplinary study. Ligament morphology and biomechanical evaluation. Am J Sports Med 23:736-45, 1995
170. Race A, Amis AA: Loading of the two bundles of the posterior cruciate ligament: an analysis of bundle function in a-P drawer. J Biomech 29:873-9, 1996
171. Li G, Gill TJ, DeFrate LE, et al: Biomechanical consequences of PCL deficiency in the knee under simulated muscle loads—an in vitro experimental study. J Orthop Res 20:887-92, 2002
172. Piziali RL, Seering WP, Nagel DA, et al: The function of the primary ligaments of the knee in anterior-posterior and medial-lateral motions. J Biomech 13:777-84, 1980
173. Li G, Papannagari R, Li M, et al: Effect of posterior cruciate ligament deficiency on in vivo translation and rotation of the knee during weight-bearing flexion. Am J Sports Med 36:474-9, 2008
174. Van Dommelen BA, Fowler PJ: Anatomy of the posterior cruciate ligament: a review. Am J Sports Med 17:24-9, 1989
175. Loredo R, Hodler J, Pedowitz R, et al: Posteromedial corner of the knee: MR imaging with gross anatomic correlation. Skeletal Radiol 28:305-11, 1999
176. Aronowitz ER, Parker RD, Gatt CJ: Arthroscopic identification of the popliteofibular ligament. Arthroscopy 17:932-9, 2001
177. Petersen W, Loerch S, Schanz S, et al: The role of the posterior oblique ligament in controlling posterior tibial translation in the posterior cruciate ligament-deficient knee. Am J Sports Med 36:495-501, 2008
178. Crespo B, James EW, Metsavaht L, et al: Injuries to posterolateral corner of the knee: a comprehensive review from anatomy to surgical treatment. Rev Bras Ortop 50:363-70, 2015
179. LaPrade RF, Ly TV, Wentorf FA, et al: The posterolateral attachments of the knee: a qualitative and quantitative morphologic analysis of the fibular collateral ligament, popliteus tendon, popliteofibular ligament, and lateral gastrocnemius tendon. Am J Sports Med 31:854-60, 2003
180. Dean RS, LaPrade RF: ACL and posterolateral corner injuries. Curr Rev Musculoskelet Med 13:123-32, 2020
181. Kawashima T, Takeishi H, Yoshitomi S, et al: Anatomical study of the fabella, fabellar complex and its clinical implications. Surg Radiol Anat 29:611-6, 2007
182. Nagasaki S, Ohkoshi Y, Yamamoto K, et al: The incidence and cross-sectional area of the meniscofemoral ligament. Am J Sports Med 34:1345-50, 2006
183. Lunden JB, Bzdusek PJ, Monson JK, et al: Current concepts in the recognition and treatment of posterolateral corner injuries of the knee. J Orthop Sports Phys Ther 40:502-16, 2010
184. Yamamoto Y, Hsu WH, Fisk JA, et al: Effect of the iliotibial band on knee biomechanics during a simulated pivot shift test. J Orthop Res 24:967-73, 2006
185. Fairclough J, Hayashi K, Toumi H, et al: The functional anatomy of the iliotibial band during flexion and extension of the knee: implications for understanding iliotibial band syndrome. J Anat 208:309-16, 2006
186. Muhle C, Ahn JM, Yeh L, et al: Iliotibial band friction syndrome: MR imaging findings in 16 patients and MR arthrographic study of six cadaveric knees. Radiology 212:103-10, 1999
187. Goh LA, Chhem RK, Wang SC, et al: Iliotibial band thickness: sonographic measurements in asymptomatic volunteers. J Clin Ultrasound 31:239-44, 2003
188. Hamill J, Miller R, Noehren B, et al: A prospective study of iliotibial band strain in runners. Clin Biomech (Bristol) 23:1018-25, 2008
189. Terry GC, Hughston JC, Norwood LA: The anatomy of the iliopatellar band and iliotibial tract. Am J Sports Med 14:39-45, 1986
190. Rauschning W: Anatomy and function of the communication between knee joint and popliteal bursae. Ann Rheum Dis 39:354-8, 1980
191. Saavedra MA, Navarro-Zarza JE, Villasenor-Ovies P, et al: Clinical anatomy of the knee. Reumatol Clin 8 Suppl 2:39-45, 2012
192. LaPrade RF: The anatomy of the deep infrapatellar bursa of the knee. Am J Sports Med 26:129-32, 1998
193. Bohnsack M, Wilharm A, Hurschler C, et al: Biomechanical and kinematic influences of a total infrapatellar fat pad resection on the knee. Am J Sports Med 32:1873-80, 2004
194. LaPrade RF, Hamilton CD: The fibular collateral ligament-biceps femoris bursa: an anatomic study. Am J Sports Med 25:439-43, 1997
195. Asano T, Akagi M, Nakamura T: The functional flexion-extension axis of the knee corresponds to the surgical epicondylar axis: in vivo analysis using a biplanar image-matching technique. J Arthroplasty 20:1060-7, 2005
196. Li G, DeFrate LE, Park SE, et al: In vivo articular cartilage contact kinematics of the knee: an investigation using dual-orthogonal fluoroscopy and magnetic resonance image-based computer models. Am J Sports Med 33:102-7, 2005
197. Fuss FK: Anatomy of the cruciate ligaments and their function in extension and flexion of the human knee joint. Am J Anat 184:165-76, 1989
198. Thompson WO, Thaete FL, Fu FH, et al: Tibial meniscal dynamics using three-dimensional reconstruction of magnetic resonance images. Am J Sports Med 19:210-5; discussion 215-6, 1991
199. Rowe PJ, Myles CM, Walker C, et al: Knee joint kinematics in gait and other functional activities measured using flexible electrogoniometry: how much knee motion is sufficient for normal daily life? Gait Posture 12:143-55, 2000
200. Hemmerich A, Brown H, Smith S, et al: Hip, knee, and ankle kinematics of high range of motion activities of daily living. J Orthop Res 24:770-81, 2006
201. Shelbourne KD, Urch SE, Gray T, et al: Loss of normal knee motion after anterior cruciate ligament reconstruction is associated with radiographic arthritic changes after surgery. Am J Sports Med 40:108-13, 2012
202. Loudon JK, Goist HL, Loudon KL: Genu recurvatum syndrome. J Orthop Sports Phys Ther 27:361-7, 1998
203. Almquist PO, Arnbjornsson A, Zatterstrom R, et al: Evaluation of an external device measuring knee joint rotation: an in vivo study with simultaneous Roentgen stereometric analysis. J Orthop Res 20:427-32, 2002
204. Markolf KL, Bargar WL, Shoemaker SC, et al: The role of joint load in knee stability. J Bone Joint Surg Am 63:570-85, 1981
205. Buchanan TS, Lloyd DG: Muscle activation at the human knee during isometric flexion-extension and varus-valgus loads. J Orthop Res 15:11-7, 1997
206. Zhang LQ, Xu D, Wang G, et al: Muscle strength in knee varus and valgus. Med Sci Sports Exerc 33:1194-9, 2001
207. Chang AH, Lee SJ, Zhao H, et al: Impaired varus-valgus proprioception and neuromuscular stabilization in medial knee osteoarthritis. J Biomech 47:360-6, 2014
208. Colle F, Lopomo N, Visani A, et al: Comparison of three formal methods used to estimate the functional axis of rotation: an extensive in-vivo analysis performed on the knee joint. Comput Methods Biomech Biomed Engin 19:484-92, 2016
209. Kim HY, Kim KJ, Yang DS, et al: Screw-home movement of the tibiofemoral joint during normal gait: three-dimensional analysis. Clin Orthop Surg 7:303-9, 2015
210. Moglo KE, Shirazi-Adl A: Cruciate coupling and screw-home mechanism in passive knee joint during extension–flexion. J Biomech 38:1075-83, 2005
211. Buford WL, Jr, Ivey FM, Jr, Nakamura T, et al: Internal/external rotation moment arms of muscles at the knee: moment arms for the normal knee and the ACL-deficient knee. Knee 8:293-303, 2001
212. Mohamed O, Perry J, Hislop H: Relationship between wire EMG activity, muscle length, and torque of the hamstrings. Clin Biomech (Bristol) 17:569-79, 2002
213. Shelburne KB, Pandy MG: A musculoskeletal model of the knee for evaluating ligament forces during isometric contractions. J Biomech 30:163-76, 1997
214. Li L, Landin D, Grodesky J, et al: The function of gastrocnemius as a knee flexor at selected knee and ankle angles. J Electromyogr Kinesiol 12:385-90, 2002
215. Powers CM, Lilley JC, Lee TQ: The effects of axial and multi-plane loading of the extensor mechanism on the patellofemoral joint. Clin Biomech (Bristol) 13:616-624, 1998
216. Lieb FJ, Perry J: Quadriceps function: an anatomical and mechanical study using amputated limbs. J Bone Joint Surg Am 50:1535-48, 1968
217. Hubbard JK, Sampson HW, Elledge JR: Prevalence and morphology of the vastus medialis oblique muscle in human cadavers. Anat Rec 249:135-42, 1997
218. Glenn LL, Samojla BG: A critical reexamination of the morphology, neurovasculature, and fiber architecture of knee extensor muscles in animal models and humans. Biol Res Nurs 4:128-41, 2002
219. Giles LS, Webster KE, McClelland JA, et al: Atrophy of the quadriceps is not isolated to the vastus medialis oblique in individuals with patellofemoral pain. J Orthop Sports Phys Ther 45:613-9, 2015
220. Im HS, Goltzer O, Sheehan FT: The effective quadriceps and patellar tendon moment arms relative to the tibiofemoral finite helical axis. J Biomech 48:3737-42, 2015
221. Kellis E, Baltzopoulos V: In vivo determination of the patella tendon and hamstrings moment arms in adult males using videofluoroscopy during submaximal knee extension and flexion. Clin Biomech (Bristol) 14:118-24, 1999
222. El-Ashker S, Carson BP, Ayala F, et al: Sex-related differences in joint-angle-specific functional hamstring-to-quadriceps strength ratios. Knee Surg Sports Traumatol Arthrosc 25:949-957, 2017
223. Escamilla RF, Fleisig GS, Zheng N, et al: Biomechanics of the knee during closed kinetic chain and open kinetic chain exercises. Med Sci Sports Exerc 30:556-69, 1998

224. Wilk KE, Escamilla RF, Fleisig GS, et al: A comparison of tibiofemoral joint forces and electromyographic activity during open and closed kinetic chain exercises. Am J Sports Med 24:518-27, 1996
225. Stuart MJ, Meglan DA, Lutz GE, et al: Comparison of intersegmental tibiofemoral joint forces and muscle activity during various closed kinetic chain exercises. Am J Sports Med 24:792-9, 1996
226. Heijne A, Fleming BC, Renstrom PA, et al: Strain on the anterior cruciate ligament during closed kinetic chain exercises. Med Sci Sports Exerc 36:935-41, 2004
227. Beynnon BD, Fleming BC: Anterior cruciate ligament strain in-vivo: a review of previous work. J Biomech 31:519-25, 1998
228. Fox AJ, Wanivenhaus F, Rodeo SA: The basic science of the patella: structure, composition, and function. J Knee Surg 25:127-41, 2012
229. Grelsamer RP, Klein JR: The biomechanics of the patellofemoral joint. J Orthop Sports Phys Ther 28:286-98, 1998
230. Komistek RD, Dennis DA, Mabe JA, et al: An in vivo determination of patellofemoral contact positions. Clin Biomech (Bristol) 15:29-36, 2000
231. Kobayashi K, Hosseini A, Sakamoto M, et al: In vivo kinematics of the extensor mechanism of the knee during deep flexion. J Biomech Eng 135:81002, 2013
232. Biyani R, Elias JJ, Saranathan A, et al: Anatomical factors influencing patellar tracking in the unstable patellofemoral joint. Knee Surg Sports Traumatol Arthrosc 22:2334-41, 2014
233. Bull AM, Katchburian MV, Shih YF, et al: Standardisation of the description of patellofemoral motion and comparison between different techniques. Knee Surg Sports Traumatol Arthrosc 10:184-93, 2002
234. Nagamine R, Otani T, White SE, et al: Patellar tracking measurement in the normal knee. J Orthop Res 13:115-22, 1995
235. van Kampen A, Huiskes R: The three-dimensional tracking pattern of the human patella. J Orthop Res 8:372-82, 1990
236. Ahmad CS, McCarthy M, Gomez JA, et al: The moving patellar apprehension test for lateral patellar instability. Am J Sports Med 37:791-6, 2009
237. Powers CM, Ward SR, Fredericson M, et al: Patellofemoral kinematics during weight-bearing and non-weight-bearing knee extension in persons with lateral subluxation of the patella: a preliminary study. J Orthop Sports Phys Ther 33:677-85, 2003
238. Lin F, Makhsous M, Chang AH, et al: In vivo and noninvasive six degrees of freedom patellar tracking during voluntary knee movement. Clin Biomech (Bristol) 18:401-9, 2003
239. Mizuno Y, Kumagai M, Mattessich SM, et al: Q-angle influences tibiofemoral and patellofemoral kinematics. J Orthop Res 19:834-40, 2001
240. Moro-oka T, Matsuda S, Miura H, et al: Patellar tracking and patellofemoral geometry in deep knee flexion. Clin Orthop Relat Res:161-8, 2002
241. Hefzy MS, Jackson WT, Saddemi SR, et al: Effects of tibial rotations on patellar tracking and patellofemoral contact areas. J Biomed Eng 14:329-43, 1992
242. Heino Brechter J, Powers CM: Patellofemoral stress during walking in persons with and without patellofemoral pain. Med Sci Sports Exerc 34:1582-93, 2002
243. Powers CM, Ho KY, Chen YJ, et al: Patellofemoral joint stress during weight-bearing and non-weight-bearing quadriceps exercises. J Orthop Sports Phys Ther 44:320-7, 2014
244. Kobayashi T, Papaioannou G, Mirzamohammadi F, et al: Early postnatal ablation of the microRNA-processing enzyme, Drosha, causes chondrocyte death and impairs the structural integrity of the articular cartilage. Osteoarthritis Cartilage 23:1214-20, 2015
245. Kernozek TW, Vannatta CN, van den Bogert AJ: Comparison of two methods of determining patellofemoral joint stress during dynamic activities. Gait Posture 42:218-22, 2015
246. Singerman R, Davy DT, Goldberg VM: Effects of patella alta and patella infera on patellofemoral contact forces. J Biomech 27:1059-65, 1994
247. Willy RW, Hoglund LT, Barton CJ, et al: Patellofemoral pain. J Orthop Sports Phys Ther 49:CPG1-95, 2019
248. Fitzgerald GK: Open versus closed kinetic chain exercise: issues in rehabilitation after anterior cruciate ligament reconstructive surgery. Phys Ther 77:1747-54, 1997
249. Mikkelsen C, Werner S, Eriksson E: Closed kinetic chain alone compared to combined open and closed kinetic chain exercises for quadriceps strengthening after anterior cruciate ligament reconstruction with respect to return to sports: a prospective matched follow-up study. Knee Surg Sports Traumatol Arthrosc 8:337-42, 2000
250. Snyder-Mackler L, Delitto A, Bailey SL, et al: Strength of the quadriceps femoris muscle and functional recovery after reconstruction of the anterior cruciate ligament: a prospective, randomized clinical trial of electrical stimulation. J Bone Joint Surg Am 77:1166-73, 1995
251. Barton CJ, Lack S, Hemmings S, et al: The "Best Practice Guide to Conservative Management of Patellofemoral Pain": incorporating level 1 evidence with expert clinical reasoning. Br J Sports Med 49:923-34, 2015
252. Crossley KM, Bennell KL, Cowan SM, et al: Analysis of outcome measures for persons with patellofemoral pain: which are reliable and valid? Arch Phys Med Rehabil 85:815-22, 2004
253. Bollier M, Fulkerson JP: The role of trochlear dysplasia in patellofemoral instability. J Am Acad Orthop Surg 19:8-16, 2011
254. Qiu L, Li J, Sheng B, et al: Patellar shape is associated with femoral trochlear morphology in individuals with mature skeletal development. BMC Musculoskelet Disord 23:56, 2022
255. Lewallen LW, McIntosh AL, Dahm DL: Predictors of recurrent instability after acute patellofemoral dislocation in pediatric and adolescent patients. Am J Sports Med 41:575-81, 2013
256. Smith TO, Bowyer D, Dixon J, et al: Can vastus medialis oblique be preferentially activated? A systematic review of electromyographic studies. Physiother Theory Pract 25:69-98, 2009
257. Livingston LA, Mandigo JL: Bilateral within-subject Q angle asymmetry in young adult females and males. Biomed Sci Instrum 33:112-7, 1997
258. Horton MG, Hall TL: Quadriceps femoris muscle angle: normal values and relationships with gender and selected skeletal measures. Phys Ther 69:897-901, 1989
259. Herrington L, Nester C: Q-angle undervalued? The relationship between Q-angle and medio-lateral position of the patella. Clin Biomech (Bristol) 19:1070-3, 2004
260. Galloway RT, Xu Y, Hewett TE, et al: Age-dependent patellofemoral pain: hip and knee risk landing profiles in prepubescent and postpubescent female athletes. Am J Sports Med 46:2761-71, 2018
261. Powers CM: The influence of altered lower-extremity kinematics on patellofemoral joint dysfunction: a theoretical perspective. J Orthop Sports Phys Ther 33:639-46, 2003
262. Dye SF, Vaupel GL, Dye CC: Conscious neurosensory mapping of the internal structures of the human knee without intraarticular anesthesia. Am J Sports Med 26:773-7, 1998

CHAPTER 12

The Ankle and Foot Complex

RobRoy L. Martin PT, PhD, CSCS |
Lindsay A. Carroll PT, DPT, PhD, OCS

CHAPTER OUTLINE

INTRODUCTION 400
DEFINITIONS OF MOTION 400
JOINT STRUCTURE 401
- **The Ankle Joint** 401
  - Proximal Articular Surfaces 401
  - Proximal Tibiofibular Joint 402
  - Distal Tibiofibular Joint 402
  - Distal Articular Surface 403
  - Capsule and Ligaments 403
- **The Subtalar Joint** 405
  - Ligaments 405
- **Transverse Tarsal Joint** 406
  - Talonavicular Joint 406
  - Calcaneocuboid Joint 407
- **Tarsometatarsal Joints** 408
- **Metatarsophalangeal Joints** 408
- **Interphalangeal Joints** 409

JOINT FUNCTION 409
- **The Ankle Joint** 409
  - Talocrural Axis 409
- **The Subtalar Joint** 412
  - The Subtalar Axis 412
  - Non–Weight-Bearing Subtalar Joint Motion 412
  - Weight-Bearing Subtalar Joint Motion 414
  - Range of Subtalar Motion and Subtalar Neutral 417
- **Transverse Tarsal Joint** 418
  - Transverse Tarsal Joint Axes 418
  - Weight-Bearing Rearfoot Pronation and Transverse Tarsal Joint Motion 421
  - Weight-Bearing Rearfoot Supination and Transverse Tarsal Joint Motion 421
- **Tarsometatarsal Joints** 423
  - Tarsometatarsal Axes 423
  - Supination Twist 423
  - Pronation Twist 424
- **Metatarsophalangeal Joints** 424
  - Metatarsophalangeal Extension and the Metatarsal Break 424
  - Metatarsophalangeal Flexion, Abduction, and Adduction 425

PLANTAR ARCHES 427
- **Structure of the Arches** 427
- **Function of the Arches** 428
  - Plantar Aponeurosis 428
  - Weight Distribution 430
- **Muscular Contribution to the Arches** 430

MUSCLES OF THE ANKLE AND FOOT 430
- **Extrinsic Musculature** 431
  - Posterior Compartment Muscles 431
  - Lateral Compartment Muscles 432
  - Anterior Compartment Muscles 432
- **Intrinsic Musculature** 433

LIFE SPAN AND CLINICAL CONSIDERATIONS 433
- **Foot and Ankle Problems Revisited** 434

SUMMARY 435
STUDY QUESTIONS 436
REFERENCES 436

ANATOMY OVERVIEW

MUSCLE ACTIONS OF THE ANKLE AND FOOT			
TABLE KEY: Primary muscle Secondary muscles			
Sagittal		**Dorsiflexion**	**Plantarflexion**
	Talocrural joint	Tibialis anterior Extensor digitorum longus Extensor hallucis longus Fibularis tertius	Gastrocnemius Soleus Plantaris Tibialis posterior Flexor hallucis longus Flexor digitorum longus Fibularis longus Fibularis brevis
		Flexion	**Extension**
	Metatarsophalangeal (MTP) joint	Lumbricals Flexor hallucis brevis Interossei Flexor digiti minimi brevis Flexor digitorum longus (digits 2–5) Flexor digitorum brevis (digits 2–5) Flexor hallucis longus (digit 1)	Extensor digitorum longus (digits 2–5) Extensor digitorum brevis Extensor hallucis longus (digit 1)
	Proximal interphalangeal (PIP) joint	Flexor digitorum longus (digits 2–5) Flexor digitorum brevis (digits 2–5) Flexor hallucis longus (digit 1)	Extensor digitorum longus (digits 2–5) Extensor digitorum brevis Extensor hallucis longus (digit 1)
	Distal interphalangeal (DIP) joint	Flexor digitorum longus (digits 2–5)	Extensor digitorum longus (digits 2–5) Extensor digitorum brevis
Frontal		**Inversion**	**Eversion**
		Tibialis anterior Tibialis posterior Flexor digitorum longus Flexor hallucis longus	Fibularis longus Fibularis brevis Fibularis tertius Extensor digitorum longus

ANATOMY OVERVIEW

FOOT AND ANKLE MUSCLE ATTACHMENTS		
Muscles	**Proximal Attachment**	**Distal Attachment**
Tibialis anterior	Lateral condyle and superior 2/3 of anterolateral surface of tibia and interosseous membrane	Medial and inferior surfaces of medial cuneiform and base of 1st metatarsal
Extensor digitorum longus	Lateral condyle of tibia and superior 3/4 of medial surface of fibula and interosseous membrane	Middle and distal phalanges of digits 2–5
Extensor hallucis longus	Middle part of anterior surface of fibula and interosseous membrane	Dorsal aspect of base of distal phalanx of digit 1 (hallux)
Fibularis longus	Head and superior 2/3 of lateral surface of tibia	Base of 1st metatarsal and medial cuneiform
Fibularis brevis	Inferior 2/3 of lateral surface of fibula	Dorsal surface of tuberosity on lateral side of base of 5th metatarsal
Fibularis tertius	Inferior 1/3 of anterior surface of fibula and interosseous membrane	Dorsum of base of 5th metatarsal

FOOT AND ANKLE MUSCLE ATTACHMENTS		
Muscles	**Proximal Attachment**	**Distal Attachment**
Gastrocnemius	Lateral head: Lateral aspect of lateral condyle of femur Medial head: Popliteal surface of femur; superior to medial femoral condyle	Posterior surface of calcaneus via calcaneal tendon
Soleus	Posterior aspect of head and superior 1/4 of posterior surface of fibula; middle third of medial border of tibia	Posterior surface of calcaneus via calcaneal tendon
Plantaris	Inferior end of lateral supracondylar line of femur; oblique popliteal ligament	Posterior surface of calcaneus via calcaneal tendon
Flexor hallucis longus	Inferior 2/3 of posterior surface of fibula and interosseous membrane	Base of distal phalanx of digit 1 (hallux)
Flexor digitorum longus	Medial part of posterior surface of tibia inferior to soleal line	Base of distal phalanges of digits 2–5
Tibialis posterior	Interosseous membrane; posterior surface of tibia inferior to soleal line; posterior surface of fibula	Tuberosity of navicular, cuneiform, cuboid, and sustentaculum tail of calcaneus; bases of 2nd, 3rd, and 4th metatarsals
Lumbricals	Tendons of flexor digitorum longus	Medial aspect of expansion (digits 2–5)
Flexor hallucis brevis	Plantar component of cuboid and lateral cuneiforms	Both sides of base of proximal phalanx (digit 1)
Plantar interossei	Plantar aspect of medial sides of shafts of metatarsals 3–5	Medial sides of bases of phalanges of digits 3–5
Dorsal interossei	Adjacent sides of shafts of metatarsals 1–5	Medial side of proximal phalanx of digit 2 Lateral sides of proximal phalanx of digits 2–4
Flexor digiti minimi brevis	Base of 5th metatarsal	Base of proximal phalanx of digit 5
Flexor digitorum brevis	Medial tubercle of tuberosity of calcaneus; plantar aponeurosis	Both sides of middle phalanges (digits 2–5)
Extensor digitorum brevis	Distal and lateral surface of calcaneus in front of groove for fibularis brevis	Long extensor tendons of digits 2–4

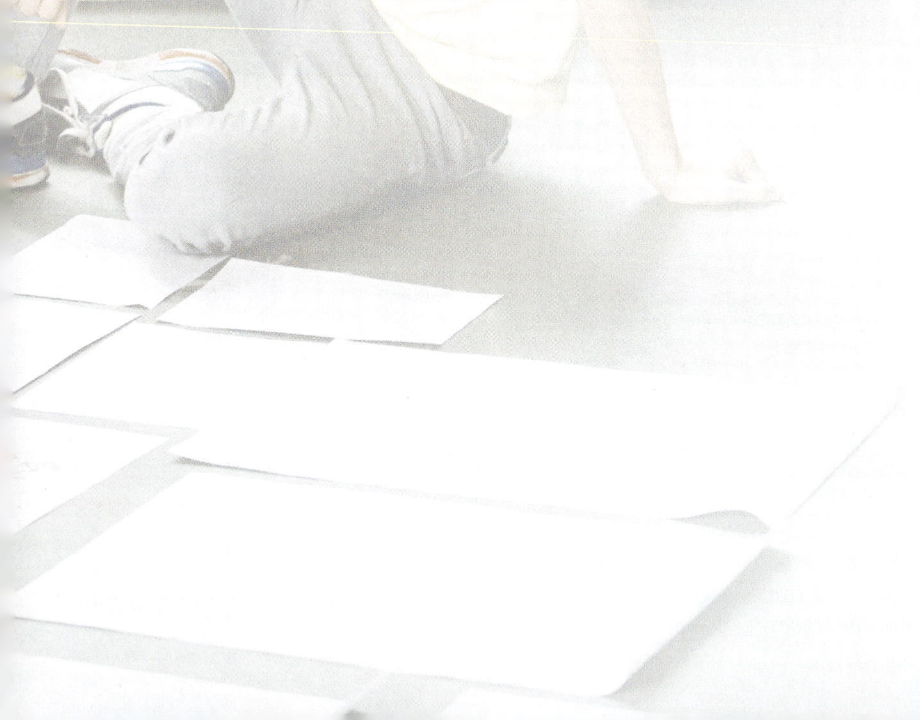

Introduction

The ankle/foot complex is structurally analogous to the wrist/hand complex of the upper extremity, with adaptations that optimize its primary role to bear weight. The ankle/foot complex permits both stability and mobility, depending on current needs. The foot is able to sustain large weight-bearing stresses while accommodating a variety of surfaces and activities. The foot must be stable to provide an adequate base of support and to function as a rigid lever for pushing off when walking, running, or jumping. In contrast, the foot must also be mobile to adapt to uneven terrain, absorb shock as the foot hits the ground, and control forces imposed by the more proximal joints of the lower extremity. The ankle/foot complex meets these diverse requirements through the integrated movements of its 28 bones that form 25 component joints. These joints include the **proximal and distal tibiofibular joints, talocrural (ankle) joint, talocalcaneal (subtalar) joint, talonavicular and calcaneocuboid joints (transverse tarsal joints)**, five **tarsometatarsal** and **metatarsophalangeal joints**, and nine **interphalangeal joints**.

To facilitate description and understanding of the ankle/foot complex, the bones of the foot are traditionally divided into three functional segments. These are the **rearfoot** (posterior segment), composed of the talus and calcaneus; the **midfoot** (middle segment), composed of the navicular, cuboid, and three cuneiform bones; and the **forefoot** (anterior segment), composed of the metatarsals and the phalanges **(Fig. 12–1)**. These terms are commonly used in descriptions of ankle/foot dysfunction or deformity and are similarly useful in understanding typical ankle and foot function.

Ankle or foot pathology can be related to the integrated multifunctional structures of the ankle/foot complex combined with the demands of stability and mobility placed upon these structures. Additionally, the ankle and foot complex respond to forces from the ground as well as from superimposed forces of the spine, pelvis, hip, and knee. Structural abnormalities can lead to altered movements between joints and contribute to excessive stresses that result in injury to the ankle/foot complex.[1]

Definitions of Motion

A unique set of terms is used to describe the motion of the foot and ankle. The same terms are used at most of the joints of the ankle and foot, and, consequently, it is useful to describe them at the outset. As we have seen at other joint complexes, few, if any, of the joint axes lie in the cardinal planes; more commonly, the joint axes are oblique and cut across all multiple planes of motion. The obliquity of the axes and implications for motion and function will be described in detail as we present individual joints.

The three motions of the ankle/foot complex that *approximate* cardinal planes and axes are dorsiflexion/plantarflexion, inversion/eversion, and abduction/adduction **(Fig. 12–2)**.

Dorsiflexion and plantarflexion are motions that occur approximately in the sagittal plane around a coronal axis. **Dorsiflexion** decreases the angle between the leg and the dorsum (top) of the foot, whereas **plantarflexion** increases

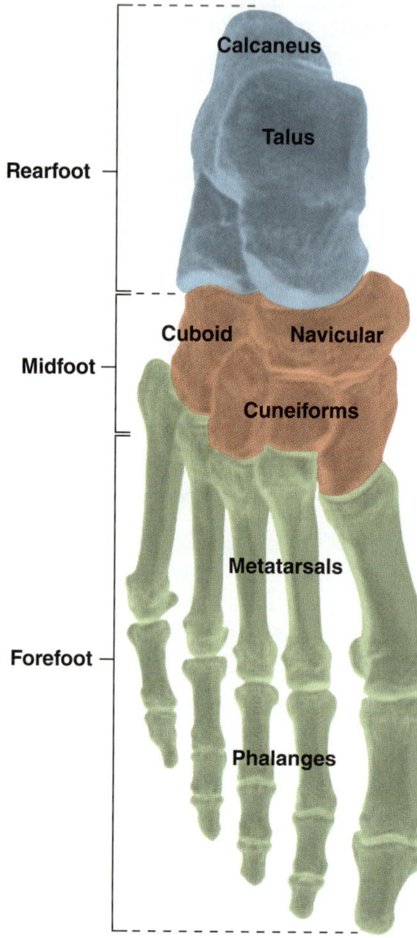

Figure 12–1 Bones of the foot divided into the functional segments of the foot.

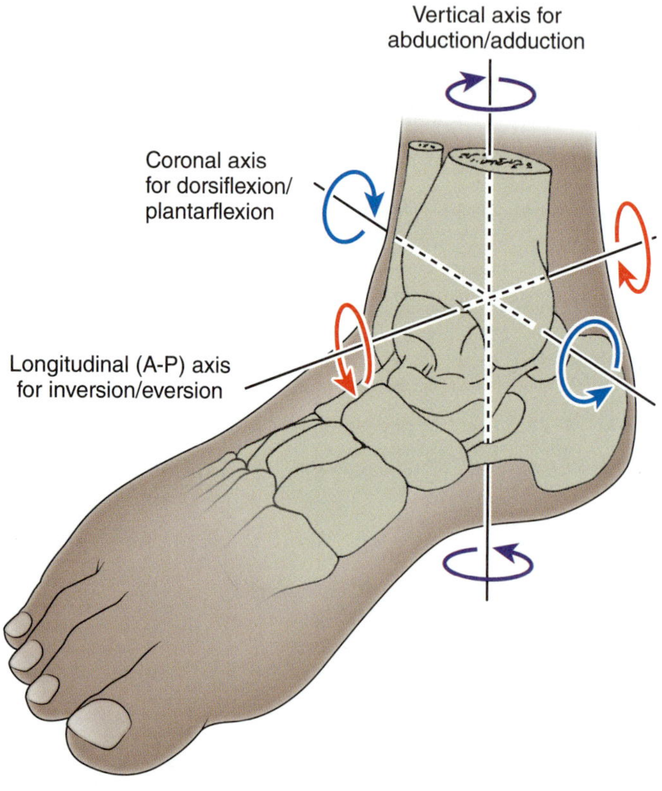

Figure 12–2 "Cardinal" axes for the motions of the ankle/foot complex.

this angle. At the toes, motion around a similar axis is termed **extension** (bringing the toes up in approximation of dorsal surfaces), whereas the opposite motion is **flexion** (bringing the toes down or curling them down). Inversion and eversion occur approximately in the frontal plane around a longitudinal (anteroposterior [A-P]) axis that runs through the length of the foot. **Inversion** occurs when the plantar surface of the segment is brought toward the midline; **eversion** is the opposite. Abduction and adduction occur approximately in the transverse plane around a vertical axis. **Abduction** is when the anterior aspect of a segment moves away from the midline of the body (or away from the midline of the foot in the case of the toes); **adduction** is the opposite.

Pronation/supination in the foot are motions that occur around an axis that lies at an angle to each of the axes for "cardinal" motions of dorsiflexion/plantarflexion, inversion/eversion, and abduction/adduction. Consequently, *pronation* and *supination* are terms used to describe "composite" motions that have components of each of the cardinal motions. In non–weight-bearing, **pronation** is motion about an axis that results in coupled motions of dorsiflexion, eversion, and abduction. Likewise, **supination** is a motion about an axis that results in coupled motions of plantarflexion, inversion, and adduction. The proportional contribution that each of the coupled motions makes to pronation/supination is dependent on and varies with the angle of the pronation/supination joint axis. This concept will be expanded on as we delve into the relevant joints.

Valgus and **varus** are terms that may be used for the ankle/foot complex in several ways, depending on the context. The definitions that we used throughout discussion of other joints in other chapters will not change. That is, valgus refers to an increase in the *medial angle* between two bones (or movement of the distal segment away from the midline); varus refers to the opposite. However, valgus and varus are sometimes used to refer to *fixed deformities* in the ankle/foot complex, whereas at other times the terms are used to describe or as synonyms for typical motions. An example of common usage is to describe the fixed or weight-bearing position of the posterior calcaneus in relation to the posterior midline of the leg, with an increase in the medial angle between these segments referred to as *valgus of the calcaneus* (or **calcaneovalgus**) and a decrease in medial angle being *varus of the calcaneus* (or **calcaneovarus**) **(Fig. 12-3)**. We will define the

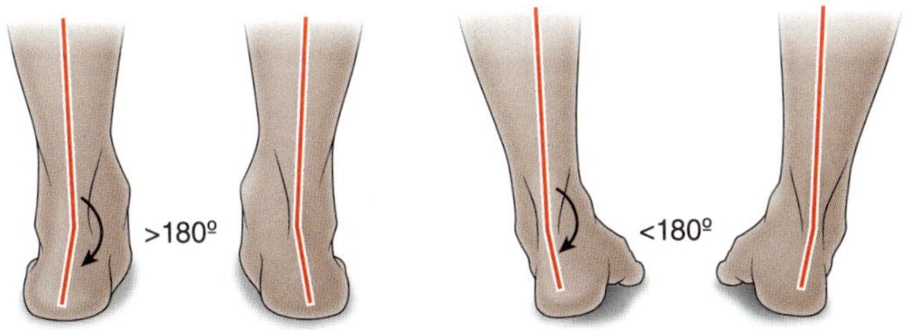

Figure 12–3 The term *valgus* (or calcaneovalgus) refers to an increase in the *medial angle* between the calcaneus and posterior leg. The term *varus* (or calcaneovarus) refers to a decrease in the *medial angle* between the calcaneus and posterior leg.

use and context as we encounter these terms in descriptions of ankle/foot structure and function.

Foundational Concepts 12–1
Ankle/Foot Terminology

As we have seen at other joints, terminology used to describe motions around a joint or of a segment is often not consistent among investigators. This is very much the case for the ankle/foot complex. Because the anterior surface of the leg and the top of the foot are embryologically dorsal surfaces, dorsiflexion may also be referred to as extension, and plantarflexion may be referred to as flexion.[2] Although the flexion/extension terminology is commonly used for the toes, it is occasionally applied to the ankle. Some sources use the term *inversion/eversion* to refer to the composite motion of *supination/pronation.* As we proceed to describe the joints and their motions, we will see that some of these terminology differences are not really as problematic as they might initially seem.

It may enhance your understanding of ankle/foot terminology if you consider the ankle and foot to be analogous to the wrist and hand. Put your hand—palm down—and forearm on a surface. Extension of the wrist or fingers is similar to dorsiflexion (extension) of the ankle and extension of the toes; abduction/adduction of the wrist is similar to abduction/adduction of the foot (vertical axis through the tibia); supination/pronation of the forearm (and hand) are similar to supination/pronation of the foot (A-P axis through the foot). This analogy helps with terminology; however, there are structural differences in the ankle/foot that, as already noted, meet the demands of its weight-bearing functions while maintaining mobility.

Joint Structure

The Ankle Joint

The term **ankle** refers specifically to the talocrural joint, defined as the articulation between the distal tibia and fibula proximally and the body of the talus distally **(Fig. 12–4A)**. The ankle is a synovial hinge joint with a joint capsule and associated ligaments.

Proximal Articular Surfaces

The proximal segment of the ankle is composed of the concave surface of the distal tibia (known as the *tibial plafond*) and of the tibial and fibular malleoli. These three facets form an almost continuous concave joint surface that extends more distally on the fibular (lateral) side than on the tibial (medial) side (see Fig. 12–4A), and more distally on the posterior margin of the tibia than on the anterior margin. The structure of the distal tibia and two malleoli resembles, and is referred to as, a *mortise*. A common example of a mortise is the gripping part of a wrench (see **Fig. 12-4B**). Either the wrench can be fixed (fitting a bolt of only one size) or it can be adjustable (permitting use of the wrench on a variety of bolt sizes). The adjustable mortise is more complex than a fixed mortise because it combines mobility and stability functions. The mortise of the ankle is adjustable, relying on the proximal and distal tibiofibular joints to both permit and control any changes in the mortise width.

The proximal and distal tibiofibular joints **(Fig. 12–5)** are anatomically distinct but functionally linked to the ankle. Unlike their upper extremity counterparts (i.e., the proximal

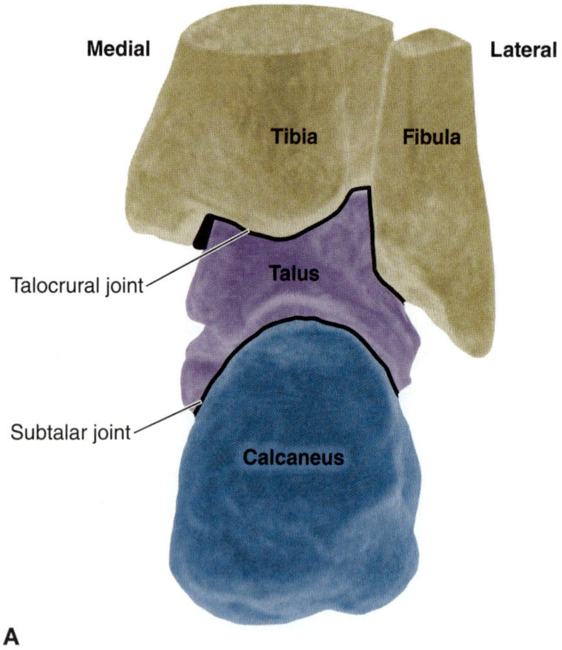

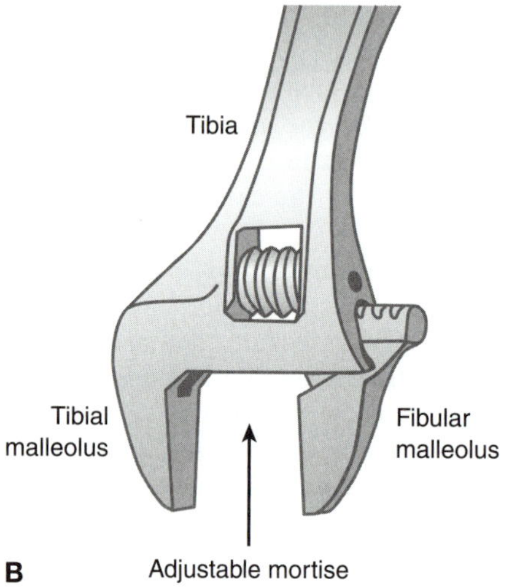

Figure 12–4 The ankle joint is formed by the tibia and fibula (mortise) proximally and by the talus distally. **A.** This posterior view shows the talocrural joint proximal to (above) the talus and the subtalar joint distal to (below) the talus. **B.** An adjustable wrench can be analogized to the tibiofibular mortise of the ankle joint.

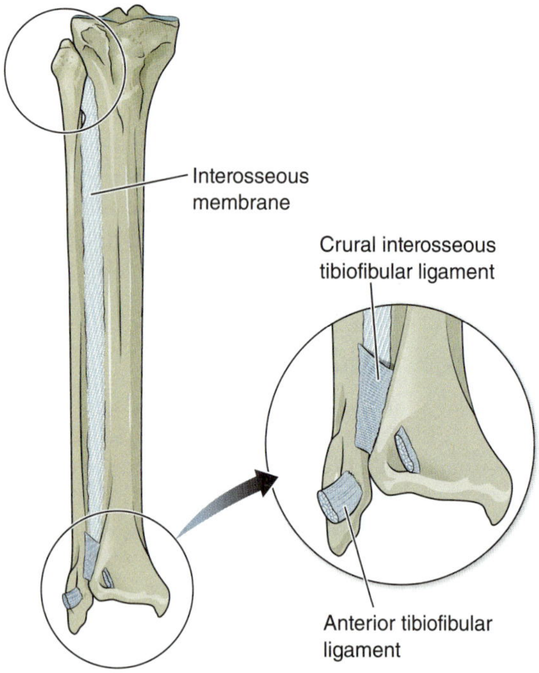

Figure 12–5 Proximal and distal tibiofibular joints.

and distal radioulnar joints), the tibiofibular joints do not add any degrees of freedom to the more distal ankle and foot. However, the tibiofibular joints do contribute to total ankle motion. Fusion of the radioulnar joints would have little effect on wrist range of motion (ROM), whereas fusion of the tibiofibular joints may impair typical ankle function.

Proximal Tibiofibular Joint

The proximal tibiofibular joint is a plane synovial joint formed by the articulation of the head of the fibula with the posterolateral aspect of the tibia. The facets of the proximal tibiofibular joint are fairly flat, but can generally be considered to have a convex tibial facet and concave fibular facet.[3] The proximal tibiofibular joint is surrounded by a joint capsule that is reinforced by anterior and posterior tibiofibular ligaments. Although the proximal tibiofibular joint is generally thought to be anatomically separate from the knee joint, communication between these joints can occur.[4] Proximal tibiofibular joint movement has shown variations with respect to fibular translation and rotation that occur with ankle motion.[5,6] However, when this joint is unstable, symptoms of pain, snapping, and/or catching can occur.[7] The relevance of motion at the proximal and distal tibiofibular joints will be seen when ankle joint motion is discussed.

Distal Tibiofibular Joint

The distal tibiofibular joint is a syndesmosis, or fibrous union, between the concave facet of the tibia and the convex facet of the fibula. The distal tibia and fibula do not actually come into contact with each other but are separated by fibroadipose tissue. Although there is no joint capsule, there are several associated ligaments. Because the proximal and distal joints are linked (the tibia, fibula, and tibiofibular joints are part of a closed chain), all the ligaments that lie between the tibia and fibula contribute to stability at both joints.

The ligaments of the distal tibiofibular joint are primarily responsible for maintaining a stable mortise. The **anterior** and **posterior tibiofibular ligaments** and **interosseous**

membrane provide support to the distal tibiofibular joint.[8] The interosseous membrane directly supports both proximal and distal tibiofibular articulations. Although the distal tibiofibular joint is an extremely strong articulation, injuries can occur when the talus is forcibly dorsiflexed and abducted within the ankle mortise.[9] These injuries can compromise the integrity of the joint, causing the fibula and tibia to separate and are diagnosed as a high or syndesmotic ankle sprain. If the force were to continue, fracture of the fibula proximal to the distal tibiofibular ligaments could result.[10]

The function of the ankle (talocrural) joint depends on adequate stability of the tibiofibular mortise. The ankle mortise would be unable to grasp and hold on to the talus if the tibia and fibula were permitted to separate or if one side of the mortise were missing. This would be similar to a wrench that could not perform its function of grasping a bolt if the two pincer segments moved apart every time a force was applied to the wrench (see Fig. 12-4B). Conversely, the ankle mortise must have some mobility for typical function. The mobility role of the mortise belongs primarily to the fibula. The fibula is generally thought to have little weight-bearing function, with one study suggesting the fibula transmits no more than 10% of weight-bearing forces.[11] However, the amount of axial load through the fibula may be related to positioning, because greater weight-bearing forces are transmitted through the fibula when the ankle is in a position of eversion.[12]

Distal Articular Surface

The body of the talus **(Fig. 12–6)** forms the distal articulation of the ankle joint. The body of the talus has three articular surfaces: a large lateral (fibular) facet, a smaller medial (tibial) facet, and a trochlear (superior) facet. The large, convex trochlear surface has a central groove that runs at a slight angle to the head and neck of the talus. The body of the talus also appears wider anteriorly than posteriorly, which gives it a wedge shape. The articular cartilage covering the trochlea is continuous with the cartilage covering the more extensive lateral facet and the smaller medial facet. In addition to the bony articulations, the structural integrity of the ankle joint is maintained throughout the ROM of the joint by a number of supportive soft tissue structures.

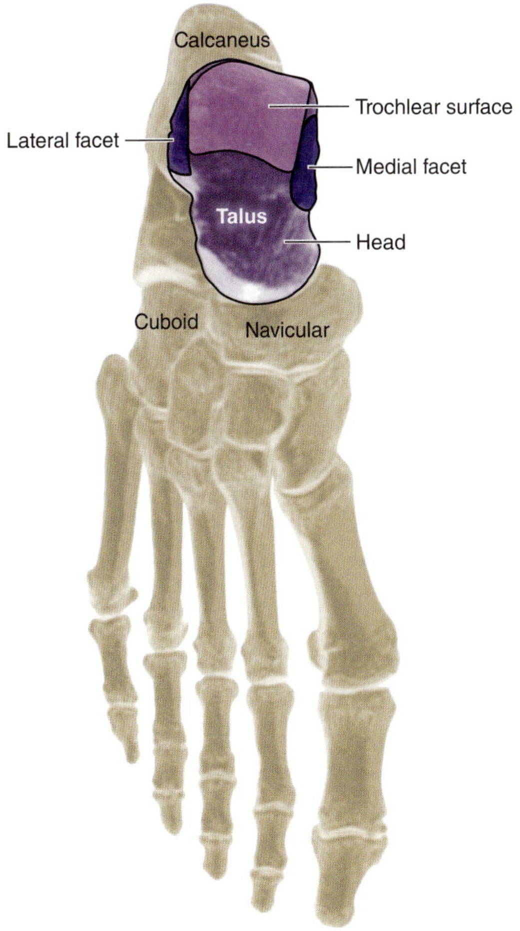

Figure 12–6 The wedge-shaped body of the talus with its trochlear (superior) surface, medial (tibial) facet, and lateral (fibular) facet form the distal segment of the ankle joint.

Capsule and Ligaments

The capsule of the ankle joint is fairly thin and especially weak anteriorly and posteriorly. Therefore, the stability of the ankle depends on an intact ligamentous structure. The ligaments that support the proximal and distal tibiofibular joints are important for stability of the mortise and, therefore, for stability of the ankle. The proximal and distal joints both have **anterior and posterior tibiofibular ligaments**; both joints are stabilized by the **tibiofibular interosseous membrane** (see Fig. 12-5) and by the **crural tibiofibular interosseous ligament** (Fig. 12-5 inset). Two other major ligament complexes maintain contact and congruence of the mortise and talus and control medial-lateral ankle joint stability. These capsular ligaments are the **medial collateral ligament** (MCL) and the **lateral collateral ligament** (LCL). Portions of these ligaments also provide support for the subtalar (or talocalcaneal) joint that they also cross.[13] Therefore, function of the collateral ligaments at the ankle joint can be difficult to separate from their function at the subtalar joint.

The MCL is commonly called the **deltoid ligament.** As its name implies, the deltoid ligament is fan shaped. It has superficial and deep fibers that arise from the borders of the medial malleolus (the base of the fan) and insert (fan out into) in a continuous line anterior to posterior on the navicular, talus, and calcaneus **(Fig. 12–7)**.[14,15] The deltoid ligament as a whole is extremely strong, which partially accounts for the relatively low prevalence of injury to these ligaments. Forceful eversion or pronation of the ankle and talus (i.e., outward rotation of the foot combined with inward rotation of the tibia) can injure the deltoid ligament.[15] However, these forces may actually fracture and displace (avulse) the medial malleolus before the deltoid ligament tears.

The LCL is composed of three distinct bands that are commonly referred to as separate ligaments. These are the **anterior** and **posterior talofibular** ligaments and the **calcaneofibular** ligament, all three of which attach proximally to the fibular malleolus **(Fig. 12–8)**. The anterior and posterior ligaments run in a fairly horizontal position, whereas the longer calcaneofibular ligament is nearly vertical.[16] Just the opposite of the MCL, the LCL helps limit excessive inversion or supination of the ankle and talus (i.e., inward rotation of

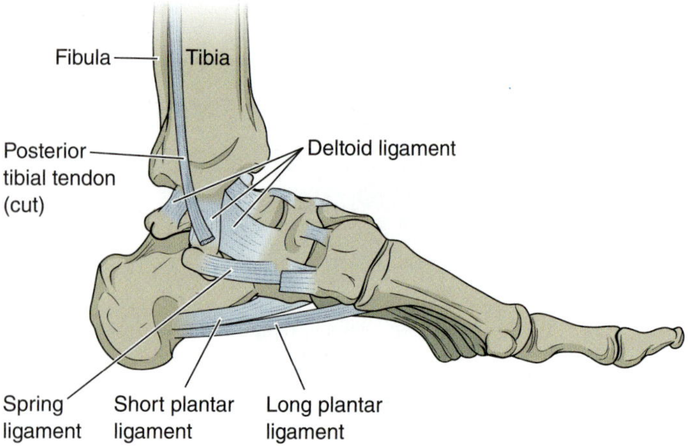

Figure 12–7 Medial ligaments of the posterior ankle/foot complex.

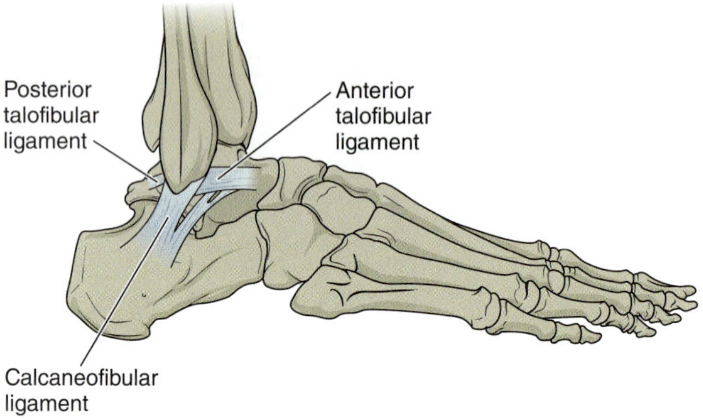

Figure 12–8 Lateral ligaments of the posterior ankle/foot complex.

the foot combined with outward rotation of the tibia).[17] The components of the LCL are weaker and more susceptible to injury than the MCL.

Clinical Application 12–1
Assessing Injury to the Ligaments of the Ankle Complex

Clinicians assess the integrity and function of a ligament by placing the ligament in a position in which it is taut and then applying stress. Findings such as excess motion, a soft "end feel," and/or symptom provocation typically suggest that the ligament has been injured. Understanding the function of each ligament allows clinicians to selectively assess each ligament for injury. Selected clinical tests for ligamentous integrity are described here as they relate to their biomechanical foundations.[18]

Testing of the Lateral Ligament Complex

The anterior talofibular ligament (*ATFL*) and calcaneofibular ligament (*CFL*) are the most commonly injured ligaments of the ankle's lateral collateral ligaments. Because these ligaments are similar in their function and location, the special tests used to assess these ligaments are similar.

Testing the ATFL

The ATFL is oriented horizontally and functions to restrain anterior translation of the talus on the mortise and to limit an inversion motion. To assess the integrity of the ATFL, the examiner must place the ankle in a position in which the ligament is taut and then apply stresses that check the ligament's ability to resist inversion or anterior translation of the talus.

The **anterior drawer test** is used to assess the ability of the ATFL to resist anterior translation of the talus. To perform this test, the patient is positioned in short sitting at the edge of a plinth with their knees flexed to about 90°. The examiner places the talocrural joint in a position of 10° to 20° of plantarflexion to put the ligament under tension, and then gently slides the talus anteriorly. If the examiner identifies increased movement of the talus (3 mm or more when compared to the uninvolved ankle), the test is positive and suggests that the ATFL has been injured.

The **inversion stress test,** also known as the **lateral talar tilt test,** can also be used to assess the ATFL. To perform this test, the ankle is placed in plantarflexion to put the ligament under tension. Then, the ligament's ability to limit inversion is assessed as the examiner inverts the talus and the calcaneus. Excess motion compared to the other ankle or symptom provocation suggest injury to the ligament.

Testing the CFL

The CFL is oriented more vertically than the ATFL and is thus maximally stressed when the foot-ankle complex is placed in slight dorsiflexion, rather than plantarflexion. The CFL can be assessed by using modified versions of the anterior drawer test and the inversion stress test/lateral talar tilt test.

To use the **anterior drawer test** to assess the CFL, the examiner first places the ankle in about 10° dorsiflexion. This places tension on the CFL and allows the examiner to focus the forces of their anterior talar slide on the CFL. Similar to the use of this test for the ATFL, the examiner then applies an anteriorly directed force on the talus/calcaneus. Excess motion or pain suggests an injury to the CFL.

The **inversion stress test/lateral talar tilt test** can also be used to assess the CFL's integrity. To apply this test to the CFL, the examiner positions the ankle in about 10° of dorsiflexion to place the ligament under tension. Then, the examiner applies an inversion stress to the joint. The presence of excess motion or pain suggests that the CFL is injured.

Testing the Medial Ligament Complex

The medial ankle ligaments function to limit eversion and are acutely injured less frequently than the lateral ligaments. The **eversion stress test** can be used to test the integrity of the medial ligament complex. To perform this test, the examiner stabilizes the tibia and everts the calcaneus and talus. Similar to the previously described tests, an increase in motion or pain constitutes a positive test and suggests that the MCL is injured.

Testing the Syndesmosis

The anterior and posterior tibiofibular ligaments and the interosseous membrane of the distal tibiofibular joint function to stabilize the proximal aspect of the talocrural joint. Because these soft tissue structures function to limit separation of the tibia and fibula, testing these structures involves attempting to separate the bones. Clinicians often use the **external rotation test,** also known as the **Kleiger test,** for this purpose. To perform this test, clinicians dorsiflex the talocrural joint to force the wider anterior portion of the talus into the mortise. Then, the talus is abducted by laterally (externally) rotating the foot into the mobile fibula. This positioning allows the talus to apply a laterally directed force into the fibula, stressing the soft tissues that hold the fibula and tibia together. Reproduction of pain at the syndesmosis is a positive test and indicates dysfunction of these tissues.

In addition to the MCL and LCL, portions of the extensor and fibular retinaculae of the ankle are also credited with contributing to stability at the ankle joint[19,20] **(Fig. 12–9)**. The inferior band of the **superior fibular retinaculum**, which lies close and parallel to the calcaneofibular ligament, appears to reinforce that ligament.[20] Because the ankle collateral ligaments and retinaculae also contribute to stability of the subtalar joint, they will be discussed again in that context.

The Subtalar Joint

The talocalcaneal, or subtalar, joint is a composite joint formed by three separate articulations between the talus superiorly and the calcaneus inferiorly; these subtalar articulations share the weight-bearing load transmitted primarily through the tibia. The subtalar joint articulating surfaces are highly variable, but the posterior articulation is consistently the largest of the three articulations found between the talus and calcaneus. The posterior articulation is formed by a concave facet on the undersurface of the body of the talus and a convex facet on the body of the calcaneus. The smaller anterior and middle talocalcaneal articulations are formed by two convex facets on the inferior body and neck of the talus and two concave facets on the calcaneus **(Fig. 12–10)**. The anterior and middle articulations, therefore, have an intra-articular configuration that is the reverse of that found at the posterior facet. Between the posterior articulation and the anterior and middle articulations, there is a bony tunnel formed by a **sulcus** (concave groove) in the inferior talus and superior calcaneus. This funnel-shaped tunnel, known as the *tarsal tunnel*, runs obliquely across the foot. Its large end (the **sinus tarsi**) lies just anterior to the lateral malleolus **(Fig. 12–11)**; its small end lies posteriorly below the medial malleolus and above a bony outcropping on the calcaneus called the **sustentaculum tali** (see Fig. 12–10). The tarsal tunnel and its associated ligaments divide the posterior articulation and the anterior and middle articulations into two separate noncommunicating synovial joint cavities. The posterior articulation has its own capsule, whereas the anterior and middle articulations share a capsule with the talonavicular joint.[21]

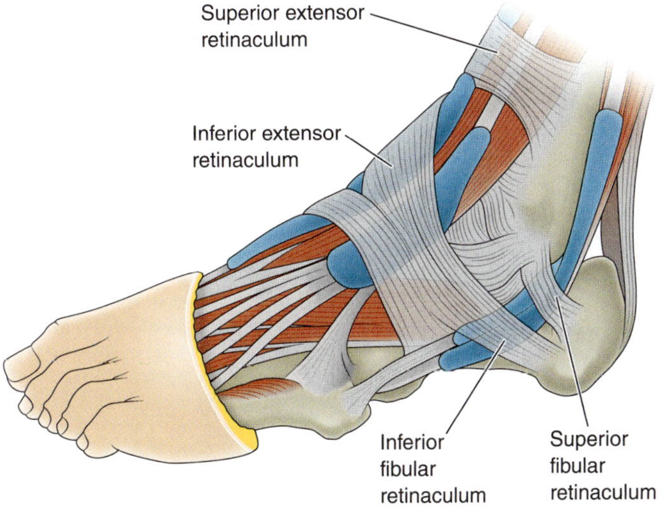

Figure 12–9 The superior and inferior extensor retinacula; the superior and inferior fibular (peroneal) retinacula.

Wang and colleagues found that the subtalar articular surfaces, although smaller than those of the ankle joint surfaces, showed a similar proportion of contact across surfaces under similar conditions.[22] These investigators found that the posterior facet received 75% of the force transmitted through the subtalar joint. Given the larger contact area of the posterior facet, it was determined that the pressure (i.e., force per area) in the posterior facet was similar to that of the middle and anterior facets. Like the ankle joint, the subtalar joint rarely undergoes degenerative change unless damaged by high stresses (e.g., fracture).

Ligaments

The subtalar joint is a stable joint that is rarely dislocated because of congruent osseous anatomy as well as strong ligamentous support. The subtalar joint receives support from the ligamentous structures that support the ankle, as well as from ligamentous structures that only cross the subtalar joint.[23] These ligaments can be divided into extrinsic and intrinsic. Extrinsic ligaments reinforce joint capsules and include the calcaneofibular ligament and **lateral talocalcaneal ligament.** Intrinsic ligaments lie within joint capsules and include the **interosseous talocalcaneal ligament** and **cervical ligament**[24] **(Fig. 12–12)**. The cervical ligament is the strongest of the talocalcaneal structures. It lies in the

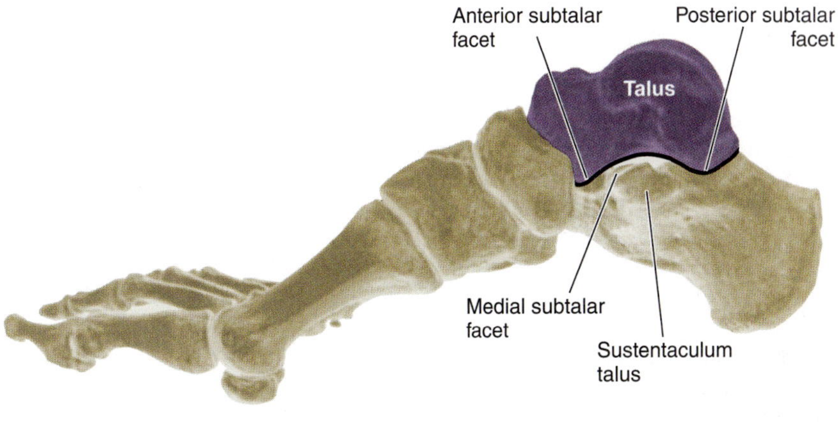

Figure 12–10 Medial view of the foot, showing the talus sitting on the calcaneus (the subtalar joint).

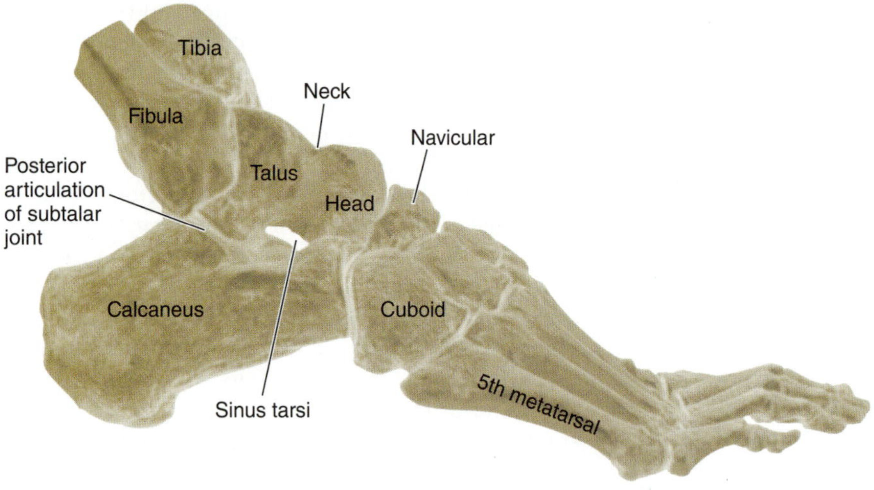

Figure 12–11 Lateral view of the foot, showing the talus sitting on the calcaneus (the subtalar joint). The sinus tarsi is the lateral opening of the tarsal canal.

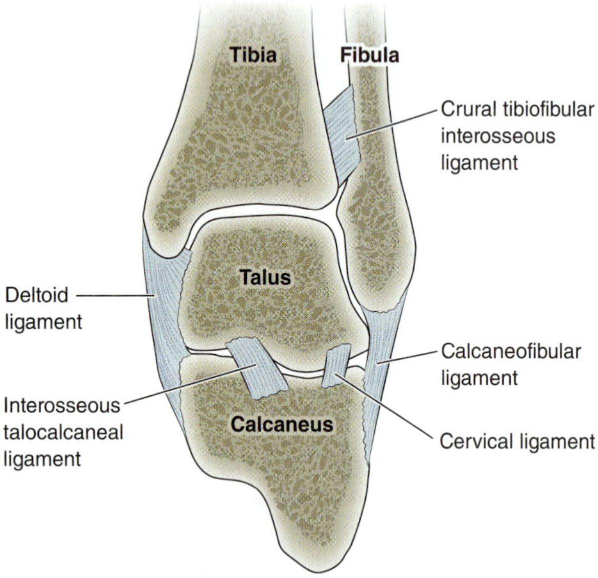

Figure 12–12 The ligaments of the subtalar joint (in a posterior cross-sectional view). The interosseous talocalcaneal ligament and the cervical ligament are intrinsic (intracapsular) while the deltoid and calcaneofibular ligaments are extracapsular.

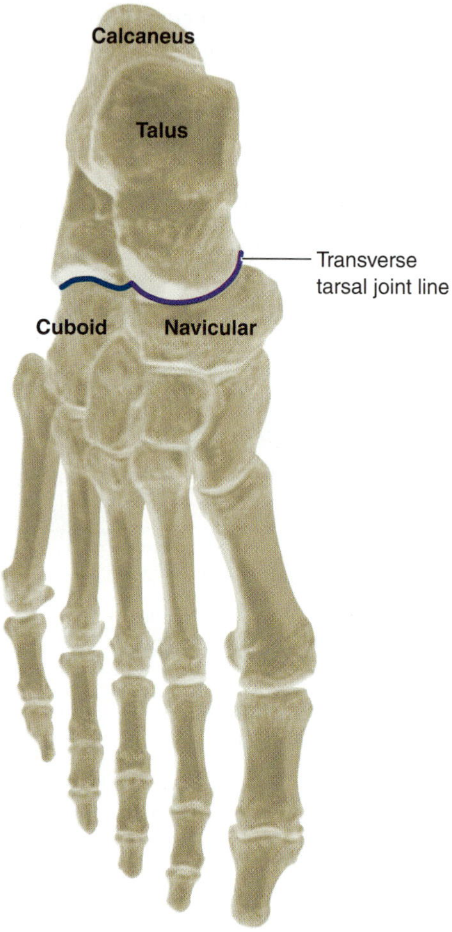

Figure 12–13 The talonavicular joint and calcaneocuboid joint form a compound joint known as the *transverse tarsal joint* line that transects the foot.

anterior sinus tarsi and joins the neck of the talus to the neck of the calcaneus (hence its name).[23] The interosseous talocalcaneal ligament lies more medially within the tarsal canal and follows an oblique path from the talus to the calcaneus (see Fig. 12–12).[25,26] Divisions of the inferior extensor retinaculum (see Fig. 12-9) also provide stability to the subtalar joint superficially as well as through connections within the tarsal canal.[25] Although the subtalar joint is considered to be very stable, instability can occur, particularly with traumatic injuries to calcaneofibular, cervical, and interosseous talocalcaneal ligaments.[24,26]

Transverse Tarsal Joint

The transverse tarsal joint, also called the *midtarsal* or *Chopart joint*, is a compound joint formed by the talonavicular and calcaneocuboid joints **(Fig. 12–13)**.

Talonavicular Joint

The proximal portion of the talonavicular articulation is formed by the anterior portion of the *head* of the talus (see Fig. 12-11), with the distal articulation formed by the concave posterior aspect of the navicular bone. We also noted earlier that the

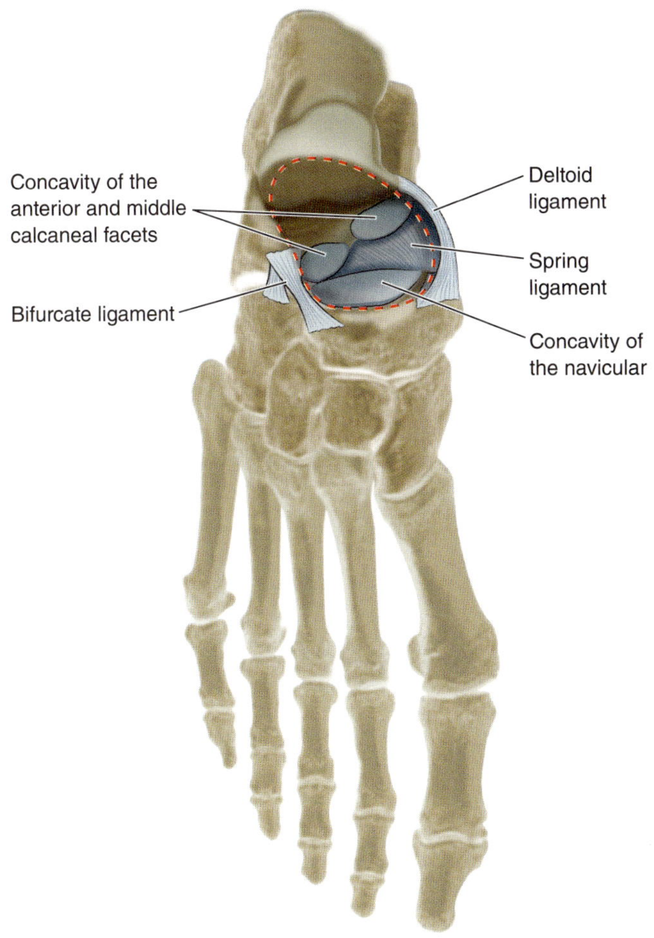

Figure 12–14 With the talus removed, this superior view shows the outlined concavity ("socket") formed by the navicular bone anteriorly, the deltoid ligament medially, the medial band of the bifurcate ligament laterally, and the spring (plantar calcaneonavicular) ligament inferiorly.

talar head articulates inferiorly with the anterior and middle facets of the calcaneus as the anterior part of the subtalar joint. A single synovial joint capsule thus encompasses the talonavicular joint facets as well as the anterior and middle facets of the subtalar joint **(Fig. 12–14)**. The inferior aspect of this joint capsule is formed by the **plantar calcaneonavicular ligament** (**spring ligament**) that spans the gap between the calcaneus and navicular immediately below the talar head. The capsule is reinforced medially by the deltoid and laterally by the **bifurcate ligament**. Given these structural relationships, the large convexity of the head of the talus can be considered the "ball" that is received by a large "socket." This "socket" is formed anteriorly by the concavity of the navicular bone, inferiorly by the concavities of the anterior and middle calcaneal facets and by the plantar calcaneonavicular ligament, medially by the deltoid ligament, and laterally by the bifurcate ligament (see Fig. 12-14).

The spring (plantar calcaneonavicular) ligament (see Figs. 12–7 and 12–14) is a triangular sheet of ligamentous connective tissue arising from the sustentaculum tali of the calcaneus and inserting on the inferior navicular bone. It combines with a portion of the deltoid ligament of the ankle medially and can be divided into three separate bands: superomedial, medioplantar oblique, and inferoplantar longitudinal.[27] The spring ligament plays an important role in supporting the head of the talus and talonavicular joint, as well as functioning as one of the main static or passive stabilizers of the medial longitudinal arch.[27,28]

We already noted that the talonavicular facets and the anteriorly located talocalcaneal facets share a joint capsule. The large posterior facet of the subtalar joint is contained within its own capsule and is physically separated from the capsule containing the talonavicular joint by the tarsal canal and the ligaments within the canal. However, the talonavicular joint and the subtalar joint are linked mechanically in the weight-bearing foot. Weight-bearing eversion/inversion and adduction/abduction of the talus on the calcaneus during subtalar supination/pronation involve simultaneous movement of the head of the talus on the relatively fixed navicular bone. In weight-bearing, therefore, the talonavicular and subtalar joints are both anatomically and functionally related.[29]

Foundational Concepts 12–2
Talar Linkages

Because of the anatomic and functional linkage of the talus to the structures below and anterior to it, the subtalar and talonavicular joints have been referred to as the **talocalcaneonavicular joint.**[2] However, it might be argued that even this compound term is incomplete. The talus, in weight-bearing, can also be considered to act as a ball bearing between three joints: (1) the tibiofibular mortise (the ankle joint) superiorly, (2) the calcaneus (the subtalar joint) inferiorly, and (3) the navicular bone (the talonavicular joint) anteriorly. In weight-bearing supination/pronation, the tibia/fibula (ankle mortise) dorsiflexes and plantarflexes on the talus. Abduction/adduction and inversion/eversion *of the talus* during supination/pronation not only occurs on the calcaneus and the navicular bone but also affects the position of the mortise as the body of the talus laterally and medially rotates.

The ligaments of the talonavicular joint include the spring and bifurcate ligaments. In addition, the talonavicular articulation is also supported by the **dorsal talonavicular ligament** and receives support from the ligaments of the subtalar joint—including the MCL and LCL, the inferior extensor retinacular structures, and the cervical and interosseous talocalcaneal ligaments. Support is also received from the ligaments that reinforce the adjacent calcaneocuboid joint, which forms the remainder of the transverse tarsal joint and to which the talonavicular joint is linked functionally.

Calcaneocuboid Joint

The calcaneocuboid joint is formed proximally by the anterior calcaneus and distally by the posterior cuboid bone (see Fig. 12–13). The articular surfaces of both the calcaneus and the cuboid bone are complex, being reciprocally concave/convex both side to side and top to bottom. The reciprocal shape makes available motion at the calcaneocuboid joint more restricted than that of the ball-and-socket–shaped talonavicular joint. The calcaneocuboid joint, like the talonavicular joint, is linked in weight-bearing to the subtalar joint.[29] In weight-bearing subtalar supination/pronation, the inversion/eversion of the calcaneus under the talus causes the calcaneus to move simultaneously on the relatively fixed cuboid bone. As the calcaneus moves at the subtalar joint during weight-bearing activities, it must meet the conflicting intra-articular demands of the opposing saddle-shaped surfaces, which results in a twisting motion.

The synovial calcaneocuboid articulation has its own capsule that is reinforced by several important ligaments. The capsule is reinforced laterally by the lateral band of the bifurcate ligament (also known as the **calcaneocuboid ligament**), dorsally by the **dorsal calcaneocuboid ligament,** and inferiorly by the **plantar calcaneocuboid (short plantar)** and the **long plantar ligaments**[30] (see Fig. 12-7). The long plantar ligament is the most important of these ligaments, because the inferiorly located long plantar ligament spans the calcaneus and the cuboid bone and then continues on distally to the bases of the second, third, and fourth metatarsals. Therefore the long plantar ligament provides support to the transverse tarsal joint as well as the lateral longitudinal arch of the foot.[31] The extrinsic muscles of the foot also provide important support for the transverse tarsal joint as they pass medial, lateral, and inferior to the joint.

Tarsometatarsal Joints

The tarsometatarsal (TMT) joints are plane synovial joints, similar to the carpometacarpal (CMC) joints of the hand. The TMTs are formed by the distal row of tarsal bones and the bases of the metatarsals **(Fig. 12–15)**. This articulation between the midfoot and forefoot is also known as the *Lisfranc joint complex*.[32] The first (medial) TMT joint is composed of the articulation between the base of the first metatarsal and the medial cuneiform bone, and has its own articular capsule. The second TMT joint is composed of the articulation of the base of the second metatarsal with a mortise formed by the middle cuneiform bone and the sides of the medial and lateral cuneiform bones. This joint is set more posteriorly than the other TMT joints with restricted motion. The third TMT joint, formed by the third metatarsal and the lateral cuneiform, shares a capsule with the second TMT joint. The bases of the fourth and fifth metatarsals, with the distal surface of the cuboid bone, form the fourth and fifth TMT joints. These two joints also share a common joint capsule. Small plane articulations exist between the bases of the metatarsals to permit motion of one metatarsal on the next. Numerous dorsal, plantar, and interosseous ligaments along with fibularis longus and tibialis tendons reinforce the Lisfranc joint complex in a stratified lattice-like arrangement that contributes to both strength and flexibility of the joint.[32] In addition, there is a deep transverse metatarsal ligament that spans the heads of the metatarsals on the plantar surface and is similar to that found in the hand.[33,34] Just as the deep transverse metacarpal ligament contributed to stability of the more proximally located CMC joints in the hand, the deep transverse metatarsal ligament contributes to stability of the proximally located TMT joints by preventing excessive motion and splaying of the metatarsal heads.[35]

Metatarsophalangeal Joints

The five metatarsophalangeal (MTP) joints, analogous to the metacarpophalangeal (MCP) joints of the hand, are condyloid synovial joints with two degrees of freedom: extension/flexion (or dorsiflexion/plantarflexion) and abduction/adduction. The MTP joints are formed proximally by the convex heads of the metatarsals and distally by the concave bases of the proximal phalanges (see Fig. 12–15).

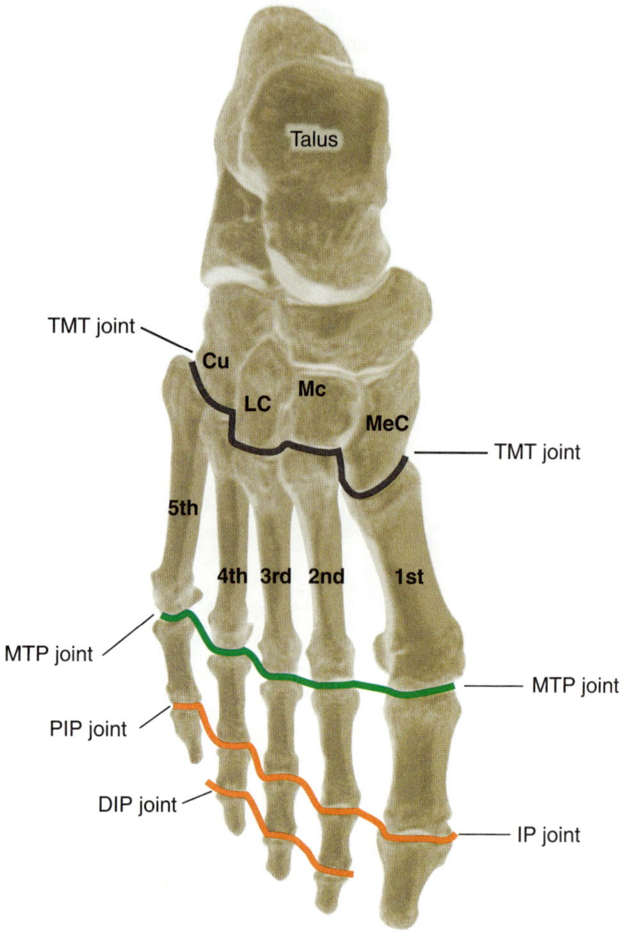

Figure 12–15 Tarsometatarsal (TMT), metatarsophalangeal (MTP), and interphalangeal (IP: PIP and DIP) joints of the foot. CU, cuboid; LC, lateral cuneiform; MC, middle cuneiform; MeC, medial cuneiform.

Expanded Concepts 12–1
Metatarsal Length

The lengths of the five metatarsals vary between individuals and are classified into three types. *Index plus* is characterized by the first metatarsal being longer than the second, with the remaining three toes progressively decreasing in length. *Index plus minus* is characterized by the first and second metatarsal being the same length, with the other remaining three metatarsals progressively decreasing in length. *Index minus*, or *Morton's foot*, is classified by the second metatarsal being longest followed progressively by the first, third, fourth, and fifth. Metatarsal bone stress injuries are common among athletes and active individuals due to repetitive loading through the foot. Risk factors for metatarsal bone stress injuries include abnormal foot biomechanics, metatarsal length, bone density, bone geometry, intrinsic muscle strength, gait pattern, and footwear.[36] A Morton's foot has been hypothesized to cause an increase in force through the second metatarsal, predisposing it to stress injuries. The relationship between metatarsal length and injury pattern, however, is unclear because the literature has not fully supported this hypothesis in athletes.[37,38]

As noted earlier, the structure of the MTP joints is analogous to the structure of the MCP joints with a few exceptions. Unlike the MCP joints, the range of MTP extension exceeds the range of MTP flexion. Because all five metatarsal heads bear weight in stance, the articular cartilage must remain clear of the weight-bearing surface on the plantar aspect of the metatarsal head. This structural requirement restricts the available range of MTP flexion. Also, in contrast to the hand, there is no opposition available at the first MTP joint; the **hallux** (first toe) moves exclusively in the same planes as the other four digits.

The first MTP joint has two sesamoid bones associated with it that are located on the plantar aspect of the first metatarsal head **(Fig. 12–16)**. These are analogous to the sesamoid bones on the volar surface of the MCP joint. In the neutral position of the first MTP joint, the sesamoid bones lie in two grooves, separated by the intersesamoid ridge, on the metatarsal head.[39] The ligaments associated with the sesamoid bones form a triangular mass that stabilizes the sesamoid bones within their grooves.[40] The sesamoid bones serve as anatomic pulleys for the **flexor hallucis brevis** muscle and protect the tendon of the **flexor hallucis longus** muscle from weight-bearing trauma. The flexor hallucis longus is protected as it passes through a tunnel formed by the sesamoid bones and the intersesamoid ligament that connects the sesamoid bones across their plantar surfaces.[40] Unlike the sesamoid bones of the thumb, the sesamoid bones of the first metatarsal absorb weight-bearing stress, along with the relatively large quadrilaterally shaped first metatarsal head.[40,41] In toe extension greater than 10°, the sesamoid bones no longer lie in their grooves and may become unstable. Chronic lateral instability of the sesamoid bones may lead to MTP deformity.[41]

Stability of the MTP joints is provided by a joint capsule, **plantar plates, collateral ligaments,** and the deep transverse metatarsal ligament. The plantar plates are structurally similar to the volar plates in the hand. These fibrocartilaginous structures in the four lesser toes are each connected to the base of the proximal phalange distally and blend with the joint capsule proximally. The plates of the four lesser toes are interconnected by the deep transverse metatarsal ligament and the **plantar aponeurosis.**[42] The collateral ligaments of the MTP joints, like those at the MCP joint, have two components: a phalangeal portion that parallels the metatarsal and phalange, and an accessory component that runs obliquely from the metatarsal head to the plantar plate.[43] The plantar plates protect the weight-bearing surface of the metatarsal heads and, with the collateral ligaments, contribute to stability of the MTP joints. Plantar plate insufficiency or atrophy can result in excessive loading and metatarsal head pain, known as *metatarsalgia*.[44,45]

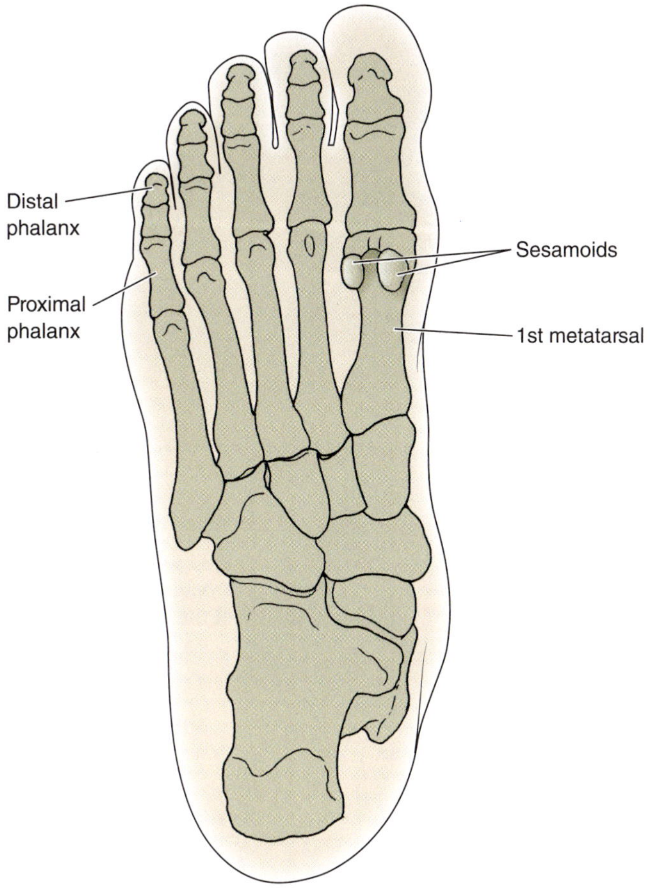

Figure 12–16 The plantar surface of the foot. The two sesamoid bones of the great toe can easily be seen sitting on the head of the first metatarsal.

Interphalangeal Joints

The interphalangeal (IP) joints of the toes are synovial hinge joints with one degree of freedom: flexion/extension. Like the thumb, the great toe has only one IP joint connecting two phalanges, whereas the four lesser toes have two IP joints (proximal and distal IP joints) connecting three phalanges (see Fig. 12–16). Each phalanx is virtually identical in structure to its counterpart in the hand, although substantially shorter in length. Consequently, the reader is referred to Chapter 9 for details on IP joint structure of the thumb and fingers to understand the structure of the IP joints of the toes. The toes function to smooth the weight shift to the opposite foot in gait and help maintain stability by pressing against the ground in standing. Injuries to the IP joints are relatively uncommon but may include dislocations and fractures.

Joint Function

The Ankle Joint

Talocrural Axis

In a neutral ankle position, the joint axis passes approximately through the lateral malleolus and the body of the talus and through or just below the medial malleolus **(Fig. 12–17)**.[46] The

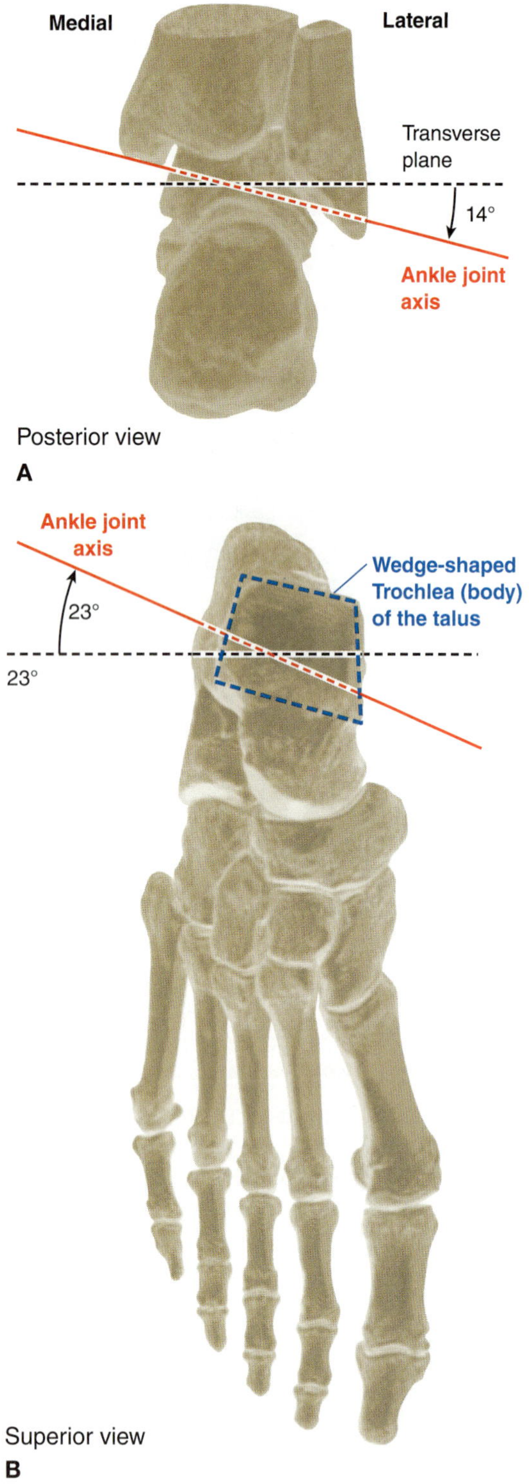

Figure 12–17 The axis of the ankle joint. **A.** Posterior view showing the mortise around the body of the talus and the average 14° inclination of the ankle axis from the transverse plane. **B.** Superior view showing the ankle axis rotated, on average, 23° from the frontal plane. Also shown is the wedge-shaped trochlea (body) of the talus, wider anteriorly than posteriorly.

lateral malleolus and its associated fibular facet on the talus are located more distally (see **Fig. 12–17A**) and posteriorly (see **Fig. 12–17B**) than the medial malleolus and its associated tibial facet. The more posterior position of the lateral malleolus is due to the typical lateral torsion or twist that exists in the distal tibia in relation to the tibia's proximal plateau. This tibial torsion (or tibiofibular torsion, because both the tibia and fibula are involved with the rotation in the transverse plane) may account for the toe-out position of the foot in typical standing.[47] The torsion in the tibia is similar to the torsion found in the shaft of the femur, although typically reversed in direction. The amount of lateral tibial torsion increases from birth until 10 years of age.[48] As tibial torsion increases, the axis of the ankle joint is positioned more laterally in the transverse plane. Although variations exist, clinical measures have reported values that approximate 19º of lateral torsion for both adult males and females.[49,50] It should be noted that larger values for tibial torsion have been reported in studies that used computerized tomography.[48]

The ankle joint classically is considered to have one degree of freedom, with dorsiflexion/plantarflexion occurring between the talus and the mortise. During open-chain (non–weight-bearing) movements at the ankle, dorsiflexion refers to a motion of the head of the talus (see Fig. 12–6) dorsally (or upward) as the body of the talus slides posteriorly in the mortise, bringing the rest of the foot with it. Plantarflexion is the opposite motion of the head and body of the talus. Because of the lower position of the lateral malleolus, the axis of the ankle is declined on the lateral side. A classic anatomic study found this downward angulation to average 14° (see Fig. 12-17A).[51] However, the amount of angulation may be highly variable between individuals. Stiehl used a simple hinged model with a level indicator to demonstrate how a single axis that is oriented more distally and more posteriorly on the lateral side will create a motion of the foot (or tibia and fibula in weight-bearing) across three planes (triplanar motion) while moving around a single fixed axis.[52] He showed that dorsiflexion of the foot around a typically oriented ankle axis will bring the foot up (dorsiflexion), but will also simultaneously bring it slightly lateral to the leg (abduction) and appear to turn the foot longitudinally away from the midline (eversion). Conversely, plantarflexion around the same single oblique ankle axis will result in the foot going down, moving medial to the leg (adduction), and appearing to turn the foot longitudinally toward the midline (inversion). When the foot is weight-bearing, the same relative pattern of motion exists when the tibia and fibula move on the fixed foot. In weight-bearing ankle dorsiflexion, the leg (tibia and fibula) will move forward and medial to the foot, as well as appear to rotate medially in the transverse plane. The opposite occurs during weight-bearing ankle plantarflexion.

It should be noted, however, that although a pure hinge model (e.g., goniometry) helps to explain ankle motion, anatomic studies have demonstrated that the instantaneous axis of rotation for the ankle joint changes throughout the ROM.[53,54] Talar rotation within the mortise—in both the transverse plane around a vertical axis (talar rotation or talar abduction/adduction) and in the frontal plane around an A-P axis (talar tilt or talar inversion/eversion)—must occur to maintain tibiotalar congruency.[55] These rotations, however, are relatively small in comparison with sagittal plane dorsiflexion and plantarflexion motion. Clearly, the majority, but not all, of the ankle motion occurs in the sagittal plane.

Expanded Concepts 12–2
Talocrural Joint Arthroplasty

Ankle replacement (total ankle arthroplasty) is being used more commonly to treat ankle arthritis. First introduced in the 1970s, the long-term results of total ankle arthroplasty demonstrated unacceptable failure rates. In the late 1980s, second-generation total ankle replacements were developed. These newer prosthetic joint replacements were designed to better represent typical ankle anatomy and joint kinematics. This included allowing rotation of the talus to occur in multiple planes.[56,57] Third- and fourth-generation implants have further evolved based on biomechanical analyses of the ankle-foot complex. These implants are divided into two main classes: fixed bearing and mobile bearing. Fixed-bearing devices appear to offer increased stability at the risk of loosening of the tibial component over time. This loosening is believed to occur due to excess stress where the tibial component articulates with the tibia. Mobile bearing implants allow the ankle to have more mobility, but this may contribute to painful impingement. Both classes of implants are considered superior to previous iterations and the type of implant that is used for a specific patient is determined by the surgeon. Current-generation implants are associated with 5- and 10-year survivorship rates (longevity of the implant) of 92% and 83.5%, respectively. This is significantly improved versus earlier generation implants, which have 5- and 10-year survivorship rates of 87% and 71%.[58,59]

A commonly referenced source notes that typical ankle joint ROM is 20° for dorsiflexion and 50° for plantarflexion.[60] Large variations in ankle motion can exist between individuals, depending on measurement technique and subject characteristics.[61] Differences in technique include the amount of force used to determine when end ROM occurs and whether or not talocrural joint motion is isolated.[62] While approximately 10° of ankle dorsiflexion ROM historically has been considered the minimal amount needed to ambulate without deviation, the amount of ROM required may depend on a number of factors including gait speed.[63]

During ankle joint dorsiflexion/plantarflexion, the shape of the body of the talus facilitates joint stability. As noted earlier, the trochlear (superior) surface of the talus is wider anterior than posterior (see Fig. 12–17B). When the foot is weight-bearing, dorsiflexion occurs by the concave tibiofibular segment rotating anteriorly over the fixed talus. The wider anterior portion of the talus will "wedge" into the mortise, spreading the tibia and fibula apart slightly to enhance stability of the ankle joint. In contrast, the loose-packed position of the ankle joint is in plantarflexion, when the narrower posterior body of the talus is in contact with the mortise. Consequently, the mortise loses some of its "grip" on the narrower portion of the trochlea. That the ankle is less stable in plantarflexion is consistent with the typical mechanism of injury to the lateral ankle ligaments (i.e., plantarflexion and inversion).[64] Additionally, the contact between the talus and the tibia/fibular mortise helps distribute weight-bearing forces. The ability of the ankle to distribute these weight-bearing forces combined with the mechanical properties of the tibiotalar articular cartilage reduces the risk of osteoarthritis at the talocrural joint.[56] However, trauma may lead to ankle arthritis not only because of direct cartilage damage but also structural changes that lead to biomechanical abnormalities. Therefore, posttraumatic arthritis is the most common type of arthritis occurring at the ankle.[65]

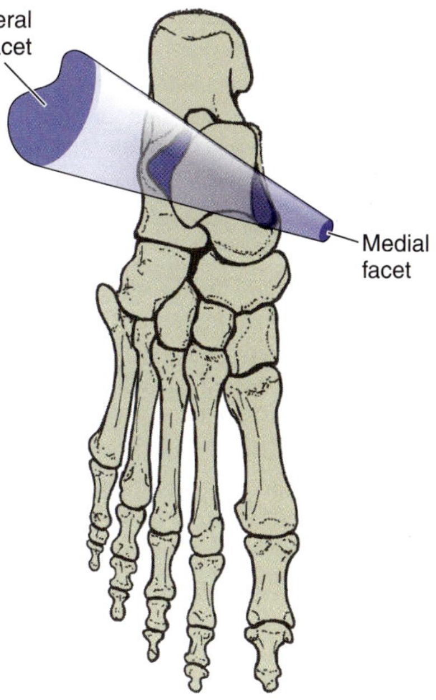

Figure 12–18 The three articular surfaces of the talus (the trochlea, smaller medial facet, and larger lateral facet) can be pictured as part of a cone-shaped surface, with ends of the cone cut off (the larger ends of the cone facing laterally).

The asymmetry in size and orientation of the lateral and medial facets of the ankle joint contributes to changes in the ankle mortise that occur during ankle dorsiflexion. The lateral (fibular) facet is substantially larger than the medial (tibial) facet, and its surface is oriented slightly obliquely to that of the medial facet (see Fig. 12–17). Inman and Mann proposed that the body of the talus can be thought of as a segment of a cone lying on its side with its base directed laterally.[66] The cone should be visualized as "truncated" or cut off on either end at slightly different angles **(Fig. 12–18)**.[47] The asymmetry in size and orientation of the facets means that the distal fibula moving on the larger lateral facet of the talus must undergo a greater displacement (in a slightly different plane) than the medial malleolus as the tibia and fibula move together during dorsiflexion. This large arc of motion of the lateral malleolus (compared to the small arc for the medial malleolus) results in superior/inferior motion and medial/lateral rotation of the fibula that requires mobility of the fibula at both the proximal and the distal tibiofibular joints.

Although fibular motion can occur in transverse, sagittal, and frontal planes with ankle plantarflexion and dorsiflexion, the amount of motion seems to be highly variable between individuals.[67,68] Differences in fibular motion may be related to orientation of the proximal tibiofibular facet, with more mobility available in the facets that are more vertical. Effectively, however, mobility of the fibula at the tibiofibular joints should be considered a component of typical ankle motion.

Expanded Concepts 12–3
Syndesmotic Injuries

Injuries to the distal tibiofibular syndesmosis (see Fig. 12-5 inset) occur when the ankle-foot complex is forcefully dorsiflexed and/or laterally rotated. These injuries can lead to instability of the talocrural joint because the mortise is no longer held together, making it unable to provide proximal stability to the joint. Surgical intervention involving placement of internal fixation implants, such as screws or a suture-button device, is often required when patients have high-grade injuries or when their function cannot be restored with conservative management. Screws are the most common devices used to surgically stabilize the distal tibiofibular joint following a syndesmotic injury, and screws are implanted so that the typically mobile fibula is now *fixed* to the stable tibia. The mortise stability that is provided by surgical fixation comes at a cost of ROM at the talocrural joint because the fibula is no longer able to move as the talus rotates into the mortise. Historically, patients underwent planned postoperative surgical removal of these screws in order to restore talocrural ROM after the syndesmosis had healed. This was believed to improve ROM because it would allow fibular mobility during talocrural ROM. Recently, however, researchers determined that the risks of scheduled removal of surgical screws outweighed the benefits for many patients. This suggests that the effect of fibular mobility on ROM and function may vary across patients.[69]

Ankle dorsiflexion and plantarflexion movements are limited primarily by soft tissue restrictions. Active or passive tension in the **triceps surae** (**gastrocnemius** and **soleus muscles**) is the primary limitation to dorsiflexion. Typically, less ankle dorsiflexion ROM is seen with the knee extended compared with a flexed knee position. This can be attributed to tension in the multi-joint gastrocnemius muscle caused by lengthening of the muscle both by ankle dorsiflexion and the extended knee.[70] Ankle dorsiflexion is limited by the soleus muscle and the posterior talocrural joint capsule when the knee is flexed (and tension in the gastrocnemius released). Tension in the **tibialis anterior, extensor hallucis longus,** and **extensor digitorum longus** muscles is the primary limit to plantarflexion. The medial and lateral collateral ankle ligaments may play some role in guiding ankle motion for typical activities but are most important for limiting motion at end-range.[71] The more critical function of these ligaments appears to be in minimizing side-to-side movement or rotation of the talus in the mortise. The ligaments are assisted in that function by the muscles that pass on either side of the ankle. The **tibialis posterior, flexor hallucis longus,** and **flexor digitorum longus** muscles help protect the medial aspect of the ankle, whereas the **fibularis (peroneus) longus** and **fibularis (peroneus) brevis** muscles protect the lateral aspect. Bony checks to any of the potential ankle motions are rarely encountered unless there is extreme hypermobility (as may be found among gymnasts or dancers) or a failure of one or more of the other restraint systems. A more complete analysis of the function of the muscles crossing the ankle will be presented later because all muscles of the ankle cross at least two and generally three or more joints of the ankle and foot.

The Subtalar Joint

Although the subtalar joint is composed of three articulations, the alternating convex-concave facets limit the potential mobility of the joint. Together, the three articulations provide a triplanar movement around a single joint axis. When the talus moves on the posterior facet of the calcaneus, the articular surface of the talus should, theoretically, slide in the *same* direction as the bone moves—a concave surface moving on a stable convex surface. However, at the middle and anterior joints, the talar surfaces (again, theoretically) should slide in a direction opposite to movement of the bone—a convex surface moving on a stable concave surface. Motion of the talus on the calcaneus, therefore, is a complex twisting or screw-like motion that can proceed only as long as the facets can accommodate simultaneous and opposite motions across the surfaces. The result is a triplanar motion of the talus around a single oblique joint axis, producing the motion of supination/pronation.

The Subtalar Axis

The axis for subtalar supination/pronation has been the subject of many investigations that indicate substantial variability, even among healthy individuals without impairments **(Fig. 12–19)**. The average subtalar axis was found to be (1) inclined 42° upward and anteriorly from a longitudinal (A-P axis)—with a broad interindividual range of 29° to 47° (see **Fig. 12–19A**), and (2) inclined medially 16° from the longitudinal axis—with a broad interindividual range of 8° to 24° (see **Fig. 12–19B**).[72] Clearly, motion about this oblique subtalar axis will cross all three planes. Supination/pronation, like the triplanar ankle joint motion, can be modeled by a single oblique hinge joint.[73] Although the triplanar motions of pronation/supination can be described by its three component (cardinal) motions, these subtalar component motions are coupled and cannot occur independently. The coupled motions must occur simultaneously because the calcaneus (or talus) twists across the subtalar joint's three articular surfaces.

To understand the components of subtalar pronation/supination, we can consider how the subtalar axis varies from the cardinal axes shown in Figure 12–2. If the subtalar joint axis were a vertical axis, the motion around that axis would produce abduction/adduction; if the subtalar axis were a longitudinal axis, the motion would be inversion/eversion; and if the subtalar axis were a coronal (medial/lateral) axis, the motion would be plantarflexion/dorsiflexion. In reality, the subtalar axis lies about halfway between being a longitudinal axis and being a vertical axis. Consequently, pronation/supination includes approximately equal magnitudes of eversion/inversion and abduction/adduction. The subtalar axis is inclined only very slightly away from a longitudinal axis and toward being a coronal axis (~16°); therefore, subtalar motion has only a small component of dorsiflexion/plantarflexion. The contribution of each of the coupled movements to composite supination/pronation will depend greatly on individual differences in inclination of the subtalar axis. As one example, if the subtalar axis is inclined upwardly only 30° (rather than the average of 42°), the relative amount of inversion/eversion will be much greater than the relative amount of adduction/abduction because the axis is closer to being longitudinal. We will now examine how subtalar joint component motions are coupled to create the complex motions of pronation/supination in both non–weight-bearing and weight-bearing positions.

Non–Weight-Bearing Subtalar Joint Motion

In non–weight-bearing supination and pronation, subtalar motion is described by motion of its distal segment (the calcaneus)

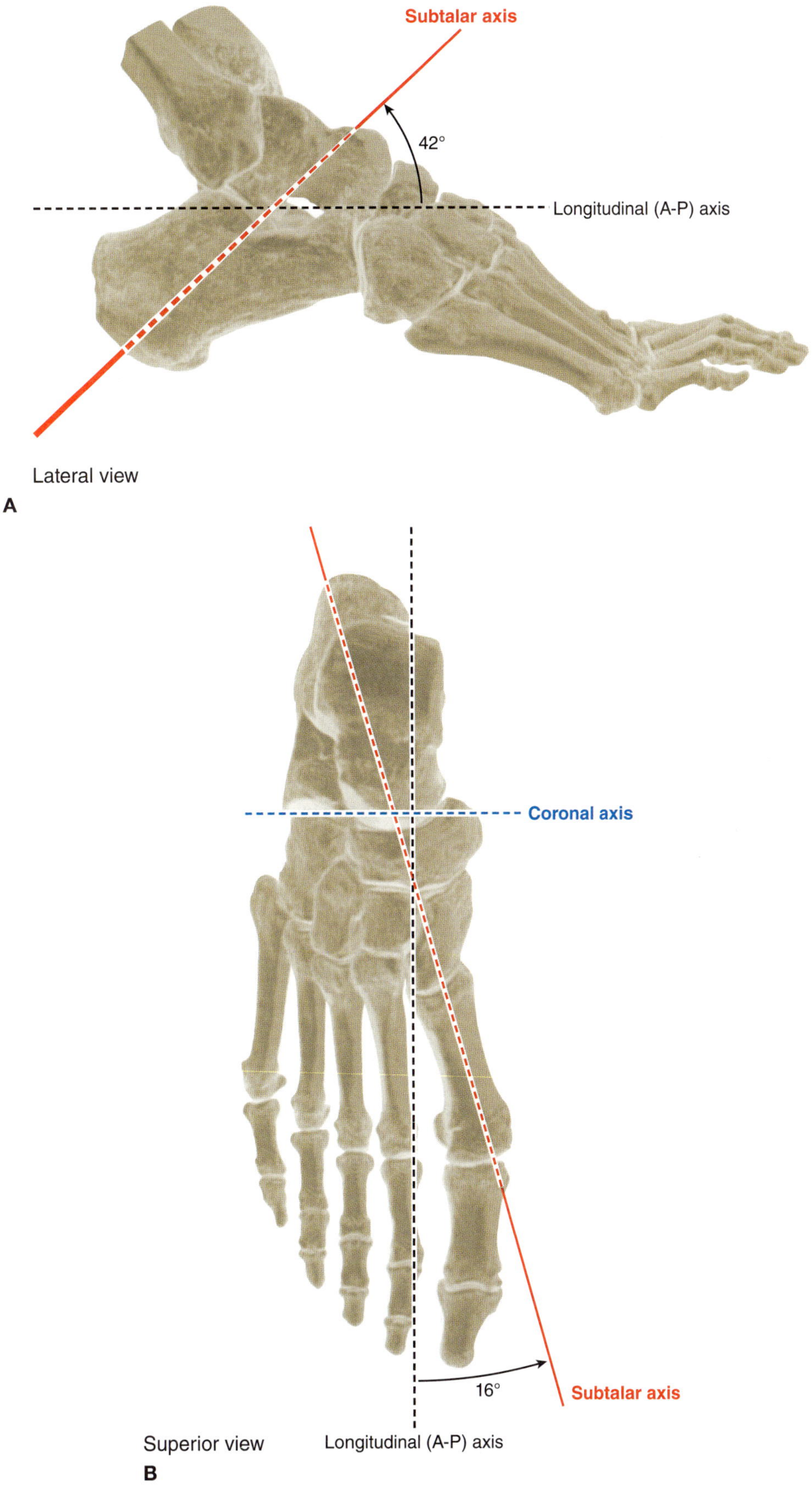

Figure 12–19 Axis of the subtalar joint is: **A.** inclined up from a longitudinal (A-P) axis approximately 42°, and **B.** inclined medially from a longitudinal (and toward a coronal) axis approximately 16°.

Table 12–1 Summary of Coupled Subtalar Motions: Coupled Movements of Subtalar Pronation/Supination

	NON–WEIGHT-BEARING	WEIGHT-BEARING
Supination	Calcaneal inversion (or varus) Calcaneal adduction Calcaneal plantarflexion	Calcaneal inversion (or varus) Talar abduction (or lateral rotation) Talar dorsiflexion Tibiofibular lateral rotation
Pronation	Calcaneal eversion (or valgus) Calcaneal abduction Calcaneal dorsiflexion	Calcaneal eversion (or valgus) Talar adduction (or medial rotation) Talar plantarflexion Tibiofibular medial rotation

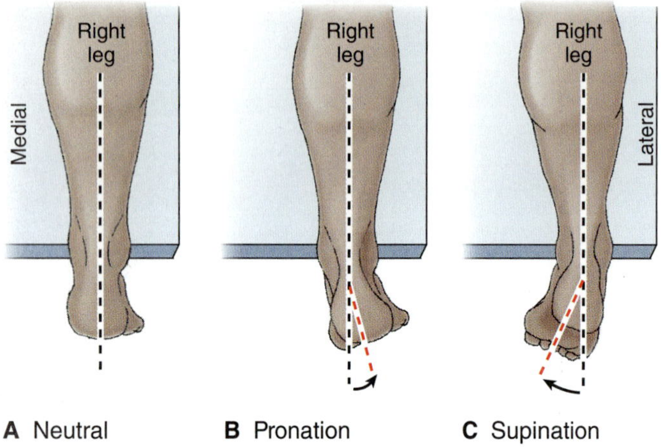

Figure 12–20 Non–weight-bearing motion at the right subtalar joint. **A.** The right rearfoot is shown in neutral. **B.** Pronation of the subtalar joint is observable as eversion (valgus movement) of the calcaneus, although the coupled motions of dorsiflexion and abduction of the calcaneus must also be occurring. **C.** Supination of the subtalar joint is observable as inversion (varus movement) of the calcaneus, although the coupled motions of plantarflexion and adduction of the calcaneus must also be occurring.

on the relatively stationary talus and lower leg, where the reference point on the calcaneus is its anteriorly located head (see Fig. 12–6). Non–weight-bearing supination is composed of the coupled calcaneal motions of adduction, inversion, and plantarflexion; pronation of the non–weight-bearing calcaneus on the fixed talus and lower leg is composed of the coupled motions of abduction, eversion, and dorsiflexion (Table 12–1). The most readily observable of the coupled motions of the calcaneus during pronation and supination are eversion and inversion, respectively. These calcaneal motions are often observed at the posterior calcaneus, with the subject prone and the foot and lower leg over the end of the plinth **(Fig. 12–20)**. Eversion (see **Fig. 12–20B**) may also be referred to as a *valgus movement of the calcaneus*, and inversion (see **Fig. 12–20C**) as a *varus movement of the calcaneus*. The eversion and inversion components of pronation/supination appear as if they are occurring in isolation. However, the coupled components of calcaneal abduction and dorsiflexion must simultaneously accompany eversion, and the coupled components of calcaneal adduction and plantarflexion must simultaneously accompany inversion.

Foundational Concepts 12–3
Terminology Revisited

Although the apparent interchangeable use of the terms *pronation/supination* and *eversion/inversion*, respectively, to describe the composite uniaxial motions of the subtalar joint appears confusing, the "disagreement" in terminology is not as discrepant as it first appears. When the composite term *pronation* (a triplanar motion) is used to describe subtalar motion, the coupled calcaneal component of *eversion* will always be part of the motion. When the component term *eversion* is used to describe subtalar motion, then the other coupled calcaneal components of *pronation* (i.e., abduction, dorsiflexion) will always be part of the motion. Consequently, *pronation* and *eversion* are invariably linked, regardless of the terminology frame of reference. The same is true of supination and inversion; whether used as a composite term or a component term, *supination* and *inversion* are invariably linked. It would certainly be less troublesome if a universal definitional framework were accepted. However, the wary reader who understands the association between supination/pronation and inversion/eversion may be able to infer definitions when they are not overtly offered by authors.

Weight-Bearing Subtalar Joint Motion

When an individual is weight-bearing, the *relative* movements between the talus and calcaneus are the same as during non--weight-bearing; however, the description of which segment is moving is different. Typically, during a weight-bearing movement, we describe the motion of the proximal segment on the distal segment. At the foot, however, when the calcaneus is on the ground, it is generally still free to move around the longitudinal axis (inversion/eversion) without leaving the ground, but limited in its ability to move around the coronal axis (plantarflexion/dorsiflexion) and vertical axis (adduction/abduction) because of the superimposed body weight and ground beneath the foot. Consequently, the coupled motions that contribute to pronation/supination cannot be accomplished exclusively by the calcaneus; instead the remaining components are described by movement of the talus on the calcaneus. The weight-bearing calcaneus will continue to contribute to the inversion/eversion component of subtalar motion; the other two coupled components of the subtalar motion (abduction/adduction and dorsiflexion/plantarflexion) will be accomplished by movement of the talus (whereby the *head* of the talus is used as the reference) on the more fixed calcaneus rather than by movement of the calcaneus on the relatively fixed talus. As a reminder, the relative motion accomplished at any joint around a given axis remains unchanged whether the distal segment of the joint moves or the proximal segment moves. In weight-bearing subtalar motion, the direction of the movement contributed by the talus in space is described as the opposite of what the calcaneus would contribute, although the same relative motion occurs between the segments. We recognize that this difference in terminology at the foot can be confusing. For the reader who has become accustomed to thinking about movements as one segment relative to another (e.g., knee flexion represents posterior roll of either the tibia on femur, or femur on tibia), it may become challenging to think about joint motion terminology being used to describe movements of one segment relative to its starting position (e.g., the talus abducts in space on a relatively fixed calcaneus to produce subtalar joint adduction). When reading further, please note whether the terminology references the movement of a segment in space (e.g., talus) or the relative movement at a joint (e.g., subtalar). This will provide important information about what is moving.

In weight-bearing supination, the calcaneus continues to contribute the component of inversion. However, the calcaneus cannot adduct and plantarflex in weight-bearing, and so the remaining coupled components of subtalar supination are accomplished by the head of the *talus* abducting and dorsiflexing in space. Weight-bearing subtalar supination (see Table 12–1), therefore, is observed as inversion (or varus movement) of the calcaneus, while the simultaneous dorsiflexion and abduction of the head of the talus in space are seen in the elevation of the medial longitudinal arch and a convexity on the dorsal lateral midfoot. Although subtalar joint supination is a typical foot motion, a foot that appears fixed in this position often is called a "supinated" or **pes cavus foot.**

Weight-bearing subtalar pronation is accomplished by the coupled component movements of eversion of the calcaneus and plantarflexion and adduction of the head of the talus in space (see Table 12–1). In standing, the calcaneus can be observed to move into eversion (or valgus movement), whereas talar adduction and plantarflexion in space are reflected in a lowering of the medial longitudinal arch and a bulging or convexity in the plantar medial midfoot. Although subtalar joint pronation is a typical foot motion, a foot that appears fixed in this position often is called "pronated," **pes planus,** or **flat foot.**

The most critical functions of the foot occur in weight-bearing. When the foot is weight-bearing and the body remains positioned over one or both feet, the joints of the lower extremity form a closed chain. Consequently, the kinematics and kinetics of the subtalar joint will affect and be affected by more proximal and distal joints. An important consequence of closed-chain subtalar function can be seen in its interdependence with lower extremity or leg rotation.

WEIGHT-BEARING SUBTALAR JOINT MOTION AND ITS EFFECT ON THE LEG

During weight-bearing subtalar supination/pronation, the coupled component motions of dorsiflexion/plantarflexion and abduction/adduction of the talar head in space require that the body of the talus move as well. The body of the talus is, of course, lodged within the superimposed mortise. Dorsiflexion of the head of the talus requires the body of the talus to slide posteriorly within the mortise **(Fig. 12–21A)**, whereas plantarflexion of the head of the talus requires the body of the talus to move anteriorly within the mortise. The tibia (leg) remains unaffected by the talar dorsiflexion/plantarflexion movement of the talus as long as the ankle joint is free to move. However, the ankle joint cannot absorb the coupled component motions of talar abduction/adduction without affecting the leg. For this reason, the tibia can be observed to medially/laterally rotate on the foot during weight-bearing adduction/abduction of the talus in space.

When the head of the talus abducts in weight-bearing subtalar supination, the body of the talus must rotate laterally in the transverse plane (see **Fig. 12–21B**). Correspondingly, the head of the talus adducts in weight-bearing subtalar pronation, with its body rotating medially in the transverse plane. Because the *body* of the talus can rotate only minimally at most within the mortise, rotation of the body of the talus can occur in weight-bearing only if the superimposed mortise moves *with* the talus. When the subtalar joint supinates in a weight-bearing position, the coupled component of talar abduction rotates the mortise (composed of the tibia and fibula) laterally, producing lateral rotation of the leg. Correspondingly, weight-bearing subtalar joint pronation consists of talar adduction, rotating the body of the talus medially and carrying the superimposed tibia and fibula into medial rotation.

As previously described, the component movements of abduction and adduction of the talus during weight-bearing subtalar joint motion directly influences the segments and joints superior to it. A weight-bearing subtalar joint maintained in pronation (e.g., a flat foot) can create a medial rotation force on the leg that, in turn, influences the knee and hip joints. Just as subtalar pronation and supination may impose rotatory forces on the leg in weight-bearing, so too may rotations of the leg influence the subtalar joint. When a lateral rotatory force is imposed on the weight-bearing leg (as when you rotate to the right around a planted right foot), the lateral motion of the leg carries the mortise and its interposed body of the talus laterally. Lateral rotation of the body of the talus (abduction of the head of the talus) cannot occur without its coupled components of talar dorsiflexion and calcaneal inversion, thus producing supination of the subtalar joint. A medial rotatory force imposed on the weight-bearing leg, likewise, will necessarily result in subtalar pronation as the talus is medially rotated (adducted) by the rotating tibiofibular mortise and carries with it the coupled components of talar plantarflexion and calcaneal eversion. The interdependence of the leg and talus were mechanically represented by Inman and Mann, who used the concept of the subtalar joint as a mitered hinge.[66] This mitered-hinge concept **(Fig. 12–22)** presents a good visualization of the concept of the interdependence of the leg and foot through the oblique subtalar axis.

The kinematic coupling in the subtalar joint is thought to play an important role in lower extremity injuries when abnormalities exist.[74,75] Although the mitered hinge model helps to understand movement between the subtalar joint and leg, in vivo studies have found a great deal of individual variability in movement coupling.[76-78]

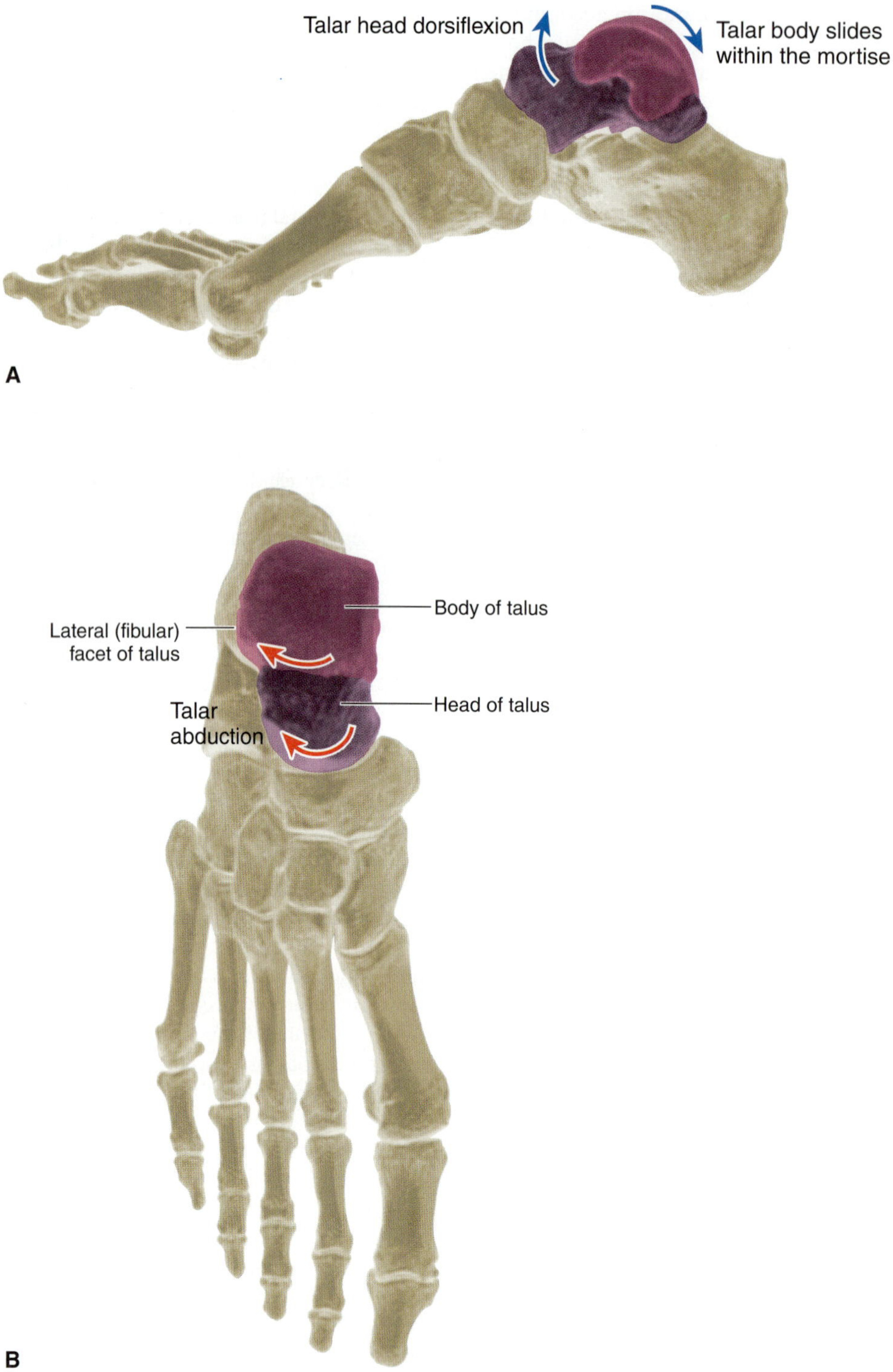

Figure 12–21 Talar motions in subtalar supination. **A.** Dorsiflexion of the head of the talus during weight-bearing subtalar supination slides the body of the talus posteriorly within the tibiofibular mortise. **B.** Abduction of the head of the talus during weight-bearing subtalar supination rotates the body of the talus laterally, typically taking the tibiofibular mortise along with it.

Patient Application 12–1

Arnold Benson is a 63-year-old man seeking intervention for right foot pain. Mr. Benson says he has "flat feet," which seem to have worsened over the past few years. In weight-bearing, it looks like Mr. Benson's foot is in a pronated foot posture. His right leg and thigh appear to be rotated medially, as well. It is possible that there is a relationship between Mr. Benson's medially rotated lower extremity and his pronated foot. While weight-bearing subtalar joint pronation can contribute to medial rotation of the leg and, subsequently, the thigh, the opposite can also occur, wherein the medially rotated lower extremity leads the subtalar joint to pronate. A thorough examination and history can help clinicians determine the factors that are contributing to Mr. Benson's standing posture and pain.

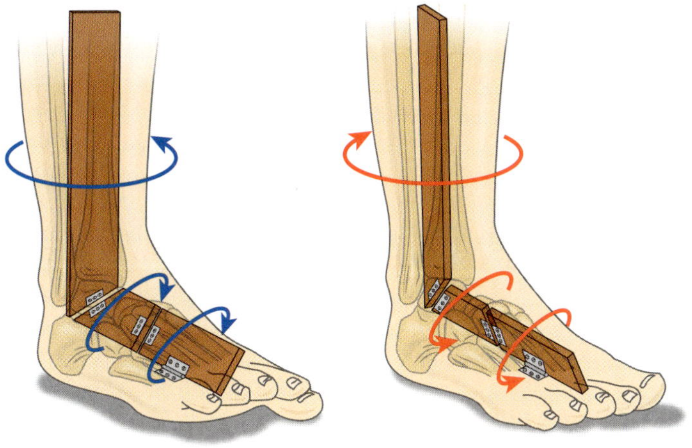

Figure 12–22 The subtalar joint can be visualized as a mitered (slanted) hinge between the leg and the foot. **A.** Medial rotation of the weight-bearing leg imposes pronation on the distally located subtalar joint. **B.** Lateral rotation of the leg proximally imposes supination on the distally located subtalar joint.

Range of Subtalar Motion and Subtalar Neutral

The range of subtalar supination and pronation is difficult to determine objectively because of the triplanar nature of the movement and because the component contributions vary with typical variations in the inclination of the subtalar axis. The calcaneal inversion/eversion (varus/valgus) component of subtalar motion can be measured in both weight-bearing and non–weight-bearing positions by using the posterior calcaneus and posterior midline of the leg as reference lines. This technique assumes that the neutral position (0°) is where the two posterior lines align to form a straight line (see Fig. 12–20A). For individuals without impairments, 5° to 10° of calcaneal eversion (valgus) from neutral, and 20° to 30° of calcaneal inversion (varus) from neutral, have been reported for a total range of 25° to 40°.[79-81] This measurement technique is problematic, however, because isolating subtalar motion from tibiotalar motion is clinically difficult and as a result, this measurement technique may have problems related to reliability.[82-86] Although the range of calcaneal inversion/eversion is not equivalent in magnitude to those of subtalar supination/pronation, the ranges should be directly proportional.

The variability in the inclination of the subtalar axis described by Manter[72] directly affects the range of the coupled components of subtalar motion. If the axis is inclined upward less than the average of 42° (see Fig. 12–19A), the subtalar axis will more closely approximate a longitudinal axis down the length of the foot; the proportion of inversion/eversion of the calcaneus that is part of subtalar motion will increase, whereas the proportion of coupled abduction/adduction of the calcaneus (or talus) will decrease. Because the change in inclination of the subtalar axis will affect both the foot and leg position in weight-bearing, a considerable amount of attention has been given to determining how an individual's subtalar axis might differ from the "average" (or standard) axis. This has led to an attempt to define an individual's **subtalar neutral** position of the subtalar joint and use this as a reference for a "typical" or "ideal" foot position. However, an individual's neutral subtalar joint position may deviate from the point at which the midlines of the posterior calcaneus and the posterior leg coincide, with a medial increase in that angle referred to as *valgus* and a decrease referred to as *varus* (see Fig. 12–3).

Expanded Concepts 12–4
Foot Posture

Clinicians use the validated and reliable Foot Posture Index-6 (FPI-6) to objectively assess and report the position of a patient's foot in static standing. Scores on the FPI-6 range from −12 to +12, with a more positive score indicating a more pronated, flattened, or pes planus foot posture and more negative score indicating a more supinated, high-arched, or pes cavus foot posture.[87,88]

The FPI-6 consists of six areas of assessment that globally assess position of the rearfoot, midfoot, and forefoot in static, bilateral stance.[87] The areas of assessment include the following:

1. *Talar head palpation:* Clinicians palpate the talar head to determine if the talus is adducted (medial side is more prominent when palpated, as in a pronated foot posture) neutral, or abducted (lateral side is more prominent, as in a supinated foot posture).
2. *Visual assessment of the curves above and below the lateral malleolus:* In a more pronated foot, the concavity below the lateral malleolus is significantly greater than the concavity created by the fibula above the malleolus. A neutral foot would have similar curves above and below the lateral malleolus. A supinated foot would present with a convex or flat curve below the lateral malleolus.
3. *Calcaneal position:* Calcaneal position is visually assessed. A calcaneus that is in eversion is associated with a more pronated foot posture, a vertical calcaneus with a neutral posture, and an inverted calcaneus with a more supinated foot posture.
4. *Talonavicular congruence:* The articulation between the talus and navicular is visually inspected to determine if it is prominent (as would occur in a pronated foot posture, as the talus adducts), flat, or concave (as would occur in a supinated foot posture, as the talus abducts).
5. *Medial longitudinal arch height:* The height of the medial longitudinal arch is assessed to determine if it is flat (as in a pronated foot posture), typical, or high (as in a supinated foot posture).
6. *Forefoot position:* The clinician is positioned behind the patient to visually assess the position of the forefoot. Visualization of only lateral toes indicates an abducted forefoot, which is most consistent with a pronated foot posture. Equal visualization of the medial and lateral toes indicates a more neutral foot posture. Visualization of only medial toes indicates an adducted forefoot and a more supinated foot posture.

A pronated or neutral foot posture is more common than a supinated foot posture. A 2022 study measured the foot posture of 102 healthy adults and found that 70% of the individuals on the FPI-6 were classified as "typical" (0–5 points) or "pronated" (6–9 points). Thirteen percent scored greater than 10 points and were classified as "highly pronated," 12% scored −1 to −4 points and were classified as "supinated," and 5% scored less than −5 and were considered to have "highly supinated" foot posture.[89] Patients with FPI-6 scores greater than 4 or less than 0 may benefit from clinical management of their abnormal pronated foot posture and abnormal supinated foot posture, respectively.[74]

The work of Cornwall and McPoil can be used to highlight some of the controversy that exists around the definition and application of the term **subtalar neutral.**[90] Cornwall and

McPoil described calcaneal motion during walking in 153 subjects between 18 and 41 years old with no history of foot impairments. They reported that the calcaneus is inverted 3.0° (±2.7°) at heel strike relative to the tibia and then everts 2.2° (±2.4°) by 55% of stance phase. After a period of eversion, the motion is reversed to 5.5° (±3.2°) of inversion just before the foot leaves the ground.[90] When looking at the overall results of the study, it was apparent that the subtalar joint does not function about a neutral position during walking but actually functions more in an everted position.[90] This finding was in agreement with their previous work.[91-93] They concluded that the "neutral" position of the weight-bearing subtalar joint was best represented by the resting position of the calcaneus (with respect to the lower leg)—instead of the *palpated* subtalar joint neutral position. The resting position of the calcaneus in relaxed bilateral stance averaged approximately 3.5° of calcaneal valgus (eversion) in a group of their subjects.[91] These findings appear to support the conclusion of Åstrom and Arvidson, who noted that the typical weight-bearing foot is more pronated than previously thought and that reliance on the palpated subtalar neutral position could lead to overdiagnosis of excessive subtalar pronation.[81] It should also be acknowledged that very few individuals may actually have an "ideal" foot position, and clinical examination may not be able to predict dynamic foot function.[94-96]

Foundational Concepts 12-4
Subtalar Joint Neutral Summary

Morton Root, a podiatrist, is credited with describing the theoretical management approach to foot and ankle problems that focused on the subtalar joint neutral position.[80] A basic premise of the approach is that the subtalar joint should be in a neutral position during midstance. The approach to intervention for several foot deformities includes use of an orthotic device to "balance the foot" and achieve a defined subtalar joint neutral position during midstance. As just described, there are a number of problems with this approach. These include contradictions that the subtalar joint is in neutral at midstance, poor reliability of measures, and inability to predict dynamic function from static measures. Additionally, although the subtalar joint position may contribute to our understanding of foot structure and function, the influence of subtalar position must be considered with other interdependent factors, including bony abnormalities (i.e., femoral or tibial rotation); extrinsic factors such as footwear, running surface, and activity level (magnitude and change); and physiological factors such as obesity or disease.

When the subtalar joint is non–weight-bearing, the motions of the subtalar joint and the leg are independent and do not influence each other. When the foot is weight-bearing, a primary function of the subtalar joint is to absorb the imposed lower extremity transverse plane rotations that occur during walking and other weight-bearing activities. Such rotations would otherwise spin the foot on the ground or damage the ankle joint by rotating the talus within the mortise. In supination, the subtalar joint surfaces are drawn together resulting in locking (close-packing) of the articular surfaces. Conversely, the adduction and plantarflexion of the talus that occur in weight-bearing pronation cause a splaying (spreading) of the adjacent tarsal bones that permits some intertarsal mobility (i.e., loose-packed position). The subtalar joint is strategically located between the ankle joint proximally and the transverse tarsal joint distally. We have already discussed how motions at the subtalar joint are associated with motions of the leg and ankle joint in weight-bearing. We will now focus our attention on motion between the talus and the navicular bone and between the calcaneus and cuboid bones. These articulations are grouped differently according to various authors, but the approach of this chapter will focus on the transverse tarsal joint as the primary functional unit accounting for motion in the midfoot. We will also see how motion at the subtalar joint influences motion at the transverse tarsal joint.

Transverse Tarsal Joint

The two joints formed by the talonavicular and calcaneocuboid together present an S-shaped joint line that transects the foot (see Fig. 12-13), dividing the rearfoot from the midfoot and forefoot. The navicular and the cuboid bones are considered, in essence, immobile in the weight-bearing foot. Transverse tarsal joint motion, therefore, is the motion of the talus and calcaneus on the relatively fixed *naviculocuboid unit*. Motion at the compound transverse tarsal joint, however, is more complex than the relatively simple joint line might suggest, and occurs synchronously with motion at the subtalar joint.[29]

Transverse Tarsal Joint Axes

Movements at the transverse tarsal joint are more difficult to study than movement at the ankle or subtalar joint, because multiple segments and axes are involved. Although the talonavicular and calcaneocuboid joints have some independent movement, motion at one is generally accompanied by at least some motion of the other because of their functional, bony, and ligamentous connections. We continue to rely on the classic works of Elftman, Manter, and Hicks, who proposed unique longitudinal and oblique axes around which the talus and calcaneus move on the relatively fixed naviculocuboid unit **(Fig. 12-23)**.[51,72,97] The longitudinal axis of the transverse tarsal joint is nearly horizontal, being inclined 15° upward from the transverse plane (see **Fig. 12-23A**), and is also angled 9° medially from the sagittal plane (see **Fig. 12-23B**).[72] This orientation of the longitudinal axis of the transverse tarsal joint results primarily in inversion/eversion movements. Nevertheless, motion around this axis is triplanar, producing supination/pronation with coupled components (small amounts of dorsiflexion/plantarflexion and abduction/adduction) similar to those seen at the subtalar joint but now simultaneously including both the talus and calcaneus segments moving on the navicular and cuboid segments.

The oblique (transverse) axis of the transverse tarsal joint also contributes to the movements observed at the transverse tarsal joint **(Fig. 12-24)**. This axis is positioned approximately 57° medial to the sagittal plane (see **Fig. 12-24B**) and 52° superior to the transverse plane (see **Fig. 12-24A**).[72] As a triplanar axis, the oblique axis also provides supination/pronation with coupled component movements of the talus and calcaneus segments moving together on the navicular and cuboid bones, but dorsiflexion/plantarflexion and abduction/adduction components predominate over inversion/eversion motions.

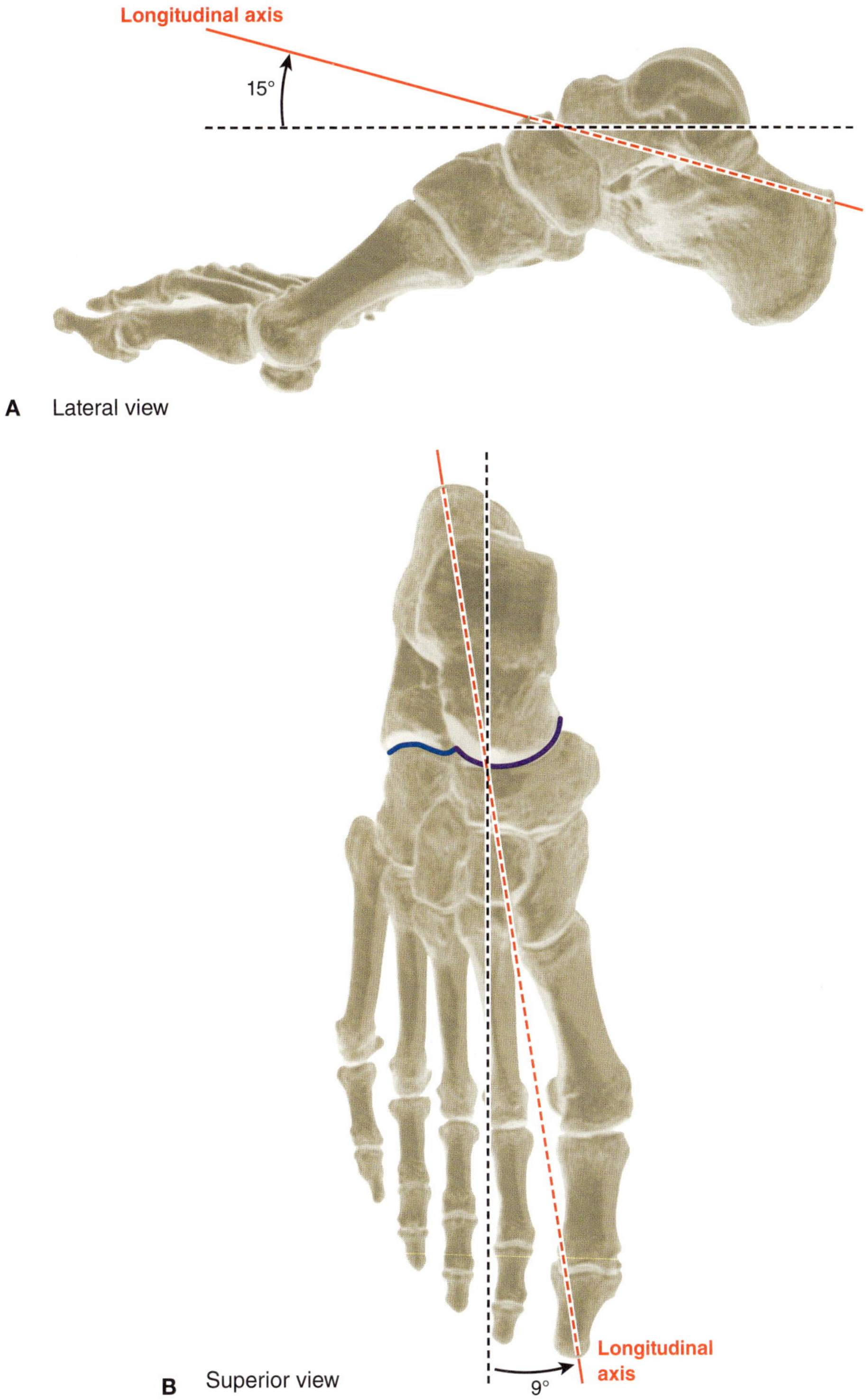

Figure 12–23 The longitudinal axis of the transverse tarsal joint is: **A.** inclined 15° superiorly from the transverse plane, and **B.** inclined 9° medially from the sagittal plane.

Motions about the longitudinal and oblique axes are difficult to separate and quantify. The longitudinal and oblique axes together provide a total range of supination/pronation of the talus and calcaneus that is about one-third to one-half of the range available at the subtalar joint.[51]

The proposed longitudinal and oblique axes for the transverse tarsal joint indicate a function similar to that of the subtalar joint. In fact, as already noted, the subtalar and transverse tarsal joints are linked mechanically so that any weight-bearing subtalar (talocalcaneal) motion causes the talonavicular and calcaneocuboid joints to move simultaneously as well. As the subtalar joint supinates, its linkage to the transverse tarsal joint causes the talonavicular and calcaneocuboid joints to begin to supinate. When the subtalar joint is fully supinated and locked (bony surfaces are drawn together), the transverse tarsal joint is also carried into full

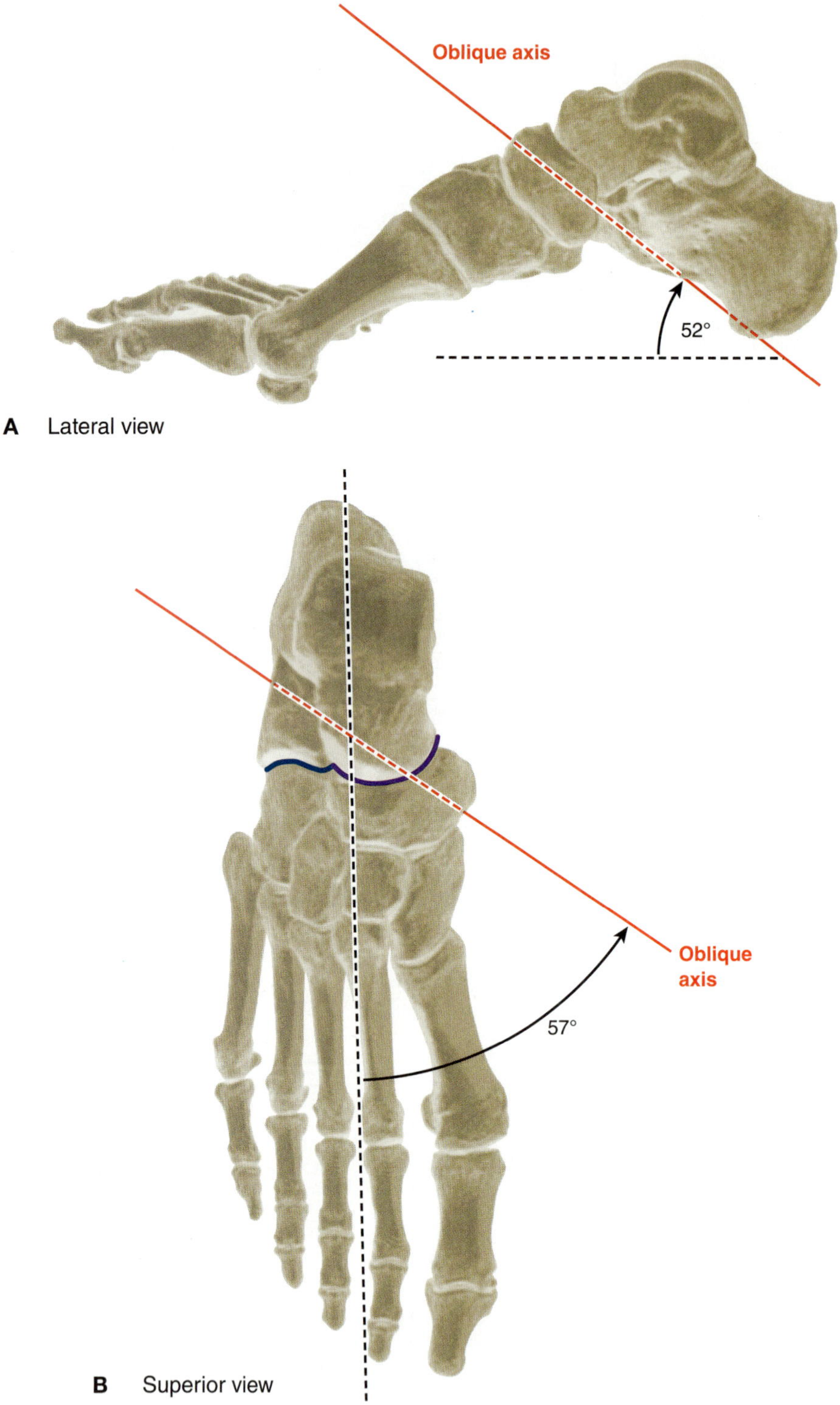

Figure 12–24 The oblique axis of the transverse tarsal joint is: **A.** inclined 52° superiorly from the transverse plane, and **B.** inclined 57° from the sagittal plane.

supination, and its bony surfaces are similarly drawn together into a locked (i.e., closed-packed) position. When the subtalar joint is pronated and loose packed, the transverse tarsal joint is also mobile and loose packed.

The transverse tarsal joint is the transitional link between the rearfoot and the forefoot, serving to (1) add to the supination/pronation range of the subtalar joint, and (2) compensate at the forefoot for rearfoot position. Compensation in this context refers to the ability of the forefoot to remain flat on the ground (relatively immobile) while the rearfoot (talus and calcaneus) pronates or supinates in response to the terrain or the rotations imposed by the leg. The first of the transverse tarsal joint functions (adding range to supination/pronation) can occur either in the weight-bearing foot or in the non–weight-bearing foot. The second function requires closer analysis.

Weight-Bearing Rearfoot Pronation and Transverse Tarsal Joint Motion

In the weight-bearing position, medial rotation of the tibia (as occurs, for example, if someone pivots on a fixed foot) imposes pronation on the subtalar joint. If the pronation force continued distally through the foot, the lateral border of the foot would tend to lift from the ground, diminishing the stability of the base of support, resulting in unequal weight-bearing, and imposing stress at multiple joints. This undesirable effect of weight-bearing subtalar joint pronation may be avoided if the forefoot remains flat on the ground. This can occur so long as the transverse tarsal joint is mobile and can effectively "absorb" the rearfoot pronation (allowing the rearfoot to move without passing the movement on to the forefoot). When the talus and calcaneus move on an essentially fixed naviculocuboid unit, there is a relative supination of the bony segments distal to the transverse tarsal joint (imposed by the rearfoot pronation), with the result that the forefoot remains relatively flat on the ground. The transverse tarsal joint maintains typical weight-bearing forces on the forefoot while allowing the rearfoot (subtalar joint) to absorb the rotation of the lower limb. Inman and Mann's mechanical model **(Fig. 12–25)** nicely represents how a medial rotatory force imposed on the leg acts through the oblique axis of the subtalar joint *and* through the transverse tarsal joint to maintain the forefoot in a relatively fixed position.[66] Note that the fixed *forefoot* has effectively moved in a direction opposite to that of the *rearfoot* segment.

Inman and Mann's model indicates that when the weight-bearing rearfoot (subtalar joint) is pronated, the transverse tarsal joint will supinate, thus moving in a direction opposite to the rearfoot (see **Fig. 12-25A**).[66] However, in reality the transverse tarsal joint is relatively free to move either into pronation or supination (depending on the demands of the terrain) as long as the subtalar joint is pronated (unlocked). In a bilateral standing position on level ground, both the subtalar joint and the transverse tarsal joints pronate slightly (see **Fig. 12–25B**), presumably to allow the foot to absorb the body's weight. As a result of the pronation, there will be a slight medial rotatory force on the leg. As a person moves into single-limb support and begins to walk, the subtalar joint will continue to pronate, but because the forefoot must remain flat on the floor, the transverse tarsal joint will assume an equal amount of relative supination to maintain proper weight-bearing in the forefoot. As a reminder, the relative supination at the transverse tarsal joint in this example arises from the movement of the talus and the calcaneus (rearfoot).

During walking on uneven terrain, as long as the rearfoot is in pronation, the forefoot can move toward either supination or pronation, depending on the demands of the terrain. If, for example, there is a rock under the medial forefoot during walking, the transverse tarsal joint may move into greater supination to maintain appropriate contact of the forefoot with the ground (see **Fig. 12–25C**). If the supination range is not available at the transverse tarsal joint, the rock may also force the rearfoot into a supinated position (putting the lateral collateral ligaments at risk for injury). With other surface demands, such as standing sideways on a steep hill, the uphill foot must pronate substantially to maintain contact with the ground. Therefore, pronation may be required at the subtalar and the transverse tarsal joints. As long as the subtalar joint is in some degree of pronation, the subtalar and transverse tarsal joints are relatively mobile and free to make compensatory changes (within the limits of the joints' ROM) to maintain contact of the foot with the ground.

Weight-Bearing Rearfoot Supination and Transverse Tarsal Joint Motion

As shown in the mechanical model of Inman and Mann, a lateral rotational force on the leg will create subtalar supination in the weight-bearing subtalar joint, with a relative pronation of the transverse tarsal joint (opposite motion of

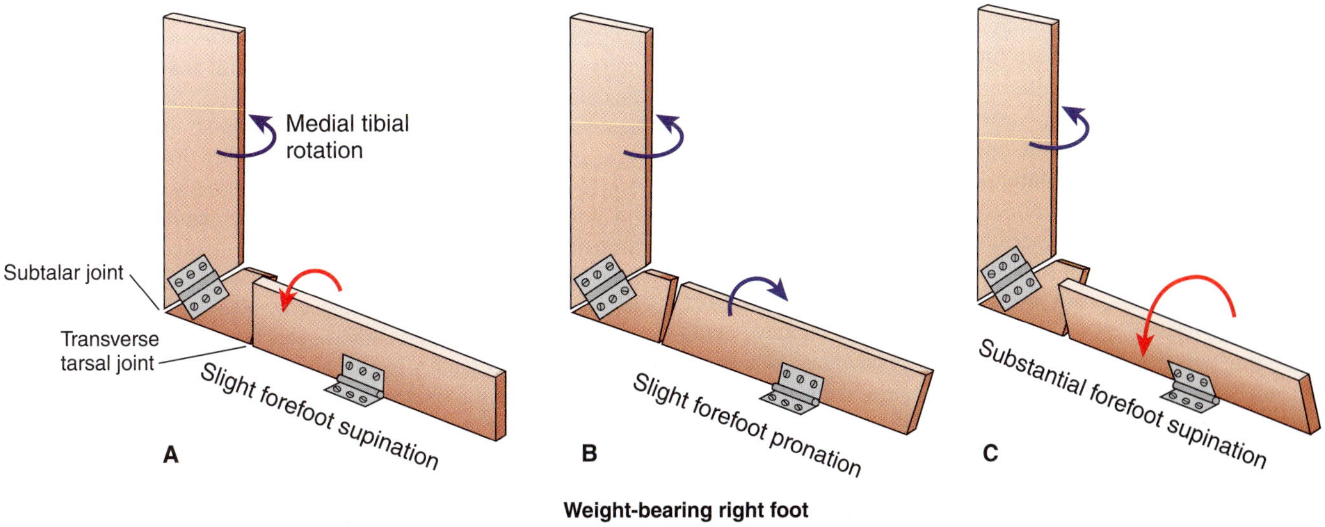

Figure 12–25 With pronation occurring at the subtalar joint through superimposed medial rotation of the right leg, the transverse tarsal joint is free to: **A.** supinate slightly to maintain the relatively fixed position of the forefoot segment; **B.** pronate slightly as occurs in typical standing; or **C.** supinate substantially to maintain appropriate weight-bearing of the forefoot segment on uneven terrain. *(Adapted from Mann RA: Biomechanics of running. In Mann RA [ed]: Surgery of the Foot [ed 5], p. 15. St. Louis, MO, CV Mosby, 1986.)*

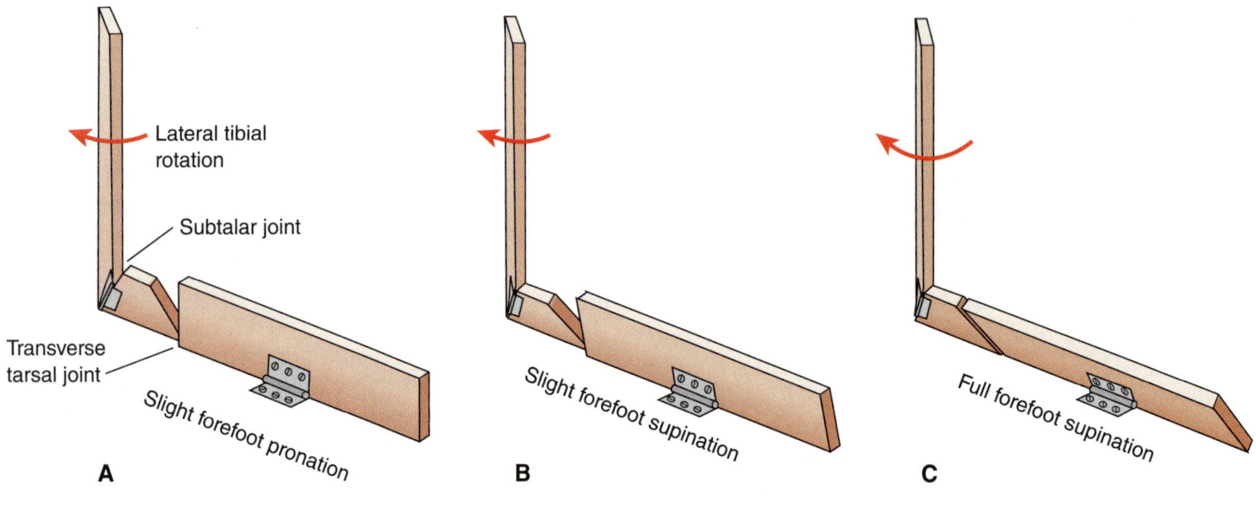

Figure 12–26 **A.** With supination occurring at the subtalar joint through lateral rotation of the right leg, the transverse tarsal joint has limited ability to pronate to maintain the relatively fixed position of the forefoot segment. **B.** The transverse tarsal joint will begin to supinate with a greater range of subtalar supination and lateral rotation of the leg or it will **C.** fully supinate along with a fully supinated subtalar joint and maximal lateral rotation of the superimposed leg and both joints are pulled into close-packed positions.

the forefoot segment) to maintain appropriate weight-bearing on a level surface **(Fig. 12–26)**.[66] Supination of the subtalar joint, however, can proceed to only a certain point before the transverse tarsal joint also begins to supinate. As bony and ligamentous structures of the subtalar joint draw the talus and calcaneus closer together (become increasingly close packed), the navicular and cuboid bones are also drawn toward the talus and calcaneus; that is, transverse tarsal joint mobility is increasingly limited as the subtalar joint moves toward full supination. With increasing supination of the subtalar joint (caused either by the terrain or by an increased lateral rotatory force on the leg), the transverse tarsal joint cannot absorb the additional rotation but begins to move toward supination as well (see **Fig. 12–26B**).

In full subtalar joint supination, such as when the tibia is maximally laterally rotated on the weight-bearing foot, supination locks not only the subtalar joint but also the transverse tarsal joint (see **Fig. 12–26C**). The fully supinated subtalar joint and transverse tarsal joint will tend to shift the weight-bearing in the forefoot fully to the lateral border of the foot. Barring other compensatory mechanisms or when the demands of the terrain exceed the foot's ability to compensate, the entire medial border of the foot may lift and, unless the muscles on the lateral side of the foot and ankle are active, a supination (often called *inversion*) sprain of the lateral ligaments may occur. When the locked subtalar and transverse tarsal joints are unable to absorb the rotation superimposed by the weight-bearing limb or by uneven ground, the forces must be dissipated at the ankle, and excessive stresses may result in injury to the ankle joint structures. The subtalar joint of a high-arched (pes cavus) foot tends to be set in a supinated position with limited pronation motion. This supinated position also limits the ability of the transverse tarsal joint to compensate. Therefore, a high-arched foot is relatively more rigid and may be more susceptible to impact injuries.

Patient Application 12–2

Jackie Montgomery is a 65-year-old woman who is complaining of right foot pain and reports that she did not always have "flat feet." She has pain with active plantarflexion and supination, with some tenderness behind her medial malleolus. Mrs. Montgomery is likely to have progressive collapsing foot deformity, which is a complex condition that results in a progressively worsening pronated foot posture, or pes planus. The cause of this condition is unclear, but it has been suggested that factors such as dysfunction of the posterior tibialis tendon, arthritic changes in the foot and ankle, neuromuscular dysfunction, and trauma may contribute.[98] When posterior tibialis tendon dysfunction contributes to the pronated foot posture, the bony, ligamentous, and capsular structures on the medial aspect of the foot are placed under increased stress, contributing to further collapse of the foot. The pronated foot posture seen in progressive collapsing foot deformity occurs at several sites in the foot/ankle complex and the changes can be flexible or rigid. When clinicians assess for this condition, they look for lengthening of the medial aspect of the rearfoot, the ability to visualize the patient's toes lateral to the patient's heel when standing directly behind the patient (midfoot/forefoot abduction), flattening of the medial longitudinal arch, instability of the subtalar joint, and instability of the talocrural joint.[99] Functionally, these deformities can cause more than a flat foot and pain. Most notably, they have been associated with decreased walking speed, decreased stride length, and decreased cadence.[100] Risk factors for this condition include obesity and a lack of flexibility of the gastrocnemius-soleus complex. Conservative treatment is very effective in the early stages and consists of techniques for decreasing inflammation, such as bracing and activity modification, followed by orthotics, and stretching and strengthening to optimize the function of the foot and ankle complex.[98] Surgical interventions may be necessary for this condition if the deformities are rigid and the pronated foot posture cannot be passively corrected to neutral.[101]

Tarsometatarsal Joints

Tarsometatarsal Axes

Each TMT joint is considered to have a unique, although not fully independent, axis of motion. Hicks examined the axes for each of the five rays.[51] A *ray* is defined as a functional unit formed by a metatarsal and (for the first through third rays) its associated cuneiform bone. The cuneiform bones are included as parts of the movement units of the TMT rays because of the small and relatively insignificant amount of motion occurring at the cuneonavicular joints. The cuneonavicular motion, therefore, becomes functionally part of the available TMT motions. The fourth and fifth rays are formed by the metatarsal alone because these metatarsals share an articulation with the cuboid bone.

According to Hicks, the first and fifth rays exhibit the most motion of the TMT joints[51] **(Fig. 12–27)**. Each axis is oblique and, therefore, triplanar. Of the TMT joints, the first has the largest ROM. The axis of the first ray is inclined so that dorsiflexion of the first ray also includes inversion and adduction, whereas plantarflexion is accompanied by eversion and abduction. The abduction/adduction components typically are minimal. Movements of the fifth ray around its axis are more restricted and occur with the opposite arrangement of components: Dorsiflexion is accompanied by eversion and abduction, and plantarflexion is accompanied by inversion and adduction.

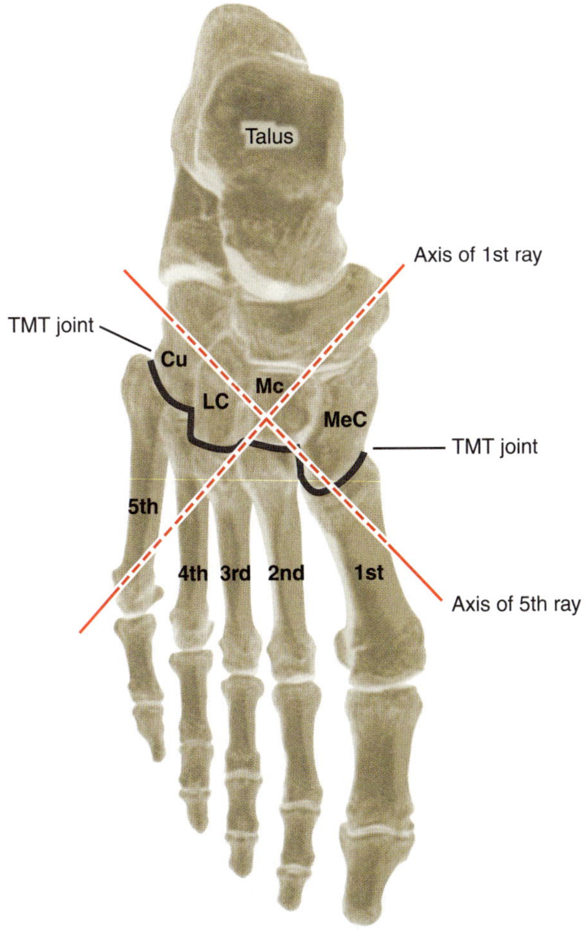

Figure 12–27 Tarsometatarsal (TMT) joint lines and axes for the 1st and 5th TMT joints.

The axis for the third ray nearly coincides with a coronal axis; the predominant motion, therefore, is dorsiflexion/plantarflexion, but is very limited. The axes for the second and fourth rays were not determined by Hicks but were considered to be intermediate between the adjacent axes for the first and fifth rays, respectively.[51] The second ray moves around an axis that is inclined toward, but is not as oblique as, the first axis. The fourth ray moves around an axis that is similar to, but not as steep as, the fifth axis. The second ray is considered to be the least mobile of the five.

The motions of the TMT joints are interdependent, as are the motions of the CMC joints in the hand. Like the CMC joints of the hand, the TMT joints contribute to hollowing and flattening of the foot. For example, as the rays of the forefoot produce inversion together, the first ray must also dorsiflex (along with the second ray to a very small extent), whereas the fifth ray (and to a small extent the fourth ray) must plantarflex. In contrast to the hand, however, the greatest relevance of TMT joint motions is found during weight-bearing. In weight-bearing, the TMT joints function primarily to augment the function of the transverse tarsal joint; that is, the TMT joints attempt to regulate position of the metatarsals and phalanges (the forefoot) in relation to the weight-bearing surface.[102] As long as transverse tarsal joint motion is adequate to compensate for the rearfoot position, considerable TMT joint motion is not required. However, when the rearfoot position is at an end point in its available ROM or the transverse tarsal joint is inadequate to provide full compensation, the TMT joints may rotate to provide further adjustment of forefoot position.[80]

Supination Twist

When the rearfoot pronates substantially in weight-bearing, the transverse tarsal joint generally will supinate to some degree to counterrotate the forefoot and keep the plantar aspect of the foot in contact with the ground. If the range of transverse tarsal supination is not sufficient to meet the demands of the pronating rearfoot (or if the transverse tarsal joint is prevented from effectively serving this function), the medial forefoot will press into the ground, and the lateral forefoot will tend to lift. The first and second ray will be pushed into dorsiflexion by the ground reaction force, and the muscles controlling the fourth and fifth rays will plantarflex the TMT joints in an attempt to maintain contact with the ground. Both dorsiflexion of the first and second rays and plantarflexion of the fourth and fifth rays include the component motion of inversion of the ray. Consequently, the entire forefoot (each ray and its associated toe) undergoes an inversion rotation around a hypothetical axis at the second ray. This rotation is referred to as *supination twist* of the TMT joints.[51]

As an example of supination twist of the forefoot, **Figure 12–28** shows the response of the segments of the foot to a strong pronation torque across the subtalar joint that may be caused either by a strong medial rotatory force from the leg or by inadequate support of the arch. In weight-bearing pronation, the calcaneus everts, and the talus plantarflexes and adducts in space. With sufficient pronation, the navicular bone is pushed

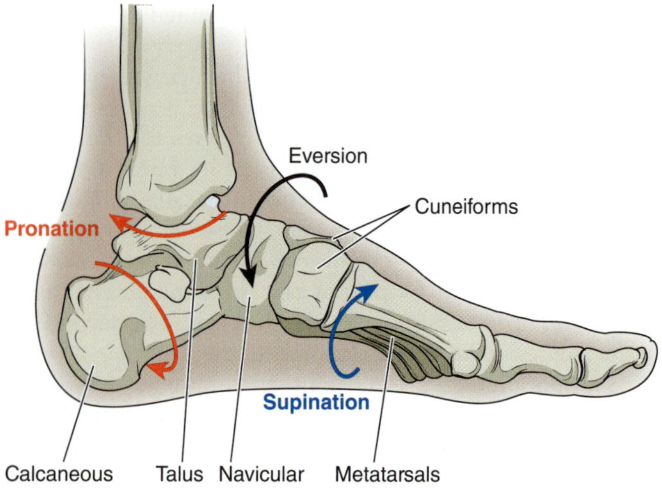

Figure 12–28 Extreme pronation at the subtalar joint is accompanied by adduction and plantarflexion of the head of the talus, eversion of the calcaneus, and (in some instances) pronation at the transverse tarsal joint as a result of the navicular bone being forced down by the talus. If the forefoot is to remain on the ground, the tarsometatarsal joints must undergo a counteracting supination twist.

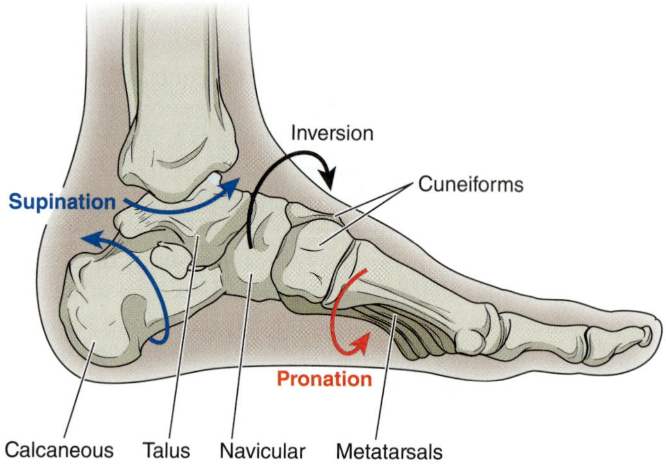

Figure 12–29 Extreme supination at the subtalar joint is accompanied by abduction and dorsiflexion of the head of the talus, inversion of the calcaneus, and forced supination of the transverse tarsal joint. If the forefoot is to remain on the ground, the tarsometatarsal joints must undergo a counteracting pronation twist.

downward by the motion of the talar head, thus limiting the ability of the transverse tarsal joint to supinate adequately. The first and second rays will dorsiflex and invert, whereas the fourth and fifth rays will plantarflex and invert. This results in a supination (inversion) twist of the TMT joints to attempt to adequately adjust the forefoot. Because the five TMT joints have some independence, the configuration of the forefoot in a supination twist can vary according to the weight-bearing needs of the foot and the terrain.

Pronation Twist

When both the rearfoot and the transverse tarsal joints are locked in supination, the adjustment of forefoot position must be left entirely to the TMT joints. With rearfoot supination, the forefoot tends to lift off the ground on its medial side and press into the ground on its lateral side. The muscles controlling the first and second rays will cause the rays to plantarflex to maintain contact with the ground, whereas the fourth and fifth rays are forced into dorsiflexion by the ground reaction force. Because eversion accompanies both plantarflexion of the first and second rays and dorsiflexion of the fourth and fifth rays, the forefoot as a whole undergoes a pronation twist.[51]

Pronation twist, like supination twist, can vary in configuration. Although the pronation twist may provide adequate counterrotation for moderate rearfoot supination, it may be inadequate to maintain forefoot stability in extreme supination. In **Figure 12–29**, subtalar supination results in calcaneal inversion, with dorsiflexion and abduction of the talus. The transverse tarsal joint will have little if any ability to pronate, given that the navicular and cuboid bones are carried along with the rearfoot motion. The first and second rays will plantarflex and evert, whereas the fourth and fifth rays will dorsiflex and evert, which results in a pronation (eversion) twist of the TMT joints in an attempt to adequately adjust the forefoot.

Pronation twist and supination twist of the TMT joints occur only when the transverse tarsal joint function is inadequate, that is, when the transverse tarsal joint is unable to counterrotate or when the transverse tarsal joint range is insufficient to fully compensate for rearfoot position.

Metatarsophalangeal Joints

Although multiple degrees of freedom might be useful to the MTP joints in rare instances, like when the foot participates in some kind of grasping activities, flexion and extension are the predominant functional movements at these joints. During the late stance phase of walking, toe extension at the MTP joints permits the foot to pass over the toes, whereas the metatarsal heads and toes help balance the superimposed body weight through activity of the intrinsic and extrinsic toe flexor muscles, coupled with the passive rigidity imposed within the supinated hindfoot. Like the MCP joints of the hand the MTP joints have two degrees of freedom, but flexion/extension motion is much greater than abduction/adduction motion, and extension exceeds flexion. It should be noted that abduction/adduction at the MTP joints are identified in reference to the defined midline of the foot—a longitudinal line through the foot and second toe **(Fig. 12–30)**. Although MTP motions can occur in weight-bearing or non–weight-bearing, the MTP joints serve primarily to allow the weight-bearing foot to rotate over the toes through MTP extension (known as the *metatarsal break*) when rising on the toes or during walking.

Metatarsophalangeal Extension and the Metatarsal Break

The metatarsal break derives its name from the hinge or *break* that occurs at the MTP joints as the heel rises and the metatarsal heads and toes remain weight-bearing. The metatarsal break occurs as MTP extension around a single oblique axis that lies through the second to fifth metatarsal heads. The axis is oblique because of the diminishing lengths of the metatarsals

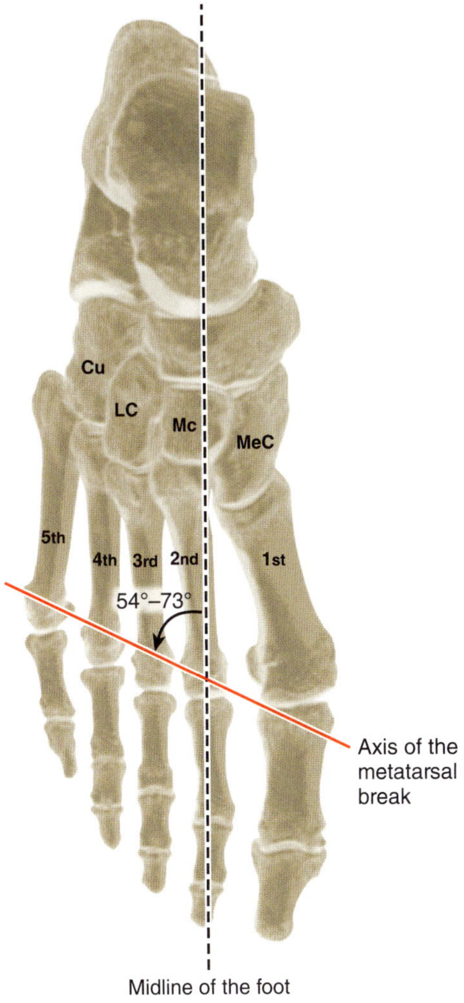

Figure 12–30 Abduction/adduction at the MTP joints are identified relative to movement away from the midline (abduction) or toward the midline (adduction). The metatarsal break occurs around an oblique axis that passes through the heads of the four lesser toes (toes 2–5), at an angle to the long axis of the foot that varies widely among studied individuals from 54° to 73°.

from the second through the fifth rays, but the orientation of this axis varies among individuals. The angle of the axis around which the metatarsal break occurs may range from 54° to 73° with respect to the long axis of the foot.[103] The range of MTP extension will vary depending on the amount of dorsiflexion/plantarflexion motion at the TMT joints, the age of the individual, and whether the motion is assessed in weight-bearing or non–weight-bearing.[104,105] Limited-extension ROM at the first MTP joint will interfere with the metatarsal break and is known as *hallux rigidus.* Limited first MTP extension can affect gait, particularly impairing typical push-off.[106,107]

For the heel to rise while weight-bearing, there must be an active contraction of ankle plantarflexor musculature. Most of the plantarflexion muscles also contribute to supination of the subtalar and transverse tarsal joints. The plantarflexion musculature typically cannot lift the heel completely unless the joints of the rearfoot and midfoot are supinated and locked so that the foot can become a rigid lever from the calcaneus through the metatarsals. This rigid lever will then rotate ("break") around the MTP axis (see Fig. 12-30). As MTP joint extension occurs, the convex metatarsal heads slide in a plantar direction on the concave phalanges and their MTP plantar plates that are stabilized by the supporting surface. The metatarsal heads and toes become the base of support, and the body's line of gravity (LoG) must move to stay within this base to remain stable. The obliquity of the axis for the metatarsal break allows weight to be distributed across the metatarsal heads and toes more evenly than would occur if the axis were truly coronal. If the body weight passed forward through the foot and the metatarsal break occurred around a *coronal* MTP axis, an excessive amount of weight would be placed on the first and second metatarsal heads. These two toes would also require a disproportionately large extension range. The obliquity of the axis of the metatarsal break shifts the weight laterally, minimizing the large load on the first two digits.

Expanded Concepts 12–5

Hammer Toe Deformity

The plantar plate provides stability to the lesser MTP joints (joints 2–5) by restricting extension motion and holding the first phalanx securely on the metatarsal head. Repetitive stress to, and subsequent breakdown of, the plantar plate can be caused by impaired control of the muscles of the foot, as with individuals with diabetic peripheral neuropathy, or by altered foot biomechanics caused by factors such as a longer second metatarsal or wearing high-heeled shoes. Breakdown of the plantar plate can result in instability of the lesser MTP joints. Initially, instability at these joints presents as a painful forefoot. As the structure of the plantar plate further deteriorates, the first phalanx can subluxate or even dislocate dorsally on the metatarsal head. This results in a hyperextension deformity, or hammer toe, at the MTP joint. When the lesser MTP joints are resting in a position of hyperextension, the function of the interosseous muscles is altered, and the interosseous muscles are now oriented to act as extensors of the MTP joints, rather than flexors. This, combined with the new orientation of the lumbricals relative to the MTP joint axis, can further exacerbate the hyperextension deformity at the MTP joint.[108]

Hammer toe deformities are especially common in individuals with diabetes and peripheral neuropathy, presumably because of impaired neuromuscular function of the intrinsic foot muscles. In this population, hammer toe deformity has been reported to be associated with increased plantar pressures during walking.[109] Increased forces during walking may contribute to increased skin breakdown and heightened risk of wounds, making a thorough foot assessment important for patients with diabetes. **Figure 12–31** shows a healthy foot and a hammer toe deformity in a patient with diabetic peripheral neuropathy.

Metatarsophalangeal Flexion, Abduction, and Adduction

Flexion ROM at the MTP joints can occur to a limited degree from neutral position but has relatively little purpose in the weight-bearing foot other than when the supporting terrain drops away distal to the metatarsal heads. Most MTP flexion occurs as a return to neutral position from extension. However, the ability to generate adequate flexor force by the toe flexor musculature is *quite important* and should be distinguished from

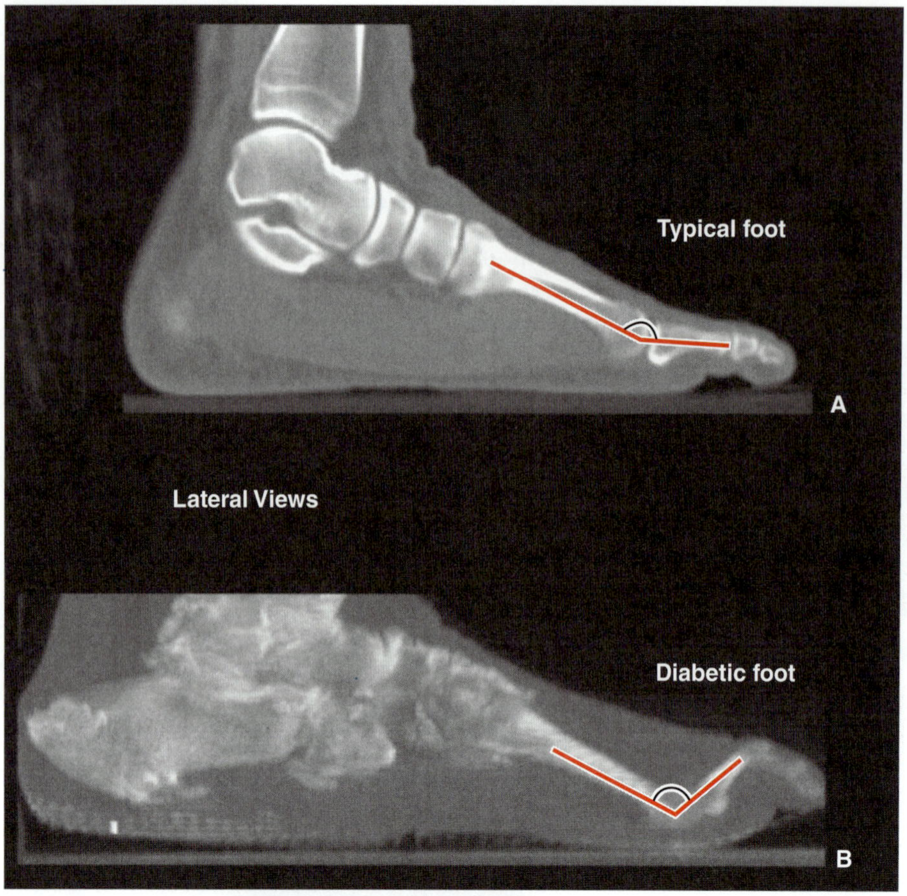

Figure 12–31 **A.** Radiographic image of a foot from a healthy subject and **B.** a foot from a person with diabetes and peripheral neuropathy. The diabetic foot shows a hammer toe deformity (hyperextension at the MTP joint and flexion at the IP joint).

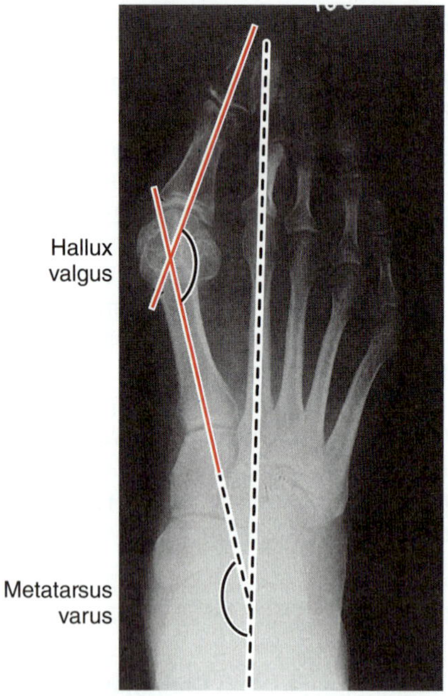

Figure 12–32 Right Foot. A radiograph showing both a hallux valgus at the first MTP joint, and a metatarsus varus at the first TMT joint. The excessive bony growth at the head of the first metatarsal is due to abnormal pressures from the malalignment.

the functionally less relevant MTP flexion ROM. Abduction and adduction of the MTP joint appear to be helpful in absorbing some of the force that would be imposed on the toes by the metatarsals as they move in a pronation or supination twist. Recalling that MTP abduction/adduction reference the midline of the foot (see Fig. 12-30), the first toe typically is abducted on the first metatarsal about 15° to 19°.[41,109] An increase in this typical valgus angulation of the first MTP joint is referred to as *hallux valgus* and may be associated with a varus angulation of the first metatarsal at the TMT joint, known as *metatarsus varus* **(Fig. 12–32)**.

Patient Application 12–3

Jared Brown recently visited his physician because of right foot pain at his first MTP joint. By inspection, he has an evident hallux valgus deformity. Hallux valgus can result in or may be associated with a reduction in first MTP joint ROM, gradual lateral subluxation of the toe flexor tendons crossing the first MTP joint, reduced weight-bearing on the great toe, and increased weight-bearing on the first metatarsal head.[110] These structural changes can lead to pain and difficulty during walking. People with a pronated foot may push off during walking with a greater-than-typical adductor moment on the great toe that pushes the toe into a valgus (MTP joint adducted) position. Localized swelling and pain at the medial or dorsal aspect of the first MTP joint may be related to an inflamed medial bursa and is commonly called a *bunion.* The etiology of hallux valgus deformities is likely multifactorial and related to repetitive forces applied to the first MTP joint.[110] The person with a flat foot deformity and excessive pronation like Mr. Brown may have instability and excessive mobility of the first ray, contributing to the hallux valgus deformity.[111] In addition to excessive pronation and first ray mobility, risk factors may include improper shoe wear, and genetic predisposition.[112,113]

Expanded Concepts 12–6
Varus/Valgus Terminology

Varus and *valgus* are consistently used to refer to a decrease or increase, respectively, in the medial angle. However, in the ankle and foot (as we've seen elsewhere), the reference lines and the resulting angles keep changing. In the rearfoot, we already noted that varus/valgus either can be synonyms for inversion/eversion of the calcaneus (see Fig. 12–20) or may refer to fixed positioning of the subtalar joint in excessive supination or pronation (see Fig. 12–3). In both cases, the reference lines are the posterior leg and a line bisecting the posterior calcaneus. *Metatarsus varus* is a deformity appropriately identified as a *decrease* in the medial angle between the long axis of the metatarsal and the long axis of the foot (or abduction of the metatarsal if referencing the midline of the foot). Metatarsus varus is typically accompanied by *hallux valgus,* a deformity identified by an *increase* in the medial angle between the long axes of the metatarsal and proximal phalanx (or adduction of the proximal phalanx toward the midline of the foot) (see Fig. 12–32). We also defined forefoot varus as a fixed supination twist of the forefoot in relation to a neutral subtalar joint. In this instance, the medial angle is formed by a line through the metatarsal heads and a line bisecting the "neutral" subtalar joint. Unfortunately, the terminology may appear contradictory because of the shift in reference lines. For example, varus/valgus at the TMT and MTP joints can be either abduction or adduction at a TMT or MTP joint depending on the reference line. *Varus* of the first metatarsal (metatarsus varus) is *abduction* of the first metatarsal away from the long axis of the foot, while a similarly named *varus* deformity of the third toe is *adduction* of the third metacarpal toward the same reference line. One must be aware of reference lines to assure correct terminology.

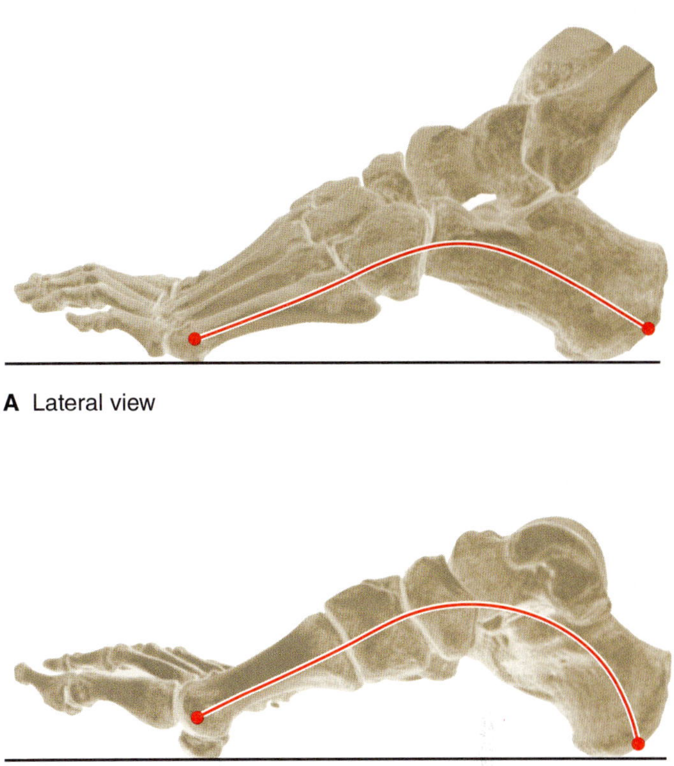

Figure 12–33 The longitudinal arch viewed from: **A.** the lateral side of the foot and **B.** the medial side of the foot. It can be seen that the lateral arch is smaller than the medial arch.

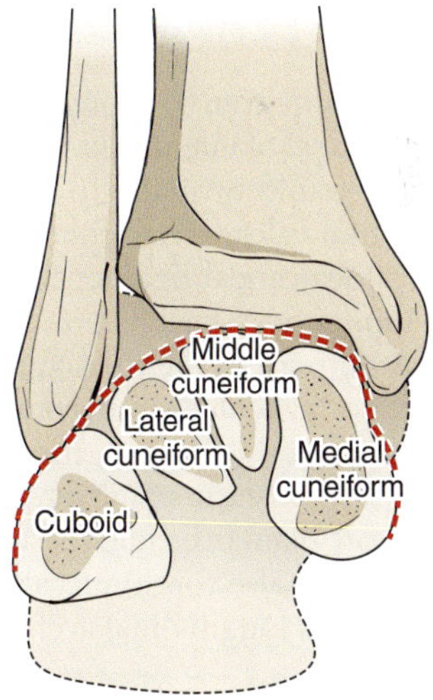

Figure 12–34 The transverse arch at the level of the middle of the tarsals.

Plantar Arches

Although we have examined the function of the joints of the foot individually and discussed the effect of each joint on contiguous joints, combined function is best investigated by looking at the behavior of the arch-like structures of the foot. The foot typically is characterized as having three arches: **medial** and **lateral longitudinal arches** and a **transverse arch**. The medial longitudinal arch is the largest and most commonly discussed. Although we may think of and refer to the three arches as if they were separate, the arches are fully integrated with one another (being more analogous to a segmented continuous vault) to enhance the dynamic function of the foot. The arches are usually not present at birth but evolve with the progression of weight-bearing. Flattened longitudinal arches are seen in younger children, less than 5 years of age. When gait parameters become similar to that of an adult (around age 5), the majority of children will develop a typical arch.[114] One study found that flat foot was prevalent in 54% of children at 3 years of age, decreasing to 25% by the age of 6, and 4% to 15% by 10 years of age.[115]

Structure of the Arches

The longitudinal arches are anchored posteriorly at the calcaneus and anteriorly at the metatarsal heads (**Fig. 12–33**). The longitudinal arch is continuous both laterally (see **Fig. 12–33A**) and medially (see **Fig. 12–33B**) through the foot. However, because the medial arch is higher than its lower lateral counterpart, the medial side usually is the side of reference. The talus rests at the top of the vault of the foot and is considered to be the "keystone" of the arch. All weight transferred from the body to the heel or the forefoot must pass through the talus.

The transverse arch, like the longitudinal arch, is a continuous structure (**Fig. 12–34**). The transverse arch can be visualized at the distal metatarsals where the second metatarsal, recessed into its mortise, is at the apex of the arch. Visualized in the

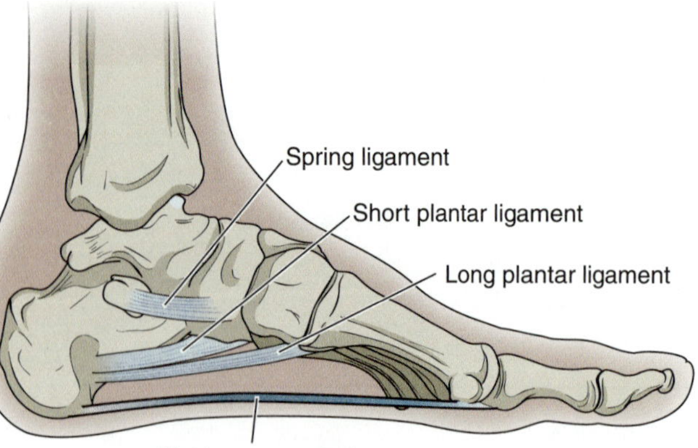

Figure 12–35 The medial longitudinal arch with its associated ligamentous support, including the plantar aponeurosis. The more laterally located short plantar ligament would not ordinarily be seen in a medial view, but it is shown here as if projected "through" the foot.

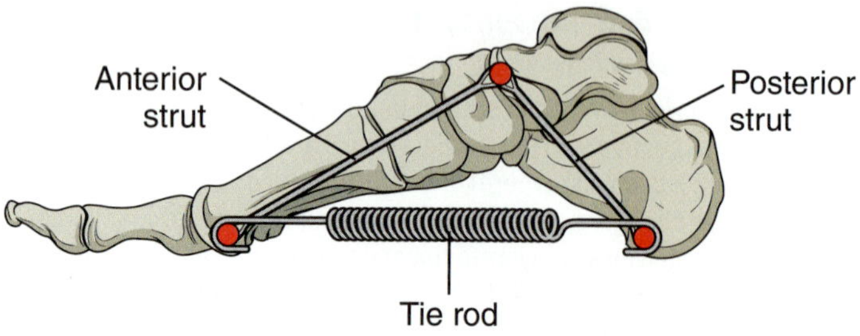

Figure 12–36 The foot can be considered to function as a truss and tie rod, with the calcaneus and talus serving as the posterior strut, the remainder of the tarsals and the metatarsals serving as the anterior strut, and the plantar aponeurosis serving as a tensed tie rod (analogous to a triangle). Weighting the foot will compress the struts (as the force on the apex of the triangle attempts to flatten it), while creating additional tension in the tie rod as the tie rod (the aponeurosis) "resists" flattening of the triangle.

midfoot at the level of the TMT joints, the middle cuneiform forms the keystone of the arch.

The shape and arrangement of the bones are partially responsible for stability of the plantar arches. As illustrated in Figure 12–34, the wedge-shaped midtarsal bones provide an inherent stability to the transverse arch. The inclination of the calcaneus and first metatarsal contribute to stability of the medial longitudinal arch, particularly in standing (see Fig. 12–33B). Although the structure of the tarsal bones provides a certain inherent stability to the arches, the arches would collapse without additional support from ligaments and muscles.

Because the three arches can be thought of as a segmented vault or one continuous set of interdependent linkages, support at one point in the system contributes to support throughout the system. The plantar calcaneonavicular (spring) ligament, the interosseous talocalcaneal ligament, deltoid ligament, and the plantar aponeurosis have been credited with providing key passive support to the medial longitudinal arch **(Fig. 12–35)**.[116,117] The "articular" (superomedial) portion of the spring ligament directly supports the head of the talus and is the most important static stabilizer.[29,116] The laterally located long and short plantar ligaments support the lateral longitudinal arch and may also contribute, although indirectly, in supporting the medial longitudinal arch.

Function of the Arches

Although the archlike structures of the foot are similar to the palmar arches of the hand, the purpose served by each of these systems is quite different. The arches of the hand are structured predominantly to facilitate grasping and manipulation, but they must also assist the hand in occasional weight-bearing functions. In contrast, the foot in most individuals is rarely called on to perform any grasping activities. The plantar arches are adapted uniquely to serve *both* mobility and stability weight-bearing functions.[118] First, the foot must accept weight during early stance phase and adapt to various surface shapes. To accomplish this weight-bearing *mobility* function, the plantar arches must be flexible enough to allow the foot to (1) dampen the impact of weight-bearing forces, (2) dampen superimposed rotational motions, and (3) adapt to changes in the supporting surface. To accomplish weight-bearing *stability* functions, the arches must allow (1) distribution of weight through the foot for proper weight-bearing and (2) conversion of the flexible foot to a rigid lever for push-off. The mobility-stability functions of the arches of the weight-bearing foot may be examined by looking at the role of the plantar aponeurosis and the distribution of weight through the foot during different activities.

Plantar Aponeurosis

The plantar aponeurosis (plantar fascia) is a dense fascia that runs nearly the entire length of the foot. It begins posteriorly on the medial tubercle of the calcaneus and continues anteriorly to attach by digitations to the plantar plates and then, via the plates, to the proximal phalanx of each toe (see Fig. 12–35).[35,119] As we shall see, the distal attachments of the aponeurosis to the plantar plates and phalanges are critical to its function. From the beginning to the end of the stance phase of gait, tension on the plantar aponeurosis increases, with maximum tension averaging 96% of body weight.[120] This increase in tension through the plantar aponeurosis arises as force is transmitted from the Achilles tendon to the forefoot.[120] In vivo experiments using radiographic fluoroscopy have shown that the plantar fascia deforms, or stretches, 9% to 12% during the stance phase of gait.[121] For this reason, the function of the aponeurosis in supporting the arches has been compared with the function of a tie rod on a truss in classic descriptions.[122] The truss and the tie rod form a triangle **(Fig. 12–36)**; the two struts of the truss form the sides of the triangle and the tie rod is the bottom. The talus and calcaneus form the posterior strut, and the remaining tarsal and metatarsals form the anterior strut. The plantar aponeurosis, as the tie rod, holds together the anterior and posterior struts when the body weight is loaded on the triangle. This structural design is efficient for the weight-bearing foot because the struts (bones) are subjected to compression forces as the body weight attempts to flatten the triangle; the tie rod (aponeurosis) is subjected to tension forces as it "resists" flattening of the triangle.

The role of the plantar aponeurosis in providing arch support is linked to the relationship between the plantar aponeurosis and the MTP joint. When the toes are extended at the MTP joints (regardless of whether the motion is active or passive, weight-bearing or non–weight-bearing), the plantar aponeurosis is pulled increasingly tight as the proximal phalanges slide dorsally in relation to the metatarsals or as the metatarsal heads slide in a relatively plantar direction on the fixed toes (e.g., during calf raises). The metatarsal heads act as pulleys around which the plantar aponeurosis is pulled and tightened. When the plantar aponeurosis is pulled and tightened with MTP extension, the added tension in the aponeurosis (tie rod) draws the heel and MTP joint toward each other, raising the arch and contributing to supination of the foot **(Fig. 12–37)**. The phenomenon of pulling the aponeurosis tighter as it wraps around the extending toes has been referred to as the *windlass mechanism*; this mechanism allows the plantar aponeurosis to increase its role in supporting the arches as the heel rises and the foot rotates around the MTP joints in weight-bearing (during the metatarsal break).[123]

The tension in the plantar aponeurosis (the tie rod) in the loaded foot is evident if active or passive MTP extension is attempted while the triangle is flattened (that is, when the subtalar and transverse tarsal joint are pronated). In this example, the range of MTP extension will be limited because the plantar aponeurosis is already loaded (lengthened by lowering the triangle), and resists further lengthening. Alternatively, raising the height of the triangle by acting on the struts can unload the tie rod. For example, when the tibia is subjected to a lateral rotatory force, the rearfoot will supinate, the posterior strut will become more oblique, the height of the medial longitudinal arch will increase, and the plantar aponeurosis (the tie rod) will be relatively *unloaded*. The reduction in tension in the plantar aponeurosis will allow an increase in the range of MTP extension.

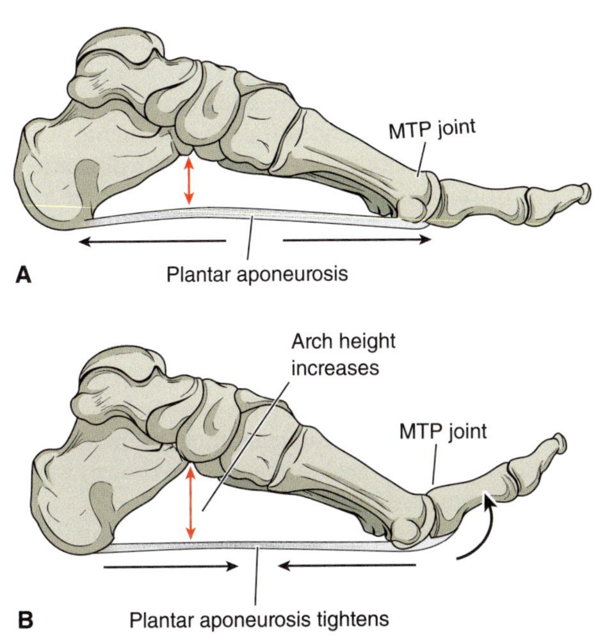

Figure 12–37 Windlass mechanism. **A.** The right foot with MTP joints in neutral. **B.** Elevation of the arch with toe extension occurs as the plantar aponeurosis *winds* around the metatarsal heads and draws the two ends of the aponeurosis toward each other.

Through the pulley effect of the MTP joints on the plantar aponeurosis, the plantar aponeurosis acts interdependently with the joints of the rearfoot to contribute to increasing the longitudinal arch (supination of the foot) as the heel rises during the metatarsal break, thus contributing to converting the foot to a rigid lever for effective push-off. The tightened plantar aponeurosis also increases the passive *flexor* force at the MTP joints, preventing excessive toe extension that might stress the MTP joint, or affect stability if the LoG moves anterior to the toes. Finally, the passive flexor force of the tensed plantar aponeurosis also assists the active toe flexor musculature in pressing the toes into the ground to support the body weight on its now limited base of support.

Foundational Concepts 12–5
Summary of Tie Rod and Truss Relations

- Tension in the plantar aponeurosis (the tie rod) caused by MTP joint extension can draw the rearfoot and forefoot (the struts) together to raise the longitudinal arch (supinate the foot).
- Supination of the weight-bearing foot through lateral rotation of the leg or by applying a varus force to the calcaneus will decrease the angle between the struts (raise the apex of the triangle) and release tension in the tie rod (plantar aponeurosis).
- Flattening of the triangle (pronation of the foot) in weight-bearing will increase tension in the plantar aponeurosis (the tie rod) and limit MTP joint extension.

Patient Application 12–4

Stacy Miller is a 40-year-old woman who has had plantar fasciitis (inflammation of the fascia/aponeurosis) for about 6 months. Her pain is worst at the medial calcaneal tubercle where the plantar aponeurosis inserts on the calcaneus, but she also feels pain along much of the plantar aspect of her foot. Stacy's symptoms are worst when she takes her first steps after being non–weight-bearing for a period of time, such as first thing in the morning, or after sitting at her desk for a few hours. After Stacy's first painful steps, her symptoms briefly ease. If she walks for more than about 5 minutes, her pain worsens again. Stacy is at risk for plantar fasciitis because of her apparent decreased ankle dorsiflexion ROM, higher body mass index, and participation in recreational running.[124] These factors may contribute to increased risk for plantar fasciitis because they apply high levels of force to the plantar aponeurosis that result in degenerative or inflammatory damage to the tissue.[1] Many of the evidence-based interventions for plantar fasciitis include strategies for decreasing the stress on the plantar aponeurosis. For example, because both the calf muscles and the plantar aponeurosis attach to the calcaneus, stretching of or applying manual therapy to the calf muscles may improve the flexibility of the calf muscles and allow them to absorb some of the excess forces that are put on Stacy's plantar aponeurosis. Stretching of the plantar aponeurosis is also supported as an intervention.[124] This may be an effective treatment because stretching applies a level of stress that is greater than that of the maintenance levels but is not sufficient to cause tissue damage. This may encourage the tissue to adapt to these increased loads and, ultimately, tolerate higher levels of stress. Applying tape to support the medial longitudinal arch is also recommended for patients with plantar fasciitis because it may help to unload the tissue while its microtears begin to heal.[124]

Weight Distribution

Because the foot is a flexible rather than fixed arch, the distribution of body weight through the foot depends on many factors, including the shape of the arch and the location of the LoG at any given moment. Distribution of superimposed body weight begins with the talus because the body of the talus receives all the weight that passes down through the leg. Therefore, each talus receives 50% and 100% of the superimposed body weight in bilateral or unilateral stance, respectively. At least 50% of the weight received by the talus passes through the large posterior subtalar articulation to the calcaneus, and 50% or less passes anteriorly through the talonavicular and calcaneocuboid joints. The pattern of weight distribution through the foot can be seen by looking at the trabeculae in the bones of the foot **(Fig. 12–38)**. Because of the more medial location of the talar head, about twice as much weight passes through the talonavicular joint as through the calcaneocuboid joint. The somewhat lesser roles of the more laterally located long and short plantar ligaments in supporting the longitudinal arch may be attributable to the reduced weight-bearing compression through the calcaneocuboid joint in comparison with the more medially located talonavicular joint.[125]

Generally during quiet standing, the rearfoot and forefoot bear a majority of the force. When comparing these two regions, a larger load was found under the rearfoot compared to forefoot.[126] The distribution of weight-bearing, however, can be variable and largely depends on foot type, whether pes planus, pes cavus, or "typical."[127]

Plantar pressures are much greater during walking than during standing, with the highest pressures typically under the metatarsal heads and occurring during the push-off phase of walking (at ~80% of the stance phase), when only the forefoot is in contact with the ground and is pushing to accelerate the body forward.[128] Plantar pressure under the foot during walking arises from a complex interaction of multiple factors. These factors include physical characteristics such as age, body weight, and height, as well as foot structure, such as arch height, hallux length, and joint motion.[129-133] Gait style and muscle action will also influence plantar pressures.[129] As walking progresses to running, plantar force and peak pressures increase. For example, maximum plantar force increased from 1.11 to 2.14 times body weight when walking was compared with running.[134] Excessive plantar pressures can contribute to pain and injury in otherwise healthy people or contribute to skin breakdown in patients with diabetes and peripheral neuropathy. Structural and functional factors such as hammer toe deformity, soft tissue thickness, hallux valgus, foot type, and walking speed have been shown to be important predictors of forefoot plantar pressures during walking in people with diabetes.[109]

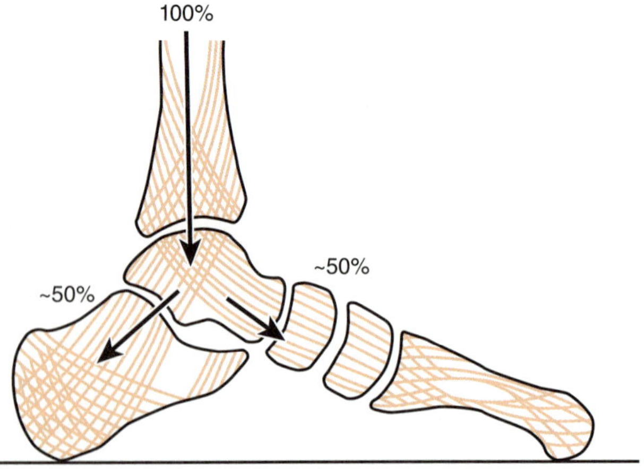

Figure 12–38 Whether in unilateral or bilateral stance, the talus receives all the weight passing through the tibia. Trabeculae of the bones on the medial aspect of the foot show trabecular density at the tibiotalar interface, as well as force distribution by trabecular lines with 50% of the received body weight passing posteriorly to the calcaneus and 50% anteriorly to the forefoot through the talonavicular and calcaneocuboid joints.

Muscular Contribution to the Arches

The role of muscle activity in maintaining and supporting the arches of the foot has not been well defined. Extrinsic muscles that include the posterior tibialis, anterior tibialis, fibularis longus, flexor digitorum longus, and fibularis tertius have all been found to play a role in dynamic arch support.[116,135,136] The posterior tibialis has been shown to have the most consistent function in medial longitudinal arch support.[116] The plantar intrinsic muscles also provide support to the arch in static standing.[137]

Muscles of the Ankle and Foot

As discussed throughout this chapter, muscle activity is critical for the dynamic stability and integration of movement at multiple joints of the foot. There are no muscles in the ankle or foot that cross and act on only one joint in isolation; all muscles act on at least two joints or joint complexes. Muscle function is dependent upon the muscle's structure and, of course, where the muscle passes in relation to each joint axis the muscle crosses. The position of the ankle/foot muscles with respect to the talocrural joint axis and subtalar joint axis is represented in **Figure 12–39**. As illustrated in this figure, all muscles that pass anterior to the talocrural (ankle) joint (in blue) will create dorsiflexion torques or moments, whereas those that pass posterior to the axis will create plantarflexion moments. Muscles that pass medial to the subtalar axis (in red) will create supination moments at the subtalar joint, and those that pass lateral to the subtalar axis will create pronation moments. A muscle, of course, can (and will) create both an ankle joint and a subtalar joint moment simultaneously. For example, the tibialis anterior muscle passes anterior to the talocrural axis *and* medial to the subtalar joint axis, consequently creating a simultaneous dorsiflexion moment at the ankle and a supination moment at the subtalar joint. An understanding of the position of the muscle with respect to the axis is critical for understanding its function.

A brief overview of muscle function is presented in this chapter with a more comprehensive description of the muscles described in Chapters 13 and 14. Extrinsic ankle/foot muscles are those that arise proximal to the ankle and insert onto the foot. Intrinsic foot muscle attachments are entirely within the foot (do not cross the ankle). Extrinsic muscles will be divided further into the three compartments based on their location in the leg: the posterior, lateral, and anterior compartments.

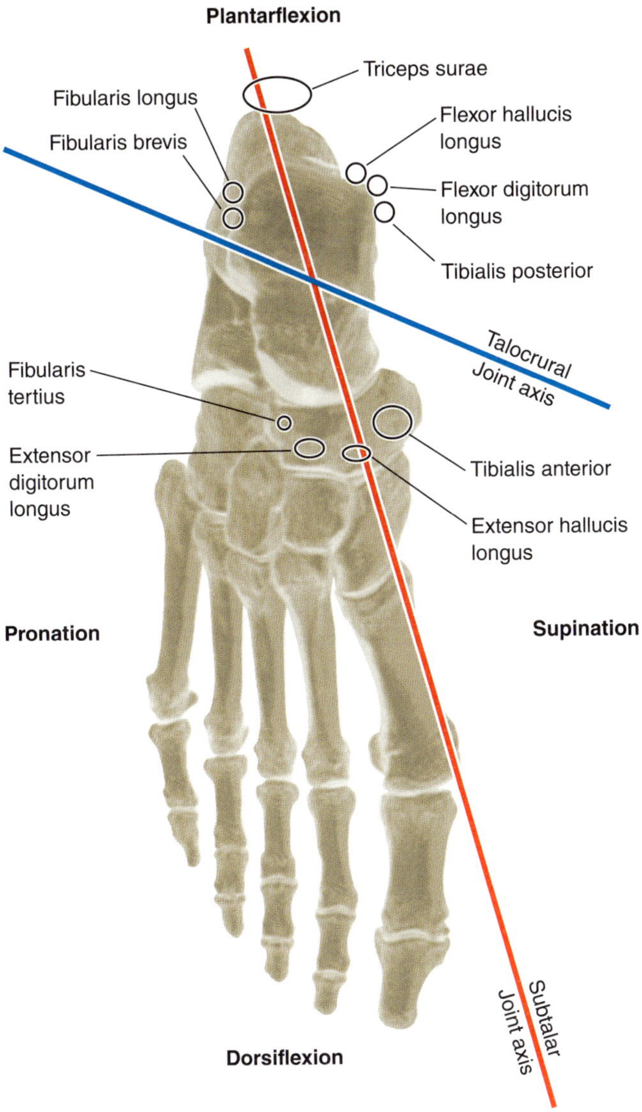

Figure 12–39 Location of muscle insertions in relation to ankle (talocrural) in blue and subtalar joint axis in red. Muscles that cross anterior to the ankle joint axis will cause dorsiflexion torques at the ankle joint, whereas those that cross posterior to the axis will cause plantarflexion torques. Muscles that cross medial to the subtalar joint axis will cause supination torques, whereas those that cross laterally will cause pronation torques.

Extrinsic Musculature

Posterior Compartment Muscles

The muscles of the posterior compartment all pass posterior to the talocrural joint axis and, therefore, are all plantarflexors. The muscles in the posterior compartment are the gastrocnemius, soleus, plantaris, tibialis posterior, flexor digitorum longus, and flexor hallucis longus muscles. The gastrocnemius muscle arises proximally from two heads on the condyles of the femur and inserts distally via the Achilles tendon into the most posterior aspect of the calcaneus. The soleus muscle is deep to the gastrocnemius, attaching proximally on the posterior tibia and fibula and inserting with the gastrocnemius into the posterior calcaneus. The two heads of the gastrocnemius and soleus muscles together are known as the *triceps surae* and are the strongest plantarflexors of the ankle. The Achilles tendon inserts perpendicularly on the calcaneus relatively far from the ankle joint axis (see Fig. 12–39). This efficient attachment provides a large moment arm to generate plantarflexion torque. The Achilles tendon function in the frontal plane may be variable and dependent on the position of the subtalar joint with respect to being in inversion or eversion given its location relative to the subtalar joint axis (see Fig. 12-39). In typical bilateral stance, the triceps surae moment arm for inversion is very small. According to one study, when the subtalar joint was *everted*, the triceps surae produced an *inversion* moment; when the subtalar joint was *inverted*, it produced an *eversion* moment.[138] The study findings reflect a shift in location of the muscular line of pull relative to the subtalar joint axis. Because the foot is typically everted near midstance, activity of the gastrocnemius and soleus on the weight-bearing foot helps to invert and lock the foot into a rigid lever both through direct supination of the subtalar joint and through indirect supination of the transverse tarsal joint. Continued plantarflexion force will raise the heel and cause elevation of the arch (potentially assisted by the increased tension in the plantar aponeurosis as the MTP joints extend).

The soleus and the gastrocnemius together eccentrically control dorsiflexion of the ankle while also supinating the subtalar joint after the foot is loaded in stance. These muscles provide supination torque, which contributes to making the foot a rigid lever for push-off, and continue to provide plantarflexion torque throughout heel rise and plantarflexion of the ankle as the ground reaction force moves to the metatarsal heads and toes.

Expanded Concepts 12–7
Shortening of the Gastrocnemius and Soleus Muscles

Because the gastrocnemius and soleus muscles pass posterior to the ankle joint, a limitation in the length of the muscles (i.e., tightness) results in limited dorsiflexion ROM. Furthermore, the gastrocnemius also passes behind the knee joint, so shortness in the gastrocnemius may limit dorsiflexion ROM even more when the knee is extended. Limited dorsiflexion ROM as a result of a short gastrocnemius muscle may cause a pulling sensation behind the knee when sitting and simultaneously extending the knee and dorsiflexing the ankle. Tight hamstring muscles also may contribute to this type of pulling sensation behind the knee and could be distinguished from a short gastrocnemius muscle by extending the hip (which relieves tension on the hamstrings but not the gastrocnemius muscle). Limited dorsiflexion ROM as a result of a short triceps surae muscle group is thought to contribute to excessive pronation at the subtalar joint and has been associated with midfoot and forefoot pain.[139]

The tendon of tibialis posterior muscle passes just behind the medial malleolus, medial to the subtalar joint (see Fig. 12–39), to insert into the navicular bone and plantar medial arch. The tibialis posterior muscle is the largest extrinsic foot muscle after the triceps surae and has a relatively large moment arm for both subtalar joint and transverse tarsal joint supination.[138] The tibialis posterior muscle is an important dynamic contributor to arch support and has a significant role in eccentrically controlling and reversing pronation of the foot that occurs during gait.[116,135,138] When the foot is being loaded early in the stance phase of walking, the tibialis posterior muscle activates eccentrically to control subtalar and transverse tarsal pronation. Tibialis posterior muscle activity continues to work concentrically as the foot moves toward supination and plantarflexion. Because of its insertion along the plantar medial longitudinal arch, tibialis posterior dysfunction is a key problem associated with acquired pes planus, or flat foot.[116,135,138]

The flexor hallucis longus and the flexor digitorum longus muscles pass posterior to the tibialis posterior muscles at the medial malleolus, spanning the medial longitudinal arch and helping support the arch during gait. Because the tendons pass medial to the subtalar joint (see Fig. 12-39), the extrinsic toe flexors also assist in subtalar joint supination. The flexor hallucis longus attaches distally to the base of the IP of the great toe. The flexor digitorum longus tendon splits into four tendons after passing around the medial malleolus, with one attaching to the distal phalanx of each of the four lesser toes. Like their analogs in the hand, the flexor pollicus long us and the flexor digitorum profundus, they flex the IP and DIP joints, respectively, as well as the immediate joints proximal to their distal attachment. Unlike the profundus tendon that passes over the wrist beneath the centrally located transverse carpal ligament, the flexor digitorum longus wraps around the medial malleolus before continuing distally, and thus has a line of pull that is oblique and, without assistance, would cause the toes to simultaneously flex and deviate toward the medial aspect of the foot. The **quadratus plantae** muscle is an intrinsic muscle arising from either side of the inferior calcaneus that inserts into the lateral border and plantar surface of the flexor digitorum longus tendon. This intrinsic muscle and the long toe flexors together form a concurrent force system with a resultant line of pull that flexes the toes with minimal deviation; there is no equivalent muscle to the quadratus plantae in the hand.

Although there is relatively little need for the toes to actually move into toe flexion, the toe flexors play an important role in balance when the LoG moves toward the metatarsal heads and toes. The toe flexors actively reinforce the passive role of the plantar aponeurosis during gait by eccentrically controlling the MTP extension (metatarsal break) at the end of stance phase, preventing the LoG from passing too far forward in the foot. In more static activities, the toes effectively lengthen the base of support for postural sway and during activities such as leaning forward to reach for or pick up objects, as long as the toe flexors are strong enough to resist MTP extension and press firmly into the ground.

Flexion of the IP joint of the hallux by the flexor hallucis longus muscle presses the toe against the ground **(Fig. 12–40A)**. Flexion of the distal and proximal IP joints of the four lesser toes by the flexor digitorum longus causes clawing (MTP extension with IP flexion) similar to what occurs in the fingers when the proximal phalanx is not stabilized by intrinsic musculature (see **Fig. 12–40B**). As is true in the hand, activity of the interossei muscles can stabilize the MTP joint and prevent MTP hyperextension that occurs with clawing. Pathologies (such as peripheral neuropathy) that cause weakness of the interossei muscles can contribute to destabilization of the MTP joint, hammer toe deformity (hyperextension at the MTP joint), and excessive stresses under the metatarsal heads.[140] These excessive stresses can contribute to pain under the metatarsal heads (i.e., **metatarsalgia**) or skin breakdown in persons who lack protective sensation (i.e., those with peripheral neuropathy).

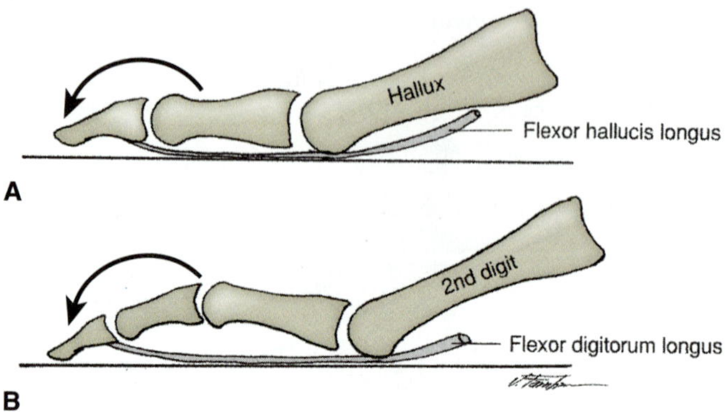

Figure 12–40 **A.** Action of the flexor hallucis longus causes the distal phalanx of the hallux to press against the ground. **B.** Activity of the flexor digitorum longus causes the four lesser toes to grip the ground.

Lateral Compartment Muscles

The fibularis (peroneus) longus and brevis muscles pass lateral to the subtalar joint and, because of their significant moment arms, are the primary pronators (everters) at the subtalar joint1[38] (see Fig. 12–39). Their tendons pass posterior but close to the ankle axis and thus are weak plantar flexors. The tendon of the fibularis longus muscle passes around the lateral malleolus, under the cuboid bone, and across the transverse arch and inserts into the middle cuneiform bone and base of the first metatarsal **(Fig. 12–41)**. Muscle contraction during late stance phase of gait facilitates transfer of weight from the lateral to the medial side of the foot and stabilizes the first ray as the ground reaction force attempts to dorsiflex it, actively facilitating pronation twist of the TMT joints while the rearfoot moves into increased supination.[141] Because of its path across the arches, the fibularis longus tendon is credited with support of the transverse and lateral longitudinal arches as it causes eversion after heel contact, and stabilizes the forefoot after heel rise.[142]

The stability of each of the fibularis tendons at the lateral malleolus depends on integrity of the superior and inferior fibular retinacula located just superior and inferior to the ankle joint, respectively (see Fig. 12–9). Sprains of the lateral ankle structures may affect the fibular retinacula that contribute to lateral ankle and subtalar support. Laxity of the superior retinaculum can lead to acute or chronic subluxation of the fibularis tendons, causing lateral ankle pain and possibly a sense of instability.[143]

Anterior Compartment Muscles

The muscles of the anterior compartment of the leg are the tibialis anterior, the extensor hallucis longus, the extensor digitorum longus, and the fibularis tertius muscles. All muscles in the anterior compartment of the lower leg pass under the

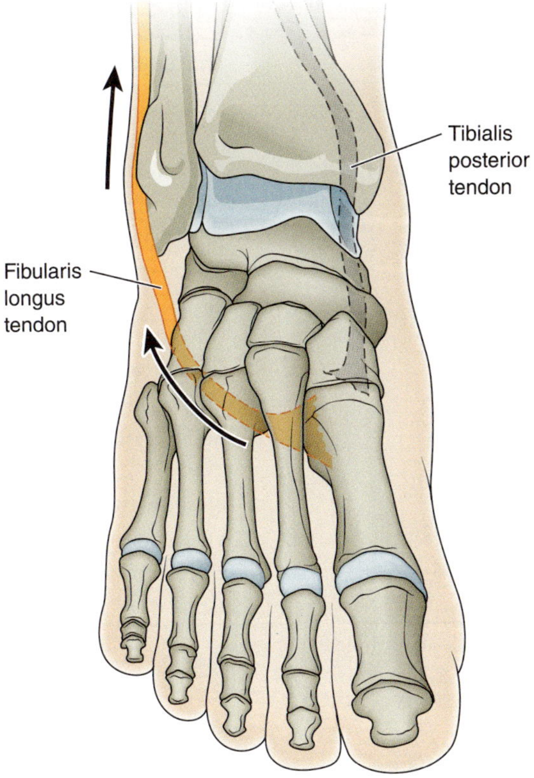

Figure 12–41 The tendon of the fibularis longus passes transversely beneath the foot to insert into the base of the first metatarsal. An active contraction of the muscle can support the transverse arch and the first ray of the foot. The tibialis posterior tendon passes medial to the joint and produces supination and eccentric control of pronation.

extensor retinaculum (see Fig. 12–9) and insert well anterior to the talocrural joint axis (see Fig. 12–39). Besides being a strong dorsiflexor muscle at the ankle joint, the tibialis anterior muscle passes medial to the subtalar axis and is a key supinator of the subtalar and transverse tarsal joints. The tibialis anterior muscle eccentrically controls rearfoot plantarflexion from heel contact to 10% stance, and pronation between 10% stance and foot flat.[142] The tendon of the extensor hallucis longus muscle crosses near the subtalar joint axis and is, at best, a weak supinator of the foot. Additionally, the extensor hallucis longus muscle is active in gait when the heel first contacts the ground to control the strong plantarflexion moment at the ankle created by the ground reaction force. Both the tibialis anterior and extensor hallucis longus muscles are active in dorsiflexing the ankle as the foot leaves the ground to hold the foot up against the plantarflexion torque of gravity.

The tendons of the extensor digitorum longus and the fibularis tertius muscles pass beneath the extensor retinaculum and insert anterior to the ankle joint axis and lateral to the subtalar joint axis; consequently, these muscles are dorsiflexors of the ankle and pronators of the rearfoot. The extensor digitorum longus muscle also extends the MTP joints of the lesser toes, working with the extensor hallucis longus muscle to hold the toes up when the foot is off the ground. The structure and function of the extensor digitorum longus muscle at the MTP and IP joints are identical to those of the extensor digitorum communis of the hand.

Intrinsic Musculature

The intrinsic muscles of the foot function to provide dynamic support to the transverse and longitudinal arches, stabilize the toes, provide proprioception, and participate in balance control.[137] The extensor mechanism of the toes is similar to that of the fingers. Activity in the lumbricals, and the dorsal and plantar interossei muscles, flex the MTP joints while producing IP extension as in the hand. This helps to stabilize the MTP joints during walking to allow the toes to remain weight-bearing and reduce loading on the metatarsal heads. Also during walking, the intrinsic foot muscles lengthen eccentrically from heel strike to midstance and then work concentrically from midstance to toe off.[137] Thereby, the intrinsic foot muscles participate in the windlass mechanism and serve to actively augment the tie-rod function of the plantar aponeurosis.[144]

Patient Application 12–5
Achy, Flat Feet

Wyatt Michaels has flat feet, and he states that his feet often ache at the end of the day. Although there can be several reasons for this type of generalized foot pain, a primary reason may be that the intrinsic muscles have to work harder and longer to stabilize the arches of the flat foot in comparison with a typical or high-arched foot. The high-arched foot receives substantial passive support from the ligaments and alignment of the bones and joints, whereas the flat foot may rely more on the active contraction of the intrinsic muscles for this support. Because Wyatt's muscles have to work to support his feet all day, his intrinsic foot muscles may be aching due to overuse and fatigue at the end of the day.

The specific function of the intrinsic muscles of the foot can be understood and appreciated by comparing each foot muscle with its corresponding hand muscle. Although most people are not able to use the muscles of the foot with the same ability that they use the muscles in the hand, the potential for similar function is limited only by the unopposable hallux and the length of the digits. Table 12–2 summarizes the specific functions of the intrinsic muscles of the foot.

Life Span and Clinical Considerations

The complex interdependency of the foot and ankle joints makes it almost impossible to have dysfunction or abnormality in only one joint or structure. Although foot and ankle disorders can occur across the life span, they are less common in the pediatric population. As children become more active and move to adolescence and young adulthood, traumatic ankle injuries, such as sprains, become more common. These injuries can cause biomechanical abnormalities and deviations that may affect both proximal and distal joints. Over time, if not treated effectively, these abnormalities can cause limitations and progressive deterioration of musculoskeletal structures as the patient ages. As an example, an individual with posttraumatic ankle arthritis may require a total ankle replacement to restore function. As the human life span continues to increase, a rise in the older adult population presenting with

Table 12–2 Intrinsic Muscles of the Foot

MUSCLE	FUNCTION	ANALOG IN HAND
Extensor digitorum brevis	Extends MTP joints	None
Abductor hallucis	Abducts and flexes MTP of hallux	Abductor pollicis brevis
Flexor digitorum brevis	Flexes PIP of four lesser toes	Flexor digitorum superficialis*
Abductor digiti minimi	Abducts and flexes small toe	Abductor digiti minimi
Quadratus plantae	Adjusts oblique pull of flexor digitorum longus into line with long axes of digits	None
Lumbricals	Flex MTPs, extend IPs of four lesser toes	Lumbricals
Flexor hallucis brevis	Flexes MTP of hallux	Flexor pollicis brevis
Adductor hallucis	Oblique head: Adducts and flexes MTP of hallux Transverse head: Adducts metatarsal heads transversely	Adductor pollicis
Flexor digiti minimi	Flexes MTP of small toe	Flexor digiti minimi
Plantar interossei	Adduct MTPs of 3rd–5th toes, flex MTPs, extend IPs of four lesser toes	Volar interossei
Dorsal interossei	Abduct MTPs of 2nd toe (either way), abduct MTPs, 3rd and 4th toes, flex MTPs, extend IPs of four lesser toes	Dorsal interossei

*The flexor digitorum superficialis is an extrinsic muscle, whereas the flexor digitorum brevis is an intrinsic foot muscle.
IP, interphalangeal; MTP, metatarsophalangeal; PIP, proximal interphalangeal.

foot and ankle injuries will likely become more prevalent. The decline of musculoskeletal function, including decreased ROM and muscle performance, increased pain and stiffness, and impaired balance, can lead to a decline in function and independence. Arthritis and bony deformities in the forefoot, midfoot, and rearfoot are prevalent in the older population.[145] The sequalae of all these foot and ankle issues may restrict activity, which has been associated with hospitalization and mortality in older adults.[146]

Foot and Ankle Problems Revisited

The large number of congenital and acquired ankle/foot problems cannot all be described, although several have been referenced in the chapter. The capsule of the ankle joint (specifically, the talocrural joint) is fairly thin and is especially weak anteriorly and posteriorly, so the stability of the ankle depends on an intact ligamentous structure. Stability of the talocrural joint begins proximally with both the proximal and distal tibiofibular joints. The soft tissue structures that support these joints are the crural tibiofibular interosseous ligament, the anterior and posterior tibiofibular ligaments, and the tibiofibular interosseous membrane. All of these are important for stability of the fibula and the mortise and therefore, for stability of the ankle joint itself. Although the distal tibiofibular joint is an extremely strong articulation, injuries can occur when the talus is forcibly dorsiflexed and laterally (externally) rotated within the ankle mortise.[147] Medially, the talocrural joint is supported by the robust deltoid ligament. Although this structure can be injured with excessive eversion or pronation of the ankle and talus,[64,148] these forces may actually fracture and displace (avulse) the medial malleolus before the deltoid ligament tears. Laterally, the ankle is stabilized by the horizontally oriented anterior and posterior talofibular ligaments and the nearly vertical calcaneofibular ligament.[149] In contrast to the medial deltoid ligament, the lateral ligamentous structures help control inversion or supination of the ankle and talus, and are weaker and more susceptible to injury.[64]

Not all injuries at the ankle joint involve excessive motion. Following prolonged periods of immobilization or surgical fixation of the distal tibiofibular joint, patients may present with a limitation in dorsiflexion ROM. These limitations may be due to decreased joint or soft tissue mobility. Limited dorsiflexion motion may also occur in patients with contractures of the gastrocnemius/soleus complex, as with patients with neuromuscular disorders, such as stroke or spinal cord injury. Patients with common conditions such as midportion Achilles tendinopathy may also present with limited ankle dorsiflexion ROM. In these patients, the tendon becomes weakened and less tolerant to stress, resulting in painful and limited dorsiflexion ROM, and impaired ability of the muscle to produce force.[150] Osteoarthritis of the ankle joint may also result in limited ROM. The most common type of arthritis occurs following physical trauma to the joint's cartilage or structural damage that leads to biomechanical abnormalities of the talocrural joint.[151]

Subtalar joint supination and pronation are foot motions that must occur for typical foot function. It has been reported that approximately 60% of individuals have an arch height considered typical, with 20% having a high arch (supinated foot posture or pes cavus) and 20% having a low arch (pronated foot posture, pes planus, or flat foot).[152,153] An excessive or insufficient amount of pronation or supination can be related to dysfunction of the foot or lower extremity. A foot that is fixed in excessive supination is one that has an elevated medial longitudinal arch, lengthening of the lateral aspect of the foot-ankle complex, and an inverted (varus) calcaneus. In some cases, the excessive inversion of the calcaneus that is involved in a supinated foot posture allows the heel pad to be observed medial to the calcaneus when the patient stands with the foot straight ahead. This has been referred to as the "peek-a-boo" sign[154] because the heel pad is not typically visible from this view. A supinated foot posture can have effects both distal and proximal to the subtalar joint. Because the subtalar joint and the transverse tarsal joint are linked, a patient with an excessively supinated foot posture will have both a supinated subtalar joint *and* transverse tarsal joint. This "locks" the foot and limits its ability to absorb shock or accommodate to uneven terrain, contributing to an increased risk of stress injuries. Proximally, a patient with a supinated foot posture may present with a laterally rotated leg and thigh, which shifts the body weight laterally and increases the risk of recurrent ankle sprains, fibularis (peroneal) tendon pathology, metatarsalgia, and fifth metatarsal stress fractures.[155] In contrast, when a foot appears to be fixed in excessive pronation, it has an everted (valgus) calcaneus and a flattened medial longitudinal arch that, in extreme instances, may result in a navicular that contacts the floor. The medial longitudinal arch is supported by the posterior tibialis tendon and dysfunction of this tendon can lead to a progressive condition called *adult-acquired flat foot* or, more recently, *progressive collapsing foot deformity*.[99] In this condition, the arch becomes progressively more flattened because the posterior tibialis tendon fails to produce enough force to support the foot. Patients with this diagnosis will have difficulty locking the transverse tarsal joint into supination during gait, limiting their ability to effectively transmit force from the plantarflexors to the floor and propel themselves forward during walking. This causes increased stress on the medial structures of the foot, such as the deltoid and spring ligaments, the joint capsule of the talonavicular joint, and the plantar fascia, which contributes to further collapse of the arch and worsened pronated foot posture.[98] Proximally, patients with excessive pronation of the foot can present with medial rotation of the leg and thigh in weight-bearing.

The structure of the forefoot can alter force distribution through the foot during typical walking and activities of daily living. The metatarsals and forefoot transmit much of the force that is responsible for propelling the body forward during typical walking. In patients with a Morton's forefoot structure (second toe longest), forces have been found to be increased under the second metatarsal head during barefoot walking.[156] Although not yet proven, this finding has led clinicians and researchers to suggest that this may be related to injuries to the plantar plate. When there is excessive loading at the head of the first metatarsal, the sesamoid bones and their supporting structures can become inflamed in a condition called *sesamoiditis*. This inflammation can progress to acute fracture, stress fracture, osteonecrosis, or chrondromalacia.[157]

The MTP joints have two degrees of freedom: flexion/extension and abduction/adduction. From a neutral position, the available ROM of extension far exceeds that of flexion. Although toe flexion ROM has relatively little purpose in the weight-bearing foot, it does contribute to walking stability when the support terrain drops away distal to the metatarsal heads. Toe flexion may be important in balance because strength of the toe flexors is important in balance, and stronger toe flexors do contribute to improved postural stability in older adults.[158] All of the toes must extend at the end-of-stance phase during typical walking, with the first MTP joint extending 60° to 75°.[159,160] A loss of this ROM is often observed in patients with bunions, or hallux valgus. In this foot deformity, the first metatarsal is angled so that the head of the metatarsal is more medial than the base, as in Figure 12–32. The first phalanx is angled in the opposite direction, with the distal end more lateral than the proximal end. Because of the altered orientation of the joint, patients with hallux valgus often have limited extension motion of the first MTP, lateral subluxation of the toe flexor tendons crossing the first MTP joint, reduced weight-bearing on the great toe, and increased weight-bearing on the first metatarsal head.[110]

Extrinsic muscles are divided into the three compartments of the lower leg: the posterior, lateral, and anterior compartments. Each compartment is susceptible to injury, which can limit function. In the posterior compartment, limited dorsiflexion ROM as a result of a short triceps surae muscle group is thought to contribute to excessive pronation at the subtalar joint and has been associated with midfoot and forefoot pain.[161] The tibialis posterior muscle works concentrically as the foot moves toward supination and plantarflexion. Because of its insertion along the plantar medial longitudinal arch, tibialis posterior dysfunction is a key problem associated with acquired pes planus, or flat foot.[116,135,138] As is true in the hand, activity of the interossei muscles can stabilize the MTP joint and prevent MTP hyperextension. Pathologies (such as peripheral neuropathy) that cause weakness of the interossei muscles can contribute to destabilization of the MTP joint, hammer toe deformity (hyperextension at the MTP joint), and excessive stresses under the metatarsal heads.[140] These excessive stresses can contribute to pain under the metatarsal heads (i.e., metatarsalgia) or skin breakdown in persons who lack protective sensation (i.e., those with more severe peripheral neuropathy). In the lateral compartment, the fibularis (peroneus) longus and brevis muscles pass lateral to the subtalar joint and, because of their significant moment arms, are the primary pronators at the subtalar joint.[138] Sprains of the lateral ankle structures may affect the peroneal retinacula that contribute to lateral ankle and subtalar support. Laxity of the superior retinaculum can lead to acute or chronic subluxation of the fibularis tendons, causing lateral ankle pain and possibly a sense of instability.[162]

SUMMARY

- The foot and ankle consist of a complex arrangement of structures and joints that allow the foot to be flexible during the midstance phase of gait, yet relatively rigid during the late-stance phase. The complexity of the interrelationships makes it easy to disrupt typical function or exceed the limitations of the active and passive tissues that make up the ankle/foot complex.
- Studies that have investigated the relationship between various foot types or alignments and lower extremity injury often show little or no correlation. This should not be surprising, given the multifactorial and complex nature of health, injury, and an individual's function.[1]
- An important point of this chapter, however, has been to consider how various structures and structural deviations can affect movement and stresses on adjacent structures and tissues. Although group studies may minimize the apparent influence of a given structural problem in dysfunction, the

problem should not be ruled out as a factor in, or even primary cause of, pain or dysfunction in an individual case.

- The kinesiology effect of a given set of alignments and apparent forces in producing maladaptive stresses should be placed in the full context of the individual person, his or her health status, and his or her activity level and participation goals.

STUDY QUESTIONS

1. Identify the proximal and distal articular surfaces that constitute the ankle (talocrural) joint. What is the joint classification?
2. Describe the proximal and distal tibiofibular joints, including classification and their composite function.
3. Identify the ligaments that support the tibiofibular joints.
4. Describe the ligaments that support the ankle joint, including the names of components when relevant.
5. Why is ankle joint motion considered triplanar?
6. Why does the fibula move during dorsiflexion/plantarflexion of the ankle?
7. What are the primary checks/stops of ankle joint motion?
8. Which muscles crossing the ankle are single-joint muscles?
9. Describe the three articular surfaces of the subtalar joint, including the capsular arrangement.
10. Which ligaments support the subtalar joint?
11. Describe the axis for subtalar motion. What movements take place around that axis, and how are these motions defined?
12. When the foot is weight-bearing, the calcaneus (the distal segment) of the subtalar joint is not free to move in all directions. Describe the movements that take place during weight-bearing subtalar supination/pronation.
13. What is the close-packed position for the subtalar joint? Which motion of the tibia will lock the weight-bearing subtalar joint?
14. Describe the relationship between the subtalar and the talonavicular joint with regard to articular surfaces, axes, and available motion.
15. Describe the articulations of the transverse tarsal joint.
16. What is the general function of the transverse tarsal joint in relation to the subtalar joint?
17. What are the TMT rays? Describe the axis for the first and fifth ray and the movements that occur around each axis.
18. What is the function of the TMT joints in relation to the subtalar and the transverse tarsal joints?
19. How does pronation twist of the TMT joints relate to supination of the subtalar joint?
20. What ligaments contribute to support of the medial longitudinal arch of the foot?
21. What is the weight distribution through the various joints from the ankle through the metatarsal heads in unilateral stance?
22. How does extension of the MTP joints contribute to stability of the foot?
23. In terms of structure, compare the MTP joints of the foot with the MCP joints of the fingers.
24. What is the metatarsal break? When does this occur, and how is it related to support of the longitudinal arch?
25. What is the role of the triceps surae muscle group at each joint it crosses?
26. What other muscles besides the triceps surae exert a plantarflexion influence at the ankle? What is the primary function of each of these muscles?
27. Which muscles may contribute to support of the arches of the foot?
28. What is the function of the quadratus plantae? What is the analog of this muscle in the hand?
29. Drawing an analogy between the foot and the hand, describe the function of each of the intrinsic and extrinsic foot muscles.
30. If a person has a pes planus, describe two possible causes for this condition.
31. Identify at least three possible effects of pes planus.
32. Identify three primary signs to identify an excessively supinated or pronated foot.

REFERENCES

1. Mueller MJ, Maluf KS: Tissue adaptation to physical stress: a proposed "Physical Stress Theory" to guide physical therapist practice, education, and research. Phys Ther 82:383-403, 2002
2. Williams P: Gray's Anatomy (ed 38). New York, NY, Churchill Livingstone, 1999
3. Espregueira-Mendes JD, da Silva MV: Anatomy of the proximal tibiofibular joint. Knee Surg Sports Traumatol Arthrosc 14:241-9, 2006
4. Bozkurt M, Yilmaz E, Atlihan D, et al: The proximal tibiofibular joint: an anatomic study. Clin Orthop Relat Res:136-40, 2003
5. Soavi R, Girolami M, Loreti I, et al: The mobility of the proximal tibiofibular joint. A Roentgen stereophotogrammetric analysis on six cadaver specimens. Foot Ankle Int 21:336-42, 2000
6. Burkhart TA, Asa B, Payne MW, et al: Anatomy of the proximal tibiofibular joint and interosseous membrane, and their contributions to joint kinematics in below-knee amputations. J Anat 226:143-9, 2015
7. Miller TL, Curatolo C: Proximal tibiofibular joint instability: an underrecognized cause of lateral knee pain and mechanical symptoms. J Am Acad Orthop Surg 31:e412-23, 2023
8. Hermans JJ, Beumer A, de Jong TA, et al: Anatomy of the distal tibiofibular syndesmosis in adults: a pictorial essay with a multimodality approach. J Anat 217:633-45, 2010
9. Tourne Y, Molinier F, Andrieu M, et al: Diagnosis and treatment of tibiofibular syndesmosis lesions. Orthop Traumatol Surg Res 105:S275-86, 2019
10. Williams GN, Jones MH, Amendola A: Syndesmotic ankle sprains in athletes. Am J Sports Med 35:1197-207, 2007
11. Takebe K, Nakagawa A, Minami H, et al: Role of the fibula in weight-bearing. Clin Orthop Relat Res:289-92, 1984
12. Funk JR, Rudd RW, Kerrigan JR, et al: The line of action in the tibia during axial compression of the leg. J Biomech 40:2277-82, 2007
13. Kong A, Cassumbhoy R, Subramaniam RM: Magnetic resonance imaging of ankle tendons and ligaments: Part I—anatomy. Australas Radiol 51:315-23, 2007
14. Koris J, Calder JDF, Dalmau-Pastor M, et al: Deltoid ligament injuries: a review of the anatomy, diagnosis and treatments. Knee Surg Sports Traumatol Arthrosc 32(12):3052-3064, 2024
15. Obionu K, Palm H, Astrup Y, et al: A clinical guide to the medial ligaments of the ankle: anatomy, function, diagnosis of injuries and treatment of instability-a narrative review. Foot Ankle Surg 30:85-91, 2024
16. Ruzik K, Gonera B, Borowski A, et al: Anatomic variations of the calcaneofibular ligament. Foot Ankle Int:10711007241241073, 2024
17. Hur ES, Bohl DD, Lee S: Lateral ligament instability: review of pathology and diagnosis. Curr Rev Musculoskelet Med 13:494-500, 2020
18. Larkins LW, Baker RT, Baker JG: Physical examination of the ankle: a review of the original orthopedic special test description and scientific validity of common tests for ankle examination. Arch Rehabil Res Clin Transl 2:100072, 2020
19. Abu-Hijleh MF, Harris PF: Deep fascia on the dorsum of the ankle and foot: extensor retinacula revisited. Clin Anat 20:186-95, 2007
20. Hatch GF, Labib SA, Rolf RH, et al: Role of the peroneal tendons and superior peroneal retinaculum as static stabilizers of the ankle. J Surg Orthop Adv 16:187-91, 2007

21. Keener BJ, Sizensky JA: The anatomy of the calcaneus and surrounding structures. Foot Ankle Clin 10:413-24, 2005
22. Wang CL, Cheng CK, Chen CW, et al: Contact areas and pressure distributions in the subtalar joint. J Biomech 28:269-79, 1995
23. Gomes TM, Oliva XM, Viridiana Sanchez E, et al: Anatomy of the ankle and subtalar joint ligaments: what we do not know about it? Foot Ankle Clin 28:201-16, 2023
24. Tan CY, Thevendran G: Subtalar instability. J Orthop Surg (Hong Kong) 31:10225536231182350, 2023
25. Li SY, Hou ZD, Zhang P, et al: Ligament structures in the tarsal sinus and canal. Foot Ankle Int 34:1729-36, 2013
26. Pereira BS, Andrade R, Espregueira-Mendes J, et al: Current concepts on subtalar instability. Orthop J Sports Med 9:23259671211021352, 2021
27. Belis AM, Foote GA: The Spring ligament complex—anatomy and function. Clin Podiatr Med Surg 39:393-403, 2022
28. Tryfonidis M, Jackson W, Mansour R, et al: Acquired adult flat foot due to isolated plantar calcaneonavicular (spring) ligament insufficiency with a normal tibialis posterior tendon. Foot Ankle Surg 14:89-95, 2008
29. Sammarco VJ: The talonavicular and calcaneocuboid joints: anatomy, biomechanics, and clinical management of the transverse tarsal joint. Foot Ankle Clin 9:127-45, 2004
30. Aoki A, Makihara Y, Tamura A, et al: Anatomical analysis of ligaments surrounding calcaneocuboid joint: implications for role in foot stability. Surg Radiol Anat 46:425-31, 2024
31. Ward KA, Soames RW: Morphology of the plantar calcaneocuboid ligaments. Foot Ankle Int 18:649-53, 1997
32. Lalwani R, Kotgirwar S, Athavale SA: Support system of Lisfranc joint complex: an anatomical investigation with an evolutionary perspective. Foot Ankle Surg 28:1089-93, 2022
33. Lee CA, Birkedal JP, Dickerson EA, et al: Stabilization of Lisfranc joint injuries: a biomechanical study. Foot Ankle Int 25:365-70, 2004
34. Kura H, Luo ZP, Kitaoka HB, et al: Mechanical behavior of the Lisfranc and dorsal cuneometatarsal ligaments: in vitro biomechanical study. J Orthop Trauma 15:107-10, 2001
35. Stainsby GD: Pathological anatomy and dynamic effect of the displaced plantar plate and the importance of the integrity of the plantar plate-deep transverse metatarsal ligament tie-bar. Ann R Coll Surg Engl 79:58-68, 1997
36. Troy KL, Davis IS, Tenforde AS: A narrative review of metatarsal bone stress injury in athletic populations: etiology, biomechanics, and management. PM R 13:1281-90, 2021
37. Drez D, Jr., Young JC, Johnston RD, et al: Metatarsal stress fractures. Am J Sports Med 8:123-5, 1980
38. Davidson G, Pizzari T, Mayes S: The influence of second toe and metatarsal length on stress fractures at the base of the second metatarsal in classical dancers. Foot Ankle Int 28:1082-6, 2007
39. Brenner E: The intersesamoidal ridge of the first metatarsal bone: anatomical basics and clinical considerations. Surg Radiol Anat 25:127-31, 2003
40. Anwar R, Anjum SN, Nicholl JE: Sesamoids of the foot. Curr Orthop 19:40-8, 2005
41. Yoshioka Y, Siu DW, Cooke TD, et al: Geometry of the first metatarsophalangeal joint. J Orthop Res 6:878-85, 1988
42. Robberecht J, Decroocq L, Schramm M, et al: Transverse laxity of the forefoot. Foot Ankle Surg 28:1-6, 2022
43. Deland JT, Lee KT, Sobel M, et al: Anatomy of the plantar plate and its attachments in the lesser metatarsal phalangeal joint. Foot Ankle Int 16:480-6, 1995
44. Waldecker U: Plantar fat pad atrophy: a cause of metatarsalgia? J Foot Ankle Surg 40:21-7, 2001
45. Waldecker U, Lehr HA: Is there histomorphological evidence of plantar metatarsal fat pad atrophy in patients with diabetes? J Foot Ankle Surg 48:648-52, 2009
46. Hockenbury RT: Forefoot problems in athletes. Med Sci Sports Exerc 31:S448-58, 1999
47. Seber S, Hazer B, Kose N, et al: Rotational profile of the lower extremity and foot progression angle: computerized tomographic examination of 50 male adults. Arch Orthop Trauma Surg 120:255-8, 2000
48. Kristiansen LP, Gunderson RB, Steen H, et al: The normal development of tibial torsion. Skeletal Radiol 30:519-22, 2001
49. Shultz SJ, Nguyen AD: Bilateral asymmetries in clinical measures of lower-extremity anatomic characteristics. Clin J Sport Med 17: 357-61, 2007
50. Nguyen AD, Shultz SJ: Sex differences in clinical measures of lower extremity alignment. J Orthop Sports Phys Ther 37:389-98, 2007
51. Hicks JH: The mechanics of the foot. I. The joints. J Anat 87:345-57, 1953
52. Stiehl J: Biomechanics of the ankle joint, in Stiehl J (ed): Inman's Joints of the Ankle (ed 2). Baltimore, MD, Williams & Wilkins, 1991
53. Sheehan FT, Seisler AR, Siegel KL: In vivo talocrural and subtalar kinematics: a non-invasive 3D dynamic MRI study. Foot Ankle Int 28:323-35, 2007
54. Yu J, Cao S, Wang C, et al: In vivo evaluation of the position and orientation of the geometric axis of the tibiotalar joint. Appl Bionics Biomech 2023:2763099, 2023
55. Barnett CH, Napier JR: The axis of rotation at the ankle joint in man: its influence upon the form of the talus and the mobility of the fibula. J Anat 86:1-9, 1952
56. Martin RL, Stewart GW, Conti SF: Posttraumatic ankle arthritis: an update on conservative and surgical management. J Orthop Sports Phys Ther 37:253-9, 2007
57. Conti S, Lalonde KA, Martin R: Kinematic analysis of the agility total ankle during gait. Foot Ankle Int 27:980-4, 2006
58. St Mart JP, Goh EL, Hay D, et al: Contemporary modern total ankle arthroplasty (TAA): a systematic review and meta-analysis of indications, survivorship and complication rates. Surgeon 22:174-81, 2024
59. Gonzalez-Alonso M, Trapote-Cubillas AR, Madera-Gonzalez FJ, et al: Fixed-bearing versus mobile-bearing total ankle replacement survivorship: a meta-analysis. Foot Ankle Surg 30:275-84, 2024
60. Surgeons AAoO: American Academy of Orthopaedic Surgeons: Joint Motion: Method of Measuring and Recording. Chicago, IL, AAOS, 1965
61. Martin RL, McPoil TG: Reliability of ankle goniometric measurements: a literature review. J Am Podiatr Med Assoc 95:564-72, 2005
62. Moseley AM, Crosbie J, Adams R: Normative data for passive ankle plantarflexion—dorsiflexion flexibility. Clin Biomech (Bristol, Avon) 16:514-21, 2001
63. Liu Q, Chen H, Song Y, et al: Running velocity and longitudinal bending stiffness influence the asymmetry of kinematic variables of the lower limb joints. Bioengineering (Basel) 9, 2022
64. Fujii T, Kitaoka HB, Luo ZP, et al: Analysis of ankle-hindfoot stability in multiple planes: an in vitro study. Foot Ankle Int 26:633-7, 2005
65. Shibuya N, McAlister JE, Prissel MA, et al: Consensus statement of the American College of Foot and Ankle Surgeons: diagnosis and treatment of ankle arthritis. J Foot Ankle Surg 59:1019-31, 2020
66. Inman V, Mann R: Biomechanics of the foot and ankle, in Mann R (ed): DuVries Surgery of the Foot (ed 4). St. Louis, MO, CV Mosby, 1978
67. Hogg-Cornejo V, Hunt KJ, Bartolomei J, et al: Normal kinematics of the syndesmosis and ankle mortise during dynamic movements. Foot Ankle Orthop 5:2473011420933007, 2020
68. Bozkurt M, Tonuk E, Elhan A, et al: Axial rotation and mediolateral translation of the fibula during passive plantarflexion. Foot Ankle Int 29:502-7, 2008
69. Acevedo D, Suarez A, Kaur K, et al: Syndesmotic screws, unscrew them, or leave them? A systematic review and meta-analysis of randomized controlled trials. J Orthop 54:136-42, 2024
70. De Monte G, Arampatzis A, Stogiannari C, et al: In vivo motion transmission in the inactive gastrocnemius medialis muscle-tendon unit during ankle and knee joint rotation. J Electromyogr Kinesiol 16:413-22, 2006
71. Kleipool RP, Blankevoort L: The relation between geometry and function of the ankle joint complex: a biomechanical review. Knee Surg Sports Traumatol Arthrosc 18:618-27, 2010
72. Manter J: Movements of the subtalar and transverse tarsal joints. Anat Rec 80:397, 1941
73. Sangeorzan B: Biomechanics of the Subtalar Joint (ed 2). Baltimore, MD, Williams & Wilkins, 1991
74. Carroll LA, Paulseth S, Martin RL: Forefoot injuries in athletes: integration of the movement system. Int J Sports Phys Ther 17:81-9, 2022
75. Riskowski JL, Dufour AB, Hagedorn TJ, et al: Associations of foot posture and function to lower extremity pain: results from a population-based foot study. Arthritis Care Res (Hoboken) 65:1804-12, 2013
76. Takabayashi T, Edama M, Inai T, et al: Shank and rearfoot coordination and its variability during running in flatfoot. J Biomech 115:110119, 2021
77. Takabayashi T, Edama M, Inai T, et al: Gender differences in coordination variability between shank and rearfoot during running. Hum Mov Sci 66:91-7, 2019
78. Koshino Y, Yamanaka M, Ezawa Y, et al: Coupling motion between rearfoot and hip and knee joints during walking and single-leg landing. J Electromyogr Kinesiol 37:75-83, 2017
79. Sarrafian SK: Biomechanics of the subtalar joint complex. Clin Orthop Relat Res:17-26, 1993
80. Root M, Orien WP, Weed JH: Normal And Abnormal Function of the Foot: Clinical Biomechanics, vol II. Los Angeles, CA, Clincial Biomechanics Corp, 1977
81. Åstrom M, Arvidson T: Alignment and joint motion in the normal foot. J Orthop Sports Phys Ther 22:216-22, 1995
82. Elveru RA, Rothstein JM, Lamb RL: Goniometric reliability in a clinical setting. Subtalar and ankle joint measurements. Phys Ther 68:672-7, 1988

83. Bovens AM, van Baak MA, Vrencken JG, et al: Variability and reliability of joint measurements. Am J Sports Med 18:58-63, 1990
84. Menadue C, Raymond J, Kilbreath SL, et al: Reliability of two goniometric methods of measuring active inversion and eversion range of motion at the ankle. BMC Musculoskelet Disord 7:60, 2006
85. Keenan AM, Bach TM: Clinicians' assessment of the hindfoot: a study of reliability. Foot Ankle Int 27:451-60, 2006
86. Buckley RE, Hunt DV: Reliability of clinical measurement of subtalar joint movement. Foot Ankle Int 18:229-32, 1997
87. Redmond AC, Crosbie J, Ouvrier RA: Development and validation of a novel rating system for scoring standing foot posture: the Foot Posture Index. Clin Biomech (Bristol, Avon) 21:89-98, 2006
88. Cornwall MW, McPoil TG, Lebec M, et al: Reliability of the modified Foot Posture Index. J Am Podiatr Med Assoc 98:7-13, 2008
89. Hunsawong T, Motantasuta P, Mato L, et al: Agreement between clinical measures to classify foot posture in asymptomatic adults. BMC Musculoskelet Disord 23:1042, 2022
90. Cornwall MW, McPoil TG: Motion of the calcaneus, navicular, and first metatarsal during the stance phase of walking. J Am Podiatr Med Assoc 92:67-76, 2002
91. McPoil T, Cornwall MW: Relationship between neutral subtalar joint position and pattern of rearfoot motion during walking. Foot Ankle Int 15:141-5, 1994
92. McPoil TG, Cornwall MW: The relationship between static lower extremity measurements and rearfoot motion during walking. J Orthop Sports Phys Ther 24:309-14, 1996
93. McPoil TG, Cornwall MW: Relationship between three static angles of the rearfoot and the pattern of rearfoot motion during walking. J Orthop Sports Phys Ther 23:370-5, 1996
94. Van Gheluwe B, Kirby KA, Roosen P, et al: Reliability and accuracy of biomechanical measurements of the lower extremities. J Am Podiatr Med Assoc 92:317-26, 2002
95. Pierrynowski MR, Smith SB, Mlynarczyk JH: Proficiency of foot care specialists to place the rearfoot at subtalar neutral. J Am Podiatr Med Assoc 86:217-23, 1996
96. Garbalosa JC, McClure MH, Catlin PA, et al: The frontal plane relationship of the forefoot to the rearfoot in an asymptomatic population. J Orthop Sports Phys Ther 20:200-6, 1994
97. Elftman H: The transverse tarsal joint and its control. Clin Orthop 16:41-6, 1960
98. Abousayed MM, Alley MC, Shakked R, et al: Adult-acquired flatfoot deformity: etiology, diagnosis, and management. JBJS Rev 5:e7, 2017
99. Myerson MS, Thordarson DB, Johnson JE, et al: Classification and nomenclature: progressive collapsing foot deformity. Foot Ankle Int 41:1271-6, 2020
100. Ness ME, Long J, Marks R, et al: Foot and ankle kinematics in patients with posterior tibial tendon dysfunction. Gait Posture 27:331-9, 2008
101. Alvarez RG, Marini A, Schmitt C, et al: Stage I and II posterior tibial tendon dysfunction treated by a structured nonoperative management protocol: an orthosis and exercise program. Foot Ankle Int 27:2-8, 2006
102. Okita N, Meyers SA, Challis JH, et al: Midtarsal joint locking: new perspectives on an old paradigm. J Orthop Res 32:110-5, 2014
103. Morris JM: Biomechanics of the foot and ankle. Clin Orthop Relat Res:10-7, 1977
104. Halstead J, Redmond AC: Weight-bearing passive dorsiflexion of the hallux in standing is not related to hallux dorsiflexion during walking. J Orthop Sports Phys Ther 36:550-6, 2006
105. Hopson MM, McPoil TG, Cornwall MW: Motion of the first metatarsophalangeal joint: reliability and validity of four measurement techniques. J Am Podiatr Med Assoc 85:198-204, 1995
106. Menz HB, Auhl M, Tan JM, et al: Centre of pressure characteristics during walking in individuals with and without first metatarsophalangeal joint osteoarthritis. Gait Posture 63:91-6, 2018
107. Allan JJ, McClelland JA, Munteanu SE, et al: First metatarsophalangeal joint range of motion is associated with lower limb kinematics in individuals with first metatarsophalangeal joint osteoarthritis. J Foot Ankle Res 13:33, 2020
108. Jastifer JR: Plantar plate repair for metatarsophalangeal joint instability of the lesser toes. Orthop Clin North Am 53:349-59, 2022
109. Mueller MJ, Hastings M, Commean PK, et al: Forefoot structural predictors of plantar pressures during walking in people with diabetes and peripheral neuropathy. J Biomech 36:1009-17, 2003
110. Easley ME, Trnka HJ: Current concepts review: hallux valgus part 1: pathomechanics, clinical assessment, and nonoperative management. Foot Ankle Int 28:654-9, 2007
111. Glasoe WM, Allen MK, Saltzman CL: First ray dorsal mobility in relation to hallux valgus deformity and first intermetatarsal angle. Foot Ankle Int 22:98-101, 2001
112. Abdalbary SA: Foot mobilization and exercise program combined with toe separator improves outcomes in women with moderate hallux valgus at 1-year follow-up (a randomized clinical trial). J Am Podiatr Med Assoc 108:478-86, 2018
113. Coughlin MJ, Jones CP: Hallux valgus: demographics, etiology, and radiographic assessment. Foot Ankle Int 28:759-77, 2007
114. Gould N, Moreland M, Alvarez R, et al: Development of the child's arch. Foot Ankle 9:241-5, 1989
115. Honig EL, Haeberle HS, Kehoe CM, et al: Pediatric orthopedic mythbusters: the truth about flexible flatfeet, tibial and femoral torsion, W-sitting, and idiopathic toe-walking. Curr Opin Pediatr 33:105-13, 2021
116. Thordarson DB, Schmotzer H, Chon J, et al: Dynamic support of the human longitudinal arch: a biomechanical evaluation. Clin Orthop Relat Res:165-72, 1995
117. Kitaoka HB, Ahn TK, Luo ZP, et al: Stability of the arch of the foot. Foot Ankle Int 18:644-8, 1997
118. Van Boerum DH, Sangeorzan BJ: Biomechanics and pathophysiology of flat foot. Foot Ankle Clin 8:419-30, 2003
119. Moraes do Carmo CC, Fonseca de Almeida Melao LI, Valle de Lemos Weber MF, et al: Anatomical features of plantar aponeurosis: cadaveric study using ultrasonography and magnetic resonance imaging. Skeletal Radiol 37:929-35, 2008
120. Erdemir A, Hamel AJ, Fauth AR, et al: Dynamic loading of the plantar aponeurosis in walking. J Bone Joint Surg Am 86-A:546-52, 2004
121. Gefen A: The in vivo elastic properties of the plantar fascia during the contact phase of walking. Foot Ankle Int 24:238-44, 2003
122. Lapidus PW: Kinesiology and mechanical anatomy of the tarsal joints. Clin Orthop Relat Res 30:20-36, 1963
123. Hicks JH: The mechanics of the foot. II. The plantar aponeurosis and the arch. J Anat 88:25-30, 1954
124. Koc TA, Jr, Bise CG, Neville C, et al: Heel pain - Plantar fasciitis: revision 2023. J Orthop Sports Phys Ther 53:CPG1-39, 2023
125. Sarrafian SK: Functional characteristics of the foot and plantar aponeurosis under tibiotalar loading. Foot Ankle 8:4-18, 1987
126. Birtane M, Tuna H: The evaluation of plantar pressure distribution in obese and non-obese adults. Clin Biomech (Bristol, Avon) 19:1055-9, 2004
127. Buldt AK, Forghany S, Landorf KB, et al: Foot posture is associated with plantar pressure during gait: a comparison of normal, planus and cavus feet. Gait Posture 62:235-40, 2018
128. Kelly VE, Mueller MJ, Sinacore DR: Timing of peak plantar pressure during the stance phase of walking: a study of patients with diabetes mellitus and transmetatarsal amputation. J Am Podiatr Med Assoc 90:18-23, 2000
129. Morag E, Cavanagh PR: Structural and functional predictors of regional peak pressures under the foot during walking. J Biomech 32:359-70, 1999
130. Weijers RE, Walenkamp GH, van Mameren H, et al: The relationship of the position of the metatarsal heads and peak plantar pressure. Foot Ankle Int 24:349-53, 2003
131. Burns J, Crosbie J, Hunt A, et al: The effect of pes cavus on foot pain and plantar pressure. Clin Biomech (Bristol, Avon) 20:877-82, 2005
132. Hessert MJ, Vyas M, Leach J, et al: Foot pressure distribution during walking in young and old adults. BMC Geriatr 5:8, 2005
133. Hills AP, Hennig EM, McDonald M, et al: Plantar pressure differences between obese and non-obese adults: a biomechanical analysis. Int J Obes Relat Metab Disord 25:1674-9, 2001
134. Chuckpaiwong B, Nunley JA, Mall NA, et al: The effect of foot type on in-shoe plantar pressure during walking and running. Gait Posture 28:405-11, 2008
135. Kitaoka HB, Luo ZP, An KN: Effect of the posterior tibial tendon on the arch of the foot during simulated weight-bearing: biomechanical analysis. Foot Ankle Int 18:43-6, 1997
136. O'Connor KM, Hamill J: The role of selected extrinsic foot muscles during running. Clin Biomech (Bristol, Avon) 19:71-7, 2004
137. Jastifer JR: Intrinsic muscles of the foot: anatomy, function, rehabilitation. Phys Ther Sport 61:27-36, 2023
138. Klein P, Mattys S, Rooze M: Moment arm length variations of selected muscles acting on talocrural and subtalar joints during movement: an in vitro study. J Biomech 29:21-30, 1996
139. DiGiovanni CW, Kuo R, Tejwani N, et al: Isolated gastrocnemius tightness. J Bone Joint Surg Am 84-A:962-70, 2002

140. Robertson DD, Mueller MJ, Smith KE, et al: Structural changes in the forefoot of individuals with diabetes and a prior plantar ulcer. J Bone Joint Surg Am 84:1395-404, 2002
141. Sumal AS, Jarvis GE, Norrish AR, et al: The role of the angle of the fibularis longus tendon in foot arch support. Clin Anat 34:651-8, 2021
142. Hunt AE, Smith RM, Torode M: Extrinsic muscle activity, foot motion and ankle joint moments during the stance phase of walking. Foot Ankle Int 22:31-41, 2001
143. Koutsogiannis P, Frane N, Aliyev T, et al: Peroneus longus and peroneus brevis: a review on pathology and updated treatments. JBJS Rev 10, 2022
144. Kelly LA, Lichtwark G, Cresswell AG: Active regulation of longitudinal arch compression and recoil during walking and running. J R Soc Interface 12:20141076, 2015
145. Lee DK, Mulder GD: Foot and ankle surgery: considerations for the geriatric patient. J Am Board Fam Med 22:316-24, 2009
146. Henderson IL, Bone RW, Stevens R, et al: The association between restricted activity and patient outcomes in older adults: systematic literature review and meta-analysis. BMC Geriatr 24:316, 2024
147. Teramoto A, Kura H, Uchiyama E, et al: Three-dimensional analysis of ankle instability after tibiofibular syndesmosis injuries: a biomechanical experimental study. Am J Sports Med 36:348-52, 2008
148. Hintermann B, Valderrabano V, Boss A, et al: Medial ankle instability: an exploratory, prospective study of fifty-two cases. Am J Sports Med 32:183-90, 2004
149. Masciocchi C, Barile A: Magnetic resonance imaging of the hindfoot with surgical correlations. Skeletal Radiol 31:131-42, 2002
150. Martin RL, Chimenti R, Cuddeford T, et al: Achilles pain, stiffness, and muscle power deficits: Midportion Achilles Tendinopathy Revision 2018. J Orthop Sports Phys Ther 48:A1-38, 2018
151. Saltzman CL, Salamon ML, Blanchard GM, et al: Epidemiology of ankle arthritis: report of a consecutive series of 639 patients from a tertiary orthopaedic center. Iowa Orthop J 25:44-6, 2005
152. Subotnick SI: The biomechanics of running: implications for the prevention of foot injuries. Sports Med 2:144-53, 1985
153. Ledoux WR, Shofer JB, Ahroni JH, et al: Biomechanical differences among pes cavus, neutrally aligned, and pes planus feet in subjects with diabetes. Foot Ankle Int 24:845-50, 2003
154. Manoli A, 2nd, Smith DG, Hansen ST, Jr: Scarred muscle excision for the treatment of established ischemic contracture of the lower extremity. Clin Orthop Relat Res:309-14, 1993
155. Manoli A, 2nd, Graham B: The subtle cavus foot, "the underpronator." Foot Ankle Int 26:256-63, 2005
156. Fleischer AE, Hshieh S, Crews RT, et al: Association between second metatarsal length and forefoot loading under the second metatarsophalangeal joint. Foot Ankle Int 39:560-7, 2018
157. Cohen BE: Hallux sesamoid disorders. Foot Ankle Clin 14:91-104, 2009
158. Quinlan S, Fong Yan A, Sinclair P, et al: The evidence for improving balance by strengthening the toe flexor muscles: a systematic review. Gait Posture 81:56-66, 2020
159. Coughlin MJ, Shurnas PS: Hallux rigidus: demographics, etiology, and radiographic assessment. Foot Ankle Int 24:731-43, 2003
160. Zammit GV, Menz HB, Munteanu SE: Structural factors associated with hallux limitus/rigidus: a systematic review of case control studies. J Orthop Sports Phys Ther 39:733-42, 2009
161. DiGiovanni CW, Kuo R, Tejwani N, et al: Isolated gastrocnemius tightness. J Bone Joint Surg Am 84:962-70, 2002
162. Ogawa BK, Thordarson DB: Current concepts review: peroneal tendon subluxation and dislocation. Foot Ankle Int 28:1034-40, 2007

SECTION 5

Integrated Function

CHAPTER 13 **Posture** 442
CHAPTER 14 **Gait** 469
CHAPTER 15 **Aquatics: Biomechanical Principles** 512

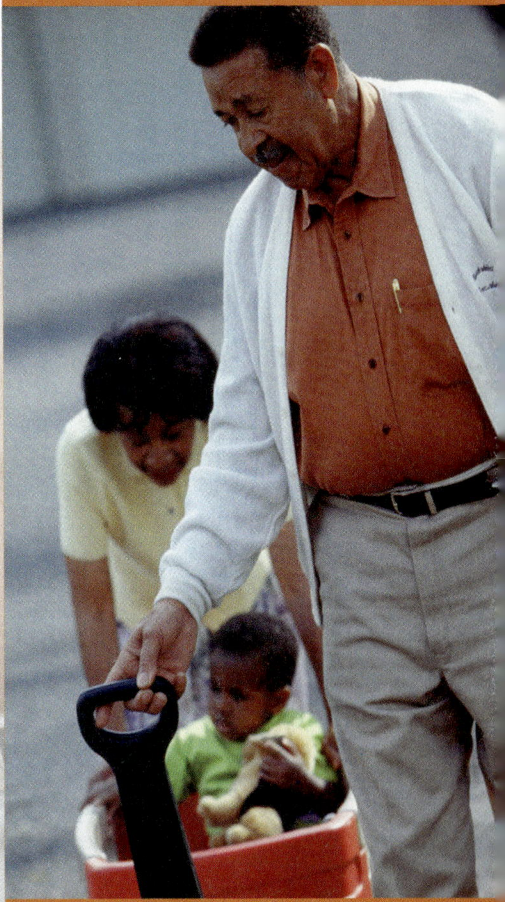